Litt's DRUG ERUPTION & REACTION MANUAL

25th EDITION

Neil H. Shear

CRC Press
Taylor & Francis Group
Boca Raton London New York

CRC Press is an imprint of the
Taylor & Francis Group, an **informa** business

CRC Press
Taylor & Francis Group
6000 Broken Sound Parkway NW, Suite 300
Boca Raton, FL 33487-2742

Printed on acid-free paper

International Standard Book Number-13: 978-0-367-03065-0 (Paperback)
International Standard Book Number-13: 978-0-367-03068-1 (Hardback)

Visit the Taylor & Francis Web site at
http://www.taylorandfrancis.com

and the CRC Press Web site at
http://www.crcpress.com

CONTENTS

Editors' introductory notes

Any drug has the potential to cause an adverse reaction. An adverse drug reaction (ADR) is an unwanted, unpleasant, noxious, or harmful consequence associated with the use of a medication that has been administered in a standard dose by the proper route, for the purpose of prophylaxis, diagnosis, or treatment. Death is the ultimate adverse drug event.

ADRs are a major problem in drug therapy. They are the most common of all iatrogenic illnesses that complicate up to 15% of therapeutic drug courses and are a leading cause of morbidity and mortality in healthcare. ADRs should therefore be considered in the differential diagnosis of a wide variety of medical disorders. Many more people – particularly the elderly – are taking more and more prescription and over-the-counter medications. In addition, new drugs are appearing in the medical marketplace on an almost daily basis. It is unsurprising, then, that more and more drug reactions and cutaneous eruptions are emerging.

Prevention, diagnosis and treatment of adverse drug events are becoming increasingly complex, and it is to be expected that physicians in all specialties are often perplexed by the nature of ADRs. To this end, I now offer a new and improved edition that has evolved from the treasured Drug Eruption Reference Manual of previous editions. I hope that you will find this new edition informative and valuable.

Enjoy!

Jerome Z. Litt M..D, Editor emeritus

What is new in 2019?

Patients frequently ask about their prescribed drug: "Is it safe?" This text is meant to help all prescribers, dispensers and patients understand what the risk of harm might be; whether it is from a drug reaction or interaction, *Litt's D.E.R.M.* is the go-to information source. How does this information help answer the unanswerable? Simply put, safety is a process, not a question. With the right information at hand a safe environment can thrive; the most up-to-date relevant data help peel away background noise from a seemingly infinite number of sources. This new edition adds additional support to a risk management environment, and we will continue to provide the most up-to-date and relevant information. I look forward to feedback and suggestions.

For this edition we are starting to add known genetic risks that are associated with drug reactions and can be screened prior to drug thearpy. This will expand annually as appropriateness of testing becomes part of practice.

Litt D.E.R.M. is more than a text. It is part of a community of resources to make prescribing safe and to help optimize therapy. To that end remember that the on-line data is almost double what you see in the text. And it too is kept up-to-date!

For me in my practice I am in love with the recently introduced Litt app – an easy portal to the online database, particularly if you are moving between various work spaces. Recently a patient on three critical drugs developed a rash on day 8 of treatment. The Litt app gave me easy access to the likelihood of an exathematous rash for each, and I could provide a clear and thoughtful direction for the immediate future.

Finally, I want to note what I call the "Drug Reaction of the Year 2019"! There are indeed new drug reactions, and for me the BIG one is "-gliptin"-induced. When you recognize this and stop the "-gliptins" (dipeptidyl-peptidase 4 inhibitors), in a diabetic patient you will see the reaction clear over the following month. The big "aha" moment for me is when I see a patient with bullous pemphigoid and start to worry about the impact of corticosteroids on their glucose. Even patients who have been on the "-gliptins" for two years will clear.

I thank Jerry Litt for this great opportunity and the awesome work of the team at CRC Press to keep on top of all new medications that are making the landscape even more complex.

And USE THE APP!!

Neil H. Shear, M.D., F.R.C.P.C., F.A.C.P.

Litt's Drug Eruption & Reaction Manual – at a glance

This 25th edition has been revised and updated throughout to present a quick clinical reference guide to adverse drug reactions (ADRs), side effects, drug interactions and other safety information for prescription and over-the-counter medications. There is also material on reactions caused by classes of drugs, enabling you to see at a glance whether a reaction is common to all the drugs in that particular class, or to a majority of them, or only to a significant few.

The aims of this edition remain:

1. To help medical practitioners make informed and safe decisions when diagnosing and prescribing, and also when generally seeking information.
2. To help healthcare professionals remain pharmacovigilant.
3. To provide all physicians, lecturers, educators and pharmacists with an easy-to-use and reliable quick reference tool.

The full and comprehensive picture for all drugs – from which our information derives – can be found at our website database (www.drugeruptiondata.com), which is updated continually. (This may now also be accessed via an app.) Space in the manual is, unfortunately, constrained, so full profiles for various generic drugs have been eliminated from this print manual because either they have been withdrawn from the marketplace or they are rarely, if ever, prescribed today; new to this edition are links to their basic profiles in the website database. Important new drugs added to this edition of the manual are noted with an asterisk.

A note on ADRs

The incidence and severity of ADRs are influenced by a number of factors:

1. Patient-related factors:

- Age – geriatric, pediatric, adolescent . . . older patients are taking more medications—hence more of a possibility of developing reactions; pediatric patients have more delicate skins; hormonal changes occur in adolescents . . . All these factors play roles in the development of possible adverse reactions.
- Gender – male or female – and if the latter, then pregnant/breast-feeding/menopausal . . .
- Disease – not only the disease being treated, but also other pre-existing health conditions and comorbid diseases. For example, atopic patients are at increased risk for serious allergic reactions. Also, there would be an increased risk for hypersensitivity drug reactions if the patient has asthma or lupus erythematosus.
- Genetics – a patient could have abnormal drug metabolism by cytochrome P450 due to inheriting abnormal alleles.
- Geography – patients living in sunny climes could develop photoxicities from photosensitizing drugs more readily than those who inhabit cooler, less sunny climates.

2. Drug-related factors:

- Type/class of drug – for example, there is a heightened risk of hypersensitivity with the use of beta-blockers (see further the tables on class reactions).
- Duration of therapy – the longer a patient maintains the therapy, the greater the possibility that he/she could develop a reaction.
- Dosage – the greater the dosage, the more likely an adverse side effect.
- Bioavailability – the extent to and rate at which the drug enters systemic circulation, thereby accessing the site of action.
- Interactions with other drugs – for example, synergistic QT prolongation can occur when two QT prolonging agents, such as erythromycin + ritonavir, are used together.
- Route of administration – intramuscular, intravenous, subcutaneous, and topical administrations are more likely to cause hypersensitivity reactions; oral medications are less likely to result in drug hypersensitivity.

The terms "drug allergy," "drug hypersensitivity," and "drug reaction" are often used interchangeably. Drug allergy specifically refers to a reaction mediated by IgE; drug hypersensitivity is an immune-mediated response to a drug agent in a sensitized patient; and drug reactions comprise all adverse events related to drug administration, regardless of etiology.

Vigilance at point of care:

While the possibilities for adverse drug reactions seem endless, we must be on the lookout for any new medication(s) the patient might be taking. A thorough, detailed history of all medications must be made in order to elicit any remote possibility that the drug in question might be the culprit for the side effect. People do not often realize that the common over-the-counter analgesics – aspirin, Tylenol, Advil, Motrin, Naprosyn, and others – are actually medications. Herbals and supplements such as St. John's wort, ginkgo biloba, and echinacea can be responsible for various hypersensitivity reactions. For example, St. John's wort, in particular, interacts adversely with SSRIs and tricyclic antidepressants.

Contents of the book, and how to use them

1. **The A–Z**

   The major portion of the manual lists in alphabetical order the 1000 most consulted and most important generic drugs, biologics, and supplements, and the adverse reactions that can arise from their use. An asterisk against the entry title indicates this drug is new to this edition. If you do not find a drug in the main A–Z listing under the name you know it by, you can turn to the concordance of synonyms and trade names to find the generic name it will be listed under.

   Trade (Brand) name(s) are then listed alphabetically. When there are many trade names, the ten (or so) most commonly recognized ones are listed.

   Following the trade names is – in parentheses – the latest name of the pharmaceutical company that markets the drug. Many of the names of the companies have changed from earlier editions of this manual because of acquisitions, mergers, and other factors in the pharmaceutical industry.

   Next appear the Indication(s), the Class in which the drug belongs, and the Half-life of each drug, where known.

   Drug interactions: many severe, hazardous drug–drug interactions are recorded. Only clinically significant drug interactions that have been reported to trigger potential harm and that could be life threatening have been included here in the profile. These interactions are predictable and well documented in controlled studies; they should be avoided.

   Pregnancy category: for new drugs approved on or after 30 June 2015 this field gives (where available) a brief summary of the full statement reflecting the risk for pregnant women as given in the prescribing guidelines; health care providers are advised to check the individual label where necessary.

   An explanation of the categories for older drugs (A, B, C, D and X) can be found on our website www.drugeruptiondata.com.

   Adverse Drug Reactions: under each drug profile is a list of related ADRs. These adverse events have been classified under the following categories: **Skin**, **Hair**, **Nails**, **Mucosal**, **Cardiovascular**, **Central Nervous System**, **Neuromuscular/Skeletal**, **Gastrointestinal/Hepatic**, **Respiratory**, **Endocrine/Metabolic**, **Genitourinary**, **Renal**, **Hematologic**, **Otic**, **Ocular**, **Local**, **Other**.

   Within each category, the reactions are listed alphabetically. Thus, the order of listing does not reflect severity or frequency in any way.

   The terminology used to list reaction patterns has been simplified as far as possible by eliminating, for the most part, tags such as "like" (as in "-Psoriasis-like"), "-reactivation," "-syndrome," "-dissemination," "-iform," etc.

   The number of reports is given for each reaction in square brackets. The incidence of the most important reactions is given in parentheses where indicated (usually from the full prescribing information for the relevant drug). For example, the profile for Amoxicillin begins:

   Skin

   AGEP [28]
   Anaphylactoid reactions/Anaphylaxis [16]
   Angioedema (<10%) [5]

   This means that we have 28 journal articles referring to occurrence of AGEP (acute generalized exanthematous pustulosis); 16 articles mentioning the occurrence of anaphylaxis; and 5 articles discussing angioedema, as reactions to Amoxicillin within the Skin category. All these articles appear on the website www.drugeruptiondata.com together with links to the article abstracts on PubMed®. Additionally, the incidence of angioedema as a reaction has been reported as up to 10%.

On some occasions, there are very few adverse reactions to a specific drug. These drugs are still included in the manual as there is a positive significance in negative findings.

2. **Important eruptions / reactions**

i) This section of the manual includes a listing of descriptions of important eruption and reaction patterns. Over 40 eruptions/reactions are described here in alphabetical order, from Acanthosis nigricans to Xerostomia.
(Descriptions of several other reactions, and lists of drugs associated with these reactions, can be found on our website – www.drugeruptiondata.com.)

ii) We then have a list of the main classes of drugs, from 5-HT1 agonists to Xanthine alkaloids, as a quick reference guide.

iii) We then have an enlarged section of tables of class reactions, enabling you to see at a glance whether a reaction is common to all the drugs in that particular class, or to a majority of them, or only to a significant few.

iv) New to this edition are tables of reported genetic associations with cutaneous adverse drug reactions and recommendations from various sources regarding genetic screening to prevent cutaneous adverse drug reactions.

3. **The Concordance**

The final part of the manual is a concordance to match synonyms (noted in italic) and trade names with the generic drug name. If you know only the synonym or trade name, you can use this list to find the corresponding generic name to look up in the main A–Z listing section of the book.

ABACAVIR

Trade names: Epzicom (ViiV), Triumeq (ViiV), Trizivir (ViiV), Ziagen (ViiV)
Indications: HIV infections in combination with other antiretrovirals
Class: Nucleoside analog reverse transcriptase inhibitor
Half-life: 1.5 hours
Clinically important, potentially hazardous interactions with: alcohol, arbutamine, argatroban, arsenic, darunavir, ganciclovir, lopinavir, methadone, phenobarbital, phenytoin, protease inhibitors, ribavirin, rifampin, tipranavir, valganciclovir
Pregnancy category: C
Important contra-indications noted in the prescribing guidelines for: nursing mothers
Note: Check for presence of HLA B*57:01
Epzicom is abacavir and lamivudine; Triumeq is abacavir, dolutegravir and lamivudine; Trizivir is abacavir, lamivudine and zidovudine.
Warning: HYPERSENSITIVITY REACTIONS, LACTIC ACIDOSIS and SEVERE HEPATOMEGALY, and EXACERBATIONS OF HEPATITIS B

Skin
- Anaphylactoid reactions/Anaphylaxis (3%) [3]
- Exanthems [2]
- Hypersensitivity (8–9%) [69]
- Lipoatrophy [2]
- Rash (5–7%) [18]
- Stevens-Johnson syndrome [2]
- Toxic epidermal necrolysis [2]

Cardiovascular
- Myocardial infarction [10]

Central Nervous System
- Abnormal dreams (10%) [2]
- Anxiety (5%)
- Chills (6%)
- Depression (6%)
- Fever (6%) [2]
- Headache (7–13%) [4]
- Insomnia [2]
- Migraine (7%)
- Neuropsychiatric disturbances [3]
- Sleep related disorder (10%)
- Vertigo (dizziness) (6%) [3]

Neuromuscular/Skeletal
- Asthenia (fatigue) (7–12%) [2]
- Bone or joint pain (5–6%)
- Myalgia/Myopathy (5–6%) [2]

Gastrointestinal/Hepatic
- Abdominal pain (6%)
- Diarrhea (7%) [3]
- Gastritis (6%)
- Hepatotoxicity [4]
- Nausea (7–19%) [5]
- Vomiting (2–10%)

Respiratory
- Bronchitis (4%)
- Cough [2]
- Pneumonia (4%)

Endocrine/Metabolic
- ALT increased (6%)
- AST increased (6%)
- Hyperamylasemia (2–4%)
- Hypertriglyceridemia (2–6%)

Renal
- Fanconi syndrome [2]

Hematologic
- Agranulocytosis [3]
- Neutropenia (2–5%)

Other
- Adverse effects [4]
- Infection (5%)

ABALOPARATIDE

Trade name: Tymlos (Radius Health)
Indications: Osteoporosis in postmenopausal women
Class: Parathyroid hormone analog
Half-life: <2 hours
Clinically important, potentially hazardous interactions with: none known
Pregnancy category: N/A (Not indicated for use in females of reproductive potential)
Important contra-indications noted in the prescribing guidelines for: pediatric patients
Warning: RISK OF OSTEOSARCOMA

Cardiovascular
- Orthostatic hypotension (<4%)
- Palpitation (5%)
- Tachycardia (2%)

Central Nervous System
- Headache (8%)
- Vertigo (dizziness) (2–10%)

Neuromuscular/Skeletal
- Asthenia (fatigue) (3%)

Gastrointestinal/Hepatic
- Abdominal pain (3%)
- Nausea (8%)

Endocrine/Metabolic
- Hypercalcemia (3%) [3]
- Hyperuricemia (25%)

Genitourinary
- Hypercalciuria (11%)
- Urolithiasis (2%)

Local
- Injection-site edema (10%)
- Injection-site erythema (58%)
- Injection-site pain (9%)

ABATACEPT

Trade name: Orencia (Bristol-Myers Squibb)
Indications: Rheumatoid arthritis, juvenile idiopathic arthritis in pediatric patients 6 years of age and older
Class: Disease-modifying antirheumatic drug (DMARD), T-cell co-stimulation modulator
Half-life: 12–23 days
Clinically important, potentially hazardous interactions with: adalimumab, anakinra, certolizumab, denosumab, echinacea, etanercept, golimumab, infliximab, lenalidomide, live vaccines, natalizumab, pimecrolimus, sipuleucel-T, tacrolimus, TNF antagonists, trastuzumab
Pregnancy category: C
Important contra-indications noted in the prescribing guidelines for: nursing mothers; pediatric patients

---

Skin
- Basal cell carcinoma [3]
- Eczema [2]
- Herpes simplex (<5%) [3]
- Herpes zoster [3]
- Hypersensitivity [2]
- Malignancies [10]
- Psoriasis [13]
- Rash (4%) [6]
- Sjögren's syndrome [4]
- Squamous cell carcinoma [5]
- Vasculitis [2]

Mucosal
- Stomatitis [3]

Cardiovascular
- Hypertension (7%) [4]
- Hypotension [2]

Central Nervous System
- Fever (5%) [2]
- Headache (5–18%) [6]
- Vertigo (dizziness) (9%) [3]

Neuromuscular/Skeletal
- Asthenia (fatigue) [2]
- Back pain (7%) [2]
- Pain in extremities (3%)

Gastrointestinal/Hepatic
- Abdominal pain (5%)
- Diarrhea (5%) [3]
- Dyspepsia (6%)
- Gastroenteritis [5]
- Nausea (5%) [2]
- Vomiting [2]

Respiratory
- Bronchitis (<13%) [4]
- Cough (5–8%)
- Influenza (5–13%) [2]
- Nasopharyngitis (12%) [6]
- Pharyngitis [3]
- Pneumonia (<5%) [7]
- Pulmonary toxicity [2]
- Rhinitis (<5%) [2]
- Sinusitis (5–13%) [3]
- Tuberculosis [2]
- Upper respiratory tract infection (>10%) [9]

Genitourinary
- Urinary tract infection (5–13%) [10]

Local
- Infusion-related reactions [4]
- Infusion-site reactions (9%) [5]
- Injection-site erythema [3]
- Injection-site hematoma [2]
- Injection-site pain [3]
- Injection-site pruritus [2]
- Injection-site reactions (3%) [8]

Other
- Adverse effects [24]
- Death [2]
- Infection (36–54%) [25]

ABEMACICLIB

Trade name: Verzenio (Lilly)
Indications: Hormone receptor-positive, human epidermal growth factor 2-negative advanced or metastatic breast cancer, either as monotherapy or in combination with fulvestrant, or as inital endocrine-based therapy with an aromatase inhibitor
Class: CDK4/6 inhibitor
Half-life: 18 hours
Clinically important, potentially hazardous interactions with: grapefruit juice, ketoconazole, strong CYP3A4 inducers or inhibitors
Pregnancy category: N/A (Can cause fetal harm)
Important contra-indications noted in the prescribing guidelines for: nursing mothers; pediatric patients

Hair
- Alopecia (12%)

Mucosal
- Stomatitis (14%)
- Xerostomia (17%)

Central Nervous System
- Anorexia [3]
- Dysgeusia (taste perversion) (12%)
- Fever (11%)
- Headache (20%)
- Vertigo (dizziness) (11%)

Neuromuscular/Skeletal
- Arthralgia (15%)
- Asthenia (fatigue) (65%) [9]

Gastrointestinal/Hepatic
- Abdominal pain (39%) [2]
- Constipation (17%)
- Diarrhea (90%) [10]
- Nausea (64%) [9]
- Vomiting (35%) [4]

Respiratory
- Cough (19%)

Endocrine/Metabolic
- ALT increased (31%)
- Appetite decreased (45%) [3]
- AST increased (30%)
- Dehydration (10%)
- Serum creatinine increased (13%) [3]
- Weight loss (14%) [2]

Hematologic
- Anemia (25%) [3]
- Leukopenia (17%) [5]
- Neutropenia (37%) [8]
- Thrombocytopenia (20%) [3]

Other
- Infection (31%)

ABIRATERONE

Trade name: Zytiga (Janssen Biotech)
Indications: Metastatic castration-resistant prostate cancer (in combination with prednisone)
Class: CYP17 inhibitor, Enzyme inhibitor
Half-life: 12 hours
Clinically important, potentially hazardous interactions with: atazanavir, carbamazepine, clarithromycin, CYP3A4 inducers or inhibitors, indinavir, itraconazole, ketoconazole, nefazodone, nelfinavir, phenobarbital, phenytoin, rifabutin, rifampin, rifapentine, ritonavir, saquinavir, telithromycin, thioridazine, voriconazole
Pregnancy category: X
Important contra-indications noted in the prescribing guidelines for: nursing mothers; pediatric patients
Note: Contra-indicated in women who are or may become pregnant.

Skin
- Edema (27%) [21]
- Hot flashes (19%) [3]

Cardiovascular
- Arrhythmias (7%)
- Atrial fibrillation [3]
- Cardiac failure (2%)
- Cardiotoxicity [6]
- Chest pain (4%)
- Hypertension (9%) [25]
- Tachycardia [3]

Central Nervous System
- Headache [2]

Neuromuscular/Skeletal
- Arthralgia [6]
- Asthenia (fatigue) [13]
- Back pain [5]
- Bone or joint pain (30%) [9]
- Myalgia/Myopathy (26%)
- Pain in extremities [3]
- Rhabdomyolysis [2]

Gastrointestinal/Hepatic
- Constipation [8]
- Diarrhea (18%) [6]
- Dyspepsia (6%)
- Hepatotoxicity (2%) [13]
- Nausea [9]
- Vomiting [2]

Respiratory
- Cough (11%)
- Dyspnea [3]
- Upper respiratory tract infection (5%) [2]

Endocrine/Metabolic
- ALT increased (11%) [5]
- AST increased (31%) [3]
- Hypercholesterolemia [2]
- Hypertriglyceridemia (63%)
- Hypokalemia [23]

Genitourinary
- Nocturia (6%)
- Urinary frequency (7%)
- Urinary tract infection (12%) [3]

Hematologic
- Anemia [6]
- Febrile neutropenia [2]
- Neutropenia [2]
- Thrombocytopenia [3]

Other
- Adverse effects [7]

ACALABRUTINIB *

Trade name: Calquence (AstraZeneca)
Indications: Treatment of adult patients with mantle cell lymphoma (MCL) who have received at least one prior therapy
Class: Bruton's tyrosine kinase (BTK) inhibitor
Half-life: <3 hours
Clinically important, potentially hazardous interactions with: antacids, famotidine, H2-receptor antagonists, itraconazole, proton pump inhibitors, ranitidine, rifampin, strong CYP3A inducers, strong or moderate CYP3A inhibitors
Pregnancy category: N/A (May cause fetal toxicity based on findings in animal studies)
Important contra-indications noted in the prescribing guidelines for: nursing mothers; pediatric patients

Skin
- Ecchymoses (21%)
- Hematoma (8%)
- Malignancies (11%)
- Petechiae (21%)
- Rash (18%)

Mucosal
- Epistaxis (nosebleed) (6%)

Cardiovascular
- Atrial fibrillation (3%)
- Atrial flutter (3%)
- Hypertension [2]

Central Nervous System
- Fever [2]
- Headache (39%) [6]

Neuromuscular/Skeletal
- Arthralgia [2]
- Asthenia (fatigue) (28%) [2]
- Myalgia/Myopathy (21%) [2]

Gastrointestinal/Hepatic
- Abdominal pain (15%)
- Constipation (15%)
- Diarrhea (31%) [5]
- Nausea (19%)
- Vomiting (13%)

Respiratory
- Pneumonia [2]

Endocrine/Metabolic
- Weight gain [4]

Hematologic
- Anemia (46%)
- Hemorrhage (8%)
- Neutropenia (36%)
- Thrombocytopenia (44%)

ACARBOSE

Trade names: Glucobay (Bayer), Precose (Bayer)
Indications: Non-insulin dependent diabetes Type II
Class: Alpha-glucosidase inhibitor, Antidiabetic
Half-life: 2 hours
Clinically important, potentially hazardous interactions with: alcohol, anabolic steroids, beta blockers, cholestyramine, corticosteroids, diazoxide, digoxin, diuretics, estrogens, hypoglycemic agents, MAO inhibitors, neomycin, orlistat, pancreatin, pegvisomant, pramlintide, progestogens, somatropin, testosterone
Pregnancy category: B
Important contra-indications noted in the prescribing guidelines for: nursing mothers; pediatric patients
Note: Contra-indicated in patients with diabetic ketoacidosis or cirrhosis; also in patients with inflammatory bowel disease, colonic ulceration, partial intestinal obstruction or in patients predisposed to intestinal obstruction.

Skin
AGEP [2]

Gastrointestinal/Hepatic
Abdominal distension [2]
Abdominal pain (19%)
Diarrhea (31%)
Flatulence (74%) [3]
Hepatitis [2]
Hepatotoxicity [3]
Pneumatosis intestinalis [8]

Other
Adverse effects [5]

ACETAMINOPHEN

Synonyms: APAP; paracetamol
Trade names: Anacin-3 (Wyeth), Darvocet-N (aaiPharma), Excedrin (Bristol-Myers Squibb), Lorcet (Forest), Panadol (GSK), Percocet (Endo), Tylenol (Ortho-McNeil), Vicodin (AbbVie)
Indications: Pain, fever
Class: Analgesic, non-narcotic
Half-life: <3 hours
Clinically important, potentially hazardous interactions with: alcohol, anticonvulsants, barbiturates, busulfan, carbamazepine, cholestyramine, conivaptan, coumarins, didanosine, dong quai, exenatide, imatinib, isoniazid, liraglutide, melatonin, metoclopramide, metyrapone, PEG-interferon, pramlintide, probenecid, St John's wort
Pregnancy category: C
Important contra-indications noted in the prescribing guidelines for: nursing mothers
Note: Acetaminophen is the active metabolite of phenacetin. [IV] = intravenous. As a general point most reactions listed are those that have developed following the normal prescribing doses for acetaminophen and the overdosing, poisoning, and other toxicities that have been reported have been excluded.

Skin
AGEP [10]
Anaphylactoid reactions/Anaphylaxis [19]
Angioedema [8]
Dermatitis [3]
Erythema [3]
Erythema multiforme [3]
Exanthems [7]
Exfoliative dermatitis [2]
Fixed eruption [41]
Hyperhidrosis [2]
Hypersensitivity [12]
Neutrophilic eccrine hidradenitis [2]
Pemphigus [2]
Pruritus [5]
Purpura [6]
Rash [IV] [2]
Stevens-Johnson syndrome [11]
Toxic epidermal necrolysis [14]
Urticaria [17]
Vasculitis [4]

Mucosal
Xerostomia [3]

Cardiovascular
Hypertension [IV] [3]
Hypotension [2]

Central Nervous System
Agitation [IV] (>5%)
Fever [IV] (5%)
Headache [IV] (10%) [5]
Insomnia [IV] (7%)
Somnolence (drowsiness) [8]
Vertigo (dizziness) [15]

Neuromuscular/Skeletal
Rhabdomyolysis [4]

Gastrointestinal/Hepatic
Abdominal distension [2]
Abdominal pain [IV] [3]
Constipation [IV] (>5%) [7]
Diarrhea [IV] [2]
Hepatotoxicity [70]
Nausea [IV] (34%) [18]
Pancreatitis [6]
Vomiting (15%) [16]

Respiratory
Asthma [3]
Pulmonary toxicity [IV] (>5%)

Endocrine/Metabolic
Acidosis [3]

Renal
Nephrotoxicity [9]
Renal failure [3]

Hematologic
Thrombocytopenia [2]

Other
Adverse effects [16]
Death [6]

ACETAZOLAMIDE

Trade name: Diamox (Duramed)
Indications: Epilepsy, glaucoma
Class: Carbonic anhydrase inhibitor, Diuretic
Half-life: 2–6 hours
Clinically important, potentially hazardous interactions with: arsenic, aspirin, ephedra, indacaterol, lisdexamfetamine, lithium, metformin, mivacurium, triamcinolone
Pregnancy category: C
Important contra-indications noted in the prescribing guidelines for: the elderly; nursing mothers; pediatric patients
Note: Acetazolamide is a sulfonamide and can be absorbed systemically. Sulfonamides can produce severe, possibly fatal, reactions such as toxic epidermal necrolysis and Stevens-Johnson syndrome.

Skin
AGEP [2]
Anaphylactoid reactions/Anaphylaxis [3]
Exanthems [2]
Pemphigus [2]
Stevens-Johnson syndrome [7]
Toxic epidermal necrolysis [2]

Central Nervous System
Depression [2]
Dysgeusia (taste perversion) (>10%) [8]
Paresthesias [6]

Neuromuscular/Skeletal
Asthenia (fatigue) [4]

Gastrointestinal/Hepatic
Diarrhea [2]
Dyspepsia [2]
Nausea [2]
Vomiting [2]

Endocrine/Metabolic
Acidosis [3]
Libido decreased [2]
Weight loss [2]

Renal
Nephrolithiasis [3]

Ocular
Choroidal detachment [2]
Corneal edema [2]
Glaucoma [5]
Myopia [2]

ACETYLCYSTEINE

Synonyms: N-acetylcysteine; L-Cysteine; NAC
Indications: Emphysema, bronchitis, tuberculosis, bronchiectasis, tracheostomy care, antidote for acetaminophen toxicity
Class: Antidote, Antioxidant
Half-life: N/A
Clinically important, potentially hazardous interactions with: carbamazepine, nitroglycerin
Pregnancy category: B
Note: As an antidote, it is difficult to differentiate side effects due to the drug from those due to the effects of the poison.

Skin
Anaphylactoid reactions/Anaphylaxis (8–18%) [14]
Angioedema [6]
Flushing (<8%) [2]
Pruritus (<4%) [3]
Rash (2–4%) [4]
Urticaria (6–8%)

Cardiovascular
Tachycardia (<4%)

Central Nervous System
Seizures [2]

Gastrointestinal/Hepatic
Diarrhea [2]
Nausea (<6%) [3]
Vomiting (2–10%) [2]

Other
Adverse effects [2]
Death [2]

ACITRETIN

Trade names: Neotigason (Actavis), Soriatane (Stiefel)
Indications: Psoriasis
Class: Retinoid
Half-life: 49 hours
Clinically important, potentially hazardous interactions with: alcohol, bexarotene, chloroquine, cholestyramine, corticosteroids, coumarins, danazol, demeclocycline, doxycycline, ethanolamine, isotretinoin, lithium, lymecycline, medroxyprogesterone, methotrexate, minocycline, oxytetracycline, phenytoin, progestins, St John's wort, tetracycline, tigecycline, vitamin A
Pregnancy category: X
Important contra-indications noted in the prescribing guidelines for: nursing mothers; pediatric patients
Note: Oral retinoids can cause birth defects, and women should avoid acitretin when pregnant or trying to conceive.
Warning: PREGNANCY

Skin
Angioedema [2]
Atrophy (10–25%)
Bromhidrosis (<10%)
Bullous dermatitis (<10%)
Clammy skin (<10%)
Dermatitis (<10%)
Diaphoresis (<10%) [2]
Edema (<10%)
Erythema (18%)
Erythroderma [3]
Exanthems (10–25%) [2]
Exfoliative dermatitis (25–50%) [3]
Fissures (<10%)
Hot flashes (<10%)
Hyperhidrosis (<10%) [2]
Palmar–plantar desquamation (20–80%) [7]
Photosensitivity [3]
Pigmentation [3]
Pruritus (10–50%) [10]
Psoriasis (aggravated) (<10%)
Purpura (<10%)
Rash (>10%)
Seborrhea (<10%)
Stickiness (3–50%) [7]
Sunburn (<10%)
Toxicity [3]
Ulcerations (<10%)
Xerosis (25–50%) [14]

Hair
Alopecia (10–75%) [21]
Curly hair [3]
Hair changes (<10%)
Hair pigmentation [2]

Nails
Brittle nails [3]
Nail changes (25–50%)
Paronychia (10–25%) [6]
Pyogenic granuloma (<10%) [4]

Mucosal
Cheilitis (>75%) [14]
Dry mucous membranes [4]
Epistaxis (nosebleed) (10–25%) [2]
Gingival bleeding (<10%)
Gingivitis (<10%)
Mucocutaneous reactions [3]
Sialorrhea (<10%)
Stomatitis (<10%) [2]
Tongue disorder (<10%)
Ulcerative stomatitis (<10%)
Xerostomia (10–60%) [7]

Cardiovascular
Capillary leak syndrome [2]

Central Nervous System
Anorexia (<10%)
Depression (<10%) [4]
Dysgeusia (taste perversion) (<10%)
Headache (<10%) [2]
Hyperesthesia (10–25%)
Insomnia (<10%)
Neurotoxicity [3]
Pain (<10%)
Paralysis (facial) (<10%)
Paresthesias (10–25%) [2]
Pseudotumor cerebri [5]
Rigors (10–25%) [2]
Somnolence (drowsiness) (<10%)
Stroke [2]
Suicidal ideation [2]

Neuromuscular/Skeletal
Arthralgia (10–25%) [2]
Asthenia (fatigue) (<10%) [3]
Back pain (<10%)
Bone or joint pain [2]
Hyperostosis [10]
Myalgia/Myopathy [4]
Osteoporosis [2]

Gastrointestinal/Hepatic
Abdominal pain (<10%)
Diarrhea (<10%) [2]
Hepatitis [5]
Hepatotoxicity [8]
Nausea (<10%) [2]
Pancreatitis [3]
Vomiting [2]

Respiratory
Laryngitis [2]
Rhinitis (25–50%) [2]
Sinusitis (<10%)

Endocrine/Metabolic
GGT increased [2]
Hyperbilirubinemia [2]
Hypercholesterolemia (25–50%) [3]
Hyperlipidemia [5]
Hypertriglyceridemia (50–75%) [4]

Genitourinary
Vulvovaginal candidiasis [2]

Otic
Ear pain (<10%)
Tinnitus (<10%)

Ocular
Blepharitis (<10%)
Cataract (<10%)
Conjunctivitis (<10%) [2]
Diplopia (<10%)
Night blindness (<10%) [2]
Ocular adverse effects [2]
Ocular itching [2]
Ocular pain (<10%)
Photophobia (<10%) [2]
Vision blurred (<10%)
Xerophthalmia (10–25%) [3]

Other
Adverse effects [9]
Dipsia (thirst) (<10%)
Infection [2]
Side effects [4]
Teratogenicity [7]

ACYCLOVIR

Synonyms: aciclovir; ACV; acycloguanosine
Trade names: Sitavig (Cipher), Zovirax (GSK)
Indications: Herpes simplex, herpes zoster
Class: Antiviral, Antiviral, topical, Guanine nucleoside analog
Half-life: 3 hours (adults)
Clinically important, potentially hazardous interactions with: cobicistat/elvitegravir/emtricitabine/tenofovir alafenamide, cobicistat/elvitegravir/emtricitabine/tenofovir disoproxil, meperidine, tenofovir disoproxil
Pregnancy category: B
Important contra-indications noted in the prescribing guidelines for: nursing mothers

---

Skin
Acneform eruption (<3%)
Dermatitis [12]
Exanthems (<5%) [5]
Facial edema (3–5%)
Peripheral edema [2]
Pruritus (<10%)
Radiation recall dermatitis [2]
Rash (<3%) [3]
Urticaria (<5%) [4]

Hair
Alopecia (<3%)

Central Nervous System
Headache (2%) [4]
Neurotoxicity [8]

Neuromuscular/Skeletal
Asthenia (fatigue) (12%)

Gastrointestinal/Hepatic
Diarrhea (2–3%)
Nausea (2–5%) [3]
Vomiting (3%)

Renal
Nephrotoxicity [13]
Renal failure [4]

Hematologic
Thrombocytopenia [2]

Ocular
Hallucinations, visual [2]
Periorbital edema (3–5%)

Local
Injection-site inflammation (>10%)
Injection-site thrombophlebitis (9%)

Other
Adverse effects [2]

ADALIMUMAB

Trade names: Amjevita (Amgen), Humira (AbbVie)
Indications: Rheumatoid arthritis, polyarticular juvenile idiopathic arthritis, psoriatic arthritis, ankylosing spondylitis, Crohn's disease, ulcerative colitis, psoriasis
Class: Cytokine inhibitor, Disease-modifying antirheumatic drug (DMARD), Monoclonal antibody, TNF inhibitor
Half-life: 10–20 days
Clinically important, potentially hazardous interactions with: abatacept, anakinra, live vaccines
Pregnancy category: B
Important contra-indications noted in the prescribing guidelines for: nursing mothers
Note: TNF inhibitors should be used in patients with heart failure only after consideration of other treatment options. TNF inhibitors are contra-indicated in patients with a personal or family history of multiple sclerosis or demyelinating disease. TNF inhibitors should not be administered to patients with moderate to severe heart failure (New York Heart Association Functional Class III/IV).
Warning: SERIOUS INFECTIONS AND MALIGNANCY

Skin
Acneform eruption [3]
Anaphylactoid reactions/Anaphylaxis [2]
Angioedema [4]
Carcinoma [2]
Cellulitis (<5%) [2]
Dermatomyositis [5]
Eczema [2]
Erysipelas (<5%)
Granulomatous reaction [5]
Henoch-Schönlein purpura [2]
Herpes zoster [10]
Hidradenitis [2]
Hypersensitivity [3]
Lesions [2]
Lichenoid eruption [5]
Lupus erythematosus [16]
Lupus syndrome [3]
Lymphoma [8]
Malignancies [6]
Melanoma [6]
Neoplasms [2]
Palmoplantar pustulosis [3]
Peripheral edema (<5%)
Pruritus [6]
Psoriasis [40]
Rash (12%) [6]
Sarcoidosis [9]
Squamous cell carcinoma [5]
Stevens-Johnson syndrome [2]
Urticaria [4]
Vasculitis [9]
Vitiligo [2]

Hair
Alopecia [5]
Alopecia areata [7]
Alopecia universalis [2]

Cardiovascular
Arrhythmias (<5%)
Cardiac arrest (<5%)
Chest pain (<5%)
Congestive heart failure (<5%) [2]
Hypertension (<5%)
Myocardial infarction (<5%)
Palpitation [2]
Pericarditis (<5%)
Tachycardia (<5%)
Thromboembolism [2]

Central Nervous System
Aseptic meningitis [2]
Confusion (<5%)
Depression [2]
Encephalitis [2]
Fever (<5%) [3]
Guillain–Barré syndrome [5]
Headache (12%) [8]
Leukoencephalopathy [3]
Multiple sclerosis (<5%) [3]
Neurotoxicity [3]
Paresthesias (<5%) [2]
Syncope (<5%)
Tremor (<5%)
Vertigo (dizziness) [2]

Neuromuscular/Skeletal
Arthralgia (<5%) [6]
Asthenia (fatigue) [2]
Back pain (6%) [3]
Tuberculous arthritis [2]

Gastrointestinal/Hepatic
Abdominal pain (7%) [2]
Cholecystitis (<5%)
Colitis [2]
Esophagitis (<5%)
Gastroenteritis (<5%)
Hepatitis [7]
Hepatotoxicity [11]
Nausea (9%) [2]
Vomiting (<5%)

Respiratory
Asthma (<5%)
Bronchitis [3]
Bronchospasm (<5%)
Dyspnea (<5%)
Flu-like syndrome (7%)
Nasopharyngitis [7]
Pleural effusion (<5%)
Pneumonia (<5%) [6]
Pneumonitis [3]
Pulmonary fibrosis [3]
Pulmonary toxicity [7]
Sinusitis (11%) [3]
Tuberculosis [10]
Upper respiratory tract infection (17%) [13]

Endocrine/Metabolic
Creatine phosphokinase increased (<5%)
Hypercholesterolemia (6%)

Genitourinary
Cystitis (<5%)
Hematuria (5%)
Pelvic pain (<5%)
Urinary tract infection (8%) [2]

Renal
Nephrotoxicity [3]

Hematologic
Agranulocytosis (<5%)
Eosinophilia [3]
Hemolytic anemia [2]
Leukopenia (<5%)
Pancytopenia [2]
Sepsis [2]

Ocular
Cataract (<5%)
Optic neuritis [5]
Uveitis [4]

Local
Infusion-related reactions [2]
Injection-site edema (15%) [2]
Injection-site erythema (15%) [3]
Injection-site pain (12%)
Injection-site reactions [30]

Other
Adverse effects [46]
Allergic reactions [2]
Death [9]
Infection (5%) [75]
Side effects [2]

ADAPALENE

Trade names: Differin (Galderma), Epiduo (Galderma)
Indications: Acne vulgaris
Class: Retinoid
Half-life: N/A
Clinically important, potentially hazardous interactions with: resorcinol, salicylates
Pregnancy category: C
Important contra-indications noted in the prescribing guidelines for: nursing mothers; pediatric patients
Note: Epiduo is adapalene and benzoyl peroxide.

Skin
Burning (38%) [7]
Erythema (38%) [9]
Pruritus (>10%) [11]
Scaling (44%) [6]
Stinging (38%) [3]
Xerosis (45%) [10]

Other
Adverse effects [3]

ADEFOVIR

Trade name: Hepsera (Gilead)
Indications: HIV infection, hepatitis B infection
Class: Antiretroviral, Nucleotide analog reverse transcriptase inhibitor
Half-life: 16–18 hours
Clinically important, potentially hazardous interactions with: amikacin, amphotericin B, cobicistat/elvitegravir/emtricitabine/tenofovir disoproxil, delavirdine, drugs causing kidney toxicity, foscarnet, gentamicin, hydroxyurea, pentamidine, tenofovir disoproxil, tobramycin
Pregnancy category: C
Important contra-indications noted in the prescribing guidelines for: the elderly; nursing mothers; pediatric patients
Warning: SEVERE ACUTE EXACERBATIONS OF HEPATITIS, NEPHROTOXICITY, HIV RESISTANCE, LACTIC ACIDOSIS AND SEVERE HEPATOMEGALY WITH STEATOSIS

Skin
Pruritus (<10%)
Rash (<10%)
Stevens-Johnson syndrome [2]

Central Nervous System
Headache (9%) [2]
Pain [2]

Neuromuscular/Skeletal
Asthenia (fatigue) (13%) [3]
Back pain (<10%)
Fractures [2]
Osteomalacia [7]

Gastrointestinal/Hepatic
Abdominal pain (9%)
Diarrhea (3%)
Dyspepsia (3%)
Flatulence (4%)
Hepatotoxicity (<25%)
Nausea (5%)
Vomiting (<10%)

Respiratory
Cough (6–8%)
Rhinitis (<5%)

Endocrine/Metabolic
Hypophosphatemia [6]

Genitourinary
Hematuria (11%)

Renal
Fanconi syndrome [11]
Nephrotoxicity [14]

ADENOSINE

Synonym: ATP
Trade names: Adenocard (Astellas), Adenocur (Sanofi-Aventis)
Indications: Paroxysmal supraventricular tachycardia, varicose vein complications with stasis dermatitis
Class: Antiarrhythmic class IV, Neurotransmitter
Half-life: <10 seconds
Clinically important, potentially hazardous interactions with: aminophylline, antiarrhythmics, beta blockers, bupivacaine, carbamazepine, dipyridamole, levobupivacaine, nicotine, prilocaine, QT prolonging agents, ropivacaine
Pregnancy category: C
Important contra-indications noted in the prescribing guidelines for: pediatric patients

---

Skin
Flushing (18–44%)

Cardiovascular
Arrhythmias [2]
Atrial fibrillation [6]
Chest pain [5]
Coronary vasospasm [2]
Torsades de pointes [2]

Central Nervous System
Headache (2–18%) [2]
Vertigo (dizziness) (2–12%)

Neuromuscular/Skeletal
Jaw pain (<15%)

Gastrointestinal/Hepatic
Abdominal pain (13%)

Respiratory
Cough (6–8%)
Dyspnea [3]
Respiratory distress (11%)

Other
Adverse effects [2]

AFATINIB

Trade name: Gilotrif (Boehringer Ingelheim)
Indications: Metastatic non-small cell lung cancer in patients whose tumors have epidermal growth factor receptor exon 19 deletions or exon 21 (L858R) substitution mutations, metastatic squamous non-small cell lung cancer progressing following platinium-based chemotherapy
Class: Tyrosine kinase inhibitor
Half-life: 37 hours
Clinically important, potentially hazardous interactions with: amiodarone, carbamazepine, cyclosporine, erythromycin, itraconazole, ketoconazole, nelfinavir, P-glycoprotein inhibitors, phenobarbital, phenytoin, quinidine, rifampin, ritonavir, saquinavir, St John's wort, tacrolimus, verapamil
Pregnancy category: D
Important contra-indications noted in the prescribing guidelines for: nursing mothers; pediatric patients

---

Skin
Acneform eruption [27]
Fissures [2]
Hand–foot syndrome [2]
Pruritus [3]
Rash [52]
Stevens-Johnson syndrome [4]
Toxicity [3]
Xerosis [8]

Nails
Nail changes [2]
Paronychia (58%) [17]

Mucosal
Epistaxis (nosebleed) [3]
Mucosal inflammation [7]
Mucositis [10]
Rhinorrhea (11%)
Stomatitis (71%) [21]

Central Nervous System
Anorexia [3]
Fever (12%)

Neuromuscular/Skeletal
Asthenia (fatigue) [18]

Gastrointestinal/Hepatic
Diarrhea (96%) [71]
Dysphagia [2]
Hepatotoxicity (10%) [5]
Nausea [16]
Vomiting [10]

Respiratory
Dyspnea [3]
Pneumonitis [2]
Pulmonary toxicity [5]

Endocrine/Metabolic
ALT increased [2]
Appetite decreased (29%) [5]
Dehydration [3]
Hypokalemia [2]

Hematologic
Anemia [3]
Febrile neutropenia [2]
Leukopenia [2]
Neutropenia [6]
Thrombocytopenia [2]

Other
Adverse effects [7]
Death [4]

AFLIBERCEPT

Synonym: ziv-aflibercept
Trade names: Eylea (Regeneron), Zaltrap (Sanofi-Aventis)
Indications: Neovascular (wet) age-related macular degeneration (Eylea), metastatic colorectal cancer (Zaltrap) in combination with FOLFIRI (fluorouracil, leucovorin and irinotecan)
Class: Fusion protein
Half-life: terminal 5–6 days
Clinically important, potentially hazardous interactions with: none known
Pregnancy category: C
Important contra-indications noted in the prescribing guidelines for: nursing mothers; pediatric patients
Note: Eylea: Contra-indicated in patients with ocular or periocular infection or active intraocular inflammation.
Warning: Zaltrap: HEMORRHAGE, GASTROINTESTINAL PERFORATION, COMPROMISED WOUND HEALING

Mucosal
Epistaxis (nosebleed) [3]
Stomatitis [6]

Cardiovascular
Hypertension [13]
Myocardial infarction (<2%)
Venous thromboembolism [2]

Central Nervous System
Anorexia [2]
Headache [2]
Stroke (<2%)

Neuromuscular/Skeletal
Asthenia (fatigue) [6]

Gastrointestinal/Hepatic
Diarrhea [6]
Gastrointestinal perforation [5]

Respiratory
Dysphonia [5]
Dyspnea [2]
Pulmonary embolism [2]

Endocrine/Metabolic
Weight loss [2]

Renal
Proteinuria [9]

Hematologic
Hemorrhage [3]
Neutropenia [11]

Ocular
Cataract (7%) [2]
Conjunctival hemorrhage (25%) [3]
Conjunctival hyperemia (4%)
Conjunctivitis [2]
Corneal erosion (4%)
Intraocular pressure increased (5%) [2]
Lacrimation (3%)
Ocular adverse effects [4]
Ocular pain (3–9%)
Vision blurred (2%)
Vitreous detachment (6%)
Vitreous floaters (6%)

Local
Injection-site pain (3%)

Other
Adverse effects [2]
Death [3]
Infection [3]

ALBENDAZOLE

Trade name: Albenza (GSK)
Indications: Nematode infections, hydatid cyst disease
Class: Anthelmintic
Half-life: 8–12 hours
Clinically important, potentially hazardous interactions with: antimalarials, conivaptan, dexamethasone, high fat foods
Pregnancy category: C
Important contra-indications noted in the prescribing guidelines for: nursing mothers

---

Skin
Fixed eruption [2]
Pruritus [4]
Urticaria [2]

Hair
Alopecia (reversible) (<2%) [4]

Central Nervous System
Fever (<2%)
Headache (<11%) [5]
Intracranial pressure increased (<2%)
Psychosis [2]
Vertigo (dizziness) (<2%) [2]

Neuromuscular/Skeletal
Dystonia [3]

Gastrointestinal/Hepatic
Abdominal pain (<7%) [7]
Hepatitis [5]
Nausea (4–6%) [3]
Vomiting (4–6%) [2]

Other
Adverse effects [5]

ALBIGLUTIDE

Trade name: Tanzeum (GSK)
Indications: To improve glycemic control in adults with Type II diabetes mellitus
Class: Glucagon-like peptide-1 (GLP-1) receptor agonist
Half-life: 5 days
Clinically important, potentially hazardous interactions with: none known
Pregnancy category: C
Important contra-indications noted in the prescribing guidelines for: nursing mothers; pediatric patients
Note: Contra-indicated in patients with a personal or family history of medullary thyroid carcinoma or in patients with multiple endocrine neoplasia syndrome Type 2.
Warning: RISK OF THYROID C-CELL TUMORS

Central Nervous System
Headache [4]
Vertigo (dizziness) [2]

Neuromuscular/Skeletal
Arthralgia (7%)
Back pain (7%) [2]

Gastrointestinal/Hepatic
Constipation [2]
Diarrhea (13%) [15]
Dyspepsia (3%)
Gastroesophageal reflux (4%)
Nausea (11%) [20]
Pancreatitis [4]
Vomiting (4%) [15]

Respiratory
Cough (7%)
Influenza (5%)
Nasopharyngitis [3]
Pneumonia (2%)
Sinusitis (6%)
Upper respiratory tract infection (14%) [4]

Endocrine/Metabolic
GGT increased (2%)
Hypoglycemia (2%) [5]

Local
Injection-site hematoma (2%)
Injection-site reactions (11%) [16]

Other
Adverse effects [4]

ALBUTEROL

Synonym: salbutamol
Trade names: AccuNeb (Mylan Specialty), Combivent (Boehringer Ingelheim), Duoneb (Mylan Specialty), Proventil (Schering), Ventolin (GSK), Volmax (Muro)
Indications: Bronchospasm associated with asthma
Class: Beta-2 adrenergic agonist, Bronchodilator, Tocolytic
Half-life: 3–6 hours
Clinically important, potentially hazardous interactions with: atomoxetine, epinephrine, insulin degludec, insulin detemir, insulin glargine, insulin glulisine
Pregnancy category: C
Important contra-indications noted in the prescribing guidelines for: nursing mothers
Note: Combivent is albuterol and ipratropium.

Skin
Dermatitis [2]
Diaphoresis (<10%)
Erythema (palmar) (with infusion) [2]
Flushing (<10%)

Mucosal
Xerostomia (<10%)

Cardiovascular
Atrial fibrillation [2]
Hypertension [2]
Myocardial infarction [2]
Palpitation [2]
Tachyarrhythmia [2]
Tachycardia [2]

Central Nervous System
Dysgeusia (taste perversion) (<10%)
Tremor [2]

Respiratory
Dyspnea [2]

Endocrine/Metabolic
Acidosis [4]

Other
Adverse effects [2]

ALDESLEUKIN

Synonyms: IL-2; interleukin-2
Trade name: Proleukin (Chiron)
Indications: Metastatic renal cell carcinoma and metastatic melanoma
Class: Biologic, Immunomodulator, Interleukin-2
Half-life: 6–85 minutes
Clinically important, potentially hazardous interactions with: acebutolol, alfuzosin, altretamine, amikacin, aminoglycosides, antineoplastics, betamethasone, bleomycin, busulfan, captopril, carboplatin, carmustine, chlorambucil, ciclesonide, cilazapril, cisplatin, corticosteroids, cyclophosphamide, cytarabine, dacarbazine, dactinomycin, daunorubicin, docetaxel, doxorubicin, enalapril, estramustine, etoposide, fludarabine, fluorouracil, fosinopril, gemcitabine, gentamicin, hydroxyurea, idarubicin, ifosfamide, indomethacin, interferon alfa, irbesartan, kanamycin, levamisole, lisinopril,

lomustine, mechlorethamine, melphalan, mercaptopurine, methotrexate, mitomycin, mitotane, mitoxantrone, neomycin, olmesartan, PEG-interferon, pentostatin, plicamycin, procarbazine, quinapril, ramipril, streptomycin, streptozocin, thioguanine, thiotepa, tobramycin, trandolapril, tretinoin, triamcinolone, uracil, vinblastine, vincristine, vinorelbine
Pregnancy category: C
Important contra-indications noted in the prescribing guidelines for: nursing mothers; pediatric patients
Note: Contra-indicated in patients with significant cardiac, pulmonary, renal, hepatic, or CNS impairment.
Warning: CAPILLARY LEAK SYNDROME

Skin
Angioedema [2]
Dermatitis [2]
Edema (47%) [3]
Erythema (41%) [5]
Erythema nodosum [3]
Erythroderma [4]
Exanthems [5]
Exfoliative dermatitis (18%)
Linear IgA bullous dermatosis [4]
Necrosis [2]
Pemphigus [2]
Peripheral edema (28%)
Petechiae (4%)
Pruritus (24%) [7]
Psoriasis [4]
Purpura (4%)
Rash (42%) [2]
Scleroderma [2]
Toxic epidermal necrolysis [2]
Toxicity [6]
Urticaria (2%) [3]
Vitiligo [3]
Xerosis (15%)

Hair
Alopecia [2]

Mucosal
Oral mucosal eruption [2]
Stomatitis (22%)

Cardiovascular
Arrhythmias (10%)
Capillary leak syndrome [12]
Cardiotoxicity (11%) [2]
Hypotension (71%) [6]
Supraventricular tachycardia (12%)
Tachycardia (23%)
Vascular leak syndrome [6]
Vasodilation (13%)

Central Nervous System
Anorexia (20%)
Anxiety (12%)
Chills (52%)
Confusion (34%)
Depression [3]
Dysgeusia (taste perversion) (7%)
Fever (29%) [8]
Neurotoxicity [3]
Pain (12%)
Rigors [3]
Somnolence (drowsiness) (22%)
Vertigo (dizziness) (11%)

Neuromuscular/Skeletal
Asthenia (fatigue) (23–27%)
Myalgia/Myopathy (6%)
Myasthenia gravis [2]

Gastrointestinal/Hepatic
Abdominal pain (11%)
Diarrhea (67%) [3]
Hepatotoxicity [2]
Nausea (35%) [9]
Vomiting (50%) [6]

Respiratory
Cough (11%)
Dyspnea (43%)
Pulmonary toxicity (11–24%) [2]
Rhinitis (10%)

Endocrine/Metabolic
Acidosis (12%)
ALP increased (10%)
AST increased (23%)
Creatine phosphokinase increased (33%) [2]
Hypocalcemia (11%)
Hypomagnesemia [2]
Hypophosphatemia [2]
Weight gain (16%)
Weight loss [2]

Genitourinary
Oliguria (63%)

Renal
Nephrotoxicity [4]

Hematologic
Anemia (29%)
Leukopenia (16%) [2]
Sepsis [3]
Thrombocytopenia (37%) [2]

Local
Injection-site inflammation [2]
Injection-site nodules [2]
Injection-site reactions (3%) [2]

Other
Adverse effects [3]
Death [5]
Infection (13%) [2]

ALECTINIB

Trade name: Alecensa (Genentech)
Indications: Anaplastic lymphoma kinase-positive, metastatic non-small cell lung cancer in patients who have progressed on, or are intolerant to, crizotinib
Class: Kinase inhibitor
Half-life: 33 hours
Clinically important, potentially hazardous interactions with: none known
Pregnancy category: N/A (Can cause fetal harm)
Important contra-indications noted in the prescribing guidelines for: nursing mothers; pediatric patients

---

Skin
Edema (30%)
Peripheral edema [6]
Photosensitivity (10%) [2]
Rash (18%) [3]

Hair
Alopecia [2]

Central Nervous System
Dysgeusia (taste perversion) [3]
Headache (17%) [3]

Neuromuscular/Skeletal
Asthenia (fatigue) (41%) [5]
Back pain (12%)
Myalgia/Myopathy (29%) [7]

Gastrointestinal/Hepatic
Constipation (34%) [8]
Diarrhea (16%) [3]
Nausea (18%) [4]
Vomiting (12%) [3]

Respiratory
Cough (19%)
Dyspnea (16%)
Pulmonary toxicity [5]

Endocrine/Metabolic
ALP increased (47%) [3]
ALT increased (34%) [6]
AST increased (51%) [7]
Creatine phosphokinase increased (43%) [7]
GGT increased [2]
Hyperbilirubinemia (39%) [6]
Hyperglycemia (36%)
Hypocalcemia (32%)
Hypokalemia (29%)
Hyponatremia (20%)
Hypophosphatemia (21%)
Serum creatinine increased (28%)
Weight gain (11%)

Hematologic
Anemia (56%) [3]
Lymphopenia (22%)
Neutropenia [6]

Ocular
Visual disturbances (10%)

Other
Adverse effects [2]

ALEMTUZUMAB

Trade names: Campath (Bayer), MabCampath (Schering)
Indications: B-cell chronic lymphcyotic leukemia, non-Hodgkin's lymphoma
Class: Biologic, Immunosuppressant, Monoclonal antibody
Half-life: 12 days
Clinically important, potentially hazardous interactions with: none known
Pregnancy category: C
Note: Prophylactic therapy against PCP pneumonia and herpes viral infections is recommended upon initiation of therapy and for at least 2 months following last dose.
Warning: CYTOPENIAS, INFUSION REACTIONS, and INFECTIONS

Skin
Carcinoma [2]
Erythema (4%)
Flushing [2]
Herpes [2]
Herpes simplex [2]

Herpes zoster [3]
Lymphoma [2]
Lymphoproliferative disease (64–70%)
Peripheral edema (13%)
Pruritus (14–24%)
Purpura (8%)
Rash (13–40%) [5]
Thrombocytopenic purpura [11]
Urticaria (16–30%) [2]

Mucosal
Stomatitis (14%)

Cardiovascular
Hypertension (11–15%)
Hypotension (15–32%) [2]
Tachycardia (10%)

Central Nervous System
Anorexia (20%)
Anxiety (8%)
Chills (53%)
Depression (7%)
Dysesthesia (15%)
Fever (69–85%) [6]
Guillain–Barré syndrome [2]
Headache (13–24%) [3]
Insomnia (10%)
Intracranial hemorrhage [2]
Leukoencephalopathy [5]
Rigors (87%)
Tremor (3%)
Vertigo (dizziness) (12%)

Neuromuscular/Skeletal
Asthenia (fatigue) (22–34%)
Bone or joint pain (24%)
Myalgia/Myopathy (11%)

Gastrointestinal/Hepatic
Abdominal pain (11%)
Diarrhea (10–22%) [2]
Nausea (47–54%) [4]
Vomiting (33–41%) [2]

Respiratory
Dyspnea (14–26%)
Flu-like syndrome [2]
Pharyngitis (12%)
Pneumonia (16%) [3]
Pneumonitis [3]
Respiratory tract infection [2]
Tuberculosis [2]

Endocrine/Metabolic
Hyperthyroidism [2]
Hypothyroidism [2]
Thyroid dysfunction [16]

Genitourinary
Cystitis [2]

Renal
Nephrotoxicity [4]

Hematologic
Anemia (76%) [4]
Cytopenia [2]
Hemolytic anemia [4]
Hemotoxicity [4]
Leukopenia [4]
Lymphopenia (97%) [2]
Neutropenia (77%) [8]
Sepsis [2]
Thrombocytopenia (71%) [11]

Local
Application-site reactions [2]
Infusion-related reactions [12]
Infusion-site reactions [5]
Injection-site pruritus (30–40%)
Injection-site reactions (90%) [5]

Other
Adverse effects [7]
Death [13]
Infection (43–74%) [52]

ALENDRONATE

Trade names: Binosto (Mission), Fosamax (Merck)
Indications: Osteoporosis in postmenopausal women, Paget's disease
Class: Bisphosphonate
Half-life: >10 years
Clinically important, potentially hazardous interactions with: none known
Pregnancy category: C
Important contra-indications noted in the prescribing guidelines for: nursing mothers; pediatric patients

---

Skin
Angioedema [2]
Erythema multiforme [2]
Hypersensitivity [3]
Rash [5]

Mucosal
Oral ulceration [9]

Central Nervous System
Headache [2]

Neuromuscular/Skeletal
Arthralgia [6]
Bone or joint pain (<6%) [5]
Fractures [20]
Osteonecrosis [12]

Gastrointestinal/Hepatic
Abdominal pain (<7%) [8]
Dyspepsia [8]
Dysphagia [4]
Esophageal perforation [2]
Esophagitis [12]
Hepatotoxicity [7]
Nausea [7]
Vomiting [4]

Endocrine/Metabolic
Hypocalcemia (18%) [5]

Renal
Nephrotoxicity [2]
Renal failure [2]

Ocular
Conjunctivitis [2]
Ocular adverse effects [2]
Ocular inflammation [2]
Scleritis [3]
Uveitis [6]

Other
Adverse effects [5]

ALFUZOSIN

Trade names: Uroxatral (Concordia), Xatral (Sanofi-Aventis)
Indications: Benign prostatic hyperplasia
Class: Adrenergic alpha-receptor antagonist
Half-life: 10 hours
Clinically important, potentially hazardous interactions with: ACE inhibitors, adrenergic neurone blockers, alcohol, aldesleukin, alprostadil, amitriptyline, angiotensin II receptor antagonists, antipsychotics, anxiolytics and hypnotics, arsenic, atazanavir, atenolol, baclofen, beta blockers, boceprevir, calcium channel blockers, cimetidine, citalopram, clonidine, conivaptan, corticosteroids, CYP3A4 inducers or inhibitors, darunavir, dasabuvir/ombitasvir/paritaprevir/ritonavir, dasatinib, deferasirox, degarelix, delavirdine, diazoxide, diltiazem, diuretics, estrogens, food, general anesthetics, hydralazine, indinavir, itraconazole, ketoconazole, lapatinib, levodopa, levofloxacin, lopinavir, MAO inhibitors, methyldopa, minoxidil, moxifloxacin, moxisylyte, moxonidine, nelfinavir, nitrates, nitroprusside, NSAIDs, pazopanib, phosphodiesterase 5 inhibitors, protease inhibitors, QT prolonging agents, ritonavir, sildenafil, St John's wort, tadalafil, telaprevir, telavancin, telithromycin, tipranavir, tizanidine, vardenafil, voriconazole, vorinostat, ziprasidone
Pregnancy category: B
Important contra-indications noted in the prescribing guidelines for: pediatric patients

---

Cardiovascular
Hypotension [2]
Orthostatic hypotension [3]
QT prolongation [2]

Central Nervous System
Headache (3%)
Pain (<2%)
Vertigo (dizziness) (6%) [19]

Neuromuscular/Skeletal
Asthenia (fatigue) (3%)

Gastrointestinal/Hepatic
Abdominal pain (<2%)
Hepatotoxicity [2]

Respiratory
Bronchitis (<2%)
Pharyngitis (<2%)
Sinusitis (<2%)
Upper respiratory tract infection (3%)

Genitourinary
Ejaculatory dysfunction [3]
Erectile dysfunction [2]

Ocular
Floppy iris syndrome [4]

Other
Adverse effects [2]

ALIROCUMAB

Trade name: Praluent (Regeneron)
Indications: Adjunct to diet and statin therapy in hypercholesterolemia or clinical atherosclerotic cardiovascular disease where additional lowering of low density lipoprotein cholesterol is required
Class: Monoclonal antibody, Proprotein convertase subtilisin kexin type 9 (PCSK9) inhibitor
Half-life: 17–20 days
Clinically important, potentially hazardous interactions with: none known
Pregnancy category: N/A (No data available but likely to cross the placenta in second and third trimester)
Important contra-indications noted in the prescribing guidelines for: pediatric patients

---

Skin
Hematoma (2%)

Cardiovascular
Cardiotoxicity [3]
Myocardial infarction [3]

Central Nervous System
Cognitive impairment [2]
Headache [4]
Neurotoxicity [4]
Stroke [2]
Vertigo (dizziness) [6]

Neuromuscular/Skeletal
Arthralgia [6]
Asthenia (fatigue) [2]
Back pain [6]
Bone or joint pain (2%) [2]
Muscle spasm (3%)
Myalgia/Myopathy (4%) [7]

Gastrointestinal/Hepatic
Diarrhea (5%) [3]
Hepatotoxicity (3%)
Nausea [2]

Respiratory
Bronchitis (4%)
Cough (3%)
Influenza (6%) [4]
Nasopharyngitis (11%) [9]
Sinusitis (3%) [2]
Upper respiratory tract infection [7]

Endocrine/Metabolic
ALT increased [3]
Creatine phosphokinase increased [3]

Genitourinary
Urinary tract infection (5%)

Ocular
Ocular adverse effects [2]

Local
Injection-site pain [2]
Injection-site reactions (7%) [19]

Other
Adverse effects [6]
Allergic reactions (9%)
Death [2]

ALITRETINOIN

Trade name: Panretin (Ligand)
Indications: Kaposi's sarcoma cutaneous lesions
Class: Retinoid
Half-life: N/A
Clinically important, potentially hazardous interactions with: ketoconazole, simvastatin, vitamin A
Pregnancy category: D
Important contra-indications noted in the prescribing guidelines for: the elderly; pediatric patients
Note: Oral alitretinoin (Toctino) is not available in the USA.

Skin
Edema (3–8%)
Erythema [2]
Exfoliative dermatitis (3–9%)
Flushing [2]
Pigmentation (3%)
Pruritus (8–11%)
Rash (25–77%)
Ulcerations (2%)
Xerosis (10%)

Hair
Curly hair [2]

Mucosal
Mucocutaneous reactions [2]

Central Nervous System
Depression [2]
Headache [7]
Paresthesias (3–22%)

Gastrointestinal/Hepatic
Nausea [2]

Endocrine/Metabolic
Creatine phosphokinase increased [2]
Hypertriglyceridemia [2]

ALLOPURINOL

Trade names: Duzallo (AstraZeneca), Zyloprim (Prometheus)
Indications: Gouty arthritis
Class: Purine analog, Xanthine oxidase inhibitor
Half-life: <3 hours
Clinically important, potentially hazardous interactions with: acenocoumarol, amoxicillin, ampicillin, ampicillin/sulbactam, azathioprine, benazepril, capecitabine, captopril, cilazapril, cyclopenthiazide, dicumarol, enalapril, fosinopril, imidapril, lisinopril, mercaptopurine, pantoprazole, quinapril, ramipril, trandolapril, uracil/tegafur, vidarabine, zofenopril
Pregnancy category: C
Note: HLA-B*58:01 confers a risk of allopurinol-induced serious skin reactions like SJS/TEN and DRESS. Should be seriously considered in patients of south Asian ancestry (see also Genetic Tables 1 and 2, pp. 356–66)
Duzallo is allopurinol and lesinurad (see separate entry).

Skin
AGEP [6]
DRESS syndrome [47]
Eosinophilic pustular folliculitis [2]
Erythema multiforme [7]
Exanthems (<5%) [20]
Exfoliative dermatitis (>10%) [15]
Fixed eruption [11]
Granuloma annulare (disseminated) [2]
Hypersensitivity [49]
Lupus erythematosus [3]
Pityriasis rosea [2]
Pruritus [7]
Purpura (>10%) [2]
Rash (>10%) [11]
Stevens-Johnson syndrome (>10%) [54]
Toxic epidermal necrolysis [73]
Toxic pustuloderma [3]
Toxicity [2]
Urticaria (>10%) [6]
Vasculitis [7]

Hair
Alopecia (<10%) [2]

Mucosal
Oral ulceration [3]
Stomatitis [2]

Cardiovascular
Polyarteritis nodosa [3]

Central Nervous System
Chills (<10%)
Fever [2]
Headache [3]
Vertigo (dizziness) [3]

Neuromuscular/Skeletal
Arthralgia [3]
Asthenia (fatigue) [2]
Back pain [2]
Bone or joint pain [2]
Joint disorder [2]
Myalgia/Myopathy [3]

Gastrointestinal/Hepatic
Diarrhea [5]
Hepatotoxicity [7]
Nausea [3]

Respiratory
Nasopharyngitis [2]
Upper respiratory tract infection [4]

Endocrine/Metabolic
ALT increased [2]
AST increased [3]

Renal
Nephrotoxicity [3]

Other
Adverse effects [13]
Allergic reactions (severe) [2]
Death [9]

ALMOTRIPTAN

Trade names: Almogran (Almirall), Axert (Ortho-McNeil)
Indications: Migraine headaches
Class: 5-HT1 agonist, Serotonin receptor agonist, Triptan
Half-life: 3–4 hours
Clinically important, potentially hazardous interactions with: conivaptan, darunavir, delavirdine, dihydroergotamine, ergotamine,

indinavir, ketoconazole, methysergide, SNRIs, SSRIs, telithromycin, triptans, voriconazole
Pregnancy category: C
Important contra-indications noted in the prescribing guidelines for: pediatric patients
Note: Contra-indicated in patients with history, symptoms, or signs of ischemic cardiac, cerebrovascular, or peripheral vascular syndromes, or with uncontrolled hypertension.

Cardiovascular
Chest pain [3]

Central Nervous System
Headache [2]
Neurotoxicity [2]
Paresthesias [4]
Somnolence (drowsiness) [5]
Vertigo (dizziness) [6]

Neuromuscular/Skeletal
Asthenia (fatigue) [4]

Gastrointestinal/Hepatic
Nausea [6]
Vomiting [3]

Respiratory
Flu-like syndrome (12%)
Upper respiratory tract infection (20%)

Other
Adverse effects [10]

ALOE VERA (GEL, JUICE, LEAF)

Family: Liliaceae
Scientific names: *Aloë africana, Aloë barbadensis, Aloë ferox, Aloë spicata*
Indications: Oral: anesthetic, antiseptic, antipyretic, antipruritic, vasodilator, anti-inflammatory, vermifuge, antifungal. antiulcer, diabetes, asthma
Topical: promote healing, cold sores, ulceration, radiations injuries, psoriasis, frostbite. Also used in cosmetics and for its moisturizing and emollient properties
Class: Anthroquinone glycoside, Anti-inflammatory
Half-life: N/A
Clinically important, potentially hazardous interactions with: arsenic
Pregnancy category: N/A
Note: One blade of aloe can be used for weeks. The severed end of the blade is self healing.
I have perfumed my bed with myrrh, aloes and cinnamon (Proverbs 7:17).
Cleopatra regarded the gel as a fountain of youth and used it to preserve her skin against the ravages of the Egyptian sun.

Skin
Contact dermatitis [2]
Henoch-Schönlein purpura [2]
Hypersensitivity [2]

Gastrointestinal/Hepatic
Diarrhea [2]
Hepatitis [6]

Endocrine/Metabolic
Hypokalemia [2]

Other
Allergic reactions [2]

ALOGLIPTIN

Trade name: Nesina (Takeda)
Indications: Type II diabetes mellitus
Class: Antidiabetic, Dipeptidyl peptidase-4 (DPP-4) inhibitor
Half-life: 21 hours
Clinically important, potentially hazardous interactions with: none known
Pregnancy category: B
Important contra-indications noted in the prescribing guidelines for: nursing mothers; pediatric patients

---

Skin
Hypersensitivity [2]
Pruritus [2]

Central Nervous System
Headache (4%) [8]
Vertigo (dizziness) [3]

Neuromuscular/Skeletal
Arthralgia [2]

Gastrointestinal/Hepatic
Constipation [2]
Diarrhea [2]
Pancreatitis [3]

Respiratory
Nasopharyngitis (4%) [8]
Upper respiratory tract infection (4%) [6]

Endocrine/Metabolic
Hypoglycemia [14]

Other
Adverse effects [6]
Infection [3]

ALPRAZOLAM

Trade name: Xanax (Pfizer)
Indications: Anxiety, depression, panic attacks
Class: Benzodiazepine
Half-life: 11–16 hours
Clinically important, potentially hazardous interactions with: alcohol, amprenavir, aprepitant, boceprevir, clarithromycin, CNS depressants, darunavir, delavirdine, digoxin, efavirenz, fluconazole, fluoxetine, fluvoxamine, grapefruit juice, indinavir, itraconazole, ivermectin, kava, ketoconazole, posaconazole, propoxyphene, ritonavir, saquinavir, St John's wort, telaprevir, tipranavir
Pregnancy category: D
Important contra-indications noted in the prescribing guidelines for: the elderly; nursing mothers; pediatric patients

---

Skin
Dermatitis (4%) [5]
Diaphoresis (16%)
Edema (5%)
Photosensitivity [4]
Pruritus (<10%) [2]
Rash (11%) [4]

Mucosal
Sialopenia (33%)
Sialorrhea (4%)
Xerostomia (15%) [6]

Cardiovascular
Hypotension (<10%)

Central Nervous System
Cognitive impairment (>10%)
Coma [2]
Depression (>10%)
Dysarthria (>10%)
Incoordination (<10%)
Memory loss [2]
Neurotoxicity [2]
Paresthesias (2%)
Restlessness [2]
Sedation [2]
Seizures (<10%) [2]
Somnolence (drowsiness) (>10%)

Neuromuscular/Skeletal
Asthenia (fatigue) (>10%) [2]

Endocrine/Metabolic
Galactorrhea [2]

Genitourinary
Micturition difficulty (>10%)

ALPROSTADIL

Synonyms: PGE; prostaglandin E_1
Trade names: Caverject (Pfizer), Edex (Schwarz), Muse (Vivus), Prostin VR (Pfizer)
Indications: Impotence, to maintain patent ductus arteriosus
Class: Prostaglandin
Half-life: 5–10 minutes
Clinically important, potentially hazardous interactions with: acebutolol, alfuzosin, captopril, cilazapril, enalapril, fosinopril, irbesartan, lisinopril, olmesartan, quinapril, ramipril
Pregnancy category: D (not indicated for use in women)
Important contra-indications noted in the prescribing guidelines for: pediatric patients
Warning: APNEA (in neonates with congenital heart defects)

Skin
Edema (<10%)
Flushing (>10%)
Penile rash (<10%)

Mucosal
Nasal congestion (<10%)

Cardiovascular
Bradycardia (<10%)
Hypertension (<10%)
Hypotension (<10%)
Tachycardia (<10%)

Central Nervous System
Fever (>10%)
Headache (>10%)
Pain (>10%)
Vertigo (dizziness) (>10%)

Neuromuscular/Skeletal
Back pain (<10%)

Gastrointestinal/Hepatic
Diarrhea (<10%)

Respiratory
Apnea (>10%)
Cough (<10%)
Flu-like syndrome (<10%)
Sinusitis (<10%)

Genitourinary
Erectile dysfunction (prolonged erection / >4 hours) (4%)
Penile pain (>10%)
Priapism (4%) [8]
Urethral burning (>10%) [2]

Local
Application-site burning [3]
Application-site erythema [3]
Application-site pain [2]
Application-site pruritus [2]
Injection-site ecchymoses (<10%)
Injection-site hematoma (3%)
Injection-site pain (2%)

ALTEPLASE

Synonym: tPA
Trade name: Activase (Genentech)
Indications: Acute myocardial infarction, acute pulmonary embolism
Class: Fibrinolytic, Plasminogen activator
Half-life: 30–45 minutes
Clinically important, potentially hazardous interactions with: defibrotide, nitroglycerin, ticlopidine
Pregnancy category: C
Important contra-indications noted in the prescribing guidelines for: the elderly; nursing mothers

---

Skin
Anaphylactoid reactions/Anaphylaxis [5]
Angioedema [12]
Ecchymoses (<10%)
Purpura (<10%)

Central Nervous System
Fever (<10%)
Intracranial hemorrhage [8]

Gastrointestinal/Hepatic
Hemorrhagic colitis (5%)

Hematologic
Bleeding [3]
Hemorrhage (4%)

Other
Death [4]

AMBRISENTAN

Trade names: Letairis (Gilead), Volibris (GSK)
Indications: Pulmonary arterial hypertension
Class: Antihypertensive, Endothelin receptor (ETR) antagonist, Vasodilator
Half-life: 9 hours
Clinically important, potentially hazardous interactions with: conivaptan, cyclosporine, CYP2C19 inducers or inhibitors, CYP3A4 inducers or inhibitors, dasatinib, deferasirox, grapefruit juice, St John's wort
Pregnancy category: X
Important contra-indications noted in the prescribing guidelines for: nursing mothers; pediatric patients
Note: Also contra-indicated in patients with idiopathic pulmonary fibrosis.
Warning: CONTRA-INDICATED IN PREGNANCY

Skin
Edema [4]
Flushing (4%)
Peripheral edema (17%) [9]

Mucosal
Nasal congestion (6%) [2]

Cardiovascular
Palpitation (5%)

Central Nervous System
Headache (15%) [4]

Gastrointestinal/Hepatic
Abdominal pain (3%)
Constipation (4%)
Hepatotoxicity [3]

Respiratory
Dyspnea (4%)
Nasopharyngitis (3%)
Sinusitis (3%)

Hematologic
Anemia [5]

AMIKACIN

Trade name: Amikacin sulfate (Bedford)
Indications: Short-term treatment of serious infections due to gram-negative bacteria
Class: Antibiotic, aminoglycoside
Half-life: 1.5–2.5 hours (adults)
Clinically important, potentially hazardous interactions with: adefovir, aldesleukin, aminoglycosides, atracurium, bumetanide, cephalexin, doxacurium, ethacrynic acid, furosemide, succinylcholine, teicoplanin, torsemide
Pregnancy category: D
Important contra-indications noted in the prescribing guidelines for: nursing mothers; pediatric patients
Note: Aminoglycosides may cause neurotoxicity and/or nephrotoxicity.

Skin
Dermatitis [3]
Exanthems [2]

Central Nervous System
Neurotoxicity (<10%)

Renal
Nephrotoxicity (<10%) [11]

Otic
Hearing loss [5]
Ototoxicity (<10%) [8]
Tinnitus [3]

Ocular
Macular infarction [3]

AMILORIDE

Trade names: Midamor (Merck), Moduretic (Merck)
Indications: Prevention of hypokalemia associated with kaliuretic diuretics, management of edema in hypertension
Class: Diuretic, potassium-sparing
Half-life: 6–9 hours
Clinically important, potentially hazardous interactions with: ACE inhibitors, benazepril, captopril, cyclosporine, enalapril, fosinopril, lisinopril, magnesium, metformin, moexipril, potassium salts, quinapril, quinidine, ramipril, spironolactone, trandolapril, zofenopril
Pregnancy category: B
Note: Moduretic is amiloride and hydrochlorothiazide. Hydrochlorothiazide is a sulfonamide and can be absorbed systemically. Sulfonamides can produce severe, possibly fatal, reactions such as toxic epidermal necrolysis and Stevens-Johnson syndrome.

Skin
Photosensitivity [4]

Central Nervous System
Headache (<10%)
Vertigo (dizziness) (<10%)

Neuromuscular/Skeletal
Asthenia (fatigue) (<10%)
Myalgia/Myopathy (<10%)

Respiratory
Cough (<10%)
Dyspnea (<10%)

Endocrine/Metabolic
Gynecomastia (<10%)
Hyperkalemia [2]

Genitourinary
Impotence (<10%)

AMINOLEVULINIC ACID

Trade names: Ameluz (Biofrontera), Levulan Kerastick (Dusa)
Indications: Non-hyperkeratotic actinic keratoses of face and scalp
Class: Photosensitizer, Protoporphyrin IX (PpIX) (wakefulness promoting agent)
Half-life: 20–40 hours
Clinically important, potentially hazardous interactions with: none known

Pregnancy category: C
Important contra-indications noted in the prescribing guidelines for: nursing mothers; pediatric patients
Note: In photodynamic therapy: to be used in conjunction with the relevant illuminator as approved by the manufacturer.

Skin
Burning (>50%) [6]
Crusting (64–71%) [2]
Dermatitis [2]
Desquamation [2]
Edema (35%) [9]
Erosions (14%) [2]
Erythema (99%) [13]
Exfoliative dermatitis (from topical treatment) [3]
Hypomelanosis (22%)
Photosensitivity [3]
Pigmentation (from topical treatment) (22%) [7]
Pruritus (25%) [2]
Pustules (<4%)
Scaling (64–71%)
Stinging (>50%) [2]
Ulcerations (4%)
Vesiculation (4%) [2]

Central Nervous System
Dysesthesia (2%)
Pain [12]

AMINOPHYLLINE

Synonym: theophylline ethylenediamine
Trade names: Elixophyllin (Forest), Phyllocontin (Napp), Quibron (Monarch)
Indications: Prevention or treatment of reversible bronchospasm
Class: Xanthine alkaloid
Half-life: 3–15 hours (in adult nonsmokers)
Clinically important, potentially hazardous interactions with: adenosine, anagrelide, arformoterol, azithromycin, BCG vaccine, caffeine, capsicum, carbimazole, cimetidine, ciprofloxacin, clorazepate, cocoa, erythromycin, eucalyptus, febuxostat, fluvoxamine, halothane, indacaterol, influenza vaccine, levofloxacin, mebendazole, methylprednisolone, moxifloxacin, nilutamide, norfloxacin, obeticholic acid, ofloxacin, oral contraceptives, prednisolone, prednisone, propranolol, rasagiline, raspberry leaf, roflumilast, ropivacaine, roxithromycin, St John's wort, torasemide, torsemide, triamcinolone, zafirlukast
Pregnancy category: C
Important contra-indications noted in the prescribing guidelines for: the elderly; nursing mothers

---

Skin
Dermatitis [7]
Exanthems [5]
Exfoliative dermatitis [6]
Hypersensitivity [6]
Pruritus [3]
Stevens-Johnson syndrome [3]
Urticaria [6]

Cardiovascular
Arrhythmias [2]
Palpitation [3]
Tachycardia [2]

Central Nervous System
Insomnia [2]
Seizures [11]
Tremor [2]

Neuromuscular/Skeletal
Rhabdomyolysis [5]

Gastrointestinal/Hepatic
Abdominal pain [2]
Nausea [5]
Vomiting [2]

Endocrine/Metabolic
SIADH [2]

Other
Adverse effects [3]
Allergic reactions [5]
Death [2]

AMIODARONE

Trade names: Cordarone (Wyeth), Pacerone (Upsher-Smith)
Indications: Ventricular fibrillation, ventricular tachycardia
Class: Antiarrhythmic, Antiarrhythmic class III, CYP1A2 inhibitor, CYP3A4 inhibitor
Half-life: 26–107 days
Clinically important, potentially hazardous interactions with: abarelix, acebutolol, acenocoumarol, afatinib, amisulpride, amitriptyline, amprenavir, anisindione, anticoagulants, arsenic, artemether/lumefantrine, asenapine, astemizole, atazanavir, atorvastatin, azoles, betrixaban, boceprevir, bosentan, carbimazole, celiprolol, cholestyramine, cimetidine, ciprofloxacin, clopidogrel, cobicistat/elvitegravir/emtricitabine/tenofovir alafenamide, cobicistat/elvitegravir/emtricitabine/tenofovir disoproxil, colchicine, cyclosporine, dabigatran, daclatasvir, darunavir, degarelix, delavirdine, dextromethorphan, dicumarol, digoxin, diltiazem, disopyramide, dronedarone, droperidol, echinacea, enoxacin, fentanyl, flecainide, fosamprenavir, gatifloxacin, grapefruit juice, indinavir, ledipasvir & sofosbuvir, lesinurad, letermovir, levofloxacin, levomepromazine, lidocaine, lomefloxacin, lopinavir, loratadine, macrolide antibiotics, methotrexate, moxifloxacin, naldemedine, nelfinavir, nevirapine, nilotinib, norfloxacin, ofloxacin, orlistat, oxprenolol, pentamidine, phenytoin, pimavanserin, procainamide, propranolol, quinidine, quinine, quinolones, ribociclib, rifabutin, rifampin, rifapentine, ritonavir, ropivacaine, rosuvastatin, simvastatin, sofosbuvir & velpatasvir, sofosbuvir/velpatasvir/voxilaprevir, sotalol, sparfloxacin, St John's wort, sulpiride, tacrolimus, telaprevir, tetrabenazine, thalidomide, tipranavir, trazodone, vandetanib, venetoclax, verapamil, warfarin, zuclopenthixol
Pregnancy category: D
Important contra-indications noted in the prescribing guidelines for: the elderly; nursing mothers; pediatric patients
Warning: PULMONARY TOXICITY

Skin
Anaphylactoid reactions/Anaphylaxis [2]
Angioedema [2]
Diaphoresis [2]
Edema (<10%)
Erythema nodosum [2]
Exanthems [5]
Facial erythema (3%) [2]
Flushing (<10%)
Iododerma [2]
Linear IgA bullous dermatosis [6]
Lupus erythematosus [5]
Myxedema [3]
Photosensitivity (10–75%) [42]
Phototoxicity [3]
Pigmentation (blue) (<10%) [68]
Pruritus (<5%) [2]
Psoriasis [2]
Purpura (2%)
Toxic epidermal necrolysis [2]
Toxicity [5]
Vasculitis [6]

Hair
Alopecia [5]

Mucosal
Sialorrhea (<10%)

Cardiovascular
Arrhythmias (<3%) [3]
Atrial fibrillation (paroxysmal) [3]
Atrioventricular block [3]
Bradycardia [18]
Cardiotoxicity [4]
Hypotension (16%) [4]
QT prolongation [25]
Tachycardia [2]
Thrombophlebitis [2]
Torsades de pointes [36]
Ventricular arrhythmia [2]

Central Nervous System
Anorexia (10–33%)
Coma [2]
Dysgeusia (taste perversion) (<10%)
Headache (3–40%)
Insomnia (3–40%)
Neurotoxicity [5]
Paresthesias (4–9%)
Parkinsonism [4]
Parosmia (<10%)
Peripheral neuropathy [4]
Syncope [2]
Tremor (3–40%) [4]
Vertigo (dizziness) (3–40%)

Neuromuscular/Skeletal
Ataxia [4]
Myoclonus [2]
Rhabdomyolysis [7]

Gastrointestinal/Hepatic
Abdominal pain (<10%)
Constipation (10–33%)
Hepatic failure [2]
Hepatic steatosis [2]
Hepatitis (<3%) [3]

Hepatotoxicity [28]
Nausea (10–33%)
Pancreatitis [5]
Vomiting (10–33%)

Respiratory
Cough [2]
Eosinophilic pneumonia [2]
Pneumonia [4]
Pneumonitis [5]
Pulmonary toxicity [25]

Endocrine/Metabolic
Hyperthyroidism (<3%) [10]
Hyponatremia [2]
Hypothyroidism (<3%) [19]
SIADH [11]
Thyroid dysfunction [26]
Thyrotoxicosis [20]

Genitourinary
Epididymitis [2]

Otic
Vestibular disorder [3]

Ocular
Corneal deposits (>90%) [2]
Keratopathy [6]
Ocular adverse effects [4]
Ocular toxicity [2]
Optic neuropathy [7]
Visual disturbances (2–9%)

Other
Adverse effects [5]
Death [9]
Side effects (12%) [4]

AMITRIPTYLINE

Trade names: Elavil (AstraZeneca), Limbitrol (Valeant)
Indications: Depression
Class: Antidepressant, tricyclic, Muscarinic antagonist
Half-life: 10–25 hours
Clinically important, potentially hazardous interactions with: adrenergic neurone blockers, alcohol, alfuzosin, altretamine, amiodarone, amphetamines, amprenavir, anticholinergics, antiepileptics, antihistamines, antimuscarinics, antipsychotics, apraclonidine, arsenic, artemether/lumefantrine, aspirin, atomoxetine, baclofen, barbiturates, brimonidine, bupropion, cannabis extract, carbamazepine, cimetidine, cinacalcet, ciprofloxacin, cisapride, clonidine, clozapine, cobicistat/elvitegravir/emtricitabine/tenofovir alafenamide, cobicistat/elvitegravir/emtricitabine/tenofovir disoproxil, conivaptan, coumarins, CYP2D6 inhibitors, desmopressin, dexmethylphenidate, diltiazem, disopyramide, disulfiram, diuretics, dronedarone, droperidol, duloxetine, entacapone, ephedra, epinephrine, estrogens, eucalyptus, flecainide, gadobutrol, general anesthetics, gotu kola, grapefruit juice, guanethidine, histamine, interferon alfa, iobenguane, isocarboxazid, isoproterenol, kava, linezolid, lithium, MAO inhibitors, methylphenidate, metoclopramide, moclobemide, moxifloxacin, moxonidine, nefopam, nicorandil, nilotinib, nitrates, NSAIDs, opioid analgesics, paroxetine hydrochloride, pentamidine, phenelzine, phenothiazines, phenytoin, pimozide, pramlintide, primidone, propafenone, propoxyphene, protease inhibitors, QT interval prolonging agents, quinidine, quinine, quinolones, rasagiline, ritonavir, saquinavir, selegiline, sibutramine, sodium oxybate, sotalol, sparfloxacin, SSRIs, St John's wort, sulfonylureas, terbinafine, tetrabenazine, thioridazine, thyroid hormones, tramadol, tranylcypromine, valerian, valproic acid, verapamil, vitamin K antagonists, yohimbine, ziprasidone
Pregnancy category: C
Important contra-indications noted in the prescribing guidelines for: the elderly; nursing mothers; pediatric patients
Note: Limbitrol is amitriptyline and chlordiazepoxide.
Warning: SUICIDALITY AND ANTIDEPRESSANT DRUGS

Skin
Diaphoresis (<10%)
DRESS syndrome [2]
Photosensitivity [3]
Pigmentation [4]
Pruritus [3]
Pseudolymphoma [2]
Purpura [2]

Mucosal
Xerostomia (>10%) [17]

Cardiovascular
Brugada syndrome [4]
Myocardial infarction [2]
Postural hypotension [2]
QT prolongation [2]

Central Nervous System
Delirium [2]
Depression [2]
Dysgeusia (taste perversion) (>10%) [2]
Hallucinations [3]
Headache [2]
Restless legs syndrome [2]
Sedation [3]
Seizures [7]
Serotonin syndrome [4]
Somnolence (drowsiness) [7]
Vertigo (dizziness) [6]

Neuromuscular/Skeletal
Asthenia (fatigue) [4]
Rhabdomyolysis [2]

Gastrointestinal/Hepatic
Cholestasis [2]
Constipation [5]
Nausea [2]

Endocrine/Metabolic
SIADH [5]
Weight gain [7]

Otic
Tinnitus [3]

Ocular
Hallucinations, visual [2]
Vision blurred [2]

Other
Adverse effects [5]
Death [3]

AMLODIPINE

Trade names: Caduet (Pfizer), Exforge (Novartis), Istin (Pfizer), Lotrel (Novartis), Norvasc (Pfizer), Prestalia (Symplmed), Tekamlo (Novartis)
Indications: Hypertension, angina
Class: Antiarrhythmic class IV, Calcium channel blocker
Half-life: 30–50 hours
Clinically important, potentially hazardous interactions with: amprenavir, carbamazepine, cobicistat/elvitegravir/emtricitabine/tenofovir alafenamide, cobicistat/elvitegravir/emtricitabine/tenofovir disoproxil, conivaptan, delavirdine, epirubicin, imatinib, phenytoin, primidone, sildenafil, simvastatin, St John's wort, tadalafil, telaprevir
Pregnancy category: C
Important contra-indications noted in the prescribing guidelines for: the elderly; nursing mothers; pediatric patients
Note: Caduet is amlodipine and atorvastatin; Exforge is amlodipine and valsartan; Lotrel is amlodipine and benazepril; Prestalia is amlodipine and perindopril; Tekamlo is amlodipine and aliskiren.

Skin
Angioedema [6]
Dermatitis (<10%)
Eczema [2]
Edema (5–14%) [20]
Erythema multiforme [2]
Exanthems (2–4%) [2]
Flushing (<10%) [5]
Peripheral edema (>10%) [45]
Pigmentation [2]
Pruritus (2–4%) [3]
Purpura [2]
Rash (<10%)
Telangiectasia (facial) [5]
Toxic epidermal necrolysis [2]
Toxicity [2]
Vasculitis [2]

Mucosal
Gingival hyperplasia/hypertrophy [31]

Cardiovascular
Bradycardia [2]
Hypotension [9]
Orthostatic hypotension [2]

Central Nervous System
Headache [12]
Parkinsonism [2]
Syncope [2]
Vertigo (dizziness) [15]

Neuromuscular/Skeletal
Asthenia (fatigue) [5]
Rhabdomyolysis [2]

Gastrointestinal/Hepatic
Diarrhea [3]
Gastritis [2]
Hepatotoxicity [3]
Nausea [5]
Vomiting [2]

Respiratory
Bronchitis [2]
Cough [3]

Upper respiratory tract infection [4]

Endocrine/Metabolic

Hyponatremia [2]

Other

Adverse effects [8]

AMODIAQUINE

Trade names: Camoquin (Pfizer), Flavoquin (Sanofi-Aventis)
Indications: Malaria
Class: Anti-inflammatory, Antimalarial
Half-life: 15.7–19.5 hours
Clinically important, potentially hazardous interactions with: none known
Pregnancy category: N/A
Important contra-indications noted in the prescribing guidelines for: pediatric patients

Skin

Pruritus [4]

Central Nervous System

Extrapyramidal symptoms [3]

Neuromuscular/Skeletal

Asthenia (fatigue) [4]

Gastrointestinal/Hepatic

Abdominal pain [3]
Diarrhea [3]
Hepatotoxicity [2]
Vomiting [8]

Hematologic

Neutropenia [2]

Other

Adverse effects [2]
Death [2]

AMOXAPINE

Trade name: Amoxapine (Watson)
Indications: Depression
Class: Antidepressant, tricyclic, Muscarinic antagonist
Half-life: 11–30 hours
Clinically important, potentially hazardous interactions with: amprenavir, artemether/lumefantrine, clonidine, dronedarone, epinephrine, fluoxetine, guanethidine, iobenguane, isocarboxazid, linezolid, MAO inhibitors, nilotinib, phenelzine, pimozide, quetiapine, quinine, quinolones, sparfloxacin, tetrabenazine, thioridazine, toremifene, tranylcypromine, vandetanib, vemurafenib, ziprasidone
Pregnancy category: C
Important contra-indications noted in the prescribing guidelines for: the elderly; nursing mothers; pediatric patients
Warning: SUICIDALITY AND ANTIDEPRESSANT DRUGS

Skin

AGEP [3]
Diaphoresis (<10%)
Edema (<10%)
Exanthems [2]
Rash (<10%)
Toxic epidermal necrolysis [2]

Mucosal

Xerostomia (14%)

Central Nervous System

Dysgeusia (taste perversion) (>10%)
Headache (<10%)
Insomnia (<10%)
Neuroleptic malignant syndrome [2]
Somnolence (drowsiness) (14%)
Vertigo (dizziness) (<10%)

Neuromuscular/Skeletal

Asthenia (fatigue) (<10%)

Gastrointestinal/Hepatic

Constipation (12%)
Nausea (<10%)

Endocrine/Metabolic

Galactorrhea [2]

Ocular

Vision blurred (7%)

Other

Side effects (5%)

AMOXICILLIN

Synonym: amoxycillin
Trade names: Amoxil (GSK), Augmentin (GSK), Prevpac (TAP), Trimox (Bristol-Myers Squibb)
Indications: Infections of the respiratory tract, skin and urinary tract
Class: Antibiotic, penicillin
Half-life: 0.7–1.4 hours
Clinically important, potentially hazardous interactions with: allopurinol, bromelain, chloramphenicol, demeclocycline, doxycycline, erythromycin, imipenem/cilastatin, methotrexate, minocycline, omeprazole, oxytetracycline, sulfonamides, tetracycline
Pregnancy category: B
Note: Augmentin is amoxicillin and clavulanic acid.

Skin

AGEP [28]
Anaphylactoid reactions/Anaphylaxis [16]
Angioedema (<10%) [5]
Baboon syndrome (SDRIFE) [11]
Bullous pemphigoid [2]
Dermatitis [4]
DRESS syndrome [6]
Edema [2]
Erythema multiforme [18]
Exanthems (>5%) [33]
Fixed eruption [10]
Hypersensitivity [5]
Jarisch-Herxheimer reaction [2]
Linear IgA bullous dermatosis [3]
Pemphigus [4]
Pruritus [7]
Pustules [8]
Rash (<10%) [14]
Serum sickness-like reaction (<10%) [6]
Stevens-Johnson syndrome [13]
Toxic epidermal necrolysis [14]
Toxic pustuloderma [2]
Urticaria (<5%) [16]

Mucosal

Stomatitis [2]

Central Nervous System

Anorexia [2]
Dysgeusia (taste perversion) [6]
Hallucinations [3]
Headache [5]
Somnolence (drowsiness) [3]
Vertigo (dizziness) [5]

Neuromuscular/Skeletal

Asthenia (fatigue) [3]
Rhabdomyolysis [2]

Gastrointestinal/Hepatic

Abdominal distension [2]
Abdominal pain [7]
Diarrhea [19]
Dyspepsia [2]
Hepatotoxicity [37]
Nausea [13]
Vomiting [9]

Genitourinary

Vaginitis [3]

Renal

Nephrotoxicity [2]

Other

Adverse effects [20]
Kounis syndrome [6]
Side effects [4]
Tooth fluorosis [2]

AMPHOTERICIN B

Trade names: Abelcet (Sigma-Tau), AmBisome (Astellas), Amphocin (Pfizer), Amphotec (Alkopharma)
Indications: Potentially life-threatening fungal infections
Class: Antifungal
Half-life: initial: 15–48 hours; terminal: 15 days
Clinically important, potentially hazardous interactions with: adefovir, aminoglycosides, arsenic, astemizole, betamethasone, cephalothin, cidofovir, cyclosporine, digoxin, ethoxzolamide, fluconazole, flucytosine, ganciclovir, griseofulvin, hydrocortisone, itraconazole, ketoconazole, micafungin, pentamidine, probenecid, sulpiride, terbinafine, triamcinolone, voriconazole
Pregnancy category: B
Important contra-indications noted in the prescribing guidelines for: nursing mothers

Skin

Anaphylactoid reactions/Anaphylaxis [4]
Diaphoresis (7%)
Exanthems [4]
Flushing (<10%) [2]
Peripheral edema (15%)
Pruritus (11%) [2]
Purpura [3]
Rash (25%)
Toxicity [2]
Urticaria [2]

Mucosal

Epistaxis (nosebleed) (15%)

Cardiovascular

Chest pain (12%)

Hypertension (8%) [4]
Hypotension (14%)
Tachycardia (13%)
Thrombophlebitis (<10%)

Central Nervous System
Anorexia (>10%)
Anxiety (14%)
Chills (48%) [6]
Confusion (11%)
Delirium (>10%)
Fever (>10%) [5]
Headache (20%)
Insomnia (17%)
Leukoencephalopathy [4]
Pain (14%)
Paresthesias (<10%)
Parkinsonism [2]
Rigors [2]

Neuromuscular/Skeletal
Asthenia (fatigue) (13%)
Back pain (12%)

Gastrointestinal/Hepatic
Abdominal pain (20%)
Diarrhea (30%)
Gastrointestinal bleeding (10%)
Hepatotoxicity [6]
Nausea (40%)
Vomiting (32%)

Respiratory
Bronchospasm [2]
Cough (18%)
Dyspnea (23%)
Hypoxia (8%)
Pleural effusion (13%)
Pulmonary toxicity (18%)
Rhinitis (11%)
Tachypnea (>10%)

Endocrine/Metabolic
ALP increased (22%)
ALT increased (15%)
AST increased (13%)
Creatine phosphokinase increased (22%)
Hyperglycemia (23%)
Hypernatremia (4%)
Hypervolemia (12%)
Hypocalcemia (18%)
Hypokalemia [2]
Hypomagnesemia (20%)

Genitourinary
Hematuria (14%)
Urinary retention (<10%)

Renal
Nephrotoxicity [51]

Hematologic
Anemia (>10%) [4]
Leukocytosis (<10%)
Sepsis (14%)

Local
Infusion-related reactions [5]
Injection-site pain (>10%)
Injection-site reactions [5]

Other
Adverse effects [5]
Death [4]
Infection (11%)

AMPICILLIN

Trade name: Totacillin (GSK)
Indications: Susceptible strains of gram-negative and gram-positive bacterial infections
Class: Antibiotic, penicillin
Half-life: 1–1.5 hours
Clinically important, potentially hazardous interactions with: allopurinol, anticoagulants, chloramphenicol, cyclosporine, demeclocycline, doxycycline, erythromycin, levodopa, methotrexate, minocycline, oxytetracycline, sulfonamides, tetracycline
Pregnancy category: B
Important contra-indications noted in the prescribing guidelines for: nursing mothers
Note: Five to 10% of people taking ampicillin develop eruptions between the 5th and 14th day following initiation of therapy. Also, there is a 95% incidence of exanthematous eruptions in patients who are treated for infectious mononucleosis with ampicillin. The allergenicity of ampicillin appears to be enhanced by allopurinol or by hyperuricemia. Ampicillin is clearly the more allergenic of the two drugs when given alone.

Skin
AGEP [9]
Anaphylactoid reactions/Anaphylaxis [10]
Angioedema [2]
Baboon syndrome (SDRIFE) [3]
Dermatitis [8]
Erythema multiforme [11]
Exanthems (>10%) [84]
Exfoliative dermatitis [3]
Fixed eruption [10]
Hypersensitivity [5]
Linear IgA bullous dermatosis [4]
Pemphigus [6]
Pruritus (<5%) [5]
Psoriasis [5]
Purpura [6]
Pustules [4]
Rash (<10%)
Stevens-Johnson syndrome [10]
Toxic epidermal necrolysis [15]
Urticaria [16]
Vasculitis [4]

Hematologic
Thrombocytopenia [2]

Local
Injection-site pain (>10%)

Other
Allergic reactions (<10%) [3]

AMPICILLIN/SULBACTAM

Trade name: Unasyn (Pfizer)
Indications: Various infections caused by susceptible organisms
Class: Antibiotic, beta-lactam, Antibiotic, penicillin
Half-life: 1 hour
Clinically important, potentially hazardous interactions with: allopurinol, probenecid
Pregnancy category: B
Important contra-indications noted in the prescribing guidelines for: nursing mothers
Note: Serious and occasionally fatal hypersensitivity (anaphylactic) reactions have been reported in patients on penicillin therapy. Contra-indicated in patients with a history of hypersensitivity reactions to any of the penicillins.

Skin
Anaphylactoid reactions/Anaphylaxis [2]
Linear IgA bullous dermatosis [3]
Rash (<10%)

Gastrointestinal/Hepatic
Diarrhea (<10%)

Local
Injection-site pain (16%)

ANAKINRA

Trade name: Kineret (Amgen)
Indications: Rheumatoid arthritis, neonatal-onset multisystem inflammatory disease
Class: Disease-modulating antirheumatoid drug, Interleukin-1 receptor antagonist (IL-IRa)
Half-life: 4–6 hours
Clinically important, potentially hazardous interactions with: abatacept, adalimumab, certolizumab, etanercept, golimumab, infliximab, lenalidomide, live vaccines
Pregnancy category: B
Important contra-indications noted in the prescribing guidelines for: nursing mothers

Central Nervous System
Fever (12%)
Headache (12–14%) [2]

Neuromuscular/Skeletal
Arthralgia (6–12%)

Gastrointestinal/Hepatic
Abdominal pain (5%)
Diarrhea (8%)
Nausea (8%)
Vomiting (14%)

Respiratory
Flu-like syndrome (6%)
Nasopharyngitis (12%)
Sinusitis (7%)
Upper respiratory tract infection (4%) [2]

Local
Injection-site edema [2]
Injection-site erythema [3]
Injection-site inflammation [2]
Injection-site pain [4]
Injection-site reactions (71%) [32]

Other
Adverse effects [6]
Infection (40%) [11]

ANASTROZOLE

Trade name: Arimidex (AstraZeneca)
Indications: Breast carcinoma (localized – advanced or metastatic)
Class: Antineoplastic, Aromatase inhibitor
Half-life: 50 hours
Clinically important, potentially hazardous interactions with: estradiol, estrogens, tamoxifen
Pregnancy category: N/A (Contra-indicated in women of premenopausal endocrine status, including pregnant women)
Important contra-indications noted in the prescribing guidelines for: nursing mothers
Note: The efficacy of anastrozole in the treatment of pubertal gynecomastia in adolescent boys and in the treatment of precocious puberty in girls with McCune-Albright syndrome has not been demonstrated.

Skin
Flushing (>5%)
Hot flashes (12–36%) [13]
Lupus erythematosus [3]
Peripheral edema (10%)
Pruritus (2–5%)
Rash (6–11%) [2]

Hair
Alopecia (2–5%)

Cardiovascular
Angina (2%)
Hypertension (2–13%)
Thrombophlebitis (2–5%)

Central Nervous System
Carpal tunnel syndrome [2]
Depression (5–13%)
Headache (9–13%) [2]
Pain (14%)
Tumor pain (>5%)

Neuromuscular/Skeletal
Arthralgia (2–5%) [8]
Asthenia (fatigue) (19%) [7]
Back pain (12%) [2]
Bone or joint pain (6–11%) [2]
Joint disorder [3]
Myalgia/Myopathy (2–5%) [2]
Osteoporosis (11%)

Gastrointestinal/Hepatic
Diarrhea [2]
Hepatitis [2]
Hepatotoxicity [5]
Nausea (11–19%)
Vomiting (8–13%)

Respiratory
Cough (11%)
Flu-like syndrome (7%)
Pharyngitis (6–14%)

Endocrine/Metabolic
Mastodynia (2–5%)

Genitourinary
Vaginal dryness (2%) [3]

Other
Infection (2–5%)

ANIDULAFUNGIN

Trade names: Ecalta (Pfizer), Eraxis (Pfizer)
Indications: Candidemia, candidal esophagitis
Class: Antimycobacterial, echinocandin
Half-life: 40–50 hours
Clinically important, potentially hazardous interactions with: none known
Pregnancy category: C
Important contra-indications noted in the prescribing guidelines for: nursing mothers; pediatric patients

---

Skin
Angioedema (<2%)
Erythema (<2%)
Flushing (<2%) [2]
Hot flashes (<2%)
Hyperhidrosis (<2%)
Peripheral edema (11%)
Pruritus (<2%)
Ulcerations (5%)
Urticaria (<2%)

Mucosal
Oral candidiasis (5%)

Cardiovascular
Atrial fibrillation (<2%)
Bundle branch block (<2%)
Chest pain (5%)
Hypertension (12%)
Hypotension (15%)
Phlebitis [2]
Thrombophlebitis (<2%)
Venous thromboembolism (10%)

Central Nervous System
Confusion (8%)
Depression (6%)
Fever (9–18%) [3]
Headache (8%) [5]
Insomnia (15%)
Rigors (<2%)
Seizures (<2%)
Vertigo (dizziness) (<2%)

Neuromuscular/Skeletal
Back pain (5%)

Gastrointestinal/Hepatic
Abdominal pain (6%)
Cholestasis (<2%)
Constipation (8%)
Diarrhea (9–18%)
Dyspepsia (aggravated) (7%)
Hepatotoxicity [4]
Nausea (7–24%) [4]
Vomiting (7–18%) [4]

Respiratory
Cough (7%)
Dyspnea (12%)
Pleural effusion (10%)
Pneumonia (6%)
Respiratory distress (6%)

Endocrine/Metabolic
ALP increased (12%)
ALT increased (2%)
Creatine phosphokinase increased (5%)
Dehydration (6%)
Hyperglycemia (6%)
Hyperkalemia (6%)
Hypoglycemia (7%)
Hypokalemia (5–15%)
Hypomagnesemia (12%)

Genitourinary
Urinary tract infection (15%)

Hematologic
Anemia (8–9%)
Coagulopathy (<2%)
Leukocytosis (5%)
Sepsis (7%)
Thrombocythemia (6%)
Thrombocytopenia (<2%)

Ocular
Ocular pain (<2%)
Vision blurred (<2%)
Visual disturbances (<2%)

Local
Infusion-related reactions [2]

Other
Adverse effects [3]
Infection (63%)

ANTHRAX VACCINE

Trade name: BioThrax (Emergent BioSolutions)
Indications: Anthrax prophylaxis
Class: Vaccine
Half-life: Requires 1 month to achieve immunity (92.5% efficient)
Clinically important, potentially hazardous interactions with: corticosteroids, immunosuppressive therapies, other vaccines
Pregnancy category: D
Important contra-indications noted in the prescribing guidelines for: the elderly; nursing mothers; pediatric patients
Note: Dr. Sue Bailey, Assistant Secretary for Health Affairs, released a statement on June 29, 1999 that 'almost one million shots given, the anthrax immunization is proving to be one of the safest vaccination programs on record.' The ADRs reported occurred for '50 service members at one installation alone.' Note that no number of military personnel was mentioned at this installation, nor did it give any percentages for the reactions reported.

Skin
Diaphoresis [2]
Edema (3%) [2]
Hypersensitivity [5]
Lupus erythematosus [2]
Pruritus (<10%) [2]
Rash [2]
Stevens-Johnson syndrome [2]
Urticaria [2]

Central Nervous System
Chills [2]
Fever [3]
Guillain-Barré syndrome [2]
Headache (4–64%) [2]

Neuromuscular/Skeletal
Arthralgia [3]
Asthenia (fatigue) (5–62%)
Myalgia/Myopathy (2–72%) [3]

Gastrointestinal/Hepatic
Diarrhea (6–8%)
Nausea (6%)

Respiratory
Flu-like syndrome [3]
Nasopharyngitis (12–15%)

Genitourinary
Dysmenorrhea (7%)

Local
Injection-site edema [4]
Injection-site nodules [2]
Injection-site pain [4]
Injection-site pruritus [2]
Injection-site reactions [6]

Other
Allergic reactions [2]

ANTIHEMOPHILIC FACTOR

Synonym: rFVIIIFc
Trade names: Afstyla (CSL Behring), Eloctate (Biogen Idec), Kovaltry (Bayer)
Indications: Control and prevention of bleeding episodes in Hemophilia A
Class: Antihemorrhagic, Recombinant fusion protein
Half-life: 20 hours (adults)
Clinically important, potentially hazardous interactions with: none known
Pregnancy category: C
Important contra-indications noted in the prescribing guidelines for: nursing mothers

---

Other
Adverse effects [2]

APIXABAN

Trade name: Eliquis (Bristol-Myers Squibb)
Indications: Reduce the risk of stroke and systemic embolism in patients with nonvalvular atrial fibrillation
Class: Anticoagulant, Direct factor Xa inhibitor
Half-life: 5–12 hours
Clinically important, potentially hazardous interactions with: carbamazepine, darunavir, phenytoin, rifampin, St John's wort, tipranavir, voriconazole
Pregnancy category: B
Important contra-indications noted in the prescribing guidelines for: nursing mothers; pediatric patients
Note: Contra-indicated in patients with active pathological bleeding.
Warning: DISCONTINUING ELIQUIS IN PATIENTS WITHOUT ADEQUATE CONTINUOUS ANTICOAGULATION INCREASES RISK OF STROKE

Gastrointestinal/Hepatic
Hepatotoxicity [2]

Hematologic
Hemorrhage [15]

Other
Adverse effects [4]

APRACLONIDINE

Trade name: Iopidine (Alcon)
Indications: Post-surgical intraocular pressure elevation
Class: Adrenergic alpha2-receptor agonist
Half-life: 8 hours
Clinically important, potentially hazardous interactions with: amitriptyline
Pregnancy category: C
Important contra-indications noted in the prescribing guidelines for: nursing mothers; pediatric patients

---

Skin
Dermatitis [3]
Pruritus (10%)

Mucosal
Xerostomia (<10%)

Central Nervous System
Dysgeusia (taste perversion) (3%)

Ocular
Conjunctivitis (<5%)
Eyelid edema (<3%)
Ocular pruritus (5–15%)
Xerophthalmia (<5%)

Other
Allergic reactions [5]

APREMILAST

Trade name: Otezla (Celgene)
Indications: Psoriatic arthritis, plaque psoriasis
Class: Phosphodiesterase inhibitor, Phosphodiesterase type 4 (PDE4) inhibitor
Half-life: 6–9 hours
Clinically important, potentially hazardous interactions with: carbamazepine, phenobarbital, phenytoin, rifampin
Pregnancy category: C
Important contra-indications noted in the prescribing guidelines for: nursing mothers; pediatric patients

---

Central Nervous System
Depression [4]
Headache (5–6%) [28]

Neuromuscular/Skeletal
Arthralgia [2]
Asthenia (fatigue) [5]

Gastrointestinal/Hepatic
Abdominal pain (<2%) [4]
Diarrhea (8–9%) [35]
Dyspepsia [2]
Nausea (7–9%) [35]
Vomiting (<3%) [10]

Respiratory
Nasopharyngitis (<3%) [19]
Upper respiratory tract infection (<4%) [16]

Endocrine/Metabolic
ALT increased [2]
Appetite decreased [2]
Weight loss (10–12%) [6]

Other
Adverse effects [5]
Infection [2]

APREPITANT

Trade name: Emend (Merck)
Indications: Prevention of postoperative and chemotherapy induced nausea and vomiting
Class: Antiemetic, CYP3A4 inhibitor, Neurokinin 1 receptor antagonist
Half-life: 9–13 hours
Clinically important, potentially hazardous interactions with: alprazolam, antifungal agents, astemizole, avanafil, betamethasone, carbamazepine, cisapride, clarithromycin, colchicine, conivaptan, corticosteroids, CYP2C9 substrates, CYP3A4 inducers or inhibitors, dasatinib, deferasirox, dexamethasone, diltiazem, docetaxel, eplerenone, estrogens, everolimus, fentanyl, grapefruit juice, halofantrine, ifosfamide, imatinib, irinotecan, itraconazole, ketoconazole, methylprednisolone, midazolam, mifepristone, naldemedine, nefazodone, neratinib, olaparib, oral contraceptives, paroxetine hydrochloride, phenobarbital, phenytoin, pimecrolimus, pimozide, progestins, ranolazine, rifampin, rifamycin derivatives, rifapentine, ritonavir, salmeterol, saxagliptin, St John's wort, telithromycin, terfenadine, tolbutamide, tolvaptan, trabectedin, triamcinolone, troleandomycin, vinblastine, vincristine, voriconazole, warfarin
Pregnancy category: N/A (Insufficient evidence to inform drug-associated risk)
Important contra-indications noted in the prescribing guidelines for: nursing mothers; pediatric patients
Note: Fosaprepitant is a prodrug of aprepitant for injection. Aprepitant treatment is given along with a 5-HT3-receptor antagonist and dexamethasone.

Skin
Pruritus (8%)

Hair
Alopecia (12%)

Mucosal
Mucocutaneous reactions (3%)
Stomatitis (3%)

Cardiovascular
Hypertension (2%)
Hypotension (6%)

Central Nervous System
Anorexia (6–10%) [3]
Encephalopathy [2]
Fever (3–6%)
Headache (5–9%) [6]
Insomnia (2–3%)
Somnolence (drowsiness) [2]
Vertigo (dizziness) (3–7%) [2]

Neuromuscular/Skeletal
Asthenia (fatigue) (5–18%) [10]

Gastrointestinal/Hepatic
Abdominal pain (5%) [3]

Constipation (9–10%) [9]
Diarrhea (<10%) [3]
Dyspepsia (5–6%)
Flatulence (4%)
Gastritis (4%)
Nausea (6–13%)
Vomiting (3–8%)

Endocrine/Metabolic
ALT increased (6%)
AST increased (3%)
Creatine phosphokinase increased (4%)
Dehydration (6%)

Genitourinary
Urinary tract infection (2%)

Renal
Proteinuria (7%)

Hematologic
Anemia (3%)
Febrile neutropenia [3]
Neutropenia (3–6%) [3]

Otic
Tinnitus (4%)

Local
Infusion-related reactions [2]
Infusion-site pain [2]

Other
Hiccups (11%) [9]
Infection [3]

ARFORMOTEROL

Trade name: Brovana (Sunovion)
Indications: Chronic obstructive pulmonary disease including chronic bronchitis and emphysema
Class: Beta-2 adrenergic agonist, Bronchodilator
Half-life: 26 hours
Clinically important, potentially hazardous interactions with: aminophylline, beta blockers, MAO inhibitors, tricyclic antidepressants
Pregnancy category: C
Important contra-indications noted in the prescribing guidelines for: nursing mothers; pediatric patients
Note: Studies in asthma patients showed that long-acting $beta_2$-adrenergic agonists may increase the risk of asthma-related death. Contra-indicated in patients with asthma without use of a long-term asthma control medication.
Warning: ASTHMA-RELATED DEATH

Skin
Abscess (<2%)
Edema (<2%)
Herpes simplex (<2%)
Herpes zoster (<2%)
Neoplasms (<2%)
Peripheral edema (3%)
Pigmentation (<2%)
Rash (4%)
Xerosis (<2%)

Mucosal
Oral candidiasis (<2%)

Cardiovascular
Arteriosclerosis (<2%)
Atrioventricular block (<2%)
Chest pain (7%) [2]
Digitalis intoxication (<2%)
QT prolongation (<2%)
Supraventricular tachycardia (<2%)

Central Nervous System
Agitation (<2%)
Fever (<2%)
Headache [2]
Hypokinesia (<2%)
Insomnia [2]
Nervousness [3]
Pain (8%)
Paresthesias (<2%)
Somnolence (drowsiness) (<2%)
Tremor (<2%) [3]

Neuromuscular/Skeletal
Arthralgia (<2%)
Back pain (6%)
Leg cramps (4%)
Neck rigidity (<2%)

Gastrointestinal/Hepatic
Nausea [2]

Respiratory
Bronchitis [3]
COPD (exacerbation) [3]
Dysphonia (<2%)
Dyspnea (4%)
Flu-like syndrome (3%)
Nasopharyngitis [3]
Sinusitis (4%) [2]

Genitourinary
Cystitis (<2%)
Nocturia (<2%)

Ocular
Glaucoma (<2%)
Visual disturbances (<2%)

Local
Injection-site pain (<2%)

Other
Adverse effects [2]
Allergic reactions (<2%)

ARIPIPRAZOLE

Trade names: Abilify (Bristol-Myers Squibb), Aristada (Alkermes)
Indications: Schizophrenia, bipolar I disorder, major depressive disorder, irritability associated with autistic disorder
Class: Antipsychotic, Mood stabilizer
Half-life: 75–94 hours
Clinically important, potentially hazardous interactions with: alcohol, atazanavir, carbamazepine, CYP3A4 inhibitors, efavirenz, itraconazole, ketoconazole, lopinavir, nelfinavir, paroxetine hydrochloride, quinidine
Pregnancy category: C
Important contra-indications noted in the prescribing guidelines for: the elderly; pediatric patients
Warning: INCREASED MORTALITY IN ELDERLY PATIENTS WITH DEMENTIA-RELATED PSYCHOSIS
SUICIDALITY AND ANTIDEPRESSANT DRUGS

Skin
Rash (6%) [2]

Mucosal
Sialorrhea (4–9%) [5]
Xerostomia (5%) [7]

Cardiovascular
Arrhythmias [2]
Hypertension [3]
QT prolongation [2]

Central Nervous System
Agitation (19%) [5]
Akathisia (8–13%) [36]
Anxiety (17%) [11]
Compulsions [2]
Dyskinesia [3]
Extrapyramidal symptoms [10]
Fever (2%)
Headache (27%) [13]
Hypersexuality [2]
Impulse control disorder [4]
Insomnia (18%) [21]
Irritability [4]
Mania [2]
Neuroleptic malignant syndrome [14]
Neurotoxicity [2]
Parkinsonism [11]
Psychosis [2]
Restlessness [8]
Schizophrenia (exacerbation) [2]
Sedation [11]
Somnolence (drowsiness) (5–11%) [13]
Stroke [2]
Suicidal ideation [6]
Tardive dyskinesia [8]
Tic disorder [2]
Tremor (3%) [9]
Vertigo (dizziness) [7]

Neuromuscular/Skeletal
Asthenia (fatigue) [5]
Ataxia [4]
Dystonia [13]
Pisa syndrome [2]

Gastrointestinal/Hepatic
Constipation (11%) [4]
Dyspepsia (9%)
Nausea (15%) [12]
Vomiting (11%) [5]

Respiratory
Cough (3%)
Nasopharyngitis [2]
Upper respiratory tract infection [3]

Endocrine/Metabolic
Appetite increased [5]
Diabetes mellitus [2]
Galactorrhea [2]
Hyperprolactinemia [2]
SIADH [2]
Weight gain (2–30%) [31]

Genitourinary
Priapism [3]
Urinary retention [2]
Vaginitis [2]

Hematologic
Neutropenia [3]

Ocular
Vision blurred (3–8%)

Local
Injection-site pain [6]

Other
Adverse effects [5]
Death [3]
Hiccups [3]
Toothache [2]

ARISTOLOCHIA

Family: Aristolochiaceae
Scientific names: *Aristolochia clematitis, Aristolochia serpentaria*
Indications: Aphrodisiac, anti-allergy, anticonvulsant, promotes menstruation
Class: Immunomodulator
Half-life: N/A
Clinically important, potentially hazardous interactions with: none known
Pregnancy category: N/A
Note: Aristolochia has been reported to cause severe kidney damage or 'Chinese herb nephropathy'. Eighteen patients developed carcinomas of the bladder, ureter and/or renal pelvis.
Aristolochia is banned in the European Union and Japan.

Skin
Carcinoma [2]
Toxicity [2]

Renal
Nephrotoxicity [9]

ARMODAFINIL

Trade name: Nuvigil (Cephalon)
Indications: Narcolepsy, obstructive sleep apnea, shift work sleep disorder
Class: Eugeroic
Half-life: 12–15 hours
Clinically important, potentially hazardous interactions with: cyclosporine
Pregnancy category: C
Important contra-indications noted in the prescribing guidelines for: the elderly; nursing mothers; pediatric patients

---

Central Nervous System
Anxiety [2]
Headache (14–23%) [10]
Insomnia (4–6%) [3]
Vertigo (dizziness) (5%) [2]

Gastrointestinal/Hepatic
Diarrhea [3]
Nausea [2]

Other
Adverse effects [2]

ARNICA

Family: Asteraceae; Compositae
Scientific names: *Arnica fulgens, Arnica montana, Arnica sororia*
Indications: Bruising, aches and sprains, insect bites, superficial phlebitis, diuretic, flavoring agent, found in hair tonic and shampoo
Class: Immunomodulator
Half-life: N/A
Clinically important, potentially hazardous interactions with: none known
Pregnancy category: N/A

Skin
Dermatitis [5]

ARTEMETHER/ LUMEFANTRINE

Trade name: Coartem (Novartis)
Indications: Acute, uncomplicated malaria infections due to *Plasmodium falciparum* in patients of 5kg bodyweight and above
Class: Antimalarial
Half-life: ~2 hours (artemether); 3–6 days (lumefantrine)
Clinically important, potentially hazardous interactions with: amiodarone, amitriptyline, amoxapine, antimalarials, antiretrovirals, arsenic, astemizole, atazanavir, atovaquone/proguanil, azithromycin, carbamazepine, ciprofloxacin, citalopram, clomipramine, conivaptan, CYP2D6 substrates, CYP3A4 inducers, inhibitors or substrates, darunavir, dasatinib, degarelix, delavirdine, disopyramide, dolasetron, duloxetine, flecainide, halofantrine, hormonal contraceptives, imipramine, indinavir, itraconazole, lapatinib, levofloxacin, levomepromazine, lopinavir, mefloquine, moxifloxacin, nelfinavir, norfloxacin, ofloxacin, paroxetine hydrochloride, pazopanib, phenytoin, pimozide, procainamide, quinidine, quinine, rifampin, risperidone, sotalol, St John's wort, telavancin, telithromycin, terfenadine, tipranavir, venlafaxine, voriconazole, vorinostat, ziprasidone, zuclopenthixol
Pregnancy category: C
Important contra-indications noted in the prescribing guidelines for: nursing mothers; pediatric patients
Note: Artemether/Lumefantrine tablets should not be used to treat severe malaria or to prevent malaria.

Skin
Abscess (<3%)
Impetigo (<3%)
Inflammation [3]
Pruritus (4%) [2]
Rash (3%) [6]
Urticaria (<3%) [2]

Cardiovascular
Palpitation (18%) [2]

Central Nervous System
Agitation (<3%)
Anorexia (40%) [6]
Chills (23%)
Fever (25–29%) [6]
Gait instability (<3%)
Headache (56%) [9]
Hypoesthesia (<3%)
Insomnia (5%) [2]
Mood changes (<3%)
Seizures [2]
Sleep disturbances (22%)
Sleep related disorder [2]
Tremor (<3%)
Vertigo (dizziness) (39%) [9]

Neuromuscular/Skeletal
Arthralgia (34%)
Asthenia (fatigue) (38%) [9]
Ataxia (<3%)
Back pain (<3%)
Myalgia/Myopathy (32%)

Gastrointestinal/Hepatic
Abdominal pain (17%) [11]
Constipation (<3%)
Diarrhea (8%) [11]
Dyspepsia (<3%)
Dysphagia (<3%)
Gastroenteritis (<3%)
Hepatomegaly (6–9%)
Nausea [8]
Peptic ulceration (<3%)
Vomiting [16]

Respiratory
Asthma (<3%)
Bronchitis (<3%)
Cough (6–23%) [2]
Influenza (<3%)
Nasopharyngitis (4%)
Pharyngolaryngeal pain (<3%)
Pneumonia (<3%)
Rhinitis (4%)
Upper respiratory tract infection (<3%)

Endocrine/Metabolic
ALT increased (<3%)
AST increased (<3%)
Hypokalemia (<3%)

Genitourinary
Hematuria (<3%)
Urinary tract infection (<3%)

Renal
Proteinuria (<3%)

Hematologic
Anemia (4–9%) [4]
Eosinophilia (<3%)
Hemolytic anemia [2]
Neutropenia [2]
Platelets decreased (<3%)

Otic
Ear infection (<3%)
Hearing impairment [2]
Tinnitus (<3%)

Ocular
Conjunctivitis (<3%)
Nystagmus (<3%)

Other
Adverse effects [3]
Infection (<3%)

ARTEMISIA

Family: Asteraceae
Scientific names: *Artemisia annua, Benflumetol, Co-artemether, Coartem, Riamet (Novartis)*
Indications: Fever, multidrug-resistant malaria, parasitemia, leukemia, colon cancer, diarrhea, schistosomiasis, worms, insect bites (topical)
Class: Antimalarial
Half-life: 10 hours
Clinically important, potentially hazardous interactions with: none known
Pregnancy category: N/A
Note: This drug profile only refers to *Artemisia annua*, NOT *Artemisia absinthium*. The latter, the main constituent of absinthe, has serious side effects, including seizures, hallucinations, and death.
Derivatives of *Artemisia annua* are often used in combination with piperaquine, or mefloquine in treatment of malaria. Benflumetol, Coartem and Co-artemether are a combination of artemether-lumefantrine (see separate profile).

Skin
Pruritus [2]
Rash [2]

Central Nervous System
Headache [2]

Local
Injection-site pain [2]

Respiratory
Cough [4]

Hematologic
Anemia [5]
Hemolysis [3]
Hemolytic anemia [2]
Neutropenia [2]

Other
Adverse effects [2]

ARTESUNATE

Trade name: Rtsun (Wiscon)
Indications: *Plasmodium falciparum* malaria
Class: Antimalarial
Half-life: 0.5 hours
Clinically important, potentially hazardous interactions with: efavirenz
Pregnancy category: N/A (Use carefully in first three trimesters of pregnancy)
Note: Artesunate therapy should be combined with other antimalarials (e.g. mefloquine) if given for less than 5 days.

Skin
Pruritus [4]

Cardiovascular
QT prolongation [2]

Central Nervous System
Anorexia [3]
Extrapyramidal symptoms [3]
Fever [3]
Headache [8]
Insomnia [2]
Vertigo (dizziness) [12]

Neuromuscular/Skeletal
Asthenia (fatigue) [6]
Myalgia/Myopathy [2]

Gastrointestinal/Hepatic
Abdominal pain [5]
Diarrhea [6]
Hepatotoxicity [2]
Nausea [6]
Vomiting [14]

ARTICHOKE

Family: Asteraceae; Compositae
Scientific names: *Cynara cardunculus, Cynara scolymus*
Indications: Dyspepsia, hyperlipidemia, nausea, hangover, irritable bowel syndrome (IBS), liver dysfunction, hypoglycemia. Flavoring, sweetener, prebiotic
Class: Antiemetic, Carminative
Half-life: N/A
Clinically important, potentially hazardous interactions with: none known
Pregnancy category: N/A
Note: Jerusalem artichoke (*Helianthus tuberosus*) is a completely different plant.

Skin
Dermatitis [3]

ASENAPINE

Trade name: Saphris (Merck)
Indications: Schizophrenia, bipolar disorder
Class: Antipsychotic
Half-life: 24 hours
Clinically important, potentially hazardous interactions with: alcohol, amiodarone, chlorpromazine, CYP2D6 substrates and inhibitors, fluvoxamine, gatifloxacin, moxifloxacin, paroxetine hydrochloride, procainamide, QT prolonging drugs, quinidine, sotalol, thioridazine, ziprasidone
Pregnancy category: C
Important contra-indications noted in the prescribing guidelines for: the elderly; nursing mothers; pediatric patients
Warning: INCREASED MORTALITY IN ELDERLY PATIENTS WITH DEMENTIA-RELATED PSYCHOSIS

Skin
Peripheral edema (3%)

Mucosal
Oral numbness [4]
Salivary hypersecretion (2%)
Xerostomia (2–3%)

Cardiovascular
Hypertension (2–3%) [2]

Central Nervous System
Akathisia (4–6%) [10]
Anxiety (4%)
Depression (2%) [3]
Dysgeusia (taste perversion) (3%) [4]
Extrapyramidal symptoms (6–10%) [11]
Headache (12%) [3]
Hypersomnia [2]
Hypoesthesia (4–5%) [7]
Insomnia (6–15%) [3]
Irritability (2%)
Sedation [9]
Somnolence (drowsiness) (13–24%) [15]
Tardive dyskinesia [2]
Vertigo (dizziness) (4–11%) [5]

Neuromuscular/Skeletal
Arthralgia (3%)
Asthenia (fatigue) (3–4%)
Pain in extremities (2%)

Gastrointestinal/Hepatic
Abdominal pain [2]
Constipation (5%)
Dyspepsia (3–4%)
Vomiting (5%)

Endocrine/Metabolic
Appetite increased (2–4%)
Weight gain (3–5%) [12]

Other
Adverse effects [4]

ASFOTASE ALFA

Trade name: Strensiq (Alexion)
Indications: Perinatal/infantile-and juvenile-onset hypophosphatasia
Class: Enzyme replacement
Half-life: 5 days
Clinically important, potentially hazardous interactions with: none known
Pregnancy category: N/A (No available data)
Important contra-indications noted in the prescribing guidelines for: the elderly; nursing mothers

Skin
Anaphylactoid reactions/Anaphylaxis (<10%)
Calcification (4%)
Erythema (<10%)
Flushing (<10%)

Central Nervous System
Chills (<10%)
Fever (<10%)
Headache (<10%)
Hypoesthesia (oral) (<10%)
Irritability (<10%)
Pain (<10%)
Rigors (<10%)

Gastrointestinal/Hepatic
Nausea (<10%)
Vomiting (5%)

Local
Injection-site bruising (8%)
Injection-site edema (13%)
Injection-site erythema (41%)
Injection-site hemorrhage (<17%)
Injection-site induration (13%)
Injection-site lipoatrophy/lipohypertrophy (5–8%)
Injection-site pain (14%)
Injection-site papules and nodules (3%)
Injection-site pigmentation (15%)
Injection-site pruritus (13%)
Injection-site reactions (9%)

Other
Adverse effects [2]

ASPARAGINASE

Synonym: L-asparaginase
Trade names: Elspar (Merck), Kidrolase (EUSA Pharma)
Indications: Acute lymphoblastic leukemia, lymphoma
Class: Antineoplastic, Enzyme
Half-life: 8–30 hours (intravenous); 34–49 hours (intramuscular)
Clinically important, potentially hazardous interactions with: none known
Pregnancy category: C
Important contra-indications noted in the prescribing guidelines for: nursing mothers

Skin
Anaphylactoid reactions/Anaphylaxis (3–40%) [4]
Angioedema [3]
Hypersensitivity (6–40%) [16]
Toxic epidermal necrolysis [2]
Toxicity [2]
Urticaria (<15%) [5]

Mucosal
Aphthous stomatitis (<10%)
Oral lesions (26%)
Stomatitis (<10%)

Central Nervous System
Chills (>10%)
Coma (25%)
Depression (>10%)
Encephalopathy [2]
Fever (>10%)
Leukoencephalopathy [3]
Neurotoxicity [4]
Seizures (10–60%) [2]
Somnolence (drowsiness) (>10%)
Stroke [2]

Gastrointestinal/Hepatic
Abdominal pain (70%)
Hepatotoxicity [3]
Pancreatitis (15%) [23]
Vomiting (50–60%)

Endocrine/Metabolic
Hyperglycemia [2]
Hyperlipidemia [2]
Hypertriglyceridemia [4]

Genitourinary
Azotemia (66%)

Hematologic
Sepsis [2]
Thrombosis [9]

Other
Adverse effects [2]
Allergic reactions (15–35%) [2]

ASPIRIN

Synonyms: acetylsalicylic acid; ASA
Trade names: Aggrenox (Boehringer Ingelheim), Anacin (Wyeth), Ascriptin (Novartis) (Wallace), Darvon Compound (aaiPharma), Durlaza (New Haven), Ecotrin (GSK), Equagesic (Women First), Excedrin (Bristol-Myers Squibb), Fiorinal (Watson), Norgesic (3M), Soma Compound (MedPointe), Talwin Compound (Sanofi-Aventis), Yosprala (Aralez)
Indications: Pain, fever, inflammation
Class: Antiplatelet, Non-steroidal anti-inflammatory (NSAID), Salicylate
Half-life: 15–20 minutes
Clinically important, potentially hazardous interactions with: acemetacin, acenocoumarol, amitriptyline, anagrelide, anticoagulants, azficel-t, bismuth, calcium hydroxylapatite, capsicum, celecoxib, cholestyramine, cilazapril, citalopram, desvenlafaxine, devil's claw, dexamethasone, dexibuprofen, dichlorphenamide, diclofenac, dicumarol, duloxetine, enoxaparin, etodolac, evening primrose, flunisolide, flurbiprofen, ginkgo biloba, ginseng, heparin, ibuprofen, iloprost, indomethacin, ketoprofen, ketorolac, lumiracoxib, meloxicam, methotrexate, methyl salicylate, methylprednisolone, milnacipran, nilutamide, NSAIDs, paroxetine hydrochloride, phellodendron, piroxicam, prednisone, resveratrol, reteplase, rivaroxaban, sermorelin, sulfites, tinzaparin, tirofiban, tolmetin, triamcinolone, urokinase, valdecoxib, valproic acid, venlafaxine, verapamil, vilazodone, warfarin, zafirlukast
Pregnancy category: D
Important contra-indications noted in the prescribing guidelines for: nursing mothers; pediatric patients
Note: NSAIDs may cause an increased risk of serious cardiovascular and gastrointestinal adverse events, which can be fatal. This risk may increase with duration of use.
Aggrenox is aspirin and dipyridamole; Yosprala is aspirin and omeprazole.

Skin
Anaphylactoid reactions/Anaphylaxis (<10%) [8]
Angioedema (<5%) [32]
Bullous dermatitis [4]
Erythema multiforme [9]
Erythema nodosum [9]
Erythroderma [2]
Exanthems [11]
Fixed eruption [22]
Hypersensitivity [5]
Lichenoid eruption [2]
Pityriasis rosea [3]
Pruritus [6]
Psoriasis [3]
Purpura [8]
Rash (<10%)
Stevens-Johnson syndrome [6]
Toxic epidermal necrolysis [9]
Urticaria (<10%) [72]
Vasculitis [2]

Mucosal
Aphthous stomatitis [3]
Epistaxis (nosebleed) [2]
Nasal polyp [4]
Oral mucosal eruption [3]
Oral ulceration [4]

Central Nervous System
Stroke [2]

Gastrointestinal/Hepatic
Black stools [3]
Gastritis [2]
Gastrointestinal bleeding [8]
Gastrointestinal ulceration [7]
Hepatotoxicity [4]
Pancreatitis [2]

Respiratory
Asthma [10]
Pulmonary toxicity [2]
Rhinitis [3]
Sinusitis [2]

Renal
Fanconi syndrome [2]

Hematologic
Bleeding [15]

Otic
Tinnitus [17]

Ocular
Periorbital edema [3]

Other
Adverse effects [9]
Allergic reactions [2]

ASTRAGALUS ROOT

Family: Fabaceae; Leguminosae
Scientific names: *Astragalus membranaceus*, *Astragalus mongholicus*
Indications: Arrhythmia, colds, upper respiratory infections, chronic fatigue syndrome, colitis, diabetes, hepatitis, hypotension, herpes simplex keratitis
Class: Antioxidant, Immune stimulant, Vasodilator
Half-life: N/A
Clinically important, potentially hazardous interactions with: none known
Pregnancy category: N/A

ATAZANAVIR

Trade names: Evotaz (Bristol-Myers Squibb), Reyataz (Bristol-Myers Squibb)
Indications: HIV infection
Class: Antiretroviral, HIV-1 protease inhibitor
Half-life: 7 hours
Clinically important, potentially hazardous interactions with: abiraterone, alfuzosin, amiodarone, antacids, aripiprazole, artemether/lumefantrine, atorvastatin, avanafil, bepridil, bosentan, buprenorphine, cabazitaxel, cabozantinib, calcifediol, cisapride, clarithromycin, colchicine, crizotinib, cyclosporine, darifenacin, dasatinib, dexlansoprazole, diltiazem, dofetilide, efavirenz, elbasvir & grazoprevir, eluxadoline, ergot derivatives, erlotinib, estrogens, etravirine, everolimus, famotidine, felodipine, fentanyl,

fesoterodine, flibanserin, fluticasone propionate, garlic, glecaprevir & pibrentasvir, indinavir, irinotecan, itraconazole, ixabepilone, ketoconazole, lapatinib, lidocaine, lopinavir, lovastatin, maraviroc, marihuana, midazolam, mifepristone, naldemedine, nevirapine, nicardipine, nifedipine, olaparib, ombitasvir/paritaprevir/ritonavir, omeprazole, oral contraceptives, paclitaxel, pantoprazole, pazopanib, pimozide, posaconazole, proton-pump inhibitors, quetiapine, quinidine, quinine, rabeprazole, raltegravir, ranolazine, rifabutin, rifampin, rilpivirine, ritonavir, rivaroxaban, romidepsin, rosuvastatin, salmeterol, saquinavir, sildenafil, simeprevir, simvastatin, sirolimus, sofosbuvir/velpatasvir/voxilaprevir, solifenacin, sonidegib, St John's wort, sunitinib, tacrolimus, tadalafil, telaprevir, telithromycin, temsirolimus, tenofovir disoproxil, ticagrelor, tipranavir, trazodone, triazolam, tricyclic antidepressants, vardenafil, vemurafenib, verapamil, voriconazole, warfarin
Pregnancy category: B
Important contra-indications noted in the prescribing guidelines for: the elderly; nursing mothers; pediatric patients
Note: Evotaz is atazanavir and cobicistat.

Skin
Jaundice (5–7%) [11]
Rash (3–20%) [7]

Cardiovascular
QT prolongation [2]
Torsades de pointes [2]

Central Nervous System
Depression (2%)
Fever (2%)
Headache (<6%) [3]
Insomnia (3%)
Neurotoxicity [2]
Pain (3%)
Vertigo (dizziness) (3%)

Neuromuscular/Skeletal
Asthenia (fatigue) (2%)
Back pain (2%)
Myalgia/Myopathy (4%)

Gastrointestinal/Hepatic
Abdominal pain (4%)
Cholelithiasis (gallstones) [4]
Diarrhea (2%) [3]
Hepatotoxicity [3]
Nausea (6–14%) [4]
Vomiting (3–4%)

Respiratory
Upper respiratory tract infection [2]

Endocrine/Metabolic
ALT increased (3%)
AST increased (3%)
Creatine phosphokinase increased (8%)
Hyperbilirubinemia [7]

Genitourinary
Urolithiasis [4]

Renal
Nephrolithiasis [5]
Nephrotoxicity [7]

Hematologic
Neutropenia (5%)

Other
Adverse effects [5]
Infection (~50%)

ATENOLOL

Trade names: Beta-Adalat (Bayer), Kalten (BPC), Tenif (AstraZeneca), Tenoret 50 (AstraZeneca), Tenoretic (AstraZeneca), Tenormin (AstraZeneca)
Indications: Angina, hypertension, acute myocardial infarction
Class: Antiarrhythmic class II, Beta adrenergic blocker, Beta blocker
Half-life: 6–7 hours (adults)
Clinically important, potentially hazardous interactions with: alfuzosin, calcium channel blockers, cisplatin, clonidine, digitalis glycosides, diltiazem, disopyramide, epinephrine, indomethacin, reserpine, verapamil
Pregnancy category: D
Important contra-indications noted in the prescribing guidelines for: the elderly; nursing mothers; pediatric patients
Note: Contra-indicated in patients with sinus bradycardia, heart block greater than first degree, cardiogenic shock, or overt cardiac failure. Beta-Adalat and Tenif are atenolol and nifedipine. Kalten, Tenoret 50 and Tenoretic are atenolol and chlorthalidone. Chlorthalidone is a sulfonamide and can be absorbed systemically. Sulfonamides can produce severe, possibly fatal, reactions such as toxic epidermal necrolysis and Stevens-Johnson syndrome.
Warning: CESSATION OF THERAPY

Skin
Anaphylactoid reactions/Anaphylaxis [2]
Lupus erythematosus [2]
Necrosis [3]
Pruritus (<5%)
Psoriasis [7]
Raynaud's phenomenon [2]
Urticaria [2]

Cardiovascular
Atrial fibrillation (5%) [2]
Atrial flutter (2%)
Bradycardia (3–18%) [8]
Cardiac arrest (2%)
Cardiac failure (19%)
Heart block (5%)
Hypotension (25%) [2]
Postural hypotension (12%)
Supraventricular tachycardia (12%)
Ventricular tachycardia (16%)

Central Nervous System
Depression (12%)
Somnolence (drowsiness) (2%)
Stroke [2]
Syncope [2]
Vertigo (dizziness) (15%)

Neuromuscular/Skeletal
Asthenia (fatigue) (26%)
Leg pain (3%)

Gastrointestinal/Hepatic
Diarrhea (3%)
Nausea (3%)

Respiratory
Dyspnea (6%)
Wheezing (3%)

Other
Adverse effects [5]

ATEZOLIZUMAB

Trade name: Tecentriq (Genentech)
Indications: Locally advanced or metastatic urothelial carcinoma in patients having disease progression following platinum-containing chemotherapy
Class: Monoclonal antibody, Programmed death-ligand (PD-L1) inhibitor
Half-life: 27 days
Clinically important, potentially hazardous interactions with: none known
Pregnancy category: N/A (Can cause fetal harm)
Important contra-indications noted in the prescribing guidelines for: nursing mothers; pediatric patients

---

Skin
Peripheral edema (18%)
Pruritus (13%) [3]
Rash (15%) [5]

Cardiovascular
Venous thromboembolism (>2%)

Central Nervous System
Fever (21%) [2]

Neuromuscular/Skeletal
Arthralgia (14%) [2]
Asthenia (fatigue) (52%) [8]
Back pain (15%)
Neck pain (15%)

Gastrointestinal/Hepatic
Abdominal pain (17%)
Colitis [5]
Constipation (21%) [2]
Diarrhea (18%) [3]
Gastric obstruction (>2%)
Hepatitis [2]
Nausea (25%) [5]
Vomiting (17%)

Respiratory
Cough (14%)
Dyspnea (16%) [3]
Hypoxia [2]
Pneumonia (>2%) [2]
Pneumonitis (3%) [3]

Endocrine/Metabolic
ALP increased (4%)
ALT increased (2%) [3]
Appetite decreased (26%) [5]
AST increased (2%) [5]
Dehydration (>2%)
Diabetes mellitus [2]
Hyperglycemia (5%)
Hyperthyroidism (2%)
Hyponatremia (10%) [2]
Hypothyroidism (6%) [2]
Serum creatinine increased (3%)

Genitourinary
Hematuria (14%)

Urinary tract infection (22%)

Renal

Nephrotoxicity (>2%)

Hematologic

Anemia (8%) [2]
Lymphopenia (10%)
Sepsis (>2%)

Local

Infusion-related reactions (3%)

Other

Adverse effects [5]
Infection (38%)

ATOMOXETINE

Trade name: Strattera (Lilly)
Indications: Attention deficit hyperactivity disorder
Class: Norepinephrine reuptake inhibitor
Half-life: 5 hours
Clinically important, potentially hazardous interactions with: albuterol, amitriptyline, cinacalcet, citalopram, delavirdine, droperidol, duloxetine, levalbuterol, levomepromazine, linezolid, lisdexamfetamine, MAO inhibitors, moxifloxacin, paroxetine hydrochloride, sotalol, terbinafine, terbutaline, tipranavir, venlafaxine, zuclopenthixol
Pregnancy category: C
Important contra-indications noted in the prescribing guidelines for: nursing mothers; pediatric patients
Warning: SUICIDAL IDEATION IN CHILDREN AND ADOLESCENTS

Skin

Pruritus (>2%)

Mucosal

Xerostomia (>5%) [9]

Cardiovascular

Cardiotoxicity [3]
Tachycardia [2]

Central Nervous System

Aggression [3]
Anorexia [5]
Depression (>2%) [3]
Headache [9]
Hypomania [2]
Insomnia [7]
Irritability [8]
Mania [2]
Mood changes [5]
Nervousness [3]
Somnolence (drowsiness) [11]
Suicidal ideation [6]
Tic disorder [7]
Tremor (>2%) [2]
Vertigo (dizziness) (>5%) [10]

Neuromuscular/Skeletal

Asthenia (fatigue) [11]

Gastrointestinal/Hepatic

Abdominal pain [12]
Constipation [2]
Dyspepsia [3]
Hepatotoxicity [12]
Nausea [18]
Vomiting [10]

Endocrine/Metabolic

Appetite decreased [27]
Weight loss [5]

Genitourinary

Erectile dysfunction [4]
Urinary hesitancy [2]

Other

Adverse effects [10]
Bruxism [2]

ATORVASTATIN

Trade names: Caduet (Pfizer), Lipitor (Pfizer), Liptruzet (Merck Sharpe & Dohme)
Indications: Hypercholesterolemia
Class: HMG-CoA reductase inhibitor, Statin
Half-life: 14 hours
Clinically important, potentially hazardous interactions with: alcohol, aliskiren, amiodarone, amprenavir, antifungals, atazanavir, azithromycin, bexarotene, boceprevir, bosentan, ciprofibrate, clarithromycin, clopidogrel, cobicistat/elvitegravir/emtricitabine/tenofovir alafenamide, cobicistat/elvitegravir/emtricitabine/tenofovir disoproxil, colchicine, conivaptan, cyclosporine, CYP3A4 inhibitors, dabigatran, danazol, daptomycin, darunavir, dasatinib, delavirdine, digoxin, diltiazem, dronedarone, efavirenz, elbasvir & grazoprevir, eltrombopag, erythromycin, estradiol, etravirine, everolimus, fenofibrate, fenofibric acid, fibrates, fluconazole, fosamprenavir, fusidic acid, gemfibrozil, glecaprevir & pibrentasvir, grapefruit juice, imatinib, imidazoles, indinavir, itraconazole, letermovir, liraglutide, lopinavir, macrolide antibiotics, midazolam, nefazodone, nelfinavir, niacin, niacinamide, norethisterone, oral contraceptives, P-glycoprotein inhibitors, posaconazole, protease inhibitors, quinine, red rice yeast, rifampin, ritonavir, rivaroxaban, saquinavir, silodosin, St John's wort, telaprevir, telithromycin, tipranavir, topotecan, trabectedin, verapamil, voriconazole, warfarin
Pregnancy category: X
Important contra-indications noted in the prescribing guidelines for: the elderly; nursing mothers; pediatric patients
Note: Caduet is atorvastatin and amlodipine; Liptruzet is atorvastatin and ezetimibe.

Skin

Acneform eruption (<2%)
Angioedema [2]
Dermatitis (<2%)
Dermatomyositis [4]
Diaphoresis (<2%)
Ecchymoses (<2%)
Eczema (<2%)
Edema (<2%)
Facial edema (<2%)
Jaundice [2]
Lupus erythematosus [2]
Petechiae (<2%)
Photosensitivity (<2%)
Pruritus (<2%)
Rash (>3%) [2]
Seborrhea (<2%)
Toxic epidermal necrolysis [2]
Toxicity [2]
Ulcerations (<2%)
Urticaria (<2%)
Xerosis (<2%)

Hair

Alopecia (<2%)

Mucosal

Cheilitis (<2%)
Glossitis (<2%)
Oral ulceration (<2%)
Stomatitis (<2%)

Cardiovascular

Hypotension [2]

Central Nervous System

Ageusia (taste loss) (<2%)
Cognitive impairment [2]
Depression [3]
Dysgeusia (taste perversion) (<2%)
Headache [4]
Neurotoxicity [2]
Paresthesias (<2%)
Parosmia (<2%)

Neuromuscular/Skeletal

Arthralgia (4–12%)
Asthenia (fatigue) [5]
Back pain [3]
Muscle spasm [2]
Myalgia/Myopathy (3–8%) [30]
Pain in extremities (6%)
Rhabdomyolysis [41]
Tendinopathy/Tendon rupture [2]

Gastrointestinal/Hepatic

Cholelithiasis (gallstones) [2]
Diarrhea (5–14%)
Hepatitis [2]
Hepatotoxicity [11]
Nausea (4–7%)
Pancreatitis [8]

Respiratory

Nasopharyngitis (4–13%)

Endocrine/Metabolic

ALT increased [3]
Creatine phosphokinase increased [5]
Diabetes mellitus [2]
Gynecomastia (<2%)

Genitourinary

Urinary tract infection (4–8%)

Renal

Nephrotoxicity [3]

Otic

Hearing loss [2]

Other

Adverse effects [10]
Allergic reactions (<2%)
Death [6]
Multiorgan failure [2]

ATOVAQUONE/ PROGUANIL

Trade name: Malarone (GSK)
Indications: Malaria prophylaxis and treatment
Class: Antimalarial
Half-life: 24 hours
Clinically important, potentially hazardous interactions with: artemether/lumefantrine, dapsone, etoposide, hypoglycemic agents, indinavir, metoclopramide, phenothiazines, rifabutin, rifampin, ritonavir, tetracycline, typhoid vaccine
Pregnancy category: C
Important contra-indications noted in the prescribing guidelines for: the elderly; nursing mothers

---

Skin
Erythema multiforme [2]
Pruritus (<10%)

Mucosal
Oral ulceration (6%) [3]

Central Nervous System
Abnormal dreams (7%)
Anorexia (5%)
Headache (10%) [4]
Insomnia (3%)
Vertigo (dizziness) (5%) [3]

Neuromuscular/Skeletal
Asthenia (fatigue) (8%)

Gastrointestinal/Hepatic
Abdominal pain (17%) [5]
Diarrhea (8%)
Dyspepsia (2%)
Gastritis (3%)
Hepatotoxicity [2]
Nausea (12%)
Vomiting (12%) [2]

Respiratory
Cough [3]

Ocular
Vision impaired (2%)

Other
Adverse effects [3]

ATROPINE SULFATE

Trade name: Lomotil (Pfizer)
Indications: Salivation, sinus bradycardia, uveitis, peptic ulcer
Class: Muscarinic antagonist
Half-life: 2–3 hours
Clinically important, potentially hazardous interactions with: anticholinergics, zuclopenthixol
Pregnancy category: C
Note: Many of the trade name drugs for atropine sulfate contain phenobarbital, scopolamine, hyoscyamine, hydrocodone, methenamine, etc.

Skin
Anaphylactoid reactions/Anaphylaxis [3]
Dermatitis [3]
Erythema multiforme [2]
Photosensitivity (<10%)

Mucosal
Xerostomia (>10%) [4]

Cardiovascular
Arrhythmias [2]
Atrial fibrillation [2]
Bradycardia [3]
Tachycardia [5]

Central Nervous System
Confusion [2]

Ocular
Amblyopia [5]
Hallucinations, visual [3]
Periocular dermatitis [3]

Local
Injection-site irritation (>10%)

Other
Allergic reactions [2]
Central anticholinergic syndrome [2]

AVANAFIL

Trade name: Stendra (Vivus)
Indications: Erectile dysfunction
Class: Phosphodiesterase type 5 (PDE5) inhibitor
Half-life: 5 hours
Clinically important, potentially hazardous interactions with: alcohol, alpha blockers, amprenavir, antihypertensives, aprepitant, atazanavir, clarithromycin, diltiazem, erythromycin, fluconazole, fosamprenavir, indinavir, itraconazole, ketoconazole, nefazodone, nelfinavir, nitrates, ritonavir, saquinavir, strong CYP3A4 inhibitors, telithromycin, verapamil
Pregnancy category: C (Not indicated for use in women)
Important contra-indications noted in the prescribing guidelines for: pediatric patients
Note: Contra-indicated in patients using any form of nitrates.

Skin
Facial flushing [2]
Flushing (3–10%) [11]
Rash (<2%)

Mucosal
Nasal congestion (<3%) [7]

Cardiovascular
Hypertension (<2%)

Central Nervous System
Headache (5–12%) [10]
Vertigo (dizziness) (<2%) [3]

Neuromuscular/Skeletal
Arthralgia (<2%)
Asthenia (fatigue) [2]
Back pain (<3%) [3]

Gastrointestinal/Hepatic
Constipation (<2%)
Diarrhea (<2%)
Dyspepsia (<2%) [5]
Nausea (<2%)

Respiratory
Bronchitis (<2%)
Influenza (<2%)
Nasopharyngitis (<5%) [5]
Sinusitis (<2%) [2]
Upper respiratory tract infection (<3%)

Other
Adverse effects [4]

AVATROMBOPAG *

Trade name: Doptelet (Akarx Inc)
Indications: treatment of thrombocytopenia in adult patients with chronic liver disease who are scheduled to undergo a procedure
Class: Thrombopoietin receptor (TPO) agonist
Half-life: ~19 hours
Clinically important, potentially hazardous interactions with: none known
Pregnancy category: N/A (may cause fetal harm)
Important contra-indications noted in the prescribing guidelines for: nursing mothers

---

Skin
Peripheral edema (3%)

Central Nervous System
Fever (10%)
Headache (6%) [3]

Neuromuscular/Skeletal
Asthenia (fatigue) (4%) [2]

Gastrointestinal/Hepatic
Abdominal pain (7%)
Nausea (7%)

AVELUMAB

Trade name: Bavencio (Merck Serono)
Indications: Metastatic Merkel cell carcinoma
Class: Monoclonal antibody, Programmed death-ligand (PD-L1) inhibitor
Half-life: 6 days
Clinically important, potentially hazardous interactions with: none known
Pregnancy category: N/A (Can cause fetal harm)
Important contra-indications noted in the prescribing guidelines for: nursing mothers; pediatric patients

---

Skin
Peripheral edema (20%)
Pruritus (10%)
Rash (22%)

Cardiovascular
Hypertension (13%)

Central Nervous System
Headache (10%)
Vertigo (dizziness) (14%)

Neuromuscular/Skeletal
Arthralgia (16%)
Asthenia (fatigue) (50%) [4]
Bone or joint pain (32%)

Gastrointestinal/Hepatic
Abdominal pain (16%)
Colitis (2%)
Constipation (17%)
Diarrhea (23%)
Nausea (22%) [2]

Vomiting (13%)

Respiratory

Cough (18%)
Dyspnea (11%)

Endocrine/Metabolic

ALT increased (20%)
Appetite decreased (20%)
AST increased (34%) [2]
Creatine phosphokinase increased [3]
Hyperamylasemia (8%)
Hyperbilirubinemia (6%)
Hyperglycemia (>10%)
Thyroid dysfunction (6%)
Weight loss (15%)

Hematologic

Anemia (35%)
Hyperlipasemia (14%)
Lymphopenia (49%)
Neutropenia (6%)
Thrombocytopenia (27%)

Local

Infusion-related reactions (22%) [4]

Other

Death [2]

AXITINIB

Trade name: Inlyta (Pfizer)
Indications: Advanced renal cell carcinoma (after failure of one prior systemic therapy)
Class: Tyrosine kinase inhibitor
Half-life: 2–6 hours
Clinically important, potentially hazardous interactions with: ketoconazole, rifampin
Pregnancy category: D
Important contra-indications noted in the prescribing guidelines for: nursing mothers; pediatric patients

---

Skin

Erythema (2%)
Hand–foot syndrome (27%) [18]
Pruritus (7%)
Rash (13%) [3]
Xerosis (10%)

Hair

Alopecia (4%) [2]

Mucosal

Mucosal inflammation (15%) [2]
Stomatitis (15%)

Cardiovascular

Hypertension (40%) [37]

Central Nervous System

Anorexia [5]
Dysgeusia (taste perversion) (11%)
Headache (14%) [4]
Leukoencephalopathy [2]

Neuromuscular/Skeletal

Arthralgia (15%) [2]
Asthenia (fatigue) (39%) [28]
Pain in extremities (13%)

Gastrointestinal/Hepatic

Abdominal pain (14%)
Constipation (20%) [2]
Diarrhea (55%) [25]
Dyspepsia (10%)
Gastrointestinal disorder [3]
Nausea (32%) [10]
Vomiting (24%) [6]

Respiratory

Cough (15%) [2]
Dysphonia (>20%) [12]
Dyspnea (15%) [4]

Endocrine/Metabolic

ALT increased (22%) [3]
Appetite decreased (34%) [7]
AST increased [2]
Dehydration [2]
Hyperthyroidism [2]
Hyponatremia [2]
Hypothyroidism (19%) [8]
Serum creatinine increased [2]
Thyroid dysfunction [2]
Weight loss (25%) [3]

Renal

Proteinuria (11%) [5]

Hematologic

Anemia [2]
Hemorrhage (16%)
Neutropenia [2]
Thrombotic complications (3%)

Other

Adverse effects [4]
Death [2]

AZACITIDINE

Trade name: Vidaza (Celgene)
Indications: Myelodysplastic syndromes, refractory anemia
Class: Antimetabolite, Antineoplastic, Cytosine analog
Half-life: 40–56 minutes
Clinically important, potentially hazardous interactions with: BCG vaccine, denosumab, echinacea, leflunomide, natalizumab, pimecrolimus, sipuleucel-T, tacrolimus, trastuzumab, vaccines
Pregnancy category: D
Important contra-indications noted in the prescribing guidelines for: nursing mothers; pediatric patients
Note: Contra-indicated in patients with advanced malignant hepatic tumors.

Skin

Anaphylactoid reactions/Anaphylaxis (<5%)
Cellulitis (8%)
Diaphoresis (11%)
Ecchymoses (31%)
Edema (14%)
Erythema (7–17%)
Hematoma (9%)
Herpes simplex (9%)
Hypersensitivity (<5%)
Induration (<5%)
Lymphoproliferative disease [2]
Neoplasms (<5%)
Nodular eruption (5%)
Pallor (16%)
Peripheral edema (19%)
Petechiae (11–24%)
Pruritus (12%)
Pyoderma gangrenosum (<5%) [2]
Rash (10–14%) [4]
Sweet's syndrome [5]
Toxicity [2]
Urticaria (6%)
Xerosis (5%)

Mucosal

Gingival bleeding (10%)
Oral bleeding (5%)
Stomatitis (8%)
Tongue ulceration (5%)

Cardiovascular

Arrhythmias [2]
Atrial fibrillation (<5%)
Cardiac failure (<5%)
Cardiomyopathy (<5%)
Cardiotoxicity [3]
Chest pain (5–16%) [4]
Congestive heart failure (<5%)
Hypertension (9%)
Hypotension (7%) [2]
Orthostatic hypotension (<5%)
QT prolongation [2]
Tachycardia [3]

Central Nervous System

Anorexia (21%)
Anxiety (5–13%)
Cerebral hemorrhage (<5%)
Depression (12%)
Fever (30–52%) [4]
Headache (22%)
Insomnia (9–11%)
Intracranial hemorrhage (<5%)
Pain (11%)
Seizures (<5%)
Syncope [2]
Vertigo (dizziness) (19%)

Neuromuscular/Skeletal

Arthralgia (22%) [2]
Asthenia (fatigue) (7–36%) [5]
Back pain (19%)
Bone or joint pain (<5%)
Myalgia/Myopathy (16%)
Neck pain (<5%)

Gastrointestinal/Hepatic

Abdominal pain (12–13%)
Black stools (<5%)
Cholecystitis (<5%)
Constipation (34–50%) [4]
Diarrhea (36%) [4]
Dyspepsia (6%)
Dysphagia (5%)
Gastrointestinal bleeding (<5%)
Loose stools (6%)
Nausea (48–71%) [7]
Vomiting (27–54%) [4]

Respiratory

Cough (30%)
Dyspnea (14–29%) [2]
Hemoptysis (<5%)
Nasopharyngitis (15%)
Pharyngolaryngeal pain (6%)
Pneumonia (11%) [2]
Pneumonitis (<5%) [2]
Pulmonary toxicity [2]
Respiratory distress (<5%)
Rhinitis (6%)
Upper respiratory tract infection (9–13%)

Endocrine/Metabolic
Dehydration (<5%)
Hypokalemia (6%)
Weight loss (8%)

Genitourinary
Hematuria (6%)
Urinary tract infection (9%)

Renal
Renal failure (<5%)

Hematologic
Agranulocytosis (<5%)
Anemia (51–70%) [4]
Bleeding [3]
Bone marrow suppression (<5%)
Cytopenia [4]
Febrile neutropenia (14–16%) [7]
Leukopenia (18–48%)
Myelosuppression [3]
Neutropenia (32–66%) [9]
Pancytopenia (<5%)
Splenomegaly (<5%)
Thrombocytopenia (66–70%) [6]

Ocular
Ocular hemorrhage (<5%)

Local
Injection-site bruising (5–14%)
Injection-site edema (5%)
Injection-site erythema (35–43%)
Injection-site hematoma (6%)
Injection-site pain (19–23%)
Injection-site pigmentation (5%)
Injection-site pruritus (7%)
Injection-site purpura (14%)
Injection-site reactions (14–29%) [7]

Other
Adverse effects [5]
Death [4]
Infection (<5%) [9]

AZATHIOPRINE

Trade names: Azasan (aaiPharma), Imuran (Prometheus)
Indications: Lupus nephritis, psoriatic arthritis, rheumatoid arthritis, autoimmune diseases, as an adjunct for the prevention of rejection in kidney transplant patients
Class: Antimetabolite, Disease-modifying antirheumatic drug (DMARD), Immunosuppressant, Purine anaolog
Half-life: 12 minutes
Clinically important, potentially hazardous interactions with: allopurinol, aminosalicylates, balsalazide, benazepril, captopril, chlorambucil, co-trimoxazole, cyclophosphamide, cyclosporine, enalapril, febuxostat, fosinopril, Hemophilus B vaccine, imidapril, lisinopril, mesalamine, mycophenolate, natalizumab, olsalazine, quinapril, ramipril, ribavirin, sulfamethoxazole, tofacitinib, trimethoprim, typhoid vaccine, vaccines, warfarin, yellow fever vaccine
Pregnancy category: D
Important contra-indications noted in the prescribing guidelines for: nursing mothers; pediatric patients
Note: Patients receiving immunosuppressants, including azathioprine, are at increased risk of developing lymphoma and other malignancies, particularly of the skin.
Warning: MALIGNANCY

Skin
Acanthosis nigricans [2]
Acneform eruption [2]
AGEP [2]
Angioedema [2]
Basal cell carcinoma [2]
Carcinoma [3]
Dermatitis [4]
Erythema gyratum repens [2]
Erythema multiforme [2]
Erythema nodosum [4]
Exanthems [10]
Herpes simplex [3]
Herpes zoster [8]
Hypersensitivity [29]
Kaposi's sarcoma [14]
Lymphoproliferative disease [4]
Malignancies [2]
Neoplasms [2]
Neutrophilic dermatosis [4]
Nevi [3]
Pellagra [2]
Porokeratosis [4]
Rash (<10%) [10]
Scabies [5]
Squamous cell carcinoma [11]
Sweet's syndrome [12]
Tinea [3]
Toxicity [3]
Tumors [8]
Urticaria [5]
Vasculitis [5]
Verrucae [3]

Hair
Alopecia [10]

Nails
Onychomycosis [2]

Mucosal
Oral ulceration [2]

Cardiovascular
Atrial fibrillation [3]

Central Nervous System
Chills (>10%)
Encephalopathy [2]
Fever [7]
Headache [3]
Leukoencephalopathy [2]

Neuromuscular/Skeletal
Arthralgia [4]
Asthenia (fatigue) [7]

Gastrointestinal/Hepatic
Abdominal pain [2]
Hepatitis [5]
Hepatotoxicity [28]
Nausea [8]
Pancreatitis [44]
Vomiting [4]

Respiratory
Flu-like syndrome [2]
Pneumonitis [2]
Pulmonary toxicity [3]

Hematologic
Bone marrow suppression [5]
Leukopenia [13]
Myelosuppression [3]
Myelotoxicity [5]
Neutropenia [2]
Pancytopenia [5]
Pure red cell aplasia [2]
Thrombocytopenia [6]

Other
Adverse effects [9]
Allergic reactions [5]
Death [2]
Infection [9]

AZITHROMYCIN

Trade names: AzaSite (Merck), Zithromax (Pfizer)
Indications: Infections of the upper and lower respiratory tract, skin infections, sexually transmitted diseases, conjunctivitis (ophthalmic preparations only)
Class: Antibacterial, Antibiotic, macrolide
Half-life: 68 hours
Clinically important, potentially hazardous interactions with: aminophylline, antacids, artemether/lumefantrine, astemizole, atorvastatin, betrixaban, bromocriptine, cabergoline, colchicine, coumarins, cyclosporine, digoxin, droperidol, ergotamine, fluvastatin, lovastatin, methysergide, mizolastine, oral typhoid vaccine, pimozide, pravastatin, quetiapine, reboxetine, rifabutin, ritonavir, simvastatin, venetoclax, warfarin
Pregnancy category: B
Important contra-indications noted in the prescribing guidelines for: nursing mothers; pediatric patients
Note: AzaSite is for topical ophthalmic use only (for reactions see [Ophth] below).

Skin
AGEP [3]
Anaphylactoid reactions/Anaphylaxis [2]
Churg-Strauss syndrome [2]
DRESS syndrome [4]
Erythema [2]
Exanthems [3]
Hypersensitivity [3]
Jarisch-Herxheimer reaction [2]
Pruritus [3]
Rash [Ophth] (2–10%) [6]
Stevens-Johnson syndrome [9]
Urticaria [Ophth] [2]

Cardiovascular
Bradycardia [2]
Cardiotoxicity [8]
QT prolongation [11]
Torsades de pointes [4]

Central Nervous System
Anorexia (2–10%)
Headache [3]
Vertigo (dizziness) [2]

Gastrointestinal/Hepatic
Abdominal pain (2–10%) [4]
Diarrhea (4–9%) [17]
Gastrointestinal disorder [3]
Hepatotoxicity [7]
Nausea (7%) [8]

Vanishing bile duct syndrome [2]
Vomiting (2–10%) [5]

Genitourinary
Vaginitis (2–10%)

Otic
Hearing loss [4]
Tinnitus [2]

Ocular
Keratitis [2]

Local
Injection-site erythema (2–10%)
Injection-site pain (2–10%) [3]

Other
Adverse effects [14]
Death [2]
Hiccups [2]
Side effects [2]

BACLOFEN

Trade names: Baclofen (Watson), Gablofen (Mallinckrodt), Lioresal (Medtronic)
Indications: Spasticity resulting from multiple sclerosis
Class: GABA receptor agonist, Skeletal muscle relaxant
Half-life: 2.5–4 hours
Clinically important, potentially hazardous interactions with: acebutolol, alcohol, alfuzosin, amitriptyline, captopril, cilazapril, diclofenac, enalapril, fosinopril, irbesartan, levodopa, lisinopril, meloxicam, olmesartan, quinapril, ramipril, trandolapril
Pregnancy category: C
Important contra-indications noted in the prescribing guidelines for: pediatric patients
Note: Children appear to be at higher risk for complications than adults when using intrathecal baclofen (ITB). ITB therapy is a safe and effective treatment for severe spasticity in the pediatric population, but does have a 31% rate of complications requiring surgical management over a 3-year treatment period.
Warning: DO NOT DISCONTINUE ABRUPTLY

Skin
Exanthems [2]
Rash (<10%)
Toxicity [2]

Cardiovascular
Bradycardia [2]
Hypertension [2]
Hypotension [3]

Central Nervous System
Coma [4]
Confusion (<10%)
Dyskinesia [2]
Encephalopathy [2]
Hallucinations [4]
Headache (<10%)
Insomnia (>10%) [2]
Seizures [11]
Sleep apnea [3]
Slurred speech (>10%)
Somnolence (drowsiness) (>10%) [7]
Vertigo (dizziness) (>10%) [7]

Neuromuscular/Skeletal
Asthenia (fatigue) (>10%) [7]

Gastrointestinal/Hepatic
Constipation (<10%)
Nausea (<10%)

Genitourinary
Polyuria (<10%)

Other
Infection [2]
Side effects (<2%)

BALSALAZIDE

Trade names: Colazal (Salix), Colazide (Almirall)
Indications: Mild to moderately active ulcerative colitis
Class: Aminosalicylate
Half-life: N/A
Clinically important, potentially hazardous interactions with: azathioprine, cardiac glycosides, folic acid, heparin, low molecular weight heparins, mercaptopurine, thiopurine analogs, varicella virus-containing vaccines
Pregnancy category: B
Important contra-indications noted in the prescribing guidelines for: nursing mothers; pediatric patients

---

Skin
Hypersensitivity [2]

Mucosal
Stomatitis (3%)

Central Nervous System
Anorexia (2%)
Fever (2–6%)
Headache (15%)
Insomnia (2%)

Neuromuscular/Skeletal
Arthralgia (4%)
Asthenia (fatigue) (2%)

Gastrointestinal/Hepatic
Abdominal pain (6–13%)
Colitis (ulcerative, exacerbation) (6%)
Diarrhea (5–9%)
Dyspepsia (2%)
Flatulence (2%)
Nausea (4%)
Vomiting (10%)

Respiratory
Cough (2–3%)
Flu-like syndrome (<4%)
Nasopharyngitis (6%)
Pharyngitis (2%)
Pharyngolaryngeal pain (3%)
Rhinitis (2%)

Genitourinary
Dysmenorrhea (3%)

BARICITINIB *

Trade name: Olumiant (Eli Lilly and Co)
Indications: treatment of adult patients with moderately to severely active rheumatoid arthritis who have had an inadequate response to one or more TNF antagonist therapies
Class: Janus kinase (JAK) inhibitor
Half-life: ~12 hours
Clinically important, potentially hazardous interactions with: none known
Pregnancy category: N/A (Insufficient data to inform a drug-associated risk for major birth defects or miscarriage)
Warning: SERIOUS INFECTIONS, MALIGNANCY, AND THROMBOSIS

Skin
Herpes simplex (1–2%)

Gastrointestinal/Hepatic
Nausea (3%)

Respiratory
Upper respiratory tract infection (15–16%) [2]

Endocrine/Metabolic
Hypercholesterolemia [2]
Serum creatinine increased [2]

Hematologic
Neutropenia [2]

Other
Adverse effects [2]
Death [2]
Infection [5]

BASILIXIMAB

Trade name: Simulect (Novartis)
Indications: Prophylaxis of organ rejection in renal transplantation
Class: Interleukin-2 receptor antagonist, Monoclonal antibody
Half-life: 7.2 days
Clinically important, potentially hazardous interactions with: cyclosporine, Hemophilus B vaccine, mycophenolate
Pregnancy category: B
Important contra-indications noted in the prescribing guidelines for: nursing mothers

---

Skin
Acneform eruption (>10%)
Candidiasis (3–10%)
Cyst (3–10%)
Edema (generalized) (3–10%)
Facial edema (3–10%)
Genital edema (3–10%)
Hematoma (3–10%)
Herpes simplex (3–10%)
Herpes zoster (3–10%)
Peripheral edema (>10%)
Pruritus (3–10%)
Rash (3–10%)
Ulcerations (3–10%)
Wound complications (>10%)

Hair
Hypertrichosis (3–10%)

Mucosal
Gingival hyperplasia/hypertrophy (3–10%)
Stomatitis (3–10%)
Ulcerative stomatitis (3–10%)

Cardiovascular
Angina (3–10%)
Arrhythmias (3–10%)
Atrial fibrillation (3–10%)
Cardiac failure (3–10%)
Chest pain (3–10%)
Hypertension (>10%)
Hypotension (3–10%)
Pulmonary edema (3–10%)
Tachycardia (3–10%)

Central Nervous System
Agitation (3–10%)
Anxiety (3–10%)
Depression (3–10%)
Fever (>10%)
Headache (>10%)
Hypoesthesia (3–10%)
Insomnia (>10%)
Pain (>10%)
Paresthesias (3–10%)
Rigors (3–10%)
Tremor (>10%)
Vertigo (dizziness) (3–10%)

Neuromuscular/Skeletal
Arthralgia (3–10%)
Asthenia (fatigue) (3–10%)
Back pain (3–10%)
Cramps (3–10%)
Fractures (3–10%)
Leg pain (3–10%)
Myalgia/Myopathy (3–10%)

Gastrointestinal/Hepatic
Abdominal distension (3–10%)
Abdominal pain (>10%)
Black stools (3–10%)
Constipation (>10%)
Diarrhea (>10%)
Dyspepsia (>10%)
Esophagitis (3–10%)
Flatulence (3–10%)
Gastroenteritis (3–10%)
Gastrointestinal bleeding (3–10%)
Gastrointestinal disorder (69%)
Hernia (3–10%)
Nausea (>10%)
Vomiting (>10%)

Respiratory
Bronchitis (3–10%)
Bronchospasm (3–10%)
Cough (3–10%)
Dyspnea (>10%)
Pharyngitis (3–10%)
Pneumonia (3–10%)
Rhinitis (3–10%)
Sinusitis (3–10%)
Upper respiratory tract infection (>10%)

Endocrine/Metabolic
Acidosis (3–10%)
Dehydration (3–10%)
Diabetes mellitus (3–10%)
Hypercalcemia (3–10%)
Hypercholesterolemia (>10%)
Hyperglycemia (>10%)
Hyperkalemia (>10%)
Hyperlipidemia (3–10%)
Hypertriglyceridemia (3–10%)
Hyperuricemia (>10%)
Hypocalcemia (3–10%)
Hypoglycemia (3–10%)
Hypokalemia (>10%)
Hypophosphatemia (>10%)
Weight gain (3–10%)

Genitourinary
Albuminuria (3–10%)
Dysuria (3–10%)
Hematuria (3–10%)
Impotence (3–10%)
Oliguria (3–10%)
Urinary frequency (3–10%)
Urinary retention (3–10%)
Urinary tract infection (>10%)

Renal
Renal tubular necrosis (3–10%)

Hematologic
Anemia (>10%)
Hemorrhage (3–10%)
Leukopenia (3–10%)
Polycythemia (3–10%)
Sepsis (3–10%)
Thrombocytopenia (3–10%)
Thrombosis (3–10%)

Ocular
Abnormal vision (3–10%)
Cataract (3–10%)
Conjunctivitis (3–10%)

Other
Infection (viral) (>10%)

BCG VACCINE

Synonym: Bacille Calmette-Guerin
Trade names: Mycobax (Sanofi-Aventis), TICE BCG (Organon)
Indications: Immunization against tuberculosis
Class: Vaccine
Half-life: N/A
Clinically important, potentially hazardous interactions with: alefacept, aminophylline, azacitidine, betamethasone, cabazitaxel, cefazolin, cefixime, ceftaroline fosamil, ceftobiprole, ciprofloxacin, demeclocycline, denileukin, docetaxel, doripenem, doxycycline, fingolimod, gefitinib, gemifloxacin, leflunomide, levofloxacin, monosodium glutamate, moxifloxacin, ofloxacin, oxaliplatin, pazopanib, sulfadiazine, telavancin, telithromycin, temsirolimus
Pregnancy category: C

Skin
Abscess [16]
Anaphylactoid reactions/Anaphylaxis [5]
Churg-Strauss syndrome [15]
Dermatitis [2]
Erythema [3]
Fixed eruption [2]
Hypersensitivity [2]
Keloid [4]
Lupus vulgaris [22]
Lymphadenitis [9]
Lymphadenopathy [92]
Papular lesions [6]
Sarcoidosis [4]
Scar [8]
Scrofuloderma [5]
Sweet's syndrome [2]
Ulcerations [6]
Vasculitis [2]

Mucosal
Mucocutaneous lymph node syndrome (Kawaski syndrom) [2]

Central Nervous System
Fever [6]
Neurotoxicity [2]

Neuromuscular/Skeletal
Arthralgia [7]
Asthenia (fatigue) [4]
Osteomyelitis [35]

Gastrointestinal/Hepatic
Hepatitis [3]
Hepatotoxicity [2]

Genitourinary
Balanitis [3]
Bladder disorder [2]
Hematuria [2]

Hematologic
Sepsis [3]

Ocular
Optic neuritis [2]
Uveitis [4]

Local
Injection-site abscess [3]
Injection-site reactions [3]
Injection-site ulceration [4]

Other
Adverse effects [4]
Cancer [3]
Death [14]
Infection [3]
Systemic reactions [2]

BECLOMETHASONE

Trade names: Beconase AQ (GSK), Qnasl (Teva), Qvar (3M), Vanceril (Schering)
Indications: Allergic rhinitis, asthma
Class: Corticosteroid, inhaled
Half-life: N/A
Clinically important, potentially hazardous interactions with: diuretics, estrogens, ketoconazole, live vaccines, oral contraceptives, phenytoin, rifampin, warfarin
Pregnancy category: C
Important contra-indications noted in the prescribing guidelines for: nursing mothers; pediatric patients

---

Skin
Bruising [3]
Candidiasis [2]

Mucosal
Epistaxis (nosebleed) (with nasally-inhaled formulation) (2%)
Nasal discomfort (5%)
Oral candidiasis [4]

Central Nervous System
Headache (2%) [2]

Neuromuscular/Skeletal
Osteoporosis [5]

Respiratory
Upper respiratory tract infection [2]

Ocular
Cataract [4]
Glaucoma [3]

Other
Adverse effects [10]

BEDAQUILINE

Trade name: Sirturo (Janssen)
Indications: Pulmonary multi-drug resistant tuberculosis
Class: Antimycobacterial, Diarylquinoline
Half-life: 5.5 months
Clinically important, potentially hazardous interactions with: ketoconazole, rifabutin, rifampin, rifapentine, strong CYP3A4 inducers or inhibitors
Pregnancy category: B
Important contra-indications noted in the prescribing guidelines for: nursing mothers; pediatric patients
Warning: INCREASED RISK OF DEATH / QT PROLONGATION

Skin
Rash (8%)

Cardiovascular
Chest pain (11%) [2]
QT prolongation [3]

Central Nervous System
Anorexia (9%)
Headache (28%) [3]
Vertigo (dizziness) [2]

Neuromuscular/Skeletal
Arthralgia (33%) [2]
Pain in extremities [2]

Gastrointestinal/Hepatic
Hepatotoxicity [2]
Nausea (38%) [4]
Vomiting [2]

Respiratory
Hemoptysis (18%)

Endocrine/Metabolic
ALT increased (<10%)
AST increased (<10%)
Hyperuricemia [2]

Otic
Hearing loss [2]

Other
Infection [3]

BELATACEPT

Trade name: Nulojix (Bristol-Myers Squibb)
Indications: Prophylaxis of organ rejection in kidney transplantation
Class: Immunosuppressant, T-cell co-stimulation blocker
Half-life: 7–10 days
Clinically important, potentially hazardous interactions with: live vaccines, mycophenolate
Pregnancy category: C
Important contra-indications noted in the prescribing guidelines for: nursing mothers; pediatric patients
Note: Contra-indicated in patients without immunity to Epstein-Barr virus.
Warning: POST-TRANSPLANT LYMPHOPROLIFERATIVE DISORDER, OTHER MALIGNANCIES, AND SERIOUS INFECTIONS

Skin
Acneform eruption (8%)
Hematoma (<10%)
Hyperhidrosis (<10%)
Lymphoproliferative disease (post-transplant) [7]
Malignancies [3]
Peripheral edema (34%)

Hair
Alopecia (<10%)

Mucosal
Aphthous stomatitis (<10%)
Stomatitis (<10%)

Cardiovascular
Atrial fibrillation (<10%)
Hypertension (32%)
Hypotension (18%)

Central Nervous System
Anxiety (10%)
Fever (28%)
Guillain–Barré syndrome (<10%)
Headache (21%)
Insomnia (15%)
Tremor (8%)
Vertigo (dizziness) (9%)

Neuromuscular/Skeletal
Arthralgia (17%)
Back pain (13%)
Bone or joint pain (<10%)

Gastrointestinal/Hepatic
Abdominal pain (9–19%)
Constipation (33%)
Diarrhea (39%)
Nausea (24%)
Vomiting (22%)

Respiratory
Bronchitis (10%)
Cough (24%)
Dyspnea (12%)
Influenza (11%)
Nasopharyngitis (13%)
Upper respiratory tract infection (15%)

Endocrine/Metabolic
Creatine phosphokinase increased (15%)
Hypercholesterolemia (11%)
Hyperglycemia (19%)
Hyperkalemia (20%)
Hyperuricemia (5%)
Hypocalcemia (13%)
Hypokalemia (21%)
Hypomagnesemia (7%)
Hypophosphatemia (19%)

Genitourinary
Dysuria (11%)
Hematuria (16%)
Urinary incontinence (<10%)
Urinary tract infection (37%) [2]

Renal
Proteinuria (16%)
Renal failure (<10%)
Renal tubular necrosis (9%)

Hematologic
Anemia (45%)
Dyslipidemia (19%)
Leukopenia (20%)
Neutropenia (<10%) [2]

Other
Graft dysfunction (25%)
Infection (<10%) [7]

BELINOSTAT

Trade name: Beleodaq (Spectrum)
Indications: Peripheral T-cell lymphoma
Class: Histone deacetylase (HDAC) inhibitor
Half-life: 1 hour
Clinically important, potentially hazardous interactions with: strong UGT1A1 inhibitors
Pregnancy category: D
Important contra-indications noted in the prescribing guidelines for: nursing mothers; pediatric patients

---

Skin
Peripheral edema (20%) [2]
Pruritus (16%)
Rash (20%)

Hair
Alopecia [2]

Cardiovascular
Hypotension (10%)
Phlebitis (10%)
QT prolongation (11%) [2]

Central Nervous System
Anorexia [2]
Chills (16%)
Fever (35%) [2]
Headache (15%) [3]
Peripheral neuropathy [2]
Vertigo (dizziness) (10%) [2]

Neuromuscular/Skeletal
Asthenia (fatigue) (37%) [11]
Myalgia/Myopathy [2]

Gastrointestinal/Hepatic
Abdominal pain (11%)
Constipation (23%) [5]
Diarrhea (23%) [6]
Nausea (42%) [10]
Vomiting (29%) [10]

Respiratory
Cough (19%)
Dyspnea (22%) [4]
Pneumonia (>2%)

Pneumonitis [2]

Endocrine/Metabolic

Appetite decreased (15%)
Creatine phosphokinase increased (>2%)
Hypokalemia (12%)

Hematologic

Anemia (32%) [5]
Leukopenia [2]
Lymphopenia [2]
Neutropenia [4]
Thrombocytopenia (16%) [3]
Thrombosis [2]

Local

Infusion-site pain (14%)
Injection-site reactions [2]

Other

Allergic reactions [2]
Hiccups [2]
Multiorgan failure (>2%)

BENAZEPRIL

Trade names: Lotensin (Novartis), Lotensin HCT (Novartis), Lotrel (Novartis)
Indications: Hypertension
Class: Angiotensin-converting enzyme (ACE) inhibitor, Antihypertensive, Vasodilator
Half-life: 10–11 hours
Clinically important, potentially hazardous interactions with: allopurinol, amifostine, amiloride, angiotensin II receptor blockers, antacids, antidiabetics, antihypertensives, azathioprine, cyclosporine, diazoxide, diuretics, eplerenone, everolimus, gold & gold compounds, herbals, lithium, MAO inhibitors, methylphenidate, NSAIDs, pentoxifylline, phosphodiesterase 5 inhibitors, potassium salts, prostacyclin analogues, rituximab, sirolimus, spironolactone, temsirolimus, tizanidine, tolvaptan, triamterene, trimethoprim, yohimbine
Pregnancy category: D
Important contra-indications noted in the prescribing guidelines for: pediatric patients
Note: Lotrel is benazepril and amlodipine. Lotensin-HCT is benazepril and hydrochlorothiazide. Hydrochlorothiazide is a sulfonamide and can be absorbed systemically. Sulfonamides can produce severe, possibly fatal, reactions such as toxic epidermal necrolysis and Stevens-Johnson syndrome.
Contra-indicated in patients with a history of angioedema with or without previous ACE inhibitor treatment.
Warning: FETAL TOXICITY

Skin

Angioedema [8]
Peripheral edema [3]

Central Nervous System

Headache (6%)
Vertigo (dizziness) (4%)

Respiratory

Cough [10]

BERGAMOT

Family: Rutaceae
Scientific name: *Citrus aurantium ssp bergamia*
Indications: Headache, bronchitis, vitiligo, mycosis fungoides, psoriasis (in conjunction with UVA), insecticide, essential oil in perfumery, cosmetics, flavoring
Class: Stimulant, mild
Half-life: N/A
Clinically important, potentially hazardous interactions with: none known
Pregnancy category: N/A
Note: Two distinct species are known by the common name of bergamot. This profile does not refer to *Monarda didyma*.
Oil of bergamot possesses photosensitive and melanogenic properties because of the presence of furocoumarins, primarily bergapten (5-methoxypsoralen [5-MOP]).
Its use is restricted or banned in many countries.

Skin

Berloque dermatitis [2]
Dermatitis [2]
Photosensitivity [3]
Phototoxicity [8]

Other

Adverse effects [2]

BETAXOLOL

Trade names: Betoptic [Ophthalmic] (Alcon), Kerlone (Pfizer)
Indications: Open-angle glaucoma, hypertension
Class: Adrenergic beta-receptor antagonist
Half-life: 14–22 hours
Clinically important, potentially hazardous interactions with: clonidine, verapamil
Pregnancy category: C
Important contra-indications noted in the prescribing guidelines for: nursing mothers; pediatric patients
Note: Cutaneous side effects of beta-receptor blockers are clinically polymorphous. They apparently appear after several months of continuous therapy.

Skin

Cold extremities (2%)
Dermatitis [3]
Diaphoresis (<2%)
Eczema (<2%)
Edema (<2%)
Erythema (<2%)
Flushing (<2%)
Lymphadenopathy (<2%)
Pruritus (<2%)
Purpura (<2%)
Rash (<2%) [3]

Hair

Alopecia (<2%)
Hypertrichosis (<2%)

Mucosal

Epistaxis (nosebleed) (<2%)
Oral ulceration (<2%)
Sialorrhea (<2%)
Xerostomia (<2%)

Cardiovascular

Angina (<2%)
Arrhythmias (<2%)
Atrioventricular block (<2%)
Bradycardia (6–8%)
Cardiac failure (<2%)
Chest pain (2–7%)
Hypertension (<2%)
Hypotension (<2%)
Myocardial infarction (<2%)
Palpitation (2%)
Peripheral ischemia (<2%)

Central Nervous System

Ageusia (taste loss) (<2%)
Amnesia (<2%)
Anorexia (<2%)
Confusion (<2%)
Dysgeusia (taste perversion) (<2%)
Emotional lability (<2%)
Fever (<2%)
Hallucinations (<2%)
Headache (7–15%)
Insomnia (<5%)
Pain (<2%)
Paresthesias (2%)
Rigors (<2%)
Stupor (<2%)
Syncope (<2%)
Tremor (<2%)
Twitching (<2%)
Vertigo (dizziness) (5–15%)

Neuromuscular/Skeletal

Arthralgia (3%)
Asthenia (fatigue) (3–10%)
Ataxia (<2%)
Bone or joint pain (5%)
Leg cramps (<2%)
Myalgia/Myopathy (3%)
Neck pain (<2%)
Tendinitis (<2%)

Gastrointestinal/Hepatic

Constipation (<2%)
Diarrhea (2%)
Dyspepsia (4–5%)
Dysphagia (<2%)
Nausea (2–6%)
Vomiting (<2%)

Respiratory

Bronchitis (<2%)
Bronchospasm (<2%)
Cough (<2%)
Dysphonia (<2%)
Dyspnea (2%)
Influenza (<2%)
Pharyngitis (2%)
Pneumonia (<2%)
Sinusitis (<2%)
Upper respiratory tract infection (3%)

Endocrine/Metabolic

Acidosis (<2%)
ALT increased (<2%)
Appetite increased (<2%)
AST increased (<2%)
Diabetes mellitus (<2%)
Gynecomastia (<2%)
Hypercholesterolemia (<2%)
Hyperglycemia (<2%)
Hyperkalemia (<2%)

Hyperuricemia (<2%)
Hypokalemia (<2%)
Libido decreased (<2%)
Mastodynia (<2%)
Menstrual irregularities (<2%)
Weight gain (<2%)
Weight loss (<2%)

Genitourinary
Cystitis (<2%)
Dysuria (<2%)
Oliguria (<2%)
Peyronie's disease (<2%)
Prostatitis (<2%)

Renal
Proteinuria (<2%)
Renal function abnormal (<2%)

Hematologic
Anemia (<2%)
Lymphocytosis (<2%)
Thrombocytopenia (<2%)
Thrombosis (<2%)

Otic
Ear pain (<2%)
Hearing loss (<2%)
Tinnitus (<2%)

Ocular
Abnormal vision (<2%)
Blepharitis (<2%)
Cataract (<2%)
Conjunctivitis (<2%)
Iritis (<2%)
Lacrimation (<2%)
Ocular hemorrhage (<2%)
Scotoma (<2%)
Xerophthalmia (<2%)

Other
Allergic reactions (<2%)
Dipsia (thirst) (<2%)

BETRIXABAN

Trade name: Bevyxxa (Portola)
Indications: Prophylaxis of venous thromboembolism in adult patients hospitalized for an acute medical illness who are at risk for thromboembolic complications
Class: Direct factor Xa inhibitor
Half-life: 19–27 hours
Clinically important, potentially hazardous interactions with: amiodarone, anticoagulants, antiplatelet drugs and thrombolytics, azithromycin, clarithromycin, ketoconazole, verapamil
Pregnancy category: N/A (Likely to increase the risk of hemorrhage during pregnancy and delivery)
Important contra-indications noted in the prescribing guidelines for: nursing mothers; pediatric patients
Note: Contra-indicated in patients with active pathological bleeding.
Warning: SPINAL/EPIDURAL HEMATOMA

Mucosal
Epistaxis (nosebleed) (2%)

Cardiovascular
Hypertension (2%)

Central Nervous System
Headache (2%)

Gastrointestinal/Hepatic
Constipation (3%)
Diarrhea (2%)
Nausea (2%)

Endocrine/Metabolic
Hypokalemia (3%)

Genitourinary
Hematuria (2%)
Urinary tract infection (3%)

Hematologic
Bleeding (<2%) [4]

BEVACIZUMAB

Trade name: Avastin (Genentech)
Indications: Colon cancer
Class: Biologic, Monoclonal antibody, Vascular endothelial growth factor antagonist
Half-life: 20 days
Clinically important, potentially hazardous interactions with: antineoplastics, irinotecan, sorafenib, sunitinib
Pregnancy category: C
Important contra-indications noted in the prescribing guidelines for: the elderly; nursing mothers; pediatric patients
Warning: GASTROINTESTINAL PERFORATIONS, SURGERY AND WOUND HEALING COMPLICATIONS, and HEMORRHAGE

Skin
Acneform eruption [6]
Hand–foot syndrome [13]
Necrosis [2]
Rash [17]
Toxicity [9]
Ulcerations [3]
Wound complications [8]

Hair
Alopecia [5]

Nails
Paronychia [2]

Mucosal
Epistaxis (nosebleed) [5]
Mucosal inflammation [2]
Mucositis [13]
Oral ulceration [2]
Stomatitis [8]

Cardiovascular
Cardiac failure [2]
Cardiotoxicity [6]
Hypertension (23–67%) [98]
Hypotension (7–15%)
Thromboembolism (<21%) [15]
Venous thromboembolism [7]

Central Nervous System
Anorexia [16]
Cerebral hemorrhage [6]
Headache [6]
Intracranial hemorrhage [2]
Leukoencephalopathy [19]
Neurotoxicity [13]
Pain [2]
Peripheral neuropathy [10]
Seizures [2]

Neuromuscular/Skeletal
Arthralgia [2]
Asthenia (fatigue) [39]
Osteonecrosis [5]

Gastrointestinal/Hepatic
Abdominal pain [4]
Colitis [3]
Diarrhea [44]
Gastrointestinal bleeding [5]
Gastrointestinal fistula [3]
Gastrointestinal perforation [28]
Hepatotoxicity [4]
Nausea [15]
Vomiting [9]

Respiratory
Hemoptysis [5]
Pulmonary embolism [5]
Pulmonary toxicity [2]

Endocrine/Metabolic
ALT increased [3]
Creatine phosphokinase increased [2]
Hyperglycemia [2]
Hypokalemia [3]
Hypomagnesemia [2]

Renal
Nephrotoxicity [2]
Proteinuria [39]

Hematologic
Anemia [16]
Bleeding [13]
Febrile neutropenia [15]
Hemorrhage [13]
Hemotoxicity [2]
Leukocytopenia [2]
Leukopenia [16]
Lymphopenia [5]
Neutropenia [49]
Thrombocytopenia [24]
Thrombosis [17]
Thrombotic complications [4]
Thrombotic microangiopathy [2]

Ocular
Hallucinations, visual [2]
Intraocular pressure increased [3]
Iritis [2]
Ocular adverse effects [2]
Uveitis [2]

Other
Adverse effects [23]
Allergic reactions [3]
Death [18]
Hiccups [2]
Infection [10]

BEXAROTENE

Trade name: Targretin (Eisai)
Indications: Cutaneous T-cell lymphoma, mycosis fungoides
Class: Antineoplastic, Retinoid
Half-life: 7 hours
Clinically important, potentially hazardous interactions with: acitretin, atorvastatin, beta-carotene, carboplatin, conivaptan, dexamethasone, dong quai, gemfibrozil,

grapefruit juice, isotretinoin, oral contraceptives, paclitaxel, saxagliptin, St John's wort, tamoxifen, tetracyclines, tretinoin, vitamin A
Pregnancy category: X
Important contra-indications noted in the prescribing guidelines for: nursing mothers; pediatric patients
Note: Retinoids can cause birth defects, and women should avoid bexarotene when pregnant or trying to conceive.
Warning: AVOID IN PREGNANCY

Skin
Acneform eruption (<10%)
Bacterial infection (<13%)
Dermatitis [2]
Erythema [2]
Exanthems (<10%)
Exfoliative dermatitis (10–28%)
Necrosis [2]
Nodular eruption (<10%)
Peripheral edema (13%)
Pruritus (20–30%) [5]
Rash (17%) [2]
Ulcerations (<10%)
Vesiculobullous eruption (<10%)
Xerosis (11%) [2]

Hair
Alopecia (4–11%)

Mucosal
Cheilitis (<10%)
Gingivitis (<10%)
Mucositis [2]
Xerostomia (<10%)

Central Nervous System
Chills (10%)
Hyperesthesia (<10%)

Neuromuscular/Skeletal
Arthralgia [2]
Asthenia (fatigue) [2]
Myalgia/Myopathy (<10%) [2]

Respiratory
Flu-like syndrome (4–13%)

Endocrine/Metabolic
Hypercholesterolemia [4]
Hyperlipidemia [4]
Hypertriglyceridemia [6]
Hypothyroidism [6]
Mastodynia (<10%)

Hematologic
Anemia [4]
Leukopenia [4]
Lymphopenia [2]
Neutropenia [6]

Other
Adverse effects [2]

BEZLOTOXUMAB

Trade name: Zinplava (Merck)
Indications: To reduce the recurrence of *Clostridium difficile* infection (CDI) in patients who are receiving antibacterial treatment of CDI and are at high risk for CDI recurrence
Class: C. difficile toxin inhibitor, Monoclonal antibody
Half-life: ~19 days
Clinically important, potentially hazardous interactions with: none known
Pregnancy category: N/A (No data available)
Important contra-indications noted in the prescribing guidelines for: nursing mothers; pediatric patients

---

Cardiovascular
Cardiac failure (2%)

Central Nervous System
Fever (5%) [2]
Headache (4%) [3]

Gastrointestinal/Hepatic
Diarrhea [4]
Nausea (7%) [4]

Local
Infusion-related reactions (10%) [2]

BICALUTAMIDE

Trade name: Casodex (AstraZeneca)
Indications: Metastatic prostatic carcinoma
Class: Androgen antagonist
Half-life: up to 10 days
Clinically important, potentially hazardous interactions with: CYP3A4 substrates
Pregnancy category: X (not indicated for use in women)
Important contra-indications noted in the prescribing guidelines for: pediatric patients

---

Skin
Diaphoresis (6%)
Edema (2–5%)
Hot flashes (49%) [9]
Peripheral edema (8%)
Pruritus (2–5%)
Rash (6%)
Xerosis (2–5%)

Hair
Alopecia (2–5%)

Mucosal
Xerostomia (2–5%)

Central Nervous System
Paresthesias (6%)

Neuromuscular/Skeletal
Asthenia (fatigue) [4]
Myalgia/Myopathy (2–5%)

Gastrointestinal/Hepatic
Constipation [2]
Hepatotoxicity [4]

Endocrine/Metabolic
Gynecomastia (38%) [34]
Mastodynia (39%) [16]

Local
Injection-site reactions (2–5%)

BIFIDOBACTERIA

Family: Actinomycetaceae
Scientific names: *Bifidobacterium adolescentis, Bifidobacterium animalis, Bifidobacterium bifidum, Bifidobacterium breve, Bifidobacterium infantis, Bifidobacterium lactis, Bifidobacterium longum*
Indications: Diarrhea, atopic eczema, candidiasis, colds and flu, hepatitis, hypercholesterolemia, lactose intolerance, ulcerative colitis, pouchitis, irritable bowel syndrome
Class: Immunomodulator, Probiotic
Half-life: N/A
Clinically important, potentially hazardous interactions with: none known
Pregnancy category: N/A
Note: Immune-deficient subjects or those with mucosal disease may experience serious adverse effects.
Bifidobacterium is often combined with *Lactobacillus, Saccharomyces* or *Streptococcus thermophilus*.

BIMATOPROST

Trade names: Latisse (Allergan), Lumigan (Allergan)
Indications: Reduction of elevated intraocular pressure in open-angle glaucoma or ocular hypertension, hypotrichosis of the eyelashes
Class: Prostaglandin analog
Half-life: 45 minutes
Clinically important, potentially hazardous interactions with: none known
Pregnancy category: C
Important contra-indications noted in the prescribing guidelines for: nursing mothers; pediatric patients

---

Skin
Pigmentation [2]

Hair
Hirsutism (<5%)
Hypertrichosis [2]

Central Nervous System
Headache (<5%)

Neuromuscular/Skeletal
Asthenia (fatigue) (<5%)

Respiratory
Nasopharyngitis [2]
Upper respiratory tract infection (10%)

Ocular
Asthenopia (<10%)
Blepharitis (<10%)
Cataract (<10%)
Choroidal detachment [2]
Conjunctival edema (<10%)
Conjunctival hemorrhage (<10%)
Conjunctival hyperemia (25–45%) [42]
Conjunctivitis (<10%)
Deepening of upper lid sulcus [9]
Eyelashes – hypertrichosis (>10%) [13]

Eyelashes – pigmentation (<10%) [3]
Eyelid erythema (3–10%) [2]
Eyelid irritation (3–10%)
Eyelid pain (3–10%)
Eyelid pigmentation (3–10%) [6]
Eyelid xerosis (3–10%)
Eyes – adverse effects [2]
Foreign body sensation (<10%)
Iris pigmentation (<10%) [4]
Keratitis [2]
Lacrimation (<10%)
Macular edema [2]
Ocular adverse effects [10]
Ocular burning (<10%)
Ocular discharge (<10%)
Ocular hyperemia [4]
Ocular itching (<10%)
Ocular pain [2]
Ocular pigmentation (<3%) [5]
Ocular pruritus (>10%) [5]
Periorbital pigmentation (<10%) [3]
Photophobia (<10%)
Punctate keratitis (<10%) [2]
Uveitis [3]

BINIMETINIB *

Trade name: Mektovi (Array Biopharma Inc)
Indications: in combination with encorafenib, for the treatment of patients with unresectable or metastatic melanoma with a BRAF V600E or V600K mutation
Class: Kinase inhibitor
Half-life: 3.5 hours
Clinically important, potentially hazardous interactions with: none known
Pregnancy category: N/A (can cause fetal harm)
Important contra-indications noted in the prescribing guidelines for: nursing mothers

---

Skin
Panniculitis (<10%)
Peripheral edema (13%)
Rash (22%) [2]

Cardiovascular
Hypertension (11%) [2]

Central Nervous System
Fever (18%)
Vertigo (dizziness) (15%)

Neuromuscular/Skeletal
Asthenia (fatigue) (43%)

Gastrointestinal/Hepatic
Abdominal pain (28%)
Colitis (<10%)
Constipation (22%)
Diarrhea (36%) [2]
Nausea (41%) [2]
Vomiting (30%)

Endocrine/Metabolic
ALP increased (21%)
ALT increased (29%)
AST increased (27%)
Creatine phosphokinase increased (58%) [3]
GGT increased (45%)
Hyponatremia (18%)
Serum creatinine increased (93%)

Hematologic
Anemia (36%)
Hemorrhage (19%)
Leukopenia (13%)
Lymphopenia (13%)
Neutropenia (13%)

Ocular
Serous retinopathy (20%)
Vision impaired (20%)

BISMUTH

Trade names: Helidac (Prometheus), Pepto-Bismol (Procter & Gamble)
Indications: As part of 'triple therapy' (antibiotics + bismuth) for eradication of *H. pylori*. Bismuth subgallate initiates clotting via activation of factor XII, and is used for bleeding during tonsillectomy and adenoidectomy. BIPP impregnated ribbon gauze is used for packing following ear surgery. Bismuth subsalicylate is in OTC products for gastrointestinal complaints and peptic ulcer disease
Class: Disinfectant, Heavy metal
Half-life: 21–72 days
Clinically important, potentially hazardous interactions with: aspirin, ciprofloxacin, demeclocycline, doxycycline, hypoglycemics, lomefloxacin, lymecycline, methotrexate, minocycline, tetracycline, warfarin
Pregnancy category: D (category C in first and second trimesters; category D in third trimester)

Skin
Dermatitis [2]
Hypersensitivity [2]
Pigmentation [5]
Pruritus (triple therapy) [2]
Rash [4]

Mucosal
Oral pigmentation [3]
Stomatitis [4]
Tongue pigmentation (>10%) [3]
Xerostomia (triple therapy) (41%)

Central Nervous System
Dysgeusia (taste perversion) (triple therapy) (46%) [9]
Encephalopathy [4]
Pain (triple therapy) (10%)
Tremor [2]
Vertigo (dizziness) [2]

Neuromuscular/Skeletal
Arthralgia [10]
Asthenia (fatigue) [2]

Gastrointestinal/Hepatic
Diarrhea [5]
Nausea [4]
Vomiting [2]

Other
Adverse effects (triple therapy) [52]
Allergic reactions [2]
Death [10]

BISOPROLOL

Trade names: Cardicor (Merck Serono), Concor (Merck Serono), Emcor (Merck Serono), Zebeta (Barr), Ziac (Barr)
Indications: Hypertension
Class: Beta adrenergic blocker, Beta blocker
Half-life: 9–12 hours
Clinically important, potentially hazardous interactions with: diltiazem, disopyramide, guanethidine, reserpine, rifampin, verapamil
Pregnancy category: C
Important contra-indications noted in the prescribing guidelines for: nursing mothers; pediatric patients
Note: Ziac is bisoprolol and hydrochlorothiazide. Hydrochlorothiazide is a sulfonamide and can be absorbed systemically. Sulfonamides can produce severe, possibly fatal, reactions such as toxic epidermal necrolysis and Stevens-Johnson syndrome.
Contra-indicated in patients with cardiogenic shock, overt cardiac failure, second or third degree AV block, and marked sinus bradycardia.

Skin
Edema (3%)
Peripheral edema (<10%)
Rash (<10%)
Raynaud's phenomenon (<10%)

Cardiovascular
Bradycardia [6]
Hypotension [3]

Central Nervous System
Headache [2]
Hyperesthesia (2%)
Vertigo (dizziness) [3]

Neuromuscular/Skeletal
Myalgia/Myopathy (<10%)

Other
Adverse effects [4]

BIVALIRUDIN

Trade name: Angiomax (The Medicines Company)
Indications: Angioplasty adjunct
Class: Thrombin inhibitor
Half-life: 25 minutes
Clinically important, potentially hazardous interactions with: anisindione, dicumarol, heparin, reteplase, streptokinase, tenecteplase, urokinase, warfarin
Pregnancy category: B

Central Nervous System
Pain (15%)

Neuromuscular/Skeletal
Back pain (42%)

Hematologic
Bleeding [5]
Thrombosis [3]

Local
Injection-site pain (8%)

BLACK COHOSH

Family: Ranunculaceae
Scientific names: *Actaea macrotys, Actaea racemosa, Cimicifuga racemosa*
Indications: Anxiety, arthritis, asthma, cardiovascular and circulatory problems, climacteric, menstrual and premenstrual disorders, colds, cough, constipation, depression, kidney disorders, malaria, sore throat, tinnitus
Class: Phytoestrogen
Half-life: N/A
Clinically important, potentially hazardous interactions with: clevidipine, salicylates
Pregnancy category: N/A
Note: In 2001, the American College of Obstetricians and Gynecologists stated that black cohosh might be helpful in the short term (6 months or less) for women with vasomotor symptoms of menopause.

Skin
Diaphoresis [2]
Rash [2]

Central Nervous System
Seizures [3]
Vertigo (dizziness) [2]

Gastrointestinal/Hepatic
Hepatic failure [2]
Hepatitis [3]
Hepatotoxicity [5]

Other
Adverse effects [4]

BLEOMYCIN

Synonyms: bleo; BLM
Trade name: Blenoxane (Mead Johnson)
Indications: Melanomas, sarcomas, lymphomas, testicular carcinoma
Class: Antibiotic, anthracycline
Half-life: 1.3–9 hours
Clinically important, potentially hazardous interactions with: aldesleukin, brentuximab vedotin
Pregnancy category: D
Important contra-indications noted in the prescribing guidelines for: nursing mothers; pediatric patients

---

Skin
Acral erythema [2]
Acral necrosis [2]
Bullous dermatitis (<5%)
Calcification [2]
Erythema [6]
Exanthems [3]
Flagellate dermatitis [10]
Flagellate erythema/pigmentation [44]
Gangrene (digital) [3]
Hand–foot syndrome [2]
Hyperkeratosis (palms and soles) [3]
Hypersensitivity (<10%) [5]
Linear streaking [4]
Lipodystrophy [2]
Neutrophilic eccrine hidradenitis [2]
Pigmentation (~50%) [21]
Pruritus (>5%) [7]
Raynaud's phenomenon (>10%) [35]
Scleroderma [16]
Stevens-Johnson syndrome [2]
Toxicity [2]

Hair
Alopecia (~50%) [8]

Nails
Nail changes [2]
Nail growth reduced [2]
Nail loss [3]
Onychodystrophy [2]
Onycholysis [3]

Mucosal
Oral ulceration [2]
Stomatitis (>10%) [8]

Central Nervous System
Chills (>10%)

Neuromuscular/Skeletal
Digital necrosis [3]

Respiratory
Pneumonitis [3]
Pulmonary fibrosis [3]
Pulmonary toxicity [7]

Endocrine/Metabolic
SIADH [2]

Hematologic
Hemolytic uremic syndrome [8]

Local
Injection-site phlebitis (<10%)

Other
Adverse effects [2]
Allergic reactions [2]

BLINATUMOMAB

Trade name: Blincyto (Amgen)
Indications: Precursor B-cell acute lymphoblastic leukemia
Class: Bispecific CD19-directed CD3 T-cell engager, Monoclonal antibody
Half-life: 1.4 hours
Clinically important, potentially hazardous interactions with: none known
Pregnancy category: C
Important contra-indications noted in the prescribing guidelines for: nursing mothers
Warning: CYTOKINE RELEASE SYNDROME and NEUROLOGICAL TOXICITIES

Skin
Edema (5%) [4]
Peripheral edema (25%) [2]
Rash (21%) [2]
Tumor lysis syndrome (4%)

Cardiovascular
Chest pain (11%)
Hypertension (8%)
Hypotension (11%)
Tachycardia (8%)

Central Nervous System
Aphasia (4%) [5]
Chills (15%)
Confusion (7%) [4]
Cytokine release syndrome (11%) [12]
Disorientation (3%) [3]
Encephalopathy (5%) [6]
Fever (62%) [9]
Headache (36%) [7]
Insomnia (15%)
Memory loss (2%)
Neurotoxicity [8]
Paresthesias (5%) [2]
Seizures (2%) [7]
Somnolence (drowsiness) [2]
Speech disorder [3]
Tremor (20%) [7]
Vertigo (dizziness) (14%) [2]

Neuromuscular/Skeletal
Arthralgia (10%)
Asthenia (fatigue) (17%) [4]
Ataxia [2]
Back pain (14%) [2]
Bone or joint pain (11%)
Pain in extremities (12%)

Gastrointestinal/Hepatic
Abdominal pain (15%)
Constipation (20%) [2]
Diarrhea (20%) [3]
Hepatotoxicity [2]
Nausea (25%) [4]
Vomiting (13%)

Respiratory
Cough (19%) [2]
Dyspnea (15%)
Pneumonia (9%) [4]

Endocrine/Metabolic
ALT increased (12%) [2]
Appetite decreased (10%)
AST increased (11%)
GGT increased (6%) [2]
Hyperbilirubinemia (8%)
Hyperglycemia (11%) [2]
Hypoalbuminemia (4%)
Hypokalemia (23%) [5]
Hypomagnesemia (12%)
Hypophosphatemia (6%)
Weight gain (11%)

Hematologic
Anemia (18%) [5]
Febrile neutropenia (25%) [8]
Leukocytosis (2%)
Leukopenia (9%) [5]
Lymphopenia [3]
Neutropenia (16%) [4]
Sepsis (7%) [3]
Thrombocytopenia (11%) [6]

Local
Catheter-related infection [2]

BLOODROOT

Family: Papaveraceae
Scientific name: *Sanguinaria canadensis*
Indications: **Oral:** emetic, cathartic, expectorant. **Topical:** debriding agent, bronchitis, asthma, croup, laryngitis, pharyngitis, scabies, eczema, athlete's foot, nasal polyps, rheumatism, fever, anemia
Class: Anti-inflammatory
Half-life: N/A
Clinically important, potentially hazardous interactions with: none known
Pregnancy category: N/A

Mucosal
Leukoplakia [2]

BLUE COHOSH

Family: Berberidaceae
Scientific name: *Caulophyllum thalictroides*
Indications: Rheumatism, dropsy, epilepsy, hysteria, uterine inflammation, thrush, menopause, headache, sexual debility, aphthous stomatitis, laxative, colic, sore throat, hiccups
Class: Diuretic, Oxytocic
Half-life: N/A
Clinically important, potentially hazardous interactions with: cardioactive drugs, clevidipine
Pregnancy category: N/A
Note: Cohosh is from the Algonquin word 'rough', referring to the appearance of the roots. It is a toxic herb and should not be confused with the safer, unrelated herb, black cohosh.

Other
Adverse effects [2]

BOCEPREVIR

Trade name: Victrelis (Merck)
Indications: Chronic hepatitis C
Class: CYP3A4 inhibitor, Direct-acting antiviral, Hepatitis C virus NS3/4A protease inhibitor
Half-life: 3 hours
Clinically important, potentially hazardous interactions with: alfuzosin, alprazolam, amiodarone, atorvastatin, bepridil, bosentan, brigatinib, budesonide, buprenorphine, cabozantinib, carbamazepine, cisapride, clarithromycin, colchicine, copanlisib, cyclosporine, dasatinib, desipramine, dexamethasone, digoxin, dihydroergotamine, drospirenone, efavirenz, ergonovine, ergotamine, estradiol, felodipine, flecainide, flibanserin, fluticasone propionate, gefitinib, itraconazole, ketoconazole, lomitapide, lovastatin, methadone, methylergonovine, midazolam, midostaurin, mifepristone, neratinib, nicardipine, nifedipine, olaparib, pazopanib, phenobarbital, phenytoin, pimozide, ponatinib, posaconazole, propafenone, quinidine, ribociclib, rifabutin, rifampin, ritonavir, ruxolitinib, salmeterol, sildenafil, simvastatin, sirolimus, St John's wort, tacrolimus, tadalafil, trazodone, triazolam, vardenafil, vorapaxar, voriconazole, warfarin
Pregnancy category: X (boceprevir is pregnancy category B but must not be used in monotherapy)
Important contra-indications noted in the prescribing guidelines for: nursing mothers; pediatric patients
Note: Must be used in combination with PEG-interferon and ribavirin (see separate entries) Combination treatment is contra-indicated in pregnant women and men whose female partners are pregnant because of the risks for birth defects and fetal death associated with ribavirin, or in coadministration with drugs that are highly dependent on CYP3A4/5 for clearance, or with potent CYP3A4/5 inducers.

Skin
Pruritus [3]
Rash [3]

Central Nervous System
Dysgeusia (taste perversion) [6]

Gastrointestinal/Hepatic
Hepatotoxicity [2]

Hematologic
Anemia [24]
Neutropenia [8]
Thrombocytopenia [8]

Other
Adverse effects [6]
Infection [2]

BORTEZOMIB

Trade name: Velcade (Millennium)
Indications: Multiple myeloma, mantle cell lymphoma
Class: Biologic, Proteasome inhibitor
Half-life: 9–15 hours
Clinically important, potentially hazardous interactions with: conivaptan, darunavir, delavirdine, efavirenz, indinavir, strong CYP3A4 inducers or inhibitors, telithromycin, thalidomide, voriconazole
Pregnancy category: D
Important contra-indications noted in the prescribing guidelines for: nursing mothers; pediatric patients
Note: Contra-indicated in patients with hypersensitivity to boron or mannitol.

Skin
Edema (23%)
Erythema [2]
Folliculitis [2]
Herpes zoster (12%) [13]
Peripheral edema [5]
Pruritus (11%)
Purpura [2]
Rash (18%) [11]
Sweet's syndrome [7]
Toxicity [4]
Tumor lysis syndrome [2]
Vasculitis [4]

Mucosal
Mucositis [2]

Cardiovascular
Arrhythmias [2]
Cardiac failure [3]
Cardiotoxicity [4]
Congestive heart failure [3]
Hypertension [3]
Hypotension (13%) [4]
QT prolongation [2]

Central Nervous System
Anorexia [2]
Anxiety (10%)
Dysesthesia (23%)
Dysgeusia (taste perversion) (13%)
Encephalopathy [3]
Fever (34%) [8]
Guillain–Barré syndrome [2]
Headache [3]
Hypoesthesia [2]
Insomnia (20%) [2]
Neurotoxicity [27]
Pain [2]
Paresthesias (22%) [3]
Peripheral neuropathy (39%) [66]
Vertigo (dizziness) (17%)

Neuromuscular/Skeletal
Arthralgia (17%) [2]
Asthenia (fatigue) (64%) [40]
Back pain (13%)
Bone or joint pain (14%) [2]
Cramps (11%)
Myalgia/Myopathy (12%)

Gastrointestinal/Hepatic
Abdominal distension [2]
Abdominal pain [3]
Colitis [2]
Constipation (41%) [7]
Diarrhea (52%) [23]
Gastrointestinal disorder [3]
Hepatotoxicity [5]
Nausea (55%) [10]
Pancreatitis [2]
Vomiting (33%) [4]

Respiratory
Cough (20%) [2]
Dyspnea (21%) [6]
Nasopharyngitis (12%)
Pneumonia (12%) [8]
Pneumonitis [4]
Pulmonary toxicity [3]
Upper respiratory tract infection (12%) [3]

Endocrine/Metabolic
Appetite decreased (36%)
Dehydration (10%) [2]
Hypocalcemia [2]
Hypokalemia [3]
Serum creatinine increased [2]
SIADH [2]
Weight loss [2]

Renal
Nephrotoxicity [2]

Hematologic
Anemia (29%) [18]
Febrile neutropenia [5]
Hemotoxicity [5]
Leukopenia [9]
Lymphopenia [11]

Myelosuppression [2]
Neutropenia (17%) [36]
Sepsis [4]
Thrombocytopenia (36%) [57]

Local

Infusion-related reactions [2]
Injection-site irritation (5%)
Injection-site reactions [4]

Other

Adverse effects [13]
Death [6]
Infection [11]

BOSENTAN

Trade name: Tracleer (Actelion)
Indications: Pulmonary arterial hypertension
Class: Antihypertensive, Endothelin receptor (ETR) antagonist, Vasodilator
Half-life: ~5 hours
Clinically important, potentially hazardous interactions with: amiodarone, amprenavir, astemizole, atazanavir, atorvastatin, boceprevir, cobicistat/elvitegravir/emtricitabine/tenofovir alafenamide, cobicistat/elvitegravir/emtricitabine/tenofovir disoproxil, cyclosporine, diltiazem, elbasvir & grazoprevir, enzalutamide, erythromycin, fluconazole, fluvastatin, glibenclamide, glyburide, indinavir, itraconazole, ketoconazole, levonorgestrel, lopinavir, lovastatin, neratinib, olaparib, oral contraceptives, palbociclib, progestogens, reboxetine, rifampin, ritonavir, sildenafil, simvastatin, St John's wort, tacrolimus, tadalafil, telaprevir, tipranavir, ulipristal, vardenafil, venetoclax, voriconazole, warfarin
Pregnancy category: X
Important contra-indications noted in the prescribing guidelines for: nursing mothers; pediatric patients
Warning: RISKS OF HEPATOTOXICITY and TERATOGENICITY

Skin

Edema (8%) [2]
Flushing (9%) [2]
Peripheral edema (8%) [5]
Pruritus (4%)

Central Nervous System

Headache [2]
Syncope [2]

Gastrointestinal/Hepatic

Hepatotoxicity [18]

Respiratory

Bronchitis [2]

Endocrine/Metabolic

AST increased [2]

Hematologic

Anemia [4]

Other

Adverse effects [7]

BOSWELLIA

Family: Burseraceae
Scientific names: *Boswellia carterii, Boswellia commiphora, Boswellia ovalifoliolata, Boswellia serrata*
Indications: Allergic rhinitis, arthritis, asthma, atherosclerosis, chronic colitis, ulcerative colitis, Crohn's disease, peritumoral brain edema, rheumatism, trypanosomiasis, ulcers
Class: Anti-inflammatory, Diuretic
Half-life: N/A
Clinically important, potentially hazardous interactions with: none known
Pregnancy category: N/A

Other

Adverse effects [2]

BOTULINUM TOXIN (A & B)

Trade names: Azzalure (Galderma), Bocouture (Merz), Botox (Allergan), Dysport (Ipsen), Myobloc (Solstice), Neurobloc (Eisai), Vistabel (Allergan), Xeomin (Merz)
Indications: Blepharospasm, hemifacial spasm, spasmodic torticollis, sialorrhea, hyperhidrosis, strabismus, oromandibular dystonia, cervical dystonia, spasmodic dysphonia, chronic migraine, urinary incontinence in people with neurologic conditions such as spinal cord injury and multiple sclerosis who have overactivity of the bladder, cosmetic application for wrinkles
Class: Acetylcholine inhibitor, Neuromuscular blocker, Ophthalmic agent, toxin
Half-life: 3–6 months
Clinically important, potentially hazardous interactions with: aminoglycosides, anticholinergics, fesoterodine, tiotropium, trospium
Pregnancy category: C
Important contra-indications noted in the prescribing guidelines for: nursing mothers; pediatric patients
Note: Distant spread of toxin effect - postmarketing reports indicate that all botulinum toxin products may spread from the area of injection to produce symptoms consistent with botulinum toxin effects. These may include asthenia, generalized muscle weakness, diplopia, ptosis, dysphagia, dysphonia, dysarthria, urinary incontinence and breathing diffculties. These symptoms have been reported hours to weeks after injection.
An antitoxin is available in the event of overdose or misinjection.
Warning: DISTANT SPREAD OF TOXIN EFFECT

Skin

Anaphylactoid reactions/Anaphylaxis [4]
Ecchymoses [4]
Erythema [2]
Granulomas [2]
Hematoma [2]
Peripheral edema (<10%)
Pruritus (<10%)
Purpura (<10%)
Rash [2]

Mucosal

Epistaxis (nosebleed) [2]
Stomatitis (<10%)
Xerostomia (3–34%) [13]

Central Nervous System

Dysgeusia (taste perversion) (<10%)
Gait instability [2]
Headache [7]
Hyperesthesia (<10%)
Neurotoxicity [3]
Pain (6–13%) [4]
Seizures [2]
Tremor (<10%)
Vertigo (dizziness) [2]

Neuromuscular/Skeletal

Arthralgia (<7%)
Asthenia (fatigue) [16]
Myasthenia gravis [2]
Neck pain [3]

Gastrointestinal/Hepatic

Constipation [3]
Diarrhea [3]
Dysphagia [18]

Respiratory

Dysphonia [2]
Dyspnea [2]
Flu-like syndrome (2–10%) [8]
Nasopharyngitis [2]
Pulmonary toxicity [3]

Genitourinary

Dysuria [2]
Hematuria [5]
Urinary incontinence [3]
Urinary retention [14]
Urinary tract infection [16]
Vulvovaginal candidiasis (<10%)

Otic

Tinnitus (<10%)

Ocular

Blepharoptosis [2]
Conjunctivitis [2]
Diplopia [10]
Eyelid edema [4]
Ocular adverse effects [2]
Ptosis (14–20%) [24]
Xerophthalmia (6%) [2]

Local

Injection-site bruising [4]
Injection-site ecchymoses [2]
Injection-site edema [8]
Injection-site erythema [3]
Injection-site pain (2–10%) [20]
Injection-site paralysis [2]
Injection-site reactions [6]

Other

Adverse effects [19]
Death [4]
Infection (13–19%)
Side effects [3]

BRENTUXIMAB VEDOTIN

Trade name: Adcetris (Seattle Genetics)
Indications: Hodgkin's lymphoma, systemic anaplastic large cell lymphoma
Class: Antibody drug conjugate (ADC), CD30-directed antibody-drug conjugate, Monoclonal antibody
Half-life: 4–6 days
Clinically important, potentially hazardous interactions with: bleomycin, efavirenz, ketoconazole, rifampin, strong CYP3A4 inhibitors
Pregnancy category: D
Important contra-indications noted in the prescribing guidelines for: the elderly; nursing mothers; pediatric patients
Warning: PROGRESSIVE MULTIFOCAL LEUKOENCEPHALOPATHY

Skin
Diaphoresis (12%)
Lymphadenopathy (11%)
Peripheral edema (4–16%)
Pruritus (19%)
Rash (31%)
Xerosis (10%)

Hair
Alopecia (14%)

Central Nervous System
Anxiety (11%)
Chills (13%)
Fever (29–38%) [4]
Headache (19%)
Insomnia (16%)
Neurotoxicity [2]
Pain (7–28%)
Peripheral neuropathy (68%) [17]
Vertigo (dizziness) (11–16%)

Neuromuscular/Skeletal
Arthralgia (9–19%)
Asthenia (fatigue) (41–49%) [4]
Back pain (14%)
Muscle spasm (10%)
Myalgia/Myopathy (17%)
Pain in extremities (10%)

Gastrointestinal/Hepatic
Abdominal pain (9–25%)
Constipation (19%)
Diarrhea (36%) [6]
Nausea (42%) [4]
Vomiting (22%)

Respiratory
Cough (17–25%)
Dyspnea (13–19%)
Pulmonary toxicity [4]
Upper respiratory tract infection (12–47%)

Endocrine/Metabolic
Appetite decreased (16%)
Weight loss (6–12%)

Hematologic
Anemia (33–52%) [2]
Neutropenia (55%) [10]
Thrombocytopenia (16–28%)

Other
Adverse effects [4]

BREWER'S YEAST

Family: Saccharomycetaceae
Scientific names: *Saccharomyces boulardii, Saccharomyces cerevisiae*
Indications: Diarrhea, rotaviral diarrhea, irritable bowel syndrome, Crohn's disease, ulcerative colitis, urinary tract infections, vaginal infections, acne, premenstrual syndrome, furunculosis
Class: Immunomodulator, Probiotic
Half-life: N/A
Clinically important, potentially hazardous interactions with: MAO inhibitors
Pregnancy category: N/A
Note: Immune-deficient subjects or those with mucosal disease may experience serious adverse effects.

BREXPIPRAZOLE

Trade name: Rexulti (Otsuka)
Indications: Schizophrenia, major depressive disorder (with antidepressants)
Class: Antipsychotic
Half-life: 86–91 hours
Clinically important, potentially hazardous interactions with: strong or moderate CYP2D6 inhibitors, strong or moderate CYP3A4 inducers or inhibitors
Pregnancy category: N/A (Neonatal risk in third trimester exposure)
Important contra-indications noted in the prescribing guidelines for: the elderly; nursing mothers; pediatric patients
Warning: INCREASED MORTALITY IN ELDERLY PATIENTS WITH DEMENTIA-RELATED PSYCHOSIS
SUICIDAL THOUGHTS AND BEHAVIORS

Central Nervous System
Agitation [3]
Akathisia (6–9%) [13]
Anxiety (3%) [2]
Headache (7%) [7]
Insomnia [5]
Psychosis [2]
Restlessness (3%) [2]
Schizophrenia [3]
Sedation (2%) [2]
Somnolence (drowsiness) (5%) [5]
Tremor (3–4%)
Vertigo (dizziness) (3%)

Neuromuscular/Skeletal
Asthenia (fatigue) (3%) [3]

Gastrointestinal/Hepatic
Constipation (2%)
Diarrhea (3%) [3]
Dyspepsia (3%)
Nausea [5]

Respiratory
Nasopharyngitis (4%)

Endocrine/Metabolic
Appetite increased (3%) [2]
Creatine phosphokinase increased (2%)
Hyperprolactinemia [2]
Weight gain (4–7%) [14]
Weight loss (10%)

Hematologic
Hemotoxicity (2%)

BRIGATINIB

Trade name: Alunbrig (Ariad)
Indications: Anaplastic lymphoma kinase-positive metastatic non-small cell lung cancer in patients who have progressed on, or are intolerant to, crizotinib
Class: Tyrosine kinase inhibitor
Half-life: 25 hours
Clinically important, potentially hazardous interactions with: boceprevir, carbamazepine, clarithromycin, cobicistat, conivaptan, CYP3A substrates and strong CYP3A inducers or inhibitors, grapefruit juice, hormonal contraceptives, indinavir, itraconazole, ketoconazole, lopinavir, nelfinavir, phenytoin, posaconazole, rifampin, ritonavir, saquinavir, St John's wort, voriconazole
Pregnancy category: N/A (May cause fetal toxicity based on findings in animal studies)
Important contra-indications noted in the prescribing guidelines for: nursing mothers; pediatric patients

---

Skin
Rash (15–24%)

Cardiovascular
Bradycardia (6–8%)
Hypertension (11–21%) [3]

Central Nervous System
Fever (6–14%)
Headache (27–28%) [2]
Insomnia (7–11%)
Peripheral neuropathy (13%)

Neuromuscular/Skeletal
Arthralgia (14%)
Asthenia (fatigue) (29–36%) [2]
Back pain (10–15%)
Muscle spasm (12–17%)
Myalgia/Myopathy (9–15%)
Pain in extremities (4–11%)

Gastrointestinal/Hepatic
Abdominal pain (10–17%)
Constipation (15–19%)
Diarrhea (19–38%) [5]
Nausea (33–40%) [4]
Vomiting (23–24%)

Respiratory
Cough (18–34%) [4]
Dyspnea (21–27%) [5]
Hypoxia (<3%) [4]
Pneumonia (5–10%) [4]
Pneumonitis (4–9%)
Pulmonary toxicity [3]

Endocrine/Metabolic
ALT increased (34–40%) [2]
Appetite decreased (15–22%)
AST increased (38–65%)
Creatine phosphokinase increased (27–48%) [2]
Hyperglycemia (38–49%)
Hypophosphatemia (15–23%)

Hematologic
Anemia (23–40%)
Hyperlipasemia (21–45%) [3]

Lymphopenia (19–27%)
Prothrombin time increased (20–22%)

Ocular
Visual disturbances (7–10%)

Other
Death [2]

BRIMONIDINE

Trade names: Alphagan P (Allergan), Mirvaso (Galderma)
Indications: Open-angle glaucoma, ocular hypertension, topical application for rosacea
Class: Adrenergic alpha2-receptor agonist
Half-life: 12 hours
Clinically important, potentially hazardous interactions with: amitriptyline, MAO inhibitors, tricyclic antidepressants
Pregnancy category: B
Important contra-indications noted in the prescribing guidelines for: nursing mothers; pediatric patients
Note: [T] = Topical.

Skin
Burning [T] (2%) [4]
Contact dermatitis [T] [2]
Dermatitis [2]
Erythema [T] (4%) [7]
Flushing [T] (3%) [3]
Hypersensitivity [3]
Irritation [3]
Pruritus [4]
Rosacea [2]
Xerosis [2]

Mucosal
Xerostomia (5–20%) [12]

Cardiovascular
Hypertension (5–20%)

Central Nervous System
Dysgeusia (taste perversion) (<10%) [4]
Somnolence (drowsiness) [2]

Neuromuscular/Skeletal
Asthenia (fatigue) [4]

Respiratory
Upper respiratory tract infection (<10%)

Ocular
Blepharitis (<10%) [2]
Conjunctival hyperemia (5–20%) [5]
Conjunctivitis (5–20%) [7]
Eyelid crusting (<10%)
Eyelid edema (<10%)
Eyelid erythema (<10%)
Intraocular pressure increased [2]
Ocular adverse effects [4]
Ocular allergy (4%) [8]
Ocular burning (<10%) [7]
Ocular hyperemia [4]
Ocular itching [2]
Ocular pain [3]
Ocular pruritus (5–20%) [5]
Ocular stinging (<10%) [6]
Periocular dermatitis [2]
Uveitis [11]
Vision blurred [T] [3]
Visual disturbances (5–20%)
Xerophthalmia [3]

Other
Adverse effects [2]
Allergic reactions [2]

BRINZOLAMIDE

Trade name: Azopt (Alcon)
Indications: Open-angle glaucoma, ocular hypertension
Class: Carbonic anhydrase inhibitor, Diuretic
Half-life: 111 days
Clinically important, potentially hazardous interactions with: conivaptan, darunavir, delavirdine, indinavir, salicylates, telithromycin, voriconazole
Pregnancy category: C
Important contra-indications noted in the prescribing guidelines for: nursing mothers
Note: Brinzolamide is a sulfonamide and can be absorbed systemically. Sulfonamides can produce severe, possibly fatal, reactions such as toxic epidermal necrolysis and Stevens-Johnson syndrome.

Skin
Dermatitis (<5%)

Mucosal
Xerostomia [4]

Central Nervous System
Dysgeusia (taste perversion) (5–10%) [14]
Headache (<5%)

Neuromuscular/Skeletal
Asthenia (fatigue) [3]

Respiratory
Rhinitis (<5%)

Endocrine/Metabolic
Acidosis [2]

Ocular
Blepharitis (<5%)
Conjunctival hyperemia [8]
Conjunctivitis [4]
Corneal abnormalities [3]
Foreign body sensation (<5%)
Lacrimation [3]
Ocular adverse effects [3]
Ocular allergy [2]
Ocular burning [4]
Ocular discharge (<5%)
Ocular hyperemia [5]
Ocular itching [6]
Ocular keratitis (<5%)
Ocular pain (<5%) [6]
Ocular pruritus (<5%) [3]
Ocular stinging [4]
Vision blurred (5–10%) [15]
Xerophthalmia (<5%) [5]

Other
Adverse effects [2]

BRIVARACETAM

Trade name: Briviact (UCB)
Indications: Epilepsy adjunct therapy
Class: Anticonvulsant, Antiepileptic
Half-life: 9 hours
Clinically important, potentially hazardous interactions with: carbamazepine, phenytoin, rifampin
Pregnancy category: C
Important contra-indications noted in the prescribing guidelines for: the elderly; nursing mothers; pediatric patients

Central Nervous System
Aggression [4]
Agitation [2]
Anxiety [2]
Balance disorder (3%)
Depression [3]
Dysgeusia (taste perversion) (<3%)
Euphoria (<3%)
Headache [12]
Impaired concentration [2]
Insomnia [2]
Irritability (3%) [8]
Neurotoxicity (13%)
Psychosis [2]
Sedation (16%)
Seizures [3]
Somnolence (drowsiness) (16%) [25]
Vertigo (dizziness) (12%) [24]

Neuromuscular/Skeletal
Asthenia (fatigue) (9%) [19]
Back pain [2]

Gastrointestinal/Hepatic
Constipation (2%)
Nausea (5%) [6]
Vomiting (5%) [3]

Respiratory
Nasopharyngitis [6]

Genitourinary
Urinary tract infection [2]

Hematologic
Leukopenia (2%)

Local
Infusion-site pain (<3%)

Other
Adverse effects [4]

BROMELAIN

Family: Bromeliaceae
Scientific names: *Ananas comosus, Ananas duckei, Ananas sativus, Bromelia ananas, Bromelia comosa*
Indications: **Oral:** inflammation, mild ulcerative colitis, osteoarthritis, sinusitis, sprains. **Topical:** burn debridement
Class: Analgesic, Anti-inflammatory
Half-life: N/A
Clinically important, potentially hazardous interactions with: amoxicillin, fluorouracil, tetracycline, vincristine
Pregnancy category: N/A

Note: Phlogenzym is rutoside, bromelain and trypsin.

Skin
Contact dermatitis [2]

Respiratory
Asthma (occupational / inhalation) [3]

Other
Adverse effects [8]

BROMOCRIPTINE

Trade name: Parlodel (Novartis)
Indications: Amenorrhea, Parkinsonism, infertility, acromegaly
Class: Dopamine receptor agonist
Half-life: initial: 6–8 hours; terminal: 50 hours
Clinically important, potentially hazardous interactions with: alcohol, antipsychotics, azithromycin, domperidone, erythromycin, isometheptene, lanreotide, levomepromazine, macrolides, memantine, methyldopa, metoclopramide, octreotide, pasireotide, pseudoephedrine, risperidone, sympathomimetics, zuclopenthixol
Pregnancy category: N/A (Contra-indicated in women who become pregnant or in the postpartum period)
Important contra-indications noted in the prescribing guidelines for: nursing mothers; pediatric patients

Skin
Flushing [2]
Livedo reticularis [3]
Raynaud's phenomenon (<10%) [8]
Scleroderma [2]

Hair
Alopecia [2]

Mucosal
Nasal congestion (3–4%)
Xerostomia (4–10%) [3]

Cardiovascular
Cardiotoxicity [2]
Coronary spasm [2]
Erythromelalgia [4]
Orthostatic hypotension (6%)
Postural hypotension (6%)

Central Nervous System
Anorexia (4%)
Hallucinations [4]
Headache (<19%) [3]
Seizures (in postpartum patients) [3]
Somnolence (drowsiness) (3%)
Syncope (<2%)
Vertigo (dizziness) (17%)

Neuromuscular/Skeletal
Asthenia (fatigue) (3–7%)

Gastrointestinal/Hepatic
Abdominal pain (4%)
Constipation (3–14%) [2]
Diarrhea (3%)
Dyspepsia (4%)
Gastrointestinal bleeding (<2%)
Nausea (18–49%) [7]
Vomiting (2–5%) [4]

Respiratory
Pleural effusion [2]
Pulmonary fibrosis [2]

Other
Adverse effects [2]

BUDESONIDE

Trade names: Pulmicort Turbuhaler (AstraZeneca), Rhinocort (AstraZeneca), Symbicort (AstraZeneca)
Indications: Asthma, rhinitis
Class: Corticosteroid, inhaled
Half-life: N/A
Clinically important, potentially hazardous interactions with: boceprevir, efavirenz, itraconazole, ketoconazole, live vaccines, oral contraceptives, telaprevir
Pregnancy category: C
Important contra-indications noted in the prescribing guidelines for: nursing mothers; pediatric patients
Note: Symbicort is budesonide and formoterol.

Skin
Acneform eruption [3]
Dermatitis [8]
Exanthems [2]
Moon face [2]
Pruritus [2]
Rash [2]

Mucosal
Oral candidiasis [2]

Central Nervous System
Fever [2]
Headache [2]
Insomnia [2]
Mood changes [2]

Respiratory
Asthma (exacerbation) [4]
Cough [2]

Endocrine/Metabolic
Adrenal insufficiency [3]
Cushing's syndrome [2]

Ocular
Cataract [2]

Other
Adverse effects [13]
Allergic reactions [3]
Infection [2]
Systemic reactions [2]

BUPRENORPHINE

Trade names: Probuphine (Braeburn), Suboxone (Reckitt Benckiser), Subutex (Reckitt Benckiser), Transtec (Napp)
Indications: Opioid dependence, moderate to severe pain
Class: Analgesic, Mixed opioid agonist/antagonist, Narcotic
Half-life: 37 hours
Clinically important, potentially hazardous interactions with: antihistamines, atazanavir, azole antifungals, benzodiazepines, boceprevir, carbamazepine, cimetidine, cobicistat/elvitegravir/emtricitabine/tenofovir alafenamide, cobicistat/elvitegravir/emtricitabine/tenofovir disoproxil, delavirdine, diazepam, efavirenz, erythromycin, HIV protease inhibitors, hydrocodone, hydromorphone, ketoconazole, ketorolac, linezolid, macrolide antibiotics, morphine, neuroleptics, oxymorphone, phenobarbital, phenytoin, rifampin, ritonavir, tapentadol, tipranavir
Pregnancy category: C
Important contra-indications noted in the prescribing guidelines for: nursing mothers; pediatric patients
Note: Suboxone contains naloxone; Probuphine is an implant for subdermal administration.
Warning: ABUSE POTENTIAL, LIFE-THREATENING RESPIRATORY DEPRESSION, and ACCIDENTAL EXPOSURE
Probuphine: IMPLANT MIGRATION, PROTRUSION, EXPULSION, and NERVE DAMAGE ASSOCIATED WITH INSERTION and REMOVAL

Skin
Abscess (2%)
Dermatitis [2]
Diaphoresis (12–14%)
Erythema [4]
Hyperhidrosis [4]
Pruritus [11]

Mucosal
Xerostomia [3]

Cardiovascular
Bradycardia [3]
Hypotension [4]
Pulmonary edema [2]
QT prolongation [2]
Vasodilation (9%)

Central Nervous System
Anxiety (12%)
Chills (6–8%)
Depression (11%)
Fever (3%)
Headache (30–36%) [6]
Insomnia (14–25%)
Nervousness (6%)
Neurotoxicity [2]
Pain (22–24%)
Seizures [3]
Somnolence (drowsiness) (5%) [4]
Vertigo (dizziness) (4%) [14]

Neuromuscular/Skeletal
Asthenia (fatigue) (7–14%) [4]
Back pain (4–14%)
Myalgia/Myopathy [2]

Gastrointestinal/Hepatic
Abdominal pain (11%) [2]
Constipation (11–12%) [12]
Diarrhea (4–5%) [2]
Dyspepsia (3%)
Hepatotoxicity [6]
Nausea (10–15%) [15]
Vomiting (5–8%) [12]

Respiratory
Cough (4%)
Flu-like syndrome (6%)
Pharyngitis (4%)
Respiratory depression [3]

Rhinitis (5–11%)

Ocular

Lacrimation (5%)

Local

Application-site reactions [3]

Other

Adverse effects [4]
Death [9]
Infection (6–20%)

BUPROPION

Trade names: Wellbutrin (GSK), Zyban (GSK)
Indications: Depression, aid to smoking cessation
Class: Antidepressant, Dopamine reuptake inhibitor
Half-life: 14 hours
Clinically important, potentially hazardous interactions with: amitriptyline, citalopram, cobicistat/elvitegravir/emtricitabine/tenofovir alafenamide, cobicistat/elvitegravir/emtricitabine/tenofovir disoproxil, cyclosporine, deutetrabenazine, efavirenz, eluxadoline, erythromycin, escitalopram, isocarboxazid, levodopa, linezolid, lopinavir, lorcaserin, methylphenidate, mifepristone, phenelzine, ritonavir, tranylcypromine, trimipramine, vortioxetine
Pregnancy category: C
Important contra-indications noted in the prescribing guidelines for: nursing mothers; pediatric patients
Warning: NEUROPSYCHIATRIC REACTIONS; AND SUICIDAL THOUGHTS AND BEHAVIORS

Skin

Acneform eruption (<10%)
AGEP [3]
Anaphylactoid reactions/Anaphylaxis [2]
Angioedema [3]
Diaphoresis (5%) [4]
Erythema multiforme [4]
Exanthems [2]
Flushing (4%)
Hypersensitivity [6]
Lupus erythematosus [2]
Peripheral edema [2]
Pruritus (4%) [3]
Psoriasis [3]
Rash (4%) [3]
Serum sickness [3]
Serum sickness-like reaction [9]
Stevens-Johnson syndrome [2]
Thrombocytopenic purpura [2]
Urticaria [9]
Xerosis (<10%)

Hair

Hirsutism (<10%)

Mucosal

Tongue edema [2]
Xerostomia (<64%) [19]

Cardiovascular

Arrhythmias [2]
Hypertension [3]
Myocardial ischemia [2]
Palpitation [2]
Tachycardia [3]

Central Nervous System

Aggression [2]
Agitation [5]
Anxiety [5]
Delirium [2]
Depression [4]
Dysgeusia (taste perversion) (4%)
Dyskinesia [2]
Hallucinations [7]
Headache [7]
Insomnia [9]
Mania [2]
Nightmares [2]
Paresthesias (2%)
Parkinsonism [2]
Psychosis [7]
Seizures [40]
Serotonin syndrome [2]
Sleep related disorder [2]
Somnolence (drowsiness) [4]
Suicidal ideation [5]
Tremor (>10%) [7]
Twitching (2%)
Vertigo (dizziness) [6]

Neuromuscular/Skeletal

Arthralgia [3]
Asthenia (fatigue) [3]
Dystonia [3]
Myalgia/Myopathy (6%) [2]
Rhabdomyolysis [3]

Gastrointestinal/Hepatic

Constipation [5]
Hepatotoxicity [3]
Nausea [15]
Vomiting [6]

Respiratory

Upper respiratory tract infection [2]

Genitourinary

Priapism [2]

Ocular

Hallucinations, visual [3]

Other

Adverse effects [2]
Congenital malformations [2]
Death [5]

BUSPIRONE

Trade name: BuSpar (Bristol-Myers Squibb)
Indications: Anxiety
Class: Anxiolytic, Serotonin antagonist
Half-life: 2–3 hours
Clinically important, potentially hazardous interactions with: citalopram, cobicistat/elvitegravir/emtricitabine/tenofovir alafenamide, cobicistat/elvitegravir/emtricitabine/tenofovir disoproxil, grapefruit juice, itraconazole, linezolid, nefazodone, paclitaxel, rifapentine, ritonavir, St John's wort, telithromycin, vilazodone, voriconazole
Pregnancy category: B

Hair

Alopecia [2]

Mucosal

Xerostomia (3%)

Central Nervous System

Serotonin syndrome [4]

BUSULFAN

Trade name: Myleran (GSK)
Indications: Chronic myelogenous leukemia, bone marrow disorders
Class: Alkylating agent
Half-life: 3.4 hours (after first dose)
Clinically important, potentially hazardous interactions with: acetaminophen, aldesleukin, itraconazole, metronidazole, voriconazole
Pregnancy category: D
Warning: LEUKEMOGENESIS and PANCYTOPENIA

Skin

Erythema (macular) (>10%)
Erythema multiforme [5]
Erythema nodosum [3]
Exanthems [2]
Pigmentation ('busulfan tan') (<10%) [13]
Urticaria (>10%) [5]
Vasculitis [3]

Hair

Alopecia (>10%) [7]

Mucosal

Mucositis [4]
Oral mucositis [2]
Stomatitis [2]

Central Nervous System

Neurotoxicity [3]
Seizures [4]

Gastrointestinal/Hepatic

Hepatotoxicity [4]

Respiratory

Pulmonary toxicity [3]

Endocrine/Metabolic

Gynecomastia [3]
Porphyria cutanea tarda [2]

Hematologic

Febrile neutropenia [3]

Other

Death [4]
Infection [3]

BUTTERBUR

Family: Asteraceae; Compositae
Scientific names: *Petasites hybridus, Petasites officinalis*
Indications: Allergic rhinitis, asthma, bronchitis, chills, cough, dysmenorrhea, hay fever, headache, heart tonic, migraine, peptic ulcer, appetite stimulant, irritable bladder, poultice for wounds or skin ulcers
Class: Anti-inflammatory
Half-life: N/A
Clinically important, potentially hazardous interactions with: none known

Pregnancy category: N/A (Contraindicated in pregnancy)
Important contra-indications noted in the prescribing guidelines for: nursing mothers
Note: Petadolex formulation has had the potentially carcinogenic pyrrolizidine alkaloids removed.

Skin
Edema [2]
Erythema [2]
Hypersensitivity [2]
Rash [2]

Gastrointestinal/Hepatic
Eructation (belching) [3]

Other
Adverse effects [2]

CABERGOLINE

Trade name: Dostinex (Pfizer)
Indications: Hyperprolactinemia, Parkinsonism
Class: Dopamine receptor agonist
Half-life: 63–69 hours
Clinically important, potentially hazardous interactions with: azithromycin, levomepromazine, risperidone, zuclopenthixol
Pregnancy category: B
Important contra-indications noted in the prescribing guidelines for: the elderly; nursing mothers; pediatric patients

---

Skin
Edema [2]
Hot flashes (3%)

Mucosal
Xerostomia (2%)

Cardiovascular
Cardiac failure [2]
Hypotension [5]
Myocardial toxicity [3]
Pericarditis [4]
Valve regurgitation [2]
Valvulopathy [9]

Central Nervous System
Dyskinesia [2]
Headache (26%) [6]
Mania [3]
Neurotoxicity [3]
Paresthesias (5%) [2]
Psychosis [3]
Somnolence (drowsiness) (<5%)
Vertigo (dizziness) (15–17%) [6]

Neuromuscular/Skeletal
Asthenia (fatigue) (6%) [5]

Gastrointestinal/Hepatic
Abdominal pain (5%)
Constipation (7–10%)
Nausea (28%) [3]

Endocrine/Metabolic
Mastodynia (2%)

CABOZANTINIB

Trade names: Carbometyx (Exelixis), Cometriq (Exelixis)
Indications: Metastatic medullary thyroid cancer (Cometriq), advanced renal cell carcinoma (Cabometyx)
Class: Tyrosine kinase inhibitor
Half-life: 55 hours (Cometriq); 99 hours (Cabometyx)
Clinically important, potentially hazardous interactions with: atazanavir, boceprevir, carbamazepine, clarithromycin, conivaptan, grapefruit juice, indinavir, itraconazole, ketoconazole, lopinavir, nefazodone, nelfinavir, phenobarbital, phenytoin, posaconazole, rifabutin, rifampin, rifapentine, ritonavir, saquinavir, St John's wort, telithromycin, voriconazole
Pregnancy category: D
Important contra-indications noted in the prescribing guidelines for: the elderly; nursing mothers; pediatric patients
Warning: PERFORATIONS AND FISTULAS, and HEMORRHAGE

Skin
Erythema (11%)
Hand–foot syndrome (50%) [20]
Hyperkeratosis (7%)
Jaundice (25%)
Rash (19%)
Toxicity [3]
Wound complications [2]
Xerosis (19%)

Hair
Alopecia (16%)
Hair changes (34%)
Hair pigmentation (34%) [2]

Mucosal
Mucosal inflammation [3]
Stomatitis (51%)

Cardiovascular
Chest pain (9%)
Hypertension (33%) [15]
Hypotension (7%)

Central Nervous System
Anorexia [3]
Anxiety (9%)
Dysgeusia (taste perversion) (34%) [2]
Headache (18%)
Paresthesias (7%)
Peripheral neuropathy (5%)
Vertigo (dizziness) (14%)

Neuromuscular/Skeletal
Arthralgia (14%)
Asthenia (fatigue) (21–41%) [22]
Muscle spasm (12%)
Pain in extremities (14%)

Gastrointestinal/Hepatic
Abdominal pain (27%)
Constipation (27%) [2]
Diarrhea (63%) [19]
Dyspepsia (11%)
Dysphagia (13%)
Gastrointestinal perforation (3%)
Hemorrhoids (9%)
Nausea (43%) [9]
Vomiting (24%) [4]

Respiratory
Cough (18%)
Dysphonia (20%)
Dyspnea (19%)
Pulmonary embolism [2]

Endocrine/Metabolic
ALP increased (52%)
ALT increased (86%) [3]
Appetite decreased (46%) [4]
AST increased (86%) [3]
Dehydration (7%)
GGT increased (27%)
Hypoalbuminemia (36%)
Hypocalcemia (52%)
Hypokalemia (18%)
Hypomagnesemia (19%)
Hyponatremia (10%)
Hypophosphatemia (28%)
Hypothyroidism [3]
Serum creatinine increased (58%)
Weight loss (48%) [8]

Renal
Proteinuria (2%)

Hematologic
Anemia [2]
Lymphopenia (53%)
Neutropenia (35%) [2]
Thrombocytopenia (35%) [2]
Thrombosis [2]

Other
Adverse effects [6]
Death (6%) [5]

CAFFEINE

Family: Rubiales
Scientific names: *Cafcit (Bedford), Coffea arabica, Coffea canephora, Coffea robusta, Cola acuminata, Thea sinensis, Theobroma cacao*
Indications: With ergotamine for migraine, with NSAIDs in analgesics, headache, respiratory depression in neonates, postprandial hypotension, enhances seizure duration in electroconvulsive therapy, ingredient in cough and cold remedies
Class: Diuretic, Xanthine alkaloid
Half-life: 2–7 hours
Clinically important, potentially hazardous interactions with: aminophylline, carbamazepine, cimetidine, clozapine, cocoa, ephedra, ferrous sulfate, fluorides, ginseng, guarana, idrocilamide, ketoconazole, ketoprofen, levomepromazine, linezolid, methoxsalen, mexiletine, norfloxacin, phenobarbital, phenylpropanolamine, phenytoin, regadenoson, terbinafine, teriflunomide, zonisamide
Pregnancy category: C
Important contra-indications noted in the prescribing guidelines for: nursing mothers
Note: Caffeine is an addictive psychoactive substance. Spontaneous abortion and low birthweight babies have occurred in pregnant women consuming 150 mg caffeine per day. Abuse can lead to cardiac damage or death. See also separate profile for guarana.
Common symptoms of caffeine withdrawal are headache; drowsiness; yawning, impaired concentration; lassitude; irritability; decreased contentedness, well-being and self-confidence;

decreased sociability; flu-like symptoms; muscle aches and stiffness; hot or cold spells; nausea or vomiting; and blurred vision. Cafcit is caffeine citrate.

Skin
Anaphylactoid reactions/Anaphylaxis [3]
Hypersensitivity [2]
Urticaria [5]

Cardiovascular
Arrhythmias [4]
Atrial fibrillation [2]
Hypertension [2]
Palpitation [2]

Central Nervous System
Anxiety [2]
Depression [2]
Headache [2]
Insomnia [2]
Psychosis [3]
Restlessness [2]
Seizures [6]
Tremor [4]

Neuromuscular/Skeletal
Rhabdomyolysis [6]

Gastrointestinal/Hepatic
Gastrointestinal disorder [2]

Other
Adverse effects [3]
Death (from abuse / overdose) [21]

CALCIFEDIOL

Synonym: calcidiol
Trade name: Rayaldee (Opko)
Indications: Hyperparathyroidism in stage 3 or 4 chronic kidney disease
Class: Vitamin D analog
Half-life: 11 days
Clinically important, potentially hazardous interactions with: anticonvulsants, atazanavir, cholestyramine, clarithromycin, indinavir, itraconazole, ketoconazole, nefazodone, nelfinavir, phenobarbital, ritonavir, saquinavir, telithromycin, thiazides, voriconazole
Pregnancy category: C
Important contra-indications noted in the prescribing guidelines for: nursing mothers; pediatric patients

Skin
Hematoma (2%)

Cardiovascular
Congestive heart failure (4%)

Neuromuscular/Skeletal
Arthralgia (2%)

Gastrointestinal/Hepatic
Constipation (3%)

Respiratory
Bronchitis (3%)
Cough (4%)
Dyspnea (4%)
Nasopharyngitis (5%)

Endocrine/Metabolic
Hyperkalemia (3%)
Hyperuricemia (2%)
Serum creatinine increased (5%)

Hematologic
Anemia (5%)

CALCIPOTRIOL

Synonym: calcipotriene
Trade name: Dovonex (Leo Pharma)
Indications: Psoriasis
Class: Antipsoriatic agent, Vitamin D analog
Half-life: ~30 minutes
Clinically important, potentially hazardous interactions with: none known
Pregnancy category: C
Important contra-indications noted in the prescribing guidelines for: nursing mothers; pediatric patients
Note: Contra-indicated in patients with acute psoriatic eruptions, hypercalcemia or vitamin D toxicity.

Skin
Burning (23%)
Contact dermatitis [8]
Erythema (<10%)
Pigmentation [3]
Pruritus (>10%) [6]
Psoriasis (<10%) [3]
Rash (11%)
Xerosis (<5%)

Respiratory
Nasopharyngitis [3]

Endocrine/Metabolic
Hypercalcemia [3]

Local
Application-site pain [3]
Application-site pruritus [2]
Application-site reactions [2]

Other
Adverse effects [3]

CALCITONIN

Trade names: Calcimar (Sanofi-Aventis), Miacalcin (Novartis)
Indications: Paget's disease of bone
Class: Parathyroid hormone antagonist
Half-life: 70–90 minutes
Clinically important, potentially hazardous interactions with: none known
Pregnancy category: C

Skin
Flushing (>10%) [5]

Gastrointestinal/Hepatic
Diarrhea [2]
Nausea [2]

Respiratory
Rhinitis (12%)

Local
Injection-site edema (>10%)
Injection-site inflammation (>10%) [2]
Injection-site reactions (10%)

CALCIUM HYDROXYLAPATITE

Trade name: Radiesse (Merz)
Indications: Correction of facial wrinkles and folds
Class: Dermal filler
Half-life: N/A
Clinically important, potentially hazardous interactions with: anticoagulants, antiplatelet drugs, aspirin

Skin
Ecchymoses [2]
Granulomas [6]
Necrosis [2]
Nodular eruption [3]

Mucosal
Oral lesions [3]

CANAGLIFLOZIN

Trade names: Invokamet (Janssen), Invokana (Janssen)
Indications: Type II diabetes mellitus
Class: Sodium-glucose co-transporter 2 (SGLT2) inhibitor
Half-life: 11–13 hours
Clinically important, potentially hazardous interactions with: digoxin, rifampin
Pregnancy category: C
Important contra-indications noted in the prescribing guidelines for: nursing mothers; pediatric patients
Note: Contra-indicated in patients with severe renal impairment, end stage renal disease, or on dialysis. Invokamet is canagliflozin and metformin.

Skin
Pruritus [2]

Cardiovascular
Postural hypotension [2]

Central Nervous System
Headache [3]
Vertigo (dizziness) [3]

Neuromuscular/Skeletal
Arthralgia [2]
Asthenia (fatigue) (2%)
Back pain [2]

Gastrointestinal/Hepatic
Abdominal pain (2%) [3]
Constipation (2%) [3]
Diarrhea [2]
Nausea (2%) [4]

Respiratory
Nasopharyngitis [2]
Upper respiratory tract infection [2]

Endocrine/Metabolic
Dehydration [3]
Diabetic ketoacidosis [2]
Hypoglycemia [8]

Genitourinary
Genital mycotic infections (4–11%) [28]
Pollakiuria [7]

Polyuria [2]
Urinary frequency (5%) [6]
Urinary tract infection (4–6%) [23]
Vulvovaginal candidiasis [2]
Vulvovaginal pruritus (2–3%) [3]

Renal
Nephrotoxicity [2]

Other
Adverse effects [4]
Death [2]
Dipsia (thirst) (2–3%) [4]

CANAKINUMAB

Trade name: Ilaris (Novartis)
Indications: Periodic fever syndromes, systemic juvenile idiopathic arthritis
Class: Interleukin-1 inhibitor, Monoclonal antibody
Half-life: 26 days
Clinically important, potentially hazardous interactions with: cytochrome P450, IL-1 blockers, lenalidomide, TNF-blockers
Pregnancy category: C
Important contra-indications noted in the prescribing guidelines for: nursing mothers; pediatric patients
Note: Interleukin-1 blockade may interfere with immune response to infections. Treatment with medications that work through inhibition of IL-1 has been associated with an increased risk of serious infections.

Central Nervous System
Headache [2]
Vertigo (dizziness) (11%) [2]

Neuromuscular/Skeletal
Myalgia/Myopathy (11%)

Gastrointestinal/Hepatic
Gastroenteritis (11%) [2]
Nausea (14%)

Respiratory
Bronchitis (11%)
Flu-like syndrome (20%)
Nasopharyngitis (34%) [3]
Pharyngitis (11%)
Rhinitis (17%)
Upper respiratory tract infection [4]

Endocrine/Metabolic
Weight gain (11%)

Hematologic
Macrophage activation syndrome [2]
Neutropenia [2]

Local
Injection-site reactions [4]

Other
Adverse effects [5]
Infection [12]

CANDESARTAN

Trade name: Atacand (AstraZeneca)
Indications: Hypertension and heart failure
Class: Angiotensin II receptor antagonist (blocker), Antihypertensive
Half-life: 9 hours
Clinically important, potentially hazardous interactions with: aliskiren
Pregnancy category: D
Important contra-indications noted in the prescribing guidelines for: nursing mothers; pediatric patients
Warning: FETAL TOXICITY

Skin
Angioedema [3]

Cardiovascular
Hypotension [5]

Central Nervous System
Dysgeusia (taste perversion) [2]
Headache [5]
Vertigo (dizziness) (4%) [6]

Neuromuscular/Skeletal
Back pain (3%) [3]

Gastrointestinal/Hepatic
Gastroenteritis [2]

Respiratory
Pharyngitis (2%)
Rhinitis (2%)
Upper respiratory tract infection (6%) [3]

Endocrine/Metabolic
Hyperkalemia (2%)

Renal
Renal failure [3]

Hematologic
Neutropenia [2]

Other
Adverse effects [4]
Fetotoxicity [2]

CANGRELOR

Trade name: Kengreal (Medicines Co)
Indications: Adjunct to percutaneous coronary intervention for reducing the risk of periprocedural myocardial infarction, repeat coronary revascularization and stent thrombosis
Class: Antiplatelet, Antiplatelet, cyclopentyl triazolo-pyrimidine (CPTP)
Half-life: 3–6 minutes
Clinically important, potentially hazardous interactions with: clopidogrel, prasugrel
Pregnancy category: C
Important contra-indications noted in the prescribing guidelines for: nursing mothers; pediatric patients
Note: Contra-indicated in patients with significant active bleeding.

Respiratory
Dyspnea [5]

Renal
Nephrotoxicity (3%)

Hematologic
Bleeding (<15%) [7]

CANNABIDIOL *

Trade name: Epidiolex (GW Research Ltd)
Indications: treatment of seizures associated with Lennox-Gastaut syndrome or Dravet syndrome in patients 2 years of age and older
Half-life: 56–61 hours
Clinically important, potentially hazardous interactions with: clobazam
Pregnancy category: N/A (may cause fetal harm)

Skin
Rash (7–13%)

Mucosal
Salivary hypersecretion (1–4%)

Central Nervous System
Aggression (3–5%)
Fever [2]
Gait instability (2–3%)
Insomnia (5–11%)
Irritability (5–9%)
Sedation (3–6%) [2]
Somnolence (drowsiness) (23–25%) [9]

Neuromuscular/Skeletal
Asthenia (fatigue) (11–12%) [3]
Ataxia [2]

Gastrointestinal/Hepatic
Abdominal pain (3%)
Diarrhea (9–20%) [5]
Gastroenteritis (4%)
Nausea [2]
Vomiting [2]

Respiratory
Hypoxia (3%)
Pneumonia (5–8%)

Endocrine/Metabolic
ALT increased (8–16%)
Appetite decreased (16–22%) [3]
AST increased (8–16%)
Weight loss (3–5%)

Hematologic
Anemia (30%)

Other
Adverse effects [2]
Infection (40–41%)

CAPECITABINE

Trade name: Xeloda (Roche)
Indications: Metastatic breast or colorectal cancer, adjuvant colon cancer
Class: Antimetabolite, Antineoplastic
Half-life: 0.5–1 hour
Clinically important, potentially hazardous interactions with: allopurinol, anticoagulants, CYP2C9 substrates, erlotinib, leucovorin, phenprocoumon, phenytoin, warfarin

Pregnancy category: D
Important contra-indications noted in the prescribing guidelines for: nursing mothers
Note: Patients receiving concomitant capecitabine and oral coumarin-derivative anticoagulants such as warfarin and phenprocoumon should have their anticoagulant response (INR or prothrombin time) monitored frequently in order to adjust the anticoagulant dose accordingly. Altered coagulation parameters and/or bleeding, including death, have been reported during concomitant use.
Contra-indicated in patients with severe renal impairment or with known hypersensitivity to fluorouracil.
Warning: XELODA - WARFARIN INTERACTION

Skin
- Acneform eruption [3]
- Actinic keratoses [3]
- Dermatitis (37%) [10]
- Edema (9%) [3]
- Exfoliative dermatitis (31–37%)
- Hand–foot syndrome (7–58%) [171]
- Jaundice [3]
- Lupus erythematosus [4]
- Photosensitivity [2]
- Pigmentation [10]
- Pruritus [2]
- Radiation recall dermatitis [6]
- Rash [14]
- Toxicity [4]
- Vitiligo [2]
- Xerosis [2]

Hair
- Alopecia [10]

Nails
- Nail changes (7%)
- Onycholysis [3]
- Onychomadesis [2]
- Paronychia [2]
- Pyogenic granuloma [2]

Mucosal
- Mucosal inflammation [2]
- Mucositis [16]
- Stomatitis (24%) [19]

Cardiovascular
- Angina [4]
- Cardiotoxicity [5]
- Chest pain [3]
- Coronary vasospasm [4]
- Hypertension [6]
- Myocardial infarction [4]
- QT prolongation [2]
- Thromboembolism [2]
- Ventricular fibrillation [2]

Central Nervous System
- Anorexia [13]
- Fever [2]
- Headache [2]
- Leukoencephalopathy [5]
- Neurotoxicity [14]
- Pain [4]
- Paresthesias (21%)
- Peripheral neuropathy [12]
- Vertigo (dizziness) [3]

Neuromuscular/Skeletal
- Asthenia (fatigue) [52]
- Ataxia [2]
- Myalgia/Myopathy (9%) [3]
- Pain in extremities [2]

Gastrointestinal/Hepatic
- Abdominal pain [9]
- Constipation [3]
- Diarrhea [74]
- Hepatotoxicity [7]
- Ileus [2]
- Nausea [39]
- Pancreatitis [2]
- Vomiting [30]

Respiratory
- Nasopharyngitis [2]

Endocrine/Metabolic
- ALT increased [5]
- Appetite decreased [2]
- AST increased [5]
- Hyperammonemia [2]
- Hyperbilirubinemia [4]
- Hyperglycemia [3]
- Hypertriglyceridemia [2]
- Hypophosphatemia [2]

Hematologic
- Anemia [26]
- Febrile neutropenia [4]
- Hemotoxicity [2]
- Leukocytopenia [3]
- Leukopenia [14]
- Neutropenia [48]
- Thrombocytopenia [22]

Other
- Adverse effects [6]
- Allergic reactions [2]
- Death [7]
- Infection [2]

CAPSICUM

Family: Solanaceae
Scientific names: *Capsicum annuum, Capsicum baccatum, Capsicum chinense, Capsicum frutescens, Capsicum pubscens*
Indications: Nausea, neuropathic pain, osteoarthritis, fibromyalgia, anticarcinogen, rheumatoid arthritis, diabetic neuropathy, postherpetic neuralgia (shingles), psoriasis, pruritus, vitiligo, dyspepsia, flatulence, ulcers, stomach cramps, hypertension, improved circulation, weight-loss
Class: Rubefacient
Half-life: N/A
Clinically important, potentially hazardous interactions with: ACE inhibitors, aminophylline, antiplatelet drugs, aspirin, latex, salicylic acid
Pregnancy category: N/A
Note: Pepper spray or gas contains 5% oleoresin capsicum (OC). It is used by police and in personal defense sprays.

Skin
- Burning [5]
- Dermatitis [3]
- Erythema [3]
- Hypersensitivity [2]
- Pruritus [2]
- Urticaria [2]

Cardiovascular
- Hypertension [2]

Central Nervous System
- Pain [5]

Ocular
- Conjunctivitis [3]

Other
- Adverse effects [6]
- Allergic reactions [3]
- Death [5]

CAPTOPRIL

Trade names: Capoten (Par), Capozide (Par)
Indications: Hypertension, congestive heart failure, to improve survival following myocardial infarction in clinically stable patients with left ventricular dysfunction, diabetic nephropathy in patients with Type I insulin-dependent diabetes mellitus and retinopathy
Class: Angiotensin-converting enzyme (ACE) inhibitor, Antihypertensive, Vasodilator
Half-life: <3 hours
Clinically important, potentially hazardous interactions with: alcohol, aldesleukin, allopurinol, alpha blockers, alprostadil, amifostine, amiloride, angiotensin II receptor antagonists, antacids, antidiabetics, antihypertensives, antipsychotics, anxiolytics and hypnotics, aprotinin, azathioprine, baclofen, beta blockers, calcium channel blockers, clonidine, cyclosporine, CYP2D6 inhibitors, darunavir, diazoxide, digoxin, diuretics, eplerenone, estrogens, everolimus, general anesthetics, gold & gold compounds, heparins, herbals, hydralazine, hypotensives, insulin, interferon alfa, levodopa, lithium, MAO inhibitors, metformin, methyldopa, methylphenidate, minoxidil, moxisylyte, moxonidine, naldemedine, nitrates, nitroprusside, NSAIDs, pentoxifylline, phosphodiesterase 5 inhibitors, potassium salts, probenecid, prostacyclin analogues, rituximab, salicylates, sirolimus, spironolactone, sulfonylureas, temsirolimus, tizanidine, tolvaptan, triamterene, trimethoprim, venetoclax, yohimbine
Pregnancy category: D (category C in first trimester; category D in second and third trimesters)
Important contra-indications noted in the prescribing guidelines for: nursing mothers; pediatric patients
Note: Capozide is captopril and hydrochlorothiazide. Hydrochlorothiazide is a sulfonamide and can be absorbed systemically. Sulfonamides can produce severe, possibly fatal, reactions such as toxic epidermal necrolysis and Stevens-Johnson syndrome.
Warning: FETAL TOXICITY

Skin
- Angioedema (<15%) [45]
- Bullous pemphigoid [2]
- Dermatitis [3]
- DRESS syndrome [2]
- Erythroderma [2]

Exanthems (4–7%) [19]
Exfoliative dermatitis (<2%) [4]
Flushing [2]
Kaposi's sarcoma [2]
Lichen planus pemphigoides [2]
Lichenoid eruption [12]
Linear IgA bullous dermatosis [5]
Lupus erythematosus [8]
Mycosis fungoides [2]
Pemphigus (<2%) [24]
Pemphigus foliaceus [2]
Penile ulceration [2]
Photosensitivity [3]
Phototoxicity (<2%)
Pigmentation [2]
Pityriasis rosea (<2%) [6]
Pruritus (<7%) [8]
Pseudolymphoma [2]
Psoriasis [8]
Rash (4–7%) [12]
Toxic epidermal necrolysis [3]
Urticaria [9]
Vasculitis [7]

Hair
Alopecia (<2%) [4]

Nails
Nail dystrophy [2]
Onycholysis [2]

Mucosal
Aphthous stomatitis (<2%) [5]
Glossitis [3]
Oral mucosal eruption [3]
Oral ulceration [4]
Sialadenitis [2]
Tongue ulceration [3]
Xerostomia (<2%)

Central Nervous System
Ageusia (taste loss) (2–4%) [11]
Dysgeusia (taste perversion) (metallic or salty taste) (2–4%) [14]
Hallucinations [2]
Paresthesias (<2%)

Gastrointestinal/Hepatic
Hepatotoxicity [3]
Nausea [2]

Respiratory
Cough [19]

Endocrine/Metabolic
Gynecomastia [3]

Renal
Nephrotoxicity [2]

Other
Adverse effects [4]
Allergic reactions [2]

CARAWAY

Family: Apiaceae Umbelliferae
Scientific names: *Apium carvi, Carum carvi*
Indications: Hypotensive, dyspepsia, hysteria, tonic, stomachic, flatulent indigestion, flatulent colic of infants, fragrance, flavoring in foods, toothpaste, and cosmetics
Class: Anti-inflammatory, Carminative
Half-life: N/A
Clinically important, potentially hazardous interactions with: none known
Pregnancy category: N/A

Other
Adverse effects [4]

CARBAMAZEPINE

Trade names: Epitol (Teva), Tegretol (Novartis)
Indications: Epilepsy, pain or trigeminal neuralgia
Class: Anticonvulsant, Antipsychotic, CYP1A2 inducer, CYP3A4 inducer, Mood stabilizer
Half-life: 18–55 hours
Clinically important, potentially hazardous interactions with: abiraterone, acetaminophen, acetylcysteine, adenosine, afatinib, amitriptyline, amlodipine, amprenavir, apixaban, apremilast, aprepitant, aripiprazole, artemether/lumefantrine, bictegravir/emtricitabine/tenofovir alafenamide, boceprevir, brigatinib, brivaracetam, buprenorphine, cabazitaxel, cabozantinib, caffeine, caspofungin, cefixime, ceritinib, charcoal, citalopram, clarithromycin, clobazam, clopidogrel, clorazepate, clozapine, cobicistat/elvitegravir/emtricitabine/tenofovir disoproxil, cobimetinib, copanlisib, crizotinib, dabigatran, daclatasvir, darunavir, dasabuvir/ombitasvir/paritaprevir/ritonavir, dasatinib, deflazacort, delavirdine, dexamethasone, diltiazem, doxacurium, doxycycline, dronedarone, efavirenz, elbasvir & grazoprevir, eliglustat, emtricitabine/rilpivirine/tenofovir alafenamide, enzalutamide, erythromycin, eslicarbazepine, estradiol, ethosuximide, etravirine, ezogabine, felodipine, fesoterodine, flibanserin, fosamprenavir, gefitinib, glecaprevir & pibrentasvir, ibrutinib, idelalisib, imatinib, indinavir, influenza vaccine, isavuconazonium sulfate, isotretinoin, itraconazole, ixabepilone, ixazomib, lacosamide, lapatinib, ledipasvir & sofosbuvir, lesinurad, levetiracetam, levomepromazine, levonorgestrel, linezolid, lopinavir, methylprednisolone, midazolam, midostaurin, mifepristone, naldemedine, nelfinavir, neratinib, nevirapine, nifedipine, nilotinib, nintedanib, olanzapine, olaparib, ombitasvir/paritaprevir/ritonavir, ondansetron, osimertinib, oxcarbazepine, oxtriphylline, paclitaxel, palbociclib, paliperidone, perampanel, pimavanserin, piracetam, ponatinib, prednisolone, propoxyphene, regorafenib, rilpivirine, riociguat, risperidone, ritonavir, rivaroxaban, roflumilast, romidepsin, rufinamide, simeprevir, simvastatin, sodium picosulfate, sofosbuvir, sofosbuvir & velpatasvir, sofosbuvir/velpatasvir/voxilaprevir, solifenacin, sonidegib, sorafenib, St John's wort, sunitinib, telaprevir, telithromycin, temsirolimus, tenofovir alafenamide, terbinafine, tezacaftor/ivacaftor, thalidomide, tiagabine, ticagrelor, tipranavir, tolvaptan, tramadol, triamcinolone, troleandomycin, ulipristal, valbenazine, vandetanib, vemurafenib, venetoclax, verapamil, vorapaxar, voriconazole, vortioxetine, ziprasidone, zuclopenthixol
Pregnancy category: D
Note: Carbamazepine is the main cause of Stevens-Johnson syndrome (SJS), toxic epidermal necrolysis (TEN), and the hypersensitivity syndrome in Han Chinese, and in peoples of other Southeast Asian countries, as a result of a strong pharmacogenetic association that has been reported in these patients between the human leukocyte antigen (HLA)-B*1502 and carbamazepine.
Warning: SERIOUS DERMATOLOGIC REACTIONS AND HLA-B*1502 ALLELE; APLASTIC ANEMIA AND AGRANULOCYTOSIS

Skin
AGEP [5]
Angioedema [5]
Anticonvulsant hypersensitivity syndrome [19]
Bullous dermatitis [4]
Dermatitis [7]
Diaphoresis (<10%)
DRESS syndrome [51]
Eczema [2]
Erythema multiforme [16]
Erythroderma [12]
Exanthems (>5%) [36]
Exfoliative dermatitis [24]
Facial edema [2]
Fixed eruption [10]
Hypersensitivity [71]
Lichen planus [2]
Lichenoid eruption [8]
Lupus erythematosus [35]
Lymphoma [2]
Lymphoproliferative disease [5]
Mycosis fungoides [3]
Pemphigus [3]
Photosensitivity [9]
Pruritus [7]
Pseudolymphoma [17]
Purpura [8]
Pustules [5]
Rash (>10%) [31]
Serum sickness [2]
Stevens-Johnson syndrome (<10%) [103]
Toxic epidermal necrolysis (<10%) [93]
Toxic pustuloderma [3]
Toxicity [2]
Urticaria [14]
Vasculitis [7]

Hair
Alopecia [7]

Mucosal
Mucocutaneous eruption [4]
Mucocutaneous lymph node syndrome (Kawasaki syndrome) [2]
Oral ulceration [2]
Tongue ulceration [2]

Cardiovascular
Bradycardia [3]
Myocarditis [2]

Central Nervous System
- Ageusia (taste loss) [3]
- Coma [3]
- Dysgeusia (taste perversion) [2]
- Headache [5]
- Memory loss [2]
- Seizures [13]
- Somnolence (drowsiness) [8]
- Tic disorder [4]
- Vertigo (dizziness) [8]

Neuromuscular/Skeletal
- Asthenia (fatigue) [3]
- Ataxia [5]
- Myasthenia gravis [2]
- Osteoporosis [2]

Gastrointestinal/Hepatic
- Diarrhea [2]
- Hepatotoxicity [11]
- Nausea [5]
- Pancreatitis [3]
- Vanishing bile duct syndrome [4]
- Vomiting [3]

Respiratory
- Respiratory depression [2]

Endocrine/Metabolic
- Acute intermittent porphyria [5]
- Hyponatremia [5]
- SIADH [17]
- Weight gain [5]

Renal
- Nephrotoxicity [2]

Hematologic
- Agranulocytosis [2]
- Eosinophilia [2]
- Leukopenia [3]
- Thrombocytopenia [3]

Otic
- Hallucinations, auditory [2]

Ocular
- Diplopia [2]

Other
- Adverse effects [8]
- Allergic reactions [9]
- Death [6]
- Side effects [3]
- Teratogenicity [12]

CARBOPLATIN

Trade name: Paraplatin (Bristol-Myers Squibb)
Indications: Various carcinomas and sarcomas
Class: Alkylating agent, Antineoplastic
Half-life: terminal: 22–40 hours
Clinically important, potentially hazardous interactions with: aldesleukin, bexarotene
Pregnancy category: D
Important contra-indications noted in the prescribing guidelines for: the elderly; nursing mothers; pediatric patients

---

Skin
- Anaphylactoid reactions/Anaphylaxis [5]
- Erythema (2%) [2]
- Exanthems [3]
- Flushing [3]
- Hand–foot syndrome [5]
- Hypersensitivity (2%) [27]
- Pigmentation [2]
- Pruritus (2%) [2]
- Radiation recall dermatitis [2]
- Rash (2%) [10]
- Scleroderma [2]
- Toxicity [6]
- Urticaria (2%) [4]

Hair
- Alopecia (3%) [18]
- Alopecia areata [2]

Mucosal
- Epistaxis (nosebleed) [2]
- Mucositis [5]
- Stomatitis (>10%) [2]

Cardiovascular
- Hypertension [9]

Central Nervous System
- Anorexia [8]
- Fever [2]
- Headache [2]
- Leukoencephalopathy [2]
- Neurotoxicity [16]
- Pain [2]
- Paresthesias [2]
- Peripheral neuropathy [9]
- Vertigo (dizziness) [2]

Neuromuscular/Skeletal
- Asthenia (fatigue) [27]
- Myalgia/Myopathy [3]

Gastrointestinal/Hepatic
- Constipation [3]
- Diarrhea [16]
- Dyspepsia [2]
- Gastrointestinal perforation [2]
- Hepatotoxicity [4]
- Nausea [17]
- Pancreatitis [2]
- Vomiting [18]

Respiratory
- Cough [2]
- Hemoptysis [3]
- Pneumonia [2]
- Pulmonary toxicity [3]

Endocrine/Metabolic
- ALT increased [4]
- AST increased [3]
- Hyperbilirubinemia [2]
- Hyperglycemia [5]
- Hyponatremia [3]
- SIADH [3]

Renal
- Nephrotoxicity [9]
- Proteinuria [3]

Hematologic
- Anemia [29]
- Febrile neutropenia [22]
- Hemolytic anemia [2]
- Hemorrhage [2]
- Hemotoxicity [8]
- Leukopenia [13]
- Lymphopenia [3]
- Myelosuppression [2]
- Myelotoxicity [2]
- Neutropenia [56]
- Pancytopenia [2]
- Thrombocytopenia [40]

Otic
- Ototoxicity [7]
- Tinnitus [3]

Local
- Injection-site pain (>10%)

Other
- Adverse effects [3]
- Allergic reactions [4]
- Death [7]
- Infection [5]

CARFILZOMIB

Trade name: Kyprolis (Onyx)
Indications: Multiple myeloma
Class: Proteasome inhibitor
Half-life: ~1 hour
Clinically important, potentially hazardous interactions with: none known
Pregnancy category: D
Important contra-indications noted in the prescribing guidelines for: nursing mothers; pediatric patients

---

Skin
- Herpes zoster (reactivation) (2%) [2]
- Peripheral edema (24%) [3]
- Tumor lysis syndrome [2]

Cardiovascular
- Cardiac failure (7%) [4]
- Cardiotoxicity [7]
- Chest pain (11%)
- Hypertension (14%) [9]

Central Nervous System
- Anorexia (12%)
- Chills (16%)
- Fever (30%) [7]
- Headache (28%) [3]
- Hypoesthesia (12%)
- Insomnia (18%) [2]
- Pain (12%)
- Peripheral neuropathy (14%) [15]
- Vertigo (dizziness) (13%)

Neuromuscular/Skeletal
- Arthralgia (16%)
- Asthenia (fatigue) (13–56%) [18]
- Back pain (20%)
- Muscle spasm (14%) [2]
- Pain in extremities (13%)

Gastrointestinal/Hepatic
- Constipation (21%) [3]
- Diarrhea (33%) [7]
- Nausea (45%) [14]
- Vomiting (22%) [4]

Respiratory
- Cough (26%) [5]
- Dyspnea (35%) [11]
- Pneumonia (13%) [7]
- Pulmonary hypertension (2%)
- Upper respiratory tract infection (28%) [5]

Endocrine/Metabolic
- AST increased (13%)
- Hypercalcemia (11%)
- Hyperglycemia (12%) [3]
- Hypokalemia (14%) [3]
- Hypomagnesemia (14%)

Hyponatremia (10%) [2]
Hypophosphatemia (11%) [3]
Serum creatinine increased [5]

Renal
Nephrotoxicity [3]
Renal failure [2]

Hematologic
Anemia (47%) [22]
Hemotoxicity [2]
Leukopenia (14%) [4]
Lymphopenia (24%) [7]
Neutropenia (21%) [10]
Thrombocytopenia (36%) [21]

Other
Adverse effects [3]

CARIPRAZINE

Trade name: Vraylar (Forest)
Indications: Schizophrenia, manic or mixed episodes associated with bipolar I disorder
Class: Antipsychotic
Half-life: 2–4 days
Clinically important, potentially hazardous interactions with: CYP3A4 inducers
Pregnancy category: N/A (Neonatal risk in third trimester exposure)
Important contra-indications noted in the prescribing guidelines for: the elderly; nursing mothers; pediatric patients
Warning: INCREASED MORTALITY IN ELDERLY PATIENTS WITH DEMENTIA-RELATED PSYCHOSIS

Skin
Rash (<2%)

Mucosal
Oropharyngeal pain (<3%)
Xerostomia (<3%)

Cardiovascular
Hypertension (2–6%)
Tachycardia (<3%)

Central Nervous System
Agitation (3–5%)
Akathisia (20–21%) [23]
Anxiety (3–6%) [3]
Extrapyramidal symptoms (15–29%) [18]
Fever (<4%) [4]
Headache (9–18%) [10]
Insomnia (8–13%) [13]
Mania (worsening) [2]
Parkinsonism (13–26%) [4]
Restlessness (4–7%) [8]
Schizophrenia (worsening) [3]
Sedation [7]
Somnolence (drowsiness) (5–10%) [4]
Tremor [10]
Vertigo (dizziness) (3–7%) [8]

Neuromuscular/Skeletal
Arthralgia (<2%)
Asthenia (fatigue) (<5%)
Back pain (<3%)
Dystonia (2–5%) [2]
Pain in extremities [2]

Gastrointestinal/Hepatic
Abdominal pain (3–8%) [2]
Constipation (6–11%) [11]
Diarrhea (<5%) [5]
Dyspepsia (4–9%) [6]
Hepatotoxicity (<3%)
Nausea (5–13%) [11]
Vomiting (4–10%) [9]

Respiratory
Cough (<4%)
Nasopharyngitis (<2%)

Endocrine/Metabolic
Appetite decreased (<4%)
Creatine phosphokinase increased (<3%)
Weight gain (2–3%) [7]

Genitourinary
Urinary tract infection (<2%)

Ocular
Vision blurred (4%) [3]

Other
Adverse effects [3]
Toothache (3–6%) [2]

CARISOPRODOL

Trade name: Soma (MedPointe)
Indications: Painful musculoskeletal disorders
Class: Central muscle relaxant
Half-life: 4–6 hours
Clinically important, potentially hazardous interactions with: CNS depressants, eucalyptus, meprobamate
Pregnancy category: C
Important contra-indications noted in the prescribing guidelines for: the elderly; nursing mothers; pediatric patients
Note: Contra-indicated in patients with acute intermittent porphyria.

Skin
Angioedema (<10%)
Fixed eruption [2]
Flushing (<10%)
Urticaria [2]

Central Nervous System
Amnesia [2]
Trembling (<10%)

Other
Death [2]

CARMUSTINE

Trade names: BiCNU (Bristol-Myers Squibb), Gliadel Wafer (Guilford)
Indications: Brain tumors, Hodgkin's disease, multiple myeloma
Class: Alkylating agent, Nitrosourea
Half-life: initial: 1.4 minutes; secondary: 20 minutes
Clinically important, potentially hazardous interactions with: aldesleukin, cimetidine, clorazepate
Pregnancy category: D
Important contra-indications noted in the prescribing guidelines for: nursing mothers; pediatric patients

---

Skin
Dermatitis [3]
Flushing (<10%) [2]
Pigmentation (on accidental contact) [2]
Telangiectasia [2]

Hair
Alopecia (<10%)

Mucosal
Stomatitis (<10%)

Central Nervous System
Intracranial hemorrhage [2]
Meningococcal infection [2]
Seizures [2]

Neuromuscular/Skeletal
Asthenia (fatigue) [2]

Gastrointestinal/Hepatic
Nausea [2]
Vomiting [2]

Hematologic
Leukopenia [2]
Thrombocytopenia [2]

Local
Injection-site burning (>10%)

CARVEDILOL

Trade name: Coreg (GSK)
Indications: Hypertension
Class: Adrenergic beta-receptor antagonist
Half-life: 7–10 hours
Clinically important, potentially hazardous interactions with: cinacalcet, delavirdine, efavirenz, irbesartan, leflunomide, propafenone, trimethoprim, venetoclax, voriconazole, zafirlukast
Pregnancy category: C
Important contra-indications noted in the prescribing guidelines for: nursing mothers; pediatric patients

---

Skin
Diaphoresis (3%)
Edema (generalized) (5–6%) [2]
Peripheral edema (<7%)
Purpura (<3%)

Cardiovascular
Angina (2–6%)
Atrial fibrillation [2]
Atrioventricular block (<3%)
Bradycardia (2–10%) [7]
Cardiac failure [2]
Congestive heart failure [2]
Extrasystoles [2]
Hypertension (<3%)
Hypotension (9–14%) [8]
Palpitation (<3%)
Postural hypotension (<3%)

Central Nervous System
Fever (<3%)
Headache (5–8%) [2]
Pain (9%)
Paresthesias (2%)
Somnolence (drowsiness) (<3%)
Syncope (3–8%)
Vertigo (dizziness) (24–32%) [5]

Neuromuscular/Skeletal
Arthralgia (<6%)
Asthenia (fatigue) (7–24%) [2]
Muscle spasm (<3%)
Myalgia/Myopathy (3%)

Gastrointestinal/Hepatic
Black stools (<3%)
Diarrhea (2–12%)
Nausea (4–9%)
Vomiting (<6%)

Respiratory
Cough (5–8%)
Dyspnea [4]
Stridor [2]

Endocrine/Metabolic
ALP increased (<3%) [2]
Creatine phosphokinase increased (<3%) [3]
Diabetes mellitus (<3%)
GGT increased (<3%)
Hypercholesterolemia (<4%)
Hyperglycemia (5–12%)
Hyperkalemia (<3%) [2]
Hyperuricemia (<3%)
Hypervolemia (<3%)
Hypoglycemia (<3%)
Hyponatremia (<3%)
Hypovolemia (<3%)
Weight gain (10–12%)
Weight loss (<3%)

Genitourinary
Albuminuria (<3%)
Hematuria (<3%)
Impotence (<3%)

Hematologic
Anemia [2]
Prothrombin time decreased (<3%)
Thrombocytopenia (<3%)

Ocular
Abnormal vision (5%)
Vision blurred (<3%)

Other
Adverse effects [8]
Infection (2%)

CASCARA

Family: Rhamnaceae
Scientific names: *Frangula purshianus, Rhamnus purshiana*
Indications: Atonic constipation, dyspepsia, colitis, diverticulitis, dyspepsia, gallstones, gout, hemorrhoids, hypertension, indigestion, insomnia, jaundice, liver disease, nervous disorders, parasites, stomach disorders
Class: Stimulant laxative
Half-life: N/A
Clinically important, potentially hazardous interactions with: antiarrhythmics, cardiac glycosides, corticosteroids, licorice, thiazide diuretics
Pregnancy category: N/A

Gastrointestinal/Hepatic
Hepatotoxicity [2]

CASPOFUNGIN

Trade name: Cancidas (Merck)
Indications: Invasive *Aspergillus* and *Candida* infections
Class: Antifungal
Half-life: beta phase: 9–11 hours; terminal: 40–50 hours
Clinically important, potentially hazardous interactions with: carbamazepine, cyclosporine, dexamethasone, efavirenz, nevirapine, phenytoin, rifampin, tacrolimus
Pregnancy category: C
Important contra-indications noted in the prescribing guidelines for: nursing mothers; pediatric patients

---

Skin
Anaphylactoid reactions/Anaphylaxis (<2%)
Edema (~3%)
Erythema (<4%)
Facial edema (3%)
Flushing (3%)
Jaundice (<5%)
Peripheral edema (11%)
Petechiae (<5%)
Pruritus (2–7%)
Rash (4–16%) [5]
Septic–toxic shock (11–13%)
Ulcerations (3%)
Urticaria (<5%)
Vasculitis (2%)

Mucosal
Epistaxis (nosebleed) (<5%)
Mucosal inflammation (6–10%)

Cardiovascular
Arrhythmias (<5%)
Atrial fibrillation (<5%)
Bradycardia (<5%)
Cardiac arrest (<5%)
Hypertension (5–10%)
Hypotension (6–12%)
Myocardial infarction (<5%)
Phlebitis (18%) [3]
Tachycardia (4–7%)
Thrombophlebitis [2]

Central Nervous System
Anxiety (<5%)
Chills (9–23%)
Confusion (<5%)
Depression (<5%)
Fever (6–29%) [8]
Headache (5–15%) [3]
Insomnia (<5%)
Pain (<5%)
Paresthesias (<3%)
Seizures (<5%)
Tremor (<2%)
Vertigo (dizziness) (<5%)

Neuromuscular/Skeletal
Arthralgia (<5%)
Asthenia (fatigue) (<5%)
Back pain (<5%)
Myalgia/Myopathy (~3%)
Pain in extremities (<5%)

Gastrointestinal/Hepatic
Abdominal distension (<5%)
Abdominal pain (7–9%)
Constipation (<5%)
Diarrhea (6–27%)
Dyspepsia (<5%)
Hepatic failure (<5%)
Hepatotoxicity (<5%) [8]
Nausea (5–15%) [2]
Vomiting (9–17%) [2]

Respiratory
Cough (6–11%)
Dyspnea (9%)
Flu-like syndrome (3%)
Hypoxia (<5%)
Pleural effusion (9%)
Pneumonia (4–11%)
Respiratory distress (8%)
Respiratory failure (6–11%)
Tachypnea (8%)

Endocrine/Metabolic
ALP increased (12–23%) [4]
ALT increased (4–18%) [4]
Appetite decreased (<5%)
AST increased (6–16%) [5]
Hypercalcemia (<5%)
Hyperglycemia (<5%)
Hypokalemia (6–8%) [3]
Hypomagnesemia (<5%)

Genitourinary
Hematuria (<5%)
Urinary tract infection (<5%)

Renal
Nephrotoxicity [5]
Renal failure (<5%)

Hematologic
Anemia (2–11%)
Coagulopathy (<5%)
Eosinophilia [2]
Febrile neutropenia (<5%)
Neutropenia (<5%)
Sepsis (5%)
Thrombocytopenia (<5%) [2]

Local
Infusion-related reactions [4]
Infusion-site pain (<5%)
Infusion-site reactions (<5%) [2]
Injection-site induration (~3%)
Injection-site reactions (2–12%) [4]

Other
Adverse effects [8]

CEFACLOR

Trade name: Ceclor (Lilly)
Indications: Various infections caused by susceptible organisms
Class: Cephalosporin, 2nd generation
Half-life: 0.6–0.9 hours
Clinically important, potentially hazardous interactions with: none known
Pregnancy category: B
Important contra-indications noted in the prescribing guidelines for: the elderly; nursing mothers; pediatric patients
Note: Penicillin and cephalosporins share a common beta-lactam structure. People who are allergic to penicillin are approximately 4 times more likely to develop an allergic reaction to a cephalosporin than those people who have no

penicillin allergy (from 5–16% of patients allergic to penicillin develop reactions to cephalosporins).

Skin
AGEP [2]
Anaphylactoid reactions/Anaphylaxis [5]
Erythema multiforme [6]
Exanthems [9]
Fixed eruption [2]
Pruritus [4]
Purpura [2]
Rash (<2%) [2]
Serum sickness [7]
Serum sickness-like reaction [23]
Urticaria [5]

Gastrointestinal/Hepatic
Diarrhea [2]

Other
Adverse effects [3]

CEFADROXIL

Trade name: Duricef (Warner Chilcott)
Indications: Various infections caused by susceptible organisms
Class: Cephalosporin, 1st generation
Half-life: 1.2–1.5 hours
Clinically important, potentially hazardous interactions with: none known
Pregnancy category: B
Important contra-indications noted in the prescribing guidelines for: nursing mothers
Note: Penicillin and cephalosporins share a common beta-lactam structure. People who are allergic to penicillin are approximately 4 times more likely to develop an allergic reaction to a cephalosporin than those people who have no penicillin allergy (from 5–16% of patients allergic to penicillin develop reactions to cephalosporins).

Skin
Urticaria [2]

Gastrointestinal/Hepatic
Diarrhea [2]
Nausea [2]

Other
Adverse effects [3]

CEFDINIR

Trade name: Omnicef (Medicis)
Indications: Community-acquired pneumonia and various infections caused by susceptible organisms
Class: Cephalosporin, 3rd generation
Half-life: 1–2 hours
Clinically important, potentially hazardous interactions with: none known
Pregnancy category: B
Important contra-indications noted in the prescribing guidelines for: pediatric patients
Note: Penicillin and cephalosporins share a common beta-lactam structure. People who are allergic to penicillin are approximately 4 times more likely to develop an allergic reaction to a cephalosporin than those people who have no penicillin allergy (from 5–16% of patients allergic to penicillin develop reactions to cephalosporins).

Skin
Rash (3%)

Gastrointestinal/Hepatic
Red stools [2]

Genitourinary
Vulvovaginal candidiasis (5%)

Other
Adverse effects [2]

CEFEPIME

Trade name: Maxipime (Elan)
Indications: Various infections caused by susceptible organisms
Class: Cephalosporin, 4th generation
Half-life: 2–2.3 hours
Clinically important, potentially hazardous interactions with: none known
Pregnancy category: B
Important contra-indications noted in the prescribing guidelines for: the elderly; nursing mothers
Note: Penicillin and cephalosporins share a common beta-lactam structure. People who are allergic to penicillin are approximately 4 times more likely to develop an allergic reaction to a cephalosporin than those people who have no penicillin allergy (from 5–16% of patients allergic to penicillin develop reactions to cephalosporins).

Skin
Exanthems (2%)
Hypersensitivity [2]
Lupus erythematosus [2]
Pruritus [3]
Rash (51%) [12]
Stevens-Johnson syndrome [2]

Central Nervous System
Encephalopathy [10]
Headache [3]
Neurotoxicity [15]
Seizures [16]
Status epilepticus [5]

Neuromuscular/Skeletal
Myoclonus [2]

Local
Injection-site reactions (3%) [2]

Other
Adverse effects [2]

CEFIXIME

Trade name: Suprax (Lupin)
Indications: Various infections caused by susceptible organisms
Class: Cephalosporin, 3rd generation
Half-life: 3–4 hours
Clinically important, potentially hazardous interactions with: aminoglycosides, anticoagulants, BCG vaccine, carbamazepine, probenecid, typhoid vaccine, warfarin
Pregnancy category: B
Important contra-indications noted in the prescribing guidelines for: nursing mothers; pediatric patients
Note: Penicillin and cephalosporins share a common beta-lactam structure. People who are allergic to penicillin are approximately 4 times more likely to develop an allergic reaction to a cephalosporin than those people who have no penicillin allergy (from 5–16% of patients allergic to penicillin develop reactions to cephalosporins).

Skin
Anaphylactoid reactions/Anaphylaxis (<2%)
Angioedema (<2%)
Erythema multiforme (<2%)
Facial edema (<2%)
Jaundice (<2%)
Pruritus (<2%)
Pruritus ani et vulvae (<2%)
Rash (<2%) [2]
Serum sickness-like reaction (<2%)
Stevens-Johnson syndrome (<2%)
Toxic epidermal necrolysis (<2%)
Urticaria (<2%) [2]

Central Nervous System
Fever (<2%)

Gastrointestinal/Hepatic
Abdominal pain (3%)
Diarrhea (16%)
Dyspepsia (3%)
Flatulence (4%)
Hepatitis (<2%)
Loose stools (6%)
Nausea (7%)
Pseudomembranous colitis (<2%)

Endocrine/Metabolic
ALP increased (<2%)
Creatine phosphokinase increased (<2%)

Genitourinary
Vaginitis (<2%)
Vulvovaginal candidiasis (<2%)

Renal
Renal failure (<2%)

CEFOTAXIME

Trade name: Claforan (Sanofi-Aventis)
Indications: Various infections caused by susceptible organisms
Class: Cephalosporin, 3rd generation
Half-life: 1 hour (adults)
Clinically important, potentially hazardous interactions with: none known
Pregnancy category: B
Important contra-indications noted in the prescribing guidelines for: nursing mothers
Note: Penicillin and cephalosporins share a common beta-lactam structure. People who are allergic to penicillin are approximately 4 times more likely to develop an allergic reaction to a cephalosporin than those people who have no penicillin allergy (from 5–16% of patients allergic to penicillin develop reactions to cephalosporins).

Skin
Anaphylactoid reactions/Anaphylaxis (2%)

DRESS syndrome [4]
Erythema multiforme [2]
Exanthems [3]
Hypersensitivity [2]
Pruritus (2%) [3]
Rash (2%) [3]
Stevens-Johnson syndrome [2]
Urticaria (2%)

Local
Injection-site inflammation (4%)
Injection-site pain (<10%)

Other
Adverse effects [2]

CEFOTETAN

Indications: Various infections caused by susceptible organisms
Class: Cephalosporin, 2nd generation
Half-life: 3–5 hours
Clinically important, potentially hazardous interactions with: none known
Pregnancy category: B
Important contra-indications noted in the prescribing guidelines for: nursing mothers; pediatric patients
Note: Penicillin and cephalosporins share a common beta-lactam structure. People who are allergic to penicillin are approximately 4 times more likely to develop an allergic reaction to a cephalosporin than those people who have no penicillin allergy (from 5–16% of patients allergic to penicillin develop reactions to cephalosporins).

Skin
Anaphylactoid reactions/Anaphylaxis [3]
Rash [2]

Hematologic
Hemolytic anemia [12]

Other
Death [5]

CEFTAROLINE FOSAMIL

Trade name: Teflaro (Forest)
Indications: Acute bacterial skin and skin structure infections, community-acquired bacterial pneumonia
Class: Antibacterial, Cephalosporin, 5th generation
Half-life: 3 hours
Clinically important, potentially hazardous interactions with: BCG vaccine, probenecid, typhoid vaccine
Pregnancy category: B
Important contra-indications noted in the prescribing guidelines for: the elderly; nursing mothers; pediatric patients
Note: Penicillin and cephalosporins share a common beta-lactam structure. People who are allergic to penicillin are approximately 4 times more likely to develop an allergic reaction to a cephalosporin than those people who have no penicillin allergy (from 5–16% of patients allergic to penicillin develop reactions to cephalosporins).

Skin
Anaphylactoid reactions/Anaphylaxis (<2%)
Hypersensitivity (<2%) [2]
Pruritus [7]
Rash (3%) [9]
Urticaria (<2%)

Cardiovascular
Bradycardia (<2%)
Hypertension [2]
Palpitation (<2%)
Phlebitis (2%) [3]

Central Nervous System
Fever (<2%)
Headache [9]
Insomnia [5]
Seizures (<2%)
Vertigo (dizziness) (<2%)

Gastrointestinal/Hepatic
Abdominal pain (<2%)
Colitis (<2%)
Constipation (2%)
Diarrhea (5%) [10]
Hepatotoxicity (<2%)
Nausea (4%) [9]
Vomiting (2%)

Respiratory
Eosinophilic pneumonia [3]

Endocrine/Metabolic
ALT increased (2%)
Hyperglycemia (<2%)
Hyperkalemia (<2%)
Hypokalemia (2%) [2]

Renal
Renal failure (<2%)

Hematologic
Anemia (<2%)
Eosinophilia (<2%) [2]
Neutropenia (<2%) [3]
Thrombocytopenia (<2%)

Other
Adverse effects [4]
Infection [2]

CEFTAZIDIME

Trade names: Ceptaz (GSK), Fortaz (Concordia), Tazicef (Hospira)
Indications: Various infections caused by susceptible organisms
Class: Cephalosporin, 3rd generation
Half-life: 1–2 hours
Clinically important, potentially hazardous interactions with: none known
Pregnancy category: B
Important contra-indications noted in the prescribing guidelines for: the elderly; nursing mothers
Note: Penicillin and cephalosporins share a common beta-lactam structure. People who are allergic to penicillin are approximately 4 times more likely to develop an allergic reaction to a cephalosporin than those people who have no penicillin allergy (from 5–16% of patients allergic to penicillin develop reactions to cephalosporins). See also separate profile for Ceftazidime & Avibactam.

Skin
Anaphylactoid reactions/Anaphylaxis (2%) [3]
Angioedema (2%)
Erythema multiforme (2%)
Hypersensitivity (2%)
Pemphigus erythematodes [2]
Pruritus (2%) [3]
Rash (2%) [5]
Stevens-Johnson syndrome (2%)
Toxic epidermal necrolysis (2%)

Central Nervous System
Encephalopathy [2]
Seizures [3]

Local
Injection-site inflammation (2%)
Injection-site reactions [2]
Injection-site thrombophlebitis (2%)

Other
Adverse effects [3]
Death [2]

CEFTAZIDIME & AVIBACTAM

Trade name: Avycaz (Cerexa)
Indications: Various infections caused by susceptible organisms
Class: Antibiotic, beta-lactam (avibactam), Cephalosporin, 3rd generation (ceftazidime)
Half-life: <3 hours
Clinically important, potentially hazardous interactions with: probenecid
Pregnancy category: B
Important contra-indications noted in the prescribing guidelines for: the elderly; nursing mothers; pediatric patients
Note: See also separate entry for ceftazidime.

Skin
Rash (<5%)

Central Nervous System
Anxiety (10%) [3]
Fever [4]
Headache [3]
Vertigo (dizziness) (6%)

Gastrointestinal/Hepatic
Abdominal pain (7%) [5]
Constipation (10%) [2]
Diarrhea [5]
Hepatotoxicity [4]
Nausea (2%) [5]
Vomiting [5]

Endocrine/Metabolic
ALP increased (3%)
ALT increased (3%) [3]
AST increased [3]
GGT increased (<5%)

Renal
Nephrotoxicity (<5%)
Renal failure (<5%) [4]

Hematologic
Eosinophilia (<5%)
Prothrombin time increased (<5%)
Thrombocytopenia (<5%)

Local
Injection-site reactions [4]
Other
Adverse effects [2]

CEFTOBIPROLE

Trade names: BAL5788 (Basilea) (Cilag AG), Zeftera (Janssen)
Indications: Bacterial infections, MRSA
Class: Cephalosporin, 5th generation
Half-life: 3 hours
Clinically important, potentially hazardous interactions with: alcohol, anticoagulants, BCG vaccine, carbenicillin, dipyridamole, heparin, pentoxifylline, plicamycin, sulfinpyrazone, ticarcillin, typhoid vaccine, valproic acid
Pregnancy category: N/A (not recommended in pregnancy)
Important contra-indications noted in the prescribing guidelines for: nursing mothers; pediatric patients
Note: Penicillin and cephalosporins share a common beta-lactam structure. People who are allergic to penicillin are approximately 4 times more likely to develop an allergic reaction to a cephalosporin than those people who have no penicillin allergy (from 5–16% of patients allergic to penicillin develop reactions to cephalosporins).

Skin
Erythema (9%)
Pruritus (9%)
Central Nervous System
Dysgeusia (taste perversion) (8%) [3]
Headache [2]
Gastrointestinal/Hepatic
Abdominal pain [2]
Diarrhea [4]
Nausea [6]
Vomiting [4]
Endocrine/Metabolic
Hyponatremia [2]
Local
Infusion-site reactions [2]
Other
Adverse effects [3]

CEFTOLOZANE & TAZOBACTAM

Trade name: Zerbaxa (Cubist)
Indications: Various infections caused by susceptible organisms
Class: Antibacterial, Antibiotic, beta-lactam, Cephalosporin, 5th generation
Half-life: <3 hours
Clinically important, potentially hazardous interactions with: none known
Pregnancy category: B
Important contra-indications noted in the prescribing guidelines for: the elderly; nursing mothers; pediatric patients

Cardiovascular
Hypertension [3]
Central Nervous System
Fever (2%) [5]
Headache (3%) [8]
Insomnia [2]
Somnolence (drowsiness) [2]
Neuromuscular/Skeletal
Myalgia/Myopathy [2]
Gastrointestinal/Hepatic
Constipation (4%) [4]
Diarrhea (2%) [10]
Nausea (3%) [11]
Vomiting [3]
Endocrine/Metabolic
ALT increased (2%)
AST increased (2%)
Hematologic
Anemia [2]
Local
Infusion-site reactions [2]

CEFTRIAXONE

Trade name: Rocephin (Roche)
Indications: Various infections caused by susceptible organisms
Class: Antibiotic, Cephalosporin, 3rd generation
Half-life: 5–9 hours
Clinically important, potentially hazardous interactions with: aminoglycosides, coumarins, histamine H_2 antagonists, oral typhoid vaccine, probenecid
Pregnancy category: B
Important contra-indications noted in the prescribing guidelines for: nursing mothers; pediatric patients
Note: Penicillin and cephalosporins share a common beta-lactam structure. People who are allergic to penicillin are approximately 4 times more likely to develop an allergic reaction to a cephalosporin than those people who have no penicillin allergy (from 5–16% of patients allergic to penicillin develop reactions to cephalosporins).

Skin
AGEP [4]
Anaphylactoid reactions/Anaphylaxis [15]
Angioedema [3]
Candidiasis (5%) [3]
Dermatitis [2]
DRESS syndrome [2]
Erythroderma [2]
Exanthems [7]
Flushing [2]
Hypersensitivity [4]
Linear IgA bullous dermatosis [2]
Pruritus [2]
Rash (2%) [5]
Serum sickness-like reaction [2]
Urticaria [4]
Mucosal
Glossitis [2]
Cardiovascular
Hypotension [2]
Phlebitis [2]
Central Nervous System
Fever [2]
Gastrointestinal/Hepatic
Cholelithiasis (gallstones) [4]
Diarrhea [6]
Hepatotoxicity [7]
Nausea [4]
Vomiting [2]
Respiratory
Dyspnea [2]
Renal
Biliary pseudolithiasis [8]
Nephrolithiasis [2]
Nephrotoxicity [6]
Renal failure [3]
Hematologic
Eosinophilia [2]
Hemolysis [9]
Hemolytic anemia [15]
Thrombocytopenia [4]
Local
Injection-site pain (<10%) [3]
Injection-site phlebitis [2]
Other
Adverse effects [7]
Death [9]
Side effects (3%) [2]

CEFUROXIME

Trade names: Ceftin (GSK), Zinacef (Concordia)
Indications: Various infections caused by susceptible organisms
Class: Cephalosporin, 2nd generation
Half-life: 1–2 hours
Clinically important, potentially hazardous interactions with: none known
Pregnancy category: B
Important contra-indications noted in the prescribing guidelines for: nursing mothers
Note: Penicillin and cephalosporins share a common beta-lactam structure. People who are allergic to penicillin are approximately 4 times more likely to develop an allergic reaction to a cephalosporin than those people who have no penicillin allergy (from 5–16% of patients allergic to penicillin develop reactions to cephalosporins).

Skin
AGEP [2]
Anaphylactoid reactions/Anaphylaxis [7]
Exanthems [2]
Hypersensitivity [4]
Serum sickness-like reaction [2]
Toxic epidermal necrolysis [2]
Urticaria [2]
Cardiovascular
Thrombophlebitis (<10%)
Gastrointestinal/Hepatic
Nausea [2]
Ocular
Ocular toxicity [2]
Other
Kounis syndrome [3]

CELECOXIB

Trade name: Celebrex (Pfizer)
Indications: Osteoarthritis, rheumatoid arthritis (adults and juveniles aged 2 years and over), ankylosing spondylitis, acute pain, primary dysmenorrhea
Class: COX-2 inhibitor, Non-steroidal anti-inflammatory (NSAID), Sulfonamide
Half-life: 11 hours
Clinically important, potentially hazardous interactions with: ACE inhibitors, aliskiren, angiotensin II receptor antagonists, aspirin, dexibuprofen, fluconazole, furosemide, lithium, NSAIDs, warfarin
Pregnancy category: D (pregnancy category C prior to 30 weeks gestation; category D starting at 30 weeks gestation)
Important contra-indications noted in the prescribing guidelines for: the elderly; nursing mothers; pediatric patients
Note: Celecoxib is a sulfonamide and can be absorbed systemically. Sulfonamides can produce severe, possibly fatal, reactions such as toxic epidermal necrolysis and Stevens-Johnson syndrome. NSAIDs may cause an increased risk of serious cardiovascular and gastrointestinal adverse events, which can be fatal. This risk may increase with duration of use.
Contra-indicated in patients with known hypersensitivity to celecoxib, aspirin, or other NSAIDs; in patients who have demonstrated allergic-type reactions to sulfonamides; in patients who have experienced asthma, urticaria, or allergic-type reactions after taking aspirin or other NSAIDs; and for the treatment of peri-operative pain in the setting of coronary artery bypass graft surgery.
Warning: CARDIOVASCULAR AND GASTROINTESTINAL RISKS

Skin
AGEP [7]
Anaphylactoid reactions/Anaphylaxis [8]
Angioedema [9]
Bacterial infection (<2%)
Candidiasis (<2%)
Dermatitis (<2%) [2]
Diaphoresis (<2%)
Edema (<2%) [5]
Erythema [2]
Erythema multiforme [3]
Exanthems (<2%) [7]
Facial edema (<2%)
Fixed eruption [2]
Herpes simplex (<2%)
Herpes zoster (<2%)
Hot flashes (<2%)
Hypersensitivity [8]
Nodular eruption (<2%)
Peripheral edema (2%) [2]
Photosensitivity (<2%)
Pruritus (<2%) [6]
Rash (2%) [11]
Stevens-Johnson syndrome [2]
Sweet's syndrome [3]
Toxic epidermal necrolysis [5]
Urticaria (<2%) [11]
Vasculitis [4]
Xerosis (<2%)

Hair
Alopecia (<2%) [3]

Nails
Nail changes (<2%)

Mucosal
Stomatitis (<2%) [4]
Xerostomia (<2%)

Cardiovascular
Cardiotoxicity [2]
Hypertension [2]
Myocardial infarction [4]

Central Nervous System
Anorexia [3]
Depression [2]
Dysgeusia (taste perversion) (<2%)
Headache [3]
Paresthesias (<2%)
Stroke [3]
Vertigo (dizziness) [3]

Neuromuscular/Skeletal
Asthenia (fatigue) [6]
Myalgia/Myopathy (<2%)
Tendinopathy/Tendon rupture (<2%)

Gastrointestinal/Hepatic
Abdominal pain [11]
Constipation [5]
Diarrhea [12]
Dyspepsia [10]
Flatulence [2]
Gastrointestinal bleeding [4]
Hepatotoxicity [3]
Nausea [15]
Vomiting [10]

Endocrine/Metabolic
Dehydration [2]
Mastodynia (<2%)

Genitourinary
Vaginitis (<2%)
Vulvovaginal candidiasis (<2%)

Renal
Nephrotoxicity [4]

Hematologic
Anemia [2]
Neutropenia [4]

Ocular
Visual disturbances [3]

Local
Application-site cellulitis (<2%)
Application-site reactions (<2%)

Other
Adverse effects [16]
Allergic reactions (<2%) [2]
Death [4]
Infection (<2%)
Tooth disorder (<2%)

CELIPROLOL

Trade names: Celectol (Winthrop), Celol (Pacific), Selectol (Sanofi-Aventis)
Indications: Hypertension, angina pectoris
Class: Beta blocker
Half-life: 5–6 hours
Clinically important, potentially hazardous interactions with: amiodarone, bepridil, diltiazem, disopyramide, floctafenine, quinidine, theophylline, verapamil
Pregnancy category: N/A
Important contra-indications noted in the prescribing guidelines for: nursing mothers

---

Central Nervous System
Headache [2]
Vertigo (dizziness) [2]

Neuromuscular/Skeletal
Asthenia (fatigue) [3]

CEPHALEXIN

Synonym: cefalexin
Trade names: Keflex (Advancis), Keftab (Biovail)
Indications: Various infections caused by susceptible organisms
Class: Cephalosporin, 1st generation
Half-life: 0.9–1.2 hours
Clinically important, potentially hazardous interactions with: amikacin, gentamicin, metformin
Pregnancy category: B
Important contra-indications noted in the prescribing guidelines for: the elderly; nursing mothers
Note: Penicillin and cephalosporins share a common beta-lactam structure. People who are allergic to penicillin are approximately 4 times more likely to develop an allergic reaction to a cephalosporin than those people who have no penicillin allergy (from 5–16% of patients allergic to penicillin develop reactions to cephalosporins).

Skin
AGEP [4]
Anaphylactoid reactions/Anaphylaxis [4]
Angioedema [2]
Bullous pemphigoid [2]
Erythema multiforme [3]
Exanthems [3]
Pemphigus [2]
Pruritus [3]
Pustules [2]
Stevens-Johnson syndrome [3]
Toxic epidermal necrolysis [4]
Urticaria [2]

Other
Adverse effects [2]
Side effects (2%) [2]

CERTOLIZUMAB

Trade name: Cimzia (Celltech) (UCB)
Indications: Crohn's disease, rheumatoid arthritis
Class: Disease-modifying antirheumatic drug (DMARD), Monoclonal antibody, TNF inhibitor
Half-life: 14 days
Clinically important, potentially hazardous interactions with: abatacept, anakinra, lenalidomide, live vaccines, natalizumab, rituximab
Pregnancy category: N/A (Limited evidence insufficient to inform drug-associated risk)
Important contra-indications noted in the prescribing guidelines for: nursing mothers; pediatric patients
Note: TNF inhibitors should be used in patients with heart failure only after consideration of other treatment options. TNF inhibitors are contra-indicated in patients with a personal or family history of multiple sclerosis or demyelinating disease. TNF inhibitors should not be administered to patients with moderate to severe heart failure (New York Heart Association Functional Class III/IV).
Warning: SERIOUS INFECTIONS AND MALIGNANCY

Skin
Herpes zoster [3]
Neoplasms [2]
Psoriasis [6]
Rash [2]

Cardiovascular
Hypertension [2]

Central Nervous System
Fever (5%) [2]
Headache (7–18%) [5]
Vertigo (dizziness) (~6%)

Neuromuscular/Skeletal
Arthralgia (6–7%) [4]
Back pain [3]

Gastrointestinal/Hepatic
Nausea [2]

Respiratory
Nasopharyngitis (4–13%) [8]
Pneumonia [2]
Pulmonary toxicity [4]
Sinusitis [2]
Upper respiratory tract infection (20%) [11]

Endocrine/Metabolic
Creatine phosphokinase increased [2]

Genitourinary
Urinary tract infection (~8%) [8]

Local
Injection-site pain [3]
Injection-site reactions (~7%) [4]

Other
Adverse effects [15]
Death [2]
Infection (14–38%) [15]

CETIRIZINE

Trade name: Zyrtec (Pfizer)
Indications: Allergic rhinitis, urticaria
Class: Histamine H1 receptor antagonist
Half-life: 8–11 hours
Clinically important, potentially hazardous interactions with: alcohol, CNS depressants, pilsicainide
Pregnancy category: B
Important contra-indications noted in the prescribing guidelines for: nursing mothers

---

Skin
Acneform eruption (<2%)
Anaphylactoid reactions/Anaphylaxis (<2%) [2]
Angioedema (<2%)
Bullous dermatitis (<2%)
Dermatitis (<2%)
Diaphoresis (<2%)
Exanthems (<2%)
Fixed eruption [7]
Flushing (<2%)
Furunculosis (<2%)
Hyperkeratosis (<2%)
Photosensitivity (<2%)
Phototoxicity (<2%)
Pruritus (<2%)
Purpura (<2%)
Rash (<2%)
Seborrhea (<2%)
Urticaria (<2%) [9]
Xerosis (<2%)

Hair
Alopecia (<2%)
Hypertrichosis (<2%)

Mucosal
Sialorrhea (<2%)
Stomatitis (<2%)
Tongue edema (<2%)
Tongue pigmentation (<2%)
Xerostomia (6%) [2]

Cardiovascular
QT prolongation [2]

Central Nervous System
Ageusia (taste loss) (<2%)
Dysgeusia (taste perversion) (<2%)
Headache [2]
Hyperesthesia (<2%)
Insomnia [2]
Paresthesias (<2%)
Parosmia (<2%)
Somnolence (drowsiness) [5]

Neuromuscular/Skeletal
Asthenia (fatigue) [3]
Dystonia [6]
Myalgia/Myopathy (<2%)

Endocrine/Metabolic
Mastodynia (<2%)

Genitourinary
Vaginitis (<2%)

Other
Adverse effects [4]

CETRORELIX

Trade name: Cetrotide (Merck)
Indications: Inhibition of premature luteinizing hormone surges in women undergoing controlled ovarian stimulation
Class: Gonadotropin-releasing hormone (GnRH) antagonist
Half-life: 5 hours
Clinically important, potentially hazardous interactions with: none known
Pregnancy category: X
Important contra-indications noted in the prescribing guidelines for: nursing mothers

---

Skin
Hot flashes [2]

Central Nervous System
Headache [2]

CETUXIMAB

Trade name: Erbitux (Bristol-Myers Squibb)
Indications: Metastatic colorectal cancer, squamous cell carcinoma of the head and neck
Class: Antineoplastic, Biologic, Epidermal growth factor receptor (EGFR) inhibitor, Monoclonal antibody
Half-life: 75–188 hours
Clinically important, potentially hazardous interactions with: none known
Pregnancy category: C
Important contra-indications noted in the prescribing guidelines for: nursing mothers; pediatric patients
Warning: SERIOUS INFUSION REACTIONS and CARDIOPULMONARY ARREST

Skin
Acneform eruption (88%) [66]
Anaphylactoid reactions/Anaphylaxis [5]
Dermatitis [4]
Desquamation (89%) [3]
Erythema [3]
Exanthems [5]
Fissures [4]
Flushing [2]
Folliculitis [13]
Hand–foot syndrome [5]
Hypersensitivity [9]
Papulopustular eruption [7]
Peripheral edema (10%)
Pruritus (40%) [9]
Radiation recall dermatitis [2]
Rash (89%) [52]
Stevens-Johnson syndrome [2]
Toxic epidermal necrolysis [4]
Toxicity [20]
Xerosis (49%) [15]

Hair
Abnormal hair growth [2]
Alopecia (5%)
Hair changes [3]
Hypertrichosis [3]

Nails
Nail changes (21%)
Nail disorder [3]

Paronychia [17]

Mucosal
Mucositis [10]
Oral mucositis [2]
Stomatitis (25%) [4]
Xerostomia (11%)

Cardiovascular
Cardiotoxicity [2]
Chest pain [2]
Thromboembolism [2]

Central Nervous System
Anorexia [2]
Anxiety (14%)
Aseptic meningitis [6]
Chills (13%) [2]
Confusion (15%)
Depression (13%)
Fever (30%) [5]
Headache (33%)
Insomnia (30%)
Pain (51%)
Peripheral neuropathy [3]
Rigors (13%)
Seizures [2]

Neuromuscular/Skeletal
Asthenia (fatigue) (89%) [29]
Back pain (11%)
Bone or joint pain (15%)

Gastrointestinal/Hepatic
Abdominal pain (59%)
Constipation (46%)
Diarrhea (39%) [21]
Dysphagia [2]
Gastrointestinal bleeding [2]
Hepatotoxicity [4]
Nausea [12]
Vomiting (37%) [8]

Respiratory
Cough (29%)
Dyspnea (48%) [6]
Pneumonia [3]
Pneumonitis [3]
Pulmonary toxicity [6]

Endocrine/Metabolic
Hypokalemia [6]
Hypomagnesemia [18]
Hyponatremia [5]

Hematologic
Anemia [6]
Febrile neutropenia [7]
Leukopenia [11]
Myelosuppression [2]
Neutropenia [25]
Sepsis (<4%)
Thrombocytopenia [5]
Thrombosis [3]

Ocular
Blepharitis [3]
Conjunctivitis (7%) [2]
Ectropion [2]
Eyelashes – hypertrichosis [3]
Trichomegaly [11]

Local
Application-site reactions (~3%)
Infusion-related reactions [7]
Infusion-site reactions (15–21%) [10]

Other
Adverse effects [9]
Allergic reactions [5]
Death [10]
Infection (13–35%) [3]

CEVIMELINE

Trade name: Evoxac (Daiichi Sankyo)
Indications: Sicca syndrome in patients with Sjøgren's syndrome
Class: Muscarinic cholinergic agonist
Half-life: 3–4 hours
Clinically important, potentially hazardous interactions with: none known
Pregnancy category: C
Important contra-indications noted in the prescribing guidelines for: nursing mothers; pediatric patients
Note: Contra-indicated in patients with uncontrolled asthma, acute iritis or narrow-angle glaucoma.

Skin
Abscess (<3%)
Candidiasis (<3%)
Diaphoresis (20%)
Edema (<3%)
Erythema (<3%)
Exanthems (<10%)
Fungal dermatitis (<10%)
Hot flashes (2%)
Hyperhidrosis (19%) [5]
Peripheral edema (<3%)
Pruritus (<3%)
Rash (4%)

Mucosal
Epistaxis (nosebleed) (<3%)
Sialadenitis (<3%)
Sialorrhea (2%)
Ulcerative stomatitis (<3%)
Xerostomia (<3%)

Cardiovascular
Chest pain (<3%)
Palpitation (<3%)

Central Nervous System
Anorexia (<3%)
Depression (<3%)
Fever (<3%)
Headache (14%)
Hypoesthesia (<3%)
Hyporeflexia (<3%)
Insomnia (2%)
Migraine (<3%)
Pain (3%)
Tremor (<3%)
Vertigo (dizziness) (4%)

Neuromuscular/Skeletal
Arthralgia (4%)
Back pain (5%)
Bone or joint pain (3%)
Hypertonia (<3%)
Leg cramps (<3%)
Myalgia/Myopathy (<3%)

Gastrointestinal/Hepatic
Abdominal pain (8%)
Constipation (<3%)
Diarrhea (10%)
Dyspepsia (8%)
Eructation (belching) (<3%)
Gastroesophageal reflux (<3%)
Nausea (14%) [3]
Vomiting (5%)

Respiratory
Bronchitis (4%)
Cough (6%)
Flu-like syndrome (<3%)
Pharyngitis (5%)
Pneumonia (<3%)
Rhinitis (11%)
Sinusitis (12%)
Upper respiratory tract infection (11%)

Genitourinary
Urinary tract infection (6%)
Vaginitis (<3%)

Hematologic
Anemia (<3%)

Otic
Ear pain (<3%)
Otitis media (<3%)

Ocular
Abnormal vision (<3%)
Conjunctivitis (4%)
Ocular pain (<3%)
Xerophthalmia (<3%)

Other
Allergic reactions (<3%)
Infection (<3%)
Tooth disorder (<3%)

CHAMOMILE

Family: Asteraceae; Compositae
Scientific names: *Chamomilla recutita, Matricaria chamomilla, Matricaria recutita*
Indications: Flatulence, travel sickness, nervous diarrhea, restlessness, menstrual cramps, hemorrhoids, mastitis, leg ulcers, inflammation of the respiratory tract. Used in flavoring, cosmetics, soaps and mouthwashes
Class: Sedative
Half-life: N/A
Clinically important, potentially hazardous interactions with: none known
Pregnancy category: N/A

Skin
Anaphylactoid reactions/Anaphylaxis [2]
Dermatitis [5]

Ocular
Ocular adverse effects [2]

Other
Adverse effects [3]
Allergic reactions (to those allergic to ragweed, marigolds, daisies) [2]

CHASTEBERRY

Family: Verbenaceae
Scientific name: *Vitex agnus-castus*
Indications: Premenstrual syndrome, abnormal uterine bleeding, mastodynia
Class: Hormone modulator
Half-life: N/A
Clinically important, potentially hazardous interactions with: dopamine-receptor antagonists
Pregnancy category: N/A
Important contra-indications noted in the prescribing guidelines for: nursing mothers
Note: Chasteberry is not a phytoestrogen; it appears to stimulate progesterone production. The Catholic Church once placed it in the pockets of neophyte monks to help them to maintain their vow of chastity.

Skin
Abscess [2]
Acneform eruption [4]
Erythema [2]
Pruritus [2]
Urticaria [3]

Mucosal
Xerostomia [3]

Central Nervous System
Headache [5]

Neuromuscular/Skeletal
Asthenia (fatigue) [3]

Gastrointestinal/Hepatic
Hepatotoxicity [4]
Nausea [4]

Endocrine/Metabolic
Menstrual irregularities [3]

Other
Adverse effects [4]

CHICORY

Family: Compositae
Scientific name: *Cichorium intybus*
Indications: Coffee substitute, jaundice, liver enlargement, gout, rheumatism, skin eruptions connected with gout, inflammation. **Topical:** leaves used for swelling and inflammation. Culinary spice, flavoring
Class: Diuretic
Half-life: N/A
Clinically important, potentially hazardous interactions with: none known
Pregnancy category: N/A

Skin
Dermatitis [2]

Other
Allergic reactions [3]

CHLORAL HYDRATE

Indications: Insomnia, sedation
Class: Anesthetic, general, Hypnotic
Half-life: 8–11 hours
Clinically important, potentially hazardous interactions with: antihistamines, azatadine, brompheniramine, buclizine, chlorpheniramine, clemastine, dexchlorpheniramine, diphenhydramine, meclizine, tripelennamine
Pregnancy category: C
Important contra-indications noted in the prescribing guidelines for: nursing mothers

Skin
Acneform eruption [2]
Angioedema [2]
Dermatitis [2]
Erythema multiforme [2]
Exanthems [3]
Fixed eruption [5]
Pruritus [2]
Purpura [2]
Rash (<10%)
Urticaria (<10%) [2]

Mucosal
Oral lesions [2]

Cardiovascular
Hypotension [2]

Central Nervous System
Agitation [2]
Sedation (prolonged) [2]

Gastrointestinal/Hepatic
Vomiting [4]

Respiratory
Apnea [2]

Other
Adverse effects [3]
Death [3]

CHLORAMPHENICOL

Indications: Various infections caused by susceptible organisms
Class: Antibiotic, CYP3A4 inhibitor
Half-life: 1.5–3.5 hours
Clinically important, potentially hazardous interactions with: amoxicillin, ampicillin, clopidogrel, clozapine, ethotoin, fosphenytoin, gliclazide, levodopa, mephenytoin, phenytoin, propyphenazone, voriconazole
Pregnancy category: C
Important contra-indications noted in the prescribing guidelines for: nursing mothers

Skin
AGEP [2]
Dermatitis [18]
Erythema multiforme [6]
Exanthems (<5%) [5]
Hypersensitivity [2]
Purpura [2]
Pustules [2]
Sensitization [2]
Toxic epidermal necrolysis [2]
Urticaria [3]

Nails
Photo-onycholysis [2]

CHLORDIAZEPOXIDE

Trade names: Libritabs (Valeant), Librium (Valeant), Limbitrol (Valeant)
Indications: Anxiety
Class: Benzodiazepine
Half-life: 6–25 hours
Clinically important, potentially hazardous interactions with: chlorpheniramine, clarithromycin, efavirenz, esomeprazole, imatinib, indinavir, ketoconazole, nelfinavir, nilutamide, ritonavir
Pregnancy category: D
Important contra-indications noted in the prescribing guidelines for: the elderly; nursing mothers; pediatric patients
Note: Limbitrol is chlordiazepoxide and amitriptyline.

Skin
Angioedema [3]
Dermatitis (<10%)
Diaphoresis (>10%)
Edema (<10%)
Erythema multiforme [5]
Erythema nodosum [2]
Exanthems [3]
Fixed eruption [7]
Lupus erythematosus [3]
Photosensitivity [6]
Purpura [5]
Rash (>10%)
Urticaria [4]
Vasculitis [2]

Hair
Alopecia [3]

Mucosal
Sialopenia (>10%)
Sialorrhea (<10%)
Xerostomia (>10%)

Endocrine/Metabolic
Galactorrhea [3]

CHLORHEXIDINE

Trade name: Hibiclens (SSL)
Indications: Skin antisepsis, gingivitis
Class: Antiseptic
Half-life: N/A
Clinically important, potentially hazardous interactions with: none known
Pregnancy category: B
Important contra-indications noted in the prescribing guidelines for: nursing mothers; pediatric patients

Skin
Anaphylactoid reactions/Anaphylaxis [29]
Dermatitis [16]
Hypersensitivity [9]
Rash [2]
Urticaria [4]

Mucosal
- Gingival pigmentation [2]
- Gingivitis [3]
- Glossitis (<10%)
- Mucosal ulceration [2]
- Oral mucosal irritation [2]
- Stomatitis (<10%)
- Tongue irritation (<10%)
- Tongue pigmentation (>10%)

Central Nervous System
- Dysgeusia (taste perversion) (>10%) [8]

Other
- Allergic reactions [6]
- Tooth pigmentation [5]

CHLOROQUINE

Trade name: Aralen (Sanofi-Aventis)
Indications: Malaria, rheumatoid arthritis, lupus erythematosus
Class: Antimalarial, Antiprotozoal, Disease-modifying antirheumatic drug (DMARD)
Half-life: 3–5 days
Clinically important, potentially hazardous interactions with: acitretin, antacids, arsenic, cholera vaccine, cholestyramine, citalopram, dapsone, dasatinib, degarelix, droperidol, ethosuximide, furazolidone, halofantrine, hydroxychloroquine, lacosamide, lanthanum, lapatinib, levofloxacin, methotrexate, methoxsalen, mivacurium, moxifloxacin, neostigmine, nilotinib, oxcarbazepine, pazopanib, penicillamine, ribociclib, sulfonamides, telavancin, telithromycin, tiagabine, typhoid vaccine, vandetanib, vigabatrin, voriconazole, vorinostat, ziprasidone
Pregnancy category: D
Important contra-indications noted in the prescribing guidelines for: nursing mothers

---

Skin
- Dermatitis [2]
- Erythema annulare centrifugum [2]
- Erythroderma [3]
- Exanthems (<5%) [3]
- Exfoliative dermatitis [4]
- Lichenoid eruption [6]
- Photosensitivity [8]
- Pigmentation [15]
- Pruritus [36]
- Psoriasis [19]
- Stevens-Johnson syndrome [4]
- Toxic epidermal necrolysis [5]
- Toxicity [2]
- Urticaria [4]
- Vitiligo [7]

Hair
- Hair pigmentation [10]
- Poliosis [3]

Nails
- Nail pigmentation [2]

Mucosal
- Mucosal membrane pigmentation [2]
- Oral pigmentation [13]

Cardiovascular
- Atrioventricular block [2]
- Cardiac failure [3]
- Cardiomyopathy [9]
- Cardiotoxicity [3]
- Congestive heart failure [2]
- Myocardial toxicity [2]
- QT prolongation [3]
- Torsades de pointes [2]

Central Nervous System
- Headache [4]
- Psychosis [4]
- Seizures [2]
- Vertigo (dizziness) [4]

Neuromuscular/Skeletal
- Myalgia/Myopathy [8]
- Myasthenia gravis [7]

Gastrointestinal/Hepatic
- Diarrhea [2]
- Nausea [3]
- Vomiting [5]

Endocrine/Metabolic
- Porphyria [7]

Ocular
- Corneal deposits [2]
- Keratopathy [2]
- Maculopathy [3]
- Ocular adverse effects [2]
- Ocular toxicity [4]
- Retinopathy [10]
- Vision blurred [2]

Other
- Adverse effects [2]
- Death [3]

CHLORPHENIRAMINE

Synonym: chlorphenamine
Trade names: Chlor-Trimeton (Schering), Triaminic (Novartis)
Indications: Allergic rhinitis, urticaria
Class: Histamine H1 receptor antagonist, Muscarinic antagonist
Half-life: 20–40 hours
Clinically important, potentially hazardous interactions with: alcohol, anticholinergics, barbiturates, benzodiazepines, butabarbital, chloral hydrate, chlordiazepoxide, chlorpromazine, clonazepam, clorazepate, diazepam, ethchlorvynol, fluphenazine, flurazepam, hypnotics, lopinavir, lorazepam, MAO inhibitors, mephobarbital, mesoridazine, midazolam, narcotics, oxazepam, pentobarbital, phenobarbital, phenothiazines, phenylbutazone, primidone, prochlorperazine, promethazine, quazepam, secobarbital, sedatives, temazepam, thioridazine, tranquilizers, trifluoperazine, zolpidem
Pregnancy category: B
Important contra-indications noted in the prescribing guidelines for: the elderly; nursing mothers; pediatric patients

---

Skin
- Angioedema (<10%)
- Dermatitis (<10%) [4]
- Photosensitivity (<10%)

Mucosal
- Xerostomia (<10%)

Central Nervous System
- Seizures [2]

CHLORPROMAZINE

Trade name: Thorazine (GSK)
Indications: Psychosis, manic-depressive disorders
Class: Antiemetic, Antipsychotic, Muscarinic antagonist, Phenothiazine
Half-life: initial: 2 hours; terminal: 30 hours
Clinically important, potentially hazardous interactions with: alcohol, antihistamines, arsenic, asenapine, chlorpheniramine, dofetilide, epinephrine, evening primrose, guanethidine, lisdexamfetamine, mivacurium, pimavanserin, propranolol, quinolones, sodium picosulfate, sparfloxacin, tetrabenazine, zolpidem
Pregnancy category: N/A
Important contra-indications noted in the prescribing guidelines for: the elderly; nursing mothers; pediatric patients
Note: The prolonged use of chlorpromazine can produce a gray-blue or purplish pigmentation over light-exposed areas. This is a result of either dermal deposits of melanin, a chlorpromazine metabolite, or to a combination of both. Chlorpromazine melanosis is seen more often in women.
Warning: INCREASED MORTALITY IN ELDERLY PATIENTS WITH DEMENTIA-RELATED PSYCHOSIS

Skin
- Exanthems (>5%) [8]
- Lupus erythematosus [12]
- Photosensitivity (<10%) [23]
- Phototoxicity [6]
- Pigmentation [16]
- Pruritus (<10%) [2]
- Purpura [6]
- Rash (<10%)
- Seborrheic dermatitis [4]
- Toxic epidermal necrolysis [2]
- Urticaria [4]
- Vasculitis [3]

Nails
- Nail pigmentation [4]

Mucosal
- Xerostomia (<10%)

Cardiovascular
- Hypotension [4]
- QT prolongation [4]
- Tachycardia [2]
- Torsades de pointes [2]

Central Nervous System
- Extrapyramidal symptoms [2]
- Neuroleptic malignant syndrome [7]
- Sedation [3]
- Seizures [2]
- Vertigo (dizziness) [2]

Endocrine/Metabolic
- Galactorrhea (<10%)
- Gynecomastia (<10%)
- Mastodynia (<10%)
- Weight gain [2]

Genitourinary
Priapism [7]
Otic
Tinnitus [2]
Ocular
Cataract [2]
Corneal opacity [2]
Eyelid edema [2]
Retinopathy [2]
Other
Adverse effects [3]

CHOLERA VACCINE

Trade name: Vaxchora (PaxVax)
Indications: Immunization against cholera for adults traveling to cholera-affected areas
Class: Vaccine
Half-life: N/A
Clinically important, potentially hazardous interactions with: antibiotics, chloroquine
Pregnancy category: N/A (Not expected to cause fetal risk)
Important contra-indications noted in the prescribing guidelines for: the elderly; pediatric patients

---

Central Nervous System
Headache (29%)
Neuromuscular/Skeletal
Asthenia (fatigue) (31%)
Gastrointestinal/Hepatic
Abdominal pain (19%)
Diarrhea (4%)
Nausea (18%)
Vomiting (18%)
Endocrine/Metabolic
Appetite decreased (17%)

CHOLESTYRAMINE

Trade name: Questran (Par)
Indications: Pruritus associated with biliary obstruction, primary hypercholesterolemia
Class: Bile acid sequestrant
Half-life: N/A
Clinically important, potentially hazardous interactions with: acarbose, acetaminophen, acitretin, amiodarone, aspirin, bezafibrate, calcifediol, chloroquine, cyclopenthiazide, cyclosporine, deferasirox, digoxin, doxepin, doxercalciferol, ergocalciferol, hydroxychloroquine, isotretinoin, leflunomide, levodopa, lovastatin, meloxicam, mycophenolate, phytonadione, propranolol, raloxifene, sulfasalazine, sulfonylureas, tetracycline, tricyclic antidepressants, troglitazone, ursodiol, valproic acid, vitamin A, vitamin E
Pregnancy category: C
Important contra-indications noted in the prescribing guidelines for: nursing mothers; pediatric patients
Note: Contra-indicated in patients with complete biliary obstruction.

Skin
Pruritus [2]
Neuromuscular/Skeletal
Osteomalacia [2]
Hematologic
Hemorrhage [2]

CHOLIC ACID

Trade name: Cholbam (Asklepion Pharmaceuticals)
Indications: Bile acid synthesis disorders, adjunctive treatment of peroxisomal disorders
Class: Bile acid
Half-life: N/A
Clinically important, potentially hazardous interactions with: cyclosporine
Pregnancy category: N/A
Important contra-indications noted in the prescribing guidelines for: the elderly; nursing mothers

---

Gastrointestinal/Hepatic
Diarrhea (2%)

CHONDROITIN

Scientific names: *Chondroitin 4- and 6-sulfate, Chondroitin 4-sulfate, Condrosulf, Structum*
Indications: Osteoarthritis (often with glucosamine), ischemic heart disease, osteoporosis, hyperlipidemia, keratoconjunctivitis, agent in cataract surgery
Class: Amino sugar, Food supplement
Half-life: N/A
Clinically important, potentially hazardous interactions with: warfarin
Pregnancy category: N/A

Gastrointestinal/Hepatic
Dyspepsia [2]
Hepatotoxicity [2]
Nausea [2]

CIDOFOVIR

Trade name: Vistide (Gilead)
Indications: Cytomegalovirus (CMV) retinitis in patients with acquired immunodeficiency syndrome (AIDS)
Class: Antiviral, nucleotide analog
Half-life: ~2.6 hours
Clinically important, potentially hazardous interactions with: amphotericin B, cobicistat/elvitegravir/emtricitabine/tenofovir alafenamide, cobicistat/elvitegravir/emtricitabine/tenofovir disoproxil, tenofovir disoproxil
Pregnancy category: C
Important contra-indications noted in the prescribing guidelines for: the elderly; nursing mothers; pediatric patients
Warning: RENAL TOXICITY and NEUTROPENIA

Skin
Acneform eruption (>10%)
Diaphoresis (<10%)
DRESS syndrome [2]
Pallor (<10%)
Pigmentation (>10%)
Pruritus (<10%) [2]
Rash (27%) [2]
Toxicity [3]
Ulcerations [2]
Urticaria (<10%)
Hair
Alopecia (22%) [2]
Mucosal
Stomatitis (<10%)
Central Nervous System
Chills (24%)
Dysgeusia (taste perversion) (<10%)
Headache [4]
Paresthesias (>10%)
Neuromuscular/Skeletal
Asthenia (fatigue) [2]
Myalgia/Myopathy [2]
Renal
Fanconi syndrome [2]
Nephrotoxicity [5]
Ocular
Intraocular inflammation [2]
Iritis [6]
Ocular hypotension [2]
Retinal detachment [3]
Uveitis [18]
Vision impaired [3]
Vision loss [3]
Local
Application-site reactions (39%) [4]
Other
Allergic reactions (<10%)

CILOSTAZOL

Trade name: Pletal (Otsuka)
Indications: Peripheral vascular disease, intermittent claudication
Class: Antiplatelet, Phosphodiesterase inhibitor, Vasodilator, peripheral
Half-life: 11–13 hours
Clinically important, potentially hazardous interactions with: anagrelide, anticoagulants, antifungals, antiplatelet agents, clarithromycin, collagenase, conivaptan, CYP2C19 inhibitors, CYP3A4 inducers or inhibitors, dasatinib, deferasirox, diltiazem, drotrecogin alfa, erythromycin, esomeprazole, fondaparinux, glucosamine, grapefruit juice, high-fat foods, ibritumomab, itraconazole, ketoconazole, macrolide antibiotics, NSAIDs, omeprazole, PEG-interferon, pentosan, pentoxifylline, prostacyclin analogues, salicylates, St John's wort, telithromycin, thrombolytic agents, tositumomab & iodine^{131}, voriconazole

Pregnancy category: C
Important contra-indications noted in the prescribing guidelines for: nursing mothers; pediatric patients
Note: Contra-indicated in patients with congestive heart failure or active pathological bleeding.
Warning: CONTRA-INDICATED IN HEART FAILURE PATIENTS

Skin
Ecchymoses (<2%)
Edema (<2%)
Facial edema (<2%)
Furunculosis (<2%)
Hypertrophy (<2%)
Peripheral edema (7–9%)
Purpura (<2%)
Rash (2%) [2]
Urticaria (<2%)
Varicosities (<2%)
Xerosis (<2%)

Mucosal
Epistaxis (nosebleed) (<2%)
Gingival bleeding (<2%)
Perioral abscess (<2%)
Rectal hemorrhage (<2%)
Tongue edema (<2%)

Cardiovascular
Arrhythmias (<2%)
Atrial fibrillation (<2%)
Atrial flutter (<2%)
Cardiac arrest (<2%)
Cardiotoxicity [4]
Congestive heart failure (<2%)
Extrasystoles (<2%)
Hypotension (<2%)
Myocardial infarction (<2%) [4]
Myocardial ischemia (<2%)
Palpitation (5–10%) [8]
Postural hypotension (<2%)
Supraventricular tachycardia (<2%)
Tachycardia (4%) [4]
Vasodilation (<2%)
Ventricular tachycardia (<2%)

Central Nervous System
Anorexia (<2%)
Anxiety (<2%)
Cerebral ischemia (<2%)
Chills (<2%)
Headache (27–34%) [20]
Hyperesthesia (2%)
Insomnia (<2%)
Neurotoxicity (<2%)
Paresthesias (2%)
Syncope (<2%)
Vertigo (dizziness) (<10%) [4]

Neuromuscular/Skeletal
Arthralgia (<2%)
Asthenia (fatigue) (<2%)
Back pain (6–7%)
Bone or joint pain (<2%)
Gouty tophi (<2%)
Myalgia/Myopathy (2–3%)

Gastrointestinal/Hepatic
Abdominal pain (4–5%)
Black stools (<2%)
Cholelithiasis (gallstones) (<2%)
Colitis (<2%)
Diarrhea (12–19%) [8]
Dyspepsia (6%)
Esophagitis (<2%)
Flatulence (2–3%)
Gastritis (<2%)
Gastroenteritis (<2%)
Gastrointestinal ulceration (<2%)
Hematemesis (<2%)
Nausea (6–7%) [4]
Peptic ulceration (<2%)
Vomiting (>2%)

Respiratory
Asthma (<2%)
Cough (3–4%) [2]
Hemoptysis (<2%)
Pharyngitis (7–10%)
Pneumonia (<2%)
Rhinitis (7–12%)
Sinusitis (<2%)

Endocrine/Metabolic
Creatine phosphokinase increased (<2%)
Diabetes mellitus (<2%)
GGT increased (<2%)
Hyperlipidemia (<2%)
Hyperuricemia (<2%)

Genitourinary
Albuminuria (<2%)
Cystitis (<2%)
Urinary frequency (<2%)
Vaginal bleeding (<2%)
Vaginitis (<2%)

Renal
Retroperitoneal bleeding (<2%)

Hematologic
Anemia (<2%)
Hemorrhage (<2%)
Polycythemia (<2%)
Thrombosis [3]

Otic
Ear pain (<2%)
Tinnitus (<2%)

Ocular
Amblyopia (<2%)
Blindness (<2%)
Conjunctivitis (<2%)
Diplopia (<2%)
Ocular hemorrhage (<2%)

Other
Adverse effects [4]
Death [3]
Infection (10–14%)

CIMETIDINE

Trade name: Tagamet (GSK)
Indications: Duodenal ulcer
Class: CYP1A2 inhibitor, CYP3A4 inhibitor, Histamine H2 receptor antagonist
Half-life: 2 hours
Clinically important, potentially hazardous interactions with: acenocoumarol, alfuzosin, aminophylline, amiodarone, amitriptyline, anisindione, anticoagulants, buprenorphine, butorphanol, caffeine, carmustine, citalopram, clobazam, clopidogrel, clozapine, cocoa, delavirdine, dicumarol, dofetilide, duloxetine, dutasteride, epirubicin, eszopiclone, fentanyl, ferrous sulfate, floxuridine, fluorouracil, galantamine, gliclazide, hydromorphone, itraconazole, ketoconazole, labetalol, levomepromazine, lidocaine, lomustine, meptazinol, metformin, metronidazole, midazolam, mizolastine, moclobemide, morphine, narcotic analgesics, neratinib, oxprenolol, oxtriphylline, oxycodone, oxymorphone, pentazocine, phenytoin, pimecrolimus, posaconazole, prednisone, propranolol, quinine, rilpivirine, risperidone, roflumilast, sertindole, sildenafil, sufentanil, tamsulosin, terbinafine, thalidomide, tolazoline, warfarin, xanthines, zaleplon, zofenopril, zolmitriptan, zolpidem
Pregnancy category: B
Important contra-indications noted in the prescribing guidelines for: nursing mothers; pediatric patients

---

Skin
Angioedema [3]
Erythema annulare centrifugum [2]
Erythema multiforme [5]
Exanthems [3]
Exfoliative dermatitis [2]
Fixed eruption [2]
Hypersensitivity [4]
Lupus erythematosus [3]
Pruritus [6]
Pseudolymphoma [2]
Psoriasis [6]
Rash (<2%)
Stevens-Johnson syndrome [3]
Toxic epidermal necrolysis [2]
Urticaria [6]
Vasculitis [3]

Hair
Alopecia [4]

Central Nervous System
Hallucinations [3]

Neuromuscular/Skeletal
Myalgia/Myopathy [2]

Endocrine/Metabolic
Gynecomastia [13]

Renal
Nephrotoxicity [3]

CIPROFLOXACIN

Trade names: Ciloxan Ophthalmic (Alcon), Cipro (Bayer), Ciproxin (Bayer)
Indications: Various infections caused by susceptible organisms, inhalational anthrax (post exposure)
Class: Antibiotic, fluoroquinolone, CYP1A2 inhibitor, CYP3A4 inhibitor
Half-life: 4 hours
Clinically important, potentially hazardous interactions with: agomelatine, aminophylline, amiodarone, amitriptyline, antacids, antineoplastics, arsenic, artemether/lumefantrine, BCG vaccine, bendamustine, bepridil, bismuth, bismuth subsalicylate, bretylium, calcium salts, citalopram, clopidogrel, clozapine, corticosteroids, cyclosporine, dairy products, dasatinib, degarelix, didanosine, disopyramide,

dolasetron, duloxetine, dutasteride, eluxadoline, erlotinib, erythromycin, flibanserin, insulin, lanthanum, lapatinib, levofloxacin, magnesium salts, meptazinol, methotrexate, methylxanthines, mifepristone, moxifloxacin, mycophenolate, neratinib, NSAIDs, olanzapine, olaparib, opiod analgesics, oral iron, oxtriphylline, P-glycoprotein inhibitors, pazopanib, pentoxifylline, phenothiazines, phenytoin, pirfenidone, probenecid, procainamide, propranolol, QT prolonging agents, quinapril, quinidine, rasagiline, ropinirole, ropivacaine, sevelamer, sotalol, St John's wort, strontium ranelate, sucralfate, sulfonylureas, telavancin, telithromycin, tizanidine, tricyclic antidepressants, typhoid vaccine, venetoclax, vitamin K antagonists, voriconazole, vorinostat, warfarin, zinc, ziprasidone, zolmitriptan
Pregnancy category: C
Important contra-indications noted in the prescribing guidelines for: the elderly; nursing mothers
Note: Fluoroquinolones are associated with an increased risk of tendinitis and tendon rupture in all ages. This risk is further increased in older patients usually over 60 years of age, in patients taking corticosteroid drugs, and in patients with kidney, heart or lung transplants.
Fluoroquinolones may exacerbate muscle weakness in persons with myasthenia gravis.
Ciprofloxacin is chemically related to nalidixic acid.
Warning: SERIOUS ADVERSE REACTIONS INCLUDING TENDINITIS, TENDON RUPTURE, PERIPHERAL NEUROPATHY, CENTRIAL NERVOUS SYSTEM EFFECTS and EXACERBATION OF MYASTHENIA GRAVIS

Skin
Acneform eruption [3]
AGEP [4]
Anaphylactoid reactions/Anaphylaxis [15]
Angioedema [8]
Candidiasis [2]
Diaphoresis [5]
Erythema multiforme [5]
Exanthems [4]
Facial edema [2]
Fixed eruption [14]
Hypersensitivity [5]
Jaundice [2]
Linear IgA bullous dermatosis [2]
Photosensitivity [20]
Phototoxicity [5]
Pruritus [11]
Purpura [4]
Rash (<10%) [14]
Serum sickness-like reaction [2]
Stevens-Johnson syndrome [10]
Toxic epidermal necrolysis [11]
Toxicity [3]
Urticaria [10]
Vasculitis [11]

Mucosal
Stomatitis [4]
Xerostomia [3]

Cardiovascular
Palpitation [2]
QT prolongation [11]
Torsades de pointes [8]

Central Nervous System
Delirium [2]
Dysgeusia (taste perversion) [3]
Fever [3]
Headache [6]
Mania [4]
Peripheral neuropathy [2]
Psychosis [6]
Seizures [5]
Syncope [2]
Tremor [2]
Vertigo (dizziness) [2]

Neuromuscular/Skeletal
Arthralgia [2]
Asthenia (fatigue) [3]
Myalgia/Myopathy [2]
Myasthenia gravis (exacerbation) [2]
Myoclonus [4]
Rhabdomyolysis [4]
Tendinitis [4]
Tendinopathy/Tendon rupture [31]

Gastrointestinal/Hepatic
Abdominal pain [2]
Constipation [2]
Flatulence [2]
Hepatitis [4]
Hepatotoxicity [7]
Nausea (3%) [4]
Pancreatitis [2]
Vomiting [2]

Genitourinary
Vaginitis [2]

Renal
Nephrotoxicity [9]
Renal failure [3]

Hematologic
Bone marrow suppression [2]
Hemolytic anemia [2]
Thrombocytopenia [4]

Otic
Hearing loss [2]

Ocular
Hallucinations, visual [6]
Vision blurred [2]

Local
Injection-site pain [2]

Other
Adverse effects [8]
Death [4]

CISPLATIN

Synonym: CDDP
Trade name: Platinol (Bristol-Myers Squibb)
Indications: Carcinomas, lymphomas
Class: Alkylating agent, Antineoplastic
Half-life: alpha phase: 25–49 minutes; beta phase: 58–73 hours
Clinically important, potentially hazardous interactions with: aldesleukin, atenolol, chlorothiazide, gadobenate, methotrexate, paclitaxel, pentamidine, rituximab, selenium, thalidomide, zinc
Pregnancy category: D
Important contra-indications noted in the prescribing guidelines for: the elderly; nursing mothers

---

Skin
Acneform eruption [7]
Anaphylactoid reactions/Anaphylaxis [10]
Angioedema [4]
Edema [3]
Erythema [3]
Exanthems [4]
Flushing [5]
Hand–foot syndrome [10]
Hypersensitivity [5]
Necrosis [2]
Peripheral edema [2]
Pigmentation [5]
Pruritus [8]
Rash [22]
Raynaud's phenomenon [14]
Thrombocytopenic purpura [2]
Toxic epidermal necrolysis [2]
Toxicity [7]
Urticaria [7]
Xerosis [2]

Hair
Alopecia (>10%) [26]

Nails
Paronychia [2]

Mucosal
Epistaxis (nosebleed) [3]
Mucositis [16]
Oral lesions [2]
Oral mucositis [2]
Stomatitis [16]

Cardiovascular
Cardiotoxicity [2]
Hypertension [8]
Thromboembolism [7]
Venous thromboembolism [4]

Central Nervous System
Anorexia [28]
Dysgeusia (taste perversion) [3]
Fever [5]
Headache [4]
Insomnia [4]
Leukoencephalopathy [10]
Neurotoxicity [15]
Pain [3]
Peripheral neuropathy [9]
Seizures [4]
Vertigo (dizziness) [2]

Neuromuscular/Skeletal
Arthralgia [2]
Asthenia (fatigue) [39]
Ataxia [2]
Myalgia/Myopathy [4]

Gastrointestinal/Hepatic
Abdominal pain [4]
Constipation [5]
Diarrhea [39]
Esophagitis [2]
Gastrointestinal bleeding [2]
Hepatotoxicity [6]
Nausea [55]
Pancreatitis [2]
Vomiting [41]

Respiratory
- Cough [4]
- Dysphonia [4]
- Dyspnea [4]
- Pneumonia [4]
- Pneumonitis [3]
- Pulmonary toxicity [5]

Endocrine/Metabolic
- ALP increased [2]
- ALT increased [7]
- Appetite decreased [7]
- AST increased [7]
- Dehydration [3]
- Hyperbilirubinemia [2]
- Hyperglycemia [4]
- Hyperkalemia [2]
- Hypocalcemia [2]
- Hypokalemia [5]
- Hypomagnesemia [14]
- Hyponatremia [19]
- Serum creatinine increased [9]
- SIADH [19]
- Weight loss [4]

Renal
- Nephrotoxicity [66]
- Proteinuria [2]
- Renal failure [3]
- Renal function abnormal [2]

Hematologic
- Anemia [53]
- Coagulopathy [2]
- Febrile neutropenia [41]
- Hemolytic uremic syndrome [12]
- Hemotoxicity [4]
- Leukopenia [35]
- Lymphopenia [5]
- Myelosuppression [8]
- Myelotoxicity [3]
- Neutropenia [98]
- Platelets decreased [2]
- Sepsis [2]
- Thrombocytopenia [50]
- Thrombosis [2]

Otic
- Hearing loss [16]
- Ototoxicity [40]
- Tinnitus [27]

Ocular
- Ocular adverse effects [2]

Local
- Injection-site cellulitis [4]

Other
- Adverse effects [16]
- Death [17]
- Hiccups [6]
- Infection [11]

CITALOPRAM

Trade names: Celexa (Forest), Cipramil (Lundbeck)
Indications: Depression, obsessive-compulsive disorder, panic disorder
Class: Antidepressant, Selective serotonin reuptake inhibitor (SSRI)
Half-life: ~35 hours
Clinically important, potentially hazardous interactions with: alcohol, alfuzosin, alpha or beta blockers, antidepressants, antiepileptics, antiplatelet agents, artemether/lumefantrine, aspirin, atomoxetine, barbiturates, bupropion, buspirone, carbamazepine, chloroquine, cimetidine, ciprofloxacin, clozapine, CNS depressants, collagenase, conivaptan, coumarins/anticoagulants, CYP2C19 inhibitors, CYP3A4 inhibitors, cyproheptadine, desmopressin, dexibuprofen, dextromethorphan, dronedarone, drotrecogin alfa, duloxetine, efavirenz, fluconazole, gadobutrol, glucosamine, haloperidol, ibritumomab, iobenguane, isocarboxazid, lithium, macrolide antibiotics, MAO inhibitors, methadone, methylphenidate, metoclopramide, mexiletine, moclobemide, nilotinib, NSAIDs, opioid anagesics, pentoxifylline, phenelzine, phenytoin, pimozide, QT prolonging agents, quinine, rasagiline, risperidone, ritonavir, salicylates, selegiline, serotonin modulators, sibutramine, SSRIs, St John's wort, sumatriptan, tetrabenazine, thioridazine, thrombolytic agents, tositumomab & iodine^{131}, tramadol, tranylcypromine, trazodone, tricyclic antidepressants, tryptophan, vitamin K antagonists, ziprasidone
Pregnancy category: C
Important contra-indications noted in the prescribing guidelines for: nursing mothers; pediatric patients
Warning: SUICIDALITY AND ANTIDEPRESSANT DRUGS

Skin
- Diaphoresis (11%) [3]
- Hyperhidrosis (11%) [2]
- Pigmentation [2]
- Pruritus (<10%) [2]
- Rash (<10%)

Mucosal
- Xerostomia (20%) [4]

Cardiovascular
- Bradycardia [2]
- Cardiotoxicity [4]
- Chest pain [2]
- Palpitation [2]
- QT prolongation [22]
- Tachycardia [3]
- Torsades de pointes [9]

Central Nervous System
- Agitation (3%)
- Akathisia [2]
- Anorexia (4%)
- Anxiety (4%) [2]
- Fever (2%)
- Headache [5]
- Incoordination [2]
- Insomnia (15%) [4]
- Nightmares [2]
- Restless legs syndrome [4]
- Sedation [2]
- Seizures (overdose) [5]
- Serotonin syndrome [19]
- Somnolence (drowsiness) (18%) [6]
- Suicidal ideation [3]
- Tremor (8%) [5]
- Vertigo (dizziness) [5]
- Yawning (2%)

Neuromuscular/Skeletal
- Arthralgia (2%)
- Asthenia (fatigue) (5%) [4]
- Dystonia [2]
- Myalgia/Myopathy (2%)

Gastrointestinal/Hepatic
- Abdominal pain (3%)
- Constipation [2]
- Diarrhea (8%) [2]
- Dyspepsia (5%)
- Nausea (21%) [4]
- Vomiting (4%) [2]

Respiratory
- Rhinitis (5%)
- Sinusitis (3%)
- Upper respiratory tract infection (5%)

Endocrine/Metabolic
- Galactorrhea [4]
- Hyponatremia [2]
- Libido decreased (2%)
- SIADH [18]
- Weight gain [3]

Genitourinary
- Dysmenorrhea (3%)
- Ejaculatory dysfunction (6%) [2]
- Impotence (3%)
- Priapism [4]
- Sexual dysfunction [5]
- Urinary frequency [2]

Otic
- Hallucinations, auditory [2]

Ocular
- Diplopia [2]
- Glaucoma [2]
- Hallucinations, visual [3]

Other
- Adverse effects [2]
- Death [8]

CLADRIBINE

Trade name: Leustatin (Janssen Biotech)
Indications: Leukemias
Class: Antimetabolite, Antineoplastic
Half-life: alpha phase: 25 minutes; beta phase: 7 hours
Clinically important, potentially hazardous interactions with: none known
Pregnancy category: D
Important contra-indications noted in the prescribing guidelines for: the elderly; nursing mothers

---

Skin
- Diaphoresis (<10%)
- Edema (6%)
- Erythema (6%)

Exanthems (27–50%) [2]
Herpes zoster [5]
Petechiae (8%)
Pruritus (6%)
Purpura (10%)
Rash (27%) [3]

Mucosal
Mucositis [2]

Neuromuscular/Skeletal
Myalgia/Myopathy (7%)

Hematologic
Lymphopenia [7]
Neutropenia [8]
Thrombocytopenia [2]

Local
Injection-site edema (9%)
Injection-site erythema (9%)
Injection-site pain (9%)
Injection-site phlebitis (2%)
Injection-site thrombosis (2%)

Other
Adverse effects [2]
Death [3]
Infection [7]

CLARITHROMYCIN

Trade name: Biaxin (AbbVie)
Indications: Various infections caused by susceptible organisms
Class: Antibiotic, macrolide, CYP3A4 inhibitor
Half-life: 5–7 hours
Clinically important, potentially hazardous interactions with: abiraterone, alprazolam, aprepitant, astemizole, atazanavir, atorvastatin, avanafil, benzodiazepines, betrixaban, boceprevir, brigatinib, cabazitaxel, cabozantinib, calcifediol, carbamazepine, chlordiazepoxide, cilostazol, clonazepam, clorazepate, cobicistat/elvitegravir/emtricitabine/tenofovir alafenamide, cobicistat/elvitegravir/emtricitabine/tenofovir disoproxil, colchicine, conivaptan, copanlisib, crizotinib, cyclosporine, dabigatran, darunavir, dasatinib, deflazacort, delavirdine, diazepam, digoxin, dihydroergotamine, disopyramide, dronedarone, efavirenz, eletriptan, eluxadoline, ergot alkaloids, estradiol, etravirine, everolimus, fesoterodine, flibanserin, fluoxetine, flurazepam, fluticasone propionate, fluvastatin, HMG-CoA reductase inhibitors, ibrutinib, imatinib, indinavir, itraconazole, ixabepilone, lapatinib, lomitapide, lopinavir, lorazepam, lovastatin, maraviroc, methylergonovine, methylprednisolone, methysergide, midazolam, midostaurin, mifepristone, naldemedine, neratinib, nevirapine, nilotinib, olaparib, omeprazole, oxazepam, oxtriphylline, paclitaxel, palbociclib, paroxetine hydrochloride, pazopanib, pimavanserin, pimozide, ponatinib, pravastatin, prednisone, quazepam, ranolazine, regorafenib, repaglinide, ribociclib, rilpivirine, rimonabant, rivaroxaban, romidepsin, ruxolitinib, sertraline, sildenafil, silodosin, simeprevir, simvastatin, solifenacin, sunitinib, tadalafil, temazepam, temsirolimus, tezacaftor/ivacaftor, ticagrelor, tipranavir, tolvaptan, trabectedin, triazolam, ulipristal, valbenazine, vandetanib, vemurafenib, venetoclax, vorapaxar, warfarin, zidovudine
Pregnancy category: C
Important contra-indications noted in the prescribing guidelines for: the elderly; nursing mothers; pediatric patients

---

Skin
Anaphylactoid reactions/Anaphylaxis [2]
Exanthems [3]
Fixed eruption [3]
Hypersensitivity [3]
Psoriasis [2]
Purpura [3]
Rash (3%) [2]
Serum sickness-like reaction [2]
Toxic epidermal necrolysis [4]
Vasculitis [3]

Mucosal
Stomatitis [2]

Cardiovascular
QT prolongation [7]
Torsades de pointes [9]

Central Nervous System
Anorexia [2]
Dysgeusia (taste perversion) (3%) [9]
Mania [4]
Neurotoxicity [4]
Psychosis [3]

Neuromuscular/Skeletal
Arthralgia [2]
Rhabdomyolysis [14]

Gastrointestinal/Hepatic
Abdominal distension [2]
Abdominal pain [5]
Diarrhea [10]
Dyspepsia [2]
Hepatotoxicity [4]
Nausea [5]
Vomiting [3]

Endocrine/Metabolic
Hypoglycemia [3]

Renal
Nephrotoxicity [2]

Ocular
Hallucinations, visual [4]

Local
Injection-site pain [2]

Other
Adverse effects [11]

CLINDAMYCIN

Trade names: Benzaclin (Dermik), Cleocin (Pfizer), Cleocin-T (Pfizer), Clindagel (Galderma), Clindets (Stiefel)
Indications: Various serious infections caused by susceptible organisms
Class: Antibiotic, lincosamide
Half-life: 2–3 hours
Clinically important, potentially hazardous interactions with: cisatracurium, erythromycin, kaolin, mivacurium, neostigmine, pyridostigmine, rocuronium, saquinavir
Pregnancy category: B
Note: See also separate entry for the combination product clindamycin/tretinoin.

Skin
AGEP [9]
Anaphylactoid reactions/Anaphylaxis [5]
Dermatitis (from topical preparations) [7]
DRESS syndrome [2]
Erythema multiforme [2]
Erythroderma [2]
Exanthems [6]
Hypersensitivity [5]
Rash (<10%) [3]
Stevens-Johnson syndrome [4]
Sweet's syndrome [2]
Toxic epidermal necrolysis [3]
Urticaria [3]
Vasculitis [2]

Mucosal
Burning mouth syndrome [2]
Xerostomia [2]

Central Nervous System
Ageusia (taste loss) [2]

Gastrointestinal/Hepatic
Colitis [2]
Diarrhea [4]
Esophagitis [2]
Hepatotoxicity [3]
Pseudomembranous colitis [5]

Hematologic
Neutropenia [2]

Otic
Tinnitus [2]

Local
Application-site erythema [3]

Other
Adverse effects [6]
Death [3]

CLOMIPRAMINE

Trade name: Anafranil (Mallinckrodt)
Indications: Obsessive-compulsive disorder
Class: Antidepressant, tricyclic, Muscarinic antagonist
Half-life: 21–31 hours
Clinically important, potentially hazardous interactions with: amprenavir, arbutamine, arsenic, artemether/lumefantrine, clonidine, duloxetine, epinephrine, formoterol, guanethidine, isocarboxazid, linezolid, MAO inhibitors, milnacipran, moclobemide, phenelzine, quinolones, sparfloxacin, tranylcypromine
Pregnancy category: C
Important contra-indications noted in the prescribing guidelines for: the elderly; nursing mothers; pediatric patients
Warning: SUICIDALITY AND ANTIDEPRESSANT DRUGS

Skin
Acneform eruption (2%)
Cellulitis (2%)
Dermatitis (2%)
Diaphoresis (29%) [2]
Edema (2%)
Flushing (8%)
Hypersensitivity [2]
Photosensitivity [3]
Pruritus (6%)

Purpura (3%)
Rash (8%)
Xerosis (2%)

Mucosal
Xerostomia (84%) [6]

Cardiovascular
QT prolongation [4]
Torsades de pointes [2]

Central Nervous System
Dysgeusia (taste perversion) (8%)
Seizures [4]
Serotonin syndrome [4]
Vertigo (dizziness) [2]

Neuromuscular/Skeletal
Myalgia/Myopathy (13%)

Gastrointestinal/Hepatic
Nausea [2]

Endocrine/Metabolic
Gynecomastia (2%)
SIADH [3]

Genitourinary
Vaginitis (2%)

Other
Adverse effects [4]
Allergic reactions (<3%)

CLONAZEPAM

Trade name: Klonopin (Roche)
Indications: Petit mal and myoclonic seizures
Class: Benzodiazepine
Half-life: 18–50 hours
Clinically important, potentially hazardous interactions with: amprenavir, chlorpheniramine, clarithromycin, cobicistat/elvitegravir/emtricitabine/tenofovir disoproxil, efavirenz, esomeprazole, imatinib, indinavir, nelfinavir, nevirapine, oxycodone, piracetam
Pregnancy category: D
Important contra-indications noted in the prescribing guidelines for: the elderly; nursing mothers; pediatric patients

---

Skin
Bullous dermatitis [2]
Dermatitis (<10%)
Diaphoresis (>10%)
Pseudolymphoma [2]
Rash (>10%)

Hair
Alopecia [2]

Mucosal
Sialopenia (>10%)
Sialorrhea (<10%)
Xerostomia (>10%)

Central Nervous System
Psychosis [2]
Seizures [2]

Other
Adverse effects [2]
Allergic reactions (<10%)

CLONIDINE

Trade name: Catapres (Boehringer Ingelheim)
Indications: Hypertension
Class: Adrenergic alpha-receptor agonist
Half-life: 6–24 hours
Clinically important, potentially hazardous interactions with: acebutolol, alfuzosin, amitriptyline, amoxapine, atenolol, betaxolol, captopril, carteolol, cilazapril, clomipramine, desipramine, dexmethylphenidate, diclofenac, doxepin, enalapril, esmolol, fosinopril, imipramine, insulin aspart, insulin degludec, insulin detemir, insulin glargine, insulin glulisine, irbesartan, levodopa, levomepromazine, lisinopril, meloxicam, metoprolol, milnacipran, nadolol, nebivolol, nortriptyline, olmesartan, oxprenolol, penbutolol, pericyazine, pindolol, propranolol, protriptyline, quinapril, ramipril, sotalol, sulpiride, timolol, trandolapril, triamcinolone, tricyclic antidepressants, trimipramine, verapamil
Pregnancy category: C
Important contra-indications noted in the prescribing guidelines for: nursing mothers; pediatric patients

---

Skin
Depigmentation [2]
Dermatitis (from patch) (20%) [23]
Eczema [2]
Erythema [2]
Lupus erythematosus [5]
Pigmentation [2]
Pityriasis rosea [2]
Pruritus (>5%) [6]
Psoriasis [2]
Rash (<10%) [4]
Ulcerations (<10%)

Mucosal
Xerostomia (40%) [13]

Cardiovascular
Bradycardia [8]
Hypotension [18]

Central Nervous System
Fever [2]
Hallucinations [3]
Headache [4]
Hyperesthesia (<10%)
Sedation [2]
Seizures [2]
Somnolence (drowsiness) [6]
Vertigo (dizziness) [4]

Neuromuscular/Skeletal
Asthenia (fatigue) [2]

Gastrointestinal/Hepatic
Nausea [2]

Other
Adverse effects [3]

CLOPIDOGREL

Trade name: Plavix (Bristol-Myers Squibb) (Sanofi-Aventis)
Indications: Acute coronary syndrome, recent myocardial infarction, recent stroke, or established peripheral arterial disease
Class: Antiplatelet, Antiplatelet, thienopyridine
Half-life: 6 hours
Clinically important, potentially hazardous interactions with: amiodarone, anisindione, anticoagulants, atorvastatin, calcium channel blockers, cangrelor, carbamazepine, chloramphenicol, cimetidine, ciprofloxacin, collagenase, dabigatran, dasatinib, delavirdine, dexlansoprazole, diclofenac, dicumarol, dipyridamole, drotrecogin alfa, efavirenz, enoxaparin, erythromycin, esomeprazole, etravirine, fluconazole, fluoxetine, fluvoxamine, fondaparinux, glucosamine, herbals with anticoagulant properties, ibritumomab, iloprost, itraconazole, ketoconazole, lansoprazole, lepirudin, macrolide antibiotics, meloxicam, miconazole, moclobemide, NSAIDs, omega-3 fatty acids, omeprazole, oxcarbazepine, pantoprazole, pentosan, pentoxifylline, polysulfate sodium, prasugrel, rabeprazole, rifapentine, rivaroxaban, salicylates, simvastatin, telithromycin, thrombolytic agents, tinzaparin, tositumomab & iodine^{131}, voriconazole, warfarin
Pregnancy category: B
Important contra-indications noted in the prescribing guidelines for: nursing mothers; pediatric patients
Note: Contra-indicated in patients with active pathological bleeding.
Warning: DIMINISHED EFFECTIVENESS IN POOR METABOLIZERS

Skin
AGEP [2]
Angioedema [4]
Bullous dermatitis (<3%)
Eczema (<3%)
Edema (3–5%)
Exanthems (<3%) [2]
Hypersensitivity [9]
Pruritus (3%) [2]
Psoriasis [2]
Purpura [18]
Rash (4%) [5]
Stevens-Johnson syndrome [2]
Thrombocytopenic purpura [9]
Ulcerations (<3%)
Urticaria (<3%) [3]

Cardiovascular
Acute coronary syndrome [2]
Myocardial infarction [2]

Central Nervous System
Ageusia (taste loss) [3]
Fever [3]
Hyperesthesia (<3%)
Intracranial hemorrhage [2]
Paresthesias (<3%)

Neuromuscular/Skeletal
Arthralgia [5]
Rhabdomyolysis [3]

Gastrointestinal/Hepatic
Gastrointestinal bleeding [3]
Hepatotoxicity [6]

Respiratory
Dyspnea [3]
Flu-like syndrome (8%)

Hematologic
Bleeding [17]
Hemolytic uremic syndrome [2]
Neutropenia [4]
Thrombocytopenia [3]
Thrombosis [2]

Ocular
Ocular hemorrhage [2]

Other
Adverse effects [2]
Allergic reactions (<3%) [2]

CLORAZEPATE

Trade name: Tranxene (Recordati)
Indications: Anxiety and panic disorders
Class: Benzodiazepine
Half-life: 48–96 hours
Clinically important, potentially hazardous interactions with: aminophylline, amprenavir, antacids, carbamazepine, carmustine, chlorpheniramine, clarithromycin, cobicistat/elvitegravir/emtricitabine/tenofovir alafenamide, cobicistat/elvitegravir/emtricitabine/tenofovir disoproxil, efavirenz, esomeprazole, imatinib, indinavir, itraconazole, ketoconazole, MAO inhibitors, midazolam, moclobemide, nelfinavir, phenytoin, sucralfate, warfarin
Pregnancy category: D
Important contra-indications noted in the prescribing guidelines for: nursing mothers; pediatric patients

---

Skin
Dermatitis (<10%)
Diaphoresis (>10%)
Rash (>10%)

Mucosal
Sialopenia (>10%)
Sialorrhea (<10%)
Xerostomia (>10%)

CLOZAPINE

Trade names: Clozaril (Novartis), Denzapine (Merz), Leponex (Novartis), Zaponex (Teva)
Indications: Treatment-resistant schizophrenia
Class: Antipsychotic
Half-life: 4–12 hours
Clinically important, potentially hazardous interactions with: alcohol, amitriptyline, antimuscarinics, arsenic, benzodiazepines, cabazitaxel, caffeine, carbamazepine, chloramphenicol, cimetidine, ciprofloxacin, citalopram, cocoa, cyclophosphamide, cytotoxics, darifenacin, dasatinib, encainide, epinephrine, erythromycin, everolimus, flecainide, fluoxetine, flupentixol, fluphenazine, fluvoxamine, gefitinib, guarana, haloperidol, insulin degludec, insulin detemir, insulin glargine, insulin glulisine, lapatinib, lithium, lomustine, lorazepam, MAO inhibitors, nilotinib, norfloxacin, ofloxacin, omeprazole, oxaliplatin, oxybutynin, paroxetine hydrochloride, pazopanib, pemetrexed, penicillamine, pipotiazine, propafenone, quinidine, rifampin, risperidone, ritonavir, saquinavir, selenium, sertraline, sorafenib, sulfonamides, sunitinib, telithromycin, temozolomide, temsirolimus, tetrazepam, tricyclic antidepressants, trospium, uracil/tegafur, valproic acid, venlafaxine, zuclopenthixol
Pregnancy category: B
Important contra-indications noted in the prescribing guidelines for: the elderly; nursing mothers; pediatric patients
Note: Contra-indicated in patients with myeloproliferative disorders, uncontrolled epilepsy, paralytic ileus, or a history of clozapine-induced agranulocytosis or severe granulocytopenia.
Warning: AGRANULOCYTOSIS / SEIZURES / MYOCARDITIS / OTHER ADVERSE CARDIOVASCULAR AND RESPIRATORY EFFECTS
INCREASED MORTALITY IN ELDERLY PATIENTS WITH DEMENTIA-RELATED PSYCHOSIS

Skin
Angioedema [2]
Diaphoresis (6%) [4]
Exanthems [2]
Lupus erythematosus [4]
Pityriasis rosea [2]
Rash (2%) [2]
Toxicity [5]

Mucosal
Parotitis [3]
Sialorrhea (31%) [77]
Xerostomia [3]

Cardiovascular
Atrial fibrillation [2]
Cardiomyopathy [15]
Cardiotoxicity [2]
Hypertension (4%) [4]
Hypotension (9%) [4]
Myocarditis [44]
Orthostatic hypotension [4]
Pericardial effusion [3]
Pericarditis [9]
QT prolongation [6]
Tachycardia (25%) [13]
Venous thromboembolism [5]

Central Nervous System
Akathisia [4]
Anxiety [2]
Compulsions [9]
Fever [8]
Headache (7%) [2]
Neuroleptic malignant syndrome [31]
Neurotoxicity [2]
Pain [2]
Restless legs syndrome [2]
Sedation (39%) [13]
Seizures [25]
Somnolence (drowsiness) [10]
Syncope [2]
Tardive dyskinesia [6]
Tic disorder [2]
Tremor (<10%) [2]
Vertigo (dizziness) (19%) [2]

Neuromuscular/Skeletal
Myoclonus [2]
Rhabdomyolysis [8]

Gastrointestinal/Hepatic
Colitis [2]
Constipation (14%) [6]
Gastric obstruction [3]
Gastrointestinal hypomotility [6]
Hepatotoxicity [6]
Ileus [6]
Pancreatitis [7]

Respiratory
Pleural effusion [4]
Pneumonia [3]
Pulmonary embolism [2]

Endocrine/Metabolic
Diabetes mellitus [7]
Diabetic ketoacidosis [2]
Galactorrhea [2]
Hyperglycemia [6]
Hyperlipidemia [3]
Metabolic syndrome [13]
Weight gain [29]

Genitourinary
Priapism [14]

Renal
Enuresis [4]
Nephrotoxicity [2]

Hematologic
Agranulocytosis [35]
Dyslipidemia [3]
Eosinophilia [10]
Granulocytopenia [2]
Hemotoxicity [2]
Leukopenia [11]
Neutropenia [19]
Pancytopenia [2]
Thrombosis [2]

Ocular
Maculopathy [2]

Other
Adverse effects [10]
Death [15]
Serositis [6]

CO-TRIMOXAZOLE

Synonyms: sulfamethoxazole-trimethoprim; SMX-TMP; SMZ-TMP; TMP-SMX; TMP-SMZ
Trade names: Bactrim (GSK), Septra (Monarch)
Indications: Various infections caused by susceptible organisms
Class: Antibiotic, sulfonamide
Half-life: 6–10 hours
Clinically important, potentially hazardous interactions with: anticoagulants, azathioprine, cyclosporine, dofetilide, isotretinoin, methotrexate, prilocaine, repaglinide, warfarin
Pregnancy category: C
Important contra-indications noted in the prescribing guidelines for: the elderly; nursing mothers; pediatric patients
Note: Co-trimoxazole is a sulfonamide and can be absorbed systemically. Sulfonamides can

produce severe, possibly fatal, reactions such as toxic epidermal necrolysis and Stevens-Johnson syndrome.
Co-trimoxazole is sulfamethoxazole and trimethoprim.

Skin
- AGEP [4]
- Anaphylactoid reactions/Anaphylaxis [6]
- Angioedema [3]
- Bullous dermatitis [2]
- Dermatitis [4]
- DRESS syndrome [10]
- Erythema multiforme [19]
- Erythema nodosum [2]
- Exanthems [35]
- Exfoliative dermatitis [5]
- Fixed eruption [51]
- Hypersensitivity [18]
- Jarisch-Herxheimer reaction [2]
- Linear IgA bullous dermatosis [4]
- Lupus erythematosus [4]
- Photosensitivity [4]
- Pruritus [10]
- Purpura [3]
- Pustules [6]
- Radiation recall dermatitis [3]
- Rash (>10%) [14]
- Stevens-Johnson syndrome (<10%) [42]
- Sweet's syndrome [9]
- Toxic epidermal necrolysis (<10%) [53]
- Toxicity [2]
- Urticaria [12]
- Vasculitis [11]

Mucosal
- Oral mucosal eruption [2]
- Oral ulceration [2]

Cardiovascular
- QT prolongation [2]
- Torsades de pointes [3]

Central Nervous System
- Aseptic meningitis [5]
- Fever [4]
- Psychosis [4]
- Tremor [4]
- Vertigo (dizziness) [2]

Neuromuscular/Skeletal
- Asthenia (fatigue) [2]
- Myalgia/Myopathy [2]
- Rhabdomyolysis [7]

Gastrointestinal/Hepatic
- Hepatotoxicity [7]
- Nausea [2]
- Pancreatitis [4]
- Vomiting [4]

Endocrine/Metabolic
- ALT increased [2]
- Hyperkalemia [4]
- Hypoglycemia [7]
- Hyponatremia [2]
- Serum creatinine increased [4]

Hematologic
- Agranulocytosis [3]
- Anemia [3]
- Methemoglobinemia [2]
- Neutropenia [5]
- Thrombocytopenia [10]

Ocular
- Glaucoma [2]
- Myopia [2]

Other
- Adverse effects [15]
- Allergic reactions [2]
- Death [4]
- Side effects [2]

COBICISTAT/ ELVITEGRAVIR/ EMTRICITABINE/ TENOFOVIR ALAFENAMIDE

Trade name: Genvoya (Gilead)
Indications: HIV-1 infection
Class: Antiretroviral, CYP3A inhibitor (cobicistat), Hepatitis B virus necleoside analog reverse transcriptase inhibitor (tenofovir alafenamide), Integrase strand transfer inhibitor (elvitegravir), Nucleoside analog reverse transcriptase inhibitor (emtricitabine)
Half-life: 3.5 hours (cobicistat); 13 hours (elvitegravir); 10 hours (emtricitabine); <1 hour (tenofovir alafenamide)
Clinically important, potentially hazardous interactions with: acyclovir, aminoglycosides, amiodarone, amitriptyline, amlodipine, antacids, antiarrhythmics, atorvastatin, benzodiazepines, bepridil, beta blockers, bosentan, buprenorphine, bupropion, buspirone, calcium channel blockers, cidofovir, clarithromycin, clorazepate, colchicine, desipramine, dexamethasone, diazepam, digoxin, diltiazem, disopyramide, drugs affecting renal function, estazolam, ethosuximide, felodipine, flecainide, flurazepam, fluticasone furoate, fluticasone propionate, ganciclovir, gentamicin, hormonal contraceptives, imipramine, immunosuppressants, itraconazole, ketoconazole, lidocaine, lorazepam, metoprolol, mexiletine, midazolam, naloxone, neuroleptics, nicardipine, nifedipine, nortriptyline, oxcarbazepine, paroxetine hydrochloride, perphenazine, propafenone, quinidine, rifabutin, rifapentine, risperidone, salmeterol, sildenafil, SSRIs, tadalafil, telithromycin, thioridazine, timolol, trazodone, tricyclic antidepressants, valacyclovir, valganciclovir, vardenafil, verapamil, voriconazole, warfarin, zolpidem
Pregnancy category: B
Important contra-indications noted in the prescribing guidelines for: nursing mothers
Note: See also separate profiles for emtricitabine and tenofovir alafenamide.
Warning: LACTIC ACIDOSIS/SEVERE HEPATOMEGALY WITH STEATOSIS and POST TREATMENT ACUTE EXACERBATION OF HEPATITIS B

Central Nervous System
- Headache (6%)

Neuromuscular/Skeletal
- Asthenia (fatigue) (5%)

Gastrointestinal/Hepatic
- Diarrhea (7%)
- Nausea (5%) [2]

Other
- Adverse effects [2]

COBICISTAT/ ELVITEGRAVIR/ EMTRICITABINE/ TENOFOVIR DISOPROXIL

Trade name: Stribild (Gilead)
Indications: HIV-1 infection
Class: Antiretroviral, CYP3A inhibitor (cobicistat), Integrase strand transfer inhibitor (elvitegravir), Nucleoside analog reverse transcriptase inhibitor (emtricitabine and tenofovir disoproxil)
Half-life: 3.5 hours (cobicistat); 13 hours (elvitegravir); 10 hours (emtricitabine); 12–18 hours (tenofovir disoproxil)
Clinically important, potentially hazardous interactions with: acyclovir, adefovir, amiodarone, amitriptyline, amlodipine, antacids, antirarrhythmics, antiretrovirals, atorvastatin, benzodiazepines, bepridil, beta blockers, bosentan, buprenorphine, bupropion, buspirone, calcium channel blockers, carbamazepine, cidofovir, clarithromycin, clonazepam, clorazepate, colchicine, cyclosporine, desipramine, dexamethasone, diazepam, digoxin, diltiazem, disopyramide, drugs affecting renal function, elbasvir & grazoprevir, emtricitabine, estazolam, ethosuximide, felodipine, flecainide, flurazepam, fluticasone propionate, ganciclovir, hormonal contraceptives, imipramine, immunosuppressants, itraconazole, ketoconazole, lamivudine, ledipasvir & sofosbuvir, lidocaine, metoprolol, mexiletine, midazolam, naloxone, neuroleptics, nicardipine, nifedipine, non-nucleoside reverse transcriptase inhibitors, nortriptyline, oxcarbazepine, paroxetine hydrochloride, perphenazine, phenobarbital, phenytoin, propafenone, protease inhibitors, quinidine, rifabutin, rifapentine, risperidone, ritonavir, salmeterol, sedatives / hypnotics, sildenafil, simeprevir, sirolimus, SSRIs, tacrolimus, tadalafil, telithromycin, tenofovir disoproxil, thioridazine, timolol, trazodone, tricyclic antidepressants, valacyclovir, valganciclovir, vardenafil, verapamil, voriconazole, warfarin, zolpidem
Pregnancy category: B
Important contra-indications noted in the prescribing guidelines for: the elderly; nursing mothers; pediatric patients
Note: See also separate profiles for emtricitabine and tenofovir disoproxil.
Warning: LACTIC ACIDOSIS/SEVERE HEPATOMEGALY WITH STEATOSIS and POST TREATMENT ACUTE EXACERBATION OF HEPATITIS B

Skin
- Rash (3%) [3]

Central Nervous System
Abnormal dreams (9%) [3]
Headache (7%) [5]
Insomnia (3%) [2]
Vertigo (dizziness) (3%) [3]

Neuromuscular/Skeletal
Asthenia (fatigue) (5%) [2]

Gastrointestinal/Hepatic
Diarrhea (12%) [6]
Flatulence (2%)
Gastrointestinal disorder [2]
Hepatotoxicity [2]
Nausea (16%) [8]

Respiratory
Upper respiratory tract infection [2]

Endocrine/Metabolic
AST increased (2%)
Serum creatinine increased [2]

Genitourinary
Hematuria (3%)

Renal
Nephrotoxicity [2]
Proteinuria (39%)

Other
Adverse effects [5]

COBIMETINIB

Trade name: Cotellic (Genentech)
Indications: Melanoma (unresectable or metastatic) in patients with BRAF V600E or V600K mutations, in combination with vemurafenib
Class: MEK inhibitor
Half-life: 23–70 hours
Clinically important, potentially hazardous interactions with: carbamazepine, efavirenz, itraconazole, phenytoin, rifampin, St John's wort, strong or moderate CYP3A4 inducers or inhibitors
Pregnancy category: N/A (Can cause fetal harm)
Important contra-indications noted in the prescribing guidelines for: nursing mothers; pediatric patients

---

Skin
Acneform eruption (16%) [3]
Basal cell carcinoma (5%)
Erythema (10%) [2]
Hyperkeratosis (11%) [3]
Keratoacanthoma [3]
Photosensitivity (46%) [8]
Rash [7]
Squamous cell carcinoma (6%) [6]

Hair
Alopecia (15%) [3]

Mucosal
Stomatitis (14%)

Cardiovascular
Hypertension (15%)

Central Nervous System
Chills (10%)
Fever (28%) [4]

Neuromuscular/Skeletal
Arthralgia [4]
Asthenia (fatigue) [6]
Myalgia/Myopathy [2]

Gastrointestinal/Hepatic
Diarrhea (60%) [8]
Gastrointestinal bleeding (4%)
Hepatotoxicity [5]
Nausea (41%) [7]
Vomiting (24%) [4]

Respiratory
Pneumonitis (<10%)

Endocrine/Metabolic
ALP increased (71%) [3]
ALT increased (68%) [3]
AST increased (73%) [3]
Creatine phosphokinase increased (79%) [4]
GGT increased (65%)
Hyperkalemia (26%)
Hypoalbuminemia (42%)
Hypocalcemia (24%)
Hypokalemia (25%)
Hyponatremia (38%)
Hypophosphatemia (68%)
Serum creatinine increased (100%)

Genitourinary
Hematuria (2%)

Hematologic
Anemia (69%) [3]
Hemorrhage (13%)
Lymphopenia (73%)
Thrombocytopenia (18%)

Ocular
Chorioretinopathy (13%) [3]
Retinal detachment (12%) [2]
Vision impaired (15%)

COCAINE

Indications: Topical anesthesia
Class: Anesthetic, local, CNS stimulant
Half-life: 75 minutes
Clinically important, potentially hazardous interactions with: epinephrine, iobenguane
Pregnancy category: C (the pregnancy category is X for non-medicinal use)

Skin
Angioedema [3]
Diaphoresis [3]
Hyperkeratosis (fingers and palms) [2]
Necrosis [6]
Purpura [4]
Raynaud's phenomenon [2]
Scleroderma (reversible) [3]
Vasculitis [14]

Mucosal
Nasal septal perforation [4]
Palatal perforation [7]

Cardiovascular
Angina [2]
Brugada syndrome [3]
Chest pain [5]
Myocardial infarction [6]
Myocardial ischemia [2]

Central Nervous System
Ageusia (taste loss) (>10%)
Anosmia (>10%)
Compulsions [2]
Hallucinations [4]
Leukoencephalopathy [3]
Psychosis [2]
Seizures [6]
Suicidal ideation [2]
Tic disorder [2]
Tremor (<10%)

Neuromuscular/Skeletal
Arthralgia [2]
Rhabdomyolysis [19]

Genitourinary
Priapism [5]

Renal
Glomerulonephritis [2]
Nephrotoxicity [2]

Hematologic
Agranulocytosis [2]
Hemolytic uremic syndrome [2]
Neutropenia [6]

Otic
Hallucinations, auditory [2]

Ocular
Hallucinations, visual [3]

Other
Death [3]

COCOA

Family: Sterculiaceae
Scientific names: *Theobroma cacao, Theobroma sativum*
Indications: Oral: asthma, bronchitis, cardiovascular disease, diarrhea. **Topical:** cosmetics, pharmaceutical preparations, foods. Chocolate is produced from cocoa powder
Class: Food supplement
Half-life: 5 hours
Clinically important, potentially hazardous interactions with: aminophylline, caffeine, cimetidine, clozapine, ephedra
Pregnancy category: N/A

Skin
Prurigo [2]

Central Nervous System
Headache [4]
Migraine [4]

CODEINE

Synonym: methylmorphine
Trade names: Halotussin (Watson), Nucofed (Monarch), Robitussin AC (Wyeth), Tussi-Organidin (MedPointe)
Indications: Pain, cough suppressant
Class: Opiate agonist
Half-life: 2.5–4 hours
Clinically important, potentially hazardous interactions with: alcohol, cinacalcet, CNS depressants, delavirdine, MAO inhibitors, mianserin, terbinafine, tipranavir

Pregnancy category: C
Important contra-indications noted in the prescribing guidelines for: the elderly; nursing mothers; pediatric patients
Warning: DEATH RELATED TO ULTRA-RAPID METABOLISM OF CODEINE TO MORPHINE

Skin
- Angioedema [2]
- Dermatitis [5]
- Erythema multiforme [4]
- Exanthems [6]
- Fixed eruption [6]
- Pruritus [3]
- Rash (<10%)
- Toxic epidermal necrolysis [2]
- Urticaria (<10%) [9]

Mucosal
- Xerostomia (<10%)

Central Nervous System
- Somnolence (drowsiness) [3]
- Vertigo (dizziness) [2]

Gastrointestinal/Hepatic
- Constipation [3]
- Nausea [2]
- Pancreatitis [5]
- Vomiting [2]

Respiratory
- Respiratory depression [4]

Local
- Injection-site pain (<10%)

Other
- Death [5]

COENZYME Q-10

Family: None
Scientific names: *Mitoquinone, Ubidecarenone, Ubiquinone*
Indications: Congestive heart failure, angina, diabetes, hypertension, breast cancer, increasing exercise tolerance, muscular dystrophy, chronic fatigue
Class: Food supplement
Half-life: N/A
Clinically important, potentially hazardous interactions with: none known
Note: CoQ-10 was first identified in 1957. It is widely used in Japan where millions of Japanese patients receive CoQ-10 as part of their treatment for congestive heart failure.

COLCHICINE

Indications: Gouty arthritis (in adults), gout, familial Mediterranean fever
Class: Alkaloid, Anti-inflammatory
Half-life: 27–31 hours (following multiple doses)
Clinically important, potentially hazardous interactions with: amiodarone, aprepitant, atazanavir, atorvastatin, azithromycin, boceprevir, clarithromycin, cobicistat/elvitegravir/emtricitabine/tenofovir alafenamide, cobicistat/elvitegravir/emtricitabine/tenofovir disoproxil, conivaptan, cyanocobalamin, cyclosporine, darunavir, dasatinib, delavirdine, digoxin, diltiazem, efavirenz, erythromycin, fenofibrate, fibrates, fluvastatin, gemfibrozil, grapefruit juice, HMG-CoA reductase inhibitors, indinavir, itraconazole, ketoconazole, lapatinib, lopinavir, ombitasvir/paritaprevir/ritonavir, P-glycoprotein inhibitors or inducers, pravastatin, protease inhibitors, ritonavir, rosuvastatin, saxagliptin, simvastatin, strong CYP3A4 inhibitors, telithromycin, troleandomycin, verapamil, voriconazole
Pregnancy category: C
Important contra-indications noted in the prescribing guidelines for: the elderly
Note: Contra-indicated in patients with renal or hepatic impairment where P-glycoprotein or strong CYP3A4 inhibitors are also prescribed.

Skin
- Pruritus [2]
- Staphylococcal scalded skin syndrome [2]
- Toxic epidermal necrolysis [3]
- Vasculitis [2]

Hair
- Alopecia (<10%) [6]

Central Nervous System
- Headache (2%)
- Neurotoxicity [3]

Neuromuscular/Skeletal
- Asthenia (fatigue) (<4%)
- Gouty tophi (4%)
- Myalgia/Myopathy [20]
- Rhabdomyolysis [18]

Gastrointestinal/Hepatic
- Abdominal pain (<20%) [2]
- Diarrhea (23%) [6]
- Gastrointestinal disorder [2]
- Hepatotoxicity [3]
- Nausea (<20%) [3]
- Vomiting (<20%) [4]

Respiratory
- Pharyngolaryngeal pain (3%)

Other
- Adverse effects [6]
- Death [3]
- Side effects (14%)

COLESEVELAM

Trade names: Cholestagel (Genzyme), Welchol (Sankyo)
Indications: Hypercholesterolemia, hyperlipidemia, Type II diabetes mellitus
Class: Bile acid sequestrant
Half-life: N/A
Clinically important, potentially hazardous interactions with: cyclosporine, deferasirox, estradiol, glyburide, levothyroxine, olmesartan, phenytoin, warfarin
Pregnancy category: B
Important contra-indications noted in the prescribing guidelines for: pediatric patients
Note: Contra-indicated in patients with a history of bowel obstruction, with serum triglyceride concentrations >500 mg/dL or with a history of hypertriglyceridemia-induced pancreatitis.

Cardiovascular
- Hypertension (3%)

Central Nervous System
- Headache [2]

Neuromuscular/Skeletal
- Myalgia/Myopathy (2%)

Gastrointestinal/Hepatic
- Abdominal pain (4%)
- Constipation (9–10%) [3]
- Diarrhea (3%)
- Dyspepsia (4–6%) [3]
- Flatulence (11%)
- Gastrointestinal disorder [4]
- Nausea (3%)

Respiratory
- Nasopharyngitis (4%)

Endocrine/Metabolic
- Hypoglycemia (3%) [3]

Other
- Adverse effects [4]

COLLAGEN (BOVINE)

Trade names: Bellafill (Suneva), Zyderm (Inamed), Zyplast (Inamed)
Indications: Cataract surgery (collagen shields), depressed cutaneous scars, facial lines, wrinkles, glottic insufficiency, phonosurgey, urinary incontinence
Class: Protein
Half-life: Several months to years
Clinically important, potentially hazardous interactions with: argatroban, avitene
Pregnancy category: N/A
Important contra-indications noted in the prescribing guidelines for: nursing mothers
Note: A reaction to the anesthetic, lidocaine, in liquid collagen injections may occur. Artecoll and Bellafill contain polymethyl-methacrylate microspheres.

Skin
- Abscess [2]
- Churg-Strauss syndrome [7]
- Dermatomyositis [3]
- Edema [2]
- Erythema [3]
- Granulomatous reaction [2]
- Hypersensitivity [10]
- Induration [3]
- Panniculitis [2]

Neuromuscular/Skeletal
- Arthralgia [2]
- Polymyositis [3]

Other
- Adverse effects [12]
- Allergic reactions [7]

COMFREY

Family: Boraginaceae
Scientific names: *Symphytum asperum, Symphytum officinale, Symphytum peregrinum, Symphytum x uplandicum*
Indications: Leaf: Gastric and duodenal ulcer, rheumatic pain, gout, arthritis. **Topical:** poultice for bruises, sprains, athlete's foot, crural ulcers, mastitis, varicose ulcers. **Root**: Gastric and duodenal ulcers, hematemesis, colitis, diarrhea. **Topical:** ulcers, wounds, fractures, hernia
Class: Carminative
Half-life: N/A
Clinically important, potentially hazardous interactions with: eucalyptus
Pregnancy category: N/A
Note: The FDA warns that comfrey contains pyrrolizidine alkaloids that can cause cirrhosis and liver failure when taken orally in high doses. Topical application is safer and more effective; allantoin in comfrey stimulates cell proliferation, accelerating wound healing.
Oral products containing comfrey are banned in the USA, UK, Australia, Canada and Germany.

Skin
Erythema [2]
Pruritus [2]

Cardiovascular
Veno-occlusive disease [4]

Gastrointestinal/Hepatic
Hepatotoxicity [3]

Local
Application-site reactions [2]

Other
Adverse effects [2]
Death [2]

CONIVAPTAN

Trade name: Vaprisol (Astellas)
Indications: Hyponatremia, SIADH
Class: CYP3A4 inhibitor, Vasopressin receptor antagonist
Half-life: 5 hours
Clinically important, potentially hazardous interactions with: acetaminophen, albendazole, alfuzosin, almotriptan, alosetron, ambrisentan, amitriptyline, amlodipine, antifungals, aprepitant, artemether/lumefantrine, atorvastatin, bexarotene, bortezomib, brigatinib, brinzolamide, bupivacaine, cabazitaxel, cabozantinib, ciclesonide, cilostazol, cinacalcet, citalopram, clarithromycin, colchicine, copanlisib, cyclobenzaprine, CYP3A4 inhibitors or substrates, darunavir, dasatinib, deferasirox, delavirdine, dienogest, digoxin, docetaxel, dronedarone, dutasteride, efavirenz, enalapril, eplerenone, estradiol, eszopiclone, everolimus, fentanyl, fesoterodine, fingolimod, flibanserin, gefitinib, guanfacine, halofantrine, indinavir, itraconazole, ixabepilone, ketoconazole, lapatinib, lomitapide, maraviroc, meloxicam, metaxalone, methylprednisolone, micafungin, midazolam, midostaurin, mifepristone, mometasone, neratinib, nilotinib, nisoldipine, oxybutynin, pantoprazole, paricalcitol, pazopanib, pimecrolimus, pioglitazone, ponatinib, prasugrel, ramelteon, ranolazine, ribociclib, ritonavir, rivaroxaban, romidepsin, rosuvastatin, ruxolitinib, salmeterol, saxagliptin, sildenafil, silodosin, simvastatin, sorafenib, St John's wort, tadalafil, tamsulosin, telithromycin, temsirolimus, terbinafine, tiagabine, tiotropium, tipranavir, tolvaptan, trimethoprim, ulipristal, vardenafil, venetoclax, vorapaxar, voriconazole, ziprasidone
Pregnancy category: C
Important contra-indications noted in the prescribing guidelines for: nursing mothers; pediatric patients

Skin
Erythema (3%)
Peripheral edema (3–8%)
Pruritus (<5%)

Mucosal
Oral candidiasis (2%)
Xerostomia (4%)

Cardiovascular
Atrial fibrillation (2–5%)
Hypertension (6–8%)
Hypotension (5–8%) [4]
Orthostatic hypotension (6–14%)
Phlebitis (32–51%)

Central Nervous System
Confusion (<5%)
Fever (5–11%) [2]
Headache (8–10%)
Insomnia (4–5%)

Gastrointestinal/Hepatic
Constipation (6–8%)
Diarrhea (<7%)
Nausea (3–5%)
Vomiting (5–7%)

Respiratory
Pharyngolaryngeal pain (<5%)
Pneumonia (2–5%)

Endocrine/Metabolic
Hypokalemia (10–22%)
Hypomagnesemia (2–5%)
Hyponatremia (6–8%)

Genitourinary
Urinary tract infection (4–5%)

Hematologic
Anemia (5–6%)

Local
Infusion-site erythema (<6%)
Infusion-site pain (<5%)
Infusion-site reactions (63–73%) [5]

Other
Dipsia (thirst) (3–6%) [2]

COPANLISIB

Trade name: Aliqopa (Bayer)
Indications: Relapsed follicular lymphoma in adult patients who have received at least two prior systemic therapies
Class: Kinase inhibitor
Half-life: 39 hours
Clinically important, potentially hazardous interactions with: boceprevir, carbamazepine, clarithromycin, cobicistat, conivaptan, danoprevir, dasabuvir/ombitasvir/paritaprevir/ritonavir, diltiazem, elvitegravir, enzalutamide, grapefruit juice, idelalisib, indinavir, itraconazole, ketoconazole, lopinavir, mitotane, nefazodone, nelfinavir, phenytoin, posaconazole, rifampin, ritonavir, saquinavir, St John's wort, strong CYP3A4 inducers or inhibitors, tipranavir, troleandomycin, voriconazole
Pregnancy category: N/A (Can cause fetal harm)
Important contra-indications noted in the prescribing guidelines for: nursing mothers; pediatric patients

Skin
Rash (15%)

Mucosal
Mucosal inflammation (8%)
Stomatitis (14%)

Cardiovascular
Hypertension (26%) [3]

Central Nervous System
Dysesthesia (7%)
Paresthesias (7%)

Neuromuscular/Skeletal
Asthenia (fatigue) (36%)

Gastrointestinal/Hepatic
Diarrhea (36%)
Nausea (26%) [2]
Vomiting (13%)

Respiratory
Pneumonitis (9%)

Endocrine/Metabolic
Hyperglycemia (54%) [5]
Hypertriglyceridemia (58%)
Hyperuricemia (25%)
Hypophosphatemia (44%)

Hematologic
Hemoglobin decreased (78%)
Hyperlipasemia (21%)
Leukopenia (36%)
Lymphopenia (78%)
Neutropenia (32%)
Thrombocytopenia (22%)

Other
Infection (21%)

CORDYCEPS

Family: Ascomycetes; Clavicipitaceae
Scientific name: *Cordyceps sinensis*
Indications: Anemia, arrhythmia, anti-aging, atherosclerosis, bronchitis, cough, dizziness, hyperlipidemia, athletic performance, lethargy, liver disorders, male sexual dysfunction, nocturia, tinnitus
Class: Immunomodulator
Half-life: N/A
Clinically important, potentially hazardous interactions with: none known
Pregnancy category: N/A

CORTISONE

Trade name: Cortone (Merck)
Indications: Arthralgia, dermatoses
Class: Corticosteroid
Half-life: N/A
Clinically important, potentially hazardous interactions with: chlorpropamide, diuretics, ethambutol, live vaccines, pancuronium, rifampin
Pregnancy category: C
Important contra-indications noted in the prescribing guidelines for: nursing mothers

---

Neuromuscular/Skeletal
Osteonecrosis [15]
Osteoporosis [10]
Tendinopathy/Tendon rupture [2]

Ocular
Cataract [5]
Glaucoma [8]

Other
Adverse effects [2]

CRANBERRY

Family: Ericaceae
Scientific name: *Vaccinium oxycoccus*
Indications: Erythema, hyperplasia, thrush, cystitis, prevention of urinary tract infections, tumor inhibition, influenza, common cold, scurvy, pleurisy
Class: Diuretic, Proanthocyanadin
Half-life: N/A
Clinically important, potentially hazardous interactions with: none known
Pregnancy category: N/A
Note: Cranberry juice contains oxalates, a common component of kidney stones, and should be limited in patients with a history of nephrolithiasis.

CREATINE

Scientific names: *N-(aminoiminomethyl)-N methyl glycine, N-amidinosarcosine*
Indications: Improve exercise performance, increase muscle mass, heart failure, neuromuscular disease, cholesterol-lowering, amyotrophic lateral sclerosis, rheumatoid arthritis, cardiac surgery (IV)
Class: Food supplement
Half-life: N/A
Clinically important, potentially hazardous interactions with: none known
Pregnancy category: N/A
Note: Creatine is found primarily in skeletal muscle (95%), also in heart, brain, testes and other tissues. The body synthesizes 1–2 grams of creatine a day.
Creatine use is widespread among amateur and professional athletes including, Mark McGuire, Sammy Sosa, John Elway and others. Americans use more than 4 million kilograms of creatine each year.

Neuromuscular/Skeletal
Myalgia/Myopathy [2]
Rhabdomyolysis [5]

Gastrointestinal/Hepatic
Hepatotoxicity [3]

Renal
Nephrotoxicity [2]

Other
Adverse effects [2]

CRISABOROLE

Trade name: Eucrisa (Pfizer)
Indications: Atopic dermatitis
Class: Phosphodiesterase type 4 (PDE4) inhibitor
Half-life: N/A
Clinically important, potentially hazardous interactions with: none known
Pregnancy category: N/A (No available data)
Important contra-indications noted in the prescribing guidelines for: nursing mothers; pediatric patients

---

Local
Application-site burning [3]
Application-site pain (4%) [4]
Application-site stinging [2]

CRIZOTINIB

Trade name: Xalkori (Pfizer)
Indications: Advanced or metastatic non-small cell lung cancer in ALK-positive patients
Class: Tyrosine kinase inhibitor
Half-life: 42 hours
Clinically important, potentially hazardous interactions with: alfentanil, atazanavir, carbamazepine, clarithromycin, cyclosporine, CYP3A4 inducers, inhibitors or substrates, dihydroergotamine, efavirenz, ergotamine, fentanyl, grapefruit juice, indinavir, itraconazole, ketoconazole, nefazodone, nelfinavir, neratinib, olaparib, phenobarbital, phenytoin, pimozide, quinidine, rifabutin, rifampin, ritonavir, saquinavir, sirolimus, St John's wort, tacrolimus, telithromycin, troleandomycin, voriconazole
Pregnancy category: D
Important contra-indications noted in the prescribing guidelines for: nursing mothers; pediatric patients

---

Skin
Edema (38%) [13]
Peripheral edema [6]
Photosensitivity [2]
Rash (16%) [4]

Mucosal
Stomatitis (11%)

Cardiovascular
Bradycardia (5%) [7]
Cardiotoxicity [2]
Chest pain (12%)
QT prolongation [9]

Central Nervous System
Dysgeusia (taste perversion) (13%) [6]
Fever (12%) [2]
Headache (13%)
Insomnia (12%)
Neurotoxicity (23%) [2]
Vertigo (dizziness) (24%) [6]

Neuromuscular/Skeletal
Arthralgia (11%)
Asthenia (fatigue) (31%) [13]
Back pain (11%)
Bone or joint pain [2]

Gastrointestinal/Hepatic
Abdominal pain (16%) [2]
Constipation (38%) [14]
Diarrhea (49%) [28]
Dyspepsia [3]
Dysphagia [3]
Esophagitis [8]
Gastroesophageal reflux [2]
Hepatitis [2]
Hepatotoxicity [14]
Nausea (57%) [26]
Vomiting (45%) [25]

Respiratory
Cough (21%)
Dyspnea (22%)
Pneumonia [2]
Pneumonitis [6]
Pulmonary toxicity [11]
Upper respiratory tract infection (20%)

Endocrine/Metabolic
ALT increased (15%) [12]
Appetite decreased (27%) [5]
AST increased (11%) [10]
Dehydration [2]
Hyperbilirubinemia [2]
Hypocalcemia [2]
Hypogonadism [6]
Hypophosphatemia [5]

Renal
Nephrotoxicity [10]

Hematologic
Anemia [3]
Leukopenia [2]
Lymphopenia (11%) [5]
Neutropenia (5%) [10]

Ocular
Diplopia [2]
Ocular adverse effects (64%) [13]
Photophobia [2]
Photopsia [3]
Reduced visual acuity [2]
Vision blurred [7]
Vision impaired [3]

Visual disturbances [17]
Vitreous floaters [2]

Other
Adverse effects [5]
Death [3]

CROFELEMER

Trade name: Fulyzaq (Salix)
Indications: Non-infectious diarrhea in adult patients with HIV/AIDS on anti-retroviral therapy
Class: Proanthocyanidin oligomer
Half-life: N/A
Clinically important, potentially hazardous interactions with: none known
Pregnancy category: C
Important contra-indications noted in the prescribing guidelines for: the elderly; nursing mothers; pediatric patients
Note: Derived from the red latex of *Croton lechleri* which is also known as Sangre de Drago or dragon's blood.

Skin
Acneform eruption (<2%)
Dermatitis (<2%)
Herpes zoster (<2%)

Mucosal
Xerostomia (<2%)

Central Nervous System
Anxiety (2%)
Depression (<2%)
Vertigo (dizziness) (<2%)

Neuromuscular/Skeletal
Arthralgia (3%)
Back pain (3%)
Bone or joint pain (2%)
Pain in extremities (<2%)

Gastrointestinal/Hepatic
Abdominal distension (2%)
Abdominal pain (<2%)
Constipation (<2%)
Dyspepsia (<2%)
Flatulence (3%)
Gastroenteritis (<2%)
Nausea (3%)

Respiratory
Bronchitis (4%)
Cough (4%)
Nasopharyngitis (2%)
Sinusitis (<2%)
Upper respiratory tract infection (6%)

Endocrine/Metabolic
ALT increased (2%)
AST increased (<2%)

Genitourinary
Pollakiuria (<2%)

Renal
Nephrolithiasis (<2%)

Hematologic
Leukopenia (<2%)

Other
Infection (giardiasis) (2%)

CYANOCOBALAMIN

Synonym: Vitamin B_{12}
Trade name: Nascobal (Nastech)
Indications: Vitamin B_{12} deficiency, pernicious anemia
Class: Vitamin
Half-life: 6 days
Clinically important, potentially hazardous interactions with: colchicine
Pregnancy category: C

Skin
Acneform eruption [8]
Anaphylactoid reactions/Anaphylaxis [6]
Dermatitis [2]
Exanthems [3]
Hypersensitivity [2]
Nicolau syndrome [2]
Pruritus (<10%)
Urticaria [7]

Other
Allergic reactions [3]

CYCLOBENZAPRINE

Trade name: Flexeril (McNeil)
Indications: Muscle spasms
Class: Central muscle relaxant
Half-life: 8–37 hours
Clinically important, potentially hazardous interactions with: acetylcholinesterase inhibitors, anticholinergics, barbiturates, cisapride, CNS depressants, conivaptan, CYP1A2 inhibitors, droperidol, levomepromazine, linezolid, MAO inhibitors, phendimetrazine, pramlintide, safinamide
Pregnancy category: B
Important contra-indications noted in the prescribing guidelines for: the elderly; nursing mothers; pediatric patients

---

Mucosal
Xerostomia (7–32%) [7]

Central Nervous System
Confusion (<3%)
Dysgeusia (taste perversion) (<3%)
Headache (5%) [3]
Irritability (<3%)
Nervousness (<3%)
Serotonin syndrome [3]
Somnolence (drowsiness) (29–39%) [8]
Vertigo (dizziness) (<11%) [8]

Neuromuscular/Skeletal
Asthenia (fatigue) (6%) [3]

Gastrointestinal/Hepatic
Abdominal pain (<3%)
Constipation (<3%) [3]
Diarrhea (<3%)
Nausea (<3%)

Respiratory
Pharyngitis (<3%)
Upper respiratory tract infection (<3%)

Ocular
Vision blurred (<3%)

Other
Adverse effects [2]

CYCLOPHOSPHAMIDE

Synonyms: CPM; CTX; CYT
Trade names: Cytoxan (Mead Johnson), Neosar (Gensia)
Indications: Lymphomas, minimal change nephrotic syndrome in pediatric patients
Class: Alkylating agent
Half-life: 3–12 hours
Clinically important, potentially hazardous interactions with: aldesleukin, azathioprine, belimumab, clozapine, cyclopenthiazide, cyclosporine, dexamethasone, etanercept, itraconazole, mycophenolate, pentostatin, prednisone, vaccines
Pregnancy category: D
Important contra-indications noted in the prescribing guidelines for: nursing mothers
Note: Contra-indicated in patients with urinary outflow obstruction.

Skin
Acral erythema [3]
Anaphylactoid reactions/Anaphylaxis [3]
Edema [5]
Exanthems [4]
Flushing (<10%)
Graft-versus-host reaction [2]
Hand–foot syndrome [10]
Herpes zoster [4]
Hypersensitivity [6]
Kaposi's sarcoma [2]
Lupus erythematosus [2]
Lymphoma [4]
Malignancies [2]
Pemphigus [2]
Pigmentation [16]
Pruritus [2]
Radiation recall dermatitis [6]
Rash (<10%) [6]
Scleroderma [2]
Squamous cell carcinoma [2]
Stevens-Johnson syndrome [2]
Toxicity [6]
Urticaria [8]
Vasculitis [2]

Hair
Alopecia [30]

Nails
Leukonychia (Mees' lines) (Muehrcke's lines) [3]
Melanonychia [2]
Nail pigmentation [16]

Mucosal
Gingival pigmentation [2]
Mucositis [4]
Oral mucositis [2]
Oral ulceration [2]
Stomatitis (10%) [6]

Cardiovascular
Atrial fibrillation [2]
Cardiotoxicity [6]
Hypotension [2]

Central Nervous System
Anorexia [3]
Dysgeusia (taste perversion) [2]
Fever [3]
Headache [3]

Leukoencephalopathy [6]
Neurotoxicity [7]
Peripheral neuropathy [8]

Neuromuscular/Skeletal
Arthralgia [2]
Asthenia (fatigue) [15]
Myalgia/Myopathy [7]

Gastrointestinal/Hepatic
Abdominal pain [2]
Constipation [2]
Diarrhea [9]
Hepatotoxicity [11]
Nausea [12]
Vomiting [12]

Respiratory
Pneumonia [4]

Endocrine/Metabolic
Amenorrhea [16]
Hyperglycemia [2]
Hyponatremia [4]
Menstrual irregularities [2]
SIADH [9]

Genitourinary
Cystitis [10]
Urinary tract infection [2]

Hematologic
Anemia [11]
Cytopenia [2]
Febrile neutropenia [16]
Hemorrhage [2]
Hemotoxicity [10]
Leukopenia [13]
Lymphopenia [3]
Myelosuppression [5]
Neutropenia [37]
Sepsis [2]
Thrombocytopenia [17]

Local
Infusion-related reactions [2]

Other
Adverse effects [17]
Allergic reactions [2]
Death [9]
Hiccups [4]
Infection [22]

CYCLOSERINE

Trade name: Seromycin (Lilly)
Indications: Tuberculosis
Class: Antibiotic
Half-life: 10 hours
Clinically important, potentially hazardous interactions with: none known
Pregnancy category: C
Important contra-indications noted in the prescribing guidelines for: nursing mothers; pediatric patients

---

Skin
Dermatitis [2]
Exanthems [4]
Lichenoid eruption [2]

Mucosal
Gingival hyperplasia/hypertrophy [3]

Central Nervous System
Depression [2]
Neurotoxicity [2]
Psychosis [7]
Seizures [4]
Suicidal ideation [2]

Renal
Nephrotoxicity [2]

Other
Adverse effects [4]

CYCLOSPORINE

Synonyms: CsA; CyA
Trade names: Neoral (Novartis), Restasis (Allergan), Sandimmune (Novartis)
Indications: Rheumatoid arthritis, prophylaxis of organ rejection in transplants, psoriasis, Restasis is indicated for patients with moderate-to-severe dry eye syndrome
Class: Calcineurin inhibitor, Disease-modifying antirheumatic drug (DMARD), Immunosuppressant
Half-life: 10–27 hours (adults)
Clinically important, potentially hazardous interactions with: afatinib, aliskiren, ambrisentan, amiloride, aminoglycosides, amiodarone, amphotericin B, ampicillin, amprenavir, anisindione, anticoagulants, armodafinil, atazanavir, atorvastatin, azathioprine, azithromycin, bacampicillin, basiliximab, benazepril, bezafibrate, boceprevir, bosentan, bupropion, captopril, carbenicillin, caspofungin, ceritinib, cholestyramine, cholic acid, choline fenofibrate, cilazapril, ciprofloxacin, clarithromycin, cloxacillin, co-trimoxazole, cobicistat/elvitegravir/emtricitabine/tenofovir disoproxil, colchicine, colesevelam, corticosteroids, crizotinib, cyclophosphamide, dabigatran, daclizumab, danazol, daptomycin, darifenacin, darunavir, dasatinib, delavirdine, dichlorphenamide, diclofenac, dicloxacillin, dicumarol, digoxin, diltiazem, disulfiram, docetaxel, doxycycline, dronedarone, echinacea, efavirenz, elbasvir & grazoprevir, eluxadoline, enalapril, enzalutamide, erythromycin, ethotoin, etoposide, etoricoxib, everolimus, ezetimibe, flunisolide, fluoxymesterone, fluvastatin, foscarnet, fosinopril, fosphenytoin, gemfibrozil, glecaprevir & pibrentasvir, grapefruit juice, Hemophilus B vaccine, HMG-CoA reductase inhibitors, imatinib, imipenem/cilastatin, indinavir, influenza vaccine, irbesartan, itraconazole, ketoconazole, lanreotide, letermovir, levofloxacin, lisinopril, lopinavir, lovastatin, meloxicam, mephenytoin, methicillin, methoxsalen, methylphenidate, methylprednisolone, methyltestosterone, mezlocillin, micafungin, mifepristone, mizolastine, moxifloxacin, mycophenolate, nafcillin, naldemedine, natalizumab, nelfinavir, neratinib, nevirapine, nifedipine, nisoldipine, norfloxacin, NSAIDs, ofloxacin, olmesartan, omeprazole, orlistat, osimertinib, oxacillin, oxcarbazepine, pasireotide, penicillins, phenytoin, pitavastatin, posaconazole, pravastatin, prednisolone, prednisone, pristinamycin, quinapril, rabeprazole, ramipril, ranolazine, ribociclib, rifabutin, rifampin, rifapentine, ritonavir, rosuvastatin, sevelamer, silodosin, simvastatin, sirolimus, sofosbuvir/velpatasvir/voxilaprevir, spironolactone, St John's wort, sulfacetamide, sulfadiazine, sulfamethoxazole, sulfisoxazole, sulfonamides, tacrolimus, telithromycin, temsirolimus, tenoxicam, terbinafine, testosterone, ticarcillin, tinidazole, tipranavir, tofacitinib, tolvaptan, trabectedin, trandolapril, triamterene, trimethoprim, troleandomycin, ursodiol, vaccines, vecuronium, venetoclax, voriconazole, warfarin, zofenopril
Pregnancy category: C
Important contra-indications noted in the prescribing guidelines for: nursing mothers; pediatric patients
Note: Restasis is an ophthalmic emulsion.

Skin
Acne keloid [2]
Acneform eruption [7]
Anaphylactoid reactions/Anaphylaxis [8]
Basal cell carcinoma [4]
Candidiasis [2]
Cyst [5]
Edema (5–14%)
Fibroadenoma [2]
Flushing (2–5%) [5]
Folliculitis [8]
Herpes simplex [4]
Herpes zoster [2]
Hot flashes [2]
Hypersensitivity [2]
Kaposi's sarcoma [5]
Keratoses [3]
Keratosis pilaris [2]
Linear IgA bullous dermatosis [2]
Lymphocytic infiltration [5]
Lymphoma [12]
Lymphoproliferative disease [2]
Malignancies [2]
Mycosis fungoides [2]
Peripheral edema [3]
Pruritus (<2%) [2]
Pseudolymphoma [6]
Psoriasis [2]
Purpura (3%) [4]
Rash (7–12%)
Raynaud's phenomenon [2]
Sebaceous hyperplasia [9]
Squamous cell carcinoma [12]
Thrombocytopenic purpura [5]
Toxicity [2]
Urticaria [2]
Vasculitis [3]

Hair
Alopecia (3–4%) [2]
Alopecia areata [6]
Hirsutism [10]
Hypertrichosis (5–19%) [35]
Pseudofolliculitis barbae [2]

Nails
Brittle nails (<2%)
Leukonychia (Mees' lines) [2]

Mucosal
Aphthous stomatitis [2]
Gingival hyperplasia/hypertrophy (2–6%) [160]
Gingivitis (3–4%)
Oral ulceration [2]
Rectal hemorrhage (<3%)
Stomatitis (5–7%)

Cardiovascular
Arrhythmias (2–5%)
Capillary leak syndrome [2]
Chest pain (4–6%)
Hypertension (8–28%) [27]

Central Nervous System
Anorexia (3%)
Depression (<6%)
Dysesthesia [2]
Encephalopathy [4]
Fever (3–6%)
Headache (14–25%) [5]
Insomnia (<4%)
Leukoencephalopathy [17]
Migraine (2–3%)
Neurotoxicity [11]
Pain (3–13%)
Paresthesias (5–11%) [8]
Parkinsonism [6]
Pseudotumor cerebri [3]
Rigors (<3%)
Seizures [4]
Tremor (7–13%) [5]
Vertigo (dizziness) (6–8%)

Neuromuscular/Skeletal
Arthralgia (<6%)
Asthenia (fatigue) (3–6%) [4]
Myalgia/Myopathy [10]
Rhabdomyolysis [13]

Gastrointestinal/Hepatic
Abdominal pain (15%) [3]
Diarrhea (5–13%) [3]
Dyspepsia (2–12%)
Flatulence (4–5%)
Gastrointestinal disorder (2–4%) [2]
Hepatotoxicity [9]
Nausea (6–23%) [2]
Vomiting (6–9%) [2]

Respiratory
Bronchitis (<3%)
Bronchospasm (5%)
Cough (3–5%)
Dyspnea (<5%)
Influenza (<10%)
Pharyngitis (3–4%)
Pneumonia (<4%)
Rhinitis (<5%)
Sinusitis (3–4%)
Upper respiratory tract infection (8–15%)

Endocrine/Metabolic
Diabetes mellitus [2]
Gynecomastia (>3%) [3]
Hypertriglyceridemia [2]
Hypomagnesemia (4–6%)
Menstrual irregularities (<3%)
Serum creatinine increased (16–43%) [4]

Genitourinary
Urinary frequency (2–4%)
Urinary tract infection (3%)

Renal
Nephrotoxicity [94]
Renal function abnormal [4]

Hematologic
Anemia [4]
Dyslipidemia [4]
Hemolytic uremic syndrome [17]
Leukopenia [2]
Neutropenia [3]

Ocular
Hallucinations, visual [2]
Ocular burning (Restasis) (17%)
Ocular pain [2]
Papilledema [2]

Other
Adverse effects [21]
Infection [6]

CYPROTERONE

Trade name: Androcur (Bayer)
Indications: Control of libido in severe hypersexuality and/or sexual deviation in the adult male
Class: Androgen antagonist, Progesterone agonist
Half-life: 1.7 days
Clinically important, potentially hazardous interactions with: alcohol, clotrimazole, fingolimod, itraconazole, ketoconazole, pazopanib, phenytoin, rifampin, ritonavir, St John's wort
Pregnancy category: X (not indicated for use in women)
Important contra-indications noted in the prescribing guidelines for: pediatric patients

---

Skin
Tumors [3]

Cardiovascular
Venous thromboembolism [2]

Neuromuscular/Skeletal
Osteoporosis [2]

Gastrointestinal/Hepatic
Hepatotoxicity [24]

Respiratory
Dyspnea [4]

CYTARABINE

Synonym: ara-C
Trade names: Cytosar-U (Sicor), DepoCyt (Pacira)
Indications: Leukemias
Class: Antimetabolite, Antineoplastic, Antiviral
Half-life: initial: 10–15 minutes
Clinically important, potentially hazardous interactions with: aldesleukin
Pregnancy category: D
Important contra-indications noted in the prescribing guidelines for: nursing mothers; pediatric patients
Note: DepoCyt is a liposomal formulation. Vasculitis, a part of the cytarabine syndrome, consists of fever, malaise, myalgia, conjunctivitis, arthralgia and a diffuse erythematous maculopapular eruption that occurs from 6–12 hours following the administration of the drug.
Warning: DepoCyt: CHEMICAL ARACHNOIDITIS ADVERSE REACTIONS

Skin
Acral erythema [16]
Anaphylactoid reactions/Anaphylaxis [3]
Ephelides (<10%)
Erythema [5]
Exanthems [7]
Hand–foot syndrome [22]
Herpes zoster [2]
Hypersensitivity [2]
Neutrophilic eccrine hidradenitis [11]
Pruritus (<10%)
Rash (>10%) [4]
Seborrheic keratoses (inflammation of) (Leser–Trélat syndrome) [2]
Toxic epidermal necrolysis [2]
Toxicity [5]
Vasculitis [3]

Hair
Alopecia (<10%) [5]

Nails
Leukonychia (Mees' lines) [2]

Mucosal
Mucositis [3]
Oral lesions [5]
Oral ulceration (>10%)
Perianal ulcerations (>10%)
Stomatitis [2]

Cardiovascular
Thrombophlebitis (>10%)

Central Nervous System
Fever [3]
Headache [4]
Leukoencephalopathy [8]
Neurotoxicity [10]
Peripheral neuropathy [2]

Neuromuscular/Skeletal
Myalgia/Myopathy (<10%)
Rhabdomyolysis [3]

Gastrointestinal/Hepatic
Diarrhea [5]
Hepatotoxicity [5]
Nausea [4]
Pancreatitis [5]
Vomiting [4]

Respiratory
Pneumonia [3]

Endocrine/Metabolic
Hypokalemia [2]

Hematologic
Anemia [2]
Bleeding [2]
Febrile neutropenia [8]
Hemotoxicity [3]
Leukopenia [2]
Myelosuppression [3]
Neutropenia [7]
Sepsis [2]
Thrombocytopenia [6]

Ocular
Ocular adverse effects [3]

Local
Injection-site cellulitis (<10%)

Other
Adverse effects [5]
Death [4]
Infection [6]

DABIGATRAN

Trade name: Pradaxa (Boehringer Ingelheim)
Indications: Prevention of venous thromboembolic events, reduce stroke risk
Class: Anticoagulant, Thrombin inhibitor
Half-life: 2.5 days
Clinically important, potentially hazardous interactions with: amiodarone, antacids, anticoagulants, atorvastatin, carbamazepine, clarithromycin, clopidogrel, collagenase, cyclosporine, darunavir, dasatinib, deferasirox, desirudin, dextran, diclofenac, dronedarone, fondaparinux, heparin, ibritumomab, itraconazole, ketoconazole, ketorolac, lapatinib, meloxicam, nandrolone, neratinib, NSAIDs, P-glycoprotein inducers and inhibitors, pantoprazole, pentosan, phenytoin, polysulfate sodium, prostacyclin analogues, proton pump inhibitors, quinidine, rifampin, rivaroxaban, salicylates, St John's wort, sulfinpyrazone, tacrolimus, telaprevir, thrombolytic agents, ticlopidine, tipranavir, tositumomab & iodine^{131}, ulipristal, verapamil, vitamin K antagonists
Pregnancy category: C
Important contra-indications noted in the prescribing guidelines for: the elderly; nursing mothers; pediatric patients
Note: Contra-indicated in patients with active pathological bleeding or with a mechanical prosthetic heart valve.
Warning: DISCONTINUING PRADAXA IN PATIENTS WITHOUT ADEQUATE CONTINUOUS ANTICOAGULATION INCREASES RISK OF STROKE

Skin
Bruising (<10%)
Exanthems [2]
Rash [2]

Mucosal
Epistaxis (nosebleed) [3]

Cardiovascular
Myocardial infarction [5]

Central Nervous System
Headache [2]
Intracranial hemorrhage [4]
Subarachnoid hemorrhage [2]

Gastrointestinal/Hepatic
Abdominal pain [2]
Dyspepsia (11%) [8]
Esophagitis [3]
Gastritis [2]
Gastrointestinal bleeding (6%) [10]

Genitourinary
Hematuria [2]

Renal
Renal failure [4]

Hematologic
Anemia (<4%)
Anticoagulation [2]
Bleeding [3]
Hemorrhage [9]
Thrombosis [3]

Other
Adverse effects [6]
Death [6]

DABRAFENIB

Trade name: Tafinlar (Novartis)
Indications: Melanoma (unresectable or metastatic) in patients with BRAF V600E mutation
Class: BRAF inhibitor, Kinase inhibitor
Half-life: 8 hours
Clinically important, potentially hazardous interactions with: strong CYP3A4 or CYP2C8 inducers or inhibitors inhibitors
Pregnancy category: D
Important contra-indications noted in the prescribing guidelines for: nursing mothers; pediatric patients

---

Skin
Acneform eruption [5]
Actinic keratoses [3]
Basal cell carcinoma [4]
Bullae (<10%)
Erythema [2]
Exanthems [2]
Hand–foot syndrome (20%) [7]
Hyperkeratosis (37%) [14]
Hypersensitivity (<10%)
Keratoacanthoma (7%) [7]
Keratosis pilaris [4]
Lesions [2]
Malignant melanoma (2%)
Panniculitis [6]
Papillomas (27%) [5]
Peripheral edema [4]
Photosensitivity [8]
Pruritus [4]
Rash (17%) [7]
Seborrheic keratoses [2]
Squamous cell carcinoma (7%) [18]
Toxicity [4]
Transient acantholytic dermatosis [4]
Xerosis [5]

Hair
Alopecia (22%) [8]
Hair changes [2]

Cardiovascular
Cardiotoxicity [2]
Chest pain [2]
Hypertension [4]

Central Nervous System
Chills [6]
Fever (28%) [26]
Headache (32%) [9]
Intracranial hemorrhage [3]

Neuromuscular/Skeletal
Arthralgia (27%) [12]
Asthenia (fatigue) [15]
Back pain (12%)
Myalgia/Myopathy (11%) [2]

Gastrointestinal/Hepatic
Abdominal pain [2]
Constipation (11%) [2]
Diarrhea [7]
Nausea [11]
Pancreatitis (<10%)
Vomiting [9]

Respiratory
Cough (12%) [3]
Nasopharyngitis (10%)

Endocrine/Metabolic
ALP increased (19%) [2]
ALT increased [4]
Appetite decreased [3]
AST increased [5]
Hyperglycemia (50%)
Hyponatremia (8%) [2]
Hypophosphatemia (37%)

Renal
Nephrotoxicity (<10%) [2]

Hematologic
Anemia [5]
Leukopenia [2]
Neutropenia [4]

Ocular
Chorioretinopathy [2]
Vision blurred [3]

Other
Adverse effects [8]

DACARBAZINE

Synonym: DIC
Trade name: DTIC-Dome (Bayer)
Indications: Malignant melanoma, carcinomas
Class: Alkylating agent, Antineoplastic
Half-life: 5 hours
Clinically important, potentially hazardous interactions with: aldesleukin
Pregnancy category: C
Important contra-indications noted in the prescribing guidelines for: nursing mothers

---

Skin
Anaphylactoid reactions/Anaphylaxis (<10%)
Flushing (<10%) [2]
Hypersensitivity [2]
Photosensitivity [10]
Rash (<10%) [2]
Urticaria [2]

Hair
Alopecia (<10%) [4]

Mucosal
Stomatitis (48%)

Central Nervous System
Dysgeusia (taste perversion) (<10%)
Peripheral neuropathy [2]

Neuromuscular/Skeletal
Asthenia (fatigue) (75%) [4]
Myalgia/Myopathy (<10%)

Gastrointestinal/Hepatic
Diarrhea [3]
Hepatotoxicity [3]
Nausea [3]
Vomiting [2]

Respiratory
Flu-like syndrome [2]
Pulmonary toxicity [2]

Endocrine/Metabolic
ALT increased [2]
AST increased [2]

Hematologic
Neutropenia [5]
Thrombocytopenia [2]

Local
Injection-site burning (>10%)
Injection-site necrosis (>10%)
Injection-site pain (>10%)

Other
Adverse effects [7]

DACLATASVIR

Trade name: Daklinza (Bristol-Myers Squibb)
Indications: Hepatitis C (in combination with sofosbuvir)
Class: Direct-acting antiviral, Hepatitis C virus NS5A inhibitor
Half-life: 12–15 hours
Clinically important, potentially hazardous interactions with: amiodarone, carbamazepine, dabigatran, phenytoin, rifampin, St John's wort
Pregnancy category: N/A (No data available)
Important contra-indications noted in the prescribing guidelines for: nursing mothers; pediatric patients
Note: See also separate entry for sofosbuvir.

Skin
Pruritus [4]
Rash [3]

Central Nervous System
Anorexia [2]
Fever [4]
Headache (14%) [22]
Insomnia [5]
Irritability [2]

Neuromuscular/Skeletal
Arthralgia [2]
Asthenia (fatigue) (14%) [19]

Gastrointestinal/Hepatic
Abdominal pain [3]
Diarrhea (5%) [12]
Hepatotoxicity [2]
Nausea (8%) [17]
Vomiting [2]

Respiratory
Nasopharyngitis [2]

Endocrine/Metabolic
ALT increased [10]
AST increased [4]

Renal
Renal failure [2]

Hematologic
Anemia [8]
Lymphopenia [2]
Neutropenia [3]
Thrombocytopenia [2]

Other
Adverse effects [8]

DACLIZUMAB

Trade names: Zenapax (Roche), Zinbryta (Biogen)
Indications: Transplant rejection (Zenapax), relapsing forms of multiple sclerosis (Zinbryta)
Class: Immunosuppressant, Monoclonal antibody
Half-life: 11–38 days
Clinically important, potentially hazardous interactions with: corticosteroids, cyclosporine, Hemophilus B vaccine, methylprednisolone, mycophenolate, prednisolone
Pregnancy category: C
Important contra-indications noted in the prescribing guidelines for: the elderly; nursing mothers; pediatric patients
Warning: Zinbryta: HEPATIC INJURY INCLUDING AUTOIMMUNE HEPATITIS and OTHER IMMUNE-MEDIATED DISORDERS

Skin
Acneform eruption (>5%)
Dermatitis [2]
Eczema [6]
Edema (>5%)
Hypersensitivity [2]
Hypohidrosis (2–5%)
Lymphadenopathy [4]
Peripheral edema (>5%)
Pruritus (2–5%)
Psoriasis [2]
Rash (2–5%) [8]
Toxicity [2]
Wound complications (>5%)

Hair
Hirsutism (2–5%)

Cardiovascular
Chest pain (>5%)
Hypertension (>5%)
Hypotension (>5%)
Pulmonary edema (>5%)
Tachycardia (>5%)

Central Nervous System
Anxiety (2–5%)
Depression (2–5%)
Fever (>5%)
Headache (>5%) [3]
Insomnia (>5%)
Pain (>5%)
Tremor (>5%)
Vertigo (dizziness) (>5%)

Neuromuscular/Skeletal
Arthralgia (2–5%)
Asthenia (fatigue) (>5%)
Back pain (>5%)
Bone or joint pain (>5%)
Myalgia/Myopathy (2–5%)

Gastrointestinal/Hepatic
Abdominal distension (>5%)
Abdominal pain (>5%)
Colitis [2]
Constipation (>5%)
Diarrhea (>5%)
Flatulence (2–5%)
Gastritis (2–5%)
Hemorrhoids (2–5%)
Hepatotoxicity [5]
Nausea (>5%)
Vomiting (>5%)

Respiratory
Cough (>5%)
Dyspnea (>5%)
Hypoxia (2–5%)
Nasopharyngitis [2]
Pharyngitis (2–5%)
Pleural effusion (2–5%)
Pneumonia [2]
Rhinitis (2–5%)
Upper respiratory tract infection [3]

Endocrine/Metabolic
ALT increased [2]
AST increased [2]
Dehydration (2–5%)
Diabetes mellitus (2–5%)

Genitourinary
Urinary retention (2–5%)
Urinary tract infection [2]

Renal
Nephrotoxicity (2–5%)

Hematologic
Hemorrhage (>5%)
Thrombosis (>5%)

Ocular
Vision blurred (2–5%)

Local
Application-site reactions (2–5%)

Other
Adverse effects [4]
Infection [7]

DACTINOMYCIN

Synonyms: ACT; actinomycin-D
Trade name: Cosmegen (Merck)
Indications: Melanomas, sarcomas
Class: Antibiotic, anthracycline
Half-life: 36 hours
Clinically important, potentially hazardous interactions with: aldesleukin
Pregnancy category: D
Important contra-indications noted in the prescribing guidelines for: the elderly; nursing mothers; pediatric patients
Note: Contra-indicated in patients with chickenpox or herpes zoster infection.

Skin
Acneform eruption (>10%) [6]
Erythema [2]
Folliculitis [2]
Pigmentation [4]
Pruritus [2]
Pustules [2]
Radiation recall dermatitis (>10%) [4]

Hair
Alopecia (>10%)

Mucosal
Oral lesions [3]
Stomatitis (ulcerative) (>5%)

Gastrointestinal/Hepatic
Nausea [2]

Hematologic
Febrile neutropenia [2]

Neutropenia [2]
Thrombocytopenia [2]

Local
Injection-site extravasation (>10%)
Injection-site necrosis (>10%)
Injection-site phlebitis (>10%)

Other
Death [2]

DALFAMPRIDINE

Synonym: 4-aminopyridine
Trade name: Ampyra (Acorda)
Indications: Multiple sclerosis (to improve walking)
Class: Potassium channel blocker
Half-life: 5–6.5 hours
Clinically important, potentially hazardous interactions with: none known
Pregnancy category: C
Important contra-indications noted in the prescribing guidelines for: nursing mothers; pediatric patients
Note: Contra-indicated in patients with a history of seizure, or with moderate or severe renal impairment.

Central Nervous System
Balance disorder (5%)
Gait instability [2]
Headache (7%) [5]
Insomnia (9%) [5]
Multiple sclerosis (relapse) (4%)
Paresthesias (4%) [2]
Seizures [5]
Vertigo (dizziness) (7%) [9]

Neuromuscular/Skeletal
Asthenia (fatigue) (7%) [3]
Back pain (5%)

Gastrointestinal/Hepatic
Constipation (3%)
Dyspepsia (2%)
Nausea (7%) [4]

Respiratory
Nasopharyngitis (4%)
Pharyngolaryngeal pain (2%)

Genitourinary
Urinary tract infection (12%) [2]

Other
Adverse effects [4]

DALTEPARIN

Trade name: Fragmin (Pfizer)
Indications: Prophylaxis of deep vein thrombosis
Class: Heparin, low molecular weight
Half-life: 4–8 hours
Clinically important, potentially hazardous interactions with: butabarbital, danaparoid
Pregnancy category: B
Important contra-indications noted in the prescribing guidelines for: nursing mothers; pediatric patients
Warning: SPINAL/EPIDURAL HEMATOMA

Skin
Anaphylactoid reactions/Anaphylaxis (<10%) [2]
Bullous dermatitis (<10%)
Pruritus (<10%)
Rash (<10%)

Hair
Alopecia [2]

Local
Injection-site hematoma (<10%)
Injection-site pain (<10%)

Other
Allergic reactions (<10%) [3]

DAN-SHEN

Family: Labiatae; Lamiaceae
Scientific name: *Salvia miltiorrhiza*
Indications: Circulation problems, ischemic stroke, angina pectoris, menstrual problems, chronic hepatitis, abdominal masses, insomnia, acne, psoriasis, eczema, bruising, hearing loss
Class: Food supplement, Platelet aggregation inhibitor
Half-life: N/A
Clinically important, potentially hazardous interactions with: none known
Pregnancy category: N/A

Hematologic
Anticoagulation [4]

Other
Adverse effects [3]

DANAZOL

Indications: Endometriosis, fibrocystic breast disease
Class: Pituitary hormone inhibitor
Half-life: ~4.5 hours
Clinically important, potentially hazardous interactions with: acenocoumarol, acitretin, atorvastatin, cyclosporine, insulin aspart, insulin degludec, insulin detemir, insulin glargine, insulin glulisine, oral contraceptives, paricalcitol, simvastatin, tacrolimus, warfarin
Pregnancy category: X
Important contra-indications noted in the prescribing guidelines for: nursing mothers; pediatric patients

Skin
Acneform eruption (>10%) [6]
Diaphoresis (3%)
Edema (>10%)
Erythema multiforme [2]
Exanthems [2]
Flushing [3]
Lupus erythematosus [4]
Rash (3%)
Seborrhea [4]

Hair
Alopecia [3]
Hirsutism (<10%) [5]

Neuromuscular/Skeletal
Rhabdomyolysis [5]

Gastrointestinal/Hepatic
Hepatotoxicity [4]

Endocrine/Metabolic
Pseudomenopause [2]
Weight gain [2]

Other
Adverse effects [3]
Death [2]

DANTROLENE

Trade names: Dantrium (Par), Ryanodex (Eagle)
Indications: Spasticity, malignant hyperthermia
Class: Skeletal muscle relaxant, hydantoin
Half-life: 8.7 hours
Clinically important, potentially hazardous interactions with: verapamil
Pregnancy category: C
Important contra-indications noted in the prescribing guidelines for: the elderly; nursing mothers; pediatric patients
Warning: HEPATOTOXICITY

Skin
Acneform eruption [3]
Rash (>10%)

Cardiovascular
Pericarditis [3]

Central Nervous System
Chills (<10%)
Vertigo (dizziness) [2]

Neuromuscular/Skeletal
Asthenia (fatigue) [2]
Myalgia/Myopathy [2]

Gastrointestinal/Hepatic
Hepatotoxicity [2]

Respiratory
Eosinophillic pleural effusion [3]
Pleural effusion [5]

Other
Adverse effects [2]
Death [4]

DAPAGLIFLOZIN

Trade names: Farxiga (AstraZeneca), Qtern (AstraZeneca), Xigduo XR (AstraZeneca)
Indications: Type II diabetes mellitus
Class: Sodium-glucose co-transporter 2 (SGLT2) inhibitor
Half-life: 13 hours
Clinically important, potentially hazardous interactions with: pioglitazone
Pregnancy category: C
Important contra-indications noted in the prescribing guidelines for: the elderly; nursing mothers; pediatric patients
Note: Contra-indicated in patients with severe renal impairment, end-stage renal disease, or undergoing dialysis. Qtern is dapagliflozin and saxagliptin; Xigduo XR is dapagliflozin and metformin.

Skin
Eczema [2]

Cardiovascular
Hypertension [2]
Hypotension [3]

Central Nervous System
Headache [3]
Vertigo (dizziness) [2]

Neuromuscular/Skeletal
Arthralgia [2]
Back pain (3–4%) [3]
Pain in extremities (2%)

Gastrointestinal/Hepatic
Constipation (2%)
Diarrhea [3]
Nausea (3%) [3]

Respiratory
Bronchitis [2]
Cough [2]
Influenza (2–3%) [2]
Nasopharyngitis (6–7%) [7]
Upper respiratory tract infection [5]

Endocrine/Metabolic
Dehydration [2]
Diabetic ketoacidosis [2]
Hypoglycemia (>10%) [14]
Hypovolemia [2]

Genitourinary
Balanitis [2]
Genital mycotic infections (particularly in women) (3–8%) [32]
Pollakiuria [2]
Urinary frequency (3–4%)
Urinary tract infection (4–6%) [36]
Vulvovaginal candidiasis [2]

Renal
Nephrotoxicity [2]
Renal failure [2]

Hematologic
Dyslipidemia (2–3%)

Other
Adverse effects [9]
Dipsia (thirst) [2]
Infection (<10%)

DAPSONE

Trade name: Aczone (Allergan)
Indications: Leprosy, dermatitis herpetiformis, acne
Class: Antibiotic, Antimycobacterial
Half-life: 10–50 hours
Clinically important, potentially hazardous interactions with: atovaquone/proguanil, chloroquine, didanosine, furazolidone, ganciclovir, hydroxychloroquine, methotrexate, pyrimethamine, rifabutin, rifampin, rifapentine, sulfonamides, trimethoprim, ursodiol
Pregnancy category: C
Important contra-indications noted in the prescribing guidelines for: nursing mothers
Note: A hypersensitivity reaction – termed the 'sulfone syndrome' or 'dapsone syndrome' – may infrequently develop during the first six weeks of treatment. This syndrome consists of exfoliative dermatitis, fever, malaise, nausea, anorexia, hepatitis, jaundice, lymphadenopathy and hemolytic anemia.

Skin
AGEP [2]
Bullous dermatitis [2]
Cyanosis [2]
Dapsone syndrome [44]
DRESS syndrome [14]
Erythema multiforme [9]
Erythema nodosum [5]
Exanthems (<5%) [12]
Exfoliative dermatitis [10]
Fixed eruption [5]
Hypersensitivity [21]
Lupus erythematosus [6]
Photosensitivity [9]
Pigmentation [6]
Rash [6]
Stevens-Johnson syndrome [5]
Toxic epidermal necrolysis [9]
Urticaria [2]

Nails
Beau's lines (transverse nail bands) [3]

Central Nervous System
Headache (4%) [2]
Insomnia [2]
Peripheral neuropathy [2]

Neuromuscular/Skeletal
Asthenia (fatigue) [2]

Gastrointestinal/Hepatic
Hepatitis [3]
Hepatotoxicity [2]
Pancreatitis [2]

Respiratory
Cough (2%)
Eosinophilic pneumonia [2]
Nasopharyngitis (5%)
Pharyngitis (2%)
Sinusitis (2%)
Upper respiratory tract infection (3%)

Hematologic
Agranulocytosis [7]
Anemia [5]
Hemolysis [7]
Hemolytic anemia [6]
Methemoglobinemia [20]

Local
Application-site erythema (13%) [2]
Application-site reactions (18%)

Other
Adverse effects [4]
Death [6]

DAPTOMYCIN

Trade name: Cubicin (Cubist)
Indications: Complicated skin and skin structure infections, *Staphylococcus aureus* bloodstream infections
Class: Antibiotic, glycopeptide
Half-life: ~8 hours
Clinically important, potentially hazardous interactions with: atorvastatin, cyclosporine, fibrates, HMG-CoA reductase inhibitors, rosuvastatin, statins, tobramycin, typhoid vaccine, warfarin
Pregnancy category: B
Important contra-indications noted in the prescribing guidelines for: the elderly; nursing mothers; pediatric patients

---

Skin
AGEP [2]
Cellulitis (<2%)
Edema (<7%)
Fungal dermatitis (3%)
Hyperhidrosis (5%)
Pruritus (3–6%)
Rash (4%)

Cardiovascular
Chest pain (7%)
Hypertension (6%)
Hypotension (2%)

Central Nervous System
Fever (2%)
Headache (5%)
Insomnia (9%)
Peripheral neuropathy [2]
Vertigo (dizziness) (2%)

Neuromuscular/Skeletal
Back pain (<2%)
Myalgia/Myopathy [8]
Rhabdomyolysis [8]

Gastrointestinal/Hepatic
Abdominal pain (<6%)
Constipation (6%)
Diarrhea (5%) [3]
Hepatotoxicity [3]
Nausea (6%) [2]
Vomiting (3%)

Respiratory
Cough (<2%)
Dyspnea (2%)
Eosinophilic pneumonia [15]
Pharyngolaryngeal pain (8%)
Pneumonia [2]

Endocrine/Metabolic
Creatine phosphokinase increased (7%) [7]

Genitourinary
Urinary tract infection (2%)

Renal
Nephrotoxicity [2]
Renal failure [2]

Hematologic
Eosinophilia [2]
Neutropenia [2]
Thrombocytopenia [2]

Local
Injection-site reactions (6%)

Other
Adverse effects [3]

DARATUMUMAB

Trade name: Darzalex (Janssen Biotech)
Indications: Multiple myeloma in patients who have received at least three prior lines of therapy including a proteasome inhibitor (PI) and an immunomodulatory agent or who are double-refractory to a PI and an immunomodulatory agent
Class: Monoclonal antibody
Half-life: 18 days
Clinically important, potentially hazardous interactions with: none known
Pregnancy category: N/A (No data available)
Important contra-indications noted in the prescribing guidelines for: pediatric patients

---

Skin
Herpes zoster (3%)

Mucosal
Nasal congestion (17%)

Cardiovascular
Chest pain (12%)
Hypertension (10%)

Central Nervous System
Chills (10%)
Cytokine release syndrome [2]
Fever (21%) [3]
Headache (12%)

Neuromuscular/Skeletal
Arthralgia (17%)
Asthenia (fatigue) (39%) [4]
Back pain (23%)
Pain in extremities (15%)

Gastrointestinal/Hepatic
Constipation (15%)
Diarrhea (16%)
Nausea (27%)
Vomiting (14%)

Respiratory
Bronchospasm (<2%) [3]
Cough (21%) [3]
Dyspnea (15%) [2]
Hypoxia (<2%)
Nasopharyngitis (15%)
Pneumonia (11%) [2]
Rhinitis (>5%)
Upper respiratory tract infection (20%) [2]

Endocrine/Metabolic
Appetite decreased (15%)

Hematologic
Anemia (45%) [7]
Lymphopenia (72%)
Neutropenia (60%) [4]
Thrombocytopenia (48%) [7]

Local
Infusion-related reactions (48%) [9]

DARBEPOETIN ALFA

Synonym: erythropoiesis stimulating protein
Trade name: Aranesp (Amgen)
Indications: Anemia associated with renal failure and chemotherapy
Class: Colony stimulating factor, Erythropoiesis-stimulating agent (ESA), Erythropoietin
Half-life: 21 hours
Clinically important, potentially hazardous interactions with: none known
Pregnancy category: C
Important contra-indications noted in the prescribing guidelines for: nursing mothers; pediatric patients
Note: There is an increased risk of death for patients suffering from chronic renal failure with this drug (6%).
Warning: ERYTHROPOIESIS-STIMULATING AGENTS (ESAs) INCREASE THE RISK OF DEATH, MYOCARDIAL INFARCTION, STROKE, VENOUS THROMBOEMBOLISM, THROMBOSIS OF VASCULAR ACCESS AND TUMOR PROGRESSION OR RECURRENCE

Skin
Edema (21%)
Peripheral edema (11%)
Pruritus (8%)
Rash (7%) [2]

Central Nervous System
Fever (9–19%)
Vertigo (dizziness) (8–14%)

Neuromuscular/Skeletal
Arthralgia (11–13%)
Asthenia (fatigue) (9–33%)
Back pain (8%)
Myalgia/Myopathy (21%)

Gastrointestinal/Hepatic
Abdominal pain (12%)

Respiratory
Cough (10%)
Flu-like syndrome (6%)
Upper respiratory tract infection (14%)

Hematologic
Thrombosis [2]

Local
Injection-site pain (7%)

Other
Adverse effects [4]

DARIFENACIN

Trade names: Emselex (Novartis), Enablex (Novartis)
Indications: Overactive bladder
Class: Anticholinergic, Antimuscarinic, Muscarinic antagonist
Half-life: 13–19 hours
Clinically important, potentially hazardous interactions with: anticholinergics, antihistamines, atazanavir, clozapine, cyclosporine, digoxin, disopyramide, domperidone, erythromycin, flecainide, fosamprenavir, haloperidol, imipramine, indinavir, itraconazole, ketoconazole, levodopa, lopinavir, MAO inhibitors, memantine, metoclopramide, nefopam, nelfinavir, nitrates (sublingual), parasympathomimetics, paroxetine hydrochloride, phenothiazines, potent CYP3A4 inhibitors, ritonavir, saquinavir, thioridazine, tipranavir, tricyclic antidepressants, verapamil
Pregnancy category: C
Important contra-indications noted in the prescribing guidelines for: nursing mothers; pediatric patients
Note: Contra-indicated in patients with, or at risk for, urinary retention, gastric retention or uncontrolled narrow-angle glaucoma.

Mucosal
Xerostomia (20%) [12]

Central Nervous System
Headache [2]

Gastrointestinal/Hepatic
Abdominal pain (2%)
Constipation [3]

DARUNAVIR

Trade names: Prezcobix (Janssen), Prezista (Janssen)
Indications: HIV infection (must be co-administered with ritonavir and with other antiretroviral agents)
Class: Antiretroviral, HIV-1 protease inhibitor
Half-life: 15 hours
Clinically important, potentially hazardous interactions with: abacavir, alfuzosin, almotriptan, alosetron, alprazolam, amiodarone, antifungals, apixaban, artemether/lumefantrine, astemizole, atorvastatin, bortezomib, brinzolamide, calcium channel blockers, captopril, carbamazepine, ciclesonide, cisapride, clarithromycin, colchicine, conivaptan, cyclosporine, CYP2D6 substrates, CYP3A4 inhibitors, inducers and substrates, dabigatran, dasatinib, deferasirox, delavirdine, didanosine, dienogest, digoxin, dihydroergotamine, dronedarone, duloxetine, dutasteride, efavirenz, elbasvir & grazoprevir, enfuvirtide, eplerenone, ergotamine, estrogens, etravirine, everolimus, fentanyl, fesoterodine, food, fusidic acid, glecaprevir & pibrentasvir, guanfacine, halofantrine, HMG-CoA reductase inhibitors, indinavir, inhaled corticosteroids, ixabepilone, ketoconazole, lidocaine, lopinavir, lovastatin, maraviroc, meperidine, methadone, methylprednisolone, midazolam, mifepristone, mometasone, nefazodone, nilotinib, nisoldipine, olaparib, P-glycoprotein substrates, paricalcitol, paroxetine hydrochloride, pazopanib, phenobarbital, phenytoin, pimecrolimus, pimozide, prasugrel, pravastatin, protease inhibitors, quetiapine, quinidine, quinine, ranolazine, rifabutin, rifampin, rilpivirine, rivaroxaban, romidepsin, rosuvastatin, salmeterol, saquinavir, saxagliptin, sertraline, sildenafil, silodosin, simeprevir, simvastatin, sirolimus, sorafenib, St John's wort, tacrolimus, tadalafil, tamsulosin, telaprevir, temsirolimus, tenofovir disoproxil, terfenadine, theophylline, tolvaptan,

topotecan, trazodone, triazolam, tricyclic antidepressants, vardenafil, voriconazole, warfarin, zidovudine
Pregnancy category: C
Important contra-indications noted in the prescribing guidelines for: nursing mothers; pediatric patients
Note: Darunavir is a sulfonamide and can be absorbed systemically. Sulfonamides can produce severe, possibly fatal, reactions such as toxic epidermal necrolysis and Stevens-Johnson syndrome.
Prezcobix is darunavir and cobicistat.

Skin
Angioedema (<2%)
Hypersensitivity (<2%) [2]
Pruritus (<2%)
Rash (6–10%) [9]
Stevens-Johnson syndrome (<2%)
Urticaria (<2%)

Central Nervous System
Abnormal dreams (<2%)
Anorexia (2%)
Headache (7%) [6]

Neuromuscular/Skeletal
Asthenia (fatigue) (2–3%)
Osteonecrosis (<2%)

Gastrointestinal/Hepatic
Abdominal distension (2%)
Abdominal pain (6%)
Diarrhea (9–14%) [10]
Dyspepsia (<3%)
Flatulence (<2%)
Gastrointestinal disorder [3]
Hepatotoxicity (<2%) [6]
Nausea (4–7%) [6]
Pancreatitis (<2%)
Vomiting (2–5%)

Endocrine/Metabolic
Diabetes mellitus (new onset or exacebated) (2%)

Other
Adverse effects [6]

DASABUVIR/ OMBITASVIR/PARITA-PREVIR/RITONAVIR

Trade name: Viekira XR (AbbVie)
Indications: Genotype 1a chronic hepatitis C virus with or without cirrhosis, genotype 1b chronic hepatitis C virus with or without cirrhosis in combination with ribavirin
Class: CYP3A4 inhibitor (ritonavir), Direct-acting antiviral, Hepatitis C virus non-nucleoside NS5B palm polymerase inhibitor (dasabuvir), Hepatitis C virus NS3/4A protease inhibitor (paritaprevir), Hepatitis C virus NS5A inhibitor (ombitasvir)
Half-life: 6 hours (dasabuvir); 21–25 hours (ombitasvir); 6 hours (paritaprevir); 4 hours (ritonavir)
Clinically important, potentially hazardous interactions with: alfuzosin, carbamazepine, cisapride, copanlisib, dihydroergotamine, dronedarone, efavirenz, ergotamine, ethinyl estradiol-containing medications, gemfibrozil, lovastatin, lurasidone, methylergonovine, midazolam, midostaurin, neratinib, phenobarbital, phenytoin, pimozide, ranolazine, rifampin, sildenafil, simvastatin, St John's wort, triazolam
Pregnancy category: N/A (Insufficient evidence to inform drug-associated risk; contra-indicated in pregnancy when given with ribavirin)
Important contra-indications noted in the prescribing guidelines for: nursing mothers; pediatric patients
Note: Contra-indicated in patients with moderate to severe hepatic impairment. See also separate entries for Ombitasvir/Paritaprevir/ Ritonavir (co-packaged with Dasabuvir as Viekira Pak) and Ribavirin.

Skin
Pruritus (7%) [4]
Rash (7%)

Central Nervous System
Headache [2]
Insomnia (5%) [4]

Neuromuscular/Skeletal
Asthenia (fatigue) (4%) [7]

Gastrointestinal/Hepatic
Hepatotoxicity [2]
Nausea (8%) [2]

Endocrine/Metabolic
ALT increased [3]
AST increased [2]
Hyperbilirubinemia (2%) [4]

DASATINIB

Trade name: Sprycel (Bristol-Myers Squibb)
Indications: Leukemia (chronic myeloid), acute lymphoblastic leukemia
Class: Antineoplastic, Biologic, Tyrosine kinase inhibitor
Half-life: 3–5 hours
Clinically important, potentially hazardous interactions with: abciximab, alfentanil, alfuzosin, ambrisentan, antacids, anticoagulants, antiplatelet agents, aprepitant, argatroban, artemether/lumefantrine, astemizole, atazanavir, atorvastatin, boceprevir, cabazitaxel, carbamazepine, chloroquine, ciclesonide, cilostazol, cinacalcet, ciprofloxacin, cisapride, clarithromycin, clopidogrel, clozapine, colchicine, conivaptan, cyclosporine, CYP3A4 inhibitors, inducers and substrates, dabigatran, darunavir, deferasirox, dexamethasone, dihydroergotamine, docetaxel, dronedarone, efavirenz, eptifibatide, ergotamine, erythromycin, eszopiclone, famotidine, fentanyl, fesoterodine, gadobutrol, gefitinib, H_2 antagonists, indinavir, itraconazole, ixabepilone, ketoconazole, lopinavir, lurasidone, maraviroc, meloxicam, nefazodone, nelfinavir, nilotinib, omeprazole, pantoprazole, phenobarbital, phenytoin, pimozide, proton pump inhibitors, QT prolonging agents, quinidine, quinine, rifampin, ritonavir, saquinavir, saxagliptin, sildenafil, simvastatin, sirolimus, St John's wort, tacrolimus, tadalafil, temsirolimus, terfenadine, tetrabenazine, thioridazine, tiagabine, tinzaparin, vardenafil, ziprasidone
Pregnancy category: D
Important contra-indications noted in the prescribing guidelines for: nursing mothers; pediatric patients

---

Skin
Acneform eruption (<10%) [2]
Dermatitis (<10%)
Eczema (<10%)
Edema (13–18%) [6]
Erythema [2]
Flushing (<10%)
Herpes (<10%)
Hyperhidrosis (<10%)
Panniculitis [4]
Peripheral edema [3]
Pruritus (<10%) [4]
Rash (11–21%) [10]
Toxicity [8]
Urticaria (<10%)
Xerosis (<10%)

Hair
Alopecia (<10%) [3]
Hair pigmentation [2]

Mucosal
Mucositis (16%)

Cardiovascular
Arrhythmias (<10%)
Cardiac failure (3%)
Congestive heart failure (2%)
Hypertension (<10%)
Palpitation (<10%)
Pericardial effusion (2–3%) [6]
QT prolongation [4]
Tachycardia (<10%)

Central Nervous System
Anorexia (<10%) [6]
Anxiety [2]
Depression (<10%)
Dysgeusia (taste perversion) (<10%)
Fever (5–39%)
Headache (12–33%) [10]
Insomnia (<10%)
Neurotoxicity (13%)
Pain (26%) [2]
Peripheral neuropathy (<10%)
Somnolence (drowsiness) (<10%)
Subdural hemorrhage [4]
Vertigo (dizziness) (<10%)

Neuromuscular/Skeletal
Arthralgia (<19%)
Asthenia (fatigue) (8%) [15]
Bone or joint pain (12–19%) [3]
Myalgia/Myopathy (6–13%) [2]

Gastrointestinal/Hepatic
Abdominal distension (<10%)
Abdominal pain (<25%) [2]
Colitis (<10%) [3]
Constipation (<10%)
Diarrhea (18–31%) [19]
Dyspepsia (<10%)
Enterocolitis (<10%)
Gastritis (<10%)
Gastrointestinal bleeding (2–8%) [3]
Hemorrhagic colitis [2]
Hepatitis [2]
Hepatotoxicity [2]
Nausea (9–23%) [11]

Vomiting (7–15%) [6]

Respiratory
Cough (<10%)
Dyspnea (20%) [5]
Pleural effusion (12–21%) [40]
Pneumonia (<10%) [4]
Pneumonitis (<10%)
Pulmonary hypertension (<10%) [16]
Pulmonary toxicity [3]
Upper respiratory tract infection (<10%)

Endocrine/Metabolic
Weight gain (<10%)
Weight loss (<10%)

Renal
Proteinuria [2]
Renal failure [3]

Hematologic
Anemia [3]
Bleeding (6–26%)
Cytopenia [3]
Febrile neutropenia (<12%)
Hemorrhage [2]
Hemotoxicity [4]
Myelosuppression [10]
Neutropenia [7]
Pancytopenia (<10%)
Thrombocytopenia [13]

Otic
Tinnitus (<10%)

Ocular
Reduced visual acuity (<10%)
Vision blurred (<10%)
Visual disturbances (<10%)
Xerophthalmia (<10%)

Other
Adverse effects [4]
Death [2]
Infection (<14%) [2]
Side effects [2]

DAUNORUBICIN

Synonyms: daunomycin; DNR; rubidomycin
Trade name: DaunoXome (Gilead)
Indications: Acute leukemias
Class: Antibiotic, anthracycline
Half-life: 14–20 hours; 4 hours (intramuscular)
Clinically important, potentially hazardous interactions with: aldesleukin, gadobenate
Pregnancy category: D
Important contra-indications noted in the prescribing guidelines for: the elderly; nursing mothers; pediatric patients
Warning: MYOCARDIAL TOXICITY / MYELOSUPPRESSION

Skin
Angioedema [4]
Dermatitis [2]
Edema (11%)
Exanthems [2]
Flushing (14%)
Folliculitis (<5%)
Hot flashes (<5%)
Hyperhidrosis (14%)
Lymphadenopathy (<5%)
Neutrophilic eccrine hidradenitis [2]
Pigmentation [3]
Pruritus (7%)
Seborrhea (<5%)
Urticaria [3]
Xerosis (<5%)

Hair
Alopecia (8%) [4]

Nails
Nail pigmentation [5]

Mucosal
Gingival bleeding (<5%)
Oral lesions [2]
Sialorrhea (<5%)
Stomatitis (10%)
Xerostomia (<5%)

Cardiovascular
Chest pain (9–14%)
Hypertension (<5%)
Myocardial toxicity [5]
Palpitation (<5%)
Tachycardia (<5%)

Central Nervous System
Amnesia (<5%)
Anorexia (23%)
Anxiety (<5%)
Cognitive impairment (<5%)
Depression (10%)
Dysgeusia (taste perversion) (<5%)
Gait instability (<5%)
Hallucinations (<5%)
Headache (25%)
Insomnia (6%)
Meningococcal infection (<5%)
Neurotoxicity (13%)
Rigors (19%)
Seizures (<5%)
Somnolence (drowsiness) (<5%)
Syncope (<5%)
Tremor (<5%)
Vertigo (dizziness) (8%)

Neuromuscular/Skeletal
Arthralgia (7%)
Asthenia (fatigue) (10%)
Ataxia (<5%)
Back pain (16%)
Hyperkinesia (<5%)
Hypertonia (<5%)
Myalgia/Myopathy (7%)

Gastrointestinal/Hepatic
Abdominal pain (23%)
Black stools (<5%)
Constipation (7%)
Diarrhea (38%)
Dysphagia (<5%)
Gastritis (<5%)
Gastrointestinal bleeding (<5%)
Hemorrhoids (<5%)
Hepatomegaly (<5%)
Nausea (54%)
Tenesmus (5%)
Vomiting (23%)

Respiratory
Cough (28%)
Dyspnea (26%)
Flu-like syndrome (5%)
Hemoptysis (<5%)
PIE syndrome (<5%)
Rhinitis (12%)
Sinusitis (8%)

Endocrine/Metabolic
Appetite increased (<5%)
Dehydration (<5%)

Genitourinary
Dysuria (<5%)
Nocturia (<5%)
Polyuria (<5%)

Hematologic
Neutropenia (15–36%)
Splenomegaly (<5%)

Otic
Ear pain (<5%)
Hearing loss (<5%)
Tinnitus (<5%)

Ocular
Abnormal vision (5%)
Conjunctivitis (<5%)
Ocular pain (<5%)

Local
Injection-site inflammation (<5%)
Injection-site necrosis (<10%) [2]
Injection-site ulceration (<10%)

Other
Dipsia (thirst) (<5%)
Hiccups (<5%)
Infection (40%)
Tooth decay (<5%)

DECITABINE

Synonym: 5-aza-2'-deoxycytidine
Trade name: Dacogen (MGI Pharma)
Indications: Myelodysplastic syndromes, leukemia
Class: Antineoplastic
Half-life: ~30 minutes
Clinically important, potentially hazardous interactions with: none known
Pregnancy category: D
Important contra-indications noted in the prescribing guidelines for: nursing mothers; pediatric patients

---

Skin
Bacterial infection (5%)
Candidiasis (10%)
Cellulitis (12%)
Ecchymoses (22%)
Edema (18%)
Erythema (14%)
Facial edema (6%)
Hematoma (5%)
Lymphadenopathy (12%)
Pallor (23%)
Peripheral edema (25%)
Petechiae (39%)
Pruritus (11%)
Rash (19%) [2]
Urticaria (6%)

Mucosal
Gingival bleeding (8%)
Glossodynia (5%)
Lip ulceration (5%)
Mucositis [2]
Oral candidiasis (6%)

Stomatitis (12%)
Tongue ulceration (7%)

Cardiovascular
Chest pain (7%)
Hypotension (6%)
Pulmonary edema (6%)
QT prolongation [2]

Central Nervous System
Anorexia (16%) [2]
Anxiety (11%)
Confusion (12%)
Fever (53%) [2]
Headache (28%)
Hypoesthesia (11%)
Insomnia (28%)
Pain (13%)
Rigors (22%)
Vertigo (dizziness) (18%)

Neuromuscular/Skeletal
Arthralgia (20%)
Asthenia (fatigue) (5–12%) [7]
Back pain (17%)
Bone or joint pain (6–19%)
Myalgia/Myopathy (5%)

Gastrointestinal/Hepatic
Abdominal distension (5%)
Abdominal pain (14%)
Ascites (10%)
Constipation (35%)
Diarrhea (34%) [2]
Dyspepsia (12%)
Dysphagia (6%)
Gastroesophageal reflux (5%)
Hemorrhoids (8%)
Hepatotoxicity [2]
Loose stools (7%)
Nausea (42%) [8]
Vomiting (25%) [5]

Respiratory
Cough (40%)
Hypoxia (10%)
Pharyngitis (16%)
Pneumonia (22%) [2]
Sinusitis (5%)

Endocrine/Metabolic
ALP increased (11%)
Appetite decreased (16%)
AST increased (10%)
Dehydration (6%)
Hyperglycemia (33%)
Hyperkalemia (13%)
Hypoalbuminemia (24%)
Hypokalemia (22%)
Hypomagnesemia (24%)
Hyponatremia (19%)

Genitourinary
Dysuria (6%)
Urinary frequency (5%)
Urinary tract infection (7%)

Hematologic
Anemia (82%) [5]
Bacteremia (5%)
Febrile neutropenia (29%) [8]
Hemotoxicity [3]
Leukopenia (28%) [2]
Lymphopenia [2]
Myelosuppression [11]
Neutropenia (90%) [13]
Thrombocytopenia (89%) [9]

Ocular
Vision blurred (6%)

Local
Injection-site edema (5%)
Injection-site erythema (5%)

Other
Adverse effects [2]
Allergic reactions [2]
Death [2]
Infection [3]

DEFERASIROX

Trade names: Exjade (Novartis), Jadenu (Novartis)
Indications: Chronic iron overload due to blood transfusions and in non-transfuson dependent thalassemia syndromes
Class: Chelator, iron
Half-life: 8–16 hours
Clinically important, potentially hazardous interactions with: alfuzosin, aluminum-containing antacids, ambrisentan, aprepitant, cabazitaxel, cholestyramine, cilostazol, colesevelam, colestipol, conivaptan, dabigatran, darunavir, dasatinib, delavirdine, docetaxel, efavirenz, enalapril, estradiol, eszopiclone, fesoterodine, gefitinib, indinavir, ixabepilone, lapatinib, lurasidone, maraviroc, pazopanib, phenobarbital, phenytoin, pioglitazone, repaglinide, rifampin, ritonavir, sildenafil, telithromycin, theophylline, tiagabine, tipranavir, trimethoprim, ulipristal
Pregnancy category: C
Important contra-indications noted in the prescribing guidelines for: the elderly; nursing mothers
Warning: RENAL FAILURE, HEPATIC FAILURE, AND GASTROINTESTINAL HEMORRHAGE

Skin
Exanthems [2]
Jaundice [2]
Rash (2–11%) [24]
Urticaria (4%)

Central Nervous System
Headache (16%) [2]

Neuromuscular/Skeletal
Arthralgia (7%)
Asthenia (fatigue) [3]
Back pain (6%)

Gastrointestinal/Hepatic
Abdominal pain (21–28%) [12]
Diarrhea (5–20%) [18]
Gastrointestinal bleeding [3]
Gastrointestinal disorder [3]
Hepatotoxicity [9]
Nausea (2–6%) [20]
Vomiting (10–21%) [7]

Respiratory
Cough (14%)
Flu-like syndrome (11%)
Upper respiratory tract infection (9%)

Endocrine/Metabolic
ALT increased [9]
Appetite decreased [2]
AST increased [4]
Serum creatinine increased [23]

Renal
Fanconi syndrome [10]
Nephrotoxicity [7]
Proteinuria [4]
Renal failure [3]
Renal function abnormal [2]

Other
Adverse effects [15]

DEFERIPRONE

Trade name: Ferriprox (ApoPharma)
Indications: Treatment of patients with transfusional iron overload due to thalassemia syndromes when current chelation therapy is inadequate
Class: Chelator, iron
Half-life: 1.9 hours
Clinically important, potentially hazardous interactions with: antacids containing iron, aluminum, zinc, diclofenac, mineral supplements, probenecid
Pregnancy category: D
Important contra-indications noted in the prescribing guidelines for: the elderly; nursing mothers; pediatric patients
Warning: AGRANULOCYTOSIS / NEUTROPENIA

Central Nervous System
Headache (3%)

Neuromuscular/Skeletal
Arthralgia (10%) [8]
Arthropathy [5]
Back pain (2%)
Bone or joint pain [2]
Pain in extremities (2%)

Gastrointestinal/Hepatic
Abdominal pain (10%) [2]
Diarrhea (3%) [2]
Dyspepsia (2%)
Gastrointestinal disorder [5]
Hepatotoxicity [3]
Nausea (13%) [4]
Vomiting (10%)

Endocrine/Metabolic
ALT increased (8%) [5]
Appetite increased (4%)
AST increased [2]
Weight gain (2%)

Renal
Chromaturia (15%)

Hematologic
Agranulocytosis (2%) [15]
Neutropenia [12]
Thrombocytopenia [2]

Other
Adverse effects [2]
Death [2]

DEFEROXAMINE

Trade name: Desferal (Novartis)
Indications: Hemochromatosis, acute iron overload
Class: Chelator, iron
Half-life: 6.1 hours
Clinically important, potentially hazardous interactions with: ascorbic acid, ferrous sulfate, zinc
Pregnancy category: C

Skin
Anaphylactoid reactions/Anaphylaxis [3]
Hypersensitivity [2]

Central Nervous System
Neurotoxicity [2]

Neuromuscular/Skeletal
Arthralgia [6]

Endocrine/Metabolic
Serum creatinine increased [2]

Otic
Hearing loss [2]
Ototoxicity [7]

Ocular
Night blindness [2]
Retinopathy [12]

Local
Injection-site inflammation (<10%)
Injection-site pain (<10%)

Other
Death [3]

DEFIBROTIDE

Trade name: Defitelio (Jazz)
Indications: Hepatic veno-occlusive disease in patients with renal or pulmonary dysfunction following hematopoietic stem-cell transplantation
Class: Oligonucleotide
Half-life: <2 hours
Clinically important, potentially hazardous interactions with: alteplase, heparin
Pregnancy category: N/A (No data available)
Important contra-indications noted in the prescribing guidelines for: nursing mothers
Note: Contra-indicated for concomitant administration with systemic anticoagulant or fibrinolytic therapy.

Skin
Graft-versus-host reaction (6%)

Mucosal
Epistaxis (nosebleed) (14%)

Cardiovascular
Hypotension (37%) [4]

Central Nervous System
Cerebral hemorrhage (2%)
Intracranial hemorrhage (3%)

Gastrointestinal/Hepatic
Diarrhea (24%)
Gastrointestinal bleeding (9%) [3]
Nausea (16%)
Vomiting (18%)

Respiratory
Alveolar hemorrhage (pulmonary) (9%)
Pneumonia (5%)
Pulmonary hemorrhage (4%)
Pulmonary toxicity (6%)

Endocrine/Metabolic
Hyperuricemia (2%)

Hematologic
Hemorrhage [2]
Sepsis (7%)

Other
Adverse effects [3]
Infection (3%)

DEFLAZACORT

Trade name: Emflaza (Marathon)
Indications: Duchenne muscular dystrophy
Class: Corticosteroid
Half-life: N/A
Clinically important, potentially hazardous interactions with: carbamazepine, clarithromycin, diltiazem, efavirenz, fluconazole, grapefruit juice, live vaccines, pancuronium, phenytoin, rifampin, verapamil
Pregnancy category: N/A (Should be used during pregnancy only if the potential benefit justifies the potential risk to the fetus)
Important contra-indications noted in the prescribing guidelines for: the elderly; nursing mothers; pediatric patients

---

Skin
Cushingoid features (33%) [3]
Erythema (8%)
Hypersensitivity [3]
Toxic epidermal necrolysis [2]

Hair
Hirsutism (10%) [2]

Mucosal
Rhinorrhea (8%)

Central Nervous System
Behavioral disturbances [2]
Irritability (8%)

Gastrointestinal/Hepatic
Abdominal pain (6%)

Respiratory
Cough (12%)
Nasopharyngitis (10%)
Upper respiratory tract infection (12%)

Endocrine/Metabolic
Appetite increased (14%) [2]
Weight gain (20%) [6]

Genitourinary
Pollakiuria (12%)

Ocular
Cataract [3]

Other
Adverse effects [3]
Side effects [2]

DELAFLOXACIN

Trade name: Baxdela (Melinta)
Indications: Acute bacterial skin and skin structure infections caused by designated susceptible bacteria
Class: Antibiotic, fluoroquinolone
Half-life: 4–9 hours
Clinically important, potentially hazardous interactions with: none known
Pregnancy category: N/A (Insufficient evidence to inform drug-associated risk)
Important contra-indications noted in the prescribing guidelines for: the elderly; nursing mothers; pediatric patients
Note: Fluoroquinolones are associated with an increased risk of tendinitis and tendon rupture in all ages. This risk is further increased in older patients usually over 60 years of age, in patients taking corticosteroid drugs, and in patients with kidney, heart or lung transplants.
Fluoroquinolones may exacerbate muscle weakness in persons with myasthenia gravis.
Warning: SERIOUS ADVERSE REACTIONS INCLUDING TENDINITIS, TENDON RUPTURE, PERIPHERAL NEUROPATHY, CENTRAL NERVOUS SYSTEM EFFECTS, and EXACERBATION OF MYASTHENIA GRAVIS

Skin
Dermatitis (<2%)
Edema (<2%)
Erythema (<2%)
Flushing (<2%)
Hypersensitivity (<2%)
Irritation (<2%)
Pruritus (<2%)
Rash (<2%)
Urticaria (<2%)

Mucosal
Oral candidiasis (<2%)

Cardiovascular
Bradycardia (<2%)
Hypertension (<2%)
Hypotension (<2%)
Palpitation (<2%)
Phlebitis (<2%)
Tachycardia (<2%)

Central Nervous System
Abnormal dreams (<2%)
Anxiety (<2%)
Dysgeusia (taste perversion) (<2%)
Headache (3%) [3]
Hypoesthesia (<2%)
Insomnia (<2%)
Paresthesias (<2%)
Presyncope (<2%)
Syncope (<2%)
Vertigo (dizziness) (<2%)

Neuromuscular/Skeletal
Myalgia/Myopathy (<2%)

Gastrointestinal/Hepatic
Abdominal pain (<2%)
Diarrhea (8%) [6]
Dyspepsia (<2%)
Nausea (8%) [6]
Vomiting (2%) [2]

Endocrine/Metabolic
ALT increased (>2%)
AST increased (>2%)
Creatine phosphokinase increased (<2%)
Hyperglycemia (<2%)
Hyperphosphatemia (<2%)
Hypoglycemia (<2%)
Serum creatinine increased (<2%)

Genitourinary
Vulvovaginal candidiasis (<2%)

Renal
Nephrotoxicity (<2%)
Renal failure (<2%)

Hematologic
Thrombosis (<2%)

Otic
Tinnitus (<2%)

Ocular
Vision blurred (<2%)

Local
Injection-site bruising (<2%)
Injection-site extravasation (<2%)

Other
Adverse effects [2]
Infection (<2%)

DENOSUMAB

Trade names: Prolia (Amgen), Xgeva (Amgen)
Indications: Osteoporosis (postmenopausal women), prevention of skeletal-related events in patients with bone metastases from solid tumors
Class: Bone resorption inhibitor, Monoclonal antibody, RANK ligand (RANKL) inhibitor
Half-life: 25–28 days
Clinically important, potentially hazardous interactions with: abatacept, alcohol, azacitidine, betamethasone, cabazitaxel, denileukin, docetaxel, fingolimod, gefitinib, immuosuppressants, leflunomide, lenalidomide, oxaliplatin, pazopanib, temsirolimus, triamcinolone
Pregnancy category: X
Important contra-indications noted in the prescribing guidelines for: nursing mothers; pediatric patients
Note: Contra-indicated in patients with hypocalcemia.

Skin
Cellulitis [9]
Dermatitis [2]
Eczema [10]
Herpes zoster (2%)
Hypersensitivity [3]
Malignancies [2]
Peripheral edema (5%)
Pruritus (2%)
Rash (3%) [4]

Cardiovascular
Angina (3%)
Atrial fibrillation (2%)
Cardiotoxicity [2]

Central Nervous System
Headache [3]
Insomnia (3%)
Pain [2]
Vertigo (dizziness) (5%)

Neuromuscular/Skeletal
Arthralgia [5]
Asthenia (fatigue) (2%) [2]
Back pain (35%) [8]
Bone or joint pain (4–8%) [3]
Fractures [10]
Myalgia/Myopathy (3%)
Osteonecrosis (jaw) [28]
Pain in extremities (12%) [6]

Gastrointestinal/Hepatic
Abdominal pain (3%)
Flatulence (2%)
Gastroesophageal reflux (2%)
Pancreatitis [2]

Respiratory
Nasopharyngitis [2]
Pharyngitis (2%)
Pneumonia (4%)
Upper respiratory tract infection (5%)

Endocrine/Metabolic
Hypercalcemia [3]
Hypercholesterolemia (7%) [2]
Hypocalcemia (2%) [35]
Hypophosphatemia [4]

Genitourinary
Cystitis (6%)

Hematologic
Anemia (3%) [2]

Other
Adverse effects [11]
Death [2]
Infection [14]

DEOXYCHOLIC ACID

Trade name: Kybella (Kythera)
Indications: Improvement in the appearance of moderate to severe convexity or fullness associated with submental fat
Class: Cytolytic
Half-life: N/A
Clinically important, potentially hazardous interactions with: none known
Pregnancy category: N/A
Important contra-indications noted in the prescribing guidelines for: the elderly; pediatric patients
Note: Contra-indicated in the presence of infection at the injection sites.

Skin
Lymphadenopathy (<2%)

Mucosal
Oropharyngeal pain (3%)

Cardiovascular
Hypertension (3%)

Central Nervous System
Headache (8%)
Syncope (<2%)

Neuromuscular/Skeletal
Neck pain (<2%)

Gastrointestinal/Hepatic
Dysphagia (2%)
Nausea (2%)

Local
Injection-site bruising (72%) [2]
Injection-site edema [2]
Injection-site erythema (27%)
Injection-site hemorrhage (<2%)
Injection-site induration (23%) [2]
Injection-site nodules (13%)
Injection-site numbness (66%) [2]
Injection-site pain (70%) [2]
Injection-site pigmentation (<2%)
Injection-site pruritus (12%)
Injection-site urticaria (<2%)

Other
Adverse effects [2]

DESLORATADINE

Trade name: Clarinex (Schering)
Indications: Allergic rhinitis, urticaria
Class: Histamine H1 receptor antagonist
Half-life: 27 hours
Clinically important, potentially hazardous interactions with: none known
Pregnancy category: C
Important contra-indications noted in the prescribing guidelines for: nursing mothers; pediatric patients

---

Skin
Urticaria [2]

Mucosal
Xerostomia [5]

Central Nervous System
Headache [7]
Somnolence (drowsiness) [7]

Neuromuscular/Skeletal
Asthenia (fatigue) [7]

Gastrointestinal/Hepatic
Diarrhea [2]
Nausea [2]

Other
Adverse effects [6]

DESMOPRESSIN

Trade names: DDAVP (Sanofi-Aventis), Minirin (Ferring), Noctiva (Serenity), Stimate (CSL Behring)
Indications: Primary nocturnal enuresis, nocturia due to nocturnal polyuria (Noctiva)
Class: Antidiuretic hormone analog
Half-life: 75 minutes
Clinically important, potentially hazardous interactions with: amitriptyline, citalopram, demeclocycline, hydromorphone, meloxicam, tapentadol
Pregnancy category: B
Important contra-indications noted in the prescribing guidelines for: the elderly; nursing mothers; pediatric patients
Warning: Noctiva: HYPONATREMIA

Skin
Flushing (<10%)

Cardiovascular
Myocardial infarction [2]
Central Nervous System
Headache [7]
Seizures [5]
Endocrine/Metabolic
Hyponatremia [13]
SIADH [2]
Local
Injection-site pain (<10%)

DESVENLAFAXINE

Trade name: Pristiq (Wyeth)
Indications: Major depressive disorder
Class: Antidepressant, Serotonin-norepinephrine reuptake inhibitor
Half-life: 11 hours
Clinically important, potentially hazardous interactions with: alcohol, aspirin, CNS-active agents, heparin, ketoconazole, linezolid, lithium, MAO inhibitors, NSAIDs, sibutramine, tramadol, venlafaxine, warfarin
Pregnancy category: C
Important contra-indications noted in the prescribing guidelines for: the elderly; nursing mothers; pediatric patients
Warning: SUICIDAL THOUGHTS AND BEHAVIORS

Skin
Hot flashes (<2%)
Hyperhidrosis (10–21%)
Hypersensitivity (2%)
Rash (<2%)
Mucosal
Epistaxis (nosebleed) (<2%)
Xerostomia (11–25%) [3]
Cardiovascular
Hypertension (<2%)
Hypotension (~2%)
Orthostatic hypotension (<2%)
Palpitation (<3%)
Tachycardia (<2%)
Central Nervous System
Abnormal dreams (2–4%)
Anorexia (5–8%) [2]
Anorgasmia (3–8%)
Anxiety (3–5%)
Chills (<4%)
Dysgeusia (taste perversion) (<2%)
Extrapyramidal symptoms (<2%)
Headache (20–29%) [3]
Impaired concentration (<2%)
Insomnia (9–12%) [3]
Irritability (2%)
Nervousness (<2%) [2]
Paresthesias (<3%)
Seizures (~2%)
Somnolence (drowsiness) (4–12%) [4]
Suicidal ideation [2]
Syncope (<2%)
Tremor (~3%)
Vertigo (dizziness) (10–16%) [5]
Yawning (<4%)
Neuromuscular/Skeletal
Asthenia (fatigue) (7–11%) [2]
Gastrointestinal/Hepatic
Constipation (9–14%)
Diarrhea (5–11%)
Nausea (22–41%) [6]
Vomiting (3–9%)
Endocrine/Metabolic
Appetite decreased (5–10%)
Libido decreased (3–6%)
Weight gain (<2%)
Weight loss (<2%)
Genitourinary
Ejaculatory dysfunction (<5%)
Erectile dysfunction (3–11%)
Sexual dysfunction (<2%)
Otic
Tinnitus (<2%)
Ocular
Mydriasis (2–6%)
Vision blurred (3–4%)

DEUTETRABENAZINE

Trade name: Austedo (Teva)
Indications: Chorea associated with Huntington's disease
Class: Vesicular monoamine transporter 2 inhibitor
Half-life: 9–10 hours
Clinically important, potentially hazardous interactions with: alcohol or other sedating drugs, bupropion, dopamine antagonists or antipsychotics, fluoxetine, MAO inhibitors, paroxetine hydrochloride, quinidine, strong CYP2D6 inhibitors, tetrabenazine
Pregnancy category: N/A (Based on animal data, may cause fetal harm)
Important contra-indications noted in the prescribing guidelines for: the elderly; nursing mothers; pediatric patients
Note: Contra-indicated in suicidal or untreated/inadequately treated depression, in hepatic impairment, or in patients taking MAO inhibitors, reserpine or tetrabenazine.
Warning: DEPRESSION AND SUICIDALITY

Skin
Hematoma (4%)
Mucosal
Xerostomia (9%)
Central Nervous System
Anxiety (4%) [2]
Depression [3]
Insomnia (7%) [3]
Somnolence (drowsiness) (11%) [6]
Vertigo (dizziness) (4%)
Neuromuscular/Skeletal
Asthenia (fatigue) (9%) [3]
Gastrointestinal/Hepatic
Constipation (4%)
Diarrhea (9%) [2]
Respiratory
Nasopharyngitis [2]
Genitourinary
Urinary tract infection (7%)

DEXAMETHASONE

Trade names: Decadron (Merck), Dexone (Solvay), Ozurdex (Allergan)
Indications: Antiemetic, arthralgias, dermatoses, diagnostic aid, macular edema following branch retinal vein occlusion (BRVO) or central retinal vein occlusion (CRVO), non-infectious uveitis affecting the posterior segment of the eye
Class: Antiemetic, Corticosteroid, systemic, Corticosteroid, topical
Half-life: N/A
Clinically important, potentially hazardous interactions with: albendazole, aminoglutethimide, amprenavir, aprepitant, aspirin, bexarotene, boceprevir, carbamazepine, caspofungin, cobicistat/elvitegravir/emtricitabine/tenofovir alafenamide, cobicistat/elvitegravir/emtricitabine/tenofovir disoproxil, cyclophosphamide, dasatinib, delavirdine, diuretics, ephedrine, imatinib, itraconazole, ixabepilone, lapatinib, lenalidomide, live vaccines, lopinavir, methotrexate, midazolam, phenobarbital, phenytoin, praziquantel, primidone, rifampin, rilpivirine, romidepsin, simeprevir, sorafenib, sunitinib, telaprevir, temsirolimus, ticagrelor, vandetanib, warfarin
Pregnancy category: C
Important contra-indications noted in the prescribing guidelines for: nursing mothers; pediatric patients

---

Skin
Acneform eruption [6]
AGEP [2]
Anaphylactoid reactions/Anaphylaxis [3]
Dermatitis [5]
Edema [4]
Erythema multiforme [3]
Exanthems [4]
Flushing [5]
Herpes zoster [2]
Hyperhidrosis [2]
Hypersensitivity [6]
Peripheral edema [8]
Pigmentation [2]
Pruritus [7]
Pruritus ani et vulvae [2]
Rash [11]
Striae [4]
Toxicity [5]
Tumor lysis syndrome [3]
Xerosis [2]
Mucosal
Oral candidiasis [2]
Cardiovascular
Bradycardia [9]
Cardiac failure [2]
Cardiotoxicity [2]
Hypertension [18]
Myocardial toxicity [11]
Tachycardia [2]
Thromboembolism [3]
Venous thromboembolism [5]
Central Nervous System
Anorexia [2]
Catatonia [2]
Dysgeusia (taste perversion) [3]
Fever [7]

Headache (<5%) [8]
Insomnia [9]
Leukoencephalopathy [2]
Neurotoxicity [11]
Paresthesias [2]
Peripheral neuropathy [27]
Somnolence (drowsiness) [2]
Vertigo (dizziness) [3]

Neuromuscular/Skeletal
Arthralgia [5]
Asthenia (fatigue) [43]
Back pain [5]
Bone or joint pain [4]
Muscle spasm [5]
Myalgia/Myopathy [6]
Osteonecrosis [15]
Osteoporosis [3]

Gastrointestinal/Hepatic
Abdominal distension [2]
Abdominal pain [5]
Constipation [11]
Diarrhea [20]
Dyspepsia [3]
Gastroesophageal reflux [2]
Gastrointestinal disorder [3]
Hepatotoxicity [4]
Nausea [12]
Pancreatitis [2]
Vomiting [7]

Respiratory
Cough [4]
Dyspnea [5]
Pneumonia [14]
Pneumonitis [2]
Upper respiratory tract infection [3]

Endocrine/Metabolic
ALT increased [2]
AST increased [2]
Cushing's syndrome [2]
Dehydration [3]
Hyperglycemia [8]
Hypokalemia [5]
Hypophosphatemia [4]
Serum creatinine increased [2]

Renal
Nephrotoxicity [2]
Renal failure [2]

Hematologic
Anemia [39]
Febrile neutropenia [7]
Hemoglobin decreased [2]
Hemotoxicity [8]
Leukopenia [11]
Lymphopenia [11]
Myelosuppression [5]
Neutropenia [51]
Sepsis [3]
Thrombocytopenia [53]
Thrombosis [2]

Otic
Ototoxicity [4]

Ocular
Cataract (<10%) [9]
Conjunctival hemorrhage (>10%)
Glaucoma [9]
Intraocular pressure increased (>10%) [13]
Ocular hypertension (<10%) [6]
Ocular pain (<10%) [6]
Vision blurred [3]

Local
Infusion-related reactions [2]
Infusion-site reactions [2]

Other
Adverse effects [20]
Allergic reactions [2]
Death [11]
Hiccups [18]
Infection [30]
Side effects [3]

DEXLANSOPRAZOLE

Trade name: Dexilant (Takeda)
Indications: Erosive esophagitis, heartburn associated with gastroesophageal reflux disease
Class: Proton pump inhibitor (PPI)
Half-life: <2 hours
Clinically important, potentially hazardous interactions with: atazanavir, clopidogrel, digoxin, emtricitabine/rilpivirine/tenofovir alafenamide, ketoconazole, tacrolimus, warfarin
Pregnancy category: B
Important contra-indications noted in the prescribing guidelines for: nursing mothers

---

Skin
Acneform eruption (<2%)
Dermatitis (<2%)
Erythema (<2%)
Hot flashes (<2%)
Lesions (<2%)
Lymphadenopathy (<2%)
Pruritus (<2%)
Rash (<2%)
Urticaria (<2%)

Mucosal
Mucosal inflammation (<2%)
Oral candidiasis (<2%)
Xerostomia (<2%)

Cardiovascular
Cardiac disorder (<2%)

Central Nervous System
Headache [2]

Gastrointestinal/Hepatic
Abdominal pain (4%) [4]
Constipation [2]
Diarrhea (5%) [4]
Flatulence (<3%) [3]
Gastrointestinal disorder (<2%)
Nausea (3%) [4]
Vomiting (<2%) [2]

Respiratory
Upper respiratory tract infection (2–3%) [3]

Hematologic
Anemia (<2%)

Otic
Ear pain (<2%)
Tinnitus (<2%)

Ocular
Ocular edema (<2%)
Ocular pruritus (<2%)

Other
Adverse effects [2]

DEXMETHYL-PHENIDATE

Trade name: Focalin (Novartis)
Indications: Attention deficit disorder
Class: CNS stimulant
Half-life: 2–4.5 hours
Clinically important, potentially hazardous interactions with: amitriptyline, clonidine, linezolid, MAO inhibitors, pantoprazole
Pregnancy category: C
Important contra-indications noted in the prescribing guidelines for: nursing mothers; pediatric patients
Note: Contra-indicated in patients with marked anxiety, tension and agitation, with glaucoma, or with motor tics or history/diagnosis of Tourette's syndrome.

Central Nervous System
Fever (5%)
Headache [4]

Gastrointestinal/Hepatic
Abdominal pain (15%) [2]

Endocrine/Metabolic
Appetite decreased [2]

DEXTRO-AMPHETAMINE

Trade names: Adderall (Shire), Dexedrine (Alliant), Mydayis (Shire)
Indications: Narcolepsy, attention deficit disorder (ADD)
Class: Amphetamine, CNS stimulant
Half-life: 10–12 hours
Clinically important, potentially hazardous interactions with: fluoxetine, fluvoxamine, MAO inhibitors, paroxetine hydrochloride, phenelzine, sertraline, tranylcypromine
Pregnancy category: C
Important contra-indications noted in the prescribing guidelines for: nursing mothers; pediatric patients
Warning: ABUSE AND DEPENDENCE

Skin
Diaphoresis (<10%)

Mucosal
Xerostomia (<10%)

Central Nervous System
Insomnia [2]

Neuromuscular/Skeletal
Rhabdomyolysis [10]

DEXTRO-METHORPHAN

Trade names: Robitussin (Wyeth), Vicks Formula 44 (Procter & Gamble)
Indications: Nonproductive cough
Class: Analgesic, narcotic, NMDA receptor antagonist
Half-life: N/A
Clinically important, potentially hazardous interactions with: amiodarone, citalopram, iloperidone, linezolid, lorcaserin, memantine, moclobemide, phenelzine, rasagiline, safinamide, sibutramine, tranylcypromine, valdecoxib
Pregnancy category: C
Important contra-indications noted in the prescribing guidelines for: nursing mothers; pediatric patients

---

Skin
Bullous dermatitis [2]
Fixed eruption [2]

Central Nervous System
Headache [2]
Serotonin syndrome [4]
Vertigo (dizziness) [3]

Gastrointestinal/Hepatic
Diarrhea [4]

Genitourinary
Urinary tract infection [2]

Other
Adverse effects [2]

DIAZEPAM

Trade names: Diastat (Xcel), Valium (Roche)
Indications: Anxiety
Class: Benzodiazepine, Skeletal muscle relaxant
Half-life: 20–70 hours
Clinically important, potentially hazardous interactions with: alcohol, amprenavir, barbiturates, buprenorphine, chlorpheniramine, clarithromycin, CNS depressants, cobicistat/elvitegravir/emtricitabine/tenofovir alafenamide, cobicistat/elvitegravir/emtricitabine/tenofovir disoproxil, efavirenz, esomeprazole, eucalyptus, fluoroquinolones, imatinib, indinavir, itraconazole, ivermectin, macrolide antibiotics, MAO inhibitors, methadone, mianserin, nalbuphine, narcotics, nelfinavir, nilutamide, olanzapine, omeprazole, phenothiazines, propranolol, ritonavir, SSRIs, voriconazole
Pregnancy category: D
Important contra-indications noted in the prescribing guidelines for: nursing mothers

---

Skin
Dermatitis (<10%) [3]
Diaphoresis (>10%)
Exanthems [6]
Exfoliative dermatitis [2]
Fixed eruption [2]
Pigmentation [2]
Purpura [4]
Rash (>10%) [2]

Mucosal
Xerostomia (>10%)

Central Nervous System
Amnesia [17]
Hallucinations [2]
Sedation [3]
Somnolence (drowsiness) [6]
Vertigo (dizziness) [2]

Neuromuscular/Skeletal
Ataxia [2]

Endocrine/Metabolic
Gynecomastia [4]
Porphyria [2]

Local
Injection-site pain [2]
Injection-site phlebitis (>10%) [2]

Other
Adverse effects [3]
Allergic reactions [2]

DICLOFENAC

Trade names: Arthrotec (Pfizer), Cataflam (Novartis), Dicolmax (Galen), Motifene (Daiichi Sankyo), Pennsaid (Mallinckrodt), Solaraze Gel (Nycomed), Voltaren (Novartis), Voltarol (Novartis), Zipsor (Depomed)
Indications: Rheumatoid and osteoarthritis, topical treatment of actinic keratosis, postoperative inflammation in patients who have undergone cataract extraction and for the temporary relief of pain and photophobia in patients undergoing corneal refractive surgery
Class: Non-steroidal anti-inflammatory (NSAID)
Half-life: 1–2 hours
Clinically important, potentially hazardous interactions with: ACE inhibitors, adrenergic neurone blockers, aldosterone antagonists, aliskiren, alpha blockers, angiotensin II receptor antagonists, anticoagulants, aspirin, baclofen, beta blockers, calcium channel blockers, cardiac glycosides, clonidine, clopidogrel, corticosteroids, coumarins, cyclosporine, dabigatran, deferiprone, diazoxide, diuretics, enoxaparin, erlotinib, furosemide, heparins, hydralazine, iloprost, ketorolac, lithium, methotrexate, methyldopa, mifamurtide, minoxidil, moxonidine, nitrates, nitroprusside, penicillamine, pentoxifylline, phenindione, potassium canrenoate, prasugrel, rifampin, ritonavir, rivaroxaban, SSRIs, sulfonylureas, tacrolimus, thiazides, tinzaparin, venlafaxine, voriconazole, warfarin, zidovudine
Pregnancy category: D (category B for topical use; category C for oral and ophthalmic use; category D in third trimester.)
Important contra-indications noted in the prescribing guidelines for: nursing mothers; pediatric patients
Note: NSAIDs may cause an increased risk of serious cardiovascular and gastrointestinal adverse events, which can be fatal. This risk may increase with duration of use.
Contra-indicated in patients who have experienced asthma, urticaria, or allergic-type reactions after taking aspirin or other NSAIDs. Severe, rarely fatal, anaphylactic-like reactions to NSAIDs have been reported in such patients.
Arthrotec is diclofenac and misoprostol.

Warning: RISK OF SERIOUS CARDIOVASCULAR AND GASTROINTESTINAL EVENTS

Skin
Anaphylactoid reactions/Anaphylaxis (<3%) [16]
Angioedema (<3%) [2]
Bullous dermatitis (<3%) [2]
Dermatitis (<3%) [10]
Dermatitis herpetiformis [2]
Eczema (<3%)
Erythema [4]
Erythema multiforme [6]
Exanthems (<5%) [6]
Fixed eruption [4]
Hypersensitivity [5]
Linear IgA bullous dermatosis [6]
Nicolau syndrome [16]
Photosensitivity (<3%) [4]
Pruritus (<10%) [6]
Purpura (<3%) [2]
Purpura fulminans [2]
Rash (>10%) [4]
Stevens-Johnson syndrome [7]
Toxic epidermal necrolysis [5]
Urticaria (<3%) [7]
Vasculitis [3]
Xerosis [3]

Hair
Alopecia (<3%)

Mucosal
Tongue edema (<3%)
Xerostomia (<3%) [2]

Cardiovascular
Atrial fibrillation [2]
Cardiotoxicity [2]
Myocardial infarction [5]

Central Nervous System
Dysgeusia (taste perversion) (<3%)
Headache [2]
Stroke [3]
Vertigo (dizziness) [4]

Neuromuscular/Skeletal
Rhabdomyolysis [3]

Gastrointestinal/Hepatic
Abdominal pain [8]
Constipation [3]
Diarrhea [4]
Dyspepsia [7]
Flatulence [2]
Gastritis [3]
Gastrointestinal bleeding [6]
Gastrointestinal ulceration [4]
Hepatotoxicity [10]
Nausea [9]
Vomiting [4]

Renal
Nephrotoxicity [4]
Renal failure [2]

Hematologic
Agranulocytosis [3]
Bleeding [2]

Local
Application-site reactions [3]

Other
Adverse effects [11]

Allergic reactions [2]
Death [6]

DICUMAROL

Indications: Atrial fibrillation, pulmonary embolism, venous thrombosis
Class: Coumarin
Half-life: 1–4 days
Clinically important, potentially hazardous interactions with: allopurinol, amiodarone, amobarbital, anabolic steroids, anti-thyroid agents, aprobarbital, aspirin, barbiturates, bivalirudin, butabarbital, butalbital, cimetidine, clofibrate, clopidogrel, cyclosporine, delavirdine, disulfiram, fenofibrate, fluconazole, gemfibrozil, glutethimide, imatinib, itraconazole, ketoconazole, levothyroxine, liothyronine, mephobarbital, methimazole, metronidazole, miconazole, penicillins, pentobarbital, phenobarbital, phenylbutazones, piperacillin, prednisone, primidone, propylthiouracil, quinidine, quinine, rifabutin, rifampin, rifapentine, rofecoxib, salicylates, secobarbital, sulfinpyrazone, sulfonamides, testosterone, zileuton
Pregnancy category: D
Important contra-indications noted in the prescribing guidelines for: nursing mothers

Skin
Dermatitis [2]
Exanthems [5]
Necrosis [10]
Purplish erythema (feet and toes) [2]
Purpura [2]
Urticaria [3]

Hair
Alopecia (<10%) [5]

Hematologic
Hemorrhage [3]

DIDANOSINE

Trade name: Videx (Bristol-Myers Squibb)
Indications: Advanced HIV infection
Class: Antiretroviral, Nucleoside analog reverse transcriptase inhibitor
Half-life: 1.5 hours
Clinically important, potentially hazardous interactions with: acetaminophen, amprenavir, ciprofloxacin, corticosteroids, dapsone, darunavir, febuxostat, gemifloxacin, indinavir, itraconazole, ketoconazole, levofloxacin, lomefloxacin, lopinavir, moxifloxacin, norfloxacin, ofloxacin, sulfones, tenofovir disoproxil, tetracycline, tipranavir, voriconazole
Pregnancy category: B
Important contra-indications noted in the prescribing guidelines for: the elderly; nursing mothers
Warning: PANCREATITIS, LACTIC ACIDOSIS and HEPATOMEGALY with STEATOSIS

Skin
Erythema multiforme [2]
Lipodystrophy [2]
Pruritus (9%)
Rash (9%)
Stevens-Johnson syndrome [3]

Mucosal
Xerostomia [4]

Cardiovascular
Myocardial infarction [2]

Central Nervous System
Neurotoxicity [4]

Gastrointestinal/Hepatic
Hepatotoxicity [2]
Non-cirrhotic portal hypertension [5]
Pancreatitis [23]

Endocrine/Metabolic
Acidosis [6]
Diabetes mellitus [2]
Gynecomastia [3]

Renal
Fanconi syndrome [5]
Nephrotoxicity [2]

Ocular
Retinopathy [3]

Other
Death [3]

DIGOXIN

Trade name: Lanoxin (Concordia)
Indications: Congestive heart failure, atrial fibrillation
Class: Antiarrhythmic class IV, Cardiac glycoside, Inotrope
Half-life: 36–48 hours
Clinically important, potentially hazardous interactions with: acarbose, alprazolam, amiodarone, amphotericin B, arbutamine, atorvastatin, azithromycin, bendroflumethiazide, benzthiazide, bisacodyl, boceprevir, bosutinib, bumetanide, canagliflozin, captopril, carbimazole, chlorothiazide, chlorthalidone, cholestyramine, clarithromycin, cobicistat/elvitegravir/emtricitabine/tenofovir alafenamide, cobicistat/elvitegravir/emtricitabine/tenofovir disoproxil, colchicine, conivaptan, cyclopenthiazide, cyclosporine, cyclothiazide, darifenacin, darunavir, demeclocycline, dexlansoprazole, dexmedetomidine, doxycycline, dronedarone, erythromycin, eslicarbazepine, esomeprazole, ethacrynic acid, etravirine, everolimus, ezogabine, fingolimod, flibanserin, flunisolide, furosemide, glycopyrrolate, glycopyrronium, hydrochlorothiazide, hydroflumethiazide, indapamide, indinavir, itraconazole, lapatinib, lenalidomide, liraglutide, lomustine, lopinavir, meloxicam, mepenzolate, metformin, methyclothiazide, metolazone, milnacipran, minocycline, mirabegron, neratinib, nifedipine, nilotinib, omeprazole, oxprenolol, oxytetracycline, pantoprazole, paricalcitol, paroxetine hydrochloride, pemetrexed, phenylbutazone, polythiazide, posaconazole, propafenone, propantheline, quinethazone, quinidine, quinine, rabeprazole, rifampin, roxithromycin, sitagliptin, sodium picosulfate, sorafenib, St John's wort, sunitinib, telaprevir, telithromycin, temozolomide, temsirolimus, teriparatide, tetracycline, thalidomide, thiazide diuretics, ticagrelor, tipranavir, tolvaptan, trichlormethiazide, trimethoprim, troglitazone, ulipristal, valbenazine, venetoclax, verapamil, zuclopenthixol
Pregnancy category: C
Important contra-indications noted in the prescribing guidelines for: the elderly; nursing mothers; pediatric patients
Note: This is the pure form of Digitalis. Contra-indicated in ventricular fibrillation.

Skin
Exanthems (2%) [2]
Psoriasis [2]
Toxicity [5]

Cardiovascular
Arrhythmias [7]
Atrial fibrillation [4]
Bradycardia [4]
Tachycardia [2]

Central Nervous System
Anorexia [2]

Neuromuscular/Skeletal
Asthenia (fatigue) [2]

Gastrointestinal/Hepatic
Nausea [4]
Vomiting [2]

Endocrine/Metabolic
Gynecomastia [2]

Ocular
Dyschromatopsia (green) [6]
Hallucinations, visual [2]

Other
Death [5]

DIHYDROCODEINE

Trade name: DHC-Continus (Napp)
Indications: Severe pain in cancer and other chronic conditions
Class: Analgesic, opioid
Half-life: 12 hours
Clinically important, potentially hazardous interactions with: CNS depressants, MAO inhibitors, phenothiazines, tranquilizers
Pregnancy category: C
Important contra-indications noted in the prescribing guidelines for: nursing mothers

Skin
AGEP [2]

Mucosal
Xerostomia [2]

Central Nervous System
Narcosis [2]
Seizures [3]
Somnolence (drowsiness) [2]

Gastrointestinal/Hepatic
Abdominal pain [2]
Constipation [2]
Nausea [2]
Vomiting [2]

Respiratory
Respiratory depression [2]

Genitourinary
Priapism [2]

Renal
Renal failure [5]

DILTIAZEM

Trade names: Cardizem (Biovail), Dilacor XR (Watson), Teczem (Sanofi-Aventis), Tiazac (Forest)
Indications: Angina, essential hypertension
Class: Antiarrhythmic class IV, Calcium channel blocker, CYP3A4 inhibitor
Half-life: 5–8 hours (for extended-release capsules)
Clinically important, potentially hazardous interactions with: acebutolol, alfuzosin, amiodarone, amitriptyline, amprenavir, aprepitant, atazanavir, atenolol, atorvastatin, avanafil, bisoprolol, bosentan, carbamazepine, celiprolol, cilostazol, cobicistat/elvitegravir/emtricitabine/tenofovir alafenamide, cobicistat/elvitegravir/emtricitabine/tenofovir disoproxil, colchicine, copanlisib, corticosteroids, cyclosporine, deflazacort, delavirdine, dronedarone, dutasteride, efavirenz, epirubicin, erythromycin, fingolimod, flibanserin, lurasidone, midostaurin, mifepristone, moricizine, naldemedine, naloxegol, neratinib, nevirapine, nifedipine, olaparib, oxprenolol, posaconazole, ranolazine, silodosin, simvastatin, sonidegib, sulpiride, telaprevir, venetoclax
Pregnancy category: C
Important contra-indications noted in the prescribing guidelines for: the elderly; nursing mothers; pediatric patients
Note: Teczem is diltiazem and enalapril.

Skin
AGEP [21]
Angioedema [3]
Diaphoresis [2]
Edema (<10%) [4]
Erythema [2]
Erythema multiforme (<31%) [11]
Exanthems [17]
Exfoliative dermatitis [6]
Flushing (<10%) [6]
Hypersensitivity [2]
Leg ulceration [2]
Lupus erythematosus [5]
Palmar–plantar desquamation [2]
Peripheral edema (5–8%)
Photosensitivity [11]
Phototoxicity [2]
Pigmentation [10]
Pruritus [6]
Psoriasis [3]
Purpura [3]
Pustules [2]
Rash [4]
Stevens-Johnson syndrome [4]
Thickening [2]
Toxic epidermal necrolysis [4]
Toxic erythema [2]
Toxicity [2]
Urticaria [5]
Vasculitis [6]

Hair
Alopecia [2]

Mucosal
Gingival hyperplasia/hypertrophy (21%) [10]
Xerostomia [2]

Cardiovascular
Atrial fibrillation [2]
Bradycardia [7]
Cardiogenic shock [2]
Hypotension [2]
QT prolongation [2]

Central Nervous System
Dysgeusia (taste perversion) [2]
Parkinsonism [3]
Somnolence (drowsiness) [2]

Neuromuscular/Skeletal
Rhabdomyolysis [4]

Other
Side effects [2]

DIMENHYDRINATE

Trade name: Dramamine (Pfizer)
Indications: Motion sickness, dizziness, nausea, vomiting
Class: Antiemetic, Cholinesterase absorption inhibitor
Half-life: N/A
Clinically important, potentially hazardous interactions with: none known
Pregnancy category: B
Important contra-indications noted in the prescribing guidelines for: nursing mothers

---

Skin
Fixed eruption [12]

Mucosal
Xerostomia (<10%)

Central Nervous System
Somnolence (drowsiness) [5]

DIMETHYL FUMARATE

Synonyms: dimethyl (E) butenedioate; BG-12
Trade names: Fumaderm (Biogen Idec), Tecfidera (Biogen Idec)
Indications: Relapsing forms of multiple sclerosis, psoriasis
Class: Fumaric acid ester
Half-life: 1 hour
Clinically important, potentially hazardous interactions with: none known
Pregnancy category: C
Important contra-indications noted in the prescribing guidelines for: the elderly; nursing mothers; pediatric patients
Note: Fumaderm is mixed dimethyl fumarate and monoethylfumarate salts.

Skin
Contact dermatitis (from topical contact) [14]
Erythema (5%) [2]
Flushing (40%) [30]
Pruritus (8%) [5]
Rash (8%) [2]

Central Nervous System
Headache [2]
Leukoencephalopathy [6]

Neuromuscular/Skeletal
Asthenia (fatigue) [3]

Gastrointestinal/Hepatic
Abdominal pain (18%) [12]
Diarrhea (14%) [10]
Dyspepsia (5%) [2]
Gastrointestinal disorder [3]
Nausea [7]
Vomiting (9%) [3]

Respiratory
Nasopharyngitis [2]

Endocrine/Metabolic
AST increased (4%) [3]

Genitourinary
Albuminuria (6%)
Urinary tract infection [2]

Renal
Proteinuria [2]

Hematologic
Hemotoxicity [2]
Lymphopenia (2%) [10]

Other
Adverse effects (gastrointestinal) [19]
Infection [2]

DINOPROSTONE

Trade names: Cervidel (Forest), Prepidil (Pfizer)
Indications: Pregnancy termination, uterine content evacuation, cervical ripening
Class: Prostaglandin
Half-life: 2.5–5 minutes
Clinically important, potentially hazardous interactions with: none known
Pregnancy category: C
Note: Dinoprostone is the naturally occurring form of Prostaglandin E2 (PGE2).

DINUTUXIMAB

Trade name: Unituxin (United Therapeutics)
Indications: High-risk neuroblastoma in combination with granulocyte-macrophage colony-stimulating factor (GM-CSF), interleukin-2 (IL-2), and isotretinoin (13-*cis*-retinoic acid), in pediatric patients who achieve at least a partial response to prior first-line multiagent, multimodality therapy
Class: GD2-binding monoclonal antibody, Monoclonal antibody
Half-life: 10 days
Clinically important, potentially hazardous interactions with: none known
Pregnancy category: N/A (May cause fetal harm)
Important contra-indications noted in the prescribing guidelines for: the elderly; nursing mothers
Warning: SERIOUS INFUSION REACTIONS AND NEUROTOXICITY

Skin
Edema (17%)
Urticaria (25–37%)

Mucosal
Nasal congestion (20%)

Cardiovascular
Capillary leak syndrome (22–40%)
Hypertension (14%)
Hypotension (60%)
Tachycardia (19%)

Central Nervous System
Fever (55–72%)
Pain (61–85%) [2]
Peripheral neuropathy (13%)

Gastrointestinal/Hepatic
Diarrhea (31–43%)
Nausea (10%)
Vomiting (33–46%)

Respiratory
Hypoxia (24%)
Wheezing (15%)

Endocrine/Metabolic
ALT increased (43–56%)
AST increased (16–28%)
Creatine phosphokinase increased (15%)
Hyperglycemia (18%)
Hypertriglyceridemia (16%)
Hypoalbuminemia (29–33%)
Hypocalcemia (20–27%)
Hypokalemia (26–43%)
Hypomagnesemia (12%)
Hyponatremia (36–58%)
Hypophosphatemia (20%)
Weight gain (10%)

Renal
Proteinuria (16%)

Hematologic
Anemia (42–51%)
Hemorrhage (17%)
Lymphopenia (54–62%)
Neutropenia (25–39%)
Sepsis (18%)
Thrombocytopenia (61–66%)

Local
Infusion-related reactions (47–60%) [2]

DIPHENHYDRAMINE

Trade name: Benadryl (Pfizer)
Indications: Allergic rhinitis, urticaria
Class: Antiemetic, Histamine H1 receptor antagonist, Muscarinic antagonist
Half-life: 2–8 hours
Clinically important, potentially hazardous interactions with: alcohol, anticholinergics, chloral hydrate, CNS depressants, glutethimide, MAO inhibitors
Pregnancy category: B
Important contra-indications noted in the prescribing guidelines for: nursing mothers

---

Skin
Anaphylactoid reactions/Anaphylaxis [4]
Contact dermatitis [2]
Dermatitis [4]
Eczema [2]
Fixed eruption [4]
Photosensitivity [3]
Pruritus [2]
Toxic epidermal necrolysis [3]
Toxicity [2]

Mucosal
Xerostomia (<10%)

Cardiovascular
QT prolongation [5]
Torsades de pointes [3]

Central Nervous System
Delirium [2]
Sedation [2]
Seizures [2]
Somnolence (drowsiness) [7]

Neuromuscular/Skeletal
Rhabdomyolysis [5]

Ocular
Hallucinations, visual [2]

Other
Death [4]

DIPHENOXYLATE

Trade name: Lomotil (Pfizer)
Indications: Diarrhea
Class: Antimotility, Opioid agonist
Half-life: 2.5 hours
Clinically important, potentially hazardous interactions with: oxybutynin
Pregnancy category: C
Important contra-indications noted in the prescribing guidelines for: nursing mothers; pediatric patients
Note: Diphenoxylate is almost always prescribed with atropine sulfate.

Mucosal
Xerostomia (3%)

DIPYRIDAMOLE

Trade names: Aggrenox (Boehringer Ingelheim), Persantine (Boehringer Ingelheim)
Indications: Thromboembolic complications following cardiac valve replacement
Class: Adenosine reuptake inhibitor, Antiplatelet
Half-life: 10–12 hours
Clinically important, potentially hazardous interactions with: adenosine, ceftobiprole, clopidogrel, enoxaparin, fondaparinux, regadenoson, reteplase, riociguat, tinzaparin
Pregnancy category: B
Important contra-indications noted in the prescribing guidelines for: nursing mothers; pediatric patients
Note: Aggrenox is dipyridamole and aspirin.

Skin
Flushing (3%)
Rash (2%)
Stevens-Johnson syndrome [2]

Central Nervous System
Headache [3]

Other
Adverse effects [3]

DISOPYRAMIDE

Trade name: Norpace (Pfizer)
Indications: Ventricular arrhythmias
Class: Antiarrhythmic, Antiarrhythmic class Ia, Muscarinic antagonist
Half-life: 4–10 hours
Clinically important, potentially hazardous interactions with: acebutolol, amiodarone, amisulpride, amitriptyline, arsenic, artemether/lumefantrine, astemizole, atenolol, bisoprolol, celiprolol, ciprofloxacin, clarithromycin, cobicistat/elvitegravir/emtricitabine/tenofovir alafenamide, cobicistat/elvitegravir/emtricitabine/tenofovir disoproxil, darifenacin, degarelix, dronedarone, droperidol, enoxacin, erythromycin, gatifloxacin, gliclazide, glycopyrrolate, glycopyrronium, insulin aspart, insulin degludec, insulin glargine, insulin glulisine, itraconazole, ketoconazole, levomepromazine, lomefloxacin, lurasidone, metformin, moxifloxacin, nevirapine, nilotinib, norfloxacin, ofloxacin, oxprenolol, oxybutynin, pimavanserin, quinine, quinolones, ribociclib, rifapentine, roxithromycin, sildenafil, sotalol, sparfloxacin, sulpiride, tadalafil, telithromycin, tiotropium, trospium, vandetanib, vardenafil, zuclopenthixol
Pregnancy category: C
Important contra-indications noted in the prescribing guidelines for: nursing mothers; pediatric patients

---

Skin
Dermatitis (<3%)
Edema (<3%)
Exanthems (<5%)
Lupus erythematosus [3]
Pruritus (<3%)
Rash (generalized) (<3%)

Mucosal
Oral lesions (40%)
Xerostomia (32%) [2]

Cardiovascular
Chest pain (<3%)
Hypotension (<3%)
QT prolongation [8]
Torsades de pointes [13]

Central Nervous System
Anorexia (<3%)
Headache (3–9%)
Nervousness (<3%)
Syncope (<3%)
Vertigo (dizziness) (3–9%)

Neuromuscular/Skeletal
Asthenia (fatigue) (3–9%)

Gastrointestinal/Hepatic
Abdominal pain (3–9%)
Constipation (11%) [2]
Diarrhea (<3%)
Nausea (3–9%)
Vomiting (<3%)

Respiratory
Dyspnea (<3%)

Endocrine/Metabolic
- Hypocalcemia [3]
- Hypoglycemia [4]
- Hypokalemia (<3%)
- Weight gain (<3%)

Genitourinary
- Impotence (<3%)
- Urinary hesitancy (14%)
- Urinary retention (3–9%)

Ocular
- Vision blurred (3–9%)
- Xerophthalmia (3–9%)

DISULFIRAM

Trade name: Antabuse (Odyssey)
Indications: Alcoholism
Class: Antialcoholism, Antioxidant
Half-life: N/A
Clinically important, potentially hazardous interactions with: acenocoumarol, alcohol, amitriptyline, anisindione, anticoagulants, benznidazole, clobazam, cyclosporine, dicumarol, dronabinol, ethanolamine, ethotoin, fosphenytoin, lopinavir, mephenytoin, metronidazole, omeprazole, oxtriphylline, phenytoin, thalidomide, tipranavir, warfarin
Pregnancy category: C
Important contra-indications noted in the prescribing guidelines for: nursing mothers; pediatric patients

---

Skin
- Acneform eruption [3]
- Bullous dermatitis [2]
- Dermatitis [17]
- Eczema [2]
- Exanthems [2]
- Fixed eruption [2]
- Flushing (with alcohol) [5]
- Rash (<10%)
- Recall reaction (nickel) [4]
- Urticaria [3]

Mucosal
- Halitosis [2]

Cardiovascular
- Hypertension [2]
- Hypotension [2]
- Polyarteritis nodosa [2]
- Tachycardia [2]

Central Nervous System
- Dysgeusia (taste perversion) (metallic or garlic aftertaste) (<10%)
- Neurotoxicity [7]
- Psychosis [5]
- Seizures [2]
- Somnolence (drowsiness) [2]
- Vertigo (dizziness) [2]

Neuromuscular/Skeletal
- Asthenia (fatigue) [2]

Ocular
- Optic neuropathy [2]

Other
- Adverse effects [2]

DOCETAXEL

Trade name: Taxotere (Sanofi-Aventis)
Indications: Metastatic breast cancer, non-small cell lung cancer, with prednisone in hormone refractory prostate cancer, with cisplatin and fluorouracil for gastric adenocarcinoma and squamous cell carcinoma of the head and neck
Class: Antineoplastic, Taxane
Half-life: 11–18 hours
Clinically important, potentially hazardous interactions with: alcohol, aldesleukin, anthracyclines, antifungals, aprepitant, BCG vaccine, conivaptan, cyclosporine, CYP3A4 inhibitors or inducers, dasatinib, deferasirox, denosumab, echinacea, erythromycin, itraconazole, ketoconazole, lapatinib, leflunomide, natalizumab, P-glycoprotein inhibitors or inducers, pimecrolimus, prednisone, ritonavir, sipuleucel-T, sorafenib, St John's wort, tacrolimus, thalidomide, trastuzumab, vaccines, voriconazole
Pregnancy category: D
Important contra-indications noted in the prescribing guidelines for: the elderly; nursing mothers; pediatric patients
Note: Contra-indicated in patients with hypersensitivity to docetaxel or polysorbate 80, or with neutrophil counts of <1500 cells/mm^3.
Warning: TOXIC DEATHS, HEPATOTOXICITY, NEUTROPENIA, HYPERSENSITIVITY REACTIONS, and FLUID RETENTION

Skin
- AGEP [2]
- Anaphylactoid reactions/Anaphylaxis [3]
- Edema (34%) [24]
- Erythema [4]
- Exanthems [3]
- Facial erythema [2]
- Flagellate erythema/pigmentation [2]
- Flushing [2]
- Hand–foot syndrome [44]
- Hypersensitivity (6%) [15]
- Peripheral edema [9]
- Photosensitivity [6]
- Pigmentation [2]
- Psoriasis [3]
- Radiation recall dermatitis [18]
- Rash [13]
- Recall reaction [2]
- Scleroderma [9]
- Stevens-Johnson syndrome [2]
- Thrombocytopenic purpura [2]
- Toxicity (20–48%) [10]
- Xerosis [2]

Hair
- Alopecia (56–76%) [32]

Nails
- Beau's lines (transverse nail bands) [2]
- Discoloration [2]
- Melanonychia [2]
- Nail changes [17]
- Nail disorder (11–41%) [2]
- Nail loss [3]
- Nail pigmentation [6]
- Onycholysis [15]
- Onychopathy [2]
- Paronychia [4]
- Pyogenic granuloma [2]
- Subungual abscess [2]
- Subungual hemorrhage [2]
- Transverse superficial loss of nail plate [2]

Mucosal
- Aphthous stomatitis [2]
- Mucositis [15]
- Oral mucositis [5]
- Stomatitis (19–53%) [19]

Cardiovascular
- Capillary leak syndrome [2]
- Cardiotoxicity [2]
- Hypertension [10]
- Hypotension (3%)
- Thromboembolism [2]

Central Nervous System
- Anorexia [13]
- Dysesthesia (4%)
- Dysgeusia (taste perversion) (6%) [7]
- Fever (31–35%) [8]
- Headache [2]
- Mood changes [2]
- Neurotoxicity [20]
- Pain [5]
- Paresthesias (4%) [3]
- Peripheral neuropathy [12]
- Vertigo (dizziness) [2]

Neuromuscular/Skeletal
- Arthralgia (3–9%) [3]
- Asthenia (fatigue) (53–66%) [63]
- Bone or joint pain [2]
- Myalgia/Myopathy (3–23%) [10]

Gastrointestinal/Hepatic
- Abdominal pain [4]
- Constipation [3]
- Diarrhea (23–43%) [50]
- Dysphagia [2]
- Hepatotoxicity [2]
- Nausea (34–42%) [29]
- Vomiting (22–23%) [21]

Respiratory
- Acute respiratory distress syndrome [2]
- Cough [2]
- Dyspnea [5]
- Pleural effusion [2]
- Pneumonia [3]
- Pneumonitis [10]
- Pulmonary embolism [2]
- Pulmonary toxicity (41%) [4]
- Respiratory failure [2]
- Upper respiratory tract infection [3]

Endocrine/Metabolic
- ALP increased (4–7%)
- ALT increased [5]
- Amenorrhea [4]
- Appetite decreased [3]
- AST increased [4]
- Dehydration [2]
- Hyperglycemia [3]
- Hypomagnesemia [2]
- Hyponatremia [4]
- Hypophosphatemia [3]

Hematologic
- Anemia (65–94%) [24]
- Febrile neutropenia (6%) [52]
- Hemolytic uremic syndrome [3]
- Hemotoxicity [3]
- Leukocytopenia [6]

Leukopenia (84–99%) [29]
Lymphopenia [4]
Myelosuppression [3]
Neutropenia (84–99%) [93]
Thrombocytopenia (8–14%) [13]

Ocular
Epiphora [8]

Local
Injection-site erythema [2]
Injection-site extravasation [3]
Injection-site pigmentation [3]
Injection-site reactions [2]

Other
Adverse effects [5]
Allergic reactions [2]
Death [17]
Infection (<34%) [9]

DOLUTEGRAVIR

Trade names: Juluca (ViiV), Tivicay (ViiV), Triumeq (ViiV)
Indications: HIV-1 infection
Class: Antiretroviral, Integrase strand transfer inhibitor
Half-life: ~14 hours
Clinically important, potentially hazardous interactions with: dofetilide
Pregnancy category: B
Important contra-indications noted in the prescribing guidelines for: nursing mothers; pediatric patients
Note: Triumeq is dolutegravir, abacavir and lamivudine. Juluca is dolutegravir and rilpivirine.

Skin
Hypersensitivity [5]
Pruritus (<2%)
Rash [3]

Central Nervous System
Abnormal dreams [2]
Headache (<2%) [17]
Insomnia (<3%) [4]
Neurotoxicity [2]

Neuromuscular/Skeletal
Asthenia (fatigue) (<2%) [3]
Myalgia/Myopathy (<2%)

Gastrointestinal/Hepatic
Abdominal pain (<2%)
Diarrhea [16]
Flatulence (<2%)
Hepatitis (<2%)
Nausea [14]
Vomiting (<2%)

Respiratory
Nasopharyngitis [4]
Upper respiratory tract infection [2]

Endocrine/Metabolic
ALT increased (<2%) [3]
AST increased (<3%)
Creatine phosphokinase increased (<4%)
Hyperglycemia (5–7%)
Serum creatinine increased [2]

Renal
Nephrotoxicity (<2%)

Other
Adverse effects [4]

DONEPEZIL

Trade names: Aricept (Eisai), Aricept Evess (Eisai)
Indications: Mild, moderate and severe dementia of the Alzheimer's type
Class: Acetylcholinesterase inhibitor, Cholinesterase inhibitor, Parasympathomimetic
Half-life: 50–70 hours
Clinically important, potentially hazardous interactions with: anticholinergics, cholinergic agonists, galantamine, non-depolarising muscle relaxants, ramelteon, succinylcholine
Pregnancy category: C
Important contra-indications noted in the prescribing guidelines for: nursing mothers; pediatric patients
Note: Contra-indicated in patients with known hypersensitivity to donepezil hydrochloride or to piperidine derivatives.

Skin
Diaphoresis [2]
Ecchymoses (4–5%)
Eczema (3%)
Purpura (<10%)

Cardiovascular
Atrioventricular block [2]
Bradycardia [7]
Chest pain (2%)
Hypertension [2]
Hypotension (3%)
QT prolongation [4]
Torsades de pointes [2]

Central Nervous System
Abnormal dreams (3%) [2]
Agitation [2]
Anorexia (4–8%) [5]
Confusion (2%) [3]
Delirium [2]
Depression (2–3%) [3]
Emotional lability (2%)
Fever (3%)
Gait instability [2]
Hallucinations (3%)
Headache (4–10%) [6]
Hostility (3%)
Insomnia (5–9%) [4]
Mania [2]
Nervousness (3%)
Neuroleptic malignant syndrome [2]
Pain (3–9%)
Parkinsonism [2]
Somnolence (drowsiness) (2%) [2]
Syncope (2%) [5]
Tremor [3]
Vertigo (dizziness) (2–8%) [6]

Neuromuscular/Skeletal
Arthralgia (2%)
Asthenia (fatigue) (5%) [3]
Back pain (3%)
Dystonia [2]
Muscle spasm [2]
Myoclonus [2]
Pisa syndrome [2]

Gastrointestinal/Hepatic
Constipation [3]
Diarrhea (10%) [12]
Hepatotoxicity [3]
Nausea (6–11%) [15]
Vomiting (5–8%) [9]

Endocrine/Metabolic
Appetite decreased [4]
Creatine phosphokinase increased (3%)
Dehydration (2%)
Hyperlipidemia (2%)
Weight loss (3%)

Genitourinary
Urinary frequency (2%) [2]
Urinary incontinence (2%)
Urinary tract infection [3]

Hematologic
Hemorrhage (2%)

Other
Adverse effects [9]
Infection (11%)

DONG QUAI

Family: Umbelliferae; Apioideae
Scientific name: *Angelica sinensis (Angelica polymorpha sinensis)*
Indications: Menopausal symptoms, PMS, menstrual disorders, anemia, constipation, insomnia, rheumatism, neuralgia, hypertension, hypopigmentation, psoriasis
Class: Immunomodulator, Phytoestrogen
Half-life: N/A
Clinically important, potentially hazardous interactions with: acetaminophen, bexarotene, demeclocycline, gemifloxacin
Pregnancy category: N/A
Note: Some recent research has questioned the efficacy of Dong Quai, and also suggested that it may be a potential carcinogen.

Endocrine/Metabolic
Gynecomastia [2]

DOPAMINE

Trade name: Intropin (Hospira)
Indications: Hemodynamic imbalances present in shock
Class: Adrenergic alpha-receptor agonist, Catecholamine, Inotropic sympathomimetic
Half-life: 2 minutes
Clinically important, potentially hazardous interactions with: ethotoin, fosphenytoin, furazolidone, lurasidone, MAO inhibitors, mephenytoin, phenelzine, phenytoin, quetiapine, tranylcypromine
Pregnancy category: C
Important contra-indications noted in the prescribing guidelines for: nursing mothers; pediatric patients

---

Cardiovascular
QT prolongation [2]

Local
Injection-site extravasation [2]
Injection-site necrosis [3]

DORAVIRINE *

Trade name: Pifeltro (Merck Sharpe & Dohme)
Indications: indicated in combination with other antiretroviral agents for the treatment of HIV-1 infection in adult patients with no prior antiretroviral treatment history
Class: Non-nucleoside reverse transcriptase inhibitor
Half-life: 15 hours
Clinically important, potentially hazardous interactions with: carbamazepine, efavirenz, enzalutamide, etravirine, mitotane, nevirapine, oxcarbazepine, phenobarbital, phenytoin, rifabutin, rifampin, rifapentine, St John's wort
Pregnancy category: N/A (No adequate data to establish risk)

Skin
Rash (2%)

Central Nervous System
Headache (6%) [2]
Vertigo (dizziness) (3%)

Neuromuscular/Skeletal
Asthenia (fatigue) (6%)

Gastrointestinal/Hepatic
Abdominal pain (5%)
Diarrhea (5%)
Nausea (7%)

DORAVIRINE/ LAMIDUVINE/ TENOFOVIR DISOPROXIL *

Trade name: Delstrigo (Merck Sharpe & Dohme)
Indications: indicated as a complete regimen for the treatment of HIV-1 infection in adult patients with no antiretroviral treatment history
Half-life: 15 hours (doravirine); 5–7 hours (lamivudine); 17 hours (tenofovir disoproxil)
Clinically important, potentially hazardous interactions with: carbamazepine, enzalutamide, ledipasvir & sofosbuvir, mitotane, oxcarbazepine, phenobarbital, phenytoin, rifabutin, rifampin, rifapentine, sofosbuvir & velpatasvir, St John's wort
Pregnancy category: N/A (insufficient data to adequately assess risk)
Important contra-indications noted in the prescribing guidelines for: nursing mothers
Note: see also separate profiles for doravirine, lamivudine and tenofovir disoproxil.
Warning: POSTTREATMENT ACUTE EXACERBATION OF HEPATITIS B

Skin
Rash (2%)

Central Nervous System
Abnormal dreams (5%)
Insomnia (4%)
Sensory disturbances (4%)
Sleep disturbances (12%)
Somnolence (drowsiness) (3%)
Vertigo (dizziness) (7%)

Gastrointestinal/Hepatic
Diarrhea (3%)
Nausea (5%)

DORZOLAMIDE

Trade names: Cosopt (Merck), Trusopt (Banyu)
Indications: Glaucoma, ocular hypertension
Class: Carbonic anhydrase inhibitor, Diuretic
Half-life: ~4 months
Clinically important, potentially hazardous interactions with: none known
Pregnancy category: C
Important contra-indications noted in the prescribing guidelines for: nursing mothers
Note: Dorzolamide is a sulfonamide and can be absorbed systemically. Sulfonamides can produce severe, possibly fatal, reactions such as toxic epidermal necrolysis and Stevens-Johnson syndrome.
Cosopt is dorzolamide and timolol.

Skin
Contact dermatitis [4]

Central Nervous System
Dysgeusia (taste perversion) (25%) [8]

Ocular
Ocular burning (33%) [5]
Ocular pain [2]
Ocular pruritus [4]
Ocular stinging [10]
Vision blurred [3]

Other
Adverse effects [2]

DOXAZOSIN

Trade name: Cardura (Pfizer)
Indications: Hypertension
Class: Adrenergic alpha-receptor antagonist
Half-life: 19–22 hours
Clinically important, potentially hazardous interactions with: tadalafil, vardenafil, zuclopenthixol
Pregnancy category: C
Important contra-indications noted in the prescribing guidelines for: the elderly; nursing mothers; pediatric patients

---

Skin
Edema (4%)
Exanthems (2%)

Mucosal
Xerostomia (2%) [2]

Cardiovascular
Hypotension [3]
Orthostatic hypotension [2]
Postural hypotension [2]

Central Nervous System
Headache [2]
Vertigo (dizziness) [9]

Neuromuscular/Skeletal
Asthenia (fatigue) [4]

Gastrointestinal/Hepatic
Abdominal pain [2]

Genitourinary
Erectile dysfunction [3]

Ocular
Floppy iris syndrome [3]

DOXEPIN

Trade names: Adapin (LGM Pharma), Silenor (Somaxon), Sinquan (Pfizer)
Indications: Mental depression, anxiety, insomnia
Class: Antidepressant, tricyclic, Muscarinic antagonist
Half-life: 6–8 hours
Clinically important, potentially hazardous interactions with: alcohol, amprenavir, arbutamine, cholestyramine, clonidine, CNS depressants, epinephrine, formoterol, guanethidine, isocarboxazid, linezolid, MAO inhibitors, phenelzine, QT prolonging agents, quinolones, ramelteon, selegiline, sparfloxacin, sympathomimetics, tranylcypromine
Pregnancy category: C (pregnancy category is B for topical use)
Important contra-indications noted in the prescribing guidelines for: nursing mothers
Warning: SUICIDALITY AND ANTIDEPRESSANT DRUGS

Skin
Dermatitis (from topical) [9]
Diaphoresis (<10%)
Pseudolymphoma [2]

Mucosal
Xerostomia (>10%) [6]

Cardiovascular
QT prolongation [2]

Central Nervous System
Dysgeusia (taste perversion) (>10%)
Headache [4]
Somnolence (drowsiness) [7]

DOXORUBICIN

Synonym: hydroxydaunomycin
Trade names: Adriamycin (Bedford), Doxil (Tibotec), Rubex (Mead Johnson)
Indications: Carcinomas, leukemias, sarcomas
Class: Antibiotic, anthracycline
Half-life: 20–48 hours
Clinically important, potentially hazardous interactions with: aldesleukin, cabazitaxel, CYP2D6 inhibitors or inducers, CYP3A4 inhibitors or inducers, gadobenate, P-glycoprotein inhibitors or inducers, paclitaxel, sorafenib, stavudine, trastuzumab, zidovudine

Pregnancy category: D
Important contra-indications noted in the prescribing guidelines for: nursing mothers
Warning: CARDIOMYOPATHY, SECONDARY MALIGNANCIES, EXTRAVASATION AND TISSUE NECROSIS, and SEVERE MYELOSUPPRESSION

Skin
- Anaphylactoid reactions/Anaphylaxis [2]
- Angioedema [5]
- Erythema [2]
- Exanthems [4]
- Exfoliative dermatitis [2]
- Flushing (<10%) [2]
- Hand–foot syndrome [61]
- Hypersensitivity [2]
- Intertrigo [3]
- Lupus erythematosus [3]
- Necrosis (local) [5]
- Palmar–plantar erythema (painful) [4]
- Pigmentation [15]
- Pruritus [2]
- Purpura [2]
- Radiation recall dermatitis [8]
- Rash [6]
- Toxicity [12]
- Urticaria [10]

Hair
- Alopecia (>10%) [41]

Nails
- Beau's lines [2]
- Melanonychia [2]
- Nail changes [2]
- Nail pigmentation [16]
- Onycholysis [5]

Mucosal
- Aphthous stomatitis [2]
- Mucositis [19]
- Oral lesions [7]
- Oral mucositis [2]
- Stomatitis (>10%) [19]
- Tongue pigmentation [3]

Cardiovascular
- Atrial fibrillation [2]
- Cardiomyopathy [6]
- Cardiotoxicity [21]
- Chest pain [2]
- Congestive heart failure [7]
- Myocardial toxicity [4]

Central Nervous System
- Anorexia [3]
- Dysgeusia (taste perversion) [2]
- Fever [5]
- Headache [3]
- Leukoencephalopathy [4]
- Neurotoxicity [4]
- Pain [2]
- Peripheral neuropathy [7]

Neuromuscular/Skeletal
- Asthenia (fatigue) [18]
- Bone or joint pain [3]
- Myalgia/Myopathy [3]

Gastrointestinal/Hepatic
- Constipation [4]
- Diarrhea [9]
- Gastrointestinal perforation [2]
- Hepatotoxicity [6]
- Nausea [15]
- Pancreatitis [2]
- Vomiting [12]

Respiratory
- Dyspnea [3]
- Pneumonia [4]
- Pneumonitis [2]

Endocrine/Metabolic
- ALT increased [3]
- Amenorrhea [2]
- Hyperglycemia [2]
- Hypokalemia [2]

Renal
- Nephrotoxicity [2]

Hematologic
- Anemia [16]
- Febrile neutropenia [18]
- Hemorrhage [2]
- Hemotoxicity [2]
- Leukopenia [4]
- Myelosuppression [2]
- Neutropenia [37]
- Thrombocytopenia [21]

Local
- Injection-site erythema [7]
- Injection-site extravasation (>10%) [12]
- Injection-site necrosis (>10%) [5]
- Injection-site reactions [2]
- Injection-site ulceration (>10%) [4]

Other
- Adverse effects [6]
- Allergic reactions [4]
- Death [11]
- Infection [5]

DOXYCYCLINE

Trade names: Adoxa (Bioglan), Doryx (Warner Chilcott), Oracea (Galderma), Vibra-Tabs (Pfizer), Vibramycin-D (Pfizer)
Indications: Various infections caused by susceptible organisms
Class: Antibiotic, tetracycline
Half-life: 12–22 hours
Clinically important, potentially hazardous interactions with: acitretin, amoxicillin, ampicillin, antacids, bacampicillin, barbiturates, BCG vaccine, bismuth, calcium salts, carbamazepine, carbenicillin, cloxacillin, corticosteroids, coumarins, cyclosporine, dairy products, digoxin, ergotamine, kaolin, methotrexate, methoxyflurane, methysergide, mezlocillin, nafcillin, oral contraceptives, oral iron, oral typhoid vaccine, oxacillin, penicillins, phenindione, phenytoin, piperacillin, primidone, quinapril, retinoids, rifampin, St John's wort, strontium ranelate, sucralfate, sulfonylureas, ticarcillin, tripotassium dicitratobismuthate, zinc
Pregnancy category: D
Important contra-indications noted in the prescribing guidelines for: nursing mothers; pediatric patients

---

Skin
- AGEP [2]
- Angioedema [2]
- Candidiasis [3]
- Erythema multiforme [4]
- Exanthems [2]
- Fixed eruption [9]
- Hypersensitivity [2]
- Photosensitivity [21]
- Phototoxicity [9]
- Pigmentation [5]
- Pruritus [3]
- Rash [5]
- Stevens-Johnson syndrome [7]
- Sweet's syndrome [2]
- Toxic epidermal necrolysis [2]
- Urticaria [6]

Nails
- Photo-onycholysis [13]

Mucosal
- Black tongue [2]
- Mucosal candidiasis [2]

Central Nervous System
- Anosmia [2]
- Fever [2]
- Headache [4]
- Intracranial pressure increased [2]
- Paresthesias [4]
- Vertigo (dizziness) [3]

Neuromuscular/Skeletal
- Myalgia/Myopathy [2]

Gastrointestinal/Hepatic
- Abdominal pain [3]
- Diarrhea [4]
- Esophagitis [3]
- Hepatotoxicity [2]
- Nausea [5]
- Pancreatitis [3]
- Ulcerative esophagitis [2]
- Vomiting [3]

Endocrine/Metabolic
- Hypoglycemia [2]

Genitourinary
- Vaginitis [2]

Other
- Adverse effects [6]
- Allergic reactions [3]
- Tooth pigmentation (>10%) [5]

DRONABINOL

Synonyms: tetrahydrocannabinol; THC
Trade names: Marinol (AbbVie), Syndros (Insys)
Indications: Chemotherapy-induced nausea, anorexia associated with weight loss in patients with AIDS
Class: Antiemetic, Cannabinoid
Half-life: 19–24 hours
Clinically important, potentially hazardous interactions with: disulfiram, metronidazole
Pregnancy category: C
Important contra-indications noted in the prescribing guidelines for: the elderly; nursing mothers; pediatric patients

---

Mucosal
- Xerostomia (<10%)

Central Nervous System
- Euphoria (<10%)
- Paranoia (<10%)

Somnolence (drowsiness) (<10%)
Vertigo (dizziness) (<10%) [5]

Gastrointestinal/Hepatic
Abdominal pain (<10%)
Nausea (<10%) [2]
Vomiting (<10%)

Other
Adverse effects [4]

DRONEDARONE

Trade name: Multaq (Sanofi-Aventis)
Indications: Atrial fibrillation and atrial flutter
Class: Antiarrhythmic, Antiarrhythmic class III
Half-life: 13–19 hours
Clinically important, potentially hazardous interactions with: amiodarone, amitriptyline, amoxapine, antiarrhythmics, antipsychotics prolonging QT interval, arsenic, atorvastatin, beta blockers, bupivacaine, calcium channel blockers, carbamazepine, citalopram, clarithromycin, conivaptan, coumarins, cyclosporine, CYP3A inducers, dabigatran, darunavir, dasabuvir/ombitasvir/paritaprevir/ritonavir, dasatinib, degarelix, delavirdine, digoxin, diltiazem, disopyramide, dolasetron, efavirenz, erythromycin, fingolimod, grapefruit juice, indinavir, itraconazole, ketoconazole, lapatinib, levobupivacaine, levofloxacin, levomepromazine, metoprolol, moxifloxacin, nefazodone, neratinib, nifedipine, ombitasvir/paritaprevir/ritonavir, oxcarbazepine, pazopanib, phenindione, phenobarbital, phenothiazines, phenytoin, posaconazole, prilocaine, propranolol, rifampin, rifapentine, ritonavir, ropivacaine, rosuvastatin, saquinavir, simvastatin, sirolimus, sotalol, St John's wort, statins, tacrolimus, telavancin, telithromycin, tricyclic antidepressants, venetoclax, verapamil, voriconazole, vorinostat, warfarin, ziprasidone
Pregnancy category: X
Important contra-indications noted in the prescribing guidelines for: nursing mothers; pediatric patients
Warning: INCREASED RISK OF DEATH, STROKE AND HEART FAILURE IN PATIENTS WITH DECOMPENSATED HEART FAILURE OR PERMANENT ATRIAL FIBRILLATION

Skin
Anaphylactoid reactions/Anaphylaxis [2]
Dermatitis (5%)
Eczema (5%)
Erythema (5%)
Pruritus (5%)
Rash (5%) [8]

Cardiovascular
Arrhythmias [3]
Bradycardia (3%) [8]
Cardiac failure (new or worsening) [9]
Cardiotoxicity [3]
Congestive heart failure [2]
QT prolongation (28%) [10]
Torsades de pointes [3]

Central Nervous System
Vertigo (dizziness) [2]

Neuromuscular/Skeletal
Asthenia (fatigue) (7%) [3]

Gastrointestinal/Hepatic
Abdominal pain (4%) [2]
Diarrhea (9%) [14]
Dyspepsia (2%)
Gastrointestinal disorder [4]
Hepatic failure [5]
Hepatotoxicity [9]
Nausea (5%) [12]
Vomiting (2%) [6]

Respiratory
Pulmonary toxicity [9]

Endocrine/Metabolic
Serum creatinine increased (51%) [6]

Renal
Nephrotoxicity [2]
Renal failure [2]

Other
Adverse effects [2]
Death [2]
Side effects [2]

DROPERIDOL

Trade names: Inapsine (Akorn), Xomolix (ProStrakan)
Indications: Tranquilizer and antiemetic in surgical procedures
Class: Antiemetic, Antipsychotic, Butyrophenone
Half-life: 2.3 hours
Clinically important, potentially hazardous interactions with: amiodarone, amisulpride, amitriptyline, arsenic, atomoxetine, azithromycin, chloroquine, CNS depressants, cyclobenzaprine, disopyramide, duloxetine, eszopiclone, fluoxetine, fluvoxamine, hydromorphone, hydroxychloroquine, levomepromazine, lurasidone, macrolides, metaxalone, milnacipran, moxifloxacin, paliperidone, pentamidine, pimozide, QT prolonging agents, quinine, ramelteon, sertraline, sotalol, sulpiride, tamoxifen, tapentadol, thiopental, tiagabine, tricyclic antidepressants
Pregnancy category: C
Important contra-indications noted in the prescribing guidelines for: nursing mothers; pediatric patients
Note: Contra-indicated in patients with known or suspected QT prolongation.
This product is not available in the European market.
Warning: QT PROLONGATION AND TORSADE DE POINTES

Skin
Anaphylactoid reactions/Anaphylaxis [3]
Angioedema [2]

Cardiovascular
Arrhythmias [2]
QT prolongation [13]
Torsades de pointes [6]

Central Nervous System
Akathisia [5]
Extrapyramidal symptoms [2]
Neuroleptic malignant syndrome [2]
Restlessness [2]
Sedation [2]

Neuromuscular/Skeletal
Dystonia [6]

Other
Death [3]

DROXIDOPA

Synonym: L-DOPS
Trade name: Northera (Chelsea Therapeutics)
Indications: Neurogenic orthostatic hypotension
Class: Amino acid analog (synthetic)
Half-life: 2.5 hours
Clinically important, potentially hazardous interactions with: none known
Pregnancy category: C
Important contra-indications noted in the prescribing guidelines for: nursing mothers; pediatric patients
Warning: SUPINE HYPERTENSION

Cardiovascular
Hypertension (2–7%)

Central Nervous System
Gait instability (15%) [2]
Headache (6–15%) [3]
Syncope (13%)
Vertigo (dizziness) (4–10%) [2]

Gastrointestinal/Hepatic
Nausea (2–9%)

Genitourinary
Urinary tract infection (15%) [2]

DULAGLUTIDE

Trade name: Trulicity (Lilly)
Indications: To improve glycemic control in adults with Type II diabetes mellitus
Class: Glucagon-like peptide-1 (GLP-1) receptor agonist
Half-life: 5 days
Clinically important, potentially hazardous interactions with: none known
Pregnancy category: C
Important contra-indications noted in the prescribing guidelines for: nursing mothers; pediatric patients
Note: Contra-indicated in patients with a personal or family history of medullary thyroid carcinoma or in patients with multiple endocrine neoplasia syndrome Type 2.
Warning: RISK OF THYROID C-CELL TUMORS

Cardiovascular
Atrioventricular block (2%)
Tachycardia (3–6%)

Central Nervous System
Headache [3]

Neuromuscular/Skeletal
Asthenia (fatigue) (4–6%)

Gastrointestinal/Hepatic
Abdominal pain (7–9%)
Constipation [4]
Diarrhea [23]
Dyspepsia (4–6%) [3]

Nausea (12–21%) [24]
Pancreatitis [2]
Vomiting (6–13%) [17]

Respiratory
Nasopharyngitis [6]

Endocrine/Metabolic
Appetite decreased (5–9%) [2]
Hypoglycemia [2]

Local
Injection-site reactions [5]

Other
Adverse effects (gastrointestinal) [4]

DULOXETINE

Trade names: Cymbalta (Lilly), Yentreve (Lilly)
Indications: Depression
Class: Antidepressant, Noradrenaline reuptake inhibitor, Serotonin reuptake inhibitor
Half-life: 8–17 hours
Clinically important, potentially hazardous interactions with: 5HT1 agonists, alcohol, amitriptyline, artemether/lumefantrine, aspirin, atomoxetine, cimetidine, ciprofloxacin, citalopram, clomipramine, CYP1A2 inducers, CYP2D6 inhibitors and substrates, darunavir, droperidol, enoxacin, fesoterodine, fluoxetine, fluvoxamine, iobenguane, levomepromazine, MAO inhibitors, meperidine, moclobemide, naratriptan, nebivolol, NSAIDs, paroxetine hydrochloride, PEG-interferon, quinidine, sibutramine, SSRIs, St John's wort, tamoxifen, teriflunomide, thioridazine, tramadol, tricyclic antidepressants, tryptophan, venlafaxine, warfarin
Pregnancy category: C
Important contra-indications noted in the prescribing guidelines for: nursing mothers; pediatric patients
Warning: SUICIDAL THOUGHTS AND BEHAVIORS

Skin
Diaphoresis (6%) [2]
Flushing (3%)
Hot flashes (>2%)
Hyperhidrosis (7%) [8]
Stevens-Johnson syndrome [2]

Mucosal
Oropharyngeal pain (>2%)
Xerostomia (13%) [24]

Cardiovascular
Palpitation (>2%)

Central Nervous System
Agitation (5%)
Anxiety (3%)
Dyskinesia [2]
Headache (14%) [11]
Insomnia (10%) [13]
Paresthesias (>2%)
Restless legs syndrome [2]
Serotonin syndrome [4]
Somnolence (drowsiness) (10%) [17]
Suicidal ideation [4]
Tardive dyskinesia [3]
Tremor (3%)
Vertigo (dizziness) (10%) [16]
Yawning (>2%) [2]

Neuromuscular/Skeletal
Arthralgia (>2%)
Asthenia (fatigue) (10%) [14]
Back pain (>2%)
Bone or joint pain (4%)
Muscle spasm (3%)

Gastrointestinal/Hepatic
Abdominal pain (>2%)
Colitis [2]
Constipation (10%) [10]
Diarrhea (9%) [6]
Hepatotoxicity (rare) [4]
Nausea (24%) [25]
Vomiting (>2%) [3]

Respiratory
Cough (>2%)
Influenza (3%)
Nasopharyngitis (5%)
Upper respiratory tract infection (4%)

Endocrine/Metabolic
ALT increased [2]
Appetite decreased (8–9%) [2]
Hyponatremia [3]
Libido decreased (4%)
SIADH [6]
Weight loss (>2%)

Genitourinary
Ejaculatory dysfunction (2–5%)
Sexual dysfunction [6]

Ocular
Vision blurred (>2%)

Other
Adverse effects [12]
Bruxism [3]
Death [2]
Side effects [2]

DURVALUMAB

Trade name: Imfinzi (AstraZeneca)
Indications: Locally advanced or metastatic urothelial carcinoma in patients having disease progression following platinum-containing chemotherapy
Class: Monoclonal antibody, Programmed death-ligand (PD-L1) inhibitor
Half-life: 17 days
Clinically important, potentially hazardous interactions with: none known
Pregnancy category: N/A (Can cause fetal harm)
Important contra-indications noted in the prescribing guidelines for: the elderly; nursing mothers; pediatric patients

---

Skin
Peripheral edema (15%)
Pruritus [3]
Rash (11%) [2]

Central Nervous System
Fever (14%)

Neuromuscular/Skeletal
Asthenia (fatigue) (39%) [5]
Bone or joint pain (24%)

Gastrointestinal/Hepatic
Abdominal pain (14%)
Colitis (13%) [2]
Constipation (21%)
Diarrhea (13%) [7]
Hepatitis [2]
Nausea (16%)

Respiratory
Cough (10%)
Dyspnea (13%)
Pneumonitis (2%) [3]

Endocrine/Metabolic
ALP increased (4%)
Appetite decreased (19%) [3]
AST increased (2%) [4]
Hypercalcemia (3%)
Hyperglycemia (3%)
Hypermagnesemia (4%)
Hyperthyroidism (5–6%)
Hyponatremia (12%)
Hypothyroidism (6–10%)

Genitourinary
Urinary tract infection (15%)

Hematologic
Anemia (8%)
Lymphopenia (11%)

Local
Infusion-related reactions (2%)

Other
Adverse effects [2]
Death [3]
Infection (30–38%)

DUTASTERIDE

Trade names: Avodart (GSK), Jalyn (GSK)
Indications: Benign prostatic hyperplasia, male pattern baldness (anecdotal)
Class: 5-alpha reductase inhibitor, Androgen antagonist
Half-life: 3–5 weeks
Clinically important, potentially hazardous interactions with: cimetidine, ciprofloxacin, conivaptan, darunavir, delavirdine, diltiazem, indinavir, ketoconazole, ritonavir, telithromycin, troleandomycin, verapamil, voriconazole
Pregnancy category: X
Important contra-indications noted in the prescribing guidelines for: nursing mothers; pediatric patients
Note: Jalyn is dutasteride and tamsulosin.

Endocrine/Metabolic
Gynecomastia [2]
Libido decreased (<3%) [3]

Genitourinary
Ejaculatory dysfunction [3]
Erectile dysfunction [8]
Impotence (<5%)
Sexual dysfunction [7]

Other
Adverse effects [2]

ECHINACEA

Family: Asteraceae; Compositae
Scientific names: *Echinacea angustifola, Echinacea pallida, Echinacea purpurea*
Indications: Colds, upper respiratory infections, peripheral vasodilator, urinary tract infections, yeast infections, ulcers, psoriasis, herpes simplex, septicemia, boils, abscesses, rheumatism, migraine, dyspepsia, eczema, bee stings and hemorrhoids
Class: Immunomodulator
Half-life: N/A
Clinically important, potentially hazardous interactions with: abatacept, alefacept, amiodarone, azacitidine, betamethasone, cabazitaxel, corticosteroids, cyclosporine, gefitinib, ketoconazole, leflunomide, methotrexate
Pregnancy category: N/A
Note: Individuals with atopy may be more likely to experience an allergic reaction when taking echinacea.

Skin
- Anaphylactoid reactions/Anaphylaxis [3]
- Angioedema [2]
- Rash [3]
- Urticaria [2]

Gastrointestinal/Hepatic
- Hepatotoxicity [2]

Ocular
- Ocular adverse effects [2]

Other
- Adverse effects [10]
- Allergic reactions [2]

ECULIZUMAB

Trade name: Soliris (Alexion)
Indications: Paroxysmal nocturnal hemoglobinuria, atypical hemolytic uremic syndrome
Class: Complement inhibitor, Monoclonal antibody
Half-life: ~12 days
Clinically important, potentially hazardous interactions with: none known
Pregnancy category: C
Important contra-indications noted in the prescribing guidelines for: nursing mothers; pediatric patients
Warning: SERIOUS MENINGOCOCCAL INFECTIONS

Skin
- Peripheral edema [2]
- Pruritus [2]

Mucosal
- Nasal congestion [2]

Cardiovascular
- Hypertension [2]

Central Nervous System
- Fever [3]
- Headache (44%) [6]
- Insomnia [2]
- Meningococcal infection [4]
- Vertigo (dizziness) [3]

Neuromuscular/Skeletal
- Asthenia (fatigue) (12%) [4]
- Back pain (19%) [3]
- Pain in extremities [2]

Gastrointestinal/Hepatic
- Abdominal pain [2]
- Diarrhea [3]
- Nausea [4]
- Vomiting [3]

Respiratory
- Cough (12%) [4]
- Nasopharyngitis (23%) [5]
- Pharyngolaryngeal pain [2]
- Upper respiratory tract infection [3]

Genitourinary
- Urinary tract infection [3]

Hematologic
- Anemia [2]
- Leukopenia [2]

EDARAVONE

Trade name: Radicava (Mitsubishi Tanabe Pharma)
Indications: Amyotrophic lateral sclerosis
Class: Antioxidant
Half-life: 4–6 hours
Clinically important, potentially hazardous interactions with: none known
Pregnancy category: N/A (May cause fetal toxicity based on findings in animal studies)
Important contra-indications noted in the prescribing guidelines for: nursing mothers; pediatric patients
Note: Radicava contains sodium bisulfite which may cause allergic type reactions.

Skin
- Dermatitis (8%) [2]
- Eczema (7%) [3]
- Hematoma (15%) [3]
- Tinea (4%) [2]

Central Nervous System
- Gait instability (13%) [3]
- Headache (10%) [3]
- Insomnia [2]

Gastrointestinal/Hepatic
- Constipation [2]
- Diarrhea [2]
- Dysphagia [3]
- Hepatotoxicity [2]

Respiratory
- Hypoxia (6%)
- Nasopharyngitis [2]
- Respiratory failure (6%) [3]

Genitourinary
- Glycosuria (4%) [3]

Renal
- Nephrotoxicity [2]

Other
- Adverse effects [2]

EDOXABAN

Trade name: Savaysa (Daiichi Sankyo)
Indications: Reduce the risk of stroke and systemic embolism in patients with nonvalvular atrial fibrillation, treatment of deep vein thrombosis and pulmonary embolism
Class: Direct factor Xa inhibitor
Half-life: 10–14 hours
Clinically important, potentially hazardous interactions with: anticoagulants, rifampin
Pregnancy category: C
Important contra-indications noted in the prescribing guidelines for: nursing mothers; pediatric patients
Note: Contra-indicated in patients with active pathological bleeding.
Warning: REDUCED EFFICACY IN NONVALVULAR ATRIAL FIBRILLATION PATIENTS WITH CRCL>95ml/min
ISCHEMIC EVENTS ON PREMATURE DISCONTINUATION
SPINAL/EDPIDURAL HEMATOMA

Skin
- Rash (4%)

Mucosal
- Epistaxis (nosebleed) (5%)
- Gingival bleeding [2]
- Oral bleeding (3%)

Gastrointestinal/Hepatic
- Diarrhea [2]
- Gastrointestinal bleeding (4%)
- Hepatotoxicity (5–8%) [2]

Genitourinary
- Hematuria (2%) [2]

Hematologic
- Anemia (2–10%)
- Bleeding (>5%) [13]

Other
- Adverse effects [4]

EFAVIRENZ

Trade names: Atripla (Gilead), Sustiva (Bristol-Myers Squibb)
Indications: HIV infection
Class: Antiretroviral, CYP1A2 inhibitor, CYP3A4 inducer, Non-nucleoside reverse transcriptase inhibitor
Half-life: 52–76 hours
Clinically important, potentially hazardous interactions with: alcohol, alprazolam, amprenavir, aripiprazole, artesunate, atazanavir, atorvastatin, atovaquone, benzodiazepines, bepridil, boceprevir, bortezomib, brentuximab vedotin, budesonide, buprenorphine, bupropion, carbamazepine, carvedilol, caspofungin, chlordiazepoxide, cisapride, citalopram, clarithromycin, clonazepam, clopidogrel, clorazepate, CNS depressants, cobimetinib, colchicine, conivaptan, crizotinib, cyclosporine, CYP2B6 inhibitors and inducers, CYP2C19 substrates, CYP2C9 substrates, CYP3A4 substrates and inducers, darunavir, dasabuvir/ombitasvir/paritaprevir/ritonavir, dasatinib,

deferasirox, deflazacort, diazepam, dihydroergotamine, diltiazem, dronedarone, elbasvir & grazoprevir, enzalutamide, eplerenone, ergot, etravirine, everolimus, exemestane, fentanyl, flurazepam, fosamprenavir, fosphenytoin, gefitinib, glecaprevir & pibrentasvir, grapefruit juice, guanfacine, halofantrine, hydroxyzine, imatinib, indinavir, itraconazole, ixabepilone, lapatinib, levomepromazine, levonorgestrel, linagliptin, lopinavir, lorazepam, lovastatin, lurasidone, maraviroc, methadone, methysergide, midazolam, mifepristone, neratinib, nevirapine, nifedipine, nilotinib, nisoldipine, olaparib, ombitasvir/paritaprevir/ritonavir, oral contraceptives, oxazepam, paclitaxel, palbociclib, pazopanib, phenytoin, pimecrolimus, pimozide, posaconazole, pravastatin, praziquantel, progestogens, propafenone, protease inhibitors, quazepam, raltegravir, ranolazine, rifabutin, rifampin, rilpivirine, ritonavir, rivaroxaban, roflumilast, romidepsin, salmeterol, saquinavir, saxagliptin, sertraline, simeprevir, simvastatin, sirolimus, sofosbuvir & velpatasvir, sofosbuvir/velpatasvir/voxilaprevir, sonidegib, sorafenib, SSRIs, St John's wort, sunitinib, tacrolimus, tadalafil, telaprevir, temazepam, ticagrelor, tipranavir, tocilizumab, tolvaptan, toremifene, triazolam, ulipristal, vandetanib, vemurafenib, venetoclax, vilazodone, vitamin K antagonists, voriconazole, warfarin, zuclopenthixol

Pregnancy category: D

Important contra-indications noted in the prescribing guidelines for: the elderly; nursing mothers; pediatric patients

Note: Atripla is efavirenz, emtricitabine and tenofovir disoproxil.

Skin
- DRESS syndrome [2]
- Eczema (<2%)
- Erythema (11%)
- Exanthems (27%) [3]
- Exfoliative dermatitis (<2%)
- Flushing (<2%)
- Folliculitis (<2%)
- Hot flashes (<2%)
- Hypersensitivity [5]
- Lipodystrophy [2]
- Peripheral edema (<2%)
- Photosensitivity [4]
- Pruritus (11%)
- Rash (26%) [16]
- Stevens-Johnson syndrome [4]
- Toxicity [2]
- Urticaria (<2%)

Hair
- Alopecia (<2%)

Mucosal
- Xerostomia (<2%)

Cardiovascular
- Thrombophlebitis (<2%)

Central Nervous System
- Abnormal dreams (<3%) [9]
- Aggression [2]
- Anorexia (<2%)
- Anxiety (13%) [4]
- Depression (19%) [9]
- Dysgeusia (taste perversion) (<2%)
- Hallucinations [2]
- Headache (2–8%) [3]
- Impaired concentration (3–5%) [5]
- Insomnia (7%) [4]
- Nervousness (7%)
- Neuropsychiatric disturbances [2]
- Neurotoxicity [14]
- Nightmares [3]
- Pain (<13%)
- Paresthesias (<2%)
- Parosmia (<2%)
- Psychosis [7]
- Sleep related disorder [2]
- Somnolence (drowsiness) (2%) [3]
- Suicidal ideation [5]
- Tremor (<2%)
- Vertigo (dizziness) (2–9%) [15]

Neuromuscular/Skeletal
- Asthenia (fatigue) (2–8%) [3]
- Myalgia/Myopathy (<2%)

Gastrointestinal/Hepatic
- Abdominal pain (2–3%)
- Diarrhea (3–14%) [2]
- Dyspepsia (4%)
- Hepatic failure [2]
- Hepatotoxicity [13]
- Nausea (2–10%) [3]
- Vomiting (3–6%)

Endocrine/Metabolic
- ALT increased [2]
- Gynecomastia [15]

Genitourinary
- Urolithiasis [3]

Hematologic
- Dyslipidemia [2]

Other
- Adverse effects [10]
- Teratogenicity [4]

EFINACONAZOLE

Trade name: Jublia (Valeant)
Indications: Onychomycosis
Class: Antifungal
Half-life: 30 hours
Clinically important, potentially hazardous interactions with: none known
Pregnancy category: C
Important contra-indications noted in the prescribing guidelines for: nursing mothers; pediatric patients

---

Nails
- Onychocryptosis (2%)

Local
- Application-site dermatitis (2%)
- Application-site reactions [4]
- Application-site vesicles (2%)

EFLORNITHINE

Trade name: Vaniqa (Women First)
Indications: Sleeping sickness, hypertrichosis
Class: Ornithine decarboxylase inhibitor
Half-life: 3–3.5 hours (intravenous); 8 hours (topical)
Clinically important, potentially hazardous interactions with: none known
Pregnancy category: C
Important contra-indications noted in the prescribing guidelines for: nursing mothers; pediatric patients

---

Skin
- Acneform eruption (24%)
- Burning (4%)
- Facial edema (3%)
- Pruritus (4%) [2]
- Rash (3%)
- Stinging (8%)
- Xerosis (2%)

Hair
- Alopecia (5–10%)
- Ingrown (2%)
- Pseudofolliculitis barbae (5–15%)

Central Nervous System
- Headache (5%)
- Paresthesias (4%)
- Seizures (7%) [2]
- Vertigo (dizziness) (<10%)

Gastrointestinal/Hepatic
- Diarrhea (<10%)
- Vomiting (<10%)

Hematologic
- Eosinophilia (<10%)

Otic
- Hearing impairment (<10%)

ELAGOLIX SODIUM *

Trade name: Orilissa (AbbVie)
Indications: indicated for the management of moderate to severe pain associated with endometriosis
Class: Gonadotropin-releasing hormone (GnRH) antagonist
Half-life: 4–6 hours
Clinically important, potentially hazardous interactions with: none known
Pregnancy category: N/A (Exposure early in pregnancy may increase the risk of early pregnancy loss.)

Skin
- Flushing (24–46%)
- Rash (6%)

Central Nervous System
- Anxiety (3–5%)
- Depression (3–6%)
- Headache (17–20%)
- Insomnia (6–9%)
- Irritability (<5%)
- Mood changes (5–6%)
- Vertigo (dizziness) (<5%)

Neuromuscular/Skeletal
Arthralgia (3–5%)

Gastrointestinal/Hepatic
Abdominal pain (<5%)
Constipation (<5%)
Diarrhea (<5%)
Nausea (11–16%)

Endocrine/Metabolic
Amenorrhea (4–7%)
Libido decreased (<5%)
Weight gain (<5%)

ELBASVIR & GRAZOPREVIR

Trade name: Zepatier (Merck)
Indications: Chronic hepatitis C virus genotypes 1 or 4 (with or without ribavirin)
Class: Direct-acting antiviral, Hepatitis C virus NS3/4A protease inhibitor (grazoprevir), Hepatitis C virus NS5A inhibitor (elbasvir)
Half-life: 24 hours (elbasvir); 31 hours (grazoprevir)
Clinically important, potentially hazardous interactions with: atazanavir, atorvastatin, bosentan, carbamazepine, cobicistat/elvitegravir/emtricitabine/tenofovir disoproxil, cyclosporine, darunavir, efavirenz, fluvastatin, ketoconazole, lopinavir, lovastatin, modafinil, moderate CYP3A inducers, nafcillin, OATP1B1/3 inhibitors, phenytoin, rifampin, rosuvastatin, saquinavir, simvastatin, strong CYP3A inducers, tacrolimus, tipranavir
Pregnancy category: N/A (No available data; contra-indicated in pregnant women and in men with pregnant partners when administered with ribavirin)
Important contra-indications noted in the prescribing guidelines for: pediatric patients
Note: Contra-indicated in patients with moderate or severe hepatic impairment (Child-Pugh B or C).

Central Nervous System
Headache (10–11%) [9]

Neuromuscular/Skeletal
Asthenia (fatigue) (5–11%) [9]

Gastrointestinal/Hepatic
Abdominal pain (2%)
Diarrhea (2%) [2]
Hepatotoxicity [2]
Nausea (11%) [8]

Hematologic
Anemia [2]

Other
Adverse effects [2]

ELETRIPTAN

Trade name: Relpax (Pfizer)
Indications: Migraine headaches
Class: 5-HT1 agonist, Serotonin receptor agonist, Triptan
Half-life: 4–5 hours
Clinically important, potentially hazardous interactions with: clarithromycin, dihydroergotamine, itraconazole, ketoconazole, methysergide, nefazodone, nelfinavir, paclitaxel, ritonavir, SNRIs, SSRIs, telithromycin, triptans, troleandomycin, voriconazole
Pregnancy category: C
Important contra-indications noted in the prescribing guidelines for: nursing mothers; pediatric patients
Note: Contra-indicated in patients with history, symptoms, or signs of ischemic cardiac, cerebrovascular, or peripheral vascular syndromes, or in patients with uncontrolled hypertension.

Skin
Flushing (2%)

Mucosal
Xerostomia (2–4%)

Cardiovascular
Chest pain (<4%) [3]

Central Nervous System
Headache (3–4%)
Neurotoxicity [2]
Paresthesias (3–4%)
Somnolence (drowsiness) (3–7%) [2]
Vertigo (dizziness) (3–7%)
Warm feeling (2%)

Neuromuscular/Skeletal
Asthenia (fatigue) (4–10%) [4]

Gastrointestinal/Hepatic
Abdominal pain (<2%)
Dyspepsia (<2%)
Dysphagia (<2%)
Nausea (3–7%) [5]
Vomiting [2]

Other
Adverse effects [2]

ELIGLUSTAT

Trade name: Cerdelga (Genzyme)
Indications: Gaucher disease
Class: Glucosylceramide synthase inhibitor
Half-life: 7–9 hours
Clinically important, potentially hazardous interactions with: carbamazepine, grapefruit juice, phenobarbital, phenytoin, rifampin, St John's wort, strong or moderate CYP2D6 inhibitors
Pregnancy category: C
Important contra-indications noted in the prescribing guidelines for: nursing mothers; pediatric patients

---

Skin
Rash (5%)

Mucosal
Oropharyngeal pain (10%)

Cardiovascular
Palpitation (5%) [3]

Central Nervous System
Headache (13–40%) [2]
Migraine (10%)
Vertigo (dizziness) (8%)

Neuromuscular/Skeletal
Asthenia (fatigue) (8–14%)
Back pain (12%)
Pain in extremities (11%)

Gastrointestinal/Hepatic
Abdominal pain (10%) [2]
Constipation (5%)
Diarrhea (12%) [2]
Dyspepsia (7%)
Flatulence (10%)
Gastroesophageal reflux (7%)
Nausea (10–12%)

Respiratory
Cough (7%)

Other
Adverse effects [2]

ELOSULFASE ALFA

Trade name: Vimizim (BioMarin)
Indications: Mucopolysaccharidosis IVA (Morquio A syndrome)
Class: Enzyme
Half-life: 8–36 minutes
Clinically important, potentially hazardous interactions with: none known
Pregnancy category: C
Important contra-indications noted in the prescribing guidelines for: nursing mothers; pediatric patients
Warning: RISK OF ANAPHYLAXIS

Skin
Anaphylactoid reactions/Anaphylaxis (8%)
Hypersensitivity (19%) [2]

Central Nervous System
Chills (10%)
Fever (33%)
Headache (26%)

Neuromuscular/Skeletal
Asthenia (fatigue) (10%)

Gastrointestinal/Hepatic
Abdominal pain (21%)
Nausea (24%)
Vomiting (31%) [2]

Local
Infusion-related reactions [2]

ELOTUZUMAB

Trade name: Empliciti (Bristol-Myers Squibb)
Indications: Multiple myeloma (in combination with lenalidomide and dexamethasone) in patients who have received one to three prior therapies
Class: Monoclonal antibody
Half-life: N/A
Clinically important, potentially hazardous interactions with: none known

Pregnancy category: N/A (Embryo-fetal toxicity with combination dosage)
Important contra-indications noted in the prescribing guidelines for: nursing mothers; pediatric patients
Note: See separate entries for dexamethasone and lenalidomide.

Skin
- Flushing [2]
- Herpes zoster (14%)
- Hyperhidrosis (>5%)
- Hypersensitivity (>5%) [2]
- Peripheral edema [5]
- Rash [2]

Mucosal
- Oropharyngeal pain (10%)

Cardiovascular
- Chest pain (>5%) [3]
- Tachycardia [2]

Central Nervous System
- Anorexia [3]
- Chills [4]
- Fever (37%) [7]
- Headache (15%) [5]
- Hypoesthesia (>5%)
- Insomnia [4]
- Mood changes (>5%)
- Neurotoxicity [2]
- Peripheral neuropathy (27%) [3]

Neuromuscular/Skeletal
- Arthralgia [2]
- Asthenia (fatigue) (62%) [11]
- Back pain [3]
- Muscle spasm [4]
- Pain in extremities (16%)

Gastrointestinal/Hepatic
- Constipation (36%) [5]
- Diarrhea (47%) [7]
- Nausea [5]
- Vomiting (15%) [4]

Respiratory
- Cough [4]
- Dyspnea [5]
- Nasopharyngitis (25%)
- Pneumonia (20%) [5]
- Upper respiratory tract infection (23%) [2]

Endocrine/Metabolic
- ALP increased (39%)
- Appetite decreased (21%)
- Hyperglycemia (89%) [2]
- Hyperkalemia (32%)
- Hypocalcemia (78%)
- Hypokalemia [4]
- Serum creatinine increased [3]
- Weight loss (14%) [2]

Hematologic
- Anemia [4]
- Leukopenia (91%) [3]
- Lymphopenia (13–99%) [6]
- Neutropenia [8]
- Thrombocytopenia (84%) [5]

Ocular
- Cataract (12%)

Local
- Infusion-related reactions (10%) [10]

ELTROMBOPAG

Trade names: Promacta (Novartis), Revolade (Novartis)
Indications: Thrombocytopenic purpura, severe aplastic anemia in patients with insufficient response to immunosuppressive therapy
Class: Thrombopoietin receptor (TPO) agonist
Half-life: 21–32 hours
Clinically important, potentially hazardous interactions with: antacids, atorvastatin, dairy products, eluxadoline, lopinavir, mineral supplements, olmesartan, rosuvastatin, selenium, zinc
Pregnancy category: C
Important contra-indications noted in the prescribing guidelines for: nursing mothers; pediatric patients
Warning: RISK FOR HEPATIC DECOMPENSATION IN PATIENTS WITH CHRONIC HEPATITIS C

Skin
- Peripheral edema (3–4%)
- Pigmentation [2]
- Rash (3–7%)

Hair
- Alopecia (2%)

Mucosal
- Oropharyngeal pain (4%)
- Xerostomia (2%)

Cardiovascular
- Myocardial infarction [2]
- Thromboembolism [5]
- Venous thromboembolism [3]

Central Nervous System
- Dysgeusia (taste perversion) (4%)
- Fever [2]
- Headache (10–21%) [12]
- Ischemic stroke [2]
- Paresthesias (3%)

Neuromuscular/Skeletal
- Arthralgia (3%) [2]
- Asthenia (fatigue) (3–4%) [5]
- Back pain (3%)
- Myalgia/Myopathy (5%)
- Pain in extremities (7%)

Gastrointestinal/Hepatic
- Abdominal pain [2]
- Constipation [2]
- Diarrhea (9%) [2]
- Hepatotoxicity [5]
- Nausea (4–9%) [5]
- Vomiting (6%)

Respiratory
- Cough (5%)
- Nasopharyngitis [3]
- Pharyngitis (4%)
- Upper respiratory tract infection (7%) [2]

Endocrine/Metabolic
- ALP increased (2%)
- ALT increased (5–6%) [5]
- AST increased (4%)

Genitourinary
- Urinary tract infection (5%)

Renal
- Renal failure [3]

Hematologic
- Bleeding [3]
- Myelotoxicity [2]
- Neutropenia [2]
- Thrombocytopenia [2]
- Thrombosis [6]

Ocular
- Cataract (5%) [3]

Other
- Adverse effects [8]

ELUXADOLINE

Trade name: Viberzi (Forest)
Indications: Irritable bowel syndrome with diarrhea
Class: Opioid mu receptor agonist
Half-life: 4–6 hours
Clinically important, potentially hazardous interactions with: alfentanil, alosetron, anticholinergics, atazanavir, bupropion, ciprofloxacin, clarithromycin, cyclosporine, dihydroergotamine, eltrombopag, ergotamine, fentanyl, fluconazole, gemfibrozil, lopinavir, opioids, paroxetine hydrochloride, paroxetine mesylate, pimozide, quinidine, rifampin, ritonavir, rosuvastatin, saquinavir, sirolimus, tacrolimus, tipranavir
Pregnancy category: N/A (Insufficient evidence to inform drug-associated risk)
Important contra-indications noted in the prescribing guidelines for: pediatric patients
Note: Contra-indicated in patients with known or suspected biliary duct obstruction, or sphincter of Oddi disease or dysfunction; alcoholism, alcohol abuse, alcohol addiction, or drink more than 3 alcoholic beverages/day; a history of pancreatitis; structural diseases of the pancreas, including known or suspected pancreatic duct obstruction; severe hepatic impairment (Child-Pugh Class C); severe constipation or sequelae from constipation, or known or suspected mechanical gastrointestinal obstruction.

Skin
- Rash (3%)

Central Nervous System
- Euphoria (<2%)
- Sedation (<2%)
- Somnolence (drowsiness) (<2%)
- Vertigo (dizziness) (3%) [2]

Gastrointestinal/Hepatic
- Abdominal distension (3%) [2]
- Abdominal pain (6–7%) [4]
- Constipation (7–8%) [7]
- Flatulence (3%)
- Gastroenteritis (<3%) [2]
- Gastroesophageal reflux (<2%)
- Nausea (7–8%) [5]
- Pancreatitis [6]
- Vomiting (4%) [3]

Respiratory
- Asthma (<2%)
- Bronchitis (3%)
- Bronchospasm (<2%)

Nasopharyngitis (3–4%) [2]
Respiratory failure (<2%)
Wheezing (<2%)

Endocrine/Metabolic
ALT increased (2–3%)
AST increased (<2%)

Other
Adverse effects [2]

EMPAGLIFLOZIN

Trade names: Glyxambi (Boehringer Ingelheim), Jardiance (Boehringer Ingelheim), Synjardy (Boehringer Ingelheim)
Indications: Type II diabetes mellitus
Class: Sodium-glucose co-transporter 2 (SGLT2) inhibitor
Half-life: 12 hours
Clinically important, potentially hazardous interactions with: none known
Pregnancy category: C
Important contra-indications noted in the prescribing guidelines for: nursing mothers; pediatric patients
Note: Contra-indicated in patients with severe renal impairment, end stage renal disease, or on dialysis. Glyxambi is empagliflozin and linagliptin; Synjardy is empagliflozin and metformin.

Central Nervous System
Headache [2]
Vertigo (dizziness) [2]

Gastrointestinal/Hepatic
Constipation [2]

Respiratory
Nasopharyngitis [4]

Endocrine/Metabolic
Hypoglycemia [5]

Genitourinary
Genital mycotic infections (2–6%) [10]
Pollakiuria [3]
Urinary frequency (3%)
Urinary tract infection (8–9%) [10]

Other
Adverse effects [7]
Death [2]
Dipsia (thirst) (2%)

EMTRICITABINE

Trade names: Atripla (Gilead), Complera (Gilead), Descovy (Gilead), Emtriva (Gilead), Truvada (Gilead)
Indications: HIV-1 infection
Class: Antiretroviral, Nucleoside analog reverse transcriptase inhibitor
Half-life: ~10 hours
Clinically important, potentially hazardous interactions with: cobicistat/elvitegravir/emtricitabine/tenofovir disoproxil, ganciclovir, lamivudine, ribavirin, valganciclovir
Pregnancy category: B
Important contra-indications noted in the prescribing guidelines for: nursing mothers
Note: Emtricitabine is a fluorinated derivative of lamivudine. Atripla is emtricitabine, efavirenz and tenofovir disoproxil; Complera is emtricitabine, rilpivirine and tenofovir disoproxil; Descovy is emtricitabine and tenofovir alafenamide; Truvada is emtricitabine and tenofovir disoproxil. See also separate profiles for emtricitabine in combination with cobicistat, elvitegravir and tenofovir disoproxil or tenofovir alafenamide.
Warning: LACTIC ACIDOSIS / SEVERE HEPATOMEGALY WITH STEATOSIS and POST TREATMENT EXACERBATION OF HEPATITIS B

Skin
Exanthems (17%)
Pigmentation (palms and soles) (32%)
Pruritus (17–30%)
Pustules (17–30%)
Rash (17–30%) [5]
Urticaria (17–30%)
Vesiculobullous eruption (17–30%)

Central Nervous System
Abnormal dreams (2–11%) [3]
Anxiety [2]
Depression (6–9%)
Fever (18%)
Headache (13–22%) [5]
Insomnia (7–16%)
Neurotoxicity [5]
Paresthesias (6%)
Peripheral neuropathy (4%)
Somnolence (drowsiness) [2]
Vertigo (dizziness) (4–25%) [4]

Neuromuscular/Skeletal
Arthralgia (3–5%)
Asthenia (fatigue) (12–16%) [4]
Myalgia/Myopathy (4–6%) [2]

Gastrointestinal/Hepatic
Abdominal pain (8–14%) [2]
Diarrhea (20–23%) [6]
Dyspepsia (4–8%)
Gastroenteritis (11%)
Hepatic failure [2]
Hepatotoxicity [2]
Nausea (13–18%) [7]
Vomiting (9–23%) [4]

Respiratory
Cough (14–28%)
Pneumonia (15%)
Rhinitis (12–20%)

Hematologic
Anemia (7%)

Otic
Otitis media (23%)

Other
Adverse effects [5]
Allergic reactions (17–30%)
Infection (44%)

EMTRICITABINE/ RILPIVIRINE/ TENOFOVIR ALAFENAMIDE

Trade name: Odefsey (Gilead)
Indications: HIV-1 infection
Class: Hepatitis B virus necleoside analog reverse transcriptase inhibitor (tenofovir alafenamide), Non-nucleoside reverse transcriptase inhibitor (rilpivirine), Nucleoside analog reverse transcriptase inhibitor (emtricitabine)
Half-life: 10 hours (emtricitabine); 50 hours (rilpivirine); <1 hour (tenofovir alafenamide)
Clinically important, potentially hazardous interactions with: carbamazepine, dexamethasone, dexlansoprazole, esomeprazole, lansoprazole, omeprazole, oxcarbazepine, pantoprazole, phenobarbital, phenytoin, rabeprazole, rifampin, rifapentine, St John's wort
Pregnancy category: N/A (Insufficient evidence to inform drug-associated risk)
Important contra-indications noted in the prescribing guidelines for: nursing mothers; pediatric patients
Warning: LACTIC ACIDOSIS/SEVERE HEPATOMEGALY WITH STEATOSIS and POST TREATMENT ACUTE EXACERBATION OF HEPATITIS B

Central Nervous System
Depression (<2%)
Headache (<2%)
Insomnia (<2%)

ENALAPRIL

Trade names: Innovace (Merck Sharpe & Dohme), Lexxel (AstraZeneca), Teczem (Sanofi-Aventis), Vaseretic (Valeant), Vasotec (Valeant)
Indications: Hypertension, symptomatic congestive heart failure, asymptomatic left ventricular dysfunction
Class: Angiotensin-converting enzyme (ACE) inhibitor, Antihypertensive, Vasodilator
Half-life: 11 hours
Clinically important, potentially hazardous interactions with: alcohol, aldesleukin, allopurinol, alpha blockers, alprostadil, amifostine, amiloride, angiotensin II receptor antagonists, antacids, antidiabetics, antihypertensives, antipsychotics, anxiolytics and hypnotics, aprotinin, azathioprine, baclofen, beta blockers, calcium channel blockers, clonidine, conivaptan, corticosteroids, cyclosporine, CYP3A4 inducers, deferasirox, diazoxide, diuretics, eplerenone, estrogens, everolimus, general anesthetics, gold & gold compounds, grapefruit juice, heparins, hydralazine, hypotensives, insulin, levodopa, lithium, MAO inhibitors, metformin, methyldopa, methylphenidate, minoxidil, moxisylyte, moxonidine, nitrates, nitroprusside, NSAIDs, pentoxifylline, phosphodiesterase 5 inhibitors, potassium salts, prostacyclin analogues, quinine, rituximab, salicylates, sirolimus, spironolactone,

sulfonylureas, tadalafil, temsirolimus, tizanidine, tolvaptan, triamterene, trimethoprim
Pregnancy category: D (category C in first trimester; category D in second and third trimesters)
Important contra-indications noted in the prescribing guidelines for: nursing mothers
Note: Lexxel is enalapril and felodipine; Teczem is enalapril and diltiazem; Vaseretic is enalapril and hydrochlorothiazide. Hydrochlorothiazide is a sulfonamide and can be absorbed systemically. Sulfonamides can produce severe, possibly fatal, reactions such as toxic epidermal necrolysis and Stevens-Johnson syndrome.
Contra-indicated in patients with a history of angioedema with or without previous ACE inhibitor treatment.
Warning: FETAL TOXICITY

Skin
- Angioedema [73]
- Bullous pemphigoid [2]
- Exanthems [9]
- Flushing [4]
- Lichenoid eruption [2]
- Lupus erythematosus [2]
- Pemphigus [11]
- Pemphigus foliaceus [2]
- Peripheral edema [2]
- Photosensitivity [2]
- Pruritus [3]
- Psoriasis [3]
- Rash [5]
- Urticaria [5]
- Vasculitis [2]

Mucosal
- Oral lesions [4]
- Oral ulceration [2]
- Tongue edema [2]

Cardiovascular
- Hypotension [2]

Central Nervous System
- Ageusia (taste loss) [4]
- Dysgeusia (taste perversion) (<10%) [7]
- Headache (5%)
- Vertigo (dizziness) (4–8%) [2]

Neuromuscular/Skeletal
- Asthenia (fatigue) (<3%)
- Pseudopolymyalgia [2]

Gastrointestinal/Hepatic
- Hepatotoxicity [3]
- Pancreatitis [2]

Respiratory
- Cough (8–23%) [40]

Endocrine/Metabolic
- Hyperkalemia [4]
- SIADH [3]

Renal
- Nephrotoxicity [2]

Other
- Adverse effects [9]
- Death [4]

ENASIDENIB

Trade name: Idhifa (Celgene)
Indications: Relapsed or refractory acute myeloid leukemia
Class: Isocitrate dehydrogenase-2 inhibitor
Half-life: 137 hours
Clinically important, potentially hazardous interactions with: none known
Pregnancy category: N/A (Can cause fetal harm)
Important contra-indications noted in the prescribing guidelines for: nursing mothers; pediatric patients
Warning: DIFFERENTIATION SYNDROME

Skin
- Differentiation syndrome (14%) [2]
- Tumor lysis syndrome (6%)

Cardiovascular
- Pulmonary edema (<10%)

Central Nervous System
- Dysgeusia (taste perversion) (12%)

Gastrointestinal/Hepatic
- Diarrhea (43%)
- Nausea (50%)
- Vomiting (34%)

Respiratory
- Acute respiratory distress syndrome (<10%)

Endocrine/Metabolic
- Appetite decreased (34%)
- Hyperbilirubinemia (81%)
- Hypocalcemia (74%)
- Hypokalemia (41%)
- Hypophosphatemia (27%)

Hematologic
- Leukocytosis (12%)

ENCORAFENIB *

Trade name: Braftovi (Array Biopharma Inc)
Indications: in combination with binimetinib, for the treatment of patients with unresectable or metastatic melanoma with a BRAF V600E or V600K mutation
Class: Kinase inhibitor
Half-life: 3.5 hours
Clinically important, potentially hazardous interactions with: none known
Pregnancy category: N/A (can cause fetal harm)
Important contra-indications noted in the prescribing guidelines for: nursing mothers

---

Skin
- Acneform eruption (3–8%)
- Erythema (7–16%)
- Hand–foot syndrome (7–51%) [2]
- Hyperkeratosis (23–57%)
- Panniculitis (<10%)
- Pruritus (13–31%)
- Rash (22–41%)
- Xerosis (16–38%)

Hair
- Alopecia (14–56%)

Central Nervous System
- Dysgeusia (taste perversion) (6–13%)
- Fever (18%)
- Headache (22%)
- Paresis (<10%)
- Peripheral neuropathy (12%)
- Vertigo (dizziness) (15%)

Neuromuscular/Skeletal
- Arthralgia (26–44%)
- Asthenia (fatigue) (43%)
- Back pain (9–15%)
- Myalgia/Myopathy (23–33%) [2]
- Pain in extremities (11%)

Gastrointestinal/Hepatic
- Abdominal pain (28%)
- Constipation (22%)
- Nausea (41%)
- Pancreatitis (<10%)
- Vomiting (30%)

Endocrine/Metabolic
- ALP increased (21%)
- ALT increased (29%)
- AST increased (27%)
- GGT increased (45%)
- Hyperglycemia (28%)
- Hypermagnesemia (10%)
- Hyponatremia (18%)
- Serum creatinine increased (93%)

Hematologic
- Anemia (36%)
- Hemorrhage (19%)
- Leukopenia (13%)
- Lymphopenia (13%)
- Neutropenia (13%)

ENFUVIRTIDE

Trade name: Fuzeon (Roche)
Indications: HIV-1 infection (in combination with other antiretroviral agents)
Class: Antiretroviral, HIV cell fusion inhibitor
Half-life: 3.8 hours
Clinically important, potentially hazardous interactions with: darunavir, indinavir, tipranavir
Pregnancy category: B
Important contra-indications noted in the prescribing guidelines for: the elderly; nursing mothers

---

Skin
- Folliculitis (2%)
- Herpes simplex (4%)
- Hypersensitivity [3]
- Papillomas (4%)
- Pruritus (62%)

Mucosal
- Xerostomia (2%)

Central Nervous System
- Anorexia (2%)
- Depression (9%)

Neuromuscular/Skeletal
- Asthenia (fatigue) (16%) [2]
- Myalgia/Myopathy (3%)
- Pain in extremities (3%)

Gastrointestinal/Hepatic
- Abdominal pain (4%)

Pancreatitis (3%)

Respiratory

Cough (4%)
Flu-like syndrome (2%)
Pneumonia (3%)
Sinusitis (6%)

Endocrine/Metabolic

ALT increased (<4%)
Appetite decreased (3%)
Creatine phosphokinase increased (3–7%)
Weight loss (7%)

Hematologic

Eosinophilia (2–9%)

Ocular

Conjunctivitis (2%)

Local

Injection-site bruising (52%)
Injection-site erythema (91%)
Injection-site induration (90%)
Injection-site nodules (80%) [4]
Injection-site pain (96%)
Injection-site pruritus (65%)
Injection-site reactions (98%) [27]
Injection-site scleroderma [2]

Other

Infection [3]

ENOXAPARIN

Trade names: Clexane (Sanofi-Aventis), Lovenox (Sanofi-Aventis)
Indications: Prevention of deep vein thrombosis, ischemic complications of unstable angina and non-Q wave myocardial infarction, treatment of acute ST-segment elevation myocardial infarction
Class: Heparin, low molecular weight
Half-life: 4.5 hours
Clinically important, potentially hazardous interactions with: ACE inhibitors, angiotensin II receptor antagonists, anticoagulants, aspirin, butabarbital, clopidogrel, danaparoid, diclofenac, dipyridamole, drotrecogin alfa, iloprost, infused nitrates, ketorolac, NSAIDs, platelet inhibitors, rivaroxaban, salicylates, sulfinpyrazone
Pregnancy category: B
Important contra-indications noted in the prescribing guidelines for: nursing mothers; pediatric patients
Note: Epidural or spinal hematomas may occur in patients who are anticoagulated with low molecular weight heparins or heparinoids and are receiving neuraxial anesthesia or undergoing spinal puncture.
Contra-indicated in patients with active major bleeding; thrombocytopenia with a positive *in vitro* test for anti-platelet antibody in the presence of enoxaparin; hypersensitivity to heparin or pork products; hypersensitivity to benzyl alcohol (multi-dose formulation only).
Warning: SPINAL/EPIDURAL HEMATOMA

Skin

Anaphylactoid reactions/Anaphylaxis [3]
Angioedema [2]
Bullous dermatitis [7]
Ecchymoses (2%)
Edema (3%)
Erythema (<10%) [2]
Exanthems [2]
Hematoma [11]
Hypersensitivity [7]
Necrosis [5]
Peripheral edema (3%)
Pruritus [2]
Purpura (<10%)

Cardiovascular

Venous thromboembolism [2]

Gastrointestinal/Hepatic

Hepatotoxicity [5]

Endocrine/Metabolic

ALT increased [4]
AST increased [3]

Genitourinary

Hematuria [2]

Hematologic

Bleeding [9]
Hemorrhage [4]
Thrombocytopenia [6]

Local

Injection-site necrosis [4]
Injection-site plaques [2]

Other

Adverse effects [4]
Death [2]

ENTACAPONE

Trade names: Comtan (Orion), Comtess (Orion), Stalevo (Orion)
Indications: Parkinsonism
Class: Catechol-O-methyl transferase inhibitor
Half-life: 2.4 hours
Clinically important, potentially hazardous interactions with: amitriptyline, MAO inhibitors, paroxetine hydrochloride, phenelzine, rasagiline, tranylcypromine, venlafaxine
Pregnancy category: C
Important contra-indications noted in the prescribing guidelines for: nursing mothers; pediatric patients

---

Skin

Diaphoresis (2%)
Purpura (2%)

Mucosal

Xerostomia (3%)

Central Nervous System

Anxiety (2%)
Dyskinesia (25%) [3]
Hyperactivity (10%)
Hypokinesia (9%)
Parkinsonism (17%)
Somnolence (drowsiness) (2%)
Vertigo (dizziness) (8%) [2]

Neuromuscular/Skeletal

Asthenia (fatigue) (8%)
Back pain (4%)

Gastrointestinal/Hepatic

Abdominal pain (8%)
Constipation (6%)
Diarrhea (10%) [3]
Dyspepsia (2%)
Flatulence (2%)
Nausea (14%) [3]
Vomiting (4%)

Respiratory

Dyspnea (3%)

Genitourinary

Melanuria (10%) [2]

ENTECAVIR

Trade name: Baraclude (Bristol-Myers Squibb)
Indications: Chronic hepatitis B virus infection
Class: Antiviral, Guanosine nucleoside analog
Half-life: ~24 hours
Clinically important, potentially hazardous interactions with: none known
Pregnancy category: C
Important contra-indications noted in the prescribing guidelines for: nursing mothers; pediatric patients
Warning: SEVERE ACUTE EXACERBATIONS OF HEPATITIS B, PATIENTS CO-INFECTED WITH HIV AND HBV, and LACTIC ACIDOSIS AND HEPATOMEGALY

Skin

Rash [2]

Hair

Alopecia [2]

Central Nervous System

Headache (2–4%) [4]
Neurotoxicity [3]
Peripheral neuropathy [2]
Vertigo (dizziness) [2]

Neuromuscular/Skeletal

Asthenia (fatigue) (<3%) [7]
Myalgia/Myopathy [3]

Gastrointestinal/Hepatic

Abdominal pain [3]
Diarrhea [2]
Nausea [2]
Pancreatitis [3]

Respiratory

Cough [2]
Upper respiratory tract infection [2]

Endocrine/Metabolic

Acidosis [6]
ALT increased (2–12%) [2]
Creatine phosphokinase increased (<2%)
Hypophosphatemia [2]

Genitourinary

Hematuria (9%)

Other

Adverse effects [4]

ENZALUTAMIDE

Trade name: Xtandi (Medivation)
Indications: Metastatic castration-resistant prostate cancer in patients who have previously received docetaxel
Class: Androgen antagonist
Half-life: 8–9 days
Clinically important, potentially hazardous interactions with: alfentanil, bosentan, carbamazepine, copanlisib, cyclosporine, dihydroergotamine, efavirenz, ergotamine, fentanyl, gemfibrozil, itraconazole, midazolam, midostaurin, modafinil, nafcillin, neratinib, omeprazole, phenobarbital, phenytoin, pimozide, quinidine, rifabutin, rifampin, rifapentine, sirolimus, St John's wort, tacrolimus, warfarin
Pregnancy category: X (not indicated for use in women)
Important contra-indications noted in the prescribing guidelines for: nursing mothers; pediatric patients

---

Skin
- Hot flashes (20%) [11]
- Peripheral edema (15%) [3]
- Pruritus (4%)
- Xerosis (4%)

Mucosal
- Epistaxis (nosebleed) (3%)

Cardiovascular
- Cardiotoxicity [2]
- Hypertension (6%) [5]

Central Nervous System
- Amnesia (>2%)
- Anxiety (7%)
- Cognitive impairment (4%)
- Gait instability [3]
- Hallucinations (2%)
- Headache (12%) [4]
- Hypoesthesia (4%)
- Insomnia (9%)
- Paresthesias (7%) [2]
- Seizures [13]
- Spinal cord compression (7%)
- Vertigo (dizziness) (10%) [2]

Neuromuscular/Skeletal
- Arthralgia (21%) [5]
- Asthenia (fatigue) (51%) [25]
- Back pain (26%) [6]
- Bone or joint pain (15%) [8]
- Fractures (4%) [2]

Gastrointestinal/Hepatic
- Constipation [4]
- Diarrhea (22%) [10]
- Hepatotoxicity [2]
- Nausea [5]

Respiratory
- Bronchitis (>2%)
- Laryngitis (>2%)
- Nasopharyngitis (>2%)
- Pharyngitis (>2%)
- Pneumonia (>2%)
- Sinusitis (>2%)
- Upper respiratory tract infection (11%) [3]

Endocrine/Metabolic
- ALT increased (10%)
- Appetite decreased [6]
- Gynecomastia [2]
- Weight loss [3]

Genitourinary
- Hematuria (7%) [2]
- Pollakiuria (5%)
- Urinary tract infection [2]

Hematologic
- Anemia [3]
- Neutropenia (15%)
- Thrombocytopenia [2]

Other
- Adverse effects [6]
- Death [3]

EPHEDRA

Family: Gnetaceae
Scientific names: *Ephedra equisetina, Ephedra intermedia, Ephedra sinica, Ephedra vulgaris*
Indications: Bronchospasm, asthma, bronchitis, allergy, appetite suppressant, colds, flu, fever, chills, edema, headache, anhidrosis, diuretic, joint and bone pain
Class: Ephedrine alkaloid, Stimulant
Half-life: N/A
Clinically important, potentially hazardous interactions with: acetazolamide, amitriptyline, caffeine, clevidipine, cocoa, corticosteroids, guanethidine, guarana, MAO inhibitors, phenelzine, selegiline, sibutramine, sodium bicarbonate
Note: Banned in the USA.

Cardiovascular
- Cardiotoxicity [2]
- Hypertension [4]
- Palpitation [2]
- Tachycardia [3]

Central Nervous System
- Seizures [7]

Other
- Adverse effects [4]
- Death [5]
- Side effects [2]

EPHEDRINE

Trade names: Rynatuss (MedPointe), Vicks Vatronol (Procter & Gamble)
Indications: Nasal congestion, acute hypotensive states, asthma
Class: Adrenergic alpha-receptor agonist, Sympathomimetic
Half-life: 3–6 hours
Clinically important, potentially hazardous interactions with: antihypertensives, dexamethasone, furazolidone, guanethidine, iobenguane, levomepromazine, MAO inhibitors, methyldopa, oxprenolol, phenelzine, phenylpropanolamine, selegiline, tranylcypromine, tricyclic antidepressants
Pregnancy category: C
Important contra-indications noted in the prescribing guidelines for: nursing mothers

---

Skin
- Dermatitis [5]
- Diaphoresis (<10%)
- Fixed eruption [6]
- Pallor (<10%)
- Urticaria [2]

Mucosal
- Xerostomia (<10%)

Central Nervous System
- Trembling (<10%)
- Tremor (<10%)

EPINEPHRINE

Synonym: adrenaline
Trade names: Adrenaclick (Amedra), Adrenalin (JHP Pharmaceuticals), Auvi-Q (Sanofi-Aventis), Epipen (Mylan)
Indications: Cardiac arrest, hay fever, asthma, anaphylaxis
Class: Catecholamine, Sympathomimetic
Half-life: N/A
Clinically important, potentially hazardous interactions with: albuterol, alpha blockers, amitriptyline, amoxapine, atenolol, beta blockers, carteolol, chlorpromazine, clomipramine, clozapine, cocaine, desipramine, doxepin, ergotamine, furazolidone, halothane, imipramine, insulin aspart, insulin degludec, insulin detemir, insulin glargine, insulin glulisine, levalbuterol, lisdexamfetamine, lurasidone, MAO inhibitors, metoprolol, milnacipran, nadolol, nortriptyline, oxprenolol, penbutolol, phenelzine, phenoxybenzamine, phenylephrine, pindolol, prazosin, propranolol, protriptyline, sympathomimetics, terbutaline, thioridazine, timolol, tranylcypromine, tricyclic antidepressants, trimipramine, vasopressors
Pregnancy category: C
Important contra-indications noted in the prescribing guidelines for: the elderly

---

Skin
- Dermatitis [4]
- Diaphoresis (<10%) [2]
- Flushing (<10%)
- Necrosis [3]
- Pemphigus (cicatricial) [2]

Cardiovascular
- Arrhythmias [3]
- Chest pain [2]
- Hypertension [3]
- Hypotension [4]
- Myocardial infarction [5]
- Palpitation [3]
- QT prolongation [2]
- Ventricular tachycardia [2]

Central Nervous System
- Anxiety [2]
- Trembling (<10%)
- Tremor [3]

Gastrointestinal/Hepatic
- Nausea [2]

EPIRUBICIN

Trade name: Ellence (Pfizer)
Indications: Adjuvant therapy in primary breast cancer
Class: Antibiotic, anthracycline
Half-life: 33 hours
Clinically important, potentially hazardous interactions with: amlodipine, bepridil, cimetidine, diltiazem, felodipine, isradipine, nicardipine, nifedipine, nimodipine, nisoldipine, verapamil
Pregnancy category: D
Important contra-indications noted in the prescribing guidelines for: nursing mothers
Warning: SEVERE OR LIFE-THREATENING HEMATOLOGICAL AND OTHER ADVERSE REACTIONS

Skin
Erythroderma (5%)
Hand–foot syndrome [5]
Hot flashes (5–39%)
Pruritus (9%)
Rash (<9%) [2]
Vasculitis [2]

Hair
Alopecia (69–95%) [18]

Mucosal
Mucositis [5]
Stomatitis [9]

Cardiovascular
Cardiotoxicity [3]
QT prolongation [3]

Central Nervous System
Anorexia [5]
Dysgeusia (taste perversion) [2]
Fever [2]
Headache [2]
Neurotoxicity [2]
Peripheral neuropathy [4]

Neuromuscular/Skeletal
Arthralgia [2]
Asthenia (fatigue) (6%) [9]
Myalgia/Myopathy (55%) [5]

Gastrointestinal/Hepatic
Abdominal pain [2]
Constipation [3]
Diarrhea [7]
Hepatotoxicity [2]
Nausea [13]
Vomiting [11]

Endocrine/Metabolic
ALT increased [2]
Amenorrhea [2]
AST increased [2]

Hematologic
Anemia [9]
Febrile neutropenia [5]
Leukopenia [4]
Neutropenia [13]
Thrombocytopenia [5]

Local
Injection-site reactions (3–20%)

Other
Allergic reactions [2]

EPOETIN ALFA

Synonyms: erythropoietin; EPO
Trade names: Epogen (Amgen), Eprex (Janssen-Cilag), Procrit (Ortho)
Indications: Anemia
Class: Erythropoiesis-stimulating agent (ESA), Erythropoietin
Half-life: 4–13 hours (in patients with chronic renal failure)
Clinically important, potentially hazardous interactions with: none known
Pregnancy category: C
Important contra-indications noted in the prescribing guidelines for: nursing mothers
Warning: ERYTHROPOIESIS-STIMULATING AGENTS (ESAs) INCREASE THE RISK OF DEATH, MYOCARDIAL INFARCTION, STROKE, VENOUS THROMBOEMBOLISM, THROMBOSIS OF VASCULAR ACCESS AND TUMOR PROGRESSION OR RECURRENCE

Skin
Angioedema (<5%)
Edema (17%)
Pruritus (12–21%) [2]
Rash (2–19%)

Cardiovascular
Hypertension (3–28%)

Central Nervous System
Fever (10–42%) [2]
Headache (5–18%)
Paresthesias (11%)

Neuromuscular/Skeletal
Arthralgia (10–16%)

Gastrointestinal/Hepatic
Constipation [2]
Nausea (35–56%)

Respiratory
Cough (4–26%)
Dyspnea [2]

Hematologic
Thrombocytopenia [2]

Ocular
Hallucinations, visual [2]

Local
Injection-site reactions (7%)

EPOPROSTENOL

Trade names: Flolan (GSK), Veletri (Actelion)
Indications: Pulmonary arterial hypertension
Class: Peripheral vasodilator
Half-life: 6 minutes
Clinically important, potentially hazardous interactions with: anticoagulants, antihypertensives, diuretics, vasodilators
Pregnancy category: B
Important contra-indications noted in the prescribing guidelines for: the elderly; nursing mothers; pediatric patients
Note: Contra-indicated in patients with heart failure induced by reduced left ventricular ejection fraction.

Skin
Diaphoresis (41%)
Flushing [6]
Pruritus (4%)
Rash (10%) [2]

Cardiovascular
Bradycardia (5%) [2]
Cardiac failure (31%)
Chest pain (11%) [2]
Hypotension (16%) [5]
Tachycardia (35%) [2]

Central Nervous System
Agitation (11%)
Anxiety (21%) [2]
Chills (25%)
Fever (25%)
Headache (83%) [13]
Insomnia (9%)
Paresthesias (12%)
Seizures (4%)
Somnolence (drowsiness) (4%)
Syncope (13%)
Tremor (21%)

Neuromuscular/Skeletal
Back pain (13%)
Jaw pain (54%) [6]
Myalgia/Myopathy (44%)

Gastrointestinal/Hepatic
Abdominal pain (14%)
Diarrhea [2]
Nausea [5]

Respiratory
Alveolar hemorrhage (pulmonary) [2]
Dyspnea (2%)
Flu-like syndrome (25%)
Pneumonia [2]

Endocrine/Metabolic
Weight loss (27%)

Hematologic
Sepsis (25%)

Local
Injection-site infection (21%)
Injection-site pain (13%)

Other
Adverse effects [3]

EPROSARTAN

Trade name: Teveten (AbbVie)
Indications: Hypertension
Class: Angiotensin II receptor antagonist (blocker), Antihypertensive
Half-life: 5–9 hours
Clinically important, potentially hazardous interactions with: none known
Pregnancy category: D (category C in first trimester; category D in second and third trimesters)
Important contra-indications noted in the prescribing guidelines for: nursing mothers; pediatric patients
Warning: FETAL TOXICITY

Central Nervous System
Dysgeusia (taste perversion) [2]
Vertigo (dizziness) [2]

Neuromuscular/Skeletal
Arthralgia (2%)
Asthenia (fatigue) (2%)

Gastrointestinal/Hepatic
Abdominal pain (2%)

Respiratory
Cough (4%) [3]
Pharyngitis (4%)
Rhinitis (4%)
Upper respiratory tract infection (8%) [2]

Other
Adverse effects [3]

EPTIFIBATIDE

Trade name: Integrilin (Merck)
Indications: Acute coronary syndrome, unstable angina
Class: Antiplatelet, Glycoprotein IIb/IIIa inhibitor
Half-life: 2.5 hours
Clinically important, potentially hazardous interactions with: anticoagulants, antiplatelet agents, collagenase, dasatinib, drotrecogin alfa, fondaparinux, glucosamine, ibritumomab, iloprost, lepirudin, NSAIDs, pentoxifylline, salicylates, thrombolytic agents, tositumomab & iodine[131]
Pregnancy category: B
Important contra-indications noted in the prescribing guidelines for: nursing mothers; pediatric patients
Note: Contra-indicated in patients with a history of bleeding diathesis, or evidence of active abnormal bleeding within the previous 30 days; severe hypertension not adequately controlled on antihypertensive therapy; major surgery within the preceding 6 weeks; history of stroke within 30 days or any history of hemorrhagic stroke; current or planned administration of another parenteral GP IIb/IIIa inhibitor; or dependency on renal dialysis.

Cardiovascular
Hypotension (7%)

Hematologic
Bleeding [3]
Hemorrhage (<10%)
Thrombocytopenia [16]
Thrombosis [3]

Other
Death [2]

ERAVACYCLINE *

Trade name: Xerava (Tetraphase Pharms Inc)
Indications: treatment of complicated intra-abdominal infections in patients 18 years of age and older
Class: Antibacterial, tetracycline
Half-life: 20 hours
Clinically important, potentially hazardous interactions with: none known
Pregnancy category: N/A (data insufficient to inform drug-associated risk of major birth defects and miscarriages.)

Gastrointestinal/Hepatic
Diarrhea (2%)
Nausea (7%) [2]
Vomiting (4%)

Local
Infusion-related reactions (8%)

ERGOMETRINE

Trade name: Ergometrine (Hameln)
Indications: Management of the third stage of labor and in the treatment of postpartum hemorrhage
Class: Amine alkaloid
Half-life: N/A
Clinically important, potentially hazardous interactions with: halothane, sympathomimetic agents
Important contra-indications noted in the prescribing guidelines for: nursing mothers

---

Cardiovascular
Myocardial infarction [4]
Myocardial ischemia [3]

ERGOTAMINE

Trade name: Wigrettes (Organon)
Indications: Migraine, migraine variants
Class: Ergot alkaloid
Half-life: 2 hours
Clinically important, potentially hazardous interactions with: acebutolol, almotriptan, amprenavir, azithromycin, boceprevir, ceritinib, chlortetracycline, crizotinib, darunavir, dasabuvir/ombitasvir/paritaprevir/ritonavir, dasatinib, delavirdine, demeclocycline, doxycycline, eluxadoline, enzalutamide, epinephrine, erythromycin, indinavir, itraconazole, letermovir, lopinavir, lymecycline, methylergonovine, mifepristone, minocycline, naratriptan, nelfinavir, nilotinib, ombitasvir/paritaprevir/ritonavir, oxytetracycline, posaconazole, propyphenazone, ribociclib, ritonavir, telaprevir, telithromycin, tetracycline, tigecycline, tipranavir, troleandomycin, voriconazole, warfarin
Pregnancy category: X
Important contra-indications noted in the prescribing guidelines for: nursing mothers
Note: Ergotamine is excreted in breast milk and may cause symptoms of vomiting, diarrhea, weak pulse and unstable blood pressure in nursing infants.

Skin
Toxicity [4]

Cardiovascular
Valvulopathy [3]

Respiratory
Pleural effusion [2]

ERIBULIN

Trade name: Halaven (Eisai)
Indications: Metastatic breast cancer in patients who have previously received at least two chemotherapeutic regimens (prior therapy should have included an anthracycline and a taxane in either the adjuvant or metastatic setting), unresectable or metastatic liposarcoma in patients who have received a prior anthracycline-containing regimen
Class: Antineoplastic, Microtubule inhibitor
Half-life: 40 hours
Clinically important, potentially hazardous interactions with: none known
Pregnancy category: N/A (No available data but caused embryo-fetal toxicity in animal studies)
Important contra-indications noted in the prescribing guidelines for: nursing mothers; pediatric patients

---

Skin
Peripheral edema (5–10%)
Rash (5–10%)

Hair
Alopecia (45%) [10]

Mucosal
Mucosal inflammation (9%)
Stomatitis (5–10%)
Xerostomia (5–10%)

Central Nervous System
Anorexia (20%) [3]
Depression (5–10%)
Dysgeusia (taste perversion) (5–10%)
Fever (21%)
Headache (19%)
Insomnia (5–10%)
Neurotoxicity [7]
Peripheral neuropathy (35%) [28]
Vertigo (dizziness) (5–10%)

Neuromuscular/Skeletal
Arthralgia (22%)
Asthenia (fatigue) (54%) [32]
Back pain (16%)
Muscle spasm (5–10%)
Myalgia/Myopathy (22%)
Pain in extremities (11%)

Gastrointestinal/Hepatic
Abdominal pain (5–10%)
Constipation (25%) [2]
Diarrhea (18%) [3]
Dyspepsia (5–10%)
Hepatotoxicity [2]
Nausea (35%) [9]
Vomiting (18%)

Respiratory
Cough (14%)
Dyspnea (16%) [2]
Upper respiratory tract infection (5–10%)

Endocrine/Metabolic
ALT increased [3]
Appetite decreased [2]
Hypokalemia (5–10%)
Weight loss (21%)

Genitourinary
Urinary tract infection (10%)

Hematologic
- Anemia (58%) [12]
- Febrile neutropenia (5%) [16]
- Leukopenia [18]
- Lymphopenia [4]
- Neutropenia (82%) [54]

Ocular
- Lacrimation (increased) (5–10%)

Other
- Adverse effects [4]
- Death [3]

ERLOTINIB

Trade name: Tarceva (OSI)
Indications: Non-small cell lung cancer, pancreatic cancer (with gemcitabine)
Class: Antineoplastic, Biologic, Epidermal growth factor receptor (EGFR) inhibitor, Tyrosine kinase inhibitor
Half-life: ~36 hours
Clinically important, potentially hazardous interactions with: atazanavir, capecitabine, carbamazepine, ciprofloxacin, clarithromycin, diclofenac, itraconazole, ketoconazole, meloxicam, nefazodone, nelfinavir, omeprazole, pantoprazole, phenobarbital, phenytoin, rifabutin, rifampin, rifapentine, ritonavir, saquinavir, St John's wort, troleandomycin, voriconazole, warfarin
Pregnancy category: D
Important contra-indications noted in the prescribing guidelines for: nursing mothers; pediatric patients

---

Skin
- Acne keloid [2]
- Acneform eruption [29]
- AGEP [2]
- Dermatitis [4]
- DRESS syndrome [2]
- Erythema (18%)
- Exanthems [3]
- Folliculitis [9]
- Hand–foot syndrome [3]
- Papulopustular eruption [9]
- Pruritus (13%) [9]
- Purpura [3]
- Rash (75%) [116]
- Rosacea [2]
- Toxicity [10]
- Xerosis (12%) [13]

Hair
- Alopecia [10]
- Hair changes [4]
- Hypertrichosis [4]

Nails
- Nail changes [3]
- Paronychia [14]

Mucosal
- Mucositis [10]
- Stomatitis (17%) [12]

Cardiovascular
- Hypertension [4]

Central Nervous System
- Anorexia [9]
- Fever [2]

Neuromuscular/Skeletal
- Asthenia (fatigue) (52%) [33]
- Rhabdomyolysis [2]

Gastrointestinal/Hepatic
- Abdominal pain (11%)
- Cholangitis [2]
- Diarrhea [70]
- Gastrointestinal bleeding [3]
- Hepatotoxicity [13]
- Nausea [18]
- Vomiting [10]

Respiratory
- Cough (33%)
- Dyspnea [4]
- Pneumonia [2]
- Pneumonitis [7]
- Pneumothorax [2]
- Pulmonary toxicity [15]

Endocrine/Metabolic
- ALT increased [3]
- Appetite decreased [4]
- AST increased [3]
- Dehydration [3]
- Hyperglycemia [3]

Hematologic
- Anemia [12]
- Febrile neutropenia [2]
- Hemotoxicity [2]
- Leukopenia [4]
- Neutropenia [14]
- Thrombocytopenia [10]

Ocular
- Conjunctivitis (12%) [3]
- Corneal perforation [2]
- Ectropion [4]
- Ocular adverse effects [3]
- Periorbital rash [2]
- Trichomegaly [13]

Other
- Adverse effects [12]
- Death [10]
- Infection (24%) [7]

ERTAPENEM

Trade name: Invanz (Merck)
Indications: Severe resistant bacterial infections caused by susceptible organisms
Class: Antibiotic, carbapenem
Half-life: 4 hours
Clinically important, potentially hazardous interactions with: probenecid
Pregnancy category: B
Important contra-indications noted in the prescribing guidelines for: the elderly; nursing mothers

---

Skin
- Edema (3%)
- Erythema (<2%)
- Pruritus (<2%)
- Rash (2–3%)
- Wound complications [2]

Cardiovascular
- Phlebitis (2%)
- Thrombophlebitis (2%)

Central Nervous System
- Delirium [2]
- Hallucinations [2]
- Seizures [7]

Gastrointestinal/Hepatic
- Nausea [2]

Respiratory
- Cough (<2%)

Genitourinary
- Vaginitis (<3%)

Local
- Injection-site extravasation (2%)

Other
- Death (2%)

ERYTHROMYCIN

Trade names: Eryc (Warner Chilcott), PCE (AbbVie)
Indications: Various infections caused by susceptible organisms
Class: Antibiotic, macrolide, CYP3A4 inhibitor
Half-life: 1.4–2 hours
Clinically important, potentially hazardous interactions with: afatinib, alfentanil, aminophylline, amisulpride, amoxicillin, ampicillin, anticonvulsants, arsenic, astemizole, atorvastatin, avanafil, benzodiazepines, bosentan, bromocriptine, buprenorphine, bupropion, carbamazepine, cilostazol, ciprofloxacin, cisapride, clindamycin, clindamycin/tretinoin, clopidogrel, clozapine, colchicine, cyclosporine, CYP3A inhibitors, darifenacin, dasatinib, digoxin, dihydroergotamine, diltiazem, disopyramide, docetaxel, doxercalciferol, dronedarone, enoxacin, eplerenone, ergotamine, estradiol, eszopiclone, everolimus, flibanserin, fluconazole, fluoxetine, fluvastatin, gatifloxacin, HMG-CoA reductase inhibitors, imatinib, indacaterol, itraconazole, ketoconazole, levodopa, lomefloxacin, lorazepam, lovastatin, methadone, methylergonovine, methylprednisolone, methysergide, midazolam, mifepristone, mizolastine, moxifloxacin, naldemedine, naloxegol, neratinib, nintedanib, nitrazepam, norfloxacin, ofloxacin, olaparib, oxtriphylline, paroxetine hydrochloride, pentamidine, pimecrolimus, pimozide, pitavastatin, pravastatin, quetiapine, quinolones, ranolazine, repaglinide, rilpivirine, rivaroxaban, roflumilast, rosuvastatin, rupatadine, sertraline, sildenafil, silodosin, simeprevir, simvastatin, sparfloxacin, sulpiride, tacrolimus, tadalafil, tamsulosin, terfenadine, tezacaftor/ivacaftor, tramadol, triamcinolone, triazolam, troleandomycin, vardenafil, venetoclax, verapamil, vilazodone, vinblastine, warfarin, zafirlukast, zaleplon, zolpidem, zuclopenthixol
Pregnancy category: B
Important contra-indications noted in the prescribing guidelines for: the elderly; nursing mothers

---

Skin
- AGEP [2]
- Anaphylactoid reactions/Anaphylaxis [2]
- Baboon syndrome (SDRIFE) [2]
- Dermatitis (systemic) [4]

Exanthems (<5%) [4]
Fixed eruption [6]
Hypersensitivity (<10%) [3]
Rash [3]
Stevens-Johnson syndrome [8]
Toxic epidermal necrolysis [8]
Urticaria [4]

Mucosal
Oral candidiasis (<10%)

Cardiovascular
QT prolongation [5]
Torsades de pointes [8]

Neuromuscular/Skeletal
Rhabdomyolysis [4]

Gastrointestinal/Hepatic
Abdominal pain [3]
Diarrhea [4]
Nausea [4]

Otic
Tinnitus [3]

Local
Injection-site phlebitis (<10%) [2]

Other
Allergic reactions (<2%) [3]

ESCITALOPRAM

Trade name: Lexapro (Forest)
Indications: Major depressive disorders, anxiety
Class: Antidepressant, Selective serotonin reuptake inhibitor (SSRI)
Half-life: 27–32 hours
Clinically important, potentially hazardous interactions with: alcohol, bupropion, MAO inhibitors, methylphenidate, omeprazole, selegiline, St John's wort, sumatriptan, telaprevir, valerian
Pregnancy category: C
Important contra-indications noted in the prescribing guidelines for: the elderly; nursing mothers; pediatric patients
Warning: SUICIDALITY AND ANTIDEPRESSANT DRUGS

Skin
Diaphoresis (5%)
Hot flashes (<10%)
Rash (<10%)

Mucosal
Oral vesiculation (<19%)
Xerostomia (6%) [6]

Cardiovascular
QT prolongation [9]
Torsades de pointes [2]

Central Nervous System
Anxiety [2]
Headache (24%) [5]
Insomnia (9–12%) [5]
Paresthesias (<10%)
Restless legs syndrome [5]
Serotonin syndrome [5]
Somnolence (drowsiness) (6–13%) [7]
Tremor (<10%)
Vertigo (dizziness) (5%) [7]

Neuromuscular/Skeletal
Asthenia (fatigue) [4]
Myalgia/Myopathy (<10%)

Gastrointestinal/Hepatic
Abdominal pain [3]
Constipation [2]
Diarrhea [4]
Dyspepsia [2]
Nausea [11]
Vomiting [3]

Respiratory
Cough (<10%)
Flu-like syndrome (5%)

Endocrine/Metabolic
Galactorrhea [2]
Hyponatremia [4]
SIADH [7]
Weight gain [3]

Genitourinary
Ejaculatory dysfunction (9–14%)
Sexual dysfunction [5]

Otic
Tinnitus (<10%)

Ocular
Glaucoma [4]

Other
Adverse effects [3]
Allergic reactions (<10%)
Toothache (<10%)

ESLICARBAZEPINE

Trade names: Aptiom (Sunovion), Zebinix (Eisai)
Indications: Partial-onset seizures
Class: Antiepileptic
Half-life: 13–20 hours
Clinically important, potentially hazardous interactions with: carbamazepine, digoxin, lamotrigine, levetiracetam, MAO inhibitors, oral contraceptives, oxcarbazepine, phenytoin, topiramate, valproic acid, warfarin
Pregnancy category: C
Important contra-indications noted in the prescribing guidelines for: nursing mothers; pediatric patients

---

Skin
Peripheral edema (<2%)
Rash (<3%) [3]

Cardiovascular
Hypertension (<2%)

Central Nervous System
Balance disorder (3%)
Depression (<3%)
Dysarthria (<2%)
Gait instability (2%)
Headache (13–15%) [13]
Incoordination [3]
Insomnia (2%)
Somnolence (drowsiness) (11–18%) [20]
Tremor (2–4%)
Vertigo (dizziness) (20–28%) [25]

Neuromuscular/Skeletal
Asthenia (fatigue) (4–7%) [9]
Ataxia (4–6%)

Gastrointestinal/Hepatic
Constipation (2%)
Diarrhea (2–4%)
Nausea (10–16%) [12]
Vomiting (6–10%) [4]

Respiratory
Cough (<2%)
Nasopharyngitis [2]

Endocrine/Metabolic
Hyponatremia (2%) [5]

Genitourinary
Urinary tract infection (2%)

Ocular
Diplopia (9–11%) [8]
Nystagmus (<2%)
Vision blurred (5–6%) [3]
Vision impaired (<2%)

Other
Adverse effects [3]

ESMOLOL

Trade name: Brevibloc (Baxter)
Indications: Tachyarrhythmias, tachycardia
Class: Adrenergic beta-receptor antagonist, Antiarrhythmic class II
Half-life: 9 minutes
Clinically important, potentially hazardous interactions with: clonidine, verapamil
Pregnancy category: C
Important contra-indications noted in the prescribing guidelines for: nursing mothers; pediatric patients

---

Skin
Diaphoresis (>10%)

Cardiovascular
Bradycardia [5]
Hypotension [12]

Local
Injection-site pain (8%)
Injection-site reactions (<10%)

Other
Death [2]

ESOMEPRAZOLE

Trade name: Nexium (AstraZeneca)
Indications: Gastroesophageal reflux disease
Class: Proton pump inhibitor (PPI)
Half-life: 1.5 hours
Clinically important, potentially hazardous interactions with: benzodiazepines, chlordiazepoxide, cilostazol, clonazepam, clopidogrel, clorazepate, diazepam, digoxin, flurazepam, lorazepam, midazolam, oxazepam, posaconazole, quazepam, rifampin, rilpivirine, St John's wort, temazepam, tipranavir, voriconazole
Pregnancy category: C
Important contra-indications noted in the prescribing guidelines for: nursing mothers; pediatric patients

---

Skin
DRESS syndrome [2]

Fixed eruption [2]
Lupus erythematosus [3]

Central Nervous System
Dysgeusia (taste perversion) [3]
Fever [2]
Headache (8–11%) [6]
Somnolence (drowsiness) [2]
Vertigo (dizziness) [3]

Neuromuscular/Skeletal
Rhabdomyolysis [2]

Gastrointestinal/Hepatic
Abdominal pain [3]
Constipation [3]
Diarrhea [7]
Nausea [5]
Vomiting [4]

Respiratory
Bronchitis (4%)

Endocrine/Metabolic
Hypomagnesemia [2]

Other
Adverse effects [6]

ESTRADIOL

Trade names: Alora (Watson), Climara (Bayer), Divigel (Upsher-Smith), Elestrin (Azur Pharma), Esclim (Women First), Estrace (Bristol-Myers Squibb) (Warner Chilcott), Estraderm (Novartis), Estring (Pharmacia & Upjohn), Estrogel (Ascend), Evamist (KV Pharm), Fempatch (Pfizer), Gynodiol (Barr), Innofem (Novo Nordisk), Menostar (Bayer), Vagifem (Novo Nordisk), Vivelle (Novartis), Vivelle-Dot (Novartis)
Indications: Menopausal symptoms, hypoestrogenism due to hypogonadism, castration or primary ovarian failure, postmenopausal osteoporosis
Class: Estrogen, Hormone
Half-life: 1.75±2.87 hours
Clinically important, potentially hazardous interactions with: alcohol, amprenavir, anastrozole, ascorbic acid, atorvastatin, boceprevir, carbamazepine, chenodiol, clarithromycin, colesevelam, conivaptan, corticosteroids, CYP1A2 inducers, CYP3A4 inducers, deferasirox, delavirdine, erythromycin, folic acid, grapefruit juice, itraconazole, ketoconazole, lopinavir, minocycline, oxtriphylline, P-glycoprotein inhibitors or inducers, PEG-interferon, phenobarbital, rifampin, ritonavir, ropinirole, saxagliptin, somatropin, St John's wort, telaprevir, thyroid products, tipranavir, ursodiol
Pregnancy category: X
Important contra-indications noted in the prescribing guidelines for: the elderly; nursing mothers; pediatric patients
Note: See also separate entry for estrogens.
Warning: ENDOMETRIAL CANCER, CARDIOVASCULAR DISORDERS, BREAST CANCER and PROBABLE DEMENTIA

Central Nervous System
Headache [2]

Gastrointestinal/Hepatic
Nausea [3]

Respiratory
Nasopharyngitis (10%)
Upper respiratory tract infection (6%)

Endocrine/Metabolic
Mastodynia (7%)

Genitourinary
Metrorrhagia (4%)

Other
Adverse effects [3]

ESTRAMUSTINE

Trade name: Emcyt (Pfizer)
Indications: Prostate carcinoma
Class: Alkylating agent, Nitrosourea
Half-life: 20 hours
Clinically important, potentially hazardous interactions with: aldesleukin
Pregnancy category: X (not indicated for use in women)

Skin
Angioedema [2]
Edema (>10%) [4]
Peripheral edema [2]
Pruritus (2%) [2]
Purpura (3%)
Xerosis (2%)

Cardiovascular
Thrombophlebitis (3%)

Neuromuscular/Skeletal
Asthenia (fatigue) [3]

Gastrointestinal/Hepatic
Diarrhea [3]
Nausea [3]

Endocrine/Metabolic
Gynecomastia (>10%) [5]
Mastodynia (66%)

Hematologic
Anemia [3]
Febrile neutropenia [2]
Leukopenia [2]
Neutropenia [5]

Local
Injection-site thrombophlebitis (<10%) [3]

Other
Allergic reactions [2]
Death [2]

ESZOPICLONE

Trade names: Imovane (Sanofi-Aventis), Lunesta (Sunovion), Zimovane (Sanofi-Aventis)
Indications: Insomnia
Class: Hypnotic, non-benzodiazepine
Half-life: 6 hours
Clinically important, potentially hazardous interactions with: alcohol, antifungals, cimetidine, CNS depressants, conivaptan, CYP3A4 inhibitors and inducers, dasatinib, deferasirox, droperidol, erythromycin, ethanol, flumazenil, ketoconazole, levomepromazine, lorazepam, nefazodone, nelfinavir, olanzapine, rifampin, ritonavir, St John's wort, telithromycin, tricyclic antidepressants, valerian, voriconazole
Pregnancy category: C
Important contra-indications noted in the prescribing guidelines for: the elderly; nursing mothers; pediatric patients

---

Skin
Pruritus (<4%)
Rash (<5%)

Mucosal
Xerostomia (3–7%) [5]

Central Nervous System
Abnormal dreams (<3%)
Amnesia [3]
Anxiety (<3%)
Confusion (<3%)
Depression (<4%)
Dysgeusia (taste perversion) (8–34%) [21]
Hallucinations (<3%)
Headache (13–21%) [8]
Nervousness (<5%)
Neurotoxicity (<3%)
Pain (4–5%)
Somnolence (drowsiness) (8–10%) [2]
Vertigo (dizziness) [3]

Gastrointestinal/Hepatic
Diarrhea (2–4%)
Dyspepsia (2–6%)
Nausea (4–5%) [2]
Vomiting (<3%)

Endocrine/Metabolic
Gynecomastia (<3%)
Libido decreased (<3%)

Genitourinary
Dysmenorrhea (<3%)
Urinary tract infection (<3%)

Other
Adverse effects [4]
Infection (3–10%)

ETANERCEPT

Trade names: Enbrel (Amgen), Erelzi (Sandoz)
Indications: Rheumatoid arthritis, polyarticular juvenile idiopathic arthritis in patients aged 2 years or older, psoriatic arthritis, ankylosing spondylitis, plaque psoriasis
Class: Cytokine inhibitor, Disease-modifying antirheumatic drug (DMARD), TNF inhibitor
Half-life: 4–13 days
Clinically important, potentially hazardous interactions with: abatacept, anakinra, cyclophosphamide, live vaccines
Pregnancy category: B
Important contra-indications noted in the prescribing guidelines for: the elderly; nursing mothers; pediatric patients
Note: TNF inhibitors should be used in patients with heart failure only after consideration of other treatment options. Contra-indicated in patients with sepsis. TNF inhibitors are contra-indicated in patients with a personal or family history of multiple sclerosis or demyelinating disease. TNF inhibitors should not be administered to patients with moderate to severe heart failure (New York Heart Association Functional Class III/IV).

Warning: SERIOUS INFECTIONS AND MALIGNANCIES

Skin
- Abscess [2]
- Anaphylactoid reactions/Anaphylaxis [2]
- Carcinoma [2]
- Cellulitis [2]
- Dermatitis [3]
- Dermatomyositis [4]
- Exanthems [2]
- Granulomas [2]
- Granulomatous reaction [5]
- Henoch-Schönlein purpura [3]
- Herpes zoster [6]
- Hidradenitis [2]
- Leprosy [2]
- Lichen planus [2]
- Lichenoid eruption [3]
- Lupus erythematosus [25]
- Lupus syndrome [4]
- Lymphoma [3]
- Malignancies (<3%) [4]
- Melanoma [2]
- Neoplasms [2]
- Nodular eruption [3]
- Pruritus (2–5%) [2]
- Psoriasis [20]
- Pustules [2]
- Rash (3–13%) [8]
- Sarcoidosis [10]
- Squamous cell carcinoma [4]
- Urticaria (2%) [2]
- Vasculitis [23]

Hair
- Alopecia [5]

Cardiovascular
- Atrial fibrillation [2]
- Cardiotoxicity [2]
- Hypertension [2]

Central Nervous System
- Demyelination [2]
- Fever (2–3%) [2]
- Headache [19]
- Leukoencephalopathy [3]
- Multiple sclerosis [2]
- Neurotoxicity [4]
- Paresthesias [2]
- Peripheral neuropathy [2]
- Vertigo (dizziness) [2]

Neuromuscular/Skeletal
- Arthralgia [2]
- Asthenia (fatigue) [7]
- Back pain [2]
- Myalgia/Myopathy [2]
- Myasthenia gravis [3]

Gastrointestinal/Hepatic
- Abdominal pain [3]
- Colitis [2]
- Crohn's disease [5]
- Diarrhea (8–16%) [5]
- Gastroenteritis [3]
- Hepatotoxicity [5]
- Inflammatory bowel disease [2]
- Nausea [5]

Respiratory
- Asthma [2]
- Bronchitis [5]
- Cough [4]
- Flu-like syndrome [3]
- Laryngitis [2]
- Nasopharyngitis [6]
- Pharyngitis [5]
- Pneumonia [6]
- Pneumonitis [2]
- Pulmonary toxicity [4]
- Rhinitis [4]
- Sinusitis [5]
- Tuberculosis [2]
- Upper respiratory tract infection (38–65%) [13]

Endocrine/Metabolic
- ALT increased [3]
- Hypertriglyceridemia [2]
- Thyroiditis [3]

Genitourinary
- Cystitis [2]
- Urinary tract infection [2]

Renal
- Nephrotoxicity [2]

Hematologic
- Leukopenia [2]
- Macrophage activation syndrome [2]
- Neutropenia [3]
- Pancytopenia [2]
- Thrombocytopenia [2]

Otic
- Otitis media [2]

Ocular
- Uveitis [13]

Local
- Injection-site reactions (37–43%) [62]

Other
- Adverse effects [37]
- Allergic reactions (<3%)
- Death [7]
- Infection (50–81%) [44]

ETELCALCETIDE

Trade name: Parsabiv (Amgen)
Indications: Secondary hyperparathyroidism in adult patients with chronic kidney disease on hemodialysis
Class: Calcimimetic
Half-life: 3–4 days
Clinically important, potentially hazardous interactions with: none known
Pregnancy category: N/A (No data available)
Important contra-indications noted in the prescribing guidelines for: nursing mothers; pediatric patients

Skin
- Facial edema (<4%)
- Hypersensitivity (4%)
- Pruritus (<4%)
- Urticaria (<4%)

Cardiovascular
- Cardiac failure (2%)
- Hypotension [2]

Central Nervous System
- Headache (8%)
- Paresthesias (6%) [2]

Neuromuscular/Skeletal
- Muscle spasm (12%) [2]
- Myalgia/Myopathy (2%)

Gastrointestinal/Hepatic
- Diarrhea (11%) [2]
- Nausea (11%) [5]
- Vomiting (9%) [6]

Endocrine/Metabolic
- Hyperkalemia (4%)
- Hypocalcemia (7–64%) [7]

ETHAMBUTOL

Trade name: Myambutol (Stat Trade)
Indications: Tuberculosis
Class: Antimycobacterial
Half-life: 3–4 hours
Clinically important, potentially hazardous interactions with: cortisone, zinc
Pregnancy category: C
Important contra-indications noted in the prescribing guidelines for: nursing mothers; pediatric patients

Skin
- Bullous dermatitis [2]
- Dermatitis [2]
- DRESS syndrome [5]
- Erythema multiforme [2]
- Exanthems (<5%) [4]
- Hypersensitivity [3]
- Lichenoid eruption [2]
- Lupus erythematosus [2]
- Pruritus [4]
- Rash [2]
- Toxic epidermal necrolysis [2]
- Urticaria [2]

Central Nervous System
- Peripheral neuropathy [2]

Renal
- Nephrotoxicity [2]

Ocular
- Amblyopia [2]
- Ocular toxicity [9]
- Optic neuritis [5]
- Optic neuropathy [9]
- Vision impaired [2]

Other
- Adverse effects [4]

ETHOSUXIMIDE

Trade name: Zarontin (Pfizer)
Indications: Absence (petit mal) seizures
Class: Antiepileptic, succinimide
Half-life: 50–60 hours
Clinically important, potentially hazardous interactions with: antipsychotics, carbamazepine, chloroquine, cobicistat/elvitegravir/emtricitabine/tenofovir alafenamide, cobicistat/elvitegravir/emtricitabine/tenofovir disoproxil, hydroxychloroquine, isoniazid, levomepromazine, lisdexamfetamine, MAO inhibitors, mefloquine, nevirapine, orlistat, phenobarbital, phenytoin, primidone, risperidone,

SSRIs, St John's wort, tricyclic antidepressants, valproic acid, zuclopenthixol
Pregnancy category: C
Important contra-indications noted in the prescribing guidelines for: nursing mothers
Note: Cases of birth defects have been reported with ethosuximide.

Skin
Exanthems (<5%) [2]
Lupus erythematosus (>10%) [22]
Raynaud's phenomenon [3]
Stevens-Johnson syndrome (>10%)
Urticaria (<5%)

Hematologic
Agranulocytosis [2]

Other
Side effects (3%)

ETIDRONATE

Trade name: Didronel (Procter & Gamble)
Indications: Paget's disease, osteoporosis
Class: Bisphosphonate
Half-life: 6 hours
Clinically important, potentially hazardous interactions with: ferrous sulfate
Pregnancy category: C
Important contra-indications noted in the prescribing guidelines for: nursing mothers; pediatric patients

---

Neuromuscular/Skeletal
Fractures [6]
Osteomalacia [3]
Pseudogout [2]
Skeletal toxicity [2]

Gastrointestinal/Hepatic
Esophagitis [2]

ETODOLAC

Trade name: Lodine (Wyeth)
Indications: Pain
Class: COX-2 inhibitor, Non-steroidal anti-inflammatory (NSAID)
Half-life: 7 hours
Clinically important, potentially hazardous interactions with: aspirin, methotrexate
Pregnancy category: C
Important contra-indications noted in the prescribing guidelines for: the elderly; nursing mothers; pediatric patients
Note: NSAIDs may cause an increased risk of serious cardiovascular and gastrointestinal adverse events, which can be fatal. This risk may increase with duration of use.

Skin
Exanthems [2]
Facial edema [2]
Fixed eruption [2]
Pruritus (<10%) [7]
Rash (>10%) [5]
Vasculitis [2]

Gastrointestinal/Hepatic
Abdominal pain [3]
Constipation [2]
Dyspepsia [4]
Nausea [3]

Other
Adverse effects [2]

ETOPOSIDE

Trade name: VePesid (Bristol-Myers Squibb)
Indications: Lymphomas, carcinomas
Class: Topoisomerase 2 inhibitor
Half-life: 4–11 hours
Clinically important, potentially hazardous interactions with: aldesleukin, atovaquone, atovaquone/proguanil, cyclosporine, gadobenate, prednisolone, St John's wort
Pregnancy category: D
Important contra-indications noted in the prescribing guidelines for: the elderly; nursing mothers; pediatric patients

---

Skin
Anaphylactoid reactions/Anaphylaxis (<2%) [3]
Erythema [3]
Exanthems [4]
Flushing [3]
Hand–foot syndrome [4]
Hypersensitivity [9]
Pigmentation [2]
Radiation recall dermatitis [3]
Rash [2]
Stevens-Johnson syndrome [3]
Toxicity [2]

Hair
Alopecia (8–66%) [10]

Mucosal
Mucositis (>10%)
Oral lesions (<5%) [2]
Stomatitis (<10%) [2]

Central Nervous System
Anorexia [3]
Leukoencephalopathy [2]
Neurotoxicity [3]

Neuromuscular/Skeletal
Asthenia (fatigue) [3]

Gastrointestinal/Hepatic
Diarrhea [3]
Hepatotoxicity [3]
Nausea [7]
Vomiting [8]

Respiratory
Pulmonary toxicity [2]

Endocrine/Metabolic
Hyponatremia [2]

Renal
Nephrotoxicity [4]

Hematologic
Anemia [8]
Febrile neutropenia [7]
Leukopenia [4]
Myeloid leukemia [2]
Neutropenia [13]
Thrombocytopenia [11]

Other
Adverse effects [3]
Allergic reactions (<2%)
Death [3]
Infection [5]

ETRAVIRINE

Trade name: Intelence (Tibotec)
Indications: HIV infection
Class: Non-nucleoside reverse transcriptase inhibitor
Half-life: 41 hours
Clinically important, potentially hazardous interactions with: atazanavir, atorvastatin, carbamazepine, clarithromycin, clopidogrel, darunavir, delavirdine, digoxin, efavirenz, fosamprenavir, indinavir, maraviroc, nelfinavir, neratinib, nevirapine, non-nucleoside reverse transcriptase inhibitors, olaparib, palbociclib, phenobarbital, phenytoin, rifabutin, rifampin, rifapentine, rilpivirine, ritonavir, sildenafil, simeprevir, St John's wort, tadalafil, telithromycin, tipranavir, vardenafil, venetoclax, voriconazole
Pregnancy category: B
Important contra-indications noted in the prescribing guidelines for: nursing mothers; pediatric patients

---

Skin
Facial edema (<2%)
Hyperhidrosis (<2%)
Lipohypertrophy (<2%)
Prurigo (<2%)
Rash (9%) [17]
Xerosis (<2%)

Mucosal
Stomatitis (<2%)
Xerostomia (<2%)

Cardiovascular
Angina (<2%)
Atrial fibrillation (<2%)
Hypertension (3%)
Myocardial infarction (<2%)

Central Nervous System
Abnormal dreams (<2%)
Amnesia (<2%)
Anorexia (<2%)
Anxiety (<2%)
Confusion (<2%)
Disorientation (<2%)
Headache (3%) [3]
Hypersomnia (<2%)
Hypoesthesia (<2%)
Insomnia (<2%)
Nervousness (<2%)
Neurotoxicity [3]
Nightmares (<2%)
Paresthesias (<2%)
Peripheral neuropathy (3%)
Seizures (<2%)
Sleep related disorder (<2%)
Somnolence (drowsiness) (<2%)
Syncope (<2%)
Tremor (<2%)
Vertigo (dizziness) (<2%)

Neuromuscular/Skeletal
Asthenia (fatigue) (3%)

Gastrointestinal/Hepatic
- Abdominal distension (<2%)
- Abdominal pain (3%)
- Constipation (<2%)
- Diarrhea [3]
- Flatulence (<2%)
- Gastritis (<2%)
- Gastroesophageal reflux (<2%)
- Hematemesis (<2%)
- Hepatic failure (<2%)
- Hepatomegaly (<2%)
- Hepatotoxicity [2]
- Nausea [4]
- Pancreatitis (<2%)
- Retching (<2%)

Respiratory
- Bronchospasm (<2%)
- Dyspnea (<2%)

Endocrine/Metabolic
- Diabetes mellitus (<2%)
- Gynecomastia (<2%)

Renal
- Renal failure (<2%)

Hematologic
- Dyslipidemia (<2%)
- Hemolytic anemia (<2%)

Ocular
- Vision blurred (<2%)

Other
- Adverse effects [6]

EUCALYPTUS

Family: Myrtacceae
Scientific names: *Eucalyptus bicostata, Eucalyptus fruticetorum, Eucalyptus globulus, Eucalyptus odorata, Eucalyptus pauciflora, Eucalyptus polybractea, Eucalyptus smithii*
Indications: Asthma, bronchitis, cough, croup, fever, joint and muscle pains, nasal congestion, sore throats, rheumatism. Flavoring, fragrance, toothpaste, substances used in root canal fillings
Class: Anti-inflammatory, Diuretic
Half-life: N/A
Clinically important, potentially hazardous interactions with: aminophylline, amitriptyline, borage, carisoprodol, coltsfoot, comfrey, diazepam, insulin, lansoprazole, nelfinavir, pantoprazole
Pregnancy category: N/A
Note: [O] = Oral.

EVENING PRIMROSE

Family: Onagraceae
Scientific names: *Oenothera biennis, Oenothera muricata, Oenothera purpurata, Oenothera rubricaulis, Oenothera suaveolens*
Indications: Mastalgia, osteoporosis, atopic dermatitis, rheumatoid arthritis, hypercholesterolemia, chronic fatigue syndrome, neurodermatitis, ulcerative colitis, irritable bowel syndrome. Used in soaps and cosmetics
Class: Anti-inflammatory, Gamma linoleic acid
Half-life: N/A
Clinically important, potentially hazardous interactions with: aspirin, chlorpromazine, fluphenazine, phenothiazine
Pregnancy category: N/A
Note: The Medicines Control Agency (MCA) has withdrawn licenses for prescription evening primrose drug products under the brand names of Epogam and Efamast. This was because there is not enough evidence that they are effective.

Other
- Adverse effects [3]

EVEROLIMUS

Trade names: Afinitor (Novartis), Certican (Novartis), Zortress (Novartis)
Indications: Prophylaxis of organ rejection in adults following kidney or liver transplant, advanced renal cell carcinoma, neuroendocrine tumors of pancreatic, gastrointestinal or lung origin, breast cancer in post-menopausal women with advanced hormone-receptor positive, HER2-negative type cancer, renal angiomyolipoma and tuberous sclerosis complex, subependymal giant cell astrocytoma associated with tuberous sclerosis
Class: Antineoplastic, Immunosuppressant, mTOR inhibitor
Half-life: ~30 hours
Clinically important, potentially hazardous interactions with: aprepitant, atazanavir, atorvastatin, benazepril, captopril, clarithromycin, clozapine, conivaptan, cyclosporine, darunavir, delavirdine, digoxin, efavirenz, enalapril, erythromycin, grapefruit juice, indinavir, itraconazole, ketoconazole, lapatinib, lisinopril, live vaccines, nelfinavir, oxcarbazepine, phenytoin, posaconazole, quinapril, ramipril, ribociclib, rifampin, rifapentine, ritonavir, saquinavir, St John's wort, telithromycin, venetoclax, verapamil, voriconazole
Pregnancy category: D
Important contra-indications noted in the prescribing guidelines for: nursing mothers; pediatric patients
Warning: In immunosuppression therapy: MALIGNANCIES AND SERIOUS INFECTIONS, KIDNEY GRAFT THROMBOSIS; NEPHROTOXICITY
In heart transplantation: MORTALITY

Skin
- Acneform eruption (3–25%) [5]
- Angioedema [4]
- Cellulitis (21%)
- Contact dermatitis (14%)
- Dermatitis [2]
- Edema (39%) [5]
- Erythema (4%)
- Exanthems [3]
- Excoriations (14%)
- Hand–foot syndrome (5%) [9]
- Hypersensitivity [2]
- Lymphedema [2]
- Peripheral edema (4–39%) [8]
- Pityriasis rosea (4%)
- Pruritus (14–21%) [5]
- Rash (18–59%) [50]
- Tinea (18%)
- Toxicity [9]
- Xerosis (13–18%)

Nails
- Nail disorder (4–22%) [2]

Mucosal
- Aphthous stomatitis [4]
- Epistaxis (nosebleed) (18–22%) [3]
- Mucosal inflammation (19%) [3]
- Mucositis [18]
- Nasal congestion (14%)
- Oral ulceration [4]
- Oropharyngeal pain (11%)
- Rhinorrhea (3%)
- Stomatitis (44–86%) [82]
- Xerostomia (8–11%)

Cardiovascular
- Chest pain (5%)
- Hypertension (4–13%) [14]
- Tachycardia (3%)

Central Nervous System
- Anorexia (25%) [12]
- Anxiety (7%)
- Chills (4%)
- Dysgeusia (taste perversion) (10–19%) [2]
- Fever (20–32%) [7]
- Headache (18–30%) [4]
- Insomnia (9%)
- Migraine (30%)
- Pain [2]
- Peripheral neuropathy [2]
- Seizures (29%)
- Somnolence (drowsiness) (7%)
- Vertigo (dizziness) (7–14%)

Neuromuscular/Skeletal
- Arthralgia (15%)
- Asthenia (fatigue) (7–45%) [63]
- Back pain (15%)
- Jaw pain (3%)
- Muscle spasm (10%)
- Pain in extremities (10–14%)

Gastrointestinal/Hepatic
- Abdominal pain (9–36%) [4]
- Constipation (11–14%)
- Diarrhea (25–50%) [36]
- Dysphagia (4%)
- Gastritis (7%)
- Gastroenteritis (18%)
- Gastrointestinal bleeding [3]
- Hemorrhoids (5%)
- Hepatotoxicity [8]
- Nausea (26–32%) [11]
- Pancreatitis [2]
- Vomiting (20–29%) [3]

Respiratory
- Cough (21–30%) [6]
- Dyspnea (20–24%) [8]
- Nasopharyngitis (25%)
- Pharyngitis (11%)
- Pharyngolaryngeal pain (4%)
- Pleural effusion (7%)
- Pneumonia [11]
- Pneumonitis (14–17%) [43]
- Pulmonary toxicity [11]
- Rhinitis (25%)
- Sinusitis (39%)
- Upper respiratory tract infection (25–82%) [2]

Endocrine/Metabolic
- ALT increased (21–48%) [4]
- Amenorrhea [2]
- Appetite decreased (30%) [5]
- AST increased (25–56%) [3]
- Diabetes mellitus (2–10%) [2]
- GGT increased [2]
- Hypercholesterolemia [7]
- Hyperglycemia [39]
- Hyperlipidemia [8]
- Hypertriglyceridemia [3]
- Hypokalemia [4]
- Hypomagnesemia [2]
- Hyponatremia [3]
- Hypophosphatemia [5]
- Hypothyroidism [2]
- Serum creatinine increased (19–50%) [4]
- Weight loss (9–28%) [3]

Genitourinary
- Urinary tract infection (15%)

Renal
- Nephrotoxicity [5]
- Proteinuria (7%) [16]
- Renal failure (3%) [3]

Hematologic
- Anemia [39]
- Cytopenia [2]
- Dyslipidemia [2]
- Febrile neutropenia [5]
- Hemoglobin decreased (86–92%) [2]
- Hemolytic uremic syndrome [2]
- Hemorrhage (3%) [3]
- Hemotoxicity [5]
- Immunosupression [2]
- Leukopenia [4]
- Lymphopenia [8]
- Neutropenia [18]
- Platelets decreased (23–45%)
- Sepsis [2]
- Thrombocytopenia [21]

Otic
- Otitis media (36%)

Ocular
- Conjunctivitis (2%)
- Eyelid edema (4%) [2]
- Ocular hyperemia (4%)

Other
- Adverse effects [31]
- Death [10]
- Infection (18%) [32]
- Side effects [2]

EVOLOCUMAB

Trade name: Repatha (Amgen)
Indications: Heterozygous or homozygous familial hypercholesterolemia where additional lowering of low density lipoprotein cholesterol is required
Class: Monoclonal antibody, Proprotein convertase subtilisin kexin type 9 (PCSK9) inhibitor
Half-life: 11–17 days
Clinically important, potentially hazardous interactions with: none known
Pregnancy category: N/A (No data available but likely to cross the placenta in second and third trimester)
Important contra-indications noted in the prescribing guidelines for: pediatric patients

Mucosal
- Nasal congestion [2]
- Oropharyngeal pain [2]

Cardiovascular
- Hypertension (2%)

Central Nervous System
- Headache (4%) [11]
- Neurotoxicity [2]
- Vertigo (dizziness) (3%)

Neuromuscular/Skeletal
- Arthralgia (2%) [9]
- Asthenia (fatigue) [3]
- Back pain (2–6%) [10]
- Bone or joint pain (3%) [4]
- Muscle spasm [7]
- Myalgia/Myopathy (3%) [11]
- Pain in extremities [5]

Gastrointestinal/Hepatic
- Diarrhea (3%) [5]
- Gastroenteritis (2%) [2]
- Hepatotoxicity [5]
- Nausea [4]

Respiratory
- Cough (<4%) [3]
- Influenza (<6%) [10]
- Nasopharyngitis (4–10%) [14]
- Pharyngitis [2]
- Sinusitis (3%) [2]
- Upper respiratory tract infection (2–6%) [11]

Endocrine/Metabolic
- Creatine phosphokinase increased [9]

Genitourinary
- Urinary tract infection (<4%)

Local
- Injection-site bruising [4]
- Injection-site edema [2]
- Injection-site erythema [3]
- Injection-site pain [7]
- Injection-site reactions (3–5%) [10]

Other
- Adverse effects [6]
- Allergic reactions (5%)

EXEMESTANE

Trade name: Aromasin (Pfizer)
Indications: Advanced breast cancer
Class: Aromatase inhibitor
Half-life: 24 hours
Clinically important, potentially hazardous interactions with: efavirenz, oxcarbazepine, rifapentine
Pregnancy category: X
Important contra-indications noted in the prescribing guidelines for: nursing mothers; pediatric patients

Skin
- Diaphoresis (6–12%) [2]
- Edema (7%)
- Hot flashes (30%) [7]
- Lymphedema (2–5%)
- Peripheral edema (9%) [2]
- Pruritus (2–5%)
- Radiation recall dermatitis [2]
- Rash (2–5%) [6]

Hair
- Alopecia (2–5%)

Mucosal
- Stomatitis [10]

Central Nervous System
- Dysgeusia (taste perversion) [2]
- Headache [3]
- Insomnia [2]
- Paresthesias (2–5%)
- Tumor pain (30%)

Neuromuscular/Skeletal
- Arthralgia [4]
- Asthenia (fatigue) [7]
- Back pain [2]
- Bone or joint pain [2]
- Myalgia/Myopathy [2]

Gastrointestinal/Hepatic
- Diarrhea [4]

Respiratory
- Dyspnea [2]
- Pneumonitis [6]
- Pulmonary toxicity [2]

Endocrine/Metabolic
- Hyperglycemia [5]

Hematologic
- Anemia [3]

Other
- Adverse effects [2]

EXENATIDE

Trade names: Bydureon (Amylin), Byetta (Amylin)
Indications: Type II diabetes mellitus
Class: Glucagon-like peptide-1 (GLP-1) receptor agonist, Incretin mimetic, Insulin secretagogue
Half-life: 2.4 hours
Clinically important, potentially hazardous interactions with: acetaminophen, alcohol, antibiotics, corticosteroids, lovastatin, oral contraceptives, pegvisomant, prandial insulin,

somatropin, sulfonylureas, thiazide diuretics, vitamin K antagonists, warfarin
Pregnancy category: C
Important contra-indications noted in the prescribing guidelines for: nursing mothers; pediatric patients
Note: Risk of thyroid C-cell tumors with exenatide extended release formulations. Bydureon is contra-indicated in patients with a personal or family history of medullary thyroid carcinoma or in patients with multiple endocrine neoplasia syndrome Type 2.

Skin
Hyperhidrosis (<10%)
Urticaria [2]

Cardiovascular
Cardiotoxicity [2]

Central Nervous System
Chills (<2%)
Headache (<10%) [9]
Vertigo (dizziness) (<10%) [4]

Neuromuscular/Skeletal
Asthenia (fatigue) (<10%)

Gastrointestinal/Hepatic
Abdominal distension (<10%)
Abdominal pain (<10%) [2]
Constipation (>5%) [2]
Diarrhea (<11%) [19]
Dyspepsia (<10%)
Flatulence (2%)
Gastroenteritis (<10%)
Gastroesophageal reflux (3%)
Nausea (<11%) [44]
Pancreatitis [10]
Vomiting (~10%) [26]

Respiratory
Nasopharyngitis [2]

Endocrine/Metabolic
Appetite decreased (<10%) [3]
Hypoglycemia (>5%) [5]

Genitourinary
Urinary tract infection [2]

Renal
Nephrotoxicity [2]
Renal failure [3]

Local
Injection-site erythema (5–7%)
Injection-site nodules (~10%) [4]
Injection-site pruritus (5–6%) [2]
Injection-site reactions [7]

Other
Adverse effects [10]
Cancer [2]

EZETIMIBE

Trade names: Ezetrol (Merck), Liptruzet (Merck Sharpe & Dohme), Vytorin (MSD), Zetia (Merck)
Indications: Hypercholesterolemia
Class: Cholesterol inhibitor
Half-life: 22 hours
Clinically important, potentially hazardous interactions with: cholestyramine, cyclosporine, fenofibrate, gemfibrozil, HMG-CoA reductase inhibitors, ritonavir
Pregnancy category: C (Pregnancy category is X when combined with a statin.)
Important contra-indications noted in the prescribing guidelines for: nursing mothers
Note: Liptruzet is ezetimibe and atorvastatin; vytorin is ezetimibe and simvastatin.

Skin
Rash [3]

Central Nervous System
Headache [5]
Vertigo (dizziness) [4]

Neuromuscular/Skeletal
Arthralgia (4%) [3]
Asthenia (fatigue) [2]
Back pain (4%) [4]
Bone or joint pain [4]
Muscle spasm [3]
Myalgia/Myopathy (5%) [16]
Pain in extremities [2]

Gastrointestinal/Hepatic
Abdominal pain (2%)
Diarrhea [4]
Hepatotoxicity [6]
Nausea [4]
Pancreatitis [3]

Respiratory
Cough (2%)
Influenza [3]
Nasopharyngitis [5]
Upper respiratory tract infection [2]

Endocrine/Metabolic
Creatine phosphokinase increased [8]

Genitourinary
Urinary tract infection [2]

Hematologic
Thrombocytopenia [2]

Local
Injection-site erythema [2]
Injection-site reactions [5]

Other
Adverse effects [6]

EZOGABINE

Synonym: retigabine
Trade names: Potiga (GSK), Trobalt (GSK)
Indications: Epilepsy
Class: Anticonvulsant, Potassium channel opener
Half-life: 7–11 hours
Clinically important, potentially hazardous interactions with: alcohol, carbamazepine, digoxin, phenytoin
Pregnancy category: C
Important contra-indications noted in the prescribing guidelines for: the elderly; nursing mothers; pediatric patients
Warning: RETINAL ABNORMALITIES AND POTENTIAL VISION LOSS

Skin
Hyperhidrosis (<2%)
Peripheral edema (<2%)
Pigmentation [2]

Mucosal
Mucosal membrane pigmentation [4]
Xerostomia (<2%)

Central Nervous System
Amnesia (2%)
Anxiety (3%)
Aphasia (4%)
Balance disorder (4%)
Confusion (9%) [6]
Disorientation (2%)
Dysarthria (4%) [3]
Dysphasia (2%)
Gait instability (4%)
Hallucinations (<2%)
Headache [6]
Hypokinesia (<2%)
Impaired concentration (6%)
Incoordination (7%)
Memory loss (6%)
Neurotoxicity [3]
Paresthesias (3%)
Somnolence (drowsiness) (22%) [14]
Speech disorder [3]
Tremor (8%) [3]
Vertigo (dizziness) (31%) [14]

Neuromuscular/Skeletal
Asthenia (fatigue) (20%) [11]
Ataxia [3]
Myoclonus (<2%)

Gastrointestinal/Hepatic
Constipation (3%)
Dyspepsia (2%)
Dysphagia (<2%)
Nausea (7%) [5]

Respiratory
Influenza (3%)

Endocrine/Metabolic
Appetite increased (<2%)
Weight gain (dose related) (3%)

Genitourinary
Dysuria (2%)
Hematuria (2%)
Urinary hesitancy (2%)
Urinary retention (<2%) [6]
Urinary tract infection [3]

Renal
Chromaturia (2%)

Ocular
Diplopia (7%) [2]
Ocular pigmentation [4]
Vision blurred (5%) [2]

Other
Adverse effects [2]

FAMCICLOVIR

Trade name: Famvir (Novartis)
Indications: Acute herpes zoster, recurrent genital herpes
Class: Antiviral, Guanine nucleoside analog
Half-life: 2–3 hours
Clinically important, potentially hazardous interactions with: none known

Pregnancy category: B
Important contra-indications noted in the prescribing guidelines for: nursing mothers; pediatric patients

Skin
Pruritus (4%)
Rash (<4%)
Vasculitis [3]

Central Nervous System
Headache (9–39%) [5]
Paresthesias (<3%)

Neuromuscular/Skeletal
Asthenia (fatigue) (<5%)

Gastrointestinal/Hepatic
Abdominal pain (<8%) [2]
Diarrhea (2–9%)
Flatulence (<5%)
Nausea (2–13%) [3]
Vomiting (<5%) [2]

Genitourinary
Dysmenorrhea (<8%)

Other
Adverse effects [4]

FAMOTIDINE

Trade names: Duexis (Horizon), Pepcid (Valeant)
Indications: Duodenal ulcer, gastric ulcer, gastroesophageal reflux disease
Class: Histamine H2 receptor antagonist
Half-life: 2.5–3.5 hours
Clinically important, potentially hazardous interactions with: acalabrutinib, atazanavir, cefditoren, dasatinib, delavirdine, rilpivirine, thalidomide
Pregnancy category: B
Important contra-indications noted in the prescribing guidelines for: nursing mothers
Note: Duexis is famotidine and ibuprofen.

Skin
Dermatitis [3]
Peripheral edema [2]
Pruritus [2]
Rash [3]
Urticaria [3]
Vasculitis [2]

Cardiovascular
Hypertension [3]

Central Nervous System
Confusion [2]
Delirium [3]
Fever [2]
Headache (5%) [4]
Neurotoxicity [2]
Somnolence (drowsiness) [2]

Neuromuscular/Skeletal
Arthralgia [2]
Back pain [2]

Gastrointestinal/Hepatic
Abdominal pain [2]
Diarrhea (2%) [3]
Dyspepsia [3]
Gastroesophageal reflux [2]
Nausea [4]
Vomiting [4]

Respiratory
Influenza [2]
Sinusitis [2]
Upper respiratory tract infection [2]

Endocrine/Metabolic
Hypomagnesemia [2]
Hypophosphatemia [2]

Genitourinary
Urinary tract infection [2]

Hematologic
Eosinophilia [2]
Thrombocytopenia [2]

FEBUXOSTAT

Trade name: Uloric (Takeda)
Indications: Hyperuricemia in gout
Class: Xanthine oxidase inhibitor
Half-life: 5–8 hours
Clinically important, potentially hazardous interactions with: aminophylline, azathioprine, didanosine, mercaptopurine, oxtriphylline, theophylline
Pregnancy category: C

Skin
Rash (2%) [7]

Cardiovascular
Cardiotoxicity [2]

Central Nervous System
Headache [5]
Vertigo (dizziness) [5]

Neuromuscular/Skeletal
Arthralgia [5]
Bone or joint pain [2]
Gouty tophi (flare) [3]
Joint disorder [2]

Gastrointestinal/Hepatic
Diarrhea [9]
Hepatotoxicity (5%) [13]
Nausea [7]
Vomiting [2]

Respiratory
Upper respiratory tract infection [2]

Other
Adverse effects [7]

FENOFIBRATE

Trade name: Tricor (AbbVie)
Indications: Hyperlipidemia
Class: Fibrate, Lipid regulator
Half-life: 20 hours
Clinically important, potentially hazardous interactions with: atorvastatin, colchicine, dicumarol, ezetimibe, lovastatin, nicotinic acid, rosuvastatin, statins, warfarin
Pregnancy category: C
Important contra-indications noted in the prescribing guidelines for: the elderly; nursing mothers; pediatric patients

Skin
Photosensitivity [11]
Phototoxicity [2]
Pruritus (4%)
Rash (2–8%) [3]

Neuromuscular/Skeletal
Myalgia/Myopathy [11]
Rhabdomyolysis [18]

Gastrointestinal/Hepatic
Hepatotoxicity [15]
Pancreatitis [3]

Endocrine/Metabolic
Gynecomastia [2]

Renal
Nephrotoxicity [3]
Renal failure [2]

Other
Adverse effects (<10%)

FENTANYL

Trade names: Actiq (Cephalon), Duragesic (Janssen)
Indications: Chronic pain
Class: Analgesic, opioid, Anesthetic
Half-life: ~7 hours
Clinically important, potentially hazardous interactions with: amiodarone, amprenavir, aprepitant, atazanavir, ceritinib, cimetidine, conivaptan, crizotinib, darunavir, dasatinib, delavirdine, efavirenz, eluxadoline, enzalutamide, indinavir, itraconazole, ketoconazole, lapatinib, letermovir, lopinavir, mifepristone, nelfinavir, nevirapine, nifedipine, osimertinib, ranitidine, ribociclib, rifapentine, ritonavir, saquinavir, telithromycin, voriconazole
Pregnancy category: C
Important contra-indications noted in the prescribing guidelines for: nursing mothers; pediatric patients
Note: Contra-indicated in opioid non-tolerant patients, and for the management of acute or postoperative pain including headache/migraines and dental pain.
Warning: ADDICTION, ABUSE, and MISUSE; LIFE-THREATENING RESPIRATORY DEPRESSION; ACCIDENTAL EXPOSURE; NEONATAL OPIOID WITHDRAWAL SYNDROME; CYTOCHROME P450 3A4 INTERACTION
EXPOSURE TO HEAT (for topical patches)

Skin
Anaphylactoid reactions/Anaphylaxis [6]
Diaphoresis (>10%) [2]
Edema (>10%)
Erythema (at application site) [3]
Flushing (3–10%)
Pruritus (3–44%) [30]
Rash [3]

Mucosal
Xerostomia (>10%) [3]

Cardiovascular
Bradycardia (>10%) [3]
Hypotension [9]
Tachycardia [2]

Central Nervous System
- Agitation [2]
- Anorexia [2]
- Coma [2]
- Confusion (>10%)
- Delirium [2]
- Depression (>10%)
- Hallucinations [2]
- Headache (>10%)
- Neuroleptic malignant syndrome [2]
- Sedation [3]
- Serotonin syndrome [4]
- Somnolence (drowsiness) [14]
- Vertigo (dizziness) [12]

Neuromuscular/Skeletal
- Asthenia (fatigue) (>10%) [2]
- Myoclonus [3]

Gastrointestinal/Hepatic
- Constipation (>10%) [11]
- Nausea (>10%) [31]
- Vomiting (>10%) [22]

Respiratory
- Cough [17]
- Respiratory depression [8]

Ocular
- Miosis (>10%)

Local
- Application-site erythema [2]

Other
- Adverse effects [7]
- Death [7]

FERUMOXYTOL

Trade name: Feraheme (AMG Pharma)
Indications: Iron deficiency anemia in adults with chronic kidney disease
Class: Iron supplement
Half-life: 15 hours
Clinically important, potentially hazardous interactions with: none known
Pregnancy category: C
Important contra-indications noted in the prescribing guidelines for: the elderly; nursing mothers; pediatric patients
Note: May cause hypersensitivity reactions, hypotension and iron overload. Feraheme may transiently affect magnetic resonance (MRI) imaging for up to 3 months following dosage. Contra-indicated in patients with evidence of iron overload or anemia not caused by iron deficiency.

Skin
- Anaphylactoid reactions/Anaphylaxis [4]
- Hypersensitivity [3]
- Pruritus [5]
- Rash [2]
- Urticaria [2]

Cardiovascular
- Hypotension (3%) [3]

Central Nervous System
- Headache [6]
- Vertigo (dizziness) (3%) [3]

Neuromuscular/Skeletal
- Asthenia (fatigue) [2]
- Back pain [2]

Gastrointestinal/Hepatic
- Abdominal pain [2]
- Nausea (3%) [6]
- Vomiting [2]

Respiratory
- Dyspnea [3]

Local
- Injection-site pain [3]

Other
- Adverse effects [2]

FESOTERODINE

Trade name: Toviaz (Pfizer)
Indications: Overactive bladder syndrome, urinary incontinence, urgency and frequency
Class: Antimuscarinic, Muscarinic antagonist
Half-life: 7 hours; 4 hours (oral)
Clinically important, potentially hazardous interactions with: alcohol, amantadine, anticholinergics, antidepressants, antimuscarinics, atazanavir, botulinum toxin (A & B), carbamazepine, cinacalcet, clarithromycin, conivaptan, CYP2D6 inhibitors, CYP3A4 inhibitors, CYP3AF inhibitors, darunavir, dasatinib, deferasirox, delavirdine, duloxetine, indinavir, itraconazole, ketoconazole, nefazodone, nelfinavir, PEG-interferon, phenobarbital, phenytoin, pramlintide, rifampin, ritonavir, saquinavir, secretin, St John's wort, telithromycin, terbinafine, tipranavir, tocilizumab, voriconazole
Pregnancy category: C
Important contra-indications noted in the prescribing guidelines for: nursing mothers; pediatric patients
Note: Contra-indicated in patients with urinary retention, gastric retention, or uncontrolled narrow-angle glaucoma.

Mucosal
- Xerostomia (19–35%) [29]

Central Nervous System
- Headache [3]

Neuromuscular/Skeletal
- Back pain (2%)

Gastrointestinal/Hepatic
- Constipation (4–6%) [17]
- Diarrhea (<10%)
- Dyspepsia (<2%) [2]
- Nausea (<2%) [2]

Respiratory
- Upper respiratory tract infection (2–3%)

Genitourinary
- Dysuria (<2%)
- Urinary retention [2]
- Urinary tract infection (3–4%) [3]

Ocular
- Vision blurred [2]
- Xerophthalmia (<4%) [2]

Other
- Adverse effects [3]

FEVERFEW

Family: Asteraceae; Compositae
Scientific names: *Chrysanthemum parthenium, Pyrethrum parthenium, Tanacetum parthenium*
Indications: Fever, headache, migraine, menstrual irregularities, arthritis, psoriasis, allergy, asthma, tinnitus, vertigo, nausea, cold, earache, orthopedic disorders, swollen feet, diarrhea, dyspepsia
Class: Antipyretic
Half-life: N/A
Clinically important, potentially hazardous interactions with: anticoagulants, NSAIDs
Pregnancy category: N/A

Skin
- Angioedema (lips) [3]
- Dermatitis [4]

Mucosal
- Oral ulceration [3]

Central Nervous System
- Ageusia (taste loss) [2]

Other
- Adverse effects [4]

FEXOFENADINE

Trade name: Allegra (Sanofi-Aventis)
Indications: Allergic rhinitis, pruritus, urticaria
Class: Histamine H1 receptor antagonist
Half-life: 14.4 hours
Clinically important, potentially hazardous interactions with: neratinib, St John's wort
Pregnancy category: C
Important contra-indications noted in the prescribing guidelines for: the elderly; nursing mothers; pediatric patients

---

Skin
- Stevens-Johnson syndrome [2]
- Urticaria [3]

Central Nervous System
- Headache (5–11%) [2]

FINAFLOXACIN

Trade name: Xtoro (Alcon)
Indications: Acute otitis externa caused by susceptible strains of *Pseudomonas aeruginosa* and *Staphylococcus aureus*
Class: Antibiotic, fluoroquinolone
Half-life: N/A
Clinically important, potentially hazardous interactions with: none known
Pregnancy category: C
Important contra-indications noted in the prescribing guidelines for: nursing mothers; pediatric patients

---

Central Nervous System
- Headache [2]

Gastrointestinal/Hepatic
- Diarrhea [2]
- Flatulence [2]

Loose stools [2]
Nausea [2]

Respiratory
Nasopharyngitis [2]
Rhinitis [2]

FINASTERIDE

Trade names: Propecia (Merck), Proscar (Merck)
Indications: Benign prostatic hypertrophy, male-pattern baldness
Class: 5-alpha reductase inhibitor, Androgen antagonist, Enzyme inhibitor
Half-life: 5–8 hours
Clinically important, potentially hazardous interactions with: none known
Pregnancy category: N/A (Contra-indicated in women)
Important contra-indications noted in the prescribing guidelines for: nursing mothers; pediatric patients

---

Skin
Folliculitis [2]
Rash [3]
Urticaria [2]
Xerosis [2]

Hair
Hirsutism [3]

Cardiovascular
Postural hypotension [2]

Central Nervous System
Depression [7]
Headache [2]
Vertigo (dizziness) (7%) [3]

Neuromuscular/Skeletal
Asthenia (fatigue) (5%) [3]
Myalgia/Myopathy (severe) [2]

Endocrine/Metabolic
Gynecomastia (<2%) [17]
Libido decreased (2–10%) [10]
Mastodynia (<2%)
Menstrual irregularities [2]

Genitourinary
Ejaculatory dysfunction [11]
Erectile dysfunction [9]
Impotence (5–19%)
Sexual dysfunction [8]

Other
Adverse effects [7]

FINGOLIMOD

Trade name: Gilenya (Novartis)
Indications: Multiple sclerosis
Class: Immunosuppressant
Half-life: 6–9 days
Clinically important, potentially hazardous interactions with: BCG vaccine, beta blockers, class Ia antiarrhythmics, class III antiarrhythmics, conivaptan, cyproterone, denosumab, digoxin, diltiazem, dronedarone, ketoconazole, leflunomide, live vaccines, natalizumab, PEG-interferon, pimecrolimus, QT prolonging drugs, roflumilast, sipuleucel-T, tacrolimus, tocilizumab, trastuzumab, typhoid vaccine, verapamil, yellow fever vaccine
Pregnancy category: C
Important contra-indications noted in the prescribing guidelines for: nursing mothers; pediatric patients
Note: Contra-indicated in patients with recent (within the last 6 months) occurrence of: myocardial infarction, unstable angina, stroke, transient ischemic attack, decompensated heart failure requiring hospitalization, or Class III/IV heart failure; history or presence of Mobitz Type II 2nd degree or 3rd degree AV block or sick sinus syndrome, unless patient has a pacemaker; baseline QT interval ≥500 ms; or is receiving treatment with Class Ia or Class III anti-arrhythmic drugs.

Skin
Basal cell carcinoma [4]
Eczema (3%)
Herpes (9%) [6]
Herpes simplex [3]
Herpes zoster [3]
Kaposi's sarcoma [2]
Lymphoma [2]
Melanoma [2]
Neoplasms [2]
Pruritus (3%)
Skin cancer [3]
Tinea (4%)
Varicella zoster [5]

Hair
Alopecia (4%)

Cardiovascular
Asystole [2]
Atrial fibrillation [2]
Atrioventricular block [19]
Bradycardia (4%) [24]
Cardiac failure [2]
Cardiotoxicity [3]
Hypertension (6%) [10]

Central Nervous System
Depression (8%)
Encephalopathy [2]
Headache (25%) [11]
Leukoencephalopathy [6]
Migraine (5%)
Paresthesias (5%)
Vertigo (dizziness) (7%)

Neuromuscular/Skeletal
Asthenia (fatigue) (3%) [5]
Back pain (12%) [5]

Gastrointestinal/Hepatic
Diarrhea (12%) [4]
Gastroenteritis (5%)
Hepatotoxicity [11]

Respiratory
Bronchitis (8%)
Cough (10%) [4]
Dyspnea (8%) [2]
Influenza (13%) [4]
Nasopharyngitis [5]
Pulmonary toxicity [4]
Respiratory tract infection [2]
Sinusitis (7%)

Endocrine/Metabolic
ALT increased (14%) [3]
AST increased (14%)
GGT increased (5%)
Weight loss (5%)

Hematologic
Leukopenia (3%)
Lymphopenia (4%) [14]

Ocular
Macular edema [23]
Ocular pain (3%)
Vision blurred (4%)

Other
Adverse effects [12]
Death [7]
Infection [18]

FISH OIL TRIGLYCERIDES *

Trade name: Omegaven (Fresenius Kabi USA)
Indications: indicated as a source of calories and fatty acids in pediatric patients with parenteral nutrition-associated cholestasis
Clinically important, potentially hazardous interactions with: none known
Pregnancy category: N/A (no available data)
Important contra-indications noted in the prescribing guidelines for: pediatric patients
Warning: Risk of Death in Preterm Infants due to Pulmonary Lipid Accumulation; Hypersensitivity Reactions; Risk of Infections, Fat Overload Syndrome, Refeeding Syndrome, and Hypertriglyceridemia; Aluminum Toxicity

---

Skin
Abscess (7%)
Erythema (12%)
Rash (8%)

Cardiovascular
Bradycardia (35%)

Central Nervous System
Agitation (35%)

Neuromuscular/Skeletal
Hypertonia (6%)

Gastrointestinal/Hepatic
Vomiting (46%)

Respiratory
Apnea (20%)

Endocrine/Metabolic
Hypertriglyceridemia (3%)

Hematologic
Bleeding (7%)
Neutropenia (7%)

Local
Infusion-site erythema (6%)

Other
Infection (16%)

FISH OILS

Scientific names: *docosahexaenoic acid (DHA), eicosapentaenoic acid (EPA), Omega-3 fatty acids*
Indications: Albuminuria, anorexia nervosa, cardiovascular disease, hypertension, lupus erythematosus, macular degeneration, osteoarthritis, otitis media, psoriasis
Class: Anti-inflammatory, Lipid regulator
Half-life: N/A
Clinically important, potentially hazardous interactions with: none known
Pregnancy category: N/A
Note: More than 25 mL or 3 g per day can decrease blood coagulation and increase the risk of bleeding. Fish oils contain a significant amount of vitamins A and D and high doses may be toxic.

Central Nervous System
Dysgeusia (taste perversion) [2]

FLECAINIDE

Trade name: Tambocor (3M)
Indications: Atrial fibrillation
Class: Antiarrhythmic, Antiarrhythmic class Ic
Half-life: 12–16 hours
Clinically important, potentially hazardous interactions with: acebutolol, amiodarone, amisulpride, amitriptyline, artemether/lumefantrine, boceprevir, cinacalcet, clozapine, cobicistat/elvitegravir/emtricitabine/tenofovir alafenamide, cobicistat/elvitegravir/emtricitabine/tenofovir disoproxil, darifenacin, delavirdine, fosamprenavir, lopinavir, mirabegron, quinine, ritonavir, telaprevir, tipranavir
Pregnancy category: C
Important contra-indications noted in the prescribing guidelines for: nursing mothers; pediatric patients

---

Skin
Diaphoresis (<3%)
Edema (4%)
Flushing (<3%)
Psoriasis [2]
Rash (<3%)

Cardiovascular
Arrhythmias [7]
Atrial fibrillation [3]
Atrial flutter [2]
Atrioventricular block [2]
Bradycardia [4]
Brugada syndrome [5]
Bundle branch block [2]
Cardiotoxicity [4]
Chest pain (5%)
Congestive heart failure [2]
Extrasystoles [2]
Hypotension [2]
Palpitation (6%)
QT prolongation [7]
Supraventricular tachycardia [2]
Tachycardia [2]
Torsades de pointes [4]

Central Nervous System
Headache (10%) [4]
Hyperesthesia (<10%)
Neurotoxicity [3]
Seizures [2]
Syncope [2]
Tremor (5%)
Vertigo (dizziness) (19%) [5]

Neuromuscular/Skeletal
Asthenia (fatigue) (5–8%)

Gastrointestinal/Hepatic
Abdominal pain (3%)
Constipation (4%)
Diarrhea (<3%) [2]
Nausea (9%) [3]

Respiratory
Dyspnea (10%)

Ocular
Vision blurred [2]
Visual disturbances (16%) [3]

Other
Adverse effects [2]

FLIBANSERIN

Trade name: Addyi (Sprout)
Indications: Hypoactive sexual desire disorder in premenopausal women
Class: Serotonin type 1A receptor agonist, Serotonin type 2A receptor antagonist
Half-life: 11 hours
Clinically important, potentially hazardous interactions with: alcohol, amprenavir, atazanavir, boceprevir, carbamazepine, ciprofloxacin, clarithromycin, conivaptan, digoxin, diltiazem, erythromycin, fluconazole, fosamprenavir, grapefruit juice, indinavir, itraconazole, ketoconazole, nefazodone, nelfinavir, phenobarbital, phenytoin, posaconazole, rifabutin, rifampin, rifapentine, ritonavir, saquinavir, St John's wort, telaprevir, telithromycin, verapamil
Pregnancy category: N/A (No data available)
Important contra-indications noted in the prescribing guidelines for: the elderly; nursing mothers; pediatric patients
Warning: HYPOTENSION AND SYNCOPE IN CERTAIN SETTINGS

Mucosal
Xerostomia (2%) [2]

Central Nervous System
Anxiety (2%)
Insomnia (5%) [4]
Sedation [2]
Somnolence (drowsiness) (11%) [10]
Vertigo (dizziness) (2%) [11]

Neuromuscular/Skeletal
Asthenia (fatigue) (9%) [5]

Gastrointestinal/Hepatic
Abdominal pain (2%)
Constipation (2%)
Nausea (10%) [7]

FLUCLOXACILLIN

Trade name: Floxapen (Actavis)
Indications: Infections due to sensitive Gram-positive organisms
Class: Antibiotic, beta-lactam
Half-life: 53 minutes
Clinically important, potentially hazardous interactions with: oral contraceptives, probenecid
Pregnancy category: N/A
Important contra-indications noted in the prescribing guidelines for: nursing mothers

---

Skin
AGEP [2]

Gastrointestinal/Hepatic
Hepatotoxicity [21]

Endocrine/Metabolic
Acidosis [2]
Hypokalemia [2]

Renal
Nephrotoxicity [4]

Hematologic
Anemia [2]

FLUCONAZOLE

Trade name: Diflucan (Pfizer)
Indications: Candidiasis
Class: Antibiotic, triazole, Antifungal, azole, CYP3A4 inhibitor
Half-life: 25–30 hours
Clinically important, potentially hazardous interactions with: alprazolam, amphotericin B, anisindione, anticoagulants, atorvastatin, avanafil, betamethasone, bosentan, celecoxib, citalopram, clobazam, clopidogrel, deflazacort, dicumarol, eluxadoline, eplerenone, erythromycin, flibanserin, irbesartan, ivacaftor, lesinurad, methadone, midazolam, mifepristone, naldemedine, neratinib, nevirapine, olaparib, ospemifene, pantoprazole, phenobarbital, phenytoin, pimecrolimus, propranolol, quetiapine, ramelteon, rifapentine, rilpivirine, ruxolitinib, simeprevir, sonidegib, sulfonylureas, temsirolimus, terbinafine, tezacaftor/ivacaftor, tipranavir, tofacitinib, trabectedin, triamcinolone, venetoclax, vinblastine, vincristine, warfarin, zidovudine
Pregnancy category: D (fluconazole is pregnancy category C for vaginal candidiasis)
Important contra-indications noted in the prescribing guidelines for: the elderly; nursing mothers

---

Skin
AGEP [3]
Erythema multiforme [3]
Exfoliative dermatitis [2]
Fixed eruption [10]
Hypersensitivity (<4%)
Rash (2%) [4]
Stevens-Johnson syndrome [6]
Toxic epidermal necrolysis [4]

Hair
Alopecia [4]
Nails
Nail changes [2]
Mucosal
Oral ulceration [2]
Cardiovascular
Hypotension [2]
QT prolongation [7]
Torsades de pointes [11]
Central Nervous System
Dysgeusia (taste perversion) [2]
Headache (2–13%) [3]
Neurotoxicity [2]
Neuromuscular/Skeletal
Rhabdomyolysis [4]
Gastrointestinal/Hepatic
Abdominal pain [2]
Diarrhea [2]
Hepatotoxicity [3]
Nausea (2–7%)
Renal
Renal failure [2]
Other
Adverse effects [5]

FLUDARABINE

Trade names: Fludara (Genzyme), Oforta (Sanofi-Aventis)
Indications: Chronic lymphocytic leukemia (B-cell)
Class: Antimetabolite, Antineoplastic
Half-life: 9 hours
Clinically important, potentially hazardous interactions with: aldesleukin, clofazimine, live vaccines, pentostatin
Pregnancy category: D
Important contra-indications noted in the prescribing guidelines for: nursing mothers; pediatric patients
Note: Severe neurologic effects, including blindness, coma, and death were observed in dose-ranging studies in patients with acute leukemia when fludarabine phosphate was administered at high doses. Instances of life-threatening and sometimes fatal autoimmune hemolytic anemia have been reported after one or more cycles of treatment with fludarabine phosphate.
Warning: CNS TOXICITY, HEMOLYTIC ANEMIA, AND PULMONARY TOXICITY

Skin
Anaphylactoid reactions/Anaphylaxis (<3%)
Diaphoresis (14%)
Edema (8–19%)
Herpes simplex (7–8%)
Herpes zoster [2]
Paraneoplastic pemphigus [4]
Peripheral edema (7%)
Pruritus (<3%)
Rash (4–15%)
Hair
Alopecia (<10%)
Mucosal
Mucositis (2%)
Stomatitis (9%)
Cardiovascular
Angina (6%)
Arrhythmias (<4%)
Chest pain (5%)
Congestive heart failure (<4%)
Myocardial infarction (<4%)
Phlebitis (<3%)
Supraventricular tachycardia (<4%)
Central Nervous System
Aneurysm (<2%)
Anorexia (7–34%)
Cerebrovascular accident (<4%)
Chills (11–19%)
Fever (11–69%) [2]
Headache (3–9%)
Leukoencephalopathy [9]
Neurotoxicity [3]
Pain (5–22%)
Paresthesias (4–12%)
Sleep related disorder (<3%)
Neuromuscular/Skeletal
Asthenia (fatigue) (6–65%)
Back pain (4–9%)
Myalgia/Myopathy (>10%)
Gastrointestinal/Hepatic
Abdominal pain (8–10%)
Cholelithiasis (gallstones) (3%)
Constipation (<3%)
Diarrhea (5–15%)
Esophagitis (3%)
Gastrointestinal bleeding (3–13%) [2]
Hepatotoxicity [2]
Nausea (<36%)
Respiratory
Bronchitis (<9%)
Cough (6–44%)
Dyspnea (<22%)
Flu-like syndrome (5–8%)
Hemoptysis (<6%)
Pharyngitis (9%)
Pneumonia (3–22%) [3]
Pneumonitis (6%)
Pulmonary toxicity [4]
Rhinitis (3–11%)
Sinusitis (<5%)
Upper respiratory tract infection (2–14%)
Endocrine/Metabolic
Hyperglycemia (<6%)
Weight loss (<6%)
Genitourinary
Dysuria (3–4%)
Hematuria (<3%)
Urinary hesitancy (3%)
Urinary tract infection (4–15%)
Hematologic
Anemia [3]
Cytopenia [2]
Febrile neutropenia [2]
Hemolytic anemia [2]
Hemotoxicity [3]
Leukopenia [2]
Myelosuppression [3]
Myelotoxicity [2]
Neutropenia [6]
Sepsis [2]
Thrombocytopenia [4]
Thrombosis (<3%)
Otic
Hearing loss (2–6%)
Ocular
Visual disturbances (3–15%)
Other
Adverse effects [2]
Death [4]
Infection (12–44%) [6]

FLUORIDES

Indications: Caries prevention (topical), osteoporosis prevention (oral)
Class: Chemical
Half-life: N/A
Clinically important, potentially hazardous interactions with: caffeine
Pregnancy category: C

Skin
Acneform eruption [2]
Burning [12]
Dermatitis [4]
Edema [2]
Erythema [2]
Hypersensitivity [6]
Necrosis [2]
Pruritus [5]
Toxicity [27]
Urticaria [7]
Mucosal
Oral ulceration [2]
Stomatitis [3]
Central Nervous System
Headache [2]
Neuromuscular/Skeletal
Arthralgia [5]
Bone or joint pain [12]
Skeletal fluorosis [35]
Gastrointestinal/Hepatic
Abdominal pain [2]
Ocular
Cataract [2]
Other
Adverse effects [9]
Death [7]
Tooth fluorosis [39]

FLUOROURACIL

Trade names: 5-fluorouracil (Taj), Carac (Valeant), Efudex (Valeant), Fluoroplex (Allergan), Fluorouracil Injection, USP (Bioniche), Tolak (Hill Dermac)
Indications: Palliative management of malignant neoplasms especially of the gastrointestinal tract, breast, liver and pancreas, topical therapy for actinic keratoses
Class: Antimetabolite, Antineoplastic
Half-life: 8–20 minutes
Clinically important, potentially hazardous interactions with: aldesleukin, bromelain, cimetidine, granulocyte colony-stimulating factor

(G-CSF), metronidazole, tinidazole
Pregnancy category: X
Important contra-indications noted in the prescribing guidelines for: nursing mothers; pediatric patients
Note: Contra-indicated in patients with dihydropyrimidine dehydrogenase deficiency. Tolak cream contains peanut oil and should be used with caution in peanut-sensitive individuals.

Skin
- Acneform eruption [3]
- Acral erythema [4]
- Actinic keratoses [4]
- Anaphylactoid reactions/Anaphylaxis [2]
- Dermatitis (>10%) [4]
- Eczema [2]
- Edema [2]
- Erythema [4]
- Erythema multiforme [3]
- Exanthems (<10%) [3]
- Folliculitis [2]
- Hand–foot syndrome (<38%) [54]
- Lupus erythematosus [6]
- Palmar–plantar pigmentation [2]
- Peripheral edema [2]
- Photosensitivity [3]
- Pigmentation [11]
- Pruritus [5]
- Radiation recall dermatitis [3]
- Rash [8]
- Recall reaction [3]
- Seborrheic dermatitis [3]
- Toxicity [5]
- Ulcerations [2]
- Xerosis (<10%) [3]

Hair
- Alopecia (>10%) [17]

Nails
- Nail pigmentation [3]
- Paronychia [2]

Mucosal
- Epistaxis (nosebleed) [2]
- Mucosal inflammation [2]
- Mucositis (<79%) [17]
- Oral mucositis [7]
- Oral ulceration [2]
- Stomatitis (>10%) [24]
- Tongue pigmentation [2]

Cardiovascular
- Angina [9]
- Bradycardia [2]
- Cardiac failure [5]
- Cardiomyopathy [4]
- Cardiotoxicity [14]
- Hypertension [11]
- Myocardial infarction [4]
- QT prolongation [4]
- Thromboembolism [2]
- Venous thromboembolism [2]
- Ventricular tachycardia [2]

Central Nervous System
- Anorexia [12]
- Dysgeusia (taste perversion) [2]
- Encephalopathy [3]
- Fever [6]
- Headache [2]
- Insomnia [2]
- Leukoencephalopathy [28]
- Neurotoxicity [12]
- Peripheral neuropathy [5]
- Vertigo (dizziness) [2]

Neuromuscular/Skeletal
- Asthenia (fatigue) [23]

Gastrointestinal/Hepatic
- Abdominal pain [4]
- Constipation [4]
- Diarrhea [36]
- Hepatotoxicity [7]
- Nausea [28]
- Vomiting [21]

Respiratory
- Dysphonia [2]
- Pneumonia [2]
- Pulmonary embolism [2]

Endocrine/Metabolic
- Acidosis [2]
- ALP increased [2]
- ALT increased [2]
- AST increased [2]
- Hyperammonemia [3]
- Hyperglycemia [3]
- Hypocalcemia [2]
- Hypokalemia [3]
- Hypomagnesemia [3]
- Hyponatremia [3]
- Serum creatinine increased [2]
- SIADH [4]
- Weight loss [2]

Renal
- Proteinuria [5]

Hematologic
- Anemia [20]
- Febrile neutropenia [21]
- Hemolytic uremic syndrome [3]
- Leukopenia [18]
- Lymphopenia [2]
- Myelosuppression [4]
- Neutropenia [54]
- Thrombocytopenia [21]

Ocular
- Ectropion [2]
- Epiphora [2]
- Ocular inflammation [2]

Local
- Application-site edema [2]
- Application-site pruritus [3]
- Injection-site burning [2]
- Injection-site desquamation [4]
- Injection-site edema [3]
- Injection-site erythema [4]
- Injection-site necrosis [2]
- Injection-site pain [2]
- Injection-site ulceration [2]

Other
- Adverse effects [8]
- Death [6]
- Infection [7]
- Side effects [2]

FLUOXETINE

Trade names: Prozac (Lilly), Sarafem (Warner Chilcott), Symbyax (Lilly)
Indications: Depression, obsessive-compulsive disorder
Class: Antidepressant, Selective serotonin reuptake inhibitor (SSRI)
Half-life: 2–3 days
Clinically important, potentially hazardous interactions with: alprazolam, amoxapine, amphetamines, astemizole, clarithromycin, clopidogrel, clozapine, desipramine, deutetrabenazine, dexibuprofen, dextroamphetamine, diethylpropion, droperidol, duloxetine, erythromycin, haloperidol, iloperidone, imipramine, insulin aspart, insulin degludec, insulin glargine, insulin glulisine, isocarboxazid, linezolid, lithium, MAO inhibitors, mazindol, meperidine, methamphetamine, midazolam, moclobemide, nifedipine, nortriptyline, olanzapine, PEG-interferon, phendimetrazine, phenelzine, phentermine, phenylpropanolamine, phenytoin, pimozide, propranolol, pseudoephedrine, rasagiline, risperidone, selegiline, serotonin agonists, sibutramine, St John's wort, sumatriptan, sympathomimetics, tramadol, tranylcypromine, trazodone, tricyclic antidepressants, troleandomycin, tryptophan, valbenazine, vortioxetine, zolmitriptan
Pregnancy category: C
Important contra-indications noted in the prescribing guidelines for: the elderly; nursing mothers; pediatric patients
Note: Increased risk of suicidal thinking and behavior in children, adolescents, and young adults taking antidepressants for Major Depressive Disorder (MDD) and other psychiatric disorders. Sarafem is not approved for use in pediatric patients with MDD and obsessive compulsive disorder. Symbyax is not approved for use in children and adolescents.
Symbyax is fluoxetine and olanzapine.
Warning: SUICIDAL THOUGHTS AND BEHAVIORS

Skin
- Diaphoresis (8%) [3]
- Exanthems (4%) [7]
- Flushing (<2%)
- Mycosis fungoides [2]
- Phototoxicity [2]
- Pruritus (2%) [4]
- Pseudolymphoma [4]
- Rash (6%) [3]
- Raynaud's phenomenon [2]
- Serum sickness-like reaction [2]
- Toxic epidermal necrolysis [2]
- Toxicity [2]
- Urticaria (4%) [5]
- Vasculitis [2]

Hair
- Alopecia [7]

Mucosal
- Black tongue [2]
- Oral ulceration [2]
- Xerostomia (12%) [7]

Cardiovascular
Orthostatic hypotension [2]
QT prolongation [7]
Torsades de pointes [2]

Central Nervous System
Akathisia [6]
Amnesia [2]
Anxiety [2]
Delirium [3]
Depression [2]
Dysgeusia (taste perversion) (2%)
Extrapyramidal symptoms [3]
Hallucinations [3]
Headache (<27%) [3]
Insomnia [3]
Neuroleptic malignant syndrome [2]
Paresthesias [2]
Restless legs syndrome [4]
Serotonin syndrome [14]
Somnolence (drowsiness) [4]
Suicidal ideation [11]
Tremor (2–10%) [2]
Vertigo (dizziness) [4]

Neuromuscular/Skeletal
Asthenia (fatigue) [3]
Rhabdomyolysis [2]

Gastrointestinal/Hepatic
Nausea [4]

Endocrine/Metabolic
Gynecomastia [2]
Libido decreased [2]
SIADH [20]
Weight gain [4]

Genitourinary
Priapism [2]
Sexual dysfunction [6]

Ocular
Hallucinations, visual [4]

Other
Adverse effects [3]
Bruxism [4]
Death [3]

FLUPHENAZINE

Trade name: Prolixin (Bristol-Myers Squibb)
Indications: Psychoses
Class: Antipsychotic, Phenothiazine
Half-life: 84–96 hours
Clinically important, potentially hazardous interactions with: antihistamines, arsenic, chlorpheniramine, clozapine, dofetilide, evening primrose, quinolones, sparfloxacin
Pregnancy category: C
Important contra-indications noted in the prescribing guidelines for: nursing mothers

---

Skin
Rash (<10%)
Vitiligo [2]

Central Nervous System
Neuroleptic malignant syndrome [14]
Parkinsonism [3]
Somnolence (drowsiness) [4]

Neuromuscular/Skeletal
Dystonia [3]

Endocrine/Metabolic
Galactorrhea (<10%)
Gynecomastia (<10%)
Mastodynia (<10%)

Genitourinary
Priapism [2]

Ocular
Maculopathy [3]

FLURBIPROFEN

Trade name: Ansaid (Pfizer)
Indications: Rheumatoid arthritis, osteoarthritis
Class: Non-steroidal anti-inflammatory (NSAID)
Half-life: 3–4 hours
Clinically important, potentially hazardous interactions with: ACE inhibitors, aspirin, furosemide, lithium, methotrexate
Pregnancy category: C
Important contra-indications noted in the prescribing guidelines for: the elderly; nursing mothers
Note: NSAIDs may cause an increased risk of serious cardiovascular and gastrointestinal adverse events, which can be fatal. This risk may increase with duration of use.
Elderly patients are at greater risk for serious gastrointestinal events.
Warning: CARDIOVASCULAR AND GASTROINTESTINAL RISKS

Skin
Eczema (3–9%)
Edema (3–9%)
Exanthems [3]
Fixed eruption [2]
Hypersensitivity [4]
Pruritus (<5%)
Rash (<3%)

Mucosal
Oral lichenoid eruption [2]

Central Nervous System
Headache [4]

Renal
Nephrotoxicity [2]

Other
Side effects (6%) [2]

FLUTAMIDE

Indications: Metastatic prostate carcinoma
Class: Androgen antagonist
Half-life: 8–10 hours
Clinically important, potentially hazardous interactions with: none known
Pregnancy category: D (not indicated for use in women)
Important contra-indications noted in the prescribing guidelines for: nursing mothers; pediatric patients
Warning: HEPATIC INJURY

Skin
Edema (4%)
Hot flashes (61%)
Photosensitivity [9]
Rash (3%)
Xerosis [2]

Central Nervous System
Paresthesias (<10%)

Gastrointestinal/Hepatic
Hepatotoxicity [13]

Endocrine/Metabolic
Gynecomastia (9%) [4]
Pseudoporphyria [3]

Local
Injection-site irritation (3%)

FLUVASTATIN

Trade name: Lescol (Novartis)
Indications: Hypercholesterolemia
Class: HMG-CoA reductase inhibitor, Statin
Half-life: 1.2 hours
Clinically important, potentially hazardous interactions with: azithromycin, bosentan, ciprofibrate, clarithromycin, colchicine, cyclosporine, delavirdine, elbasvir & grazoprevir, erythromycin, gemfibrozil, imatinib, letermovir, mifepristone, red rice yeast
Pregnancy category: X
Important contra-indications noted in the prescribing guidelines for: nursing mothers

---

Skin
Lupus erythematosus [2]
Rash (3%)

Central Nervous System
Headache (9%)

Neuromuscular/Skeletal
Asthenia (fatigue) (3%)
Myalgia/Myopathy (5%) [4]
Rhabdomyolysis [13]

Gastrointestinal/Hepatic
Diarrhea (5%)
Dyspepsia (8%)
Hepatotoxicity [5]

Respiratory
Sinusitis (3%)
Upper respiratory tract infection (16%)

Endocrine/Metabolic
Creatine phosphokinase increased [2]

Other
Allergic reactions (3%)

FLUVOXAMINE

Trade name: Luvox (Solvay)
Indications: Obsessive-compulsive disorder, depression
Class: Antidepressant, CYP1A2 inhibitor, CYP3A4 inhibitor, Selective serotonin reuptake inhibitor (SSRI)
Half-life: 15 hours
Clinically important, potentially hazardous interactions with: alosetron, alprazolam, aminophylline, amphetamines, anagrelide, asenapine, astemizole, bendamustine, clobazam, clopidogrel, clozapine, dextroamphetamine,

diethylpropion, droperidol, duloxetine, isocarboxazid, linezolid, MAO inhibitors, mazindol, methadone, methamphetamine, neratinib, olanzapine, oxtriphylline, phendimetrazine, phenelzine, phentermine, phenylpropanolamine, pirfenidone, propranolol, pseudoephedrine, ramelteon, rasagiline, roflumilast, ropivacaine, selegiline, sibutramine, St John's wort, sumatriptan, sympathomimetics, tacrine, tasimelteon, tizanidine, tramadol, tranylcypromine, trazodone, troleandomycin, tryptophan, zolmitriptan
Pregnancy category: C
Important contra-indications noted in the prescribing guidelines for: the elderly; nursing mothers; pediatric patients
Warning: SUICIDALITY AND ANTIDEPRESSANT DRUGS

Skin
Diaphoresis (<7%)
Photosensitivity [3]

Mucosal
Oral lesions (10%)
Xerostomia (<14%) [2]

Cardiovascular
Chest pain (3%)
Palpitation (3%)
QT prolongation [3]

Central Nervous System
Anorexia (6–14%)
Anxiety (5–8%)
Dysgeusia (taste perversion) (3%)
Headache (22–35%)
Insomnia (21–35%)
Neuroleptic malignant syndrome [2]
Pain (10%)
Seizures [2]
Serotonin syndrome [6]
Somnolence (drowsiness) (22–27%)
Tremor (5–8%)
Vertigo (dizziness) (11–15%)
Yawning (2–5%)

Neuromuscular/Skeletal
Asthenia (fatigue) (14–26%) [3]
Myalgia/Myopathy (5%)

Gastrointestinal/Hepatic
Diarrhea (16–18%)
Dyspepsia (8–10%)
Nausea (34–40%)

Respiratory
Pharyngitis (6%)
Upper respiratory tract infection (9%)

Endocrine/Metabolic
Galactorrhea [2]
Libido decreased (2–10%)
SIADH [2]

Genitourinary
Ejaculatory dysfunction (8–11%)
Sexual dysfunction [2]

FOLIC ACID

Synonyms: folacin; folate; vitamin B_9
Indications: Anemias
Class: Vitamin
Half-life: N/A
Clinically important, potentially hazardous interactions with: balsalazide, estradiol, raltitrexed
Pregnancy category: A

Skin
Anaphylactoid reactions/Anaphylaxis [3]
Exanthems [2]
Pruritus [2]
Urticaria [2]

FONDAPARINUX

Trade name: Arixtra (Mylan)
Indications: Prophylaxis of deep vein thrombosis
Class: Anticoagulant, Heparinoid
Half-life: 17–21 hours
Clinically important, potentially hazardous interactions with: abciximab, anagrelide, anticoagulants, cilostazol, clopidogrel, dabigatran, dipyridamole, eptifibatide, nandrolone, salicylates, ticlopidine, tirofiban
Pregnancy category: B
Important contra-indications noted in the prescribing guidelines for: the elderly; nursing mothers; pediatric patients
Warning: SPINAL/EPIDURAL HEMATOMAS

Skin
Bullous dermatitis (3%)
Edema (9%)
Hematoma [2]
Hypersensitivity [4]
Purpura (4%)
Rash (8%)

Central Nervous System
Pain (2%)

Gastrointestinal/Hepatic
Hepatotoxicity [2]

Local
Injection-site bleeding (<10%)
Injection-site pruritus (<10%)

FORMOTEROL

Trade names: Dulera (Merck Sharpe & Dohme), Foradil (Novartis), Perforomist (Mylan), Symbicort (AstraZeneca)
Indications: Asthma, bronchospasm
Class: Beta-2 adrenergic agonist, Bronchodilator
Half-life: 10–14 hours
Clinically important, potentially hazardous interactions with: beta blockers, clomipramine, desipramine, doxepin, imipramine, iobenguane, nortriptyline, protriptyline, trimipramine
Pregnancy category: C
Important contra-indications noted in the prescribing guidelines for: nursing mothers; pediatric patients
Note: Dulera is formoterol and mometasone; Symbicort is formoterol and budesonide.
Warning: ASTHMA-RELATED DEATH

Skin
Pruritus (2%)

Mucosal
Xerostomia (<3%) [4]

Cardiovascular
Atrial fibrillation [2]
Chest pain (2%)
Hypertension [2]
Myocardial infarction [2]
Palpitation [2]

Central Nervous System
Anxiety (2%)
Fever (2%)
Headache [9]
Insomnia (2%)
Tremor (2%) [7]
Vertigo (dizziness) (2–3%) [3]

Neuromuscular/Skeletal
Back pain (4%)
Cramps (2%)
Leg cramps (2%)
Muscle spasm [2]

Gastrointestinal/Hepatic
Diarrhea (5%) [2]
Nausea (5%)
Vomiting (2%)

Respiratory
Asthma (exacerbation) [3]
Bronchitis (5%)
Cough [6]
Dysphonia [2]
Dyspnea (2%) [2]
Nasopharyngitis [8]
Pharyngitis (4%) [2]
Pneumonia [2]
Rhinitis [2]
Upper respiratory tract infection (7%) [3]

Genitourinary
Urinary tract infection [2]

Other
Adverse effects [3]
Death [2]
Infection (17%)

FOSAMPRENAVIR

Trade name: Lexiva (ViiV)
Indications: HIV infections (in combination with other antiretrovirals)
Class: Antiretroviral, HIV-1 protease inhibitor
Half-life: 7.7 hours
Clinically important, potentially hazardous interactions with: amiodarone, atorvastatin, avanafil, bepridil, carbamazepine, darifenacin, delavirdine, dihydroergotamine, efavirenz, etravirine, flecainide, flibanserin, itraconazole, ketoconazole, lidocaine, lopinavir, lovastatin, midazolam, mifepristone, nevirapine, olaparib,

phenobarbital, phenytoin, pimozide, posaconazole, propafenone, quinidine, quinine, rifabutin, rifampin, rilpivirine, ritonavir, rivaroxaban, rosuvastatin, sildenafil, simeprevir, simvastatin, St John's wort, tadalafil, telaprevir, telithromycin, tipranavir, triazolam, vardenafil, warfarin
Pregnancy category: C
Important contra-indications noted in the prescribing guidelines for: the elderly; nursing mothers; pediatric patients
Note: Fosamprenavir is a sulfonamide and can be absorbed systemically. Sulfonamides can produce severe, possibly fatal, reactions such as toxic epidermal necrolysis and Stevens-Johnson syndrome.
Fosamprenavir is a prodrug of amprenavir (see separate entry).

Skin
Hypersensitivity [2]
Pruritus (7%)
Rash (~19%) [5]

Central Nervous System
Depression (8%)
Headache (19%)
Paresthesias (oral) (2%)

Neuromuscular/Skeletal
Asthenia (fatigue) (10%)

Gastrointestinal/Hepatic
Abdominal pain (5%)
Diarrhea [2]
Hepatotoxicity [2]
Vomiting [2]

Respiratory
Bronchitis [2]
Cough [2]
Nasopharyngitis [3]
Rhinitis [2]
Upper respiratory tract infection [2]

Other
Adverse effects [3]

FOSINOPRIL

Trade name: Monopril (Bristol-Myers Squibb)
Indications: Hypertension, heart failure
Class: Angiotensin-converting enzyme (ACE) inhibitor, Antihypertensive, Vasodilator
Half-life: 12 hours
Clinically important, potentially hazardous interactions with: alcohol, aldesleukin, allopurinol, alpha blockers, alprostadil, amifostine, amiloride, angiotensin II receptor blocking agents, antacids, antidiabetics, antihypertensives, antipsychotics, anxiolytics and hypnotics, azathioprine, baclofen, beta blockers, calcium channel blockers, clonidine, corticosteroids, cyclosporine, diazoxide, diuretics, estrogens, general anesthetics, gold & gold compounds, heparins, hydralazine, hypotensives, insulin, levodopa, lithium, MAO inhibitors, metformin, methyldopa, minoxidil, moxisylyte, moxonidine, nitrates, nitroprusside, NSAIDs, pentoxifylline, phosphodiesterase 5 inhibitors, potassium salts, prostacyclin analogues, rituximab, sirolimus, spironolactone, sulfonylureas, temsirolimus, tizanidine, tolvaptan, triamterene, trimethoprim
Pregnancy category: D (category C in first trimester; category D in second and third trimesters)
Important contra-indications noted in the prescribing guidelines for: nursing mothers
Warning: USE IN PREGNANCY

Skin
Angioedema [3]

Respiratory
Cough [3]

FUROSEMIDE

Trade name: Lasix (Sanofi-Aventis)
Indications: Edema
Class: Diuretic, loop
Half-life: ~2 hours
Clinically important, potentially hazardous interactions with: acemetacin, aliskiren, amikacin, amyl nitrite, celecoxib, diclofenac, digoxin, flurbiprofen, gentamicin, hyaluronic acid, hydrocortisone, kanamycin, mivacurium, neomycin, piroxicam, probenecid, streptomycin, tobramycin, tolmetin
Pregnancy category: C
Important contra-indications noted in the prescribing guidelines for: the elderly; nursing mothers; pediatric patients
Note: Furosemide is a sulfonamide and can be absorbed systemically. Sulfonamides can produce severe, possibly fatal, reactions such as toxic epidermal necrolysis and Stevens-Johnson syndrome.

Skin
AGEP [2]
Anaphylactoid reactions/Anaphylaxis [2]
Bullous dermatitis [16]
Bullous pemphigoid [11]
Erythema multiforme [3]
Exanthems (12%) [7]
Exfoliative dermatitis [3]
Lichenoid eruption [2]
Linear IgA bullous dermatosis [2]
Photosensitivity (<10%) [2]
Phototoxicity [4]
Pruritus [2]
Purpura [3]
Pustules [3]
Stevens-Johnson syndrome [4]
Sweet's syndrome [2]
Urticaria [3]
Vasculitis [7]

Mucosal
Xerostomia [3]

Cardiovascular
Hypotension [2]

Gastrointestinal/Hepatic
Pancreatitis [3]

Endocrine/Metabolic
Porphyria cutanea tarda [3]

Otic
Hearing loss [2]
Ototoxicity [3]

Other
Adverse effects [3]
Side effects [2]

GABAPENTIN

Trade names: Horizant (GSK), Neurontin (Pfizer)
Indications: Postherpetic neuralgia in adults, seizures
Class: Anticonvulsant
Half-life: 5–7 hours
Clinically important, potentially hazardous interactions with: none known
Pregnancy category: C
Important contra-indications noted in the prescribing guidelines for: the elderly; nursing mothers; pediatric patients

---

Skin
Anticonvulsant hypersensitivity syndrome [2]
Bullous pemphigoid [2]
Edema [5]
Exanthems [2]
Peripheral edema (8%) [13]
Rash [2]
Stevens-Johnson syndrome [2]

Hair
Alopecia [2]

Mucosal
Xerostomia (5%)

Central Nervous System
Aggression [2]
Coma [3]
Confusion [4]
Delirium [2]
Fever (10%)
Gait instability (2%) [4]
Headache (3%) [9]
Incoordination (2%)
Neurotoxicity [4]
Psychosis [2]
Sedation [5]
Seizures [4]
Somnolence (drowsiness) (21%) [40]
Tremor [3]
Vertigo (dizziness) (17–28%) [51]

Neuromuscular/Skeletal
Asthenia (fatigue) (6%) [13]
Ataxia (3%) [10]
Dystonia [2]
Myalgia/Myopathy [4]
Myasthenia gravis [3]
Myoclonus [5]
Rhabdomyolysis [4]

Gastrointestinal/Hepatic
Abdominal pain (3%)
Constipation (4%) [2]
Diarrhea (6%)
Flatulence (2%) [2]
Nausea (4%) [5]
Vomiting (3%) [3]

Respiratory
Respiratory depression [2]

Endocrine/Metabolic
Weight gain (2%) [8]

Genitourinary
Sexual dysfunction [5]

Otic
Hearing loss [2]

Ocular
Diplopia [2]
Hallucinations, visual [2]
Nystagmus [2]
Vision blurred (3%)

Other
Adverse effects [7]
Infection (5%)

GALANTAMINE

Trade names: Razadyne (Janssen), Reminyl (Janssen)
Indications: Alzheimer's disease
Class: Acetylcholinesterase inhibitor, Cholinesterase inhibitor
Half-life: ~7 hours
Clinically important, potentially hazardous interactions with: bethanechol, cimetidine, donepezil, edrophonium, paroxetine hydrochloride, physostigmine, pilocarpine, rivastigmine, succinylcholine, tacrine
Pregnancy category: C
Important contra-indications noted in the prescribing guidelines for: nursing mothers; pediatric patients
Note: Originally derived from snowdrop (*Galanthus* sp) bulbs.

Skin
Peripheral edema (>2%)
Purpura (>2%)

Cardiovascular
Bradycardia (2%) [5]
QT prolongation [5]

Central Nervous System
Anorexia (7–9%) [2]
Depression (7%)
Headache (8%) [2]
Insomnia (5%)
Somnolence (drowsiness) (4%)
Syncope (2%) [3]
Tremor (3%)
Vertigo (dizziness) (9%) [4]

Neuromuscular/Skeletal
Asthenia (fatigue) (5%)

Gastrointestinal/Hepatic
Abdominal pain (5%)
Diarrhea (6–12%) [5]
Dyspepsia (5%)
Nausea (6–24%) [7]
Vomiting (4–13%) [7]

Respiratory
Rhinitis (4%)
Upper respiratory tract infection (>2%)

Endocrine/Metabolic
Weight loss (5–7%)

Genitourinary
Hematuria (3%)
Urinary tract infection (8%)

Hematologic
Anemia (3%)

Other
Adverse effects [3]

GARLIC

Family: Liliaceae
Scientific name: *Allium sativum*
Indications: Hypertension, hypercholesterolemia, atherosclerosis, earache, menstrual disorders, allergy, flu, arthritis, diarrhea, bacterial and fungal infections, tinea corporis, tinea pedis, onychomycosis, vaginitis
Class: Immunomodulator
Half-life: N/A
Clinically important, potentially hazardous interactions with: arsenic, atazanavir, chlorpropamide, HIV medications, tipranavir
Pregnancy category: N/A

Skin
Anaphylactoid reactions/Anaphylaxis [2]
Burning [9]
Dermatitis [20]
Hypersensitivity [2]

Gastrointestinal/Hepatic
Esophagitis [2]

Hematologic
Bleeding [2]

Other
Adverse effects [4]
Allergic reactions [4]

GEFITINIB

Trade name: Iressa (AstraZeneca)
Indications: Advanced non-small cell lung cancer
Class: Antineoplastic, Biologic, Epidermal growth factor receptor (EGFR) inhibitor, Tyrosine kinase inhibitor
Half-life: 48 hours
Clinically important, potentially hazardous interactions with: antifungals, BCG vaccine, boceprevir, carbamazepine, cardiac glycosides, clozapine, conivaptan, CYP3A4 inhibitors and inducers, dasatinib, deferasirox, denosumab, echinacea, efavirenz, grapefruit juice, itraconazole, leflunomide, natalizumab, phenobarbital, phenytoin, pimecrolimus, ranitidine, rifampin, rifapentine, sipuleucel-T, St John's wort, tacrolimus, topotecan, trastuzumab, vaccines, vitamin K antagonists, voriconazole, warfarin
Pregnancy category: D
Important contra-indications noted in the prescribing guidelines for: nursing mothers; pediatric patients

---

Skin
Acneform eruption (25–33%) [34]
Desquamation (39%) [2]
Exanthems [3]
Folliculitis [4]
Hand–foot syndrome [2]
Papulopustular eruption [3]
Peripheral edema (2%)
Pruritus (8–9%) [6]
Rash (43–54%) [67]
Seborrhea [2]
Toxic epidermal necrolysis [2]
Toxicity [10]
Ulcerations [2]
Xerosis (13–26%) [13]

Hair
Alopecia [6]
Hypertrichosis [2]

Nails
Nail changes (17%)
Paronychia (6%) [14]
Pyogenic granuloma [2]

Mucosal
Mucositis [4]
Stomatitis [8]

Cardiovascular
Hypertension [2]

Central Nervous System
Anorexia (7–10%) [2]

Neuromuscular/Skeletal
Asthenia (fatigue) [12]

Gastrointestinal/Hepatic
Abdominal pain [3]
Diarrhea (48–67%) [40]
Gastrointestinal perforation [2]
Hepatotoxicity [27]
Nausea (13–18%) [11]
Vomiting (9–12%) [6]

Respiratory
Dyspnea (2%)
Pneumonia [2]
Pneumonitis [4]
Pulmonary toxicity [16]

Endocrine/Metabolic
ALT increased [8]
Appetite decreased [3]
AST increased [7]
Dehydration [2]
Weight loss (3–5%)

Genitourinary
Cystitis [2]

Renal
Nephrotoxicity [2]

Hematologic
Anemia [5]
Neutropenia [7]
Thrombocytopenia [3]

Ocular
Amblyopia (2%)
Blepharitis [2]
Conjunctivitis [2]

Other
Adverse effects [12]
Death [8]

GEMCITABINE

Trade name: Gemzar (Lilly)
Indications: Pancreatic carcinoma as a single agent, ovarian cancer (with carboplatin), breast cancer (with paclitaxel), non-small cell lung cancer (with cisplatin)
Class: Antimetabolite, Antineoplastic
Half-life: 42–94 minutes for short infusions; 4–11 hours for longer infusions
Clinically important, potentially hazardous interactions with: aldesleukin
Pregnancy category: D
Important contra-indications noted in the prescribing guidelines for: nursing mothers; pediatric patients

---

Skin
Acneform eruption [3]
Bullous dermatitis [2]
Cellulitis [5]
Dermatitis [6]
Eczema (13%)
Edema (13%) [4]
Exanthems [2]
Hand–foot syndrome [19]
Hypersensitivity [3]
Livedo reticularis [2]
Necrosis [2]
Peripheral edema (20%) [4]
Petechiae (16%)
Pruritus (13%) [2]
Radiation recall dermatitis (<74%) [17]
Rash (30%) [35]
Raynaud's phenomenon [3]
Thrombocytopenic purpura [6]
Toxic epidermal necrolysis [3]
Toxicity [6]
Vasculitis [3]

Hair
Alopecia (15%) [15]

Mucosal
Mucositis [7]
Stomatitis (11%) [13]

Cardiovascular
Arrhythmias [3]
Atrial fibrillation [4]
Capillary leak syndrome [9]
Cardiotoxicity [3]
Hypertension [3]
Hypotension [2]
Myocardial infarction [3]
Thromboembolism [2]
Venous thromboembolism [4]

Central Nervous System
Anorexia [13]
Fever (41%) [13]
Leukoencephalopathy [4]
Neurotoxicity [11]
Pain [2]
Paresthesias (10%) [2]
Peripheral neuropathy [7]
Somnolence (drowsiness) (11%)

Neuromuscular/Skeletal
Asthenia (fatigue) (18%) [49]
Myalgia/Myopathy (>10%) [6]

Gastrointestinal/Hepatic
Abdominal pain [2]
Cholangitis [2]
Constipation [3]
Diarrhea (19%) [26]
Gastrointestinal bleeding [2]
Hepatic disorder [2]
Hepatotoxicity [11]
Nausea (69%) [27]
Vomiting (69%) [21]

Respiratory
Dyspnea (10–23%) [2]
Flu-like syndrome (19%) [2]
Pneumonitis [5]
Pulmonary toxicity [11]

Endocrine/Metabolic
ALT increased [6]
Appetite decreased [2]
AST increased [6]
Dehydration [2]
Hyperglycemia [2]
Hypomagnesemia [7]
Hyponatremia [2]

Genitourinary
Hematuria (30%)

Renal
Nephrotoxicity [5]
Renal failure [2]

Hematologic
Anemia (70%) [40]
Febrile neutropenia [19]
Hemolytic uremic syndrome [32]
Hemotoxicity [7]
Leukocytopenia [3]
Leukopenia (62%) [25]
Myelosuppression [7]
Myelotoxicity [3]
Neutropenia (61%) [91]
Thrombocytopenia (30%) [65]
Thrombosis [3]
Thrombotic microangiopathy [5]

Local
Injection-site reactions (4%)

Other
Adverse effects [9]
Allergic reactions (4%)
Death [12]
Infection (16%) [11]

GEMFIBROZIL

Trade name: Lopid (Pfizer)
Indications: Hyperlipidemia
Class: Fibrate, Lipid regulator
Half-life: 2 hours
Clinically important, potentially hazardous interactions with: atorvastatin, bexarotene, colchicine, cyclosporine, dasabuvir/ombitasvir/paritaprevir/ritonavir, dicumarol, eluxadoline, enzalutamide, ezetimibe, fluvastatin, interferon alfa, lovastatin, nicotinic acid, paclitaxel, pioglitazone, pitavastatin, pravastatin, repaglinide, rosiglitazone, rosuvastatin, roxithromycin, selexipag, simvastatin, treprostinil, warfarin
Pregnancy category: C
Important contra-indications noted in the prescribing guidelines for: nursing mothers; pediatric patients
Note: Contra-indicated in patients with preexisting gallbladder disease.

Skin
Eczema (2%)
Exanthems (3%) [2]
Psoriasis [3]
Rash (2%)

Central Nervous System
Headache [3]

Neuromuscular/Skeletal
Asthenia (fatigue) (2%)
Compartment syndrome [2]
Myalgia/Myopathy [5]
Rhabdomyolysis [35]

Gastrointestinal/Hepatic
Abdominal pain (10%)
Dyspepsia (20%)
Hepatotoxicity [2]
Pancreatitis [2]

Other
Death [2]

GENTAMICIN

Trade names: Garamycin (Schering), Genoptic (Allergan)
Indications: Various infections caused by susceptible organisms
Class: Antibiotic, aminoglycoside
Half-life: 2–4 hours
Clinically important, potentially hazardous interactions with: adefovir, aldesleukin, aminoglycosides, atracurium, bumetanide, carbenicillin, cephalexin, cephalothin, cobicistat/elvitegravir/emtricitabine/tenofovir alafenamide, doxacurium, ethacrynic acid, furosemide, methoxyflurane, non-polarizing muscle relaxants, pancuronium, pipecuronium, polypeptide antibiotics, rocuronium, succinylcholine, teicoplanin, torsemide, tubocurarine, vecuronium
Pregnancy category: C
Important contra-indications noted in the prescribing guidelines for: the elderly; nursing mothers
Note: Aminoglycosides may cause neurotoxicity and/or nephrotoxicity.

Skin
Anaphylactoid reactions/Anaphylaxis [2]
Dermatitis [8]
Edema (<10%)
Erythema (<10%)
Exanthems [5]
Photosensitivity [2]
Pruritus (<10%)

Hair
Alopecia [2]

Renal
Fanconi syndrome [2]
Nephrotoxicity [15]

Otic
- Ototoxicity [12]
- Tinnitus [4]

Local
- Injection-site necrosis [5]

GINGER

Family: Zingiberaceae
Scientific name: *Zingiber officinale*
Indications: Colic, dyspepsia, flatulence, rheumatoid arthritis, loss of appetite, nausea, vomiting, upper respiratory infections, cough, bronchitis, burns, tinnitus, flavoring agent, fragrance component
Class: Carminative, Oleoresin
Half-life: N/A
Clinically important, potentially hazardous interactions with: arsenic, clevidipine, squill
Pregnancy category: N/A

Gastrointestinal/Hepatic
- Diarrhea [2]
- Nausea [2]

GINKGO BILOBA

Family: Ginkgoaceae
Scientific name: *Ginkgo biloba (Mericon)*
Indications: Dementia, memory loss, headache, tinnitus, dizziness, mood disturbances, hearing disorders, intermittent claudication, attention deficit hyperactivity disorder, premenstrual syndrome, heart disease
Class: Food supplement, Vascular stimulant
Half-life: N/A
Clinically important, potentially hazardous interactions with: anticoagulants, aspirin, diuretics, NSAIDs, platelet inhibitors, SSRIs, St John's wort, thiazide diuretics, trazodone
Pregnancy category: N/A
Note: *Ginkgo biloba* is the oldest living tree species in the world. Ginkgo is the most frequently prescribed herbal medicine in Germany.

Skin
- Dermatitis [3]
- Exanthems [2]
- Fixed eruption [2]

Cardiovascular
- Hypertension [2]

Central Nervous System
- Cerebral hemorrhage [2]
- Seizures [5]

Hematologic
- Bleeding [2]

Ocular
- Ocular adverse effects [2]

Other
- Adverse effects [9]

GINSENG

Family: Araliaceae; oriental ginseng
Scientific name: *Panax ginseng*
Indications: General tonic, improving stamina, cognitive function, concentration, diuretic, antidepressant, gastritis, neurasthenia, impotence, fever, hangover, cancer, cardiovascular diseases
Class: Immunomodulator
Half-life: N/A
Clinically important, potentially hazardous interactions with: alcohol, arsenic, aspirin, caffeine, clevidipine, phenelzine, squill, tamoxifen
Pregnancy category: N/A
Note: Ginseng has been used for medicinal purposes for more than 2000 years. Approximately 6,000,000 Americans use it regularly.

Skin
- Stevens-Johnson syndrome [2]

Cardiovascular
- Hypertension [2]

Central Nervous System
- Insomnia [2]
- Mania [4]

Gastrointestinal/Hepatic
- Hepatotoxicity [2]

Endocrine/Metabolic
- Mastodynia [3]

Other
- Adverse effects [8]
- Side effects [2]

GLATIRAMER

Synonym: copolymer-1
Trade names: Copaxone (Teva), Glatopa (Novartis)
Indications: Multiple sclerosis
Class: Immunomodulator
Half-life: N/A
Clinically important, potentially hazardous interactions with: Hemophilus B vaccine
Pregnancy category: B
Important contra-indications noted in the prescribing guidelines for: the elderly; nursing mothers; pediatric patients

---

Skin
- Acneform eruption (>2%)
- Anaphylactoid reactions/Anaphylaxis [3]
- Cyst (2%)
- Diaphoresis (15%)
- Ecchymoses (8%)
- Eczema (8%)
- Edema (8%)
- Erythema (4%)
- Facial edema (6%)
- Flushing [6]
- Herpes simplex (4%)
- Hyperhidrosis (15%)
- Hypersensitivity (3%)
- Lipoatrophy [3]
- Nicolau syndrome [3]
- Nodular eruption (2%)
- Panniculitis [2]
- Peripheral edema (7%)
- Pruritus (4%)
- Purpura (8%)
- Rash (18%)
- Urticaria [2]

Hair
- Alopecia (>2%)

Nails
- Nail changes (>2%)

Mucosal
- Oral vesiculation (6%)
- Xerostomia (>2%)

Cardiovascular
- Chest pain (13%) [3]
- Palpitation (7%) [7]
- Vasodilation (20%) [2]

Central Nervous System
- Anxiety (13%) [4]
- Chills (4%)
- Depression (>2%)
- Dysgeusia (taste perversion) (>2%)
- Fever (6%)
- Hyperesthesia (>2%)
- Migraine (4%)
- Pain (28%) [3]
- Paresthesias (>2%) [2]
- Tremor (7%)
- Vertigo (dizziness) (>2%)

Neuromuscular/Skeletal
- Arthralgia (24%)
- Asthenia (fatigue) (19%)
- Myalgia/Myopathy (>2%)

Gastrointestinal/Hepatic
- Hepatotoxicity [3]
- Nausea (15%) [2]
- Vomiting (7%)

Respiratory
- Cough (>2%)
- Dyspnea [4]
- Flu-like syndrome (26%)
- Sinusitis (>2%)

Endocrine/Metabolic
- Mastodynia (>2%)

Genitourinary
- Urinary tract infection [2]
- Vaginitis (4%)

Otic
- Tinnitus (>2%)

Local
- Injection-site bleeding (5%)
- Injection-site ecchymoses (>2%)
- Injection-site edema [2]
- Injection-site erythema (66%) [4]
- Injection-site induration (13%) [3]
- Injection-site inflammation (49%)
- Injection-site lipoatrophy/lipohypertrophy [2]
- Injection-site pain (73%) [3]
- Injection-site pruritus (40%) [3]
- Injection-site reactions (6–67%) [15]
- Injection-site urticaria (5%)

Other
- Adverse effects [5]
- Infection (50%) [2]

GLIMEPIRIDE

Trade names: Amaryl (Sanofi-Aventis), Avandaryl (GSK)
Indications: Non-insulin dependent diabetes Type II
Class: Sulfonylurea
Half-life: 5–9 hours
Clinically important, potentially hazardous interactions with: none known
Pregnancy category: C
Important contra-indications noted in the prescribing guidelines for: the elderly; nursing mothers; pediatric patients
Note: Glimepiride is a sulfonamide and can be absorbed systemically. Sulfonamides can produce severe, possibly fatal, reactions such as toxic epidermal necrolysis and Stevens-Johnson syndrome
Avandaryl is glimepiride and rosiglitazone.

Central Nervous System
Headache [4]
Vertigo (dizziness) [2]

Neuromuscular/Skeletal
Arthralgia [2]

Gastrointestinal/Hepatic
Diarrhea [5]
Dyspepsia [2]
Nausea [4]
Pancreatitis [2]

Endocrine/Metabolic
Hypoglycemia [8]
Weight gain [3]

Genitourinary
Genital mycotic infections [3]
Urinary tract infection [3]

Other
Adverse effects [5]

GLIPIZIDE

Trade names: Glucotrol (Pfizer), Metaglip (Bristol-Myers Squibb)
Indications: Non-insulin dependent diabetes Type II
Class: Sulfonylurea
Half-life: 2–4 hours
Clinically important, potentially hazardous interactions with: none known
Pregnancy category: C
Important contra-indications noted in the prescribing guidelines for: the elderly; nursing mothers; pediatric patients
Note: Glipizide is a sulfonamide and can be absorbed systemically. Sulfonamides can produce severe, possibly fatal, reactions such as toxic epidermal necrolysis and Stevens-Johnson syndrome.

Skin
Photosensitivity (<10%)
Pruritus (<3%)
Rash (<10%)
Stevens-Johnson syndrome [2]
Urticaria (<10%)

Central Nervous System
Hyperesthesia (<3%)
Paresthesias (<3%)

Neuromuscular/Skeletal
Myalgia/Myopathy (<3%)

Endocrine/Metabolic
Hypoglycemia [3]

Other
Adverse effects [2]

GLUCAGON

Trade name: Glucagon Emergency Kit (Lilly)
Indications: Hypoglycemic reactions
Class: Hormone, polypeptide
Half-life: 3–10 minutes
Clinically important, potentially hazardous interactions with: insulin degludec, insulin glargine, insulin glulisine, warfarin
Pregnancy category: B

Skin
Erythema necrolyticum migrans [2]
Exanthems [7]
Folliculitis [2]
Pyoderma gangrenosum [3]
Rash [2]
Sweet's syndrome [7]
Urticaria (<10%) [2]
Vasculitis [9]

Local
Injection-site reactions [3]

GLUCOSAMINE

Trade names: Arthro-Aid (NutraSense), Glucosamine sulfate (Rottapharm)
Indications: Arthritis, osteoarthritis, cartilage repair and maintenance, strained joints, improving joint function and range of motion, alleviating joint pain
Class: Amino sugar, Food supplement
Half-life: N/A
Clinically important, potentially hazardous interactions with: abciximab, cilostazol, citalopram, clopidogrel, eptifibatide, meloxicam
Pregnancy category: C

Mucosal
Oral vesiculation (7%)

Central Nervous System
Depression (6%)

Neuromuscular/Skeletal
Asthenia (fatigue) (9%) [2]

Gastrointestinal/Hepatic
Dyspepsia [2]
Hepatotoxicity [3]
Nausea [2]

Other
Adverse effects (6%) [4]
Allergic reactions (4%) [2]

GLYBURIDE

Synonyms: glibenclamide; glybenclamide
Trade names: Diabeta (Sanofi-Aventis), Glucovance (Bristol-Myers Squibb), Glynase (Pfizer), Micronase (Pfizer)
Indications: Non-insulin dependent diabetes Type II
Class: Sulfonylurea
Half-life: 5–16 hours
Clinically important, potentially hazardous interactions with: bosentan, colesevelam, letermovir, norfloxacin
Pregnancy category: C
Note: Glyburide is a sulfonamide and can be absorbed systemically. Sulfonamides can produce severe, possibly fatal, reactions such as toxic epidermal necrolysis and Stevens-Johnson syndrome.
Glucovance is glyburide and metformin.

Skin
Erythema (<5%)
Exanthems (<5%) [3]
Flushing [2]
Linear IgA bullous dermatosis [2]
Pemphigus [2]
Photosensitivity (<10%) [5]
Pruritus (<10%) [3]
Psoriasis [2]
Purpura [2]
Rash (<10%)
Urticaria (<5%) [4]
Vasculitis [5]

Endocrine/Metabolic
Hypoglycemia [2]
Weight gain [2]

Other
Adverse effects [2]

GLYCOPYRROLATE

Synonym: glycopyrronium bromide
Trade names: Cuvposa (Shionogi), Robinul (Forte), Seebri Neohaler (Novartis), Utibron Neohaler (Novartis)
Indications: Duodenal ulcer, irritable bowel syndrome, hyperhidrosis
Class: Anticholinergic, Muscarinic antagonist, Non-depolarizing muscle relaxant
Half-life: N/A
Clinically important, potentially hazardous interactions with: anticholinergics, arbutamine, belladonna alkaloids, digoxin, disopyramide, meperidine, phenothiazines, procainamide, quinidine, ritodrine, tricyclic antidepressants
Pregnancy category: C
Important contra-indications noted in the prescribing guidelines for: the elderly; nursing mothers; pediatric patients
Note: Utibron Neohaler is glycopyrrolate and indacaterol.

Skin
Flushing (30%)
Photosensitivity (<10%)
Rash [2]

Xerosis (>10%)

Mucosal
Nasal congestion (30%)
Xerostomia (40%) [10]

Cardiovascular
Bradycardia [2]

Central Nervous System
Headache (15%) [2]

Gastrointestinal/Hepatic
Constipation (35%) [2]
Vomiting (40%)

Respiratory
Sinusitis (15%)
Upper respiratory tract infection (15%)

Genitourinary
Urinary retention (15%)

Ocular
Mydriasis [2]

Local
Injection-site irritation (>10%)

GOLDENSEAL

Family: Ranunculaceae
Scientific name: *Hydrastis canadensis*
Indications: Oral: Anorexia, fever, hemorrhoids, hemorrhage, liver disorders, menstrual disorders, rhinitis, upper respiratory tract infections, urinary tract infections. **Topical:** Acne, conjunctivitis, dandruff, earache, eczema, eye inflammation, herpes, itching, mouthwash, rash, ringworm, tinnitus, wounds
Class: Immunomodulator, Isoquinolone alkaloid
Half-life: N/A
Clinically important, potentially hazardous interactions with: clevidipine
Pregnancy category: N/A

GOLIMUMAB

Trade name: Simponi (Centocor)
Indications: Rheumatoid arthritis, psoriatic arthritis, ankylosing spondylitis, ulcerative colitis
Class: Disease-modifying antirheumatic drug (DMARD), Monoclonal antibody, TNF inhibitor
Half-life: 2 weeks
Clinically important, potentially hazardous interactions with: abatacept, anakinra, live vaccines
Pregnancy category: B
Important contra-indications noted in the prescribing guidelines for: nursing mothers; pediatric patients
Note: TNF inhibitors should be used in patients with heart failure only after consideration of other treatment options. TNF inhibitors are contra-indicated in patients with a personal or family history of multiple sclerosis or demyelinating disease. TNF inhibitors should not be administered to patients with moderate to severe heart failure (New York Heart Association Functional Class III/IV).
Warning: SERIOUS INFECTIONS AND MALIGNANCY

Skin
Lupus erythematosus [3]
Malignancies [5]
Psoriasis [2]
Rash [3]

Cardiovascular
Hypertension [2]

Central Nervous System
Headache [7]

Neuromuscular/Skeletal
Arthralgia [3]
Asthenia (fatigue) [2]

Gastrointestinal/Hepatic
Colitis [2]
Diarrhea [4]
Nausea [6]

Respiratory
Cough [2]
Nasopharyngitis (6%) [7]
Pneumonia [4]
Pulmonary toxicity [2]
Tuberculosis [2]
Upper respiratory tract infection (7%) [7]

Endocrine/Metabolic
ALT increased [4]
AST increased [3]

Genitourinary
Urinary tract infection [2]

Hematologic
Sepsis [4]

Local
Injection-site erythema [7]
Injection-site reactions (6%) [7]

Other
Adverse effects [13]
Death [3]
Infection (28%) [18]

GRAPEFRUIT JUICE

Family: Rutaceae
Scientific names: *Citrus decumana, Citrus maxima, Citrus paradisi*
Indications: Atherosclerosis, anti-cancer agent, cholesterol reduction, psoriasis, weight reduction, source of potassium, vitamin C, and fiber
Class: CYP3A4 inhibitor, Food supplement
Half-life: N/A
Clinically important, potentially hazardous interactions with: abemaciclib, alprazolam, ambrisentan, amiodarone, amitriptyline, aprepitant, astemizole, atorvastatin, bexarotene, brigatinib, buspirone, cabazitaxel, cabozantinib, ceritinib, cilostazol, colchicine, copanlisib, corticosteroids, crizotinib, cyclosporine, deflazacort, dronedarone, efavirenz, eliglustat, enalapril, eplerenone, estradiol, everolimus, felodipine, flibanserin, gefitinib, ibrutinib, indinavir, itraconazole, ivacaftor, ixabepilone, lapatinib, lercanidipine, lomitapide, lovastatin, midazolam, midostaurin, mifepristone, naloxegol, neratinib, nifedipine, nilotinib, nisoldipine, olaparib, palbociclib, pazopanib, pimozide, ponatinib, prednisolone, prednisone, propafenone, ranolazine, red rice yeast, regorafenib, repaglinide, ribociclib, rosiglitazone, rupatadine, ruxolitinib, sildenafil, simvastatin, sunitinib, tacrolimus, tadalafil, temsirolimus, terfenadine, tezacaftor/ivacaftor, tolvaptan, vardenafil, venetoclax, voriconazole, warfarin
Pregnancy category: N/A

Skin
Toxicity [2]

Central Nervous System
Headache [3]

Neuromuscular/Skeletal
Rhabdomyolysis [3]

Other
Adverse effects [2]

GREEN TEA

Family: Theaceae
Scientific names: *Camellia sinensis, Camellia thea, Camellia theifera, Thea bohea, Thea sinensis, Thea viridis*
Indications: Improving cognitive performance, stomach disorders, nausea, vomiting, diarrhea, anticancer, headaches, Crohn's disease. **Topical**: soothe sunburn, bleeding gums, reduce sweating
Class: Food supplement, TNF inhibitor, Xanthine alkaloid
Half-life: N/A
Clinically important, potentially hazardous interactions with: none known
Pregnancy category: N/A
Note: Tea is consumed as a beverage.

Gastrointestinal/Hepatic
Hepatotoxicity [9]

Other
Adverse effects [5]

GRISEOFULVIN

Trade names: Fulvicin (Schering), Grifulvin V (Ortho), Gris-PEG (Pedinol)
Indications: Fungal infections of the skin, hair and nails
Class: Antifungal
Half-life: 9–24 hours
Clinically important, potentially hazardous interactions with: alcohol, levonorgestrel, liraglutide, midazolam, thalidomide, ulipristal
Pregnancy category: C
Important contra-indications noted in the prescribing guidelines for: nursing mothers; pediatric patients

---

Skin
Angioedema [3]
Bullous dermatitis [2]
Cold urticaria [2]
Erythema multiforme [6]
Exanthems [6]
Exfoliative dermatitis [2]
Fixed eruption [7]
Lichenoid eruption [2]
Lupus erythematosus [14]
Petechiae [2]
Photosensitivity (<10%) [18]

Pigmentation [2]
Pruritus [4]
Rash (>10%)
Serum sickness-like reaction [3]
Stevens-Johnson syndrome [3]
Toxic epidermal necrolysis [4]
Urticaria (>10%) [5]
Vasculitis [2]

Mucosal
Oral candidiasis (<10%)

Central Nervous System
Dysgeusia (taste perversion) [3]

Endocrine/Metabolic
Gynecomastia [2]
Porphyria [12]

Other
Adverse effects [2]
Allergic reactions (<5%)

GUARANA

Family: Sapindaceae
Scientific names: *Paullinia cupana, Paullinia sorbilis*
Indications: Aphrodisiac, diarrhea, fatigue, fever, heart problems, headache, mental alertness, neuralgia, weight loss. Cosmetic products, anti-cellulite creams, shampoo for hair loss. Flavoring
Class: Stimulant, mild
Half-life: N/A
Clinically important, potentially hazardous interactions with: caffeine, clozapine, ephedra, MAO inhibitors
Pregnancy category: N/A
Note: The main constituent of guarana is caffeine. It contains more than twice as much caffeine as coffee or tea. Excessive consumption of caffeine is contraindicated for persons with high blood pressure, cardiac disorders, diabetes, ulcers, and epilepsy. See also separate profile for caffeine.

Central Nervous System
Seizures [2]

Other
Adverse effects [7]

GUSELKUMAB

Trade name: Tremfya (Janssen Biotech)
Indications: Moderate-to-severe plaque psoriasis
Class: Interleukin-23 inhibitor, Monoclonal antibody
Half-life: 15–18 days
Clinically important, potentially hazardous interactions with: live vaccines
Pregnancy category: N/A (Insufficient evidence to inform drug-associated risk)
Important contra-indications noted in the prescribing guidelines for: nursing mothers; pediatric patients

---

Skin
Pruritus [2]

Central Nervous System
Headache (5%) [8]

Neuromuscular/Skeletal
Arthralgia (3%) [2]
Back pain [3]

Gastrointestinal/Hepatic
Diarrhea (2%)
Hepatotoxicity (3%)

Respiratory
Nasopharyngitis [15]
Upper respiratory tract infection (14%) [10]

Local
Injection-site erythema [2]
Injection-site reactions (5%) [2]

Other
Infection [6]

HALOPERIDOL

Trade name: Haldol (Ortho-McNeil)
Indications: Schizophrenia, Tourette's disorder
Class: Antiemetic, Antipsychotic
Half-life: 20 hours
Clinically important, potentially hazardous interactions with: acemetacin, arsenic, benztropine, citalopram, clozapine, darifenacin, fluoxetine, itraconazole, lisdexamfetamine, lithium, meloxicam, methotrexate, moxifloxacin, nilotinib, oxybutynin, propranolol, quinine, ribociclib, sotalol, sulpiride, tetrabenazine, tiotropium, trospium, vandetanib, venlafaxine
Pregnancy category: C
Important contra-indications noted in the prescribing guidelines for: the elderly; pediatric patients
Warning: INCREASED MORTALITY IN ELDERLY PATIENTS WITH DEMENTIA-RELATED PSYCHOSIS

Skin
Cellulitis [2]
Diaphoresis [2]
Photosensitivity [3]
Seborrheic dermatitis [2]

Hair
Alopecia areata [2]

Mucosal
Xerostomia [4]

Cardiovascular
Arrhythmias [2]
QT prolongation [23]
Torsades de pointes [12]

Central Nervous System
Agitation [4]
Akathisia [9]
Delirium [3]
Extrapyramidal symptoms [9]
Headache [2]
Insomnia [4]
Neuroleptic malignant syndrome [36]
Parkinsonism [8]
Sedation [3]
Somnolence (drowsiness) [6]
Tardive dyskinesia (<37%) [5]
Tremor [7]
Vertigo (dizziness) [3]

Neuromuscular/Skeletal
Dystonia [3]
Myoclonus [2]
Rhabdomyolysis [7]

Gastrointestinal/Hepatic
Constipation [2]
Pancreatitis [2]

Respiratory
Pneumonia [2]

Endocrine/Metabolic
Galactorrhea [4]
Hyperprolactinemia [2]
Hypoglycemia [2]
SIADH [3]
Weight gain [2]

Genitourinary
Priapism [3]
Urinary retention [3]

Local
Injection-site reactions [3]

Other
Adverse effects [5]
Death [7]

HAWTHORN (FRUIT, LEAF, FLOWER EXTRACT)

Family: Rosaceae
Scientific names: *Crataegus laevigata, Crataegus monogyna, Crataegus oxyacantha, Crataegus pentagyna*
Indications: Amenorrhea, arrhythmias, atherosclerosis, diuretic, hyperlipidemia, hypertension, hypotension, sedative, appetite stimulant, arthritis, enteritis, indigestion, sore throats. **Topical:** boils, sores and ulcers
Class: Cardio-stimulant
Half-life: N/A
Clinically important, potentially hazardous interactions with: clevidipine, squill, vasodilators
Pregnancy category: N/A
Note: The American Herbal Products Association (AHPA) gives hawthorn a class I safety rating, indicating that it is very safe. However, hawthorn should be used with caution in patients with heart disease.

Skin
Hypersensitivity [2]
Rash (hands) [4]

Cardiovascular
Circulatory collapse [2]
Palpitation [2]

Central Nervous System
Headache [2]
Migraine [2]
Vertigo (dizziness) [4]

Gastrointestinal/Hepatic
Hepatotoxicity [2]

Other
Adverse effects [2]

HEMOPHILUS B VACCINE

Trade names: ActHIB (Sanofi-Aventis), Comvax (Merck), HibTITER (Lederle), OmniHIB (GSK), PedivaxHIB (Merck), ProHIBIT (Connaught)
Indications: Hemophilus B immunization
Class: Vaccine
Half-life: N/A
Clinically important, potentially hazardous interactions with: azathioprine, basiliximab, corticosteroids, cyclosporine, daclizumab, glatiramer, mycophenolate, sirolimus, tacrolimus
Pregnancy category: C

Skin
Erythema [2]

HENNA

Family: Lythraceae
Scientific names: *Lawsonia alba, Lawsonia inermis*
Indications: Analgesic, antipyretic, seborrheic dermatitis, fungal infections, gastrointestinal ulcers, sunscreen, dandruff, scabies, headache, jaundice, decorative tattoos, Used in cosmetics, body paint, hair dyes, hair care products
Class: Anti-inflammatory
Half-life: N/A
Clinically important, potentially hazardous interactions with: none known
Pregnancy category: N/A
Note: Black Henna is henna plus paraphenylenediamine (PPD). PPD is added to henna to make it stain black. PPD is a transdermal toxin and may be used alone as hair dye or to stain skin black. Other products called 'black henna' may have indigo or food dyes added, and are generally not harmful to the skin.
Adverse side effects to pure henna are rare; those reported above may be due to additives. Henna tattoos were popularized by the singer, Madonna. Her black patterns, however, were created with body paint, not henna.

Skin
Angioedema [3]
Dermatitis [34]
Edema [3]
Erythema [3]
Hypersensitivity [10]
Lichenoid eruption [4]
Pigmentation [3]
Pruritus [3]
Urticaria [3]

Other
Adverse effects [2]
Allergic reactions [3]
Death [3]

HEPARIN

Trade names: Hep-Flush (Wyeth), Viaflex (Baxter)
Indications: Venous thrombosis, pulmonary embolism, intravascular coagulation, peripheral arterial embolism
Class: Anticoagulant, Heparinoid
Half-life: 2 hours
Clinically important, potentially hazardous interactions with: acenocoumarol, aliskiren, antihistamines, aspirin, balsalazide, bivalirudin, butabarbital, ceftobiprole, dabigatran, danaparoid, defibrotide, desvenlafaxine, iloprost, nandrolone, nicotine, nitroglycerin, palifermin, piperacillin/tazobactam, salicylates, tirofiban, warfarin
Pregnancy category: C
Important contra-indications noted in the prescribing guidelines for: the elderly
Note: A higher incidence of bleeding has been reported in patients over 60 years of age, especially women. Contra-indicated in patients with severe thrombocyopenia.

Skin
Anaphylactoid reactions/Anaphylaxis [4]
Bullous dermatitis [4]
Dermatitis [6]
Ecchymoses [3]
Erythema [2]
Exanthems [2]
Hypersensitivity [17]
Lesions [2]
Livedo reticularis [2]
Necrosis [56]
Petechiae [2]
Purpura (>10%)
Toxic epidermal necrolysis [2]
Urticaria [6]
Vasculitis [6]

Hair
Alopecia [2]

Mucosal
Gingivitis (>10%)

Genitourinary
Priapism [6]

Hematologic
Bleeding [2]
Hemorrhage [7]
Thrombocytopenia [102]
Thrombosis [9]

Local
Injection-site eczematous eruption [5]
Injection-site induration [4]
Injection-site necrosis [4]
Injection-site plaques [2]

Other
Allergic reactions (<10%) [3]
Death [6]

HEPATITIS A VACCINE

Trade names: Avaxim (Sanofi Pasteur), Havrix (GSK), Vaqta (Merck)
Indications: Hepatitis A immunization
Class: Vaccine
Half-life: >2 years
Clinically important, potentially hazardous interactions with: none known
Pregnancy category: C

Skin
Rash (<10%)

Central Nervous System
Anorexia (<10%)
Chills (<10%)
Fever (>10%) [2]
Guillain–Barré syndrome [2]
Headache (>10%) [3]
Somnolence (drowsiness) (>10%)

Neuromuscular/Skeletal
Arm pain (<10%)
Asthenia (fatigue) (<10%)
Back pain (<10%)

Gastrointestinal/Hepatic
Constipation (<10%)
Diarrhea (<10%)
Nausea (<10%)
Vomiting (<10%)

Respiratory
Cough (<10%)
Nasopharyngitis (<10%)
Pharyngitis (<10%)
Rhinitis (<10%)
Upper respiratory tract infection (<10%)

Otic
Otitis media (<10%)

Ocular
Conjunctivitis (<10%)

Local
Injection-site erythema [2]
Injection-site pain (<10%) [7]
Injection-site reactions [5]

Other
Adverse effects [2]

HEPATITIS B VACCINE

Trade names: Comvax (Merck), Engerix B (GSK), Pediatrix (GSK), Recombivax HB (Merck), Twinrix (GSK)
Other common trade names: Heptavax-B
Indications: For immunization of infection caused by all known subtypes of hepatitis B virus
Class: Vaccine
Half-life: N/A
Clinically important, potentially hazardous interactions with: none known
Pregnancy category: C

Skin
Anaphylactoid reactions/Anaphylaxis [6]
Churg-Strauss syndrome [2]
Dermatomyositis [2]
Erythema multiforme [2]

Erythema nodosum [3]
Gianotti–Crosti syndrome [2]
Granuloma annulare [2]
Lichen planus [18]
Lichenoid eruption [4]
Lupus erythematosus [9]
Pemphigus [2]
Pseudolymphoma [2]
Purpura [6]
Raynaud's phenomenon [2]
Urticaria [3]
Vasculitis [11]

Hair
Alopecia [2]

Cardiovascular
Polyarteritis nodosa [5]

Central Nervous System
Guillain–Barré syndrome [4]
Neurotoxicity [2]

Neuromuscular/Skeletal
Arthralgia [4]

Ocular
Optic neuropathy [3]
Uveitis [2]

Local
Injection-site edema [2]
Injection-site erythema [2]
Injection-site pain (22%) [3]

Other
Adverse effects [2]
Death [2]

HOPS

Family: Cannabaceae
Scientific name: *Humulus lupulus*
Indications: Insomnia, anxiety, diuretic, appetite stimulant. Flavoring in foods and beverages
Class: Cannabinoid, Phytoestrogen, Sedative
Half-life: N/A
Clinically important, potentially hazardous interactions with: none known
Pregnancy category: N/A

Skin
Urticaria [2]

HORSE CHESTNUT (BARK, FLOWER, LEAF, SEED)

Family: Hippocastanaceae
Scientific name: *Aesculus hippocastanum*
Indications: Oral: malaria, dysentery, tinnitus, pancreatitis, cough, arthritis, rheumatism, chronic venous insufficiency. **Topical:** lupus, skin ulcers eczema, phlebitis, varicose veins, hemorrhoids, rectal problems
Class: Diuretic
Half-life: N/A
Clinically important, potentially hazardous interactions with: NSAIDs
Pregnancy category: N/A
Note: The active ingredient is a toxic glycoside, escin.

Other
Adverse effects (mild) [2]

HORSETAIL

Family: Equisetaceae
Scientific names: *Equisetum arvense, Equisetum myriochaetum, Equisetum ramosissimum, Equisetum telmateia*
Indications: Oral: Alopecia, diabetes, hepatitis, bacterial infections, osteoarthritis, pressure ulcers, urinary tract infections. **Topical:** burns
Class: Anti-inflammatory, Antioxidant, Diuretic
Half-life: N/A
Clinically important, potentially hazardous interactions with: diuretics, nicotine
Pregnancy category: N/A

Gastrointestinal/Hepatic
Hepatotoxicity [2]

HUMAN PAPILLOMA-VIRUS (HPV) VACCINE

Synonym: HPV4
Trade names: Gardasil (Merck), Silgard (Merck)
Indications: For prevention of HPV genital warts, cervical cancers and vulvar dysplasias (against Types 6, 11, 16 and 18 human papillomavirus)
Class: Vaccine
Half-life: N/A
Clinically important, potentially hazardous interactions with: immunosuppressants
Pregnancy category: B
Important contra-indications noted in the prescribing guidelines for: the elderly; nursing mothers; pediatric patients

Mucosal
Oropharyngeal pain (3%)

Central Nervous System
Cognitive impairment [2]
Fever (13%) [4]
Headache (28%) [9]
Myelitis [2]
Vertigo (dizziness) (<4%) [2]

Neuromuscular/Skeletal
Asthenia (fatigue) [5]
Myalgia/Myopathy [2]

Gastrointestinal/Hepatic
Diarrhea (3–4%)
Nausea (2–7%) [2]
Vomiting (<2%)

Respiratory
Cough (2%)
Nasopharyngitis (3%)
Upper respiratory tract infection (2%)

Local
Injection-site bruising (3%)
Injection-site edema (14–25%) [3]
Injection-site erythema (17–25%) [3]
Injection-site pain (61–84%) [5]
Injection-site pruritus (3%)
Injection-site reactions [6]

Other
Adverse effects [4]
Toothache (2%)

HUMAN PAPILLOMA-VIRUS VACCINE (BIVALENT)

Trade name: Cervarix (GSK)
Indications: Prevention of human papillomavirus (HPV) types 16 and 18 in females aged 10–25 years old
Class: Vaccine
Half-life: N/A
Clinically important, potentially hazardous interactions with: immunosuppressants
Pregnancy category: B
Important contra-indications noted in the prescribing guidelines for: the elderly; nursing mothers; pediatric patients

Skin
Anaphylactoid reactions/Anaphylaxis (3%) [2]
Erythema (<10%) [4]
Pruritus (<10%)
Rash (<10%)
Urticaria (7%)

Central Nervous System
Fever (13%) [3]
Headache (53%) [2]

Neuromuscular/Skeletal
Arthralgia (21%)
Asthenia (fatigue) (55%)
Myalgia/Myopathy (49%)

Gastrointestinal/Hepatic
Abdominal pain (28%)
Diarrhea (28%)
Nausea (28%)
Vomiting (28%)

Local
Injection-site edema (44%) [3]
Injection-site erythema (48%)
Injection-site pain (92%) [9]
Injection-site reactions [5]

Other
Adverse effects [2]

HYALURONIC ACID

Synonym: hyaluronidase
Trade names: Euflexxa (Ferring), Hyalgan (Sanofi-Aventis), Hylan G-F 20 (Synvisc), Juvederm (Allergan), Perlane (Q-Med AB), Restylane Fine Lines (Medicis), Vitrase (ISTA Pharma)
Indications: Oral: joint disorders **Injection**: adjunct in eye surgery, viscosupplementation in orthopedics, cosmetic surgery **Topical**: wounds, burns, skin ulcers, stomatitis
Class: Food supplement, Glycoaminoglycan
Half-life: 2.5–5.5 minutes
Clinically important, potentially hazardous interactions with: furosemide, local anesthetics, NSAIDs, oral anticoagulants
Pregnancy category: C
Important contra-indications noted in the prescribing guidelines for: nursing mothers; pediatric patients
Note: Most reported reactions relate to orthopedic use.

Skin
- Acneform eruption (<29%)
- Anaphylactoid reactions/Anaphylaxis [2]
- Angioedema [6]
- Churg-Strauss syndrome [12]
- Dermatitis (24%)
- Ecchymoses [3]
- Edema [9]
- Erythema [6]
- Erythema multiforme [2]
- Facial edema [3]
- Granulomatous reaction [2]
- Hematoma [2]
- Herpes simplex [2]
- Hypersensitivity [6]
- Induration [2]
- Inflammation [7]
- Necrosis [4]
- Nodular eruption [2]
- Pigmentation [2]
- Pruritus [4]

Cardiovascular
- Arterial occlusion [2]
- Hypertension (4%)

Central Nervous System
- Pain [4]

Neuromuscular/Skeletal
- Arthralgia [9]
- Back pain (5%)
- Chondritis (<11%) [2]
- Gouty tophi [3]
- Tendinitis (2%)

Gastrointestinal/Hepatic
- Nausea (2%)

Ocular
- Orbital inflammation [2]

Local
- Injection-site bruising [4]
- Injection-site ecchymoses [2]
- Injection-site edema (20%) [13]
- Injection-site erythema (47%) [9]
- Injection-site granuloma [2]
- Injection-site nodules [3]
- Injection-site pain (8–47%) [16]
- Injection-site pruritus [2]
- Injection-site reactions (<11%) [12]

Other
- Adverse effects [14]
- Infection [2]

HYDRALAZINE

Trade names: Apresazide (Novartis), Apresoline (Novartis), Ser-Ap-Es (Novartis)
Indications: Hypertension
Class: Vasodilator
Half-life: 3–7 hours
Clinically important, potentially hazardous interactions with: acebutolol, alfuzosin, captopril, cilazapril, diclofenac, enalapril, fosinopril, levodopa, levomepromazine, lisinopril, meloxicam, olmesartan, quinapril, ramipril, trandolapril, triamcinolone, trifluoperazine, zuclopenthixol
Pregnancy category: C
Note: Apresazide is hydralazine and hydrochlorothiazide; Ser-Ap-Es is hydralazine, reserpine and hydrochlorothiazide.
Hydrochlorothiazide is a sulfonamide and can be absorbed systemically. Sulfonamides can produce severe, possibly fatal, reactions such as toxic epidermal necrolysis and Stevens-Johnson syndrome.

Skin
- Edema [2]
- Exanthems [4]
- Flushing (>10%)
- Lupus erythematosus (7%) [114]
- Photosensitivity [2]
- Purpura [3]
- Sweet's syndrome [6]
- Toxic epidermal necrolysis [2]
- Ulcerations [2]
- Vasculitis [14]

Mucosal
- Oral ulceration [2]
- Orogenital ulceration [2]

Gastrointestinal/Hepatic
- Hepatitis [2]
- Hepatotoxicity [2]

Respiratory
- Alveolar hemorrhage (pulmonary) [2]

Renal
- Glomerulonephritis [5]

HYDROCHLOROTHIAZIDE

Trade names: Accuretic (Pfizer), Aldactazide (Pfizer), Aldoril (Merck), Atacand HCT (AstraZeneca), Avalide (Bristol-Myers Squibb), Capozide (Par), Diovan HCT (Novartis), Dyazide (GSK), Hyzaar (Merck), Inderide (Wyeth), Lopressor (Novartis), Lotensin (Novartis), Lotensin HCT (Novartis), Micardis (Boehringer Ingelheim), Microzide (Watson), Moduretic (Merck), Prinzide (Merck), Tekturna HCT (Novartis), Teveten HCT (Biovail), Uniretic (Schwarz), Vaseretic (Biovail), Zestoretic (AstraZeneca), Ziac (Barr)
Indications: Edema
Class: Diuretic, thiazide
Half-life: 5.6–14.8 hours
Clinically important, potentially hazardous interactions with: digoxin, dofetilide, lithium, zinc
Pregnancy category: B
Important contra-indications noted in the prescribing guidelines for: nursing mothers; pediatric patients
Note: Hydrochlorothiazide is a sulfonamide and can be absorbed systemically. Sulfonamides can produce severe, possibly fatal, reactions such as toxic epidermal necrolysis and Stevens-Johnson syndrome.
Hydrochlorothiazide is often used in combination, e.g. with aliskiren (Tekturna HCT); amiloride (Moduretic); benazepril (Lotensin HCT); bisoprolol (Ziac); captopril (Capozide); enalapril (Vaseretic); irbesartan (Avalide); lisinopril (Prinzide and Zestoretic); losartan (Hyzaar); methyldopa (Aldoril); moexipril (Uniretic); spironolactone (Aldactazide); triamterene (Dyazide and Maxzide).

Skin
- Dermatitis [2]
- Diaphoresis [2]
- Edema [2]
- Erythema annulare centrifugum [2]
- Lichenoid eruption [5]
- Lupus erythematosus [16]
- Peripheral edema [5]
- Photosensitivity [20]
- Phototoxicity [5]
- Purpura [7]
- Rash [2]
- Toxic epidermal necrolysis [2]
- Vasculitis [3]

Cardiovascular
- Hypotension [6]
- Orthostatic hypotension [2]

Central Nervous System
- Headache [7]
- Vertigo (dizziness) [9]

Neuromuscular/Skeletal
- Asthenia (fatigue) [3]

Gastrointestinal/Hepatic
- Diarrhea [2]
- Nausea [2]
- Pancreatitis [4]

Respiratory
Upper respiratory tract infection [3]

Endocrine/Metabolic
Hyponatremia [4]
Serum creatinine increased [2]
SIADH [4]

Renal
Nephrotoxicity [2]

Ocular
Glaucoma [2]

Other
Adverse effects [5]
Death [2]

HYDROCODONE

Trade names: Duratuss (UCB), Entex HC (Andrx), Hycotuss (Endo), Hydromet (Actavis), Hysingla ER (Purdue), Lortab (UCB), Maxidone (Watson), Norco (Watson), Tussionex (Celltech), Vicodin (AbbVie), Vicoprofen (AbbVie), Zohydro ER (Pernix), Zydone (Endo)
Indications: Acute pain, coughing
Class: Opiate agonist
Half-life: 3.8 hours
Clinically important, potentially hazardous interactions with: alcohol, buprenorphine, butorphanol, CYP3A4 inhibitors or inducers, MAO inhibitors, nalbuphine, pentazocine
Pregnancy category: C
Important contra-indications noted in the prescribing guidelines for: nursing mothers; pediatric patients
Note: Hydrocodone is included in many combination drugs. Other medications that can be included in these preparations include: phenylpropanolamine, phenylephrine, pyrilamine, pseudoephedrine, acetaminophen, ibuprofen, and others. Zohydro ER is the first extended-release, single-entity hydrocodone-containing drug product approved by the FDA and reflects the newly updated labeling requirements recently announced by the FDA.
Warning: ADDICTION, ABUSE, AND MISUSE; LIFE-THREATENING RESPIRATORY DEPRESSION; ACCIDENTAL INGESTION; NEONATAL OPIOID WITHDRAWAL SYNDROME; INTERACTION WITH ALCOHOL; and CYTOCHROME P450 3A4 INTERACTION

Skin
Hot flashes (<10%)
Hyperhidrosis (<10%)
Peripheral edema (<3%)
Pruritus (3%) [2]
Rash (<10%)

Mucosal
Xerostomia (3%)

Cardiovascular
Chest pain (<10%)

Central Nervous System
Fever (<10%)
Headache [2]
Migraine (<10%)
Paresthesias (<10%)
Somnolence (drowsiness) (<5%) [4]
Tremor (3%)
Vertigo (dizziness) (2–3%) [4]

Neuromuscular/Skeletal
Arthralgia (<10%)
Asthenia (fatigue) (<4%)
Back pain (<4%) [2]
Bone or joint pain (<10%)
Muscle spasm (<3%)
Myalgia/Myopathy (<10%)
Neck pain (<10%)
Pain in extremities (<10%)

Gastrointestinal/Hepatic
Abdominal pain (2–3%)
Constipation (8–11%) [7]
Gastroesophageal reflux (<10%)
Nausea (7–10%) [9]
Vomiting [8]

Respiratory
Cough (<10%)
Dyspnea (<10%)
Respiratory depression [2]
Upper respiratory tract infection (<3%)

Endocrine/Metabolic
Dehydration (<10%)
GGT increased (<10%)
Hypokalemia (<10%)

Genitourinary
Urinary tract infection (<5%)

HYDROMORPHONE

Trade names: Dilaudid (AbbVie), Exalgo (Mallinckrodt), Jurnista (Janssen-Cilag), Palladone (Napp)
Indications: Pain
Class: Opiate agonist
Half-life: 1–3 hours; 2 hours (IV)
Clinically important, potentially hazardous interactions with: alcohol, alvimopan, ammonium chloride, amphetamines, anticholinergics, anxiolytics and hypnotics, buprenorphine, butorphanol, cimetidine, CNS depressants, desmopressin, domperidone, droperidol, linezolid, MAO inhibitors, metoclopramide, moclobemide, nalbuphine, pegvisomant, pentazocine, phenothiazines, sodium oxybate, SSRIs, St John's wort, succinylcholine, thiazide diuretics
Pregnancy category: C
Important contra-indications noted in the prescribing guidelines for: nursing mothers; pediatric patients
Note: OROS hydromorphone prolonged release (Jurnista) is a once-daily formulation of hydromorphone that utilizes OROS (osmotic-controlled release oral delivery system) technology to deliver the drug at a near constant rate.
Warning: ADDICTION, ABUSE, AND MISUSE; LIFE-THREATENING RESPIRATORY DEPRESSION; ACCIDENTAL INGESTION; NEONATAL OPIOID WITHDRAWAL SYNDROME; and INTERACTION WITH ALCOHOL

Skin
Flushing (<10%)
Pruritus (<11%) [12]

Mucosal
Xerostomia (<10%)

Cardiovascular
Bradycardia [2]
Hypotension [2]

Central Nervous System
Agitation [3]
Dysgeusia (taste perversion) [3]
Headache [5]
Hyperalgesia [3]
Somnolence (drowsiness) [6]
Tremor [2]
Vertigo (dizziness) [10]

Neuromuscular/Skeletal
Asthenia (fatigue) [5]
Myoclonus [3]

Gastrointestinal/Hepatic
Constipation [11]
Nausea [18]
Vomiting [11]

Endocrine/Metabolic
Appetite decreased [2]

Other
Adverse effects [7]

HYDROQUINONE

Trade names: Ambi (Johnson & Johnson), Lustra (Taro)
Indications: Ultraviolet induced dyschromia and discoloration resulting from the use of oral contraceptives, pregnancy, hormone replacement therapy, or skin trauma
Class: Depigmentation agent
Half-life: N/A
Clinically important, potentially hazardous interactions with: none known
Pregnancy category: C
Important contra-indications noted in the prescribing guidelines for: nursing mothers; pediatric patients

---

Skin
Acneform eruption [2]
Burning [2]
Contact dermatitis (localized) [2]
Depigmentation [2]
Erythema [4]
Ochronosis [15]
Peeling [2]
Pigmentation [3]
Pruritus [2]
Scaling [2]
Striae [2]
Xerosis [2]

Other
Adverse effects [3]

HYDROXY-CHLOROQUINE

Trade name: Plaquenil (Sanofi-Aventis)
Indications: Malaria, lupus erythematosus, rheumatoid arthritis
Class: Antimalarial, Antiprotozoal, Disease-modifying antirheumatic drug (DMARD)
Half-life: 32–50 days
Clinically important, potentially hazardous interactions with: chloroquine, cholestyramine, dapsone, droperidol, ethosuximide, lacosamide, lanthanum, moxifloxacin, neostigmine, oxcarbazepine, penicillamine, tiagabine, typhoid vaccine, vigabatrin, yellow fever vaccine
Pregnancy category: C
Important contra-indications noted in the prescribing guidelines for: nursing mothers; pediatric patients

---

Skin
AGEP [23]
Bullous dermatitis [2]
DRESS syndrome [3]
Erythema annulare centrifugum [3]
Erythema multiforme [2]
Erythroderma [3]
Exanthems (<5%) [4]
Exfoliative dermatitis [3]
Lichenoid eruption [4]
Photosensitivity [6]
Phototoxicity [3]
Pigmentation (<10%) [19]
Pruritus (>10%) [13]
Psoriasis (exacerbation) [14]
Rash (<10%) [4]
Thrombocytopenic purpura [2]
Toxic epidermal necrolysis [3]
Urticaria [2]

Hair
Alopecia [2]
Hair pigmentation (bleaching) (<10%) [8]

Nails
Nail pigmentation [3]

Mucosal
Oral pigmentation [7]
Stomatitis [2]

Cardiovascular
Cardiomyopathy [8]
Cardiotoxicity [4]
QT prolongation [3]

Central Nervous System
Anorexia [2]
Dysgeusia (taste perversion) [2]
Headache [2]
Neurotoxicity [3]

Neuromuscular/Skeletal
Asthenia (fatigue) [3]
Myalgia/Myopathy [8]

Gastrointestinal/Hepatic
Diarrhea [5]
Dysphagia [2]
Nausea [6]
Vomiting [4]

Endocrine/Metabolic
Hypoglycemia [4]
Porphyria [7]
Weight loss [2]

Hematologic
Anemia [3]
Neutropenia [2]
Thrombocytopenia [4]

Otic
Hearing loss [2]

Ocular
Maculopathy [5]
Ocular adverse effects [2]
Ocular toxicity [9]
Reduced visual acuity [2]
Retinopathy [30]
Vision blurred [3]

Other
Adverse effects [8]
Death [3]

HYDROXYUREA

Synonym: hydroxycarbamide
Trade names: Droxia (Bristol-Myers Squibb), Hydrea (Bristol-Myers Squibb)
Indications: Leukemia, malignant tumors
Class: Antineoplastic, Antiretroviral
Half-life: 3–4 hours
Clinically important, potentially hazardous interactions with: adefovir, aldesleukin
Pregnancy category: D

Skin
Acral erythema [8]
Atrophy [4]
Dermatitis [3]
Dermatomyositis [29]
Exanthems (<10%)
Fixed eruption [4]
Ichthyosis [3]
Keratoses [2]
Leg ulceration (29%) [20]
Lichen planus [3]
Lichenoid eruption [3]
Lupus erythematosus [3]
Palmar–plantar desquamation [6]
Pigmentation (<58%) [18]
Poikiloderma [3]
Pruritus [3]
Purpura [2]
Radiation recall dermatitis [2]
Squamous cell carcinoma [2]
Telangiectasia [2]
Tumors [5]
Ulcerations [27]
Vasculitis [6]
Xerosis (<10%) [7]

Hair
Alopecia (<10%) [8]

Nails
Atrophic nails [3]
Melanonychia [7]
Nail changes [4]
Nail dystrophy [2]
Nail pigmentation [18]
Onycholysis [2]

Mucosal
Oral lesions [2]
Oral pigmentation [2]
Oral squamous cell carcinoma [2]
Oral ulceration [8]
Stomatitis (>10%) [4]
Tongue pigmentation (<29%) [3]

Gastrointestinal/Hepatic
Pancreatitis [2]

Other
Adverse effects [2]
Death [2]
Side effects (7–35%) [3]

HYDROXYZINE

Trade names: Atarax (Pfizer), Vistaril (Pfizer)
Indications: Anxiety and tension, pruritus
Class: Histamine H1 receptor antagonist, Muscarinic antagonist
Half-life: 3–7 hours
Clinically important, potentially hazardous interactions with: alcohol, barbiturates, CNS depressants, efavirenz, lurasidone, narcotics, non-narcotic analgesics
Pregnancy category: C
Important contra-indications noted in the prescribing guidelines for: nursing mothers

---

Skin
AGEP [3]
Anaphylactoid reactions/Anaphylaxis [2]
Angioedema [3]
Erythema multiforme [2]
Exanthems [3]
Fixed eruption [3]
Urticaria [4]

Mucosal
Xerostomia (12%) [4]

Central Nervous System
Somnolence (drowsiness) [5]

Gastrointestinal/Hepatic
Vomiting [2]

HYOSCYAMINE

Trade names: IB-Stat (InKline), Levbid (Schwarz), Levsin (Schwarz), Levsin/SL (Schwarz), Levsinex (Schwarz), Nulev (Schwarz)
Indications: Treatment of gastrointestinal tract disorders caused by spasm, adjunctive therapy for peptic ulcers, cystitis, Parkinsonism, biliary and renal colic
Class: Anticholinergic, Muscarinic antagonist
Half-life: N/A
Clinically important, potentially hazardous interactions with: anticholinergics, arbutamine
Pregnancy category: C
Important contra-indications noted in the prescribing guidelines for: the elderly; nursing mothers; pediatric patients

---

Skin
Photosensitivity (<10%)
Xerosis (>10%)

Mucosal
Xerostomia (>10%)

Cardiovascular
Tachycardia [2]

Local
Injection-site inflammation (>10%)

IBANDRONATE

Synonym: ibandronic acid
Trade names: Bondronat (Roche), Boniva (Roche)
Indications: Postmenopausal osteoporosis
Class: Bisphosphonate
Half-life: 37–157 hours
Clinically important, potentially hazardous interactions with: alcohol, aminoglycosides, antacids, calcium salts, food, magnesium salts, NSAIDs, oral iron
Pregnancy category: C
Important contra-indications noted in the prescribing guidelines for: nursing mothers; pediatric patients

---

Skin
Rash (<2%)

Cardiovascular
Hypertension (6–7%)

Central Nervous System
Fever (~9%) [4]
Headache (3–7%)
Vertigo (dizziness) (<4%)

Neuromuscular/Skeletal
Arthralgia (3–6%) [2]
Asthenia (fatigue) (4%) [3]
Back pain (4–14%)
Bone or joint pain [3]
Cramps (2%)
Joint disorder (4%)
Myalgia/Myopathy (<6%)
Osteonecrosis [13]
Pain in extremities (<8%)

Gastrointestinal/Hepatic
Abdominal pain (5–8%)
Constipation (3–4%)
Diarrhea (4–7%) [2]
Dyspepsia (6–12%) [4]
Gastritis (2%)
Gastrointestinal disorder [3]
Nausea (5%) [4]
Vomiting (3%) [4]

Respiratory
Bronchitis (3–10%)
Flu-like syndrome (<4%) [7]
Nasopharyngitis (4%)
Pharyngitis (3%)
Pneumonia (6%)
Upper respiratory tract infection (2–34%)

Endocrine/Metabolic
Hypercholesterolemia (5%)
Hypocalcemia [3]
Hypophosphatemia [2]

Genitourinary
Urinary tract infection (2–6%)

Other
Adverse effects [5]
Allergic reactions (3%)
Infection (4%)
Tooth disorder (4%)

IBRUTINIB

Trade name: Imbruvica (Pharmacyclics)
Indications: Mantle cell lymphoma
Class: Bruton's tyrosine kinase (BTK) inhibitor
Half-life: 4–6 hours
Clinically important, potentially hazardous interactions with: carbamazepine, clarithromycin, grapefruit juice, itraconazole, ketoconazole, phenytoin, posaconazole, rifampin, St John's wort, strong or moderate CYP3A inhibitors or inducers, telithromycin, voriconazole
Pregnancy category: D
Important contra-indications noted in the prescribing guidelines for: nursing mothers; pediatric patients

---

Skin
Cellulitis [3]
Ecchymoses (30%) [4]
Panniculitis [2]
Peripheral edema (35%) [3]
Petechiae (11%)
Rash (25%) [5]
Toxicity (14%) [3]
Tumor lysis syndrome [3]

Mucosal
Epistaxis (nosebleed) (11%)
Stomatitis (17%)

Cardiovascular
Atrial fibrillation [14]
Hypertension [7]
Hypotension [2]

Central Nervous System
Fever (18%) [5]
Headache (13%) [2]
Peripheral neuropathy [2]
Vertigo (dizziness) (14%)

Neuromuscular/Skeletal
Arthralgia (11%) [4]
Asthenia (fatigue) (14–41%) [21]
Bone or joint pain (37%)
Muscle spasm (14%) [2]

Gastrointestinal/Hepatic
Abdominal pain (24%)
Constipation (25%)
Diarrhea (51%) [28]
Dyspepsia (11%)
Hepatotoxicity [2]
Nausea (31%) [16]
Vomiting (24%) [4]

Respiratory
Cough (19%) [3]
Dyspnea (27%)
Pneumonia (14%) [8]
Sinusitis (13%) [2]
Upper respiratory tract infection (34%) [6]

Endocrine/Metabolic
Appetite decreased (21%)
Dehydration (12%) [2]
Hyperuricemia (15%)
Hypokalemia [2]

Genitourinary
Urinary tract infection (14%) [2]

Hematologic
Anemia [12]
Bleeding [12]
Cytopenia [3]
Febrile neutropenia [3]
Hemorrhage [4]
Lymphocytosis [2]
Neutropenia [15]
Sepsis [2]
Thrombocytopenia [14]

Other
Adverse effects [2]
Death [2]
Infection [9]

IBUPROFEN

Trade names: Advil (Wyeth), Motrin (McNeil), Vicoprofen (AbbVie)
Indications: Arthritis, pain
Class: Non-steroidal anti-inflammatory (NSAID)
Half-life: 2–4 hours
Clinically important, potentially hazardous interactions with: aspirin, ciprofibrate, diuretics, methotrexate, methyl salicylate, NSAIDs, oxycodone hydrochloride, salicylates, tacrine, tacrolimus, urokinase, voriconazole
Pregnancy category: D (category C prior to 30 weeks gestation; category D starting at 30 weeks gestation)
Note: NSAIDs may cause an increased risk of serious cardiovascular and gastrointestinal adverse events, which can be fatal. This risk may increase with duration of use.

Skin
AGEP [5]
Anaphylactoid reactions/Anaphylaxis [5]
Angioedema [8]
Bullous dermatitis [3]
Bullous pemphigoid [2]
Dermatitis [5]
DRESS syndrome [4]
Erythema multiforme [11]
Erythema nodosum (<5%)
Exanthems [9]
Fixed eruption [15]
Hypersensitivity [5]
Lupus erythematosus [5]
Nicolau syndrome [2]
Peripheral edema [2]
Photosensitivity [6]
Pruritus (<5%) [6]
Psoriasis (palms) [2]
Rash (>10%) [3]
Stevens-Johnson syndrome [12]
Toxic epidermal necrolysis [9]
Urticaria (>10%) [10]
Vasculitis [8]
Vesiculobullous eruption [2]

Hair
Alopecia [2]

Cardiovascular
Cardiotoxicity [2]
Hypertension [4]

Central Nervous System
- Aseptic meningitis [16]
- Headache [4]
- Somnolence (drowsiness) [2]

Neuromuscular/Skeletal
- Arthralgia [2]
- Back pain [2]
- Rhabdomyolysis [3]

Gastrointestinal/Hepatic
- Abdominal pain [6]
- Constipation [4]
- Diarrhea [4]
- Dyspepsia [5]
- Gastroesophageal reflux [2]
- Gastrointestinal bleeding [2]
- Gastrointestinal disorder [2]
- Hepatotoxicity [3]
- Nausea [7]
- Pancreatitis [2]
- Vanishing bile duct syndrome [2]
- Vomiting [5]

Respiratory
- Influenza [2]
- Sinusitis [2]
- Upper respiratory tract infection [2]

Endocrine/Metabolic
- Pseudoporphyria [2]

Genitourinary
- Urinary tract infection [2]

Renal
- Nephrotoxicity [4]

Hematologic
- Thrombocytopenia [5]

Otic
- Hearing loss [2]
- Tinnitus [2]

Ocular
- Amblyopia [2]
- Optic neuritis [2]
- Periorbital edema [3]
- Visual disturbances [2]

Other
- Adverse effects [13]
- Kounis syndrome [4]

IBUTILIDE

Trade name: Corvert (Pfizer)
Indications: Atrial fibrillation and flutter
Class: Antiarrhythmic, Antiarrhythmic class III
Half-life: 2–12 hours
Clinically important, potentially hazardous interactions with: degarelix
Pregnancy category: C
Important contra-indications noted in the prescribing guidelines for: nursing mothers; pediatric patients

---

Cardiovascular
- Bradycardia [4]
- Hypotension [2]
- QT prolongation [5]
- Tachycardia (3%)
- Torsades de pointes [10]
- Ventricular arrhythmia [4]
- Ventricular tachycardia [6]

Central Nervous System
- Headache (4%)

Gastrointestinal/Hepatic
- Nausea (2%) [3]

IDARUBICIN

Synonyms: 4-demethoxydaunorubicin; 4-DMDR
Trade name: Idamycin (Pfizer)
Indications: Acute myeloid leukemia
Class: Antibiotic, anthracycline
Half-life: 14–35 hours (oral)
Clinically important, potentially hazardous interactions with: aldesleukin
Pregnancy category: D
Important contra-indications noted in the prescribing guidelines for: nursing mothers; pediatric patients

---

Skin
- Rash (>10%) [4]
- Urticaria (>10%)

Hair
- Alopecia (77%) [8]

Mucosal
- Mucositis (50%) [5]
- Stomatitis (>10%)

Gastrointestinal/Hepatic
- Diarrhea [3]
- Hepatotoxicity [2]
- Nausea [2]
- Vomiting [2]

Hematologic
- Febrile neutropenia [2]
- Neutropenia [2]

Other
- Infection [2]

IDARUCIZUMAB

Trade name: Praxbind (Boehringer Ingelheim)
Indications: Reversal of the anticoagulant effects of dabigatran in patients requiring emergency or urgent surgery or with life-threatening or uncontrolled bleeding
Class: Monoclonal antibody, Reversal agent for dabigatran
Half-life: 10 hours
Clinically important, potentially hazardous interactions with: none known
Pregnancy category: N/A (No data available)
Important contra-indications noted in the prescribing guidelines for: nursing mothers; pediatric patients
Note: Risk of serious adverse reactions in patients with hereditary fructose intolerance due to sorbitol excipient.

Skin
- Irritation [2]

Central Nervous System
- Delirium (7%)
- Fever (6%)
- Headache [2]

Neuromuscular/Skeletal
- Back pain [2]

Gastrointestinal/Hepatic
- Constipation (7%)

Respiratory
- Nasopharyngitis [2]
- Pneumonia (6%)

Endocrine/Metabolic
- Hypokalemia (7%)

IDELALISIB

Trade name: Zydelig (Gilead)
Indications: Relapsed chronic lymphocytic leukemia (with rituximab), follicular B-cell non-Hodgkin lymphoma, small lymphocytic lymphoma
Class: Phosphoinositide 3-kinase (PI3K) inhibitor
Half-life: 8 hours
Clinically important, potentially hazardous interactions with: carbamazepine, copanlisib, midostaurin, neratinib, phenytoin, rifampin, St John's wort, strong CYP3A inducers and substrates
Pregnancy category: D
Important contra-indications noted in the prescribing guidelines for: nursing mothers; pediatric patients
Warning: FATAL AND SERIOUS TOXICITIES: HEPATIC, SEVERE DIARRHEA, COLITIS, PNEUMONITIS, and INTESTINAL PERFORATION

Skin
- Diaphoresis (12%)
- Peripheral edema (10%)
- Rash (21%) [8]
- Toxicity [2]

Central Nervous System
- Chills [5]
- Fever [9]
- Headache (11%)
- Insomnia (12%)

Neuromuscular/Skeletal
- Asthenia (fatigue) (30%) [8]

Gastrointestinal/Hepatic
- Abdominal pain (26%)
- Colitis [6]
- Constipation [2]
- Diarrhea (47%) [16]
- Gastrointestinal perforation [2]
- Hepatotoxicity [10]
- Nausea (29%) [8]
- Vomiting (15%) [3]

Respiratory
- Cough (29%) [5]
- Dyspnea (17%)
- Pneumonia (25%) [9]
- Pneumonitis [5]
- Upper respiratory tract infection (12%) [3]

Endocrine/Metabolic
- ALT increased (50%) [8]
- Appetite decreased (16%) [2]
- AST increased (41%) [8]

Hematologic
- Anemia [6]
- Febrile neutropenia [6]

Neutropenia [8]
Thrombocytopenia [6]

Other
Adverse effects [3]
Infection [2]
Side effects [2]

IFOSFAMIDE

Trade name: Ifex (Bristol-Myers Squibb)
Indications: Cancers, sarcomas, leukemias, lymphomas
Class: Alkylating agent
Half-life: 4–15 hours
Clinically important, potentially hazardous interactions with: aldesleukin, aprepitant
Pregnancy category: D

Skin
Dermatitis (<10%)
Pigmentation (<10%) [2]
Toxicity [2]

Hair
Alopecia (50–100%) [5]

Nails
Ridging (<10%)

Cardiovascular
Phlebitis (2%)

Central Nervous System
Confusion [2]
Delirium [2]
Encephalopathy [10]
Neurotoxicity [11]
Seizures [2]

Neuromuscular/Skeletal
Osteomalacia [2]

Gastrointestinal/Hepatic
Hepatotoxicity [2]
Nausea [6]
Pancreatitis [2]
Vomiting [6]

Endocrine/Metabolic
SIADH [2]

Renal
Fanconi syndrome [4]
Nephrotoxicity [34]

Hematologic
Anemia [3]
Febrile neutropenia [2]
Leukopenia [2]
Myelosuppression [2]
Neutropenia [4]
Thrombocytopenia [4]

Other
Allergic reactions (<10%)
Death [2]
Infection [2]

ILOPERIDONE

Trade name: Fanapt (Vanda)
Indications: Schizophrenia
Class: Antipsychotic
Half-life: 18–33 hours
Clinically important, potentially hazardous interactions with: alcohol, dextromethorphan, fluoxetine, itraconazole, ketoconazole, paroxetine hydrochloride, QT prolonging agents
Pregnancy category: C
Important contra-indications noted in the prescribing guidelines for: the elderly; nursing mothers; pediatric patients
Warning: INCREASED MORTALITY IN ELDERLY PATIENTS WITH DEMENTIA-RELATED PSYCHOSIS

Skin
Rash (2%)

Mucosal
Nasal congestion (8%) [2]
Xerostomia (10%) [9]

Cardiovascular
Hypotension (3%)
Orthostatic hypotension (3%) [4]
QT prolongation [8]
Tachycardia (12%) [4]

Central Nervous System
Akathisia (2%) [3]
Anxiety [2]
Headache [3]
Insomnia (18%) [3]
Sedation [3]
Somnolence (drowsiness) (15%) [8]
Tremor (3%)
Vertigo (dizziness) (20%) [11]

Neuromuscular/Skeletal
Arthralgia (3%)
Asthenia (fatigue) (6%) [2]

Gastrointestinal/Hepatic
Diarrhea (7%)
Dyspepsia [3]
Nausea (10%) [2]

Respiratory
Dyspnea (2%)
Nasopharyngitis (3%)
Upper respiratory tract infection (3%)

Endocrine/Metabolic
Weight gain (9%) [10]

Genitourinary
Ejaculatory dysfunction (2%) [2]

IMATINIB

Trade name: Gleevec (Novartis)
Indications: Chronic myeloid leukemia
Class: Antineoplastic, Biologic, CYP3A4 inhibitor, Tyrosine kinase inhibitor
Half-life: 18 hours
Clinically important, potentially hazardous interactions with: acetaminophen, amlodipine, anisindione, anticoagulants, aprepitant, atorvastatin, barbiturates, benzodiazepines, butabarbital, carbamazepine, chlordiazepoxide, clarithromycin, clonazepam, clorazepate, corticosteroids, cyclosporine, dexamethasone, diazepam, dicumarol, efavirenz, erythromycin, ethotoin, felodipine, flurazepam, fluvastatin, fosphenytoin, isradipine, itraconazole, ketoconazole, lorazepam, lovastatin, mephenytoin, mephobarbital, midazolam, mifepristone, neratinib, nicardipine, nifedipine, nimodipine, nisoldipine, olaparib, oxazepam, oxcarbazepine, pentobarbital, phenobarbital, phenytoin, pimozide, pravastatin, primidone, quazepam, rifampin, rifapentine, safinamide, secobarbital, simvastatin, St John's wort, temazepam, voriconazole, warfarin
Pregnancy category: D
Important contra-indications noted in the prescribing guidelines for: nursing mothers

---

Skin
Acneform eruption [3]
AGEP [7]
Diaphoresis (13%)
DRESS syndrome [3]
Edema (<5%) [36]
Erythema (<10%) [5]
Erythema multiforme [2]
Erythroderma [3]
Exanthems [9]
Exfoliative dermatitis [4]
Facial edema (<10%) [3]
Hand–foot syndrome [3]
Hypomelanosis [5]
Lichen planus [5]
Lichenoid eruption [11]
Mycosis fungoides [2]
Neutrophilic eccrine hidradenitis [3]
Panniculitis [3]
Peripheral edema (<10%) [5]
Petechiae (<10%)
Photosensitivity (<10%) [3]
Pigmentation [14]
Pityriasis rosea [5]
Pruritus (6–10%) [3]
Pseudolymphoma [3]
Psoriasis [3]
Rash (32–39%) [26]
Squamous cell carcinoma [2]
Stevens-Johnson syndrome [15]
Sweet's syndrome [4]
Toxic epidermal necrolysis [2]
Toxicity [9]
Urticaria [3]
Vasculitis [2]
Xerosis (<10%) [2]

Hair
Alopecia (10–15%) [2]
Follicular mucinosis [2]

Nails
Nail dystrophy [2]
Nail pigmentation [2]

Mucosal
Mucositis [2]
Oral lichenoid eruption [3]
Oral pigmentation [4]
Oral ulceration [3]

Cardiovascular
Cardiotoxicity [2]
Congestive heart failure [2]
QT prolongation [2]

Central Nervous System
Anorexia [4]
Chills (11%)
Depression (15%) [2]
Fever (13–41%) [2]
Headache (19–37%) [4]
Hypoesthesia (<10%)
Insomnia (10–19%)
Subdural hemorrhage [2]
Vertigo (dizziness) [2]

Neuromuscular/Skeletal
Arthralgia (21–26%) [4]
Asthenia (fatigue) (29–75%) [20]
Bone or joint pain (11–31%) [13]
Muscle spasm [9]
Myalgia/Myopathy (16–62%) [11]
Osteonecrosis [3]

Gastrointestinal/Hepatic
Abdominal pain [5]
Ascites [2]
Constipation (9–16%) [2]
Diarrhea (25–59%) [17]
Dyspepsia [2]
Gastrointestinal bleeding [5]
Hepatotoxicity (6–12%) [20]
Nausea (42–73%) [15]
Vomiting (23–58%) [13]

Respiratory
Cough (11–27%)
Dyspnea (21%)
Nasopharyngitis (10–31%)
Pharyngitis (10–15%)
Pleural effusion [3]
Pneumonitis (4–13%) [2]
Pulmonary toxicity [2]
Rhinitis (17%)
Upper respiratory tract infection (3–21%)

Endocrine/Metabolic
Creatine phosphokinase increased [2]
Gynecomastia [4]
Hypophosphatemia [2]
Hypothyroidism [2]
Porphyria cutanea tarda [3]
Pseudoporphyria [5]
Weight gain (5–32%) [3]

Renal
Fanconi syndrome [2]
Nephrotoxicity [2]
Renal failure [2]

Hematologic
Anemia [10]
Febrile neutropenia [2]
Hemotoxicity [4]
Leukopenia [3]
Myelosuppression [2]
Neutropenia [13]
Thrombocytopenia [11]

Otic
Hearing loss [4]

Ocular
Epiphora (25%)
Eyelid edema [2]
Optic edema [3]
Periorbital edema (33%) [11]

Other
Adverse effects [14]
Death [3]
Side effects [2]

IMIPRAMINE

Trade name: Tofranil (Mallinckrodt)
Indications: Depression
Class: Antidepressant, tricyclic, Muscarinic antagonist
Half-life: 6–18 hours
Clinically important, potentially hazardous interactions with: amprenavir, arbutamine, artemether/lumefantrine, clonidine, cobicistat/elvitegravir/emtricitabine/tenofovir alafenamide, cobicistat/elvitegravir/emtricitabine/tenofovir disoproxil, darifenacin, epinephrine, fluoxetine, formoterol, guanethidine, iobenguane, isocarboxazid, labetalol, linezolid, MAO inhibitors, phenelzine, propranolol, quinolones, ropivacaine, sparfloxacin, tranylcypromine, zaleplon, zolpidem
Pregnancy category: D
Warning: SUICIDALITY AND ANTIDEPRESSANT DRUGS

Skin
Diaphoresis (<25%) [8]
Exanthems (<6%) [6]
Exfoliative dermatitis [4]
Photosensitivity [3]
Pigmentation [13]
Pruritus (3%) [6]
Purpura [3]
Urticaria [6]

Hair
Alopecia [2]

Mucosal
Glossitis [2]
Oral lesions [3]
Stomatitis [2]
Xerostomia (>10%) [16]

Cardiovascular
QT prolongation [3]
Tachycardia [2]

Central Nervous System
Dysgeusia (taste perversion) (metallic taste) (>10%) [2]
Parkinsonism (<10%)

Neuromuscular/Skeletal
Asthenia (fatigue) [2]

Endocrine/Metabolic
SIADH [4]

Otic
Tinnitus [4]

IMIQUIMOD

Trade names: Aldara (3M), Zyclara (Graceway)
Indications: External genital and perianal warts, actinic keratoses
Class: Antiviral, Immunomodulator
Half-life: N/A
Clinically important, potentially hazardous interactions with: none known
Pregnancy category: C
Important contra-indications noted in the prescribing guidelines for: nursing mothers; pediatric patients

---

Skin
Angioedema [2]
Burning (9–31%) [7]
Crusting [3]
Depigmentation [3]
Eczema (<10%)
Edema (12–17%) [2]
Erosions (10–32%) [5]
Erythema (33–85%) [14]
Erythema multiforme [2]
Excoriations (18–25%) [2]
Flaking (18–67%) [3]
Fungal dermatitis (<10%)
Herpes simplex (<10%)
Hypomelanosis [2]
Induration (5%)
Lichen planus [3]
Lupus erythematosus [3]
Lymphadenopathy (2%)
Pemphigus [4]
Pemphigus foliaceus [3]
Pigmentation [3]
Pruritus (22–75%) [10]
Psoriasis [4]
Scabbing (4%)
Scar [3]
Seborrheic keratoses (<10%)
Tenderness (local) (12%) [2]
Ulcerations (5–10%) [5]
Vesiculation (2–3%)
Vitiligo [7]

Hair
Alopecia (<10%)
Poliosis [2]

Cardiovascular
Chest pain (<10%)

Central Nervous System
Anorexia (<10%)
Anxiety (<10%)
Fever (<10%) [2]
Headache (<10%) [4]
Neurotoxicity [2]
Pain (2–11%) [6]
Rigors (<10%)
Vertigo (dizziness) (<10%)

Neuromuscular/Skeletal
Asthenia (fatigue) (<10%) [2]
Back pain (<10%)
Myalgia/Myopathy (<10%) [2]

Gastrointestinal/Hepatic
Nausea (<10%) [2]
Vomiting (<10%)

Respiratory
Cough (<10%)
Flu-like syndrome (<3%) [2]
Pharyngitis (<10%)
Rhinitis (<10%)
Sinusitis (<10%)
Upper respiratory tract infection (<10%)

Genitourinary
Urinary tract infection (<10%)

Hematologic
Lymphopenia [2]

Local
Application-site burning (<10%)
Application-site edema (<10%) [4]
Application-site erythema (<10%) [3]
Application-site pruritus (<10%) [5]

Application-site reactions [9]

Other

Adverse effects [6]

IMMUNE GLOBULIN IV

Synonyms: IGIV; IVIG
Trade names: Gamimune (Bayer), Gammagard (Baxter), Gammar PIV (ZLB Behring), Gamunex (Bayer), Iveegam (Baxter), Venoglobulin (Alpha Therapeutics)
Indications: Immunodeficiency in patients unable to produce sufficient amounts of IgG antibodies
Class: Immunomodulator
Half-life: N/A
Clinically important, potentially hazardous interactions with: live vaccines
Pregnancy category: C
Important contra-indications noted in the prescribing guidelines for: nursing mothers
Warning: THROMBOSIS, RENAL DYSFUNCTION and ACUTE RENAL FAILURE

Skin

Anaphylactoid reactions/Anaphylaxis [5]
Eczema [3]
Flushing [2]
Lichenoid eruption [2]
Pompholyx [3]
Rash [2]
Vasculitis [4]

Cardiovascular

Hypertension [4]
Myocardial infarction [2]
Palpitation [2]
Thromboembolism [4]

Central Nervous System

Aseptic meningitis [6]
Chills [4]
Fever [12]
Headache [19]

Neuromuscular/Skeletal

Arthralgia [3]
Asthenia (fatigue) [5]
Back pain [3]
Bone or joint pain [2]
Myalgia/Myopathy [4]

Gastrointestinal/Hepatic

Abdominal pain [2]
Diarrhea [2]
Nausea [10]
Vomiting [2]

Respiratory

Cough [2]
Dyspnea [2]
Pulmonary embolism [2]

Renal

Nephrotoxicity [6]
Renal failure [3]

Hematologic

Anemia [2]
Hemolysis [2]
Hemolytic anemia [5]
Thrombosis [3]

Local

Application-site pain (16%)
Infusion-related reactions [6]
Injection-site edema [2]
Injection-site erythema [2]

Other

Adverse effects [9]

IMMUNE GLOBULIN SC

Synonym: SCIG
Trade names: Cuvitru (Shire), Hizentra (CSL Behring), Vivaglobin (CSL Behring)
Indications: Primary immune deficiency
Class: Immunomodulator
Half-life: N/A
Clinically important, potentially hazardous interactions with: none known
Pregnancy category: C
Warning: THROMBOSIS

Skin

Pruritus [2]
Rash (<3%)

Mucosal

Oropharyngeal pain (17%)

Cardiovascular

Tachycardia (<3%)

Central Nervous System

Fever (<3%) [2]
Headache (2–32%) [3]

Neuromuscular/Skeletal

Asthenia (fatigue) (<5%)

Gastrointestinal/Hepatic

Gastrointestinal disorder (<5%)
Nausea (<11%)

Respiratory

Bronchitis [2]
Cough (10%)
Upper respiratory tract infection [2]

Local

Injection-site reactions (49–92%) [5]

Other

Adverse effects [2]
Allergic reactions (11%)

INDACATEROL

Trade names: Arcapta Neohaler (Novartis), Onbrez Breezhaler (Novartis), Utibron Neohaler (Novartis)
Indications: Long term, once-daily maintenance bronchodilator treatment of airflow obstruction in chronic obstructive pulmonary disease (COPD), including chronic bronchitis and/or emphysema
Class: Beta-2 adrenergic agonist, Bronchodilator
Half-life: 40–56 hours
Clinically important, potentially hazardous interactions with: acetazolamide, adrenergics, aminophylline, arsenic, corticosteroids, diuretics, erythromycin, ketoconazole, MAO inhibitors, pazopanib, QT prolonging agents, ritonavir, steroids, telavancin, theophylline, tricyclic antidepressants, verapamil, xanthine derivatives
Pregnancy category: C
Important contra-indications noted in the prescribing guidelines for: nursing mothers; pediatric patients
Note: Studies in asthma patients showed that long-acting $beta_2$-adrenergic agonists may increase the risk of asthma-related death. Contra-indicated in patients with asthma without use of a long-term asthma control medication. Utibron Neohaler is indacaterol and glycopyrrolate.
Warning: ASTHMA-RELATED DEATH

Mucosal

Oropharyngeal pain [2]

Cardiovascular

Prolonged QT interval [2]

Central Nervous System

Headache (5%) [4]
Pain (oropharyngeal) (2%)

Gastrointestinal/Hepatic

Nausea (2%)

Respiratory

Asthma [2]
COPD (exacerbation) [8]
Cough (7%) [10]
Dyspnea [2]
Influenza [2]
Nasopharyngitis (5%) [7]
Upper respiratory tract infection [4]

Endocrine/Metabolic

Hyperglycemia [2]

Other

Adverse effects [6]
Death [2]

INDAPAMIDE

Trade name: Lozol (Sanofi-Aventis)
Indications: Edema
Class: Diuretic, thiazide
Half-life: 14–18 hours
Clinically important, potentially hazardous interactions with: digoxin, lithium, zinc
Pregnancy category: B
Important contra-indications noted in the prescribing guidelines for: the elderly; nursing mothers; pediatric patients
Note: Indapamide is a sulfonamide and can be absorbed systemically. Sulfonamides can produce severe, possibly fatal, reactions such as toxic epidermal necrolysis and Stevens-Johnson syndrome.

Skin

Angioedema [3]
Erythema multiforme [2]
Flushing (<5%)
Pemphigus foliaceus [2]
Peripheral edema (<5%) [2]
Pruritus (<5%) [2]
Rash (<5%) [4]
Toxic epidermal necrolysis [3]
Urticaria (<5%)
Vasculitis (<5%)

Mucosal
Xerostomia (<5%) [2]

Cardiovascular
QT prolongation [5]

Central Nervous System
Paresthesias (<5%)
Vertigo (dizziness) [2]

Endocrine/Metabolic
Hypokalemia [2]
Hyponatremia [2]

INDINAVIR

Trade name: Crixivan (Merck)
Indications: HIV infection
Class: Antiretroviral, CYP3A4 inhibitor, HIV-1 protease inhibitor
Half-life: ~1.8 hours
Clinically important, potentially hazardous interactions with: abiraterone, alfuzosin, almotriptan, alosetron, alprazolam, amiodarone, amprenavir, antacids, antiarrhythmics, antifungal agents, artemether/lumefantrine, astemizole, atazanavir, atorvastatin, atovaquone, atovaquone/proguanil, avanafil, bepridil, bortezomib, bosentan, brigatinib, brinzolamide, cabazitaxel, cabozantinib, calcifediol, calcium channel blockers, carbamazepine, chlordiazepoxide, ciclesonide, cisapride, clarithromycin, clonazepam, clorazepate, colchicine, conivaptan, copanlisib, corticosteroids, crizotinib, cyclosporine, CYP3A4 inducers and substrates, darifenacin, darunavir, dasatinib, deferasirox, delavirdine, diazepam, didanosine, dienogest, digoxin, dihydroergotamine, dronedarone, dutasteride, efavirenz, enfuvirtide, eplerenone, ergot derivatives, ergotamine, estazolam, estrogens, etravirine, everolimus, felodipine, fentanyl, fesoterodine, flibanserin, flurazepam, fluticasone propionate, food, fusidic acid, grapefruit juice, guanfacine, H_2-antagonists, halazepam, halofantrine, HMG-CoA reductase inhibitors, itraconazole, ixabepilone, ketoconazole, lapatinib, lidocaine, lomitapide, lopinavir, lovastatin, maraviroc, meperidine, methylergonovine, methylprednisolone, methysergide, midazolam, midostaurin, mifepristone, mometasone, nefazodone, nelfinavir, neratinib, nevirapine, nicardipine, nifedipine, nilotinib, nisoldipine, olaparib, P-glycoprotein inhibitors and inducers, paclitaxel, palbociclib, pantoprazole, paricalcitol, pazopanib, PEG-interferon, phenobarbital, phenytoin, pimavanserin, pimecrolimus, pimozide, ponatinib, prasugrel, protease inhibitors, proton pump inhibitors, quazepam, quinidine, quinine, ranolazine, ribociclib, rifabutin, rifampin, rifapentine, rilpivirine, rivaroxaban, romidepsin, rosuvastatin, ruxolitinib, salmeterol, saxagliptin, sildenafil, silodosin, simeprevir, simvastatin, sirolimus, solifenacin, sorafenib, St John's wort, sunitinib, tacrolimus, tadalafil, tamsulosin, telithromycin, temsirolimus, tenofovir disoproxil, theophylline, ticagrelor, tolvaptan, trazodone, triazolam, tricyclic antidepressants, valproic acid, vardenafil, vemurafenib, venetoclax, venlafaxine, vorapaxar, zidovudine
Pregnancy category: C
Important contra-indications noted in the prescribing guidelines for: nursing mothers; pediatric patients
Note: Protease inhibitors cause dyslipidemia which includes elevated triglycerides and cholesterol and redistribution of body fat centrally to produce the so-called 'protease paunch', breast enlargement, facial atrophy, and 'buffalo hump'.

Skin
Bromhidrosis (<2%)
Dermatitis (<2%)
Diaphoresis (<2%)
Flushing (<2%)
Folliculitis (<2%)
Herpes simplex (<2%)
Herpes zoster (<2%)
Jaundice (2%)
Lipodystrophy [8]
Lipomatosis [2]
Pruritus [2]
Rash [2]
Seborrhea (<2%)
Stevens-Johnson syndrome [2]
Xerosis [2]

Hair
Alopecia [5]

Nails
Onychocryptosis [2]
Paronychia [5]
Pyogenic granuloma [3]

Mucosal
Aphthous stomatitis (<2%)
Cheilitis [4]
Gingivitis (<2%)

Central Nervous System
Anorexia (3%)
Dysesthesia (<2%)
Dysgeusia (taste perversion) (3%)
Fever (2%)
Headache (5%)
Hyperesthesia (<2%)
Paresthesias (<2%)
Somnolence (drowsiness) (2%)
Vertigo (dizziness) (3%)

Neuromuscular/Skeletal
Asthenia (fatigue) (2%)
Back pain (8%)
Myalgia/Myopathy with lovastatin or simvastatin (<2%)

Gastrointestinal/Hepatic
Abdominal pain (17%) [2]
Diarrhea (3%)
Dyspepsia (2%)
Nausea (12%)
Vomiting (8%)

Respiratory
Cough (2%)

Endocrine/Metabolic
ALT increased (5%)
Appetite increased (2%)
AST increased (4%)
Creatine phosphokinase increased [2]
Diabetes mellitus [2]
Gynecomastia [4]
Porphyria (acute) [2]

Genitourinary
Crystalluria [2]
Dysuria (2%)

Renal
Nephrolithiasis (9%) [4]
Nephrotoxicity [14]

Ocular
Eyelid edema (<2%)

Other
Bruxism (<2%)

INDOMETHACIN

Synonym: indometacin
Indications: Arthritis
Class: Non-steroidal anti-inflammatory (NSAID)
Half-life: 4.5 hours
Clinically important, potentially hazardous interactions with: aldesleukin, aspirin, atenolol, cyclopenthiazide, diflunisal, diuretics, methotrexate, NSAIDs, prednisolone, prednisone, sermorelin, tiludronate, torsemide, triamterene, urokinase
Pregnancy category: C
Important contra-indications noted in the prescribing guidelines for: nursing mothers; pediatric patients
Note: NSAIDs may cause an increased risk of serious cardiovascular and gastrointestinal adverse events, which can be fatal. This risk may increase with duration of use.
Warning: RISK OF SERIOUS CARDIOVASCULAR AND GASTROINTESTINAL EVENTS

Skin
Angioedema [2]
Bullous dermatitis [2]
Dermatitis [5]
Dermatitis herpetiformis (exacerbation) [2]
Edema (3–9%)
Exanthems (<5%) [7]
Fixed eruption [3]
Pruritus (<10%) [3]
Psoriasis [7]
Purpura [5]
Rash (>10%)
Toxic epidermal necrolysis [6]
Urticaria [7]
Vasculitis [5]

Mucosal
Oral lesions (<7%) [2]
Oral ulceration [4]

Central Nervous System
Psychosis [3]

Gastrointestinal/Hepatic
Gastrointestinal bleeding [2]
Gastrointestinal perforation [3]
Gastrointestinal ulceration [3]
Pancreatitis [2]

Otic
Tinnitus [2]

Ocular
Periorbital edema [2]

Other
Adverse effects [8]

INFLIXIMAB

Trade names: Inflectra (Celltrion) ((Remsima)), Remicade (Centocor), Renflexis (Samsung Bioepsis)
Indications: Crohn's disease, ulcerative colitis, rheumatoid arthritis, ankylosing spondylitis, psoriatic arthritis, plaque psoriasis
Class: Cytokine inhibitor, Disease-modifying antirheumatic drug (DMARD), Monoclonal antibody, TNF inhibitor
Half-life: 8–10 days
Clinically important, potentially hazardous interactions with: abatacept, anakinra, live vaccines, methotrexate, tocilizumab
Pregnancy category: B
Important contra-indications noted in the prescribing guidelines for: the elderly; nursing mothers
Note: TNF inhibitors should be used in patients with heart failure only after consideration of other treatment options.
Contra-indicated in patients with a personal or family history of multiple sclerosis or demyelinating disease. TNF inhibitors should not be administered to patients with moderate to severe heart failure (New York Heart Association Functional Class III/IV).
Warning: SERIOUS INFECTIONS and MALIGNANCY

Skin
Abscess [4]
Acneform eruption [6]
AGEP [2]
Anaphylactoid reactions/Anaphylaxis [11]
Angioedema [2]
Candidiasis (5%) [4]
Cellulitis [5]
Dermatitis [4]
Eczema [5]
Edema [3]
Erythema multiforme [2]
Exanthems [4]
Flushing [2]
Folliculitis [2]
Hand–foot syndrome [2]
Herpes [2]
Herpes simplex [4]
Herpes zoster [11]
Hypersensitivity [11]
Leukocytoclastic vasculitis [2]
Lichen planus [2]
Lichenoid eruption [3]
Lupus erythematosus [35]
Lupus syndrome [12]
Lymphoma [9]
Malignancies [2]
Molluscum contagiosum [2]
Neoplasms [2]
Nevi [2]
Palmar–plantar pustulosis [3]
Pityriasis lichenoides chronica [2]
Pruritus (7%) [8]
Pseudolymphoma [2]
Psoriasis [57]
Pustules [5]
Rash (10%) [13]
Sarcoidosis [5]
Serum sickness [2]
Serum sickness-like reaction (<3%) [5]
Toxic epidermal necrolysis [2]
Toxicity [2]
Urticaria [6]
Vasculitis [18]
Vitiligo [4]

Hair
Alopecia [6]
Alopecia areata [3]

Cardiovascular
Cardiotoxicity [2]
Chest pain [4]
Hypertension (7%) [3]
Palpitation [2]
Pericarditis [2]
Tachycardia [2]

Central Nervous System
Aseptic meningitis [2]
Chills (5–9%) [2]
Demyelination [4]
Fever (7%) [10]
Headache (18%) [12]
Leukoencephalopathy [2]
Neurotoxicity [8]
Pain (8%) [3]
Paresthesias (<4%) [2]
Peripheral neuropathy [7]
Seizures [2]
Vertigo (dizziness) [3]

Neuromuscular/Skeletal
Arthralgia (<8%) [16]
Asthenia (fatigue) (9%) [5]
Back pain (8%)
Myalgia/Myopathy (5%) [7]
Polymyositis [2]

Gastrointestinal/Hepatic
Abdominal pain (12%) [4]
Crohn's disease (26%)
Diarrhea (12%)
Dyspepsia (10%)
Hepatitis [11]
Hepatotoxicity [17]
Nausea (21%) [3]
Pancreatitis [2]

Respiratory
Bronchitis (10%)
Cough (12%) [3]
Dyspnea (6%) [4]
Pharyngitis (12%)
Pneumonia [12]
Pulmonary toxicity [6]
Rhinitis (8%)
Sinusitis (14%) [5]
Tuberculosis [14]
Upper respiratory tract infection (32%) [7]

Endocrine/Metabolic
ALT increased [2]

Genitourinary
Cystitis [2]
Urinary tract infection (8%) [2]

Renal
Nephrotoxicity [2]

Hematologic
Hemolytic anemia [2]
Neutropenia [5]
Sepsis [2]
Thrombocytopenia [5]

Ocular
Optic neuritis [3]
Uveitis [2]

Local
Application-site reactions (mild) (<4%) [6]
Infusion-related reactions [25]
Infusion-site reactions (20%) [12]
Injection-site reactions (6%) [9]

Other
Adverse effects [45]
Allergic reactions [8]
Death [13]
Infection (36%) [62]
Nocardiosis [3]
Side effects [2]
Systemic reactions [2]

INFLUENZA VACCINE

Trade names: Afluria (Seqirus), Agrippal (Chiron), Comvax (Merck), Fluad (Novartis), Fluarix (GSK), FluMist (Medimmune) (Wyeth), Flurix (GSK), Fluviral (Shire), Inflexal V (Berna Biotech), Invivac (Solvay), Vaxigrip (Sanofi-Aventis)
Indications: Influenza prevention
Class: Vaccine
Half-life: N/A
Clinically important, potentially hazardous interactions with: aminophylline, carbamazepine, cyclosporine, mercaptopurine, phenobarbital, phenytoin, prednisone, vincristine, warfarin
Pregnancy category: C
Important contra-indications noted in the prescribing guidelines for: pediatric patients
Note: Inactivated influenza vaccine should not be given to persons with anaphylactic hypersensitivity to eggs or other components of the vaccine. For current data on influenza in the USA consult the Centers for Disease Control and Protection website (www.cdc.gov/flu).

Skin
Anaphylactoid reactions/Anaphylaxis (rare) [4]
Henoch–Schönlein purpura [2]
Hypersensitivity [2]
Linear IgA bullous dermatosis [2]
Purpura [2]
Rash [3]
Serum sickness-like reaction [2]
Vasculitis [10]

Central Nervous System
Fever [13]
Guillain–Barré syndrome [11]
Headache [9]
Seizures [3]
Syncope [2]

Neuromuscular/Skeletal
Arthralgia [2]
Asthenia (fatigue) [7]
Myalgia/Myopathy [11]
Polymyositis [4]

Gastrointestinal/Hepatic
Abdominal pain [2]

Respiratory
- Asthma [2]
- Cough [2]

Hematologic
- Thrombocytopenia [2]

Ocular
- Oculorespiratory syndrome [15]
- Optic neuritis [2]

Local
- Injection-site edema [4]
- Injection-site erythema [7]
- Injection-site induration [5]
- Injection-site inflammation [3]
- Injection-site pain (20–28%) [15]
- Injection-site reactions [3]

Other
- Adverse effects [8]
- Side effects [4]
- Systemic reactions (injection site) [5]

INGENOL MEBUTATE

Trade name: Picato (Leo Pharma)
Indications: Actinic keratosis
Class: Cell death inducer
Half-life: N/A
Clinically important, potentially hazardous interactions with: none known
Pregnancy category: C
Important contra-indications noted in the prescribing guidelines for: pediatric patients

---

Skin
- Crusting [4]
- Erythema [4]
- Flaking [4]
- Scaling [3]

Central Nervous System
- Headache (2%) [4]

Respiratory
- Nasopharyngitis (2%) [2]

Ocular
- Eyelid edema [2]
- Periorbital edema (3%) [2]

Local
- Application-site erythema [2]
- Application-site infection (3%) [2]
- Application-site pain (2–15%) [6]
- Application-site pruritus (8%) [4]
- Application-site reactions [3]

INSULIN ASPART

Trade names: NovoLog (Novo Nordisk), NovoRapid (Novo Nordisk), Ryzodeg (Novo Nordisk)
Indications: Diabetes mellitus
Class: Hormone, polypeptide
Half-life: 81 minutes
Clinically important, potentially hazardous interactions with: ACE inhibitors, alcohol, atypical antipsychotics, beta blockers, clonidine, corticosteroids, danazol, disopyramide, diuretics, epinephrine, estrogens, fibrates, fluoxetine, isoniazid, isoniazid, lithium salts, MAO inhibitors, niacin, octreotide, oral contraceptives, pentamidine, phenothiazine derivatives, pramlintide, propoxyphene, salbutamol, salicylates, somatropin, sulfonamide antibiotics, terbutaline, thyroid hormones
Pregnancy category: B
Important contra-indications noted in the prescribing guidelines for: the elderly; pediatric patients
Note: Ryzodeg is insulin aspart and insulin degludec; various forms of insulin are available - see other insulin profiles for reaction details.

Skin
- Lipodystrophy (>5%)
- Peripheral edema (>5%)

Nails
- Onychomycosis (10%)

Cardiovascular
- Chest pain (5%)

Central Nervous System
- Headache (12%) [3]
- Hyporeflexia (11%)

Gastrointestinal/Hepatic
- Abdominal pain (5%)
- Diarrhea (5%)
- Nausea (7%)

Respiratory
- Nasopharyngitis [3]
- Sinusitis (5%)

Endocrine/Metabolic
- Diabetic ketoacidosis [2]
- Hypoglycemia (75%) [6]
- Weight gain (>5%)

Genitourinary
- Urinary tract infection (8%)

INSULIN DEGLUDEC

Trade names: Ryzodeg (Novo Nordisk), Tresiba (Novo Nordisk), Xultophy (Novo Nordisk)
Indications: Diabetes mellitus
Class: Human insulin analog, long-acting
Half-life: 25 hours
Clinically important, potentially hazardous interactions with: ACE inhibitors, albuterol, alcohol, angiotensin II receptor blocking agents, beta blockers, clonidine, clozapine, corticosteroids, danazol, DDP-4-inhibitors, disopyramide, diuretics, epinephrine, estrogens, fibrates, fluoxetine, GLP-1 receptor agonists, glucagon, guanethidine, isoniazid, lithium, MAO inhibitors, niacin, octreotide, olanzapine, oral contraceptives, pentamidine, pentoxifylline, phenothiazines, pramlintide, propoxyphene, protease inhibitors, reserpine, salicylates, SGLT-2 inhibitors, somatropin, sulfonamide antibiotics, terbutaline, thyroid hormones
Pregnancy category: C
Important contra-indications noted in the prescribing guidelines for: the elderly; nursing mothers; pediatric patients
Note: Contra-indicated during episodes of hypoglycemia. Ryzodeg is insulin degludec and insulin aspart; Xultophy is insulin degludec and liraglutide; various forms of insulin are available - see other insulin profiles for reaction details.

Skin
- Hypersensitivity [2]
- Peripheral edema (<3%)

Central Nervous System
- Headache (9–12%) [11]

Gastrointestinal/Hepatic
- Diarrhea (6%) [6]
- Gastroenteritis (5%)
- Nausea [7]
- Vomiting [2]

Respiratory
- Nasopharyngitis (13–24%) [12]
- Sinusitis (5%)
- Upper respiratory tract infection (8–12%) [3]

Endocrine/Metabolic
- Diabetic ketoacidosis [2]
- Hypoglycemia [10]

Ocular
- Retinopathy [2]

Local
- Injection-site reactions (4%) [6]

Other
- Adverse effects [4]

INSULIN DETEMIR

Trade name: Levemir (Novo Nordisk)
Indications: Diabetes (Type I or II)
Class: Human insulin analog, long-acting
Half-life: 5–7 hours
Clinically important, potentially hazardous interactions with: albuterol, alcohol, antipsychotics, beta blockers, clonidine, clozapine, corticosteroids, danazol, diuretics, epinephrine, estrogens, guanethidine, isoniazid, lithium, niacin, olanzapine, oral antidiabetics, oral contraceptives, pentamidine, phenothiazines, propranolol, protease inhibitors, reserpine, somatropin, terbutaline, thiazolidinediones, thyroid hormones
Pregnancy category: B
Important contra-indications noted in the prescribing guidelines for: the elderly; nursing mothers; pediatric patients
Note: Various forms of insulin are available - see other insulin profiles for reaction details.

Central Nervous System
- Fever (10%)
- Headache (7–31%) [3]

Neuromuscular/Skeletal
- Back pain (8%)

Gastrointestinal/Hepatic
- Abdominal pain (6–13%)
- Gastroenteritis (6–17%)
- Nausea (7%)
- Vomiting (7%)

Respiratory
- Bronchitis (5%)
- Cough (8%)
- Flu-like syndrome (6–14%)
- Pharyngitis (10–17%)
- Rhinitis (7%)
- Upper respiratory tract infection (13–36%)

Endocrine/Metabolic
- Hyperglycemia [2]
- Hypoglycemia [4]

Local
- Injection-site reactions (3–4%) [4]

Other
- Allergic reactions [3]
- Infection (viral) (7%)

INSULIN GLARGINE

Trade names: Basaglar (Lilly), Lantus (Sanofi-Aventis), Soliqua (Sanofi-Aventis)
Indications: Diabetes (Type I or II)
Class: Hormone analog, polypeptide
Half-life: N/A
Clinically important, potentially hazardous interactions with: ACE inhibitors, albuterol, alcohol, beta blockers, clonidine, clozapine, corticosteroids, danazol, disopyramide, diuretics, epinephrine, estrogens, fibrates, fluoxetine, glucagon, guanethidine, isoniazid, lithium, MAO inhibitors, niacin, olanzapine, oral antidiabetic products, oral contraceptives, pentamidine, pentoxifylline, phenothiazine derivatives, pramlintide, propoxyphene, propranolol, protease inhibitors, reserpine, salicylates, somatostain analogs, somatropin, sulfonamide antibiotics, terbutaline, thyroid hormones
Pregnancy category: C
Important contra-indications noted in the prescribing guidelines for: nursing mothers; pediatric patients
Note: Soliqua is insulin glargine and lixisenatide; various forms of insulin are available - see other insulin profiles for reaction details.

Skin
- Lipoatrophy [2]
- Peripheral edema (20%)

Central Nervous System
- Depression (11%)
- Headache (6–10%) [4]

Neuromuscular/Skeletal
- Arthralgia (14%)
- Back pain (13%)
- Pain in extremities (13%)

Gastrointestinal/Hepatic
- Diarrhea (11%) [6]
- Nausea [5]
- Vomiting [4]

Respiratory
- Bronchitis (15%)
- Cough (12%)
- Influenza (19%)
- Nasopharyngitis [6]
- Pharyngitis (8%)
- Rhinitis (5%)
- Sinusitis (19%)
- Upper respiratory tract infection (11–29%) [3]

Endocrine/Metabolic
- Hypoglycemia [5]

Genitourinary
- Urinary tract infection (11%)

Ocular
- Cataract (18%)
- Retinopathy [2]

Local
- Injection-site pain (3%)
- Injection-site reactions [4]

Other
- Adverse effects [6]
- Infection (9–14%)

INSULIN GLULISINE

Trade name: Apidra (Sanofi-Aventis)
Indications: Diabetes
Class: Insulin analog
Half-life: 13–42 minutes
Clinically important, potentially hazardous interactions with: ACE inhibitors, albuterol, alcohol, anitpsychotics, beta blockers, clonidine, clozapine, corticosteroids, danazol, disopyramide, diuretics, epinephrine, fibrates, fluoxetine, glucagon, guanethidine, isoniazid, lithium, MAO inhibitors, niacin, oral antidiabetic agents, oral contraceptives, pentamidine, pentoxifylline, phenothiazine derivatives, pramlintide, propoxyphene, propranolol, protease inhibitors, reserpine, salicylates, somatostatin analogs, somatropin, sulfonamide antibiotics, terbutaline, thyroid hormones
Pregnancy category: C
Important contra-indications noted in the prescribing guidelines for: nursing mothers; pediatric patients
Note: Various forms of insulin are available - see other insulin profiles for reaction details.

Skin
- Peripheral edema (8%)

Cardiovascular
- Hypertension (4%)

Central Nervous System
- Headache (7%)

Neuromuscular/Skeletal
- Arthralgia (6%)

Respiratory
- Influenza (4–6%)
- Nasopharyngitis (8–11%)
- Upper respiratory tract infection (7–11%)

Endocrine/Metabolic
- Hypoglycemia (6–7%) [3]

Local
- Injection-site reactions (10%) [2]

INTERFERON ALFA

Synonyms: IFN; INF
Trade names: Infergen (Intermune), Intron A (Schering), Rebetron (Schering), Roferon-A (Roche)
Indications: Chronic hepatitis C virus infection, hairy cell leukemia
Class: Biologic, Immunomodulator, Interferon
Half-life: 2 hours
Clinically important, potentially hazardous interactions with: aldesleukin, amitriptyline, captopril, gemfibrozil, metaxalone, methadone, ribavirin, telbivudine, theophylline, theophylline derivatives, zafirlukast, zidovudine
Pregnancy category: C (pregnancy category will be X when used in combination with ribavirin)
Important contra-indications noted in the prescribing guidelines for: nursing mothers; pediatric patients
Note: Many of the adverse reactions depend on the nature of the disease being treated. Either hairy cell leukemia [L] or AIDS-related Kaposi's sarcoma [K].

Skin
- Angioedema [3]
- Bullous dermatitis [4]
- Dermatitis (6%)
- Eczema [6]
- Edema [L] (11%) [2]
- Erythema [2]
- Exanthems [3]
- Herpes simplex [2]
- Kaposi's sarcoma [2]
- Lichen planus [8]
- Linear IgA bullous dermatosis [3]
- Livedo reticularis [2]
- Lupus erythematosus [17]
- Lupus syndrome [2]
- Necrosis [6]
- Pemphigus [2]
- Photosensitivity [2]
- Pigmentation [3]
- Pruritus 13% [L] 5–7% [K] (13%) [4]
- Psoriasis [24]
- Purpura [2]
- Rash 44% [L] 11% [K] [5]
- Raynaud's phenomenon [11]
- Sarcoidosis [47]
- Seborrheic dermatitis [2]
- Sjögren's syndrome [4]
- Thrombocytopenic purpura [2]
- Toxicity [4]
- Urticaria [K] (<3%) [3]
- Vasculitis [7]
- Vitiligo [9]

Hair
- Alopecia (23%) [16]
- Hair pigmentation [3]
- Hypertrichosis [3]
- Straight hair [2]

Mucosal
- Aphthous stomatitis [2]
- Oral lichen planus [7]
- Stomatitis (<10%)
- Xerostomia (>10%) [4]

Cardiovascular
Cardiotoxicity [2]
Hypertension [3]
Hypotension [2]

Central Nervous System
Ageusia (taste loss) [2]
Anorexia [5]
Anosmia [4]
Anxiety [3]
Chills [4]
Depression (5–15%) [25]
Dysgeusia (taste perversion) [K] (25%) [2]
Fever (37%) [7]
Headache (54%) [6]
Impaired concentration [2]
Insomnia (19%)
Irritability [3]
Neurotoxicity [4]
Paresthesias 8% [L] (12%)
Parkinsonism [3]
Restless legs syndrome [2]
Rigors (35%)
Seizures [2]
Suicidal ideation [6]
Tremor [2]
Vertigo (dizziness) (16%) [2]

Neuromuscular/Skeletal
Arthralgia (28%) [4]
Asthenia (fatigue) (56%) [11]
Back pain (9%)
Myalgia/Myopathy 69% [L] 71% [K] [11]
Myasthenia gravis [11]
Rhabdomyolysis [3]

Gastrointestinal/Hepatic
Abdominal pain (15%)
Constipation [2]
Diarrhea (24%) [6]
Hepatotoxicity [2]
Nausea (24%) [8]
Pancreatitis [7]
Vomiting [5]

Respiratory
Cough [2]
Dyspnea (13%) [2]
Flu-like syndrome (>10%) [11]
Pulmonary hypertension [3]

Endocrine/Metabolic
ALT increased [2]
AST increased [2]
Hyperglycemia [2]
Hyperthyroidism [3]
Thyroid dysfunction [5]
Thyroiditis [3]
Weight loss (16%) [5]

Genitourinary
Impotence [2]

Renal
Nephrotoxicity [3]
Proteinuria [2]

Hematologic
Anemia (11%) [8]
Febrile neutropenia [2]
Hemolytic uremic syndrome [6]
Leukopenia [6]
Lymphopenia (14%)
Neutropenia (21%) [5]
Thrombocytopenia [8]

Otic
Tinnitus [4]

Ocular
Eyelashes – hypertrichosis [3]
Optic neuropathy [4]
Retinopathy [6]
Vision blurred (4%)

Local
Injection-site alopecia [2]
Injection-site erythema [2]
Injection-site induration [3]
Injection-site necrosis [16]

Other
Adverse effects [6]
Infection [4]
Vogt-Koyanagi-Harada syndrome [6]

INTERFERON BETA

Trade names: Avonex (Biogen), Betaferon (Bayer), Betaseron (Bayer), Plegridy (Biogen), Rebif (Merck)
Indications: Relapsing multiple sclerosis, cancers
Class: Immunomodulator, Interferon
Half-life: 10 hours
Clinically important, potentially hazardous interactions with: theophylline, theophylline derivatives, zidovudine
Pregnancy category: C
Important contra-indications noted in the prescribing guidelines for: nursing mothers; pediatric patients

---

Skin
Cyst (4%)
Diaphoresis (23%)
Edema (generalized) (8%)
Herpes simplex (2–3%)
Herpes zoster (3)
Hypersensitivity (3%)
Lipoatrophy [2]
Lupus erythematosus [8]
Nevi (3%)
Nicolau syndrome [2]
Psoriasis [2]
Rash [2]
Raynaud's phenomenon [2]
Sarcoidosis [2]
Thrombocytopenic purpura [4]
Urticaria (5%)
Vasculitis [4]

Hair
Alopecia (4%)

Mucosal
Mucosal bleeding (12–38%)

Cardiovascular
Capillary leak syndrome [3]

Central Nervous System
Chills (21%)
Depression [8]
Fever [4]
Headache [5]
Multiple sclerosis [2]
Pain (52%)
Paresthesias [2]
Psychosis [2]
Seizures (2%) [2]
Vertigo (dizziness) (35%)

Neuromuscular/Skeletal
Arthralgia [2]
Asthenia (fatigue) [3]
Myalgia/Myopathy (44%)
Rhabdomyolysis [2]

Gastrointestinal/Hepatic
Hepatotoxicity [6]

Respiratory
Flu-like syndrome (61%) [15]
Upper respiratory tract infection (31%)

Endocrine/Metabolic
Mastodynia (7%)
Thyroid dysfunction [4]

Genitourinary
Vaginitis (4%)

Renal
Nephrotoxicity [2]

Hematologic
Hemolytic uremic syndrome [3]
Thrombotic microangiopathy [4]

Ocular
Retinopathy [3]

Local
Injection-site ecchymoses (2%)
Injection-site erythema [2]
Injection-site inflammation (3%)
Injection-site necrosis [3]
Injection-site purpura (2%)
Injection-site reactions (4%) [10]

Other
Adverse effects [4]
Death [4]
Infection (11%) [3]

INTERFERON GAMMA

Trade name: Actimmune (Horizon)
Indications: Chronic granulomatous disease, severe malignant osteopetrosis
Class: Immunomodulator, Interferon
Half-life: 6 hours
Clinically important, potentially hazardous interactions with: tasonermin, typhoid vaccine
Pregnancy category: N/A (May cause fetal toxicity based on findings in animal studies)
Important contra-indications noted in the prescribing guidelines for: nursing mothers; pediatric patients

---

Skin
Rash (17%)

Central Nervous System
Chills (14%) [3]
Fever (52%) [8]
Headache (33%) [3]

Neuromuscular/Skeletal
Arthralgia (2%)
Asthenia (fatigue) (14%) [3]
Myalgia/Myopathy (6%)

Gastrointestinal/Hepatic
Diarrhea (14%)
Nausea (10%)
Vomiting (13%)

Respiratory
Flu-like syndrome [4]

Hematologic
Lymphopenia [2]

Local
Injection-site erythema (14%) [2]

IPILIMUMAB

Trade name: Yervoy (Bristol-Myers Squibb)
Indications: Melanoma
Class: Biologic, CTLA-4-blocking monoclonal antibody, Monoclonal antibody
Half-life: 15 days
Clinically important, potentially hazardous interactions with: none known
Pregnancy category: C
Important contra-indications noted in the prescribing guidelines for: nursing mothers; pediatric patients
Warning: IMMUNE-MEDIATED ADVERSE REACTIONS

Skin
Dermatitis (12%) [14]
Dermatomyositis [2]
Erythema [5]
Erythema multiforme [2]
Exanthems [6]
Granulomas [5]
Lymphadenopathy [3]
Pruritus (21–31%) [22]
Rash (19–29%) [29]
Sarcoidosis [4]
Stevens-Johnson syndrome [3]
Toxic epidermal necrolysis [3]
Toxicity [4]
Transient acantholytic dermatosis [2]
Urticaria (2%) [3]
Vasculitis [3]
Vitiligo [3]

Hair
Alopecia [3]

Cardiovascular
Atrial fibrillation [2]
Cardiotoxicity [3]
Myocarditis [4]
Pericarditis [2]

Central Nervous System
Anorexia [3]
Chills [2]
Encephalitis [3]
Encephalopathy [4]
Fever [4]
Guillain–Barré syndrome [6]
Headache (14%) [3]
Neurotoxicity [6]

Neuromuscular/Skeletal
Arthralgia [5]
Asthenia (fatigue) (34–41%) [12]
Myalgia/Myopathy [5]
Myasthenia gravis [6]
Rhabdomyolysis [2]

Gastrointestinal/Hepatic
Abdominal pain [3]
Colitis (5–8%) [56]
Constipation [2]
Diarrhea (32–37%) [47]
Enterocolitis (7%) [7]
Gastritis [2]
Gastrointestinal perforation [5]
Hepatitis [16]
Hepatotoxicity (<2%) [19]
Ileus [2]
Nausea [5]
Pancreatitis [4]
Vomiting [2]

Respiratory
Dyspnea [2]
Pneumonia [5]
Pneumonitis [9]

Endocrine/Metabolic
Adrenal insufficiency [4]
ALT increased [12]
AST increased [10]
Diabetes mellitus [3]
Hyperthyroidism [4]
Hyponatremia [3]
Hypophysitis [39]
Hypopituitarism (<4%)
Hypothyroidism [14]
Thyroid dysfunction [4]
Thyroiditis [16]
Thyrotoxicosis [3]
Weight loss [2]

Renal
Nephrotoxicity [7]
Renal failure [4]

Hematologic
Anemia [3]
Hyperlipasemia [3]
Neutropenia [6]
Thrombocytopenia [6]

Ocular
Iridocyclitis [3]
Ocular adverse effects [3]
Orbital inflammation [4]
Retinitis [2]
Uveitis [9]
Xerophthalmia [2]

Local
Infusion-related reactions [4]
Injection-site reactions [2]

Other
Adverse effects [32]
Death [15]

IPRATROPIUM

Trade names: Atrovent (Boehringer Ingelheim), Combivent (Boehringer Ingelheim), Duoneb (Mylan Specialty), Ipratropium Steri-Neb (Ivax), Rinatec (Boehringer Ingelheim)
Indications: Bronchospasm
Class: Anticholinergic, Muscarinic antagonist
Half-life: 2 hours
Clinically important, potentially hazardous interactions with: anticholinergics
Pregnancy category: B
Important contra-indications noted in the prescribing guidelines for: nursing mothers
Note: Combivent is ipratropium and albuterol.

Mucosal
Oral lesions (<5%)
Oral ulceration [2]
Xerostomia (3%) [3]

Central Nervous System
Dysgeusia (taste perversion) [2]
Trembling (<10%)

Ocular
Mydriasis [2]

Other
Adverse effects [2]

IRBESARTAN

Trade names: Aprovel (Bristol-Myers Squibb), Avalide (Bristol-Myers Squibb), Avapro (Sanofi-Aventis)
Indications: Hypertension, diabetic nephropathy
Class: Angiotensin II receptor antagonist (blocker), Antihypertensive
Half-life: 11–15 hours
Clinically important, potentially hazardous interactions with: ACE inhibitors, adrenergic neurone blockers, alcohol, aldesleukin, aldosterone antagonists, aliskiren, alpha blockers, alprostadil, amifostine, antihypertensives, antipsychotics, anxiolytics and hypnotics, baclofen, beta blockers, calcium channel blockers, carvedilol, clonidine, corticosteroids, cyclosporine, CYP2C8 and CYP2C9 substrates, diazoxide, diuretics, eplerenone, fluconazole, general anesthetics, heparins, hypotensives, levodopa, lithium, MAO inhibitors, methyldopa, methylphenidate, moxisylyte, moxonidine, nitrates, NSAIDs, pentoxifylline, phosphodiesterase 5 inhibitors, potassium salts, prostacyclin analogues, rifamycin derivatives, rituximab, tacrolimus, tizanidine, tolvaptan, trimethoprim
Pregnancy category: D (category C in first trimester; category D in second and third trimesters)
Important contra-indications noted in the prescribing guidelines for: nursing mothers; pediatric patients
Note: Avalide is irbesartan and hydrochlorothiazide. Hydrochlorothiazide is a sulfonamide which can be absorbed systemically. Sulfonamides can produce severe, possibly fatal, reactions such as toxic epidermal necrolysis and Stevens-Johnson syndrome.
Warning: FETAL TOXICITY

Skin
Angioedema [3]
Edema (<10%)
Peripheral edema [2]
Rash (<10%)

Gastrointestinal/Hepatic
Pancreatitis [2]

Respiratory
Cough [2]

IRINOTECAN

Trade names: Camptosar (Pfizer), Onivyde (Merrimack)
Indications: Metastatic colorectal carcinoma (Camptosar), metastatic adenocarcinoma of the pancreas (Onivyde - in combination with fluorouracil and leucovorin)
Class: Antineoplastic, Topoisomerase I inhibitor
Half-life: 6–10 hours
Clinically important, potentially hazardous interactions with: aprepitant, atazanavir, bevacizumab, ketoconazole, lapatinib, safinamide, sorafenib, St John's wort, strong CYP3A4 inhibitors, voriconazole
Pregnancy category: D
Important contra-indications noted in the prescribing guidelines for: the elderly; nursing mothers; pediatric patients
Warning: DIARRHEA and MYELOSUPPRESSION (Camptosar)
SEVERE NEUTROPENIA and SEVERE DIARRHEA (Onivyde)

Skin
Acneform eruption [4]
Exfoliative dermatitis (14%)
Flushing (11%)
Hand–foot syndrome [6]
Pruritus [4]
Rash (46%) [7]
Toxicity [4]

Hair
Alopecia (13–61%) [24]

Mucosal
Mucositis (30%) [3]
Stomatitis (<14%) [6]

Cardiovascular
Bradycardia [2]
Hypertension [10]
Hypotension (5%)
Thrombophlebitis (<10%)
Vasodilation (6%)

Central Nervous System
Anorexia (44%) [19]
Chills (14%)
Confusion (3%)
Dysarthria [2]
Fever (44%) [3]
Insomnia [2]
Neurotoxicity [5]
Pain (23%)
Somnolence (drowsiness) (9%)
Vertigo (dizziness) (21%)

Neuromuscular/Skeletal
Asthenia (fatigue) (69%) [22]

Gastrointestinal/Hepatic
Abdominal pain (68%) [3]
Constipation (32%) [3]
Diarrhea (83%) [47]
Hepatotoxicity [3]
Nausea (82%) [22]
Vomiting (63%) [19]

Respiratory
Cough (20%)
Dyspnea (22%)
Pneumonia (4%) [5]

Endocrine/Metabolic
Dehydration [4]

Renal
Proteinuria [5]

Hematologic
Anemia (97%) [18]
Febrile neutropenia [15]
Leukopenia (96%) [12]
Lymphopenia [2]
Neutropenia (96%) [49]
Thrombocytopenia (96%) [10]

Other
Adverse effects [3]
Allergic reactions (9%)
Death [7]
Infection (14%) [4]

ISAVUCONAZONIUM SULFATE

Trade name: Cresemba (Astellas)
Indications: Invasive aspergillosis, mucormycosis
Class: Antifungal, azole
Half-life: 130 hours
Clinically important, potentially hazardous interactions with: carbamazepine, ketoconazole, rifampin, ritonavir, St John's wort, strong CYP3A4 inducers or inhibitors
Pregnancy category: C
Important contra-indications noted in the prescribing guidelines for: nursing mothers; pediatric patients
Note: Contra-indicated in patients with familial short QT syndrome.

Skin
Dermatitis (<5%)
Erythema (<5%)
Exfoliative dermatitis (<5%)
Hypersensitivity (<5%)
Peripheral edema (15%)
Petechiae (<5%)
Pruritus (8%)
Rash (9%)
Urticaria (<5%)

Hair
Alopecia (<5%)

Mucosal
Gingivitis (<5%)
Stomatitis (<5%)

Cardiovascular
Atrial fibrillation (<5%)
Atrial flutter (<5%)
Bradycardia (<5%)
Cardiac arrest (<5%)
Chest pain (9%)
Extrasystoles (<5%)
Hypotension (8%)
Palpitation (<5%)
QT interval shortening (<5%)
Thrombophlebitis (<5%)

Central Nervous System
Anxiety (8%)
Chills (<5%)
Confusion (<5%)
Delirium (9%)
Depression (<5%)
Dysgeusia (taste perversion) (<5%)
Encephalopathy (<5%)
Gait instability (<5%)
Hallucinations (<5%)
Headache (17%)
Hypoesthesia (<5%)
Insomnia (11%)
Migraine (<5%)
Paresthesias (<5%)
Peripheral neuropathy (<5%)
Seizures (<5%)
Somnolence (drowsiness) (<5%)
Stupor (<5%)
Syncope (<5%)
Tremor (<5%)
Vertigo (dizziness) (<5%)

Neuromuscular/Skeletal
Asthenia (fatigue) (11%)
Back pain (10%)
Bone or joint pain (<5%)
Myalgia/Myopathy (<5%)
Neck pain (<5%)

Gastrointestinal/Hepatic
Abdominal distension (<5%)
Abdominal pain (17%)
Cholecystitis (<5%)
Cholelithiasis (gallstones) (<5%)
Constipation (14%)
Diarrhea (24%) [3]
Dyspepsia (6%)
Gastritis (<5%)
Hepatic failure (<5%)
Hepatomegaly (<5%)
Hepatotoxicity (17%)
Nausea (28%) [3]
Vomiting (25%)

Respiratory
Bronchospasm (<5%)
Dyspnea (17%)
Respiratory failure (7%)
Tachypnea (<5%)

Endocrine/Metabolic
Appetite decreased (9%)
Hypoalbuminemia (<5%)
Hypoglycemia (<5%)
Hypokalemia (19%)
Hypomagnesemia (5%)
Hyponatremia (<5%)

Genitourinary
Hematuria (<5%)

Renal
Proteinuria (<5%)
Renal failure (10%)

Hematologic
Agranulocytosis (<5%)
Leukopenia (<5%)
Pancytopenia (<5%)

Otic
Tinnitus (<5%)

Ocular
Optic neuropathy (<5%)

Local
Injection-site reactions (6%)

Other
Adverse effects [3]

ISONIAZID

Synonym: INH
Trade names: Rifamate (Sanofi-Aventis), Rifater (Sanofi-Aventis)
Indications: Tuberculosis
Class: Antibiotic, Antimycobacterial
Half-life: <4 hours
Clinically important, potentially hazardous interactions with: acetaminophen, betamethasone, ethosuximide, insulin aspart, insulin degludec, insulin detemir, insulin glargine, insulin glulisine, itraconazole, levodopa, metformin, phenytoin, prednisolone, propranolol, rifampin, rifapentine, safinamide, triamcinolone
Pregnancy category: C

Skin
- Acneform eruption [7]
- AGEP [2]
- Angioedema [2]
- Bullous dermatitis [2]
- Dermatitis [3]
- DRESS syndrome [7]
- Erythema multiforme [2]
- Exanthems [4]
- Exfoliative dermatitis [5]
- Hypersensitivity [7]
- Lichenoid eruption [3]
- Lupus erythematosus [58]
- Peripheral edema [22]
- Photosensitivity [5]
- Pruritus [3]
- Purpura [7]
- Pustules [3]
- Stevens-Johnson syndrome [5]
- Toxic epidermal necrolysis [9]
- Toxicity [2]
- Urticaria (<5%) [4]
- Vasculitis [2]

Hair
- Alopecia [3]

Mucosal
- Oral lesions [2]

Central Nervous System
- Fever [3]
- Hallucinations [3]
- Neurotoxicity [2]
- Peripheral neuropathy [2]
- Psychosis [2]
- Seizures [9]

Neuromuscular/Skeletal
- Arthralgia [2]
- Rhabdomyolysis (3%) [4]

Gastrointestinal/Hepatic
- Hepatotoxicity [33]
- Pancreatitis [4]

Respiratory
- Pleural effusion [2]

Endocrine/Metabolic
- Gynecomastia [4]

Renal
- Nephrotoxicity [2]

Ocular
- Hallucinations, visual [2]
- Optic neuritis [3]

Other
- Adverse effects [6]
- Death [3]
- Side effects (2%) [2]

ISOSORBIDE

Indications: Acute angle-closure glaucoma
Class: Diuretic
Half-life: 5–9.5 hours
Clinically important, potentially hazardous interactions with: sildenafil
Pregnancy category: C
Note: Various forms of isosorbide are available – see other isosorbide profiles for reaction details.

Central Nervous System
- Headache [10]

ISOSORBIDE DINITRATE

Trade names: Dilatrate-SR (Schwarz), Isordil (Wyeth), Sorbitrate (AstraZeneca)
Indications: Angina pectoris
Class: Nitrate, Vasodilator
Half-life: 4 hours (oral)
Clinically important, potentially hazardous interactions with: sildenafil
Pregnancy category: C
Important contra-indications noted in the prescribing guidelines for: the elderly; nursing mothers; pediatric patients
Note: Various forms of isosorbide are available – see other isosorbide profiles for reaction details.

Skin
- Flushing (>10%)

Central Nervous System
- Headache [3]

ISOSORBIDE MONONITRATE

Trade names: Imdur (Schering), Monoket (Schwarz)
Indications: Angina pectoris
Class: Nitrate, Vasodilator
Half-life: ~4 hours
Clinically important, potentially hazardous interactions with: sildenafil
Pregnancy category: B
Important contra-indications noted in the prescribing guidelines for: the elderly; nursing mothers; pediatric patients
Note: Various forms of isosorbide are available – see other isosorbide profiles for reaction details.

Skin
- Flushing (>10%) [2]

Cardiovascular
- Palpitation [2]

Central Nervous System
- Headache [7]
- Vertigo (dizziness) [2]

Other
- Adverse effects [2]

ISOTRETINOIN

Synonym: 13-*cis*-retinoic acid
Trade names: Accutane (Roche), Amnesteem (Genpharm), Claravis (Barr), Roaccutane (Roche)
Indications: Cystic acne
Class: Retinoid
Half-life: 21–24 hours
Clinically important, potentially hazardous interactions with: acitretin, alcohol (ethyl), antacids, bexarotene, carbamazepine, cholestyramine, co-trimoxazole, corticosteroids, dairy products, minocycline, oral contraceptives, phenytoin, retinoids, St John's wort, tetracycline, tetracyclines, vitamin A
Pregnancy category: X
Important contra-indications noted in the prescribing guidelines for: nursing mothers; pediatric patients
Note: Oral retinoids can cause birth defects, and women should avoid isotretinoin when pregnant or trying to conceive.

Skin
- Abscess [3]
- Acneform eruption [20]
- Angioedema [3]
- Desquamation (palms and soles) (5%)
- Diaphoresis [2]
- Edema (subcutaneous, recurrent) [2]
- Erythema nodosum [3]
- Exfoliative dermatitis (<10%)
- Facial edema (<10%)
- Facial erythema [3]
- Fragility [3]
- Granulation tissue [4]
- Keloid [5]
- Pallor (<10%)
- Photosensitivity (>10%) [7]
- Pigmentation [2]
- Pityriasis rosea [2]
- Pruritus (<5%) [5]
- Pyoderma gangrenosum [3]
- Rash [3]
- Sweet's syndrome [2]
- Urticaria [2]
- Vasculitis [4]
- Xanthomas [2]
- Xerosis (>10%) [12]

Hair
- Alopecia (16%) [3]
- Curly hair [3]

Nails
- Brittle nails [2]
- Elkonyxis [2]
- Median canaliform dystrophy [3]
- Onycholysis [3]
- Paronychia [4]
- Pyogenic granuloma [8]

Mucosal
- Cheilitis (>90%) [17]
- Epistaxis (nosebleed) [2]

Mucositis [2]
Xerostomia (>10%) [5]

Central Nervous System
Depression [7]
Headache [7]
Pseudotumor cerebri [4]

Neuromuscular/Skeletal
Arthralgia [4]
Asthenia (fatigue) [2]
Myalgia/Myopathy [8]
Rhabdomyolysis [2]
Sacroiliitis [3]
Stiff person syndrome [2]

Gastrointestinal/Hepatic
Abdominal pain [3]
Hepatotoxicity [3]
Pancreatitis [3]

Endocrine/Metabolic
Amenorrhea [2]
Gynecomastia [2]
Hypercholesterolemia [2]
Hyperlipidemia [2]
Hypertriglyceridemia [5]

Hematologic
Neutropenia [2]

Ocular
Myopia [2]
Ocular adverse effects [2]
Photophobia [2]
Xerophthalmia [2]

Other
Adverse effects [10]
Side effects [2]
Teratogenicity [8]

ISRADIPINE

Trade name: DynaCirc (Reliant)
Indications: Hypertension
Class: Calcium channel blocker
Half-life: 8 hours
Clinically important, potentially hazardous interactions with: amprenavir, delavirdine, epirubicin, imatinib, phenytoin
Pregnancy category: C

Skin
Edema (7%) [6]
Exanthems (2%)
Flushing (2–9%) [9]
Pruritus (<6%)
Rash (2%)

Mucosal
Oral lesions (6%)

Cardiovascular
QT prolongation [2]

Central Nervous System
Headache (9%)
Vertigo (dizziness) (9%)

ITRACONAZOLE

Trade names: Onmel (Merz), Sporanox (Janssen)
Indications: Onychomycosis, deep mycoses, oropharyngeal candidiasis (oral solution only)
Class: Antibiotic, triazole, Antifungal, azole, CYP3A4 inhibitor
Half-life: 21 hours
Clinically important, potentially hazardous interactions with: abiraterone, acalabrutinib, afatinib, alfentanil, alfuzosin, aliskiren, alprazolam, amphotericin B, amprenavir, anisindione, antacids, aprepitant, aripiprazole, artemether/lumefantrine, astemizole, atazanavir, atorvastatin, avanafil, boceprevir, bosentan, brigatinib, budesonide, buspirone, busulfan, cabazitaxel, cabozantinib, calcifediol, calcium channel blockers, carbamazepine, cerivastatin, ciclesonide, cilostazol, cimetidine, cinacalcet, cisapride, clarithromycin, clopidogrel, clorazepate, cobicistat/elvitegravir/emtricitabine/tenofovir alafenamide, cobicistat/elvitegravir/emtricitabine/tenofovir disoproxil, cobimetinib, colchicine, conivaptan, copanlisib, corticosteroids, coumarins, crizotinib, cyclophosphamide, cyclosporine, cyproterone, dabigatran, darifenacin, dasatinib, dexamethasone, diazepam, dicumarol, didanosine, digoxin, dihydroergotamine, dihydropyridines, disopyramide, docetaxel, dofetilide, dronedarone, efavirenz, eletriptan, enzalutamide, eplerenone, ergotamine, erlotinib, erythromycin, estradiol, ethotoin, everolimus, felodipine, fentanyl, fesoterodine, flibanserin, fluticasone propionate, fosamprenavir, fosphenytoin, gefitinib, grapefruit juice, halofantrine, haloperidol, histamine H_2-antagonists, HMG-CoA reductase inhibitors, ibrutinib, iloperidone, imatinib, indinavir, irinotecan, isoniazid, ivabradine, ixabepilone, lapatinib, lercanidipine, levomethadyl, lomitapide, lopinavir, lovastatin, lurasidone, mephenytoin, methadone, methylergonovine, methylprednisolone, methysergide, micafungin, midazolam(oral), midostaurin, mifepristone, mizolastine, naldemedine, neratinib, nevirapine, nilotinib, nisoldipine, olaparib, omeprazole, oral hypoglycemics, osimertinib, paclitaxel, palbociclib, paliperidone, pantoprazole, pazopanib, phenobarbital, phenytoin, pimavanserin, pimecrolimus, pimozide, ponatinib, prednisolone, prednisone, proton pump inhibitors, quetiapine, quinidine, ranolazine, reboxetine, regorafenib, repaglinide, ribociclib, rifabutin, rifampin, rilpivirine, rimonabant, ritonavir, rivaroxaban, romidepsin, ruxolitinib, saquinavir, sildenafil, silodosin, simeprevir, simvastatin, sirolimus, solifenacin, sonidegib, sunitinib, tacrolimus, tadalafil, telaprevir, telithromycin, temsirolimus, terfenadine, tezacaftor/ivacaftor, ticagrelor, tolterodine, tolvaptan, triamcinolone, triazolam, trimetrexate, ulipristal, valbenazine, vardenafil, vemurafenib, venetoclax, vinblastine, vincristine, vinflunine, vinorelbine, vorapaxar, warfarin
Pregnancy category: C
Important contra-indications noted in the prescribing guidelines for: nursing mothers
Note: Contra-indicated in patients with evidence of ventricular dysfunction such as congestive heart failure (CHF) or a history of CHF except for the treatment of life-threatening or other serious infections.
Warning: CONGESTIVE HEART FAILURE, CARDIAC EFFECTS AND DRUG INTERACTIONS

Skin
AGEP [3]
Angioedema [2]
Diaphoresis (3%)
Edema (<4%) [11]
Exanthems (<3%) [7]
Peripheral edema (4%)
Phototoxicity [2]
Pruritus (<3%) [8]
Rash (8%) [10]
Urticaria [3]

Hair
Alopecia [3]

Mucosal
Xerostomia [3]

Cardiovascular
Cardiac arrest [2]
Cardiac failure [4]
Congestive heart failure [4]
Hypertension (3%) [3]
QT prolongation [5]
Torsades de pointes [2]

Central Nervous System
Fever [2]
Headache (4%) [3]
Neurotoxicity [5]
Peripheral neuropathy [4]
Seizures [2]
Tremor [2]
Vertigo (dizziness) [2]

Neuromuscular/Skeletal
Asthenia (fatigue) [3]
Back pain [2]
Rhabdomyolysis [7]

Gastrointestinal/Hepatic
Abdominal pain (2–6%) [5]
Constipation [2]
Diarrhea [4]
Hepatitis [2]
Hepatotoxicity [8]
Nausea (5–7%) [8]
Pancreatitis [2]
Vomiting [3]

Respiratory
Cough (4%)
Dyspnea (2%)
Flu-like syndrome [2]
Pneumonia (2%)

Endocrine/Metabolic
ALT increased [2]
AST increased [2]
Hyperbilirubinemia [2]
Hypertriglyceridemia [2]
Hypokalemia [6]

Renal
Renal failure [2]

Hematologic
Leukopenia [2]
Thrombocytopenia [2]

Other
Adverse effects [8]
Death [3]
Side effects [2]

IVABRADINE

Trade names: Corlanor (Amgen), Procoralan (Servier)
Indications: Chronic stable angina pectoris
Class: Cardiotonic agent, HCN channel blocker
Half-life: 2 hours
Clinically important, potentially hazardous interactions with: azole antifungals, clarithromycin, CYP3A4 inducers, diltiazem, grapefruit juice, itraconazole, ketoconazole, macrolide antibiotics, nefazodone, nelfinavir, pentamidine, phenytoin, rifampin, ritonavir, sotalol, St John's wort, strong or moderate CYP3A4 inhibitors, telithromycin, verapamil
Pregnancy category: N/A
Important contra-indications noted in the prescribing guidelines for: nursing mothers; pediatric patients

---

Cardiovascular
Atrial fibrillation (8%) [3]
Atrioventricular block (<10%)
Bradycardia (10%) [6]
Hypertension (9%)

Central Nervous System
Headache (2–5%) [2]
Vertigo (dizziness) (<10%) [3]

Neuromuscular/Skeletal
Myalgia/Myopathy (<10%)

Gastrointestinal/Hepatic
Nausea [2]

Ocular
Luminous phenomena (14%) [5]
Vision blurred (<10%) [3]
Visual disturbances [3]

IVACAFTOR

Trade name: Kalydeco (Vertex)
Indications: Cystic fibrosis in patients aged 6 years and older who have a *G551D* mutation in the *CFTR* gene
Class: CFTR potentiator
Half-life: 12 hours
Clinically important, potentially hazardous interactions with: CYP3A inducers or inhibitors, fluconazole, grapefruit juice, ketoconazole, rifampin, St John's wort
Pregnancy category: B
Important contra-indications noted in the prescribing guidelines for: nursing mothers; pediatric patients
Note: See also separate profiles for lumacaftor/ivacaftor and tezacaftor/ivacaftor.

Skin
Acneform eruption (4–7%)
Rash (13%) [6]

Mucosal
Nasal congestion (20%) [7]
Oropharyngeal pain (22%) [7]

Cardiovascular
Chest pain (4–7%)

Central Nervous System
Fever [2]
Headache (24%) [8]
Vertigo (dizziness) (9%) [4]

Neuromuscular/Skeletal
Arthralgia (4–7%)
Myalgia/Myopathy (4–7%)

Gastrointestinal/Hepatic
Abdominal pain (16%) [4]
Diarrhea (13%) [6]
Hepatotoxicity [3]
Nausea (12%) [3]
Vomiting [2]

Respiratory
Cough [5]
Hemoptysis [2]
Nasopharyngitis (15%) [4]
Rhinitis (4–7%)
Upper respiratory tract infection (22%) [7]
Wheezing (4–7%)

Endocrine/Metabolic
AST increased (4–7%)

Otic
Otitis media [2]

Other
Adverse effects [4]

IVERMECTIN

Trade names: Sklice (Sanofi Pasteur), Soolantra (Galderma), Stromectol (Merck)
Indications: Various infections caused by susceptible helmintic organisms
Class: Anthelmintic
Half-life: 16–35 hours
Clinically important, potentially hazardous interactions with: alprazolam, barbiturates, benzodiazepines, diazepam, midazolam, valproic acid
Pregnancy category: C
Important contra-indications noted in the prescribing guidelines for: nursing mothers; pediatric patients

---

Skin
Edema (10–53%) [7]
Exanthems (<34%) [3]
Facial edema [3]
Pruritus (38–71%) [14]
Rash (<93%) [6]
Urticaria (23%)

Cardiovascular
Tachycardia (4%)

Central Nervous System
Fever (23%) [2]
Headache [3]
Psychosis [2]
Vertigo (dizziness) (3%) [3]

Neuromuscular/Skeletal
Arthralgia (9%)
Myalgia/Myopathy (20%) [3]

Gastrointestinal/Hepatic
Abdominal pain [3]

Other
Adverse effects [4]
Side effects (mild) [3]

IVOSIDENIB *

Trade name: Tibsovo (Agios Pharmaceuticals Inc)
Indications: treatment of adult patients with relapsed or refractory acute myeloid leukemia (AML) with a susceptible IDH1 mutation as detected by an FDA-approved test
Class: isocitrate dehydrogenase-1 inhibitor
Half-life: 93 hours
Clinically important, potentially hazardous interactions with: none known
Pregnancy category: N/A (may cause fetal harm when administered to a pregnant woman)
Warning: DIFFERENTIATION SYNDROME

Skin
Edema (32%)
Rash (26%)
Tumor lysis syndrome (8%)

Mucosal
Mucositis (28%)

Cardiovascular
Chest pain (16%)
Hypotension (12%)
Prolonged QT interval [2]
QT prolongation (26%)

Central Nervous System
Fever (23%)
Headache (16%)
Peripheral neuropathy (12%)

Neuromuscular/Skeletal
Arthralgia (36%)
Asthenia (fatigue) (39%)
Myalgia/Myopathy (18%)

Gastrointestinal/Hepatic
Abdominal pain (16%)
Constipation (20%)
Diarrhea (34%)
Nausea (31%)
Vomiting (18%)

Respiratory
Cough (22%)
Dyspnea (33%)
Pleural effusion (13%)

Endocrine/Metabolic
ALP increased (27%)
ALT increased (15%)
Appetite decreased (18%)
AST increased (27%)
Hyperbilirubinemia (16%)
Hypermagnesemia (38%)
Hyperuricemia (32%)
Hypophosphatemia (25%)
Serum creatinine increased (23%)

Hematologic
Hemoglobin decreased (60%)
Leukocytosis (38%)

IXAZOMIB

Trade name: Ninlaro (Millennium)
Indications: Multiple myeloma (in combination with lenalidomide and dexamethasone) in patients who have received at least one prior therapy
Class: Proteasome inhibitor
Half-life: 10 days
Clinically important, potentially hazardous interactions with: carbamazepine, phenytoin, rifampin, St John's wort, strong CYP3A inducers
Pregnancy category: N/A (Can cause fetal harm)
Important contra-indications noted in the prescribing guidelines for: nursing mothers; pediatric patients
Note: See separate profiles for dexamethasone and lenalidomide.

Skin
Acneform eruption [3]
Erythema [4]
Erythema multiforme [2]
Exanthems [8]
Exfoliative dermatitis [4]
Facial edema [2]
Hyperhidrosis [4]
Peripheral edema (25%) [4]
Petechiae [3]
Pigmentation [3]
Pruritus [4]
Rash (19%) [10]
Urticaria [2]
Xerosis [3]

Hair
Alopecia [2]

Central Nervous System
Chills [2]
Fever [4]
Insomnia [2]
Peripheral neuropathy (28%) [11]

Neuromuscular/Skeletal
Asthenia (fatigue) [10]
Back pain (21%)

Gastrointestinal/Hepatic
Abdominal pain [2]
Constipation (34%) [3]
Diarrhea (42%) [12]
Nausea (26%) [11]
Vomiting (22%) [10]

Respiratory
Dyspnea [2]
Pneumonia [3]
Upper respiratory tract infection (19%)

Endocrine/Metabolic
Appetite decreased [4]
Dehydration [3]
Hypokalemia [2]

Renal
Renal failure [2]

Hematologic
Anemia [9]
Leukopenia [3]
Lymphopenia [5]
Neutropenia (67%) [12]
Platelets decreased [3]
Thrombocytopenia (78%) [17]

Ocular
Conjunctivitis (6%)
Vision blurred (6%)
Xerophthalmia (5%)

Other
Adverse effects [4]

IXEKIZUMAB

Trade name: Taltz (Lilly)
Indications: Moderate-to-severe plaque psoriasis, active psoriatic arthritis
Class: Interleukin-17A (IL-17A) antagonist, Monoclonal antibody
Half-life: 13 days
Clinically important, potentially hazardous interactions with: live vaccines
Pregnancy category: N/A (Insufficient evidence to inform drug-associated risk)
Important contra-indications noted in the prescribing guidelines for: pediatric patients

---

Skin
Candidiasis [3]
Hypersensitivity [6]
Peripheral edema [2]
Pruritus [2]
Tinea [2]
Urticaria [2]

Central Nervous System
Headache [8]

Neuromuscular/Skeletal
Arthralgia [2]

Gastrointestinal/Hepatic
Colitis [3]
Crohn's disease [4]
Nausea (2%)

Respiratory
Nasopharyngitis [12]
Upper respiratory tract infection (14%) [12]

Endocrine/Metabolic
ALT increased [2]
AST increased [2]

Hematologic
Neutropenia (11%) [4]
Thrombocytopenia (3%)

Otic
Ear infection (2%)

Local
Injection-site erythema [3]
Injection-site pain [2]
Injection-site reactions (17%) [15]

Other
Adverse effects [3]
Death [4]
Infection [7]

JAPANESE ENCEPHALITIS VACCINE

Trade name: Ixiaro (Novartis)
Indications: Active immunization against Japanese encephalitis for adults
Class: Vaccine
Half-life: N/A
Clinically important, potentially hazardous interactions with: immunosuppressants
Pregnancy category: C
Important contra-indications noted in the prescribing guidelines for: nursing mothers; pediatric patients

---

Skin
Edema (4%)
Pruritus (4%)
Rash (<10%)

Central Nervous System
Fever [5]
Headache (28%) [5]
Seizures [2]

Neuromuscular/Skeletal
Asthenia (fatigue) (11%) [2]
Myalgia/Myopathy (16%)

Gastrointestinal/Hepatic
Diarrhea (<10%)
Nausea (<10%)
Vomiting (<10%)

Respiratory
Flu-like syndrome (12%)

Local
Injection-site edema (<10%)
Injection-site erythema (<10%)
Injection-site induration (<10%)
Injection-site pain (33%) [4]
Injection-site pruritus (<10%)

Other
Adverse effects [5]

JOJOBA OIL

Family: Simmondsiaceae
Scientific names: *Buxus chinensis, Simmondsia chinensis*
Indications: Moisturizer in cosmetics and hair care products, edible oil
Half-life: N/A
Clinically important, potentially hazardous interactions with: none known
Pregnancy category: N/A

Skin
Dermatitis [2]

JUNIPER

Family: Cupressaceae
Scientific names: *Juniperus communis, Juniperus oxycedrus, Juniperus phoenicea, Juniperus virginiana*
Indications: Cystitis, urethritis, urinary tract infections, flatulent colic, rheumatism, arthritis, gout, leucorrhea, blenorrhea, scrofula. **Topical:** joint pain, muscle pain, neuralgia, chronic eczema. **Inhalant:** bronchitis, lung infections. Condiment, flavor component (gin, Chartreuse, bitters), perfume
Class: Anti-inflammatory
Half-life: N/A
Clinically important, potentially hazardous interactions with: loop diuretics, thiazide diuretics
Pregnancy category: N/A

KANAMYCIN

Indications: Various infections caused by susceptible organisms
Class: Antibiotic, aminoglycoside
Half-life: 2–4 hours
Clinically important, potentially hazardous interactions with: aldesleukin, atracurium, bacitracin, bumetanide, doxacurium, ethacrynic acid, furosemide, methoxyflurane, neostigmine, non-depolarizing muscle relaxants, pancuronium, polypeptide antibiotics, rocuronium, succinylcholine, teicoplanin, torsemide, vecuronium
Pregnancy category: D
Important contra-indications noted in the prescribing guidelines for: nursing mothers
Note: Aminoglycosides may cause neurotoxicity and/or nephrotoxicity.

Skin
- Edema (>10%)
- Pruritus (<10%)
- Rash (<10%)

Renal
- Nephrotoxicity [2]

Otic
- Hearing loss [2]
- Ototoxicity [8]

KAVA

Family: Piperaceae
Scientific name: *Piper methysticum*
Indications: Psychosis, depression, headache, migraines, colds, rheumatism, cystitis, vaginal prolapse, otitis, abscesses, antistress, analgesic, local anesthetic, anticonvulsant
Class: Anxiolytic
Half-life: N/A
Clinically important, potentially hazardous interactions with: alcohol, alprazolam, amitriptyline, benzodiazepines
Pregnancy category: N/A
Note: Products containing kava have been implicated in cases of severe liver toxicity. Serious adverse effects include hepatitis, cirrhosis and liver failure. At least one patient required a liver transplant. Kava has now been banned in many countries
Kava was discovered by Captain Cook, who named the plant ?intoxicating pepper.? In the South Pacific, kava is a popular social drink, similar to alcohol in Western societies.

Central Nervous System
- Coma [2]

Gastrointestinal/Hepatic
- Hepatotoxicity [13]

Other
- Adverse effects [8]
- Side effects [3]

KETAMINE

Trade name: Ketalar (Monarch)
Indications: Induction of anesthesia
Class: Anesthetic
Half-life: 2–3 hours
Clinically important, potentially hazardous interactions with: memantine, mivacurium
Pregnancy category: D

Skin
- Pruritus [3]
- Rash (<10%)

Mucosal
- Sialorrhea [2]

Cardiovascular
- Bradycardia [4]
- Hypertension [5]
- Hypotension [5]
- Tachycardia [2]

Central Nervous System
- Agitation [5]
- Amnesia [2]
- Hallucinations [14]
- Headache [3]
- Mania [2]
- Nightmares [2]
- Sedation [4]
- Tremor (>10%)
- Vertigo (dizziness) [5]

Gastrointestinal/Hepatic
- Hepatotoxicity [2]
- Nausea [8]
- Vomiting [11]

Respiratory
- Apnea [3]
- Hypoxia [3]
- Laryngospasm [4]

Genitourinary
- Cystitis [3]

Ocular
- Vision blurred [2]

Local
- Injection-site pain (<10%)

Other
- Adverse effects [4]

KETOCONAZOLE

Trade name: Nizoral (Janssen)
Indications: Fungal infections
Class: Antibiotic, imidazole, Antifungal, azole, CYP3A4 inhibitor
Half-life: initial: 2 hours; terminal: 8 hours
Clinically important, potentially hazardous interactions with: abemaciclib, abiraterone, afatinib, alcohol, alfuzosin, aliskiren, alitretinoin, almotriptan, alprazolam, amphotericin B, amprenavir, anisindione, anticoagulants, aprepitant, aripiprazole, astemizole, atazanavir, avanafil, axitinib, beclomethasone, bedaquiline, benzodiazepines, betrixaban, boceprevir, bosentan, bosutinib, brentuximab vedotin, brigatinib, budesonide, buprenorphine, cabazitaxel, cabozantinib, caffeine, calcifediol, ceritinib, chlordiazepoxide, ciclesonide, cilostazol, cimetidine, cinacalcet, cisapride, clopidogrel, clorazepate, cobicistat/elvitegravir/emtricitabine/tenofovir alafenamide, cobicistat/elvitegravir/emtricitabine/tenofovir disoproxil, colchicine, conivaptan, copanlisib, crizotinib, cyclosporine, cyproterone, dabigatran, darifenacin, darunavir, dasatinib, desvenlafaxine, dexlansoprazole, dicumarol, didanosine, disopyramide, docetaxel, dofetilide, domperidone, doxercalciferol, dronedarone, dutasteride, echinacea, elbasvir & grazoprevir, eletriptan, eplerenone, erlotinib, erythromycin, estradiol, eszopiclone, everolimus, fentanyl, fesoterodine, fingolimod, flibanserin, flunisolide, fluticasone propionate, fosamprenavir, gastric alkanizers, halofantrine, HMG-CoA reductase inhibitors, ibrutinib, iloperidone, imatinib, indacaterol, indinavir, irinotecan, isavuconazonium sulfate, ivabradine, ivacaftor, ixabepilone, lanthanum, lapatinib, levomilnacipran, lomitapide, lopinavir, lurasidone, macitentan, maraviroc, mefloquine, methadone, methylergonovine, methylprednisolone, midazolam, midostaurin, mizolastine, mometasone, naldemedine, neratinib, nevirapine, nilotinib, nisoldipine, non-sedating antihistamines, olaparib, omeprazole, ospemifene, oxybutynin, paclitaxel, palbociclib, pantoprazole, paricalcitol, pazopanib, pimavanserin, pimecrolimus, pimozide, pomalidomide, ponatinib, prednisolone, prednisone, proton-pump inhibitors, quetiapine, quinidine, rabeprazole, ramelteon, ranolazine, reboxetine, regorafenib, ribociclib, rifampin, rilpivirine, rimonabant, ritonavir, rivaroxaban, roflumilast, romidepsin, ropivacaine, rupatadine, ruxolitinib, saquinavir, saxagliptin, sildenafil, silodosin, simeprevir, simvastatin, solifenacin, sonidegib, sucralfate, sunitinib, tacrolimus, tadalafil, tamsulosin, tasimelteon, telaprevir, telithromycin, temsirolimus, tezacaftor/ivacaftor, ticagrelor, tiotropium, tofacitinib, tolterodine, tolvaptan, trabectedin, tramadol, triamcinolone, triazolam, trospium, ulipristal, valbenazine, vardenafil, vemurafenib, venetoclax, venlafaxine, vilazodone, vinblastine, vincristine, vorapaxar, warfarin, zaleplon, ziprasidone, zolpidem, zotarolimus

Pregnancy category: C
Warning: HEPATOTXICITY, QT PROLONGATION AND DRUG INTERACTIONS LEADING TO QT PROLONGATION

Skin
- Anaphylactoid reactions/Anaphylaxis [3]
- Angioedema [3]
- Dermatitis [3]
- Exanthems (<9%) [7]
- Exfoliative dermatitis [2]
- Fixed eruption [2]
- Hypersensitivity [3]
- Pigmentation [3]
- Pruritus (<9%) [5]
- Purpura [2]
- Rash (<3%) [3]
- Urticaria (<3%) [2]
- Xerosis [3]

Hair
- Alopecia (<4%) [4]

Mucosal
- Gingivitis [2]
- Oral lesions (<5%) [3]
- Oral lichenoid eruption [2]
- Oral pigmentation [2]

Cardiovascular
- QT prolongation [4]

Central Nervous System
- Chills (<3%)
- Fever [2]
- Neurotoxicity [3]

Neuromuscular/Skeletal
- Asthenia (fatigue) [3]
- Rhabdomyolysis [3]

Gastrointestinal/Hepatic
- Hepatotoxicity [18]
- Nausea (3–10%) [4]
- Vomiting (3–10%)

Endocrine/Metabolic
- Gynecomastia (<3%) [8]

Hematologic
- Eosinophilia [2]

Other
- Adverse effects [5]
- Death [5]

KETOPROFEN

Trade names: Orudis (Sanofi-Aventis), Oruvail (Wyeth)
Indications: Arthritis
Class: Non-steroidal anti-inflammatory (NSAID)
Half-life: 1.5–4 hours
Clinically important, potentially hazardous interactions with: aspirin, caffeine, methotrexate, probenecid
Pregnancy category: C
Important contra-indications noted in the prescribing guidelines for: nursing mothers; pediatric patients
Note: NSAIDs may cause an increased risk of serious cardiovascular and gastrointestinal adverse events, which can be fatal. This risk may increase with duration of use.

Skin
- Anaphylactoid reactions/Anaphylaxis [4]
- Contact dermatitis [5]
- Dermatitis [29]
- Eczema [3]
- Erythema [4]
- Exanthems [3]
- Peripheral edema (<3%)
- Photoallergic reaction [2]
- Photocontact dermatitis [5]
- Photosensitivity [36]
- Pruritus (<10%) [4]
- Rash (>10%)
- Urticaria [6]

Gastrointestinal/Hepatic
- Abdominal pain (3–9%) [2]
- Constipation [2]
- Diarrhea (3–9%)
- Dyspepsia (11%) [2]
- Gastrointestinal bleeding [2]
- Nausea (3–9%) [2]
- Pancreatitis [3]

Endocrine/Metabolic
- Pseudoporphyria [2]

Renal
- Renal function abnormal (3–9%)

Local
- Application-site reactions [2]

Other
- Adverse effects [11]
- Allergic reactions [2]

KETOROLAC

Trade names: Acular (Allergan), Toradol (Roche)
Indications: Pain, relief of inflammation following cataract surgery (ophthalmic solution)
Class: Analgesic, non-opioid, Non-steroidal anti-inflammatory (NSAID)
Half-life: 2–8 hours
Clinically important, potentially hazardous interactions with: aspirin, buprenorphine, dabigatran, diclofenac, enoxaparin, meloxicam, methotrexate, probenecid, rivaroxaban, salicylates, tiagabine, tinzaparin
Pregnancy category: C
Important contra-indications noted in the prescribing guidelines for: nursing mothers; pediatric patients
Warning: GASTROINTESTINAL, CARDIOVASCULAR, RENAL, AND BLEEDING RISK

Skin
- Anaphylactoid reactions/Anaphylaxis [3]
- Dermatitis (3–9%)
- Diaphoresis (<10%) [2]
- Edema (<10%)
- Exanthems (3–9%)
- Hematoma [2]
- Hypersensitivity [2]
- Pruritus (<10%)
- Purpura (<10%)
- Rash (<10%)

Mucosal
- Stomatitis (<10%)
- Xerostomia [2]

Cardiovascular
- Hypertension (<10%)

Central Nervous System
- Headache (>10%) [4]
- Somnolence (drowsiness) [3]
- Vertigo (dizziness) [4]

Gastrointestinal/Hepatic
- Abdominal pain (>10%)
- Constipation (<10%)
- Diarrhea (7%) [2]
- Dyspepsia (>10%)
- Flatulence (<10%)
- Gastrointestinal bleeding [6]
- Gastrointestinal ulceration (<10%) [2]
- Nausea (>10%) [12]
- Vomiting (<10%) [8]

Renal
- Renal function abnormal (<10%)

Hematologic
- Anemia (<10%)
- Prothrombin time increased (<10%)

Otic
- Tinnitus (<10%)

Ocular
- Corneal melting [4]
- Ocular burning [2]

Local
- Injection-site pain (<10%)

Other
- Adverse effects [10]
- Death [2]
- Side effects [2]

LABETALOL

Trade name: Trandate (Prometheus)
Indications: Hypertension
Class: Adrenergic beta-receptor antagonist, Antiarrhythmic class II
Half-life: 3–8 hours
Clinically important, potentially hazardous interactions with: cimetidine, halothane, imipramine, iobenguane, tricyclic antidepressants
Pregnancy category: C
Important contra-indications noted in the prescribing guidelines for: nursing mothers; pediatric patients
Note: Cutaneous side effects of beta-receptor blockers are clinically polymorphous. They apparently appear after several months of continuous therapy.

Skin
- Anaphylactoid reactions/Anaphylaxis [2]
- Edema (<2%)
- Exanthems (<5%) [4]
- Flushing (19%)
- Lichenoid eruption [4]
- Lupus erythematosus [4]
- Pityriasis rubra pilaris [2]
- Pruritus (<10%) [3]
- Psoriasis (exacerbation) [3]
- Scalp tingling [3]

Cardiovascular
- Hypotension [4]

Central Nervous System
Dysgeusia (taste perversion) (<10%)
Paresthesias (7%) [2]

Neuromuscular/Skeletal
Myalgia/Myopathy [4]

Other
Side effects (6%) [2]

LACOSAMIDE

Trade name: Vimpat (UCB Pharma)
Indications: Partial-onset seizures
Class: Anticonvulsant, Antiepileptic
Half-life: 13 hours
Clinically important, potentially hazardous interactions with: alcohol, antipsychotics, carbamazepine, chloroquine, fosphenytoin, hydroxychloroquine, lamotrigine, MAO inhibitors, mefloquine, orlistat, phenobarbital, phenytoin, pregabalin, SSRIs, St John's wort, tricyclic antidepressants
Pregnancy category: C
Important contra-indications noted in the prescribing guidelines for: the elderly; nursing mothers; pediatric patients

---

Skin
Angioedema [2]
Pruritus (2%)
Rash [4]

Cardiovascular
Atrioventricular block [4]
Bradycardia [3]
Hypotension [3]

Central Nervous System
Balance disorder (4%)
Depression (2%) [2]
Gait instability (2%) [4]
Headache (13%) [17]
Incoordination [2]
Irritability [2]
Memory loss (2%)
Sedation [4]
Seizures [5]
Somnolence (drowsiness) (7%) [12]
Tremor (7%) [4]
Vertigo (dizziness) (31%) [38]

Neuromuscular/Skeletal
Asthenia (fatigue) (2–9%) [9]
Ataxia (8%) [10]

Gastrointestinal/Hepatic
Diarrhea (4%)
Nausea (11%) [19]
Pancreatitis [2]
Vomiting (9%) [9]

Respiratory
Nasopharyngitis [2]
Upper respiratory tract infection [2]

Endocrine/Metabolic
Weight gain [2]

Ocular
Abnormal vision [3]
Diplopia (11%) [15]
Nystagmus (5%)
Vision blurred (8%) [4]

Local
Injection-site pain (2%)

Other
Adverse effects [8]

LACTOBACILLUS

Family: Lactobacillaceae
Scientific names: *Lactobacillus acidophilus, Lactobacillus amylovorus, Lactobacillus brevis, Lactobacillus bulgaricus, Lactobacillus casei, Lactobacillus crispatus, Lactobacillus delbrueckii, Lactobacillus fermentum, Lactobacillus gallinarum, Lactobacillus johnsonii, Lactobacillus paracasei, Lactobacillus plantarum, Lactobacillus reuteri, Lactobacillus rhamnosus, Lactobacillus salivarius, Lactobacillus sporogenes*
Indications: Oral: Acne, allergic rhinitis, atopic allergy, diarrhea, *Helicobacter pylori* infection, irritable bowel syndrome, rotavirus, ulcerative colitis, urinary tract infections. **Suppository**: vaginitis, urinary tract infections
Class: Immunomodulator, Probiotic
Half-life: N/A
Clinically important, potentially hazardous interactions with: none known
Note: Immune-deficient subjects or those with mucosal disease may experience serious adverse effects.

LAMIVUDINE

Synonym: 3TC
Trade names: Combivir (ViiV), Epivir (ViiV), Epzicom (ViiV), Triumeq (ViiV), Trizivir (ViiV)
Indications: HIV progression
Class: Antiretroviral, Nucleoside analog reverse transcriptase inhibitor
Half-life: 5–7 hours
Clinically important, potentially hazardous interactions with: cobicistat/elvitegravir/emtricitabine/tenofovir disoproxil, emtricitabine, trimethoprim
Pregnancy category: C
Note: Combivir is lamivudine and zidovudine; Epzicom is lamivudine and abacavir; Triumeq is abacavir, dolutegravir and lamivudine; Trizivir is lamivudine, abacavir and zidovudine,.

Skin
Angioedema [2]
Exanthems [2]
Hypersensitivity [4]
Jaundice [2]
Pigmentation [2]
Pruritus [3]
Rash (9%) [10]
Stevens-Johnson syndrome [3]
Toxic epidermal necrolysis [3]

Hair
Alopecia [3]

Central Nervous System
Abnormal dreams [2]
Chills (<10%)
Headache [6]
Insomnia [3]
Neurotoxicity [2]
Paresthesias (>10%)
Peripheral neuropathy [3]
Vertigo (dizziness) [4]

Neuromuscular/Skeletal
Asthenia (fatigue) [5]
Myalgia/Myopathy (8%)
Rhabdomyolysis [3]

Gastrointestinal/Hepatic
Abdominal pain [4]
Diarrhea [4]
Hepatotoxicity [3]
Nausea [6]
Pancreatitis [4]
Vomiting [2]

Respiratory
Upper respiratory tract infection [2]

Endocrine/Metabolic
Acidosis [3]

Renal
Nephrotoxicity [2]

Hematologic
Anemia [2]

Other
Adverse effects [9]

LAMOTRIGINE

Trade name: Lamictal (GSK)
Indications: Epilepsy
Class: Anticonvulsant, Antiepileptic, Mood stabilizer
Half-life: 24 hours
Clinically important, potentially hazardous interactions with: eslicarbazepine, lacosamide, oral contraceptives, rufinamide
Pregnancy category: C
Important contra-indications noted in the prescribing guidelines for: the elderly; nursing mothers
Warning: SERIOUS SKIN RASHES

Skin
Angioedema (<10%)
Anticonvulsant hypersensitivity syndrome [17]
DRESS syndrome [18]
Erythema (<10%) [2]
Erythema multiforme [4]
Exanthems (<10%) [19]
Hot flashes (<10%)
Hypersensitivity (<10%) [29]
Lupus erythematosus [4]
Photosensitivity [2]
Pruritus (3%) [3]
Rash (10–20%) [54]
Stevens-Johnson syndrome (<10%) [53]
Toxic epidermal necrolysis [54]

Hair
Alopecia [2]

Mucosal
Xerostomia (6%)

Central Nervous System
Agitation [2]
Aseptic meningitis [4]
Fever [2]
Hallucinations [3]

Headache [6]
Insomnia (5–10%)
Nervousness [2]
Neuroleptic malignant syndrome [2]
Pain (5%)
Seizures [9]
Somnolence (drowsiness) (9%) [8]
Suicidal ideation [2]
Tic disorder [2]
Tremor [5]
Vertigo (dizziness) [9]

Neuromuscular/Skeletal
Asthenia (fatigue) (8%) [3]
Ataxia (2–5%) [3]
Rhabdomyolysis [3]

Gastrointestinal/Hepatic
Abdominal pain (6%)
Hepatotoxicity [4]
Nausea [4]

Respiratory
Cough (5%)
Flu-like syndrome (7%)
Pharyngitis (5%)
Rhinitis (7%)

Endocrine/Metabolic
SIADH [2]

Genitourinary
Urinary frequency (<5%)
Vaginitis (4%)

Renal
Nephrotoxicity [3]

Hematologic
Agranulocytosis [3]

Ocular
Abnormal vision (2–5%)
Diplopia [5]
Hallucinations, visual [2]
Nystagmus (2–5%)

Other
Adverse effects [7]
Allergic reactions [2]
Death [6]
Multiorgan failure [2]
Side effects [2]
Teratogenicity [6]

LANREOTIDE

Trade names: Somatuline Autogel (Ipsen), Somatuline Depot (Ipsen), Somatuline LA (Ipsen)
Indications: Acromegaly, carcinoid syndrome, thyrotrophic adenoma
Class: Somatostatin analog
Half-life: 2 hours (immediate release) 5 days (sustained release).
Clinically important, potentially hazardous interactions with: antidiabetics, bromocriptine, cyclosporine, insulin, metformin, repaglinide, sulfonylureas
Pregnancy category: C
Important contra-indications noted in the prescribing guidelines for: nursing mothers; pediatric patients

---

Hair
Alopecia [2]

Cardiovascular
Bradycardia (5–18%)
Hypertension (5%)

Central Nervous System
Headache (7%)
Pain (7%)

Neuromuscular/Skeletal
Arthralgia (7%) [2]
Asthenia (fatigue) [2]

Gastrointestinal/Hepatic
Abdominal pain (7–19%) [7]
Cholelithiasis (gallstones) (2–17%) [2]
Constipation (8%)
Diarrhea (31–65%) [7]
Flatulence (6–14%) [4]
Loose stools (6%)
Nausea (11%) [3]
Steatorrhea [2]
Vomiting (7%)

Endocrine/Metabolic
Diabetes mellitus (7%)
Hyperglycemia (7%)
Hypoglycemia (7%)
Weight loss (5–11%)

Hematologic
Anemia (5–14%)

Local
Injection-site induration [3]
Injection-site pain (4%) [4]
Injection-site reactions (6–22%) [2]

Other
Adverse effects [2]

LANSOPRAZOLE

Trade name: Prevacid (TAP)
Indications: Active duodenal ulcer
Class: Proton pump inhibitor (PPI)
Half-life: 2 hours
Clinically important, potentially hazardous interactions with: bosutinib, clopidogrel, delavirdine, eucalyptus, neratinib, prednisone, rilpivirine, sucralfate
Pregnancy category: C
Important contra-indications noted in the prescribing guidelines for: nursing mothers

---

Skin
Anaphylactoid reactions/Anaphylaxis [6]
Erythema multiforme [2]
Facial edema [2]
Hypersensitivity [3]
Lupus erythematosus [3]
Peripheral edema [2]
Pruritus (3–10%)
Rash (3–10%)
Toxic epidermal necrolysis [4]
Urticaria [3]

Mucosal
Stomatitis [2]

Central Nervous System
Dysgeusia (taste perversion) [3]
Headache (3%) [4]
Vertigo (dizziness) [2]

Gastrointestinal/Hepatic
Abdominal pain [2]
Colitis [2]
Constipation [2]
Diarrhea (<5%) [6]
Hepatitis [2]
Nausea [2]

Endocrine/Metabolic
Gynecomastia [2]

Renal
Nephrotoxicity [2]

Other
Death [2]

LAPATINIB

Trade name: Tykerb (Novartis)
Indications: Breast cancer
Class: Antineoplastic, Biologic, Epidermal growth factor receptor (EGFR) inhibitor, Tyrosine kinase inhibitor
Half-life: 24 hours
Clinically important, potentially hazardous interactions with: alfuzosin, artemether/lumefantrine, atazanavir, carbamazepine, chloroquine, ciprofloxacin, clarithromycin, clozapine, colchicine, conivaptan, CYP2C8 substrates, CYP3A4 inhibitors or inducers, dabigatran, deferasirox, dexamethasone, digoxin, docetaxel, dronedarone, efavirenz, eplerenone, everolimus, fentanyl, food, gadobutrol, grapefruit juice, histamine H_2-antagonists, indinavir, irinotecan, itraconazole, ketoconazole, nefazodone, nelfinavir, nilotinib, omeprazole, P-glycoprotein inducers, paclitaxel, pantoprazole, pazopanib, phenobarbital, phenytoin, pimecrolimus, pimozide, posaconazole, proton pump inhibitors, QT prolonging agents, quinine, repaglinide, rifabutin, rifampin, rifapentin, ritonavir, rivaroxaban, safinamide, salmeterol, saquinavir, saxagliptin, silodosin, St John's wort, telithromycin, tetrabenazine, thioridazine, tolvaptan, topotecan, voriconazole, ziprasidone
Pregnancy category: D
Important contra-indications noted in the prescribing guidelines for: nursing mothers; pediatric patients
Note: Lapitinib is used in conjunction with capecitabine.
Warning: HEPATOXICITY

Skin
Acneform eruption (90%) [4]
Depigmentation (21%)
Hand-foot syndrome (53%) [10]
Inflammation (15%)
Pruritus [3]
Rash (28%) [26]
Toxicity [7]
Xerosis (10%)

Hair
Alopecia [2]

Nails
Paronychia [4]

Mucosal
Mucosal inflammation (15%)
Mucositis [2]
Stomatitis (14%)

Cardiovascular
- Hypertension [2]

Central Nervous System
- Anorexia (24%) [2]
- Fever [2]
- Insomnia (10%)
- Vertigo (dizziness) [2]

Neuromuscular/Skeletal
- Asthenia (fatigue) (12%) [21]
- Back pain (11%)
- Bone or joint pain [2]
- Pain in extremities (12%)

Gastrointestinal/Hepatic
- Abdominal pain (15%)
- Diarrhea (65%) [46]
- Dyspepsia (11%)
- Hepatotoxicity [11]
- Nausea (44%) [11]
- Vomiting (26%) [8]

Respiratory
- Dyspnea (12%) [2]

Endocrine/Metabolic
- ALT increased (37%) [6]
- AST increased (49%) [5]
- Hyperbilirubinemia [5]
- Hypoalbuminemia [2]

Hematologic
- Anemia [6]
- Febrile neutropenia [2]
- Leukopenia [5]
- Lymphopenia [2]
- Neutropenia [9]
- Thrombocytopenia [2]

Otic
- Tinnitus (14%)

Other
- Adverse effects [11]
- Death [2]

LATANOPROST

Trade name: Xalatan (Pfizer)
Indications: Reduction of elevated intraocular pressure in open angle glaucoma or ocular hypertension
Class: Prostaglandin analog
Half-life: 17 minutes
Clinically important, potentially hazardous interactions with: thimerosal
Pregnancy category: C
Important contra-indications noted in the prescribing guidelines for: nursing mothers; pediatric patients

---

Skin
- Pigmentation [2]
- Pruritus [2]
- Rash (<10%)

Cardiovascular
- Angina (<10%)
- Chest pain (<10%)

Central Nervous System
- Headache [3]
- Vertigo (dizziness) [2]

Neuromuscular/Skeletal
- Arthralgia (<10%)
- Back pain (<10%)
- Myalgia/Myopathy (<10%)

Respiratory
- Flu-like syndrome (<10%)
- Upper respiratory tract infection (<10%)

Ocular
- Conjunctival hyperemia [19]
- Deepening of upper lid sulcus [5]
- Eyelashes – hypertrichosis [15]
- Eyelashes – pigmentation [9]
- Eyelid edema (<4%)
- Eyelid erythema (<4%)
- Eyelid pain (<10%)
- Eyelid pigmentation [4]
- Eyelid pruritus (2%)
- Foreign body sensation [5]
- Iris pigmentation [7]
- Keratitis [3]
- Macular edema [7]
- Ocular adverse effects [7]
- Ocular hyperemia [4]
- Ocular itching [8]
- Ocular pigmentation (5%) [13]
- Periorbitopathy [2]
- Uveitis [5]
- Vision blurred [3]
- Xerophthalmia (<10%)

Other
- Allergic reactions (<10%)

LAVENDER

Family: Lamiaceae
Scientific names: *Lavandula angustifolia, Lavandula dentata, Lavandula spica, Lavandula vera*
Indications: Restlessness, insomnia, loss of appetite, flatulence, colic, giddiness, nervous headache, migraine, toothache, sprains, neuralgia, rheumatism, acne, pimples, nausea, vomiting. Flavoring, fragrance, insect repellent
Class: Anxiolytic
Half-life: N/A
Clinically important, potentially hazardous interactions with: none known
Pregnancy category: N/A

Skin
- Dermatitis [4]

Endocrine/Metabolic
- Gynecomastia [2]

LEDIPASVIR & SOFOSBUVIR

Trade name: Harvoni (Gilead)
Indications: Hepatitis C
Class: Hepatitis C virus NS5A inhibitor (ledipasvir), Hepatitis C virus nucleotide analog NS5B polymerase inhibitor (sofosbuvir)
Half-life: 47 hours (ledipasvir); <27 hours (sofosbuvir)
Clinically important, potentially hazardous interactions with: amiodarone, carbamazepine, cobicistat/elvitegravir/emtricitabine/tenofovir disoproxil, oxcarbazepine, phenobarbital, phenytoin, rifabutin, rifampin, rifapentine, ritonavir, rosuvastatin, simeprevir, St John's wort, tenofovir disoproxil
Pregnancy category: N/A (Insufficient evidence to inform drug-associated risk; contra-indicated in pregnancy when given with ribavirin)
Important contra-indications noted in the prescribing guidelines for: nursing mothers; pediatric patients
Note: See also separate entry for sofosbuvir.

Skin
- Pruritus [7]
- Rash [5]

Cardiovascular
- Bradycardia [3]

Central Nervous System
- Headache (11–17%) [40]
- Insomnia (3–6%) [14]
- Irritability [5]
- Vertigo (dizziness) [3]

Neuromuscular/Skeletal
- Arthralgia [3]
- Asthenia (fatigue) (7–18%) [38]
- Muscle spasm [2]
- Myalgia/Myopathy [3]

Gastrointestinal/Hepatic
- Constipation [2]
- Diarrhea (3–7%) [14]
- Hepatotoxicity [3]
- Nausea (6–9%) [22]

Respiratory
- Cough [4]
- Dyspnea [3]
- Nasopharyngitis [3]
- Upper respiratory tract infection [7]

Endocrine/Metabolic
- Hypophosphatemia [2]

Renal
- Nephrotoxicity [3]

Hematologic
- Anemia [8]

Other
- Adverse effects [6]
- Infection [2]

LEMON BALM

Family: Labiatae
Scientific name: *Melissa officinalis*
Indications: Oral: Alzheimer's disease, anxiety, attention deficit disorder, colic, dementia, depression, hyperactivity, hyperthyroidism, insomnia, menstrual cramps, fevers, headache. **Topical:** genital herpes, herpes simplex, insect bites, insect repellent, muscle tension, skin irritation
Class: Carminative, Immunomodulator
Half-life: N/A
Clinically important, potentially hazardous interactions with: none known
Pregnancy category: N/A

Other
Adverse effects [2]

LENALIDOMIDE

Trade name: Revlimid (Celgene)
Indications: Transfusion-dependent anemia due to myeloplastic syndromes, multiple myeloma (in combination with dexamethasone)
Class: Biologic, Immunomodulator, Thalidomide analog
Half-life: 3–5 hours
Clinically important, potentially hazardous interactions with: abatacept, anakinra, canakinumab, certolizumab, denosumab, dexamethasone, digoxin, erythropoietin stimulating agents, estrogen containing therapies, leflunomide, natalizumab, pimecrolimus, rilonacept, sipuleucel-T, tacrolimus, trastuzumab, vaccines
Pregnancy category: X
Important contra-indications noted in the prescribing guidelines for: nursing mothers; pediatric patients
Warning: FETAL RISK, HEMATOLOGIC TOXICITY, and DEEP VEIN THOMBOSIS AND PULMONARY EMBOLISM

Skin
Cellulitis (5%)
DRESS syndrome [3]
Ecchymoses (5–8%)
Edema (10%)
Erythema (5%)
Exanthems [3]
Folliculitis [2]
Graft-versus-host reaction [2]
Hyperhidrosis (7%) [2]
Malignancies (secondary) [6]
Peripheral edema (26%) [5]
Pigmentation [2]
Pruritus (42%) [3]
Rash (36%) [18]
Stevens-Johnson syndrome [6]
Sweet's syndrome [3]
Toxicity [6]
Tumor lysis syndrome [3]
Tumors [5]
Xerosis (14%) [2]

Mucosal
Epistaxis (nosebleed) (15%)
Xerostomia (7%)

Cardiovascular
Cardiac failure [2]
Cardiotoxicity [2]
Chest pain (5%)
Hypertension (6%) [2]
Palpitation (5%)
Thromboembolism [5]
Venous thromboembolism [13]

Central Nervous System
Anorexia (10%)
Depression (5%)
Dysgeusia (taste perversion) (6%)
Fever (21%) [4]
Headache (20%)
Hypoesthesia (7%)
Insomnia (10%) [4]
Neurotoxicity (7%) [8]
Pain (7%)
Peripheral neuropathy (5%) [14]
Rigors (6%)
Somnolence (drowsiness) [2]
Tremor (21%)
Vertigo (dizziness) (20%)

Neuromuscular/Skeletal
Arthralgia (21%) [4]
Asthenia (fatigue) (15–31%) [36]
Back pain (21%) [4]
Bone or joint pain (14%)
Cramps (33%)
Muscle spasm [5]
Myalgia/Myopathy (18%) [3]
Pain in extremities (12%)

Gastrointestinal/Hepatic
Abdominal pain (8–12%)
Constipation (24%) [10]
Diarrhea (49%) [18]
Gastrointestinal disorder [4]
Hepatotoxicity [3]
Loose stools (6%)
Nausea (24%) [9]
Vomiting (10%) [5]

Respiratory
Acute respiratory distress syndrome [2]
Alveolar hemorrhage (pulmonary) [2]
Bronchitis (11%)
Cough (20%) [6]
Dyspnea (7–17%) [4]
Nasopharyngitis (23%)
Pharyngitis (16%)
Pneumonia (12%) [10]
Pneumonitis [7]
Pulmonary toxicity [3]
Rhinitis (7%)
Sinusitis (8%)
Upper respiratory tract infection (15%) [3]

Endocrine/Metabolic
ALT increased (8%) [3]
Appetite decreased (7%)
Hyperglycemia [2]
Hypocalcemia (9%)
Hypokalemia (11%) [4]
Hypomagnesemia (6%)
Hyponatremia [2]
Hypophosphatemia [3]
Hypothyroidism (7%)
Weight loss (20%)

Genitourinary
Urinary tract infection (11%)

Renal
Nephrotoxicity [3]

Hematologic
Anemia (31%) [27]
Cytopenia [3]
Febrile neutropenia (5%) [8]
Hemotoxicity [13]
Leukopenia (8%) [12]
Lymphopenia (5%) [8]
Myelosuppression [6]
Neutropenia (59%) [60]
Thrombocytopenia (62%) [52]
Thrombosis [4]

Ocular
Vision blurred (17%)

Local
Infusion-related reactions [2]
Infusion-site reactions [2]
Injection-site reactions [2]

Other
Adverse effects [14]
Cancer [2]
Death [4]
Infection [20]
Teratogenicity [2]

LENVATINIB

Trade name: Lenvima (Eisai)
Indications: Differentiated thyroid cancer, renal cell cancer (in combination with everolimus)
Class: Tyrosine kinase inhibitor
Half-life: 28 hours
Clinically important, potentially hazardous interactions with: none known
Pregnancy category: N/A (Can cause fetal harm)
Important contra-indications noted in the prescribing guidelines for: nursing mothers; pediatric patients

---

Skin
Exanthems (21%)
Hand–foot syndrome (32%) [3]
Hyperkeratosis (7%)
Peripheral edema (21%) [3]
Rash (21%)
Toxicity [3]

Hair
Alopecia (12%)

Mucosal
Aphthous stomatitis (41%)
Epistaxis (nosebleed) (12%)
Gingivitis (10%)
Glossitis (41%)
Glossodynia (25%)
Mucosal inflammation (41%)
Oral ulceration (41%)
Oropharyngeal pain (25%)
Parotitis (10%)
Stomatitis (41%) [3]
Xerostomia (17%)

Cardiovascular
Hypertension (73%) [22]

Hypotension (9%)
QT prolongation (9%)

Central Nervous System
Anorexia [3]
Dysgeusia (taste perversion) (18%)
Headache (38%) [4]
Insomnia (12%)
Vertigo (dizziness) (15%)

Neuromuscular/Skeletal
Arthralgia (62%)
Asthenia (fatigue) (67%) [11]
Back pain (62%)
Bone or joint pain (62%)
Myalgia/Myopathy (62%)
Pain in extremities (62%)

Gastrointestinal/Hepatic
Abdominal pain (31%) [2]
Constipation (29%) [3]
Diarrhea (67%) [12]
Dyspepsia (13%)
Nausea (47%) [7]
Vomiting (36%) [5]

Respiratory
Cough (24%)
Dysphonia (31%) [2]
Nasopharyngitis [2]

Endocrine/Metabolic
ALP increased (>5%)
ALT increased (4%) [2]
Appetite decreased (54%) [7]
AST increased (5%) [2]
Creatine phosphokinase increased (3%)
Dehydration (9%)
Hyperbilirubinemia (>5%)
Hypercalcemia (>5%)
Hypercholesterolemia (>5%)
Hyperkalemia (>5%)
Hypoalbuminemia (>5%)
Hypocalcemia (9%)
Hypoglycemia (>5%)
Hypokalemia (6%)
Hypomagnesemia (>5%)
Hypothyroidism [2]
Weight loss (51%) [5]

Genitourinary
Hematuria [2]
Urinary tract infection (11%)

Renal
Proteinuria (34%) [10]

Hematologic
Leukopenia [2]
Platelets decreased (2%)
Thrombocytopenia [4]

Other
Adverse effects [4]
Death [2]
Tooth disorder (10%)

LESINURAD

Trade names: Duzallo (AstraZeneca), Zurampic (AstraZeneca)
Indications: Gout-associated hyperuricemia (in combination with a xanthine oxidase inhibitor)
Class: URAT1 inhibitor
Half-life: 5 hours
Clinically important, potentially hazardous interactions with: amiodarone, carbamazepine, CYP2C9 inducers or inhibitors, CYP3A substrates, fluconazole, rifampin, valproic acid
Pregnancy category: N/A (No available data)
Important contra-indications noted in the prescribing guidelines for: nursing mothers; pediatric patients
Note: Contra-indicated in patients with severe renal impairment (including end stage renal disease, kidney transplant recipients or patients on dialysis), tumor lysis syndrome or Lesch-Nylan syndrome. Duzallo is lesinurad and allopurinol (see separate entry).
Warning: RISK OF ACUTE RENAL FAILURE, MORE COMMON WHEN USED WITHOUT A XANTHINE OXIDASE INHIBITOR

Cardiovascular
Cardiotoxicity (<2%)

Central Nervous System
Headache (5%) [2]
Vertigo (dizziness) [2]

Neuromuscular/Skeletal
Back pain [2]

Gastrointestinal/Hepatic
Diarrhea [2]
Gastroesophageal reflux (3%)

Respiratory
Influenza (5%)
Nasopharyngitis [2]

Endocrine/Metabolic
Serum creatinine increased (4–8%) [3]

Renal
Nephrolithiasis (<3%)
Renal failure (<4%)

LETROZOLE

Trade name: Femara (Novartis)
Indications: Breast cancer
Class: Aromatase inhibitor
Half-life: ~2 days
Clinically important, potentially hazardous interactions with: none known
Pregnancy category: X
Important contra-indications noted in the prescribing guidelines for: nursing mothers; pediatric patients

---

Skin
Exanthems (5%)
Hot flashes (6%) [9]
Hyperhidrosis (<5%)
Leukocytoclastic vasculitis [2]
Pruritus (2%)
Psoriasis (5%)
Rash (<10%) [7]
Vesiculation (5%)

Hair
Alopecia (<5%) [4]

Mucosal
Stomatitis [3]

Cardiovascular
Cardiac failure [2]
Hypertension [5]
Myocardial toxicity [2]

Central Nervous System
Anorexia [3]
Depression [3]
Fever [3]
Headache [4]
Insomnia [2]
Mood changes [2]
Vertigo (dizziness) [2]

Neuromuscular/Skeletal
Arthralgia [11]
Asthenia (fatigue) [12]
Back pain [4]
Bone or joint pain [4]
Myalgia/Myopathy [7]
Osteoporosis [7]

Gastrointestinal/Hepatic
Constipation [3]
Diarrhea [9]
Nausea [10]
Vomiting [5]

Respiratory
Cough [2]
Dyspnea [3]

Endocrine/Metabolic
ALT increased [2]
AST increased [3]
Hypercholesterolemia [3]
Hyperglycemia [4]

Genitourinary
Vaginal dryness [4]

Hematologic
Anemia [4]
Febrile neutropenia [2]
Leukopenia [5]
Neutropenia [8]
Thrombocytopenia [2]

Other
Adverse effects [2]
Infection [4]

LEUCOVORIN

Synonyms: citrovorum factor; folinic acid
Indications: Overdose of methotrexate, in combination with fluorouracil in the palliative treatment of patients with colorectal cancer
Class: Adjuvant
Half-life: 15 minutes
Clinically important, potentially hazardous interactions with: capecitabine, glucarpidase, trimethoprim
Pregnancy category: C

Skin
Hand–foot syndrome [3]
Rash [6]

Toxicity [3]

Hair

Alopecia [2]

Mucosal

Mucositis [7]
Stomatitis [6]

Cardiovascular

Hypertension [7]

Central Nervous System

Anorexia [7]
Neurotoxicity [5]
Peripheral neuropathy [4]

Neuromuscular/Skeletal

Asthenia (fatigue) [12]

Gastrointestinal/Hepatic

Abdominal pain [2]
Constipation [2]
Diarrhea [27]
Nausea [15]
Vomiting [12]

Respiratory

Pneumonia [2]

Endocrine/Metabolic

ALP increased [2]

Renal

Proteinuria [4]

Hematologic

Anemia [10]
Febrile neutropenia [8]
Leukopenia [7]
Neutropenia [31]
Thrombocytopenia [6]

Other

Adverse effects [2]
Death [3]
Infection [3]

LEUPROLIDE

Trade names: Eligard (Sanofi-Aventis), Lupron (TAP), Lupron Depot-Ped (AbbVie), Viadur (Bayer)
Indications: Prostate carcinoma, endometriosis
Class: Gonadotropin-releasing hormone (GnRH) agonist
Half-life: 3–4 hours
Clinically important, potentially hazardous interactions with: none known
Pregnancy category: X
Important contra-indications noted in the prescribing guidelines for: nursing mothers

---

Skin

Anaphylactoid reactions/Anaphylaxis [3]
Dermatitis (5%)
Dermatitis herpetiformis [2]
Ecchymoses (<5%)
Edema (<10%)
Flushing (61%) [3]
Granulomas [2]
Hot flashes (12%) [6]
Peripheral edema (4–12%)
Pigmentation (<5%)
Pruritus (<5%)
Rash (<10%)
Vasculitis [2]
Xerosis (<5%)

Hair

Alopecia (<5%)

Cardiovascular

Thrombophlebitis (2%)

Central Nervous System

Dysgeusia (taste perversion) (<5%)
Paresthesias (<5%)

Neuromuscular/Skeletal

Myalgia/Myopathy [2]

Endocrine/Metabolic

Gynecomastia (7%)
Mastodynia (7%)

Ocular

Diplopia [2]

Local

Injection-site granuloma [6]
Injection-site inflammation (2%)
Injection-site pain [2]
Injection-site reactions (24%)

LEVETIRACETAM

Trade names: Elepsia XR (Sun Pharma), Keppra (UCB)
Indications: Partial onset seizures
Class: Anticonvulsant
Half-life: 7 hours
Clinically important, potentially hazardous interactions with: carbamazepine, eslicarbazepine
Pregnancy category: C
Important contra-indications noted in the prescribing guidelines for: nursing mothers

---

Skin

DRESS syndrome [7]
Erythema [2]
Erythema multiforme [2]
Rash [5]
Stevens-Johnson syndrome [4]
Toxic epidermal necrolysis [2]
Urticaria [2]

Central Nervous System

Aggression [8]
Agitation [5]
Anorexia [2]
Behavioral disturbances [5]
Compulsions [2]
Depression [9]
Encephalopathy [4]
Fever [2]
Headache (25%) [12]
Irritability [11]
Nervousness [2]
Neurotoxicity [3]
Paresthesias (2%)
Psychosis [3]
Seizures [4]
Sleep related disorder [2]
Somnolence (drowsiness) [19]
Suicidal ideation [4]
Vertigo (dizziness) (9–18%) [22]

Neuromuscular/Skeletal

Asthenia (fatigue) (<22%) [20]
Osteoporosis [2]
Rhabdomyolysis [3]

Gastrointestinal/Hepatic

Abdominal pain [2]
Diarrhea [2]
Hepatotoxicity [3]
Nausea [4]
Vomiting [4]

Respiratory

Influenza [2]
Nasopharyngitis [5]

Endocrine/Metabolic

Creatine phosphokinase increased [3]
Libido decreased [2]
Weight gain [4]

Genitourinary

Sexual dysfunction [2]

Renal

Nephrotoxicity [2]

Hematologic

Hemotoxicity [2]
Pancytopenia [2]
Thrombocytopenia [2]

Other

Adverse effects [9]
Death [2]
Infection (13–26%) [7]

LEVOCETIRIZINE

Trade name: Xyzal (UCB Pharma)
Indications: Allergic rhinitis, chronic idiopathic urticaria
Class: Histamine H1 receptor antagonist
Half-life: 6–10 hours
Clinically important, potentially hazardous interactions with: none known
Pregnancy category: B
Important contra-indications noted in the prescribing guidelines for: the elderly; nursing mothers; pediatric patients

---

Skin

Fixed eruption [3]

Mucosal

Xerostomia (2–3%)

Central Nervous System

Headache [2]
Sedation [2]
Somnolence (drowsiness) (5–6%)

Neuromuscular/Skeletal

Asthenia (fatigue) (<4%)

Gastrointestinal/Hepatic

Hepatotoxicity [2]

Respiratory

Nasopharyngitis (4–6%)
Pharyngitis (<2%)

LEVODOPA

Synonyms: L-dopa; carbidopa
Trade names: Duopa (Abbvie), Rytary (Impax), Sinemet (Bristol-Myers Squibb), Stalevo (Orion)
Indications: Parkinsonism
Class: Dopamine precursor
Half-life: 1–3 hours
Clinically important, potentially hazardous interactions with: ACE inhibitors, acebutolol, alfuzosin, alpha blockers, amisulpride, ampicillin, angiotensin II receptor antagonists, antihypertensives, antimuscarinics, antipsychotics, baclofen, benzodiazepines, beta blockers, bupropion, calcium channel blockers, captopril, chloramphenicol, cholestyramine, cilazapril, clobazam, clonidine, darifenacin, diazoxide, diuretics, dopamine D_2 receptor antagonists, enalapril, erythromycin, fosinopril, hydralazine, irbesartan, iron salts, isoniazid, levomepromazine, linezolid, lisinopril, MAO inhibitors, memantine, methyldopa, metoclopramide, minoxidil, moclobemide, moxonidine, nitrates, olanzapine, olmesartan, oral iron, oxybutynin, paliperidone, papaverine, pericyazine, phenelzine, phenytoin, probenecid, pyridoxine, quetiapine, quinapril, ramipril, rifampin, risperidone, sapropterin, selegiline, sodium nitroprusside, sulpiride, tetrabenazine, tiotropium, trandolapril, tranylcypromine, tricyclic antidepressants, trospium, volatile liquid general anesthetics, ziprasidone, zuclopenthixol, zuclopenthixol acetate, zuclopenthixol decanoate, zuclopenthixol dihydrochloride
Pregnancy category: C
Important contra-indications noted in the prescribing guidelines for: nursing mothers; pediatric patients
Note: Levodopa is always used in conjuntion with carbidopa. Stalevo is levodopa, carbidopa and entacapone. Contra-indicated in patients with narrow-angle glaucoma or those with a history of melanoma.

Skin
Chromhidrosis (<10%)
Edema [2]
Exanthems [2]
Lupus erythematosus [2]
Melanoma [28]
Rash [3]

Hair
Hair pigmentation [2]

Nails
Nail growth [2]

Mucosal
Xerostomia (<10%) [2]

Cardiovascular
Hypotension [2]
Orthostatic hypotension [4]

Central Nervous System
Agitation [2]
Anosmia [2]
Anxiety [2]
Confusion [3]
Delusions [2]
Depression [3]
Dyskinesia [47]
Gait instability [4]
Hallucinations [12]
Insomnia [6]
Narcolepsy [2]
Neuroleptic malignant syndrome [7]
Neurotoxicity [3]
Psychosis [6]
Restless legs syndrome [5]
Somnolence (drowsiness) [5]
Suicidal ideation [2]
Tardive dyskinesia [2]
Vertigo (dizziness) [5]

Neuromuscular/Skeletal
Arthralgia [2]
Asthenia (fatigue) [2]
Back pain [2]

Gastrointestinal/Hepatic
Abdominal pain [2]
Constipation [5]
Diarrhea [3]
Hepatotoxicity [2]
Nausea [11]
Vomiting [5]

Endocrine/Metabolic
Weight loss [3]

Ocular
Hallucinations, visual [2]
Ocular adverse effects [2]

Other
Adverse effects [4]
Hiccups [2]

LEVOFLOXACIN

Trade names: Iquix (Santen), Levaquin (Ortho-McNeil), Quixin (Johnson & Johnson), Tavanic (Sanofi-Aventis)
Indications: Various infections caused by susceptible organisms, inhalational anthrax (post exposure)
Class: Antibiotic, fluoroquinolone
Half-life: 6–8 hours
Clinically important, potentially hazardous interactions with: alfuzosin, aminophylline, amiodarone, antacids, antidiabetics, arsenic, artemether/lumefantrine, BCG vaccine, chloroquine, ciprofloxacin, corticosteroids, cyclosporine, didanosine, dronedarone, gadobutrol, insulin, lanthanum, mycophenolate, nilotinib, NSAIDs, oral iron, oral typhoid vaccine, phenindione, pimozide, probenecid, QT prolonging agents, quinine, strontium ranelate, sucralfate, sulfonylureas, tetrabenazine, thioridazine, vitamin K antagonists, warfarin, zinc, ziprasidone, zolmitriptan
Pregnancy category: C
Important contra-indications noted in the prescribing guidelines for: the elderly; nursing mothers
Note: Fluoroquinolones are associated with an increased risk of tendinitis and tendon rupture in all ages. This risk is further increased in older patients usually over 60 years of age, in patients taking corticosteroid drugs, and in patients with kidney, heart or lung transplants. Fluoroquinolones may exacerbate muscle weakness in persons with myasthenia gravis.

Warning: SERIOUS ADVERSE REACTIONS INCLUDING TENDINITIS, TENDON RUPTURE, PERIPHERAL NEUROPATHY, CENTRIAL NERVOUS SYSTEM EFFECTS and EXACERBATION OF MYASTHENIA GRAVIS

Skin
Anaphylactoid reactions/Anaphylaxis [6]
Erythema [2]
Erythema nodosum (<3%)
Exanthems [2]
Hypersensitivity [5]
Photosensitivity [3]
Phototoxicity [5]
Pruritus (2%) [3]
Purpura [3]
Radiation recall dermatitis [2]
Rash (2%) [2]
Stevens-Johnson syndrome [3]
Toxic epidermal necrolysis [6]
Vasculitis [3]

Cardiovascular
Myocardial infarction [2]
Palpitation [2]
QT prolongation [5]
Torsades de pointes [6]

Central Nervous System
Anorexia [2]
Delirium [5]
Depression [2]
Dysgeusia (taste perversion) [2]
Headache (6%) [6]
Insomnia (4%) [3]
Peripheral neuropathy [3]
Psychosis [3]
Seizures [9]
Vertigo (dizziness) [6]

Neuromuscular/Skeletal
Arthralgia [4]
Myalgia/Myopathy [4]
Myasthenia gravis (exacerbation) [3]
Rhabdomyolysis [4]
Tendinitis [2]
Tendinopathy/Tendon rupture [35]

Gastrointestinal/Hepatic
Abdominal pain [3]
Constipation (3%)
Diarrhea (5%) [4]
Hepatotoxicity [4]
Nausea (7%) [6]
Vomiting [3]

Endocrine/Metabolic
ALT increased [3]
AST increased [3]
Hypoglycemia [3]

Genitourinary
Vaginitis (2%)

Renal
Nephrotoxicity [5]

Hematologic
Thrombocytopenia [5]

Other
Adverse effects [14]
Death [5]
Side effects [2]

LEVOMILNACIPRAN

Trade name: Fetzima (Forest)
Indications: Major depressive disorder
Class: Antidepressant, Serotonin-norepinephrine reuptake inhibitor
Half-life: 12 hours
Clinically important, potentially hazardous interactions with: ketoconazole, MAO inhibitors, NSAIDs
Pregnancy category: C
Important contra-indications noted in the prescribing guidelines for: nursing mothers; pediatric patients
Warning: SUICIDAL THOUGHTS AND BEHAVIORS

Skin
- Hyperhidrosis (9%) [9]
- Pruritus (<2%)
- Rash (2%)
- Urticaria (<2%)
- Xerosis (<2%)

Mucosal
- Xerostomia [4]

Cardiovascular
- Angina (<2%)
- Extrasystoles (<2%)
- Hypertension (3%) [2]
- Hypotension (3%)
- Palpitation (5%) [5]
- Tachycardia (6%) [9]

Central Nervous System
- Aggression (<2%)
- Agitation (<2%)
- Extrapyramidal symptoms (<2%)
- Headache [5]
- Insomnia [3]
- Migraine (<2%)
- Panic attack (<2%)
- Paresthesias (<2%)
- Syncope (<2%)
- Vertigo (dizziness) [4]
- Yawning (<2%)

Gastrointestinal/Hepatic
- Abdominal pain (<2%)
- Constipation (9%) [9]
- Flatulence (<2%)
- Nausea (17%) [10]
- Vomiting (5%) [5]

Respiratory
- Upper respiratory tract infection [2]

Endocrine/Metabolic
- Appetite decreased (3%)

Genitourinary
- Ejaculatory dysfunction (5%) [4]
- Erectile dysfunction (6%) [7]
- Hematuria (<2%)
- Pollakiuria (<2%)
- Testicular pain (4%)
- Urinary hesitancy (4%) [3]

Renal
- Proteinuria (<2%)

Ocular
- Conjunctival hemorrhage (<2%)
- Vision blurred (<2%)
- Xerophthalmia (<2%)

Other
- Adverse effects [2]
- Bruxism (<2%)

LEVONORGESTREL

Trade names: Kyleena (Bayer), Mirena (Bayer), Plan B (Duramed)
Indications: Intrauterine contraception, treatment of heavy menstrual bleeding, emergency contraception
Class: Hormone, Progestogen
Half-life: 17 hours
Clinically important, potentially hazardous interactions with: barbiturates, bosentan, carbamazepine, CYP3A4 inducers and inhibitors, efavirenz, felbamate, griseofulvin, nevirapine, oxcarbazepine, phenytoin, rifabutin, rifampin, St John's wort, topiramate, ulipristal
Pregnancy category: X
Important contra-indications noted in the prescribing guidelines for: the elderly; nursing mothers; pediatric patients

---

Central Nervous System
- Headache (17%) [7]
- Vertigo (dizziness) (11%)

Neuromuscular/Skeletal
- Asthenia (fatigue) (17%)

Gastrointestinal/Hepatic
- Abdominal pain (18%)
- Diarrhea (5%)
- Nausea (23%) [7]
- Vomiting (6%) [3]

Endocrine/Metabolic
- Amenorrhea [3]
- Mastodynia (11%) [2]
- Menstrual irregularities (26%) [7]

Genitourinary
- Metrorrhagia [2]
- Vaginal bleeding [4]

Other
- Adverse effects [3]

LEVOTHYROXINE

Synonyms: L-thyroxine sodium; T_4
Trade names: Levothyroid (Forest), Levoxyl (Monarch), Synthroid (AbbVie), Unithroid (Watson)
Indications: Hypothyroidism
Class: Thyroid hormone, synthetic
Half-life: 6–7 days
Clinically important, potentially hazardous interactions with: colesevelam, dicumarol, lanthanum, oral anticoagulants, orlistat, propranolol, raloxifene, red rice yeast, ritonavir, warfarin
Pregnancy category: A

Skin
- Angioedema [2]
- Urticaria [3]

Cardiovascular
- Circulatory collapse [2]

Central Nervous System
- Restless legs syndrome [2]

Neuromuscular/Skeletal
- Bone loss [2]
- Fractures [2]

Endocrine/Metabolic
- Thyrotoxicosis [3]

Other
- Adverse effects [2]
- Side effects [2]

LICORICE

Family: Fabaceae; Leguminosae
Scientific names: *Glycyrrhiza glabra*, *Glycyrrhiza uralensis*
Indications: Upper respiratory tract infection, gastric and duodenal ulcers, bronchitis, colic, dry cough, arthritis, lupus, sore throat, malaria, sores, abscesses, contact dermatitis. Flavoring in foods, beverages and tobacco
Class: Anti-inflammatory
Half-life: N/A
Clinically important, potentially hazardous interactions with: alclometasone, cascara, clevidipine, squill
Pregnancy category: N/A

Skin
- Edema [2]

Cardiovascular
- Hypertension [10]

Neuromuscular/Skeletal
- Rhabdomyolysis [22]

Endocrine/Metabolic
- Hypokalemia [5]

Ocular
- Ocular adverse effects [2]

Other
- Adverse effects [2]

LIDOCAINE

Synonyms: lignocaine; xylocaine
Trade names: Anamantle HC (Doak), ELA-Max (Ferndale), EMLA (AstraZeneca), Lidoderm (Endo), Xylocaine (AstraZeneca)
Indications: Ventricular arrhythmias, topical anesthesia
Class: Anesthetic, local, Antiarrhythmic, Antiarrhythmic class Ib
Half-life: terminal: 1.5–2 hours
Clinically important, potentially hazardous interactions with: amiodarone, amprenavir, antiarrhythmics, atazanavir, cimetidine, cobicistat/elvitegravir/emtricitabine/tenofovir alafenamide, cobicistat/elvitegravir/emtricitabine/tenofovir disoproxil, darunavir, delavirdine, fosamprenavir, indinavir, lopinavir, mivacurium, nevirapine, nilutamide, oxprenolol, propranolol, telaprevir
Pregnancy category: B
Important contra-indications noted in the prescribing guidelines for: nursing mothers; pediatric patients

---

Skin
Anaphylactoid reactions/Anaphylaxis [7]
Angioedema [3]
Dermatitis [27]
Eczema [3]
Edema [2]
Erythema [3]
Erythema multiforme [2]
Exanthems [2]
Exfoliative dermatitis [2]
Fixed eruption [2]
Hypersensitivity [9]
Pruritus [3]
Toxicity [3]
Urticaria [5]

Cardiovascular
Bradycardia [2]

Central Nervous System
Hoigne's syndrome [2]
Seizures [14]
Shivering (<10%)

Hematologic
Methemoglobinemia [4]

Otic
Tinnitus [3]

Local
Application-site erythema [2]
Application-site reactions [3]
Injection-site pain [2]

Other
Adverse effects [3]
Death [3]

LIFITEGRAST

Trade name: Xiidra (Shire)
Indications: Ophthalmic solution for dry eye disease
Class: Lymphocyte function-associated antigen-1 (LFA-1) antagonist
Half-life: N/A
Clinically important, potentially hazardous interactions with: none known
Pregnancy category: N/A (No data available)
Important contra-indications noted in the prescribing guidelines for: nursing mothers; pediatric patients

---

Central Nervous System
Dysgeusia (taste perversion) (5–25%) [6]
Headache (<5%)

Respiratory
Sinusitis (<5%)

Ocular
Conjunctival hyperemia (<5%)
Lacrimation (<5%)
Ocular adverse effects [2]
Ocular burning [2]
Ocular discharge (<5%)
Ocular pruritus (5–25%) [2]
Reduced visual acuity (5–25%) [2]
Vision blurred (<5%)
Xerophthalmia [2]

Local
Application-site irritation [4]
Application-site pain [2]
Application-site reactions [7]

LINACLOTIDE

Trade name: Linzess (Forest)
Indications: Irritable bowel syndrome with constipation and chronic idiopathic constipation
Class: Amino acid, Guanylate cyclase-C agonist
Half-life: N/A
Clinically important, potentially hazardous interactions with: none known
Pregnancy category: C
Important contra-indications noted in the prescribing guidelines for: nursing mothers; pediatric patients
Note: Contra-indicated in patients with known or suspected mechanical gastrointestinal obstruction.
Warning: PEDIATRIC RISK

Central Nervous System
Headache (4%)

Neuromuscular/Skeletal
Asthenia (fatigue) (<2%)

Gastrointestinal/Hepatic
Abdominal distension (2–3%)
Abdominal pain (7%) [4]
Diarrhea (16–20%) [21]
Dyspepsia (<2%)
Flatulence (4–6%) [4]
Gastroenteritis (3%)
Gastroesophageal reflux (<2%)
Vomiting (<2%)

Respiratory
Sinusitis (3%)
Upper respiratory tract infection (5%)

LINAGLIPTIN

Trade names: Glyxambi (Boehringer Ingelheim), Tradjenta (Boehringer Ingelheim)
Indications: Type II diabetes mellitus
Class: Antidiabetic, Dipeptidyl peptidase-4 (DPP-4) inhibitor
Half-life: 12 hours
Clinically important, potentially hazardous interactions with: efavirenz, rifampin
Pregnancy category: B
Important contra-indications noted in the prescribing guidelines for: nursing mothers; pediatric patients
Note: Linagliptin should not be used in patients with Type I diabetes or for the treatment of diabetic ketoacidosis, and has not been studied in combination with insulin. Glyxambi is linagliptin and empagliflozin.

Cardiovascular
Cardiotoxicity [3]
Hypertension [2]

Central Nervous System
Headache [5]

Neuromuscular/Skeletal
Arthralgia [2]
Back pain [3]
Pain in extremities [2]

Gastrointestinal/Hepatic
Diarrhea [2]
Nausea [3]

Respiratory
Cough [4]
Nasopharyngitis [8]
Upper respiratory tract infection [5]

Endocrine/Metabolic
Hyperglycemia [2]
Hyperlipidemia [2]
Hypertriglyceridemia [2]
Hypoglycemia [16]

Genitourinary
Urinary tract infection [4]

Other
Adverse effects [17]
Infection [3]

LINCOMYCIN

Trade name: Lincocin (Pfizer)
Indications: Various infections caused by susceptible organisms
Class: Antibiotic, lincosamide
Half-life: 2–11.5 hours
Clinically important, potentially hazardous interactions with: mivacurium
Pregnancy category: C
Important contra-indications noted in the prescribing guidelines for: nursing mothers; pediatric patients

---

Skin
AGEP [3]
Dermatitis [2]

Other
Allergic reactions (<5%)

LINDANE

Synonyms: hexachlorocyclohexane; gamma benzene hexachloride
Indications: Scabies, pediculosis capitis, pediculosis pubis
Class: Chemical, Scabicide
Half-life: 17–22 hours
Clinically important, potentially hazardous interactions with: oil-based hair dressings
Pregnancy category: C
Important contra-indications noted in the prescribing guidelines for: nursing mothers; pediatric patients

---

Skin
Dermatitis [5]
Erythema (2%) [2]
Pruritus (2%) [5]
Toxicity [2]
Urticaria [2]

Central Nervous System
Neurotoxicity [3]
Pseudotumor cerebri [2]
Seizures [11]

Neuromuscular/Skeletal
Rhabdomyolysis [3]

Other
Adverse effects [4]
Death [18]

LINEZOLID

Trade name: Zyvox (Pfizer)
Indications: Various infections caused by susceptible organisms
Class: Antibiotic, oxazolidinone
Half-life: 4–5 hours
Clinically important, potentially hazardous interactions with: alcohol, alpha blockers, altretamine, amitriptyline, amoxapine, amphetamines, anilidopiperidine opioids, antihypertensives, atomoxetine, beta blockers, buprenorphine, bupropion, buspirone, caffeine, carbamazepine, clomipramine, cyclobenzaprine, desipramine, desvenlafaxine, dexmethylphenidate, dextromethorphan, diethylpropion, doxapram, doxepin, fluoxetine, fluvoxamine, hydromorphone, imipramine, levodopa, lithium, MAO inhibitors, maprotiline, meperidine, methadone, methyldopa, methylphenidate, mirtazapine, nortriptyline, oral typhoid vaccine, paroxetine hydrochloride, propoxyphene, protriptyline, reserpine, rifampin, safinamide, serotonin 5-HT1D receptor agonists, serotonin/norepinephrine reuptake inhibitors, sertraline, sibutramine, SSRIs, tapentadol, tetrabenazine, tetrahydrozoline, tramadol, trazodone, tricyclic antidepressants, trimipramine, tryptophan, venlafaxine
Pregnancy category: C
Important contra-indications noted in the prescribing guidelines for: nursing mothers

---

Skin
Cellulitis [2]
Edema (2%)
Fungal dermatitis (2%)
Pruritus [2]
Rash (<7%) [3]

Mucosal
Black tongue [2]

Central Nervous System
Dysgeusia (taste perversion) (<2%)
Fever (2–14%)
Headache (<11%) [6]
Insomnia (3%)
Neurotoxicity [5]
Peripheral neuropathy [12]
Seizures (3%)
Serotonin syndrome [27]
Vertigo (dizziness) (2%)

Gastrointestinal/Hepatic
Abdominal pain (<2%)
Constipation (2%) [2]
Diarrhea (3–11%) [11]
Gastrointestinal bleeding (2%)
Gastrointestinal disorder [2]
Loose stools (<2%)
Nausea (3–10%) [11]
Pancreatitis [2]
Vomiting (<10%) [4]

Respiratory
Apnea (2%)
Cough (<2%)
Dyspnea (3%)
Pneumonia (3%)
Upper respiratory tract infection (4%)

Endocrine/Metabolic
Acidosis [7]
ALP increased (<4%)
ALT increased (2–10%)
AST increased (2–5%)
Hypoglycemia [3]
Hypokalemia (3%)
Hyponatremia [2]

Genitourinary
Candidal vaginitis (<2%)

Renal
Nephrotoxicity [2]

Hematologic
Anemia (<6%) [6]
Leukopenia [2]
Myelosuppression [8]
Pancytopenia [5]
Sepsis (8%)
Thrombocytopenia (<5%) [20]

Ocular
Optic neuropathy [15]

Local
Injection-site reactions (3%)

Other
Adverse effects (4%) [16]
Allergic reactions (4%)
Death [2]

LINSEED

Family: Linaceae
Scientific name: *Linum usitatissimum*
Indications: Dry mouth, menopause, osteoporosis, heart disease, catarrh, bronchitis, furunculosis, pleuritic pains, constipation, high cholesterol, benign prostatic hyperplasia, bladder inflammation, gastritis, enteritis, irritable bowel syndrome. **Topical:** poultice for skin inflammation. **Ophthalmologic:** oil used for removal of foreign bodies from the eye
Class: Anti-inflammatory
Half-life: N/A
Clinically important, potentially hazardous interactions with: none known
Pregnancy category: N/A
Note: Linum is cultivated for both its stem fibers (the source of linen and some paper) and its seeds (oil used in cooking and in margarine). The oil is used in paints and varnishes and the seed residues are used in cattle cake.

Skin
Anaphylactoid reactions/Anaphylaxis [3]

LIOTHYRONINE

Synonym: T_3 sodium
Trade names: Cytomel (Pfizer), Triostat (Par)
Indications: Hypothyroidism
Class: Thyroid hormone, synthetic
Half-life: 16–49 hours
Clinically important, potentially hazardous interactions with: anticoagulants, dicumarol, warfarin
Pregnancy category: A

Skin
Urticaria [3]

LIRAGLUTIDE

Trade names: Saxenda (Novo Nordisk), Victoza (Novo Nordisk), Xultophy (Novo Nordisk)
Indications: To improve glycemic control in adults with Type II diabetes mellitus (Victoza), adjunct to diet and exercise for chronic weight management (Saxenda)
Class: Glucagon-like peptide-1 (GLP-1) receptor agonist
Half-life: 13 hours
Clinically important, potentially hazardous interactions with: acetaminophen, atorvastatin, digoxin, griseofulvin, lisinopril, warfarin
Pregnancy category: C
Important contra-indications noted in the prescribing guidelines for: nursing mothers; pediatric patients
Note: Contra-indicated in patients with a personal or family history of medullary thyroid carcinoma or in patients with multiple endocrine neoplasia syndrome Type 2. Xultophy is liraglutide and insulin degludec.
Warning: RISK OF THYROID C-CELL TUMORS

Cardiovascular
Cardiotoxicity [2]
Hypertension (3%)

Central Nervous System
Headache (~5%) [7]
Vertigo (dizziness) (6%) [2]

Neuromuscular/Skeletal
Asthenia (fatigue) [3]
Back pain (5%) [3]

Gastrointestinal/Hepatic
Abdominal pain [3]
Cholelithiasis (gallstones) [3]
Constipation (10%) [12]
Diarrhea (17%) [32]
Dyspepsia [3]
Gastrointestinal disorder [4]
Nausea (28%) [63]
Pancreatitis [11]
Vomiting (11%) [31]

Respiratory
Influenza (7%)
Nasopharyngitis (5%) [6]
Sinusitis (6%)
Upper respiratory tract infection (10%) [3]

Endocrine/Metabolic
Appetite decreased [6]

Hypoglycemia [11]
Weight loss [6]

Genitourinary
Urinary tract infection (6%)

Renal
Nephrotoxicity [2]

Local
Injection-site reactions (2%) [3]

Other
Adverse effects [13]
Malignant neoplasms (11%)

LISDEXAMFETAMINE

Trade name: Vyvanse (Shire)
Indications: Attention-deficit hyperactivity disorder (ADHD)
Class: CNS stimulant, Dextroamphetamine prodrug
Half-life: 1 hour
Clinically important, potentially hazardous interactions with: acetazolamide, ammonium chloride, analgesics, antacids, antihistamines, antihypertensives, antipsychotics, atomoxetine, cannabinoids, carbonic anhydrase inhibitors, chlorpromazine, epinephrine, ethosuximide, haloperidol, iobenguane, lithium, MAO inhibitors, meperidine, methenamine, phenobarbital, phenytoin, propoxyphene, sympathomimetics, tricyclic antidepressants, urinary alkalinizing agents
Pregnancy category: C
Important contra-indications noted in the prescribing guidelines for: nursing mothers; pediatric patients
Warning: ABUSE AND DEPENDENCE

Skin
Hyperhidrosis (3%)
Rash (3%)

Mucosal
Xerostomia (4–26%) [23]

Cardiovascular
Hypertension (3%) [2]
Tachycardia [3]

Central Nervous System
Agitation (3%)
Anorexia (5%) [3]
Anxiety [9]
Fever (2%)
Headache [32]
Insomnia (13–23%) [31]
Irritability (10%) [21]
Restlessness (3%)
Sleep related disorder [2]
Somnolence (drowsiness) (2%) [2]
Tic disorder (2%) [2]
Vertigo (dizziness) (5%) [6]

Neuromuscular/Skeletal
Asthenia (fatigue) [3]
Back pain [2]
Muscle spasm [2]

Gastrointestinal/Hepatic
Abdominal pain (12%) [12]
Constipation [2]
Diarrhea (7%)
Nausea (6–7%) [10]
Vomiting (9%) [3]

Respiratory
Dyspnea (2%)
Influenza [2]
Nasopharyngitis [6]
Sinusitis [2]
Upper respiratory tract infection [12]

Endocrine/Metabolic
Appetite decreased (27–39%) [30]
Libido decreased (<2%)
Weight loss (9%) [9]

Genitourinary
Erectile dysfunction (<2%)

Other
Adverse effects [6]

LISINOPRIL

Trade names: Prinivil (Merck), Prinzide (Merck), Zestoretic (AstraZeneca), Zestril (AstraZeneca)
Indications: Hypertension, as adjunctive therapy in the management of heart failure, short-term treatment following myocardial infarction in hemodynamically stable patients
Class: Angiotensin-converting enzyme (ACE) inhibitor
Half-life: 12 hours
Clinically important, potentially hazardous interactions with: alcohol, aldesleukin, allopurinol, alpha blockers, alprostadil, amifostine, amiloride, angiotensin II receptor antagonists, antacids, antidiabetics, antihypertensives, antipsychotics, anxiolytics and hypnotics, aprotinin, azathioprine, baclofen, beta blockers, calcium channel blockers, clonidine, corticosteroids, cyclosporine, diazoxide, diuretics, eplerenone, estrogens, everolimus, general anesthetics, gold & gold compounds, heparins, hydralazine, hypotensives, insulin, levodopa, liraglutide, lithium, MAO inhibitors, metformin, methyldopa, methylphenidate, minoxidil, moxisylyte, moxonidine, nitrates, nitroprusside, NSAIDs, pentoxifylline, phosphodiesterase 5 inhibitors, potassium salts, prostacyclin analogues, rituximab, salicylates, sirolimus, spironolactone, sulfonylureas, temsirolimus, tizanidine, tolvaptan, triamterene, trimethoprim, yohimbine
Pregnancy category: D (category C in first trimester; category D in second and third trimesters)
Important contra-indications noted in the prescribing guidelines for: nursing mothers; pediatric patients
Note: Prinzide and Zestoretic are lisinopril and hydrochlorothiazide. Hydrochlorothiazide is a sulfonamide and can be absorbed systemically. Sulfonamides can produce severe, possibly fatal, reactions such as toxic epidermal necrolysis and Stevens-Johnson syndrome.
Contra-indicated in patients with a history of angioedema related to previous treatment with an ACE inhibitor and in patients with hereditary or idiopathic angioedema.
Warning: FETAL TOXICITY

Skin
Angioedema [43]
Edema of lip [2]
Exanthems (3%) [4]
Exfoliative dermatitis [2]
Flushing [2]
Kaposi's sarcoma [2]
Lichenoid eruption [2]
Pemphigus foliaceus [2]
Pityriasis rosea [2]
Purpura [2]
Rash (2%) [5]
Urticaria [2]

Mucosal
Tongue edema [2]

Cardiovascular
Hypotension (<4%) [3]

Central Nervous System
Headache (4–6%)
Vertigo (dizziness) (5–12%)

Neuromuscular/Skeletal
Asthenia (fatigue) (3%)

Gastrointestinal/Hepatic
Hepatotoxicity [2]
Intestinal angioedema [3]
Pancreatitis [10]

Respiratory
Cough (4–9%) [15]
Upper respiratory tract infection (<2%)

Endocrine/Metabolic
Hyperkalemia [3]

Other
Death [3]

LITHIUM

Trade names: Eskalith (GSK), Lithobid (Solvay)
Indications: Manic-depressive states
Class: Antipsychotic, Mood stabilizer
Half-life: 18–24 hours
Clinically important, potentially hazardous interactions with: aceclofenac, acemetacin, acetazolamide, acitretin, amitriptyline, arsenic, benazepril, bendroflumethiazide, benzthiazide, captopril, celecoxib, chlorothiazide, chlorthalidone, cilazapril, citalopram, clozapine, cyclopenthiazide, desvenlafaxine, dichlorphenamide, diclofenac, enalapril, ethoxzolamide, etoricoxib, fluoxetine, flurbiprofen, fosinopril, haloperidol, hydrochlorothiazide, hydroflumethiazide, indapamide, insulin degludec, insulin detemir, insulin glargine, insulin glulisine, irbesartan, levomepromazine, linezolid, lisdexamfetamine, lisinopril, lorcaserin, lurasidone, meloxicam, meperidine, mesoridazine, methyclothiazide, metolazone, metronidazole, milnacipran, neostigmine, olanzapine, olmesartan, paliperidone, paroxetine hydrochloride, pericyazine, phenylbutazone, piroxicam, polythiazide, quinapril, quinethazone, ramipril, rocuronium, rofecoxib, sibutramine, sulpiride, tenoxicam, tetrabenazine, thalidomide, thiazides, tinidazole, tolmetin, trandolapril, trichlormethiazide, trifluoperazine, valdecoxib, venlafaxine, xipamide, ziprasidone, zofenopril, zuclopenthixol

Pregnancy category: D

Skin
Acneform eruption [21]
Angioedema [2]
Atopic dermatitis (3%)
Darier's disease [3]
Dermatitis [4]
Dermatitis herpetiformis [3]
Edema [3]
Erythema [2]
Exanthems [11]
Exfoliative dermatitis [3]
Follicular keratosis [3]
Folliculitis [5]
Hidradenitis [3]
Ichthyosis [2]
Keratosis pilaris [2]
Linear IgA bullous dermatosis [4]
Lupus erythematosus [5]
Myxedema [10]
Papulo-nodular lesions (elbows) [2]
Pruritus [9]
Psoriasis (2%) [59]
Purpura [2]
Pustules [2]
Rash (<10%)
Seborrheic dermatitis [3]
Toxicity [2]
Ulcerations (lower extremities) [5]
Urticaria [3]
Vasculitis [4]

Hair
Alopecia (10–19%) [18]
Alopecia areata (2%) [3]

Nails
Nail dystrophy [2]

Mucosal
Lichenoid stomatitis [3]
Oral ulceration [4]
Sialorrhea [4]
Stomatitis [2]
Xerostomia [5]

Cardiovascular
Brugada syndrome [5]
QT prolongation [4]

Central Nervous System
Amnesia [2]
Coma [2]
Dysgeusia (taste perversion) (>10%)
Hallucinations [2]
Neuroleptic malignant syndrome [7]
Neurotoxicity [3]
Parkinsonism [8]
Pseudohallucinations [2]
Restless legs syndrome [4]
Serotonin syndrome [5]
Somnambulism [3]
Tardive dyskinesia [2]
Tremor [5]

Neuromuscular/Skeletal
Myasthenia gravis [2]
Rhabdomyolysis [3]

Endocrine/Metabolic
Diabetes insipidus [5]
Hypercalcemia [4]
Hyperparathyroidism [6]
Hyperthyroidism [2]
Hypothyroidism [4]
Thyroid dysfunction [2]
Thyrotoxicosis [2]
Weight gain [4]

Genitourinary
Polyuria [3]
Priapism [5]

Renal
Nephrogenic diabetes insipidus [2]
Nephrotoxicity [15]

Other
Adverse effects [5]
Dipsia (thirst) [2]
Side effects (23–33%) [4]
Teratogenicity [3]

LIXISENATIDE

Trade names: Adlyxin (Sanofi-Aventis), Lyxumia (Sanofi-Aventis), Soliqua (Sanofi-Aventis)
Indications: To improve glycemic control in adults with Type II diabetes mellitus
Class: Glucagon-like peptide-1 (GLP-1) receptor agonist
Half-life: 3 hours
Clinically important, potentially hazardous interactions with: none known
Pregnancy category: N/A (Use during pregnancy only if the potential benefit justifies the potential risk to the fetus)
Important contra-indications noted in the prescribing guidelines for: nursing mothers; pediatric patients
Note: Soliqua is lixisenatide and insulin glargine.

Central Nervous System
Headache (9%) [3]
Vertigo (dizziness) (7%) [2]

Gastrointestinal/Hepatic
Abdominal distension (2%)
Abdominal pain (2%)
Constipation (3%)
Diarrhea (8%) [10]
Dyspepsia (3%)
Nausea (25%) [24]
Vomiting (10%) [23]

Endocrine/Metabolic
Hypoglycemia (3%) [8]

Local
Injection-site reactions (4%) [2]

Other
Adverse effects [3]
Allergic reactions [2]

LOFEXIDINE *

Trade names: BritLofex (Britannia), Lucemyra (US WorldMeds, LLC)
Indications: mitigation of opioid withdrawal symptoms to facilitate abrupt opioid discontinuation in adults
Class: Adrenergic alpha2-receptor agonist
Half-life: ~12 hours
Clinically important, potentially hazardous interactions with: methadone, naltrexone
Pregnancy category: N/A (The safety of lofexidine in pregnant women has not been established.)

Mucosal
Xerostomia (10–11%) [3]

Cardiovascular
Bradycardia (24–32%) [2]
Hypotension (30%) [7]
Orthostatic hypotension (29–42%)

Central Nervous System
Insomnia (51–55%) [2]
Sedation (12–13%) [4]
Somnolence (drowsiness) (11–13%) [3]
Syncope (<5%)
Vertigo (dizziness) (19–23%) [3]

Otic
Tinnitus (<5%)

Other
Adverse effects [2]

LOMITAPIDE

Trade name: Juxtapid (Aegerion)
Indications: Homozygous familial hypercholesterolemia
Class: Lipid regulator
Half-life: 39.7 hours
Clinically important, potentially hazardous interactions with: bile acid sequestrants, boceprevir, clarithromycin, conivaptan, grapefruit juice, indinavir, itraconazole, ketoconazole, lopinavir, lovastatin, mibefradil, nefazodone, nelfinavir, oral contraceptives, P-glycoprotein substrates, posaconazole, ritonavir, saquinavir, simvastatin, strong or moderate CYP3A4 inhibitors, telaprevir, telithromycin, voriconazole, warfarin
Pregnancy category: X
Important contra-indications noted in the prescribing guidelines for: nursing mothers; pediatric patients
Warning: RISK OF HEPATOTOXICITY

Mucosal
Nasal congestion (10%)

Cardiovascular
Angina (10%)
Chest pain (24%)
Palpitation (10%)

Central Nervous System
Fever (10%)
Headache (10%)
Vertigo (dizziness) (10%)

Neuromuscular/Skeletal
Asthenia (fatigue) (17%)
Back pain (14%)

Gastrointestinal/Hepatic
Abdominal pain (21–34%)
Constipation (21%)
Defecation (urgency) (10%)
Diarrhea (79%) [3]
Dyspepsia (38%) [3]
Flatulence (21%)
Gastroenteritis (14%)
Gastroesophageal reflux (10%)

Hepatotoxicity [6]
Nausea (65%) [2]
Tenesmus (10%)
Vomiting (34%) [3]

Respiratory
Influenza (21%)
Nasopharyngitis (17%)
Pharyngolaryngeal pain (14%)

Endocrine/Metabolic
ALT increased (17%) [3]
Weight loss (24%)

Other
Adverse effects [6]

LOPERAMIDE

Trade names: Imodium (McNeil), Maalox (Novartis)
Indications: Diarrhea
Class: Opiate agonist
Half-life: 9–14 hours
Clinically important, potentially hazardous interactions with: St John's wort
Pregnancy category: B
Important contra-indications noted in the prescribing guidelines for: nursing mothers; pediatric patients

---

Cardiovascular
Torsades de pointes [2]

Gastrointestinal/Hepatic
Abdominal pain [2]
Constipation [3]
Nausea [2]

LOPINAVIR

Trade name: Kaletra (AbbVie)
Indications: HIV-1 infected children above the age of 2 years and adults, in combination with other antiretroviral agents
Class: Antiretroviral, HIV-1 protease inhibitor
Half-life: 5–6 hours
Clinically important, potentially hazardous interactions with: abacavir, alfuzosin, amiodarone, amprenavir, aripiprazole, artemether/lumefantrine, atazanavir, atorvastatin, atovaquone, bepridil, bosentan, brigatinib, bupropion, cabozantinib, carbamazepine, chlorpheniramine, cisapride, clarithromycin, colchicine, copanlisib, cyclosporine, darifenacin, darunavir, dasatinib, delavirdine, dexamethasone, didanosine, digoxin, disulfiram, efavirenz, elbasvir & grazoprevir, eltrombopag, eluxadoline, ergotamine, estradiol, felodipine, fentanyl, flecainide, fluticasone propionate, fosamprenavir, glecaprevir & pibrentasvir, indinavir, itraconazole, ketoconazole, lidocaine, lidocaine, lomitapide, lovastatin, maraviroc, methadone, methylergonovine, metronidazole, midazolam, midostaurin, mifepristone, nelfinavir, neratinib, nevirapine, nicardipine, nifedipine, nilotinib, olaparib, ombitasvir/paritaprevir/ritonavir, palbociclib, phenobarbital, phenytoin, pimozide, pitavastatin, ponatinib, primidone, quinidine, ranolazine, ribociclib, rifabutin, rifampin, rilpivirine, rivaroxaban, rosuvastatin, ruxolitinib, salmeterol, saquinavir, sildenafil, simeprevir, simvastatin, sirolimus, sofosbuvir/velpatasvir/voxilaprevir, St John's wort, tacrolimus, tadalafil, telithromycin, tenofovir disoproxil, tipranavir, tolterodine, trazodone, triazolam, vardenafil, venetoclax, vinblastine, vincristine, voriconazole, warfarin, zidovudine
Pregnancy category: C
Important contra-indications noted in the prescribing guidelines for: nursing mothers
Note: Kaletra is lopinavir and ritonavir.

Skin
Acneform eruption (<10%)
Lipodystrophy (<10%)
Rash (<10%) [5]

Hair
Alopecia [3]

Central Nervous System
Vertigo (dizziness) [2]

Neuromuscular/Skeletal
Asthenia (fatigue) (<10%) [2]

Gastrointestinal/Hepatic
Diarrhea (>10%) [5]
Flatulence (<10%)
Nausea (<10%) [4]
Pancreatitis [2]
Vomiting (<10%) [3]

Renal
Nephrolithiasis [2]
Nephrotoxicity [2]

LORATADINE

Trade names: Alavert (Wyeth), Claritin (Schering), Claritin-D (Schering)
Indications: Allergic rhinitis, urticaria
Class: Histamine H1 receptor antagonist
Half-life: 3–20 hours
Clinically important, potentially hazardous interactions with: amiodarone
Pregnancy category: B

Skin
Anaphylactoid reactions/Anaphylaxis (>2%)
Angioedema (>2%)
Dermatitis (>2%)
Diaphoresis (>2%)
Erythema multiforme (>2%)
Fixed eruption [3]
Flushing (>2%)
Peripheral edema (>2%)
Photosensitivity (>2%)
Pruritus (>2%)
Purpura (>2%)
Rash (>2%)
Urticaria (>2%) [4]
Xerosis (>2%)

Hair
Alopecia (>2%)
Dry hair (>2%)

Mucosal
Sialorrhea (>2%)
Stomatitis (>2%)
Xerostomia (>10%) [9]

Cardiovascular
QT prolongation [2]
Torsades de pointes [4]

Central Nervous System
Dysgeusia (taste perversion) (>2%)
Headache (12%) [3]
Hyperesthesia (>2%)
Paresthesias (>2%)
Somnolence (drowsiness) [2]

Neuromuscular/Skeletal
Asthenia (fatigue) (4%) [2]
Myalgia/Myopathy (>2%)

Respiratory
Pharyngitis [2]

Endocrine/Metabolic
Gynecomastia (>2%)
Mastodynia (<10%)

Genitourinary
Vaginitis (>2%)

LORAZEPAM

Trade name: Ativan (Valeant)
Indications: Anxiety, depression
Class: Benzodiazepine
Half-life: 10–20 hours
Clinically important, potentially hazardous interactions with: alcohol, amprenavir, barbiturates, chlorpheniramine, clarithromycin, clozapine, CNS depressants, cobicistat/elvitegravir/emtricitabine/tenofovir alafenamide, efavirenz, erythromycin, esomeprazole, eszopiclone, imatinib, MAO inhibitors, narcotics, nelfinavir, phenothiazines, valproate
Pregnancy category: D

Skin
Dermatitis (<10%)
Diaphoresis (>10%)
Pseudolymphoma [2]
Rash (>10%)

Mucosal
Nasal congestion (<10%)
Sialopenia (>10%)
Xerostomia (>10%)

Cardiovascular
Hypotension [2]

Central Nervous System
Agitation [2]
Akathisia (<10%)
Amnesia (<10%) [18]
Catatonia [2]
Confusion (<10%)
Delirium [2]
Depression (<10%)
Hallucinations [2]
Headache (<10%)
Somnolence (drowsiness) (<10%) [3]
Tremor (<10%)
Vertigo (dizziness) (<10%) [2]

Respiratory
Apnea (<10%)
Hyperventilation (<10%)

Ocular
Visual disturbances (<10%)

Local
Injection-site pain (>10%)
Injection-site phlebitis (>10%)

Other
Adverse effects [2]

LORCASERIN

Trade name: Belviq (Arena)
Indications: Obesity in adults who have at least one weight-related health condition, such as high blood pressure, Type II diabetes, or high cholesterol
Class: Serotonin receptor agonist
Half-life: ~11 hours
Clinically important, potentially hazardous interactions with: antipsychotics, bupropion, dextromethorphan, lithium, MAO inhibitors, SNRIs, SSRIs, St John's wort, tramadol, tricyclic antidepressants, triptans
Pregnancy category: X
Important contra-indications noted in the prescribing guidelines for: nursing mothers; pediatric patients

---

Skin
Peripheral edema (5%)
Rash (2%)

Mucosal
Nasal congestion (3%)
Oropharyngeal pain (4%)
Xerostomia (5%) [2]

Cardiovascular
Hypertension (5%)
Valvulopathy (2–3%) [5]

Central Nervous System
Anxiety (4%)
Cognitive impairment (2%) [2]
Depression (2%) [2]
Euphoria [3]
Headache (15–17%) [11]
Insomnia (4%)
Vertigo (dizziness) (7–9%) [9]

Neuromuscular/Skeletal
Asthenia (fatigue) (7%) [3]
Back pain (6–12%) [2]
Bone or joint pain (2%)
Muscle spasm (5%)

Gastrointestinal/Hepatic
Constipation (6%)
Diarrhea (7%)
Gastroenteritis (3%)
Nausea (8–9%) [9]
Vomiting (4%)

Respiratory
Cough (4%)
Nasopharyngitis (11–13%) [2]
Upper respiratory tract infection (14%)

Endocrine/Metabolic
Appetite decreased (2%)
Diabetes mellitus (exacerbation) (3%)
Hypoglycemia (29%) [4]

Genitourinary
Urinary tract infection (7–9%)

Other
Toothache (3%)

LOSARTAN

Trade names: Cozaar (Merck), Hyzaar (Merck)
Indications: Hypertension
Class: Angiotensin II receptor antagonist (blocker), Antihypertensive
Half-life: 2 hours
Clinically important, potentially hazardous interactions with: aliskiren, rifampin, voriconazole
Pregnancy category: D (category C in first trimester; category D in second and third trimesters)
Important contra-indications noted in the prescribing guidelines for: nursing mothers
Note: Hyzaar is losartan and hydrochlorothiazide. Hydrochlorothiazide is a sulfonamide and can be absorbed systemically. Sulfonamides can produce severe, possibly fatal, reactions such as toxic epidermal necrolysis and Stevens-Johnson syndrome.
Warning: USE IN PREGNANCY

Skin
Anaphylactoid reactions/Anaphylaxis [2]
Angioedema [11]
Photosensitivity [2]
Purpura [2]

Mucosal
Nasal congestion (2%)

Central Nervous System
Ageusia (taste loss) [2]
Vertigo (dizziness) (3%)

Neuromuscular/Skeletal
Back pain (2%)

Respiratory
Upper respiratory tract infection (8%)

Endocrine/Metabolic
Hyperkalemia [7]

Other
Adverse effects [7]

LOVASTATIN

Trade names: Advicor (Kos), Altoprev (Shionogi), Mevacor (Merck)
Indications: Hypercholesterolemia
Class: HMG-CoA reductase inhibitor, Statin
Half-life: 1–2 hours
Clinically important, potentially hazardous interactions with: amprenavir, atazanavir, azithromycin, boceprevir, bosentan, cholestyramine, clarithromycin, cyclosporine, darunavir, dasabuvir/ombitasvir/paritaprevir/ritonavir, delavirdine, efavirenz, elbasvir & grazoprevir, erythromycin, exenatide, fenofibrate, fosamprenavir, gemfibrozil, glecaprevir & pibrentasvir, grapefruit juice, imatinib, indinavir, itraconazole, letermovir, lomitapide, lopinavir, mifepristone, nelfinavir, ombitasvir/paritaprevir/ritonavir, paclitaxel, posaconazole, red rice yeast, tacrolimus, telaprevir, telithromycin, ticagrelor, tipranavir, tolvaptan, verapamil
Pregnancy category: X
Important contra-indications noted in the prescribing guidelines for: nursing mothers

---

Skin
Exanthems (<5%) [3]
Lupus erythematosus [4]
Pruritus (5%) [2]
Rash (5%) [3]

Central Nervous System
Parkinsonism [2]

Neuromuscular/Skeletal
Asthenia (fatigue) [2]
Myalgia/Myopathy (<10%) [6]
Rhabdomyolysis [41]

Gastrointestinal/Hepatic
Hepatotoxicity [2]
Pancreatitis [2]

Endocrine/Metabolic
Gynecomastia (<10%)

LOXAPINE

Trade names: Adasuve (Teva), Loxitane (Watson)
Indications: Psychoses
Class: Antipsychotic
Half-life: 12–19 hours (terminal)
Clinically important, potentially hazardous interactions with: none known
Pregnancy category: N/A (May cause fetal harm based on animal studies)
Important contra-indications noted in the prescribing guidelines for: the elderly; nursing mothers; pediatric patients
Warning: BRONCHOSPASM and INCREASED MORTALITY IN ELDERLY PATIENTS WITH DEMENTIA-RELATED PSYCHOSIS

Skin
Rash (<10%)

Mucosal
Xerostomia (>10%)

Central Nervous System
Dysgeusia (taste perversion) (14%) [8]
Neuroleptic malignant syndrome [3]
Sedation (12%) [4]
Somnolence (drowsiness) [3]
Vertigo (dizziness) [2]

Neuromuscular/Skeletal
Rhabdomyolysis [3]

Gastrointestinal/Hepatic
Dysphagia [2]

Respiratory
Bronchospasm [3]
Pulmonary toxicity [3]

Endocrine/Metabolic
Gynecomastia (<10%)

LUBIPROSTONE

Trade name: Amitiza (Takeda)
Indications: Constipation, irritable bowel syndrome
Class: Chloride channel activator
Half-life: 0–1.4 hours
Clinically important, potentially hazardous interactions with: none known
Pregnancy category: C
Important contra-indications noted in the prescribing guidelines for: nursing mothers; pediatric patients
Note: Contra-indicated in patients with known or suspected mechanical gastrointestinal obstruction.

Skin
Peripheral edema (4%)

Central Nervous System
Headache (13%) [7]

Neuromuscular/Skeletal
Arthralgia (3%)
Asthenia (fatigue) (2%)
Back pain (2%)

Gastrointestinal/Hepatic
Abdominal distension [5]
Abdominal pain (7%) [8]
Diarrhea [20]
Flatulence [3]
Nausea [21]
Vomiting [7]

Respiratory
Dyspnea [4]
Flu-like syndrome (2%)
Sinusitis (5%)
Upper respiratory tract infection (4%)

Other
Adverse effects [3]

LULICONAZOLE

Trade name: Luzu (Medicis)
Indications: Interdigital tinea pedis, tinea cruris, and tinea corporis caused by the organisms *Trichophyton rubrum* and *Epidermophyton floccosum*
Class: Antifungal, azole
Half-life: N/A
Clinically important, potentially hazardous interactions with: none known
Pregnancy category: C
Important contra-indications noted in the prescribing guidelines for: nursing mothers; pediatric patients

---

Skin
Contact dermatitis [2]

LUMACAFTOR/ IVACAFTOR

Trade name: Orkambi (Vertex)
Indications: Cystic fibrosis in patients aged 12 years and older who are homozygous for the *F508del* mutation in the *CFTR* gene
Class: CFTR potentiator, CYP3A4 inducer
Half-life: 26 hours
Clinically important, potentially hazardous interactions with: rifampin, St John's wort
Pregnancy category: B
Important contra-indications noted in the prescribing guidelines for: nursing mothers; pediatric patients
Note: See also separate profile for ivacaftor.

Skin
Rash (7%) [3]

Mucosal
Rhinorrhea (6%)

Neuromuscular/Skeletal
Asthenia (fatigue) (9%) [2]

Gastrointestinal/Hepatic
Diarrhea (12%)
Flatulence (7%)
Nausea (13%) [2]

Respiratory
Dyspnea (13%) [4]
Influenza (5%)
Nasopharyngitis (13%)
Upper respiratory tract infection (10%)

Endocrine/Metabolic
Creatine phosphokinase increased (7%) [2]
Menstrual irregularities (10%)

Other
Adverse effects [2]

LURASIDONE

Trade name: Latuda (Sunovion)
Indications: Schizophrenia, depressive epidodes associated with bipolar I disorder
Class: Antipsychotic
Half-life: 18 hours
Clinically important, potentially hazardous interactions with: alcohol, amphetamines, CNS depressants, dasabuvir/ombitasvir/paritaprevir/ritonavir, dasatinib, deferasirox, diltiazem, disopyramide, dopamine, dopamine agonists, droperidol, efavirenz, epinephrine, hydroxyzine, ketoconazole, levomepromazine, lithium, MAO inhibitors, methylphenidate, metoclopramide, ombitasvir/paritaprevir/ritonavir, pimozide, procainamide, quinagolide, quinidine, rifampin, strong CYP3A4 inducers or inhibitors, tetrabenazine, tocilizumab
Pregnancy category: B
Important contra-indications noted in the prescribing guidelines for: the elderly; nursing mothers; pediatric patients
Warning: INCREASED MORTALITY IN ELDERLY PATIENTS WITH DEMENTIA-RELATED PSYCHOSIS

Mucosal
Sialorrhea (2%)

Central Nervous System
Agitation (5%)
Akathisia (13%) [21]
Anxiety (5%)
Extrapyramidal symptoms [2]
Insomnia (10%) [2]
Parkinsonism (10%) [5]
Restlessness (2%) [2]
Sedation [10]
Somnolence (drowsiness) (17%) [16]
Vertigo (dizziness) (4%) [3]

Neuromuscular/Skeletal
Dystonia (5%) [2]

Gastrointestinal/Hepatic
Dyspepsia (6%)
Nausea (10%) [14]
Vomiting (8%) [4]

Endocrine/Metabolic
Hyperprolactinemia [2]
Weight gain (5%) [5]

Other
Adverse effects [3]

LUSUTROMBOPAG *

Trade name: Mulpleta (Shionogi)
Indications: indicated for the treatment of thrombocytopenia in adult patients with chronic liver disease who are scheduled to undergo a procedure
Class: Thrombopoietin receptor (TPO) agonist
Half-life: ~27 hours
Clinically important, potentially hazardous interactions with: none known
Pregnancy category: N/A (no available data to inform the drug-associated risk)

Central Nervous System
Headache (5%)

Hematologic
Platelets increased [4]

LYCOPENE

Scientific names: *All-Trans-Lycopene, Psi-Psi-Carotene*
Indications: Cancer (prevention), cardiovascular disease (prevention), asthma
Class: Antioxidant
Half-life: N/A
Clinically important, potentially hazardous interactions with: none known
Note: Cooking increases bioavailability of lycopene. Major dietary sources are tomato paste, juice, and ketchup.

Skin
Pigmentation [2]

Other
Adverse effects [2]

MACITENTAN

Trade name: Opsumit (Actelion)
Indications: Pulmonary arterial hypertension
Class: Endothelin receptor (ETR) antagonist
Half-life: 16 hours
Clinically important, potentially hazardous interactions with: ketoconazole, rifampin, ritonavir, strong CYP3A4 inducers or inhibitors
Pregnancy category: X
Important contra-indications noted in the prescribing guidelines for: nursing mothers; pediatric patients
Note: Contra-indicated in pregnancy.
Warning: EMBRYO-FETAL TOXICITY

Skin
Peripheral edema [3]

Central Nervous System
Headache (14%) [6]

Gastrointestinal/Hepatic
Hepatotoxicity [5]

Respiratory
Bronchitis (12%) [2]
Influenza (6%)
Nasopharyngitis (20%) [6]
Pharyngitis (20%)
Upper respiratory tract infection [2]

Genitourinary
Urinary tract infection (9%)

Hematologic
Anemia (13%) [8]

MARAVIROC

Trade names: Celsentri (ViiV), Selzentry (ViiV)
Indications: HIV infection
Class: Antiretroviral, CCR5 co-receptor antagonist
Half-life: 14–18 hours
Clinically important, potentially hazardous interactions with: atazanavir, clarithromycin, conivaptan, CYP3A4 inhibitors or inducers, darunavir, dasatinib, deferasirox, delavirdine, efavirenz, etravirine, indinavir, ketoconazole, lopinavir, nelfinavir, oxcarbazepine, rifampin, rifapentine, ritonavir, saquinavir, St John's wort, telithromycin, voriconazole
Pregnancy category: B
Important contra-indications noted in the prescribing guidelines for: the elderly; nursing mothers; pediatric patients
Warning: HEPATOTOXICITY

Skin
Dermatitis (5%)
Folliculitis (5%)
Lipodystrophy (5%)
Pruritus (6%) [2]
Rash (17%) [2]

Mucosal
Stomatitis (4%)

Cardiovascular
Postural hypotension [2]

Central Nervous System
Depression (6%)
Fever (21%) [2]
Headache [3]
Pain (8%)
Paresthesias (8%)
Peripheral neuropathy (5%)
Sleep disturbances (12%)
Vertigo (dizziness) (14%)

Neuromuscular/Skeletal
Asthenia (fatigue) [2]
Myalgia/Myopathy (5%)

Gastrointestinal/Hepatic
Abdominal pain (14%)
Diarrhea [2]
Hepatotoxicity [2]

Respiratory
Cough (22%) [2]
Flu-like syndrome (3%)
Nasopharyngitis [2]
Pneumonia (4%)
Upper respiratory tract infection (37%) [2]

Genitourinary
Urinary tract infection (4%)

Other
Adverse effects [6]

MARIHUANA

Synonyms: marijuana; grass; hashish; pot; cannabis
Indications: Nausea and vomiting, substance abuse drug
Class: Antiemetic, Cannabinoid, Hallucinogen
Half-life: N/A
Clinically important, potentially hazardous interactions with: atazanavir
Pregnancy category: N/A
Note: Marihuana is the popular name for the dried flowering leaves of the hemp plant, *cannabis sativa*. It contains tetrahydrocannabinols.

Mucosal
Xerostomia [2]

Cardiovascular
Cardiotoxicity [4]
Myocardial infarction [2]

Central Nervous System
Amnesia [2]
Hallucinations [3]
Neurotoxicity [2]
Schizophrenia [3]
Seizures [2]
Stroke [2]

Gastrointestinal/Hepatic
Pancreatitis [2]

Genitourinary
Priapism [2]

Ocular
Hallucinations, visual [2]

Other
Adverse effects [2]

MDMA

Synonym: 3,4-methylenedioxymethamphetamine; ecstasy; E; X; molly; club drug
Indications: N/A
Class: Amphetamine
Half-life: N/A
Clinically important, potentially hazardous interactions with: none known

---

Skin
Diaphoresis [4]

Mucosal
Xerostomia [5]

Cardiovascular
Cardiotoxicity [2]
Myocardial infarction [2]

Central Nervous System
Amnesia [2]
Confusion [2]
Depression (37%) [14]
Hallucinations [4]
Headache [2]
Hyperthermia [3]
Memory loss [3]
Neuroleptic malignant syndrome [4]
Neurotoxicity [5]
Parkinsonism [4]
Psychosis [4]
Seizures [3]
Serotonin syndrome [6]

Neuromuscular/Skeletal
Myalgia/Myopathy [2]
Rhabdomyolysis [34]

Gastrointestinal/Hepatic
Hepatitis [2]
Hepatotoxicity [4]
Nausea [2]

Endocrine/Metabolic
Hyponatremia [5]
SIADH [8]

Genitourinary
Priapism [2]

Hematologic
Coagulopathy [2]

Ocular
Hallucinations, visual [2]

Other
Bruxism [8]
Death [47]
Dipsia (thirst) [2]
Multiorgan failure [2]

MEADOWSWEET

Family: Rosaceae
Scientific names: *Filipendula ulmaria, Spiraea ulmaria*
Indications: Colds, fevers, cough, bronchitis, dyspepsia, heartburn, peptic ulcer, gout, rheumatic disorders
Class: Anti-inflammatory, Diuretic
Half-life: N/A
Clinically important, potentially hazardous interactions with: salicylates
Pregnancy category: N/A

MEBENDAZOLE

Trade name: Vermox (Janssen)
Indications: Parasitic worm infestations
Class: Anthelmintic, Antibiotic, imidazole
Half-life: 1–12 hours
Clinically important, potentially hazardous interactions with: aminophylline
Pregnancy category: C

Skin
Stevens-Johnson syndrome [2]

Hair
Alopecia [3]

Central Nervous System
Headache [2]
Vertigo (dizziness) [2]

Gastrointestinal/Hepatic
Abdominal pain [4]

Other
Adverse effects [2]

MECHLORETHAMINE

Synonyms: mustine; nitrogen mustard
Indications: Hodgkin's disease, mycosis fungoides
Class: Alkylating agent
Half-life: <1 minute
Clinically important, potentially hazardous interactions with: aldesleukin, vaccines
Pregnancy category: D

Skin
Anaphylactoid reactions/Anaphylaxis (<10%) [4]
Bullous dermatitis [3]
Dermatitis [28]
Herpes zoster (>10%)
Hypersensitivity (<10%)
Pigmentation [10]
Pruritus [3]
Squamous cell carcinoma [3]
Urticaria [3]

Hair
Alopecia (<10%)

Central Nervous System
Dysgeusia (taste perversion) (<10%)

Local
Injection-site extravasation (<10%)
Injection-site thrombophlebitis (<10%) [2]

MEDROXY-PROGESTERONE

Trade names: Depo-Provera (Pfizer), Lunelle (Pfizer), Premphase (Wyeth), Prempro (Wyeth), Provera (Pfizer)
Indications: Secondary amenorrhea, renal or endometrial carcinoma
Class: Progestogen
Half-life: 30 days
Clinically important, potentially hazardous interactions with: acitretin, dofetilide
Pregnancy category: X

Skin
Acneform eruption (<5%)
Chloasma (<10%)
Diaphoresis (<31%)
Edema (>10%)
Flushing (12%)
Melasma (<10%)
Pruritus (<10%)
Rash (<5%)

Hair
Alopecia (<5%)

Cardiovascular
Thrombophlebitis (<10%)

Neuromuscular/Skeletal
Osteoporosis [2]

Endocrine/Metabolic
Amenorrhea [3]
Galactorrhea [2]
Mastodynia (<5%)
Weight gain [3]

Genitourinary
Vaginitis (<5%)

Local
Injection-site pain (>10%)

MEFENAMIC ACID

Trade name: Ponstel (First Horizon)
Indications: Pain, dysmenorrhea
Class: Non-steroidal anti-inflammatory (NSAID)
Half-life: 3.5 hours
Clinically important, potentially hazardous interactions with: methotrexate
Pregnancy category: C
Important contra-indications noted in the prescribing guidelines for: nursing mothers; pediatric patients
Note: NSAIDs may cause an increased risk of serious cardiovascular and gastrointestinal adverse events, which can be fatal. This risk may increase with duration of use.
Warning: CARDIOVASCULAR AND GASTROINTESTINAL RISK

Skin
Anaphylactoid reactions/Anaphylaxis [2]
Erythema multiforme [2]
Fixed eruption [12]
Pruritus (<10%)
Rash (>10%)
Toxic epidermal necrolysis [2]

Cardiovascular
Myocardial infarction [2]

Central Nervous System
Seizures [2]

Gastrointestinal/Hepatic
Hepatotoxicity [2]

Renal
Renal failure [2]

Ocular
Glaucoma [2]

MEFLOQUINE

Trade name: Lariam (Roche)
Indications: Malaria
Class: Antimalarial, Antiprotozoal
Half-life: 21–22 days
Clinically important, potentially hazardous interactions with: acebutolol, artemether/lumefantrine, ethosuximide, halofantrine, ketoconazole, lacosamide, moxifloxacin, oxcarbazepine, quinine, tiagabine, typhoid vaccine, vigabatrin
Pregnancy category: C
Important contra-indications noted in the prescribing guidelines for: nursing mothers
Warning: NEUROPSYCHIATRIC ADVERSE REACTIONS

Skin
Anaphylactoid reactions/Anaphylaxis [2]
Erythema [2]
Exanthems (30%)
Pruritus (4–10%) [2]
Psoriasis [2]
Rash (<10%)
Stevens-Johnson syndrome [2]
Toxic epidermal necrolysis [2]
Vasculitis [3]

Cardiovascular
Palpitation [3]
Tachycardia [2]

Central Nervous System
Abnormal dreams [3]
Aggression [2]
Amnesia [2]
Anorexia [2]
Anxiety [5]
Chills (<10%)
Confusion [2]
Delusions [2]
Depression [7]
Fever (<10%) [2]
Hallucinations [3]
Headache (<10%) [5]
Insomnia [3]
Mania [4]
Neurotoxicity [8]
Psychosis [8]
Seizures [6]
Sleep disturbances [2]
Suicidal ideation [2]

Vertigo (dizziness) (<10%) [20]

Neuromuscular/Skeletal
Arthralgia [2]
Asthenia (fatigue) (<10%) [2]
Myalgia/Myopathy (<10%) [2]

Gastrointestinal/Hepatic
Abdominal pain [4]
Diarrhea [4]
Nausea [8]
Vomiting [14]

Otic
Tinnitus (<10%)

Ocular
Maculopathy [2]

Other
Adverse effects [2]
Death [3]

MELATONIN

Family: None
Scientific name: *N-acetyl-5-methoxytryptamine*
Indications: Jet lag, sleep disorders, Alzheimer's disease, free radical scavenger, chemotherapy adjunct, tinnitus, depression, migraine, cluster headache, hypertension, hyperpigmentation, osteoporosis, antioxidant. Skin protectant against sunburn
Class: Hormone
Half-life: N/A
Clinically important, potentially hazardous interactions with: acetaminophen, NSAIDs, setraline
Pregnancy category: N/A

Skin
Fixed eruption [2]

Central Nervous System
Somnolence (drowsiness) [2]

MELOXICAM

Trade name: Mobic (Boehringer Ingelheim)
Indications: Osteoarthritis
Class: COX-2 inhibitor, Non-steroidal anti-inflammatory (NSAID)
Half-life: 15–20 hours
Clinically important, potentially hazardous interactions with: ACE inhibitors, adrenergic neurone blockers, alcohol, aliskiren, alpha blockers, angiotensin II receptor antagonists, anticoagulants, antidepressants, antiplatelet agents, aspirin, baclofen, beta blockers, bile acid sequestrants, calcium channel blockers, cardiac glycosides, cholestyramine, clonidine, clopidogrel, collagenase, conivaptan, corticosteroids, coumarins, cyclosporine, dabigatran, dasatinib, desmopressin, diazoxide, digoxin, diuretics, drotrecogin alfa, eplerenone, erlotinib, glucosamine, haloperidol, heparins, hydralazine, ibritumomab, iloprost, ketorolac, lithium, methotrexate, methyldopa, mifamurtide, minoxidil, moxonidine, nitrates, nitroprusside, NSAIDs, pemetrexed, penicillamine, pentosan, pentoxifylline, phenindione, pralatrexate, prasugrel, probenecid, prostacyclin analogues, quinolones, ritonavir, serotonin/norepinephrine reuptake inhibitors, SSRIs, sulfonylureas, tacrolimus, thrombolytic agents, tositumomab & iodine^{131}, treprostinil, vancomycin, venlafaxine, vitamin K antagonists, voriconazole, zidovudine
Pregnancy category: C (category D from 30 weeks gestation)
Important contra-indications noted in the prescribing guidelines for: the elderly; nursing mothers
Note: NSAIDs may cause an increased risk of serious cardiovascular and gastrointestinal adverse events, which can be fatal. This risk may increase with duration of use.
Warning: CARDIOVASCULAR AND GASTROINTESTINAL RISKS

Skin
Anaphylactoid reactions/Anaphylaxis (<2%)
Angioedema (<2%) [3]
Bullous dermatitis (<2%)
Edema (2–5%)
Erythema [2]
Erythema multiforme (<2%)
Exanthems (<2%)
Facial edema (<2%)
Hematoma [3]
Hot flashes (<2%)
Hyperhidrosis (<2%)
Hypersensitivity [2]
Photosensitivity (<2%)
Pruritus (<2%) [3]
Purpura (<2%)
Rash (<3%) [3]
Stevens-Johnson syndrome (<2%)
Toxic epidermal necrolysis (<2%)
Urticaria (<2%) [4]
Vasculitis (<2%)

Hair
Alopecia (<2%)

Mucosal
Ulcerative stomatitis (<2%)
Xerostomia (<2%)

Cardiovascular
Angina (<2%)
Arrhythmias (<2%)
Cardiac failure (<2%)
Hypertension (<2%)
Hypotension (<2%)
Myocardial infarction (<2%)
Palpitation (<2%)
Tachycardia (<2%)

Central Nervous System
Abnormal dreams (<2%)
Anxiety (<2%)
Confusion (<2%)
Depression (<2%)
Dysgeusia (taste perversion) (<2%)
Fever (<2%)
Headache (2–6%) [2]
Insomnia (<4%)
Nervousness (<2%)
Pain (4%)
Paresthesias (<2%)
Seizures (<2%)
Somnolence (drowsiness) (<2%)
Syncope (<2%)
Tremor (<2%)
Vertigo (dizziness) (<3%)

Neuromuscular/Skeletal
Arthralgia (<5%)
Asthenia (fatigue) [2]
Back pain (<3%)
Bone or joint pain (2%)

Gastrointestinal/Hepatic
Abdominal pain (2–5%) [2]
Black stools (<2%)
Colitis (<2%)
Constipation (<3%) [2]
Diarrhea (2–6%) [2]
Dyspepsia (4–10%) [2]
Eructation (belching) (<2%)
Esophagitis (<2%)
Flatulence (<3%)
Gastritis (<2%)
Gastroesophageal reflux (<2%)
Gastrointestinal bleeding [2]
Gastrointestinal perforation (<2%) [2]
Gastrointestinal ulceration (<2%) [3]
Hematemesis (<2%)
Hepatitis (<2%)
Hepatotoxicity [6]
Nausea (3–7%) [4]
Pancreatitis (<2%)
Vomiting (<3%)

Respiratory
Asthma (<2%)
Bronchospasm (<2%)
Cough (<2%)
Dyspnea (<2%)
Flu-like syndrome (2–3%)
Upper respiratory tract infection (<8%)

Endocrine/Metabolic
ALT increased (<2%)
Appetite increased (<2%)
AST increased (<2%)
Dehydration (<2%)
GGT increased (<2%)
Weight gain (<2%)
Weight loss (<2%)

Genitourinary
Albuminuria (<2%)
Hematuria (<2%)
Urinary frequency (<2%)
Urinary tract infection (<7%)

Renal
Nephrotoxicity [2]
Renal failure (<2%)

Hematologic
Anemia (<4%)
Leukopenia (<2%)

Otic
Tinnitus (<2%)

Ocular
Abnormal vision (<2%)
Conjunctivitis (<2%)

Other
Adverse effects (18%) [6]
Allergic reactions (<2%)

MELPHALAN

Trade names: Alkeran (GSK), Evomela (Spectrum)
Indications: Multiple myeloma, carcinomas
Class: Alkylating agent
Half-life: 90 minutes
Clinically important, potentially hazardous interactions with: aldesleukin, PEG-interferon, tasonermin
Pregnancy category: D
Important contra-indications noted in the prescribing guidelines for: the elderly; nursing mothers; pediatric patients
Warning: SEVERE BONE MARROW SUPPRESSION, HYPERSENSITIVITY, and LEUKEMOGENICITY

Skin
- Anaphylactoid reactions/Anaphylaxis [2]
- Angioedema [2]
- Dermatitis [2]
- Exanthems (4%) [4]
- Hypersensitivity (<10%)
- Pruritus (<10%)
- Rash (<10%)
- Toxicity [3]
- Urticaria [3]
- Vasculitis (<10%)
- Vesiculation (<10%)

Hair
- Alopecia (<10%) [2]

Nails
- Beau's lines (transverse nail bands) [4]

Mucosal
- Mucositis [8]
- Oral mucositis [4]
- Stomatitis (<10%) [2]

Cardiovascular
- Atrial fibrillation [2]

Central Nervous System
- Peripheral neuropathy [3]

Neuromuscular/Skeletal
- Rhabdomyolysis [2]

Gastrointestinal/Hepatic
- Diarrhea [3]
- Hepatotoxicity [2]
- Nausea [2]

Hematologic
- Febrile neutropenia [2]
- Neutropenia [5]
- Thrombocytopenia [5]

Other
- Death [2]

MEMANTINE

Trade names: Ebixa (Lundbeck), Namenda (Forest)
Indications: Alzheimer's disease, vascular dementia
Class: Adamantane, NMDA receptor antagonist
Half-life: 60–80 hours
Clinically important, potentially hazardous interactions with: amantadine, bromocriptine, darifenacin, dextromethorphan, ketamine, levodopa, levomepromazine, oxybutynin, risperidone, rotigotine, tiotropium, trimethoprim, trospium, zuclopenthixol
Pregnancy category: B
Important contra-indications noted in the prescribing guidelines for: nursing mothers; pediatric patients

---

Skin
- Peripheral edema (>2%)

Central Nervous System
- Agitation [2]
- Confusion [3]
- Depression (>2%)
- Gait instability [3]
- Headache (6%) [3]
- Vertigo (dizziness) (7%) [6]

Neuromuscular/Skeletal
- Arthralgia (>2%)
- Asthenia (fatigue) (2%)
- Back pain (3%)
- Myoclonus [2]

Gastrointestinal/Hepatic
- Constipation [2]
- Diarrhea [2]
- Vomiting [2]

Respiratory
- Cough (4%)
- Flu-like syndrome (>2%)
- Nasopharyngitis [2]

Genitourinary
- Urinary tract infection [2]

Ocular
- Hallucinations, visual [2]

Other
- Adverse effects [3]

MENINGOCOCCAL GROUP B VACCINE

Trade names: Bexsero (Novartis), Trumenba (Wyeth)
Indications: Immunization to prevent invasive disease caused by *Neisseria meningitidis* serogroup B
Class: Vaccine
Half-life: N/A
Clinically important, potentially hazardous interactions with: none known
Pregnancy category: B
Important contra-indications noted in the prescribing guidelines for: the elderly; nursing mothers; pediatric patients

---

Central Nervous System
- Chills (18–30%)
- Fever (2–8%) [4]
- Headache (41–57%)

Neuromuscular/Skeletal
- Arthralgia (16–22%)
- Asthenia (fatigue) (44–65%)
- Myalgia/Myopathy (35–41%)

Gastrointestinal/Hepatic
- Diarrhea (9–15%)
- Vomiting (2–8%)

Respiratory
- Upper respiratory tract infection [2]

Local
- Injection-site edema (18–22%)
- Injection-site erythema (15–20%)
- Injection-site pain (85–93%) [3]
- Injection-site reactions [2]

MENINGOCOCCAL GROUPS C & Y & HAEMOPHILUS B TETANUS TOXOID CONJUGATE VACCINE

Synonym: HibMenCY
Trade name: Menhibrix (GSK)
Indications: Immunization to prevent invasive disease caused by *Neisseria meningitidis* serogroups C and Y and *Haemophilus influenzae* Type B
Class: Vaccine
Half-life: N/A
Clinically important, potentially hazardous interactions with: immunosuppressants
Pregnancy category: C
Important contra-indications noted in the prescribing guidelines for: pediatric patients

---

Central Nervous System
- Fever (11–26%)
- Irritability (62–71%)
- Sedation (49–63%)

Endocrine/Metabolic
- Appetite decreased (30–34%)

Local
- Injection-site edema (15–25%) [2]
- Injection-site erythema (21–36%)
- Injection-site pain (42–46%) [2]

MEPERIDINE

Synonym: pethidine
Trade name: Demerol (Sanofi-Aventis)
Indications: Pain
Class: Opiate agonist
Half-life: 3–4 hours
Clinically important, potentially hazardous interactions with: acyclovir, alcohol, amphetamines, barbiturates, CNS depressants, darunavir, duloxetine, fluoxetine, furazolidone, general anesthetics, glycopyrrolate,

glycopyrronium, indinavir, isocarboxazid, linezolid, lisdexamfetamine, lithium, MAO inhibitors, moclobemide, phenelzine, phenobarbital, phenothiazines, phenytoin, rasagiline, ritonavir, safinamide, selegiline, sibutramine, SSRIs, tipranavir, tranquilizers, tranylcypromine, tricyclic antidepressants, valacyclovir
Pregnancy category: C
Important contra-indications noted in the prescribing guidelines for: the elderly; nursing mothers; pediatric patients

---

Skin
Pruritus [3]

Mucosal
Xerostomia (<10%)

Central Nervous System
Catatonia [2]
Delirium [2]
Seizures [2]
Serotonin syndrome [7]

Local
Injection-site erythema [2]
Injection-site pain (<10%)

MEPOLIZUMAB

Trade name: Nucala (GSK)
Indications: Adjunctive treatment for severe eosinophilic asthma
Class: Interleukin-5 antagonist, Monoclonal antibody
Half-life: 16–22 days
Clinically important, potentially hazardous interactions with: none known
Pregnancy category: N/A (Insufficent evidence to inform drug-associated risk)
Important contra-indications noted in the prescribing guidelines for: nursing mothers; pediatric patients

---

Skin
Eczema (3%)
Pruritus (3%)
Rash (>3%)

Mucosal
Nasal congestion (>3%)

Central Nervous System
Fever (>3%)
Headache (19%) [4]
Vertigo (dizziness) (>3%)

Neuromuscular/Skeletal
Asthenia (fatigue) (5%) [2]
Back pain (5%)
Bone or joint pain (>3%)
Muscle spasm (3%)

Gastrointestinal/Hepatic
Abdominal pain (3%)
Gastroenteritis (>3%)
Nausea (>3%) [2]
Vomiting (>3%)

Respiratory
Asthma [2]
Bronchitis (>3%) [2]
Dyspnea (>3%)
Influenza (3%)
Nasopharyngitis (>3%) [3]
Pharyngitis (>3%)
Rhinitis (>3%)
Sinusitis [2]
Upper respiratory tract infection [2]

Genitourinary
Cystitis (>3%)
Urinary tract infection (3%)

Otic
Ear infection (>3%)

Local
Injection-site reactions (8%) [2]

Other
Infection (>3%)
Toothache (>3%)

MERCAPTOPURINE

Synonyms: 6-mercaptopurine; 6-MP
Trade name: Purinethol (Gate)
Indications: Leukemias
Class: Antimetabolite, Antineoplastic
Half-life: triphasic: 45 minutes; 2.5 hours; 10 hours
Clinically important, potentially hazardous interactions with: aldesleukin, allopurinol, balsalazide, febuxostat, influenza vaccine, mycophenolate, natalizumab, olsalazine, trimethoprim, typhoid vaccine, vaccines, yellow fever vaccine
Pregnancy category: D

Skin
Dermatitis (2%)
Hand–foot syndrome [3]
Hypersensitivity [2]
Neoplasms [2]
Peripheral edema [2]
Photosensitivity [2]
Pigmentation (<10%)
Rash (<10%) [2]

Hair
Alopecia [2]

Mucosal
Mucositis (<10%)
Oral lesions (<5%) [2]
Stomatitis (<10%)

Central Nervous System
Fever [3]

Gastrointestinal/Hepatic
Hepatotoxicity [5]
Nausea [2]
Pancreatitis [9]

Hematologic
Leukopenia [2]
Myelosuppression [2]
Myelotoxicity [3]

Other
Death [2]

MEROPENEM

Trade name: Meronem (AstraZeneca)
Indications: Aerobic and anaerobic infections, febrile neutropenia
Class: Antibiotic, carbapenem, Thienamycin
Half-life: 4–6 hours
Clinically important, potentially hazardous interactions with: oral contraceptives, probenecid, valproic acid
Pregnancy category: B

Skin
AGEP [2]
Hypersensitivity [3]
Rash (2%) [6]

Central Nervous System
Fever [2]
Headache (2%)
Seizures [7]

Gastrointestinal/Hepatic
Diarrhea [4]
Hepatotoxicity [3]
Nausea [2]
Vomiting [2]

Endocrine/Metabolic
ALT increased [3]
AST increased [3]

Local
Injection-site pain [3]

Other
Adverse effects [14]
Death [2]

MESALAMINE

Synonyms: 5-aminosalicylic acid; 5-ASA; fisalamine; mesalazine
Trade names: Asacol (Procter & Gamble), Canasa (Aptalis), Lialda (Shire), Pentasa (Shire), Rowasa (Solvay)
Indications: Ulcerative colitis
Class: Aminosalicylate
Half-life: 0.5–1.5 hours
Clinically important, potentially hazardous interactions with: azathioprine, NSAIDs, pantoprazole
Pregnancy category: B
Important contra-indications noted in the prescribing guidelines for: the elderly; nursing mothers

---

Skin
Diaphoresis (3%)
Exanthems [3]
Hypersensitivity [8]
Lupus erythematosus [2]
Photosensitivity [3]
Psoriasis [2]
Rash (3%) [6]

Hair
Alopecia [6]

Cardiovascular
Cardiotoxicity [3]
Myocarditis [7]
Myopericarditis [2]

Pericarditis [5]

Central Nervous System

Fever (<6%) [6]
Headache (2–25%) [5]
Pain (14%)
Vertigo (dizziness) (2–8%)

Neuromuscular/Skeletal

Myalgia/Myopathy (3%)

Gastrointestinal/Hepatic

Abdominal pain (<18%) [6]
Colitis (ulcerative / exacerbation) [4]
Diarrhea (2–8%) [4]
Eructation (belching) (16%)
Flatulence (<6%) [2]
Hepatotoxicity [2]
Nausea (3–13%) [3]
Pancreatitis [21]
Vomiting (<5%) [2]

Respiratory

Eosinophilic pneumonia [4]
Pharyngitis (11%)
Pneumonia [5]
Pneumonitis [2]
Pulmonary toxicity [10]

Renal

Nephrotoxicity [7]

Hematologic

Anemia [2]
Eosinophilia [3]

Otic

Tinnitus (<3%)

Other

Adverse effects [11]
Allergic reactions [2]
Kounis syndrome [2]

METAXALONE

Trade name: Skelaxin (Elan)
Indications: Muscle spasm
Class: Central muscle relaxant
Half-life: 4–14 hours
Clinically important, potentially hazardous interactions with: alcohol, barbiturates, conivaptan, droperidol, interferon alfa, levomepromazine, St John's wort, tricyclic antidepressants
Pregnancy category: B
Important contra-indications noted in the prescribing guidelines for: nursing mothers; pediatric patients
Note: Contra-indicated in patients with known tendency to drug-induced, hemolytic, or other anemias, or significantly impaired renal or hepatic function.

Cardiovascular

Tachycardia [2]

Central Nervous System

Agitation [2]
Serotonin syndrome [3]
Somnolence (drowsiness) [3]
Vertigo (dizziness) [3]

Gastrointestinal/Hepatic

Nausea [2]
Vomiting [2]

METFORMIN

Trade names: Avandamet (GSK), Fortamet (Andrx), Glucophage (Merck Serono), Glucovance (Merck Serono), Invokamet (Janssen), Janumet (Merck Sharpe & Dohme), Synjardy (Boehringer Ingelheim), Xigduo XR (AstraZeneca)
Indications: Diabetes
Class: Antidiabetic, Biguanide
Half-life: 6 hours
Clinically important, potentially hazardous interactions with: ACE inhibitors, acetazolamide, alcohol, amiloride, anabolic steroids, beta blockers, bictegravir/emtricitabine/tenofovir alafenamide, calcium channel blockers, captopril, cephalexin, cilazapril, cimetidine, corticosteroids, diazoxide, dichlorphenamide, digoxin, disopyramide, diuretics, enalapril, estrogens, fosinopril, iodinated contrast agents, isoniazid, ketotifen, lanreotide, lisinopril, luteinizing hormone releasing hormone analogs, MAO inhibitors, morphine, nicotinic acid, octreotide, oral contraceptives, pegvisomant, phenothiazines, phenytoin, procainamide, progestogens, quinapril, quinidine, quinine, ramipril, ranitidine, somatropin, sympathomimetics, testosterone, thiazides, thyroid products, topiramate, trandolapril, triamterene, trimethoprim, trospium, vancomycin, zonisamide
Pregnancy category: B
Important contra-indications noted in the prescribing guidelines for: the elderly; nursing mothers; pediatric patients
Note: Lactic acidosis is a rare, but serious, metabolic complication that can occur due to metformin accumulation.
Avandamet is metformin and rosiglitazone; Glucovance is metformin and glyburide; Invokamet is metformin and canagliflozin; Janumet is metformin and sitagliptin; Synjardy is metformin and empagliflozin; Xigduo XR is metformin and dapagliflozin.
Warning: LACTIC ACIDOSIS

Skin

Angioedema [2]
Bullous pemphigoid [2]
Erythema (transient) [3]
Fixed eruption [2]
Flushing (<10%)
Lichenoid eruption [2]
Peripheral edema [5]
Photosensitivity (<10%)
Rash (<10%) [4]
Urticaria (<10%) [4]
Vasculitis [2]

Cardiovascular

Hypertension [3]
Palpitation (<10%)

Central Nervous System

Chills (<10%)
Dysgeusia (taste perversion) (3%)
Headache (6%) [10]
Vertigo (dizziness) (<10%) [6]

Neuromuscular/Skeletal

Arthralgia [5]
Asthenia (fatigue) (9%) [2]
Back pain [5]
Myalgia/Myopathy (<10%)

Gastrointestinal/Hepatic

Abdominal pain (6%) [5]
Constipation [3]
Diarrhea (10–35%) [31]
Dyspepsia [5]
Flatulence [2]
Gastroenteritis [2]
Hepatotoxicity [6]
Nausea (7–26%) [25]
Pancreatitis [5]
Vomiting (7–26%) [12]

Respiratory

Bronchitis [3]
Dyspnea (<10%)
Influenza [2]
Nasopharyngitis [6]
Respiratory tract infection (<10%)
Sinusitis [2]
Upper respiratory tract infection [6]

Endocrine/Metabolic

Acidosis [23]
Appetite decreased [5]
Hypoglycemia [15]
Weight gain [2]
Weight loss [5]

Genitourinary

Genital mycotic infections [9]
Pollakiuria [3]
Urinary tract infection [12]

Renal

Nephrotoxicity [5]

Hematologic

Anemia [2]

Other

Adverse effects [24]
Death [2]
Vitamin B-12 deficiency [5]

METHADONE

Trade names: Dolophine (Roxane), Methadose (Mallinckrodt)
Indications: Pain, narcotic addiction
Class: Opiate agonist
Half-life: 15–25 hours
Clinically important, potentially hazardous interactions with: abacavir, amprenavir, boceprevir, citalopram, darunavir, delavirdine, diazepam, efavirenz, erythromycin, fluconazole, fluvoxamine, interferon alfa, ketoconazole, linezolid, lofexidine, lopinavir, nelfinavir, nilotinib, paroxetine hydrochloride, PEG-interferon, quetiapine, ribociclib, rifapentine, rilpivirine, safinamide, St John's wort, tipranavir, vandetanib, voriconazole, zidovudine, zuclopenthixol
Pregnancy category: C
Important contra-indications noted in the prescribing guidelines for: pediatric patients
Note: Methadone is not licensed for use in children though it can be employed for the management of neonatal opiate withdrawal syndrome.

Skin

Diaphoresis (<48%) [4]

Pruritus [2]

Mucosal

Xerostomia (<10%)

Cardiovascular

Arrhythmias [2]
QT prolongation [37]
Torsades de pointes [27]
Ventricular arrhythmia [2]

Central Nervous System

Hallucinations [2]
Hyperalgesia [2]
Neurotoxicity [2]
Serotonin syndrome [2]
Somnolence (drowsiness) [2]
Syncope [2]

Neuromuscular/Skeletal

Rhabdomyolysis [4]

Respiratory

Respiratory depression [4]

Genitourinary

Sexual dysfunction [2]

Local

Injection-site pain (<10%)

Other

Adverse effects [2]
Death [15]

METHAMPHETAMINE

Trade name: Desoxyn (Recordati)
Indications: Attention deficit disorder, obesity
Class: Amphetamine
Half-life: 4–5 hours
Clinically important, potentially hazardous interactions with: fluoxetine, fluvoxamine, MAO inhibitors, paroxetine hydrochloride, phenelzine, sertraline, tranylcypromine
Pregnancy category: C
Important contra-indications noted in the prescribing guidelines for: nursing mothers; pediatric patients
Warning: POTENTIAL FOR ABUSE

Skin

Diaphoresis (<10%)

Mucosal

Xerostomia (<10%) [5]

Cardiovascular

Polyarteritis nodosa [2]

Central Nervous System

Depression [2]
Hallucinations [4]
Insomnia [2]
Neurotoxicity [6]
Paranoia [2]
Parkinsonism [2]
Psychosis [11]

Neuromuscular/Skeletal

Rhabdomyolysis (43%) [5]

Other

Bruxism [4]
Death [3]
Dental disease [2]

METHIMAZOLE

Synonym: thiamazole
Trade name: Tapazole (Paladin)
Indications: Hyperthyroidism
Class: Antithyroid, hormone modifier
Half-life: 4–13 hours
Clinically important, potentially hazardous interactions with: anticoagulants, dicumarol, warfarin
Pregnancy category: D

Skin

Aplasia cutis congenita [4]
Exanthems (<15%) [5]
Hypersensitivity [2]
Lupus erythematosus (<10%) [10]
Pruritus (<5%) [4]
Rash (>10%)
Urticaria (>5%) [2]
Vasculitis [6]

Central Nervous System

Ageusia (taste loss) (<10%)

Neuromuscular/Skeletal

Arthralgia [4]

Gastrointestinal/Hepatic

Hepatotoxicity [11]
Pancreatitis [3]

Respiratory

Pulmonary toxicity [2]

Hematologic

Agranulocytosis [11]
Neutropenia [2]

Other

Side effects (in high dosages) (28%) [2]
Teratogenicity [2]

METHOTREXATE

Synonyms: amethopterin; MTX
Trade names: Rasuvo (Medac), Rheumatrex (Stada)
Indications: Carcinomas, leukemias, lymphomas, psoriasis, rheumatoid arthritis
Class: Antimetabolite, Disease-modifying antirheumatic drug (DMARD), Folic acid antagonist
Half-life: 3–10 hours
Clinically important, potentially hazardous interactions with: acemetacin, acitretin, aldesleukin, aminoglycosides, amiodarone, amoxicillin, ampicillin, aspirin, bacampicillin, bismuth, carbenicillin, chloroquine, ciprofloxacin, cisplatin, cloxacillin, co-trimoxazole, cyclopenthiazide, dapsone, demeclocycline, dexamethasone, diclofenac, dicloxacillin, doxycycline, echinacea, etodolac, etoricoxib, etretinate, fenoprofen, flurbiprofen, folic acid antagonists, gadobenate, haloperidol, hydrocortisone, ibuprofen, indomethacin, infliximab, ketoprofen, ketorolac, leflunomide, magnesium trisalicylate, meclofenamate, mefenamic acid, meloxicam, methicillin, mezlocillin, minocycline, nabumetone, nafcillin, naproxen, natalizumab, NSAIDs, omeprazole, oxacillin, oxaprozin, oxtriphylline, oxytetracycline, pantoprazole, paromomycin, penicillin G, penicillin V, penicillins, phenylbutazone, piperacillin, piperacillin/tazobactam, piroxicam, polypeptide antibiotics, prednisolone, prednisone, pristinamycin, probenecid, procarbazine, rofecoxib, salicylates, salsalate, sapropterin, sulfadiazine, sulfamethoxazole, sulfapyridine, sulfasalazine, sulfisoxazole, sulindac, taxobactam, tenoxicam, tetracycline, ticarcillin, tolmetin, trimethoprim, vaccines
Pregnancy category: X
Important contra-indications noted in the prescribing guidelines for: the elderly; nursing mothers; pediatric patients
Warning: SEVERE TOXIC REACTIONS, INCLUDING EMBRYOFETAL TOXICITY AND DEATH

Skin

Abscess (peritoneal) [2]
Acral erythema [13]
Anaphylactoid reactions/Anaphylaxis (<10%) [9]
Bullous acral erythema [2]
Bullous dermatitis [4]
Capillaritis [2]
Carcinoma [2]
Dermatitis [2]
Edema [2]
Erosion of psoriatic plaques [8]
Erythema (>10%)
Erythema multiforme [4]
Erythroderma [2]
Exanthems (15%) [5]
Folliculitis [2]
Hand–foot syndrome [3]
Herpes simplex [2]
Herpes zoster [7]
Hypersensitivity [4]
Lymphoma [5]
Malignancies [2]
Malignant lymphoma [4]
Molluscum contagiosum [2]
Necrosis [6]
Neoplasms [2]
Nodular eruption [15]
Non-Hodgkin's lymphoma [2]
Photosensitivity (5%) [9]
Pigmentation (<10%)
Pruritus (<5%)
Pseudolymphoma [10]
Radiation recall dermatitis [8]
Rash (<3%) [13]
Squamous cell carcinoma [2]
Stevens-Johnson syndrome [4]
Sunburn (reactivation) [6]
Toxic epidermal necrolysis [8]
Toxicity [9]
Ulceration of psoriatic plaques [4]
Ulcerations [12]
Urticaria [4]
Vasculitis (>10%) [9]

Hair

Alopecia (<6%) [28]

Nails

Nail pigmentation [2]
Paronychia [2]

Mucosal

Aphthous stomatitis [2]

Gingivitis (>10%)
Glossitis (>10%)
Mucocutaneous reactions [2]
Mucositis [11]
Nasal septal perforation [2]
Oral mucositis [8]
Oral ulceration [11]
Stomatitis (3–10%) [19]

Cardiovascular
Hypertension [2]
Pericardial effusion [2]
Pericarditis [3]

Central Nervous System
Encephalopathy [5]
Fever [6]
Headache [17]
Leukoencephalopathy [62]
Migraine [2]
Neurotoxicity [12]
Vertigo (dizziness) [2]

Neuromuscular/Skeletal
Arthralgia [5]
Asthenia (fatigue) [14]
Back pain [2]
Bone or joint pain [2]

Gastrointestinal/Hepatic
Abdominal pain [9]
Colitis [2]
Diarrhea [13]
Dyspepsia [3]
Gastroenteritis [2]
Hepatic steatosis [2]
Hepatitis [3]
Hepatotoxicity [57]
Nausea [30]
Vomiting [13]

Respiratory
Cough [3]
Nasopharyngitis [6]
Pharyngitis [2]
Pneumonia [8]
Pneumonitis [8]
Pulmonary toxicity [9]
Upper respiratory tract infection [9]

Endocrine/Metabolic
ALT increased [7]
AST increased [3]
Diabetes mellitus [2]
Gynecomastia [8]
Hypoalbuminemia [2]
Weight gain [2]

Genitourinary
Urinary tract infection [4]

Renal
Nephrotoxicity [28]
Renal failure [2]

Hematologic
Anemia [9]
Febrile neutropenia [3]
Hemotoxicity [2]
Leukopenia [11]
Myelosuppression [7]
Myelotoxicity [4]
Neutropenia [10]
Pancytopenia [10]
Thrombocytopenia [9]

Ocular
Cotton wool spots [2]
Optic neuropathy [2]

Local
Injection-site reactions [3]

Other
Adverse effects [40]
Death [17]
Hodgkin's disease (nodular sclerosing) [2]
Infection [25]
Side effects [3]
Teratogenicity [3]

METHOXSALEN

Trade name: Oxsoralen (Valeant)
Indications: Psoriasis, vitiligo
Class: CYP1A2 inhibitor, Psoralen, Repigmenting agent
Half-life: 1.1 hours
Clinically important, potentially hazardous interactions with: caffeine, chloroquine, cyclosporine, fluoroquinolones, phenothiazines, sulfonamides
Pregnancy category: C
Important contra-indications noted in the prescribing guidelines for: pediatric patients
Note: Potential hazards of long-term therapy include the possibilities of carcinogenicity and cataractogenicity.

Skin
Anaphylactoid reactions/Anaphylaxis [2]
Basal cell carcinoma [3]
Bullous dermatitis (with UVA) [4]
Burning (<10%) [3]
Carcinoma [5]
Dermatitis [4]
Edema (<10%)
Ephelides (<10%) [5]
Erythema (<10%)
Exanthems [2]
Herpes zoster [2]
Hypomelanosis (<10%)
Lupus erythematosus [3]
Photosensitivity [9]
Phototoxicity [7]
Pigmentation [3]
Porokeratosis (actinic) [3]
Pruritus (>10%)
Rash (<10%)
Squamous cell carcinoma [4]
Tumors [2]
Vitiligo [2]

Hair
Hypertrichosis [3]

Nails
Nail pigmentation [5]
Photo-onycholysis [5]

Mucosal
Cheilitis (<10%)

Central Nervous System
Pain [2]

Ocular
Ocular toxicity [2]

METHYLDOPA

Trade name: Aldoclor (Merck)
Indications: Hypertension
Class: Adrenergic alpha-receptor agonist
Half-life: 1.7 hours
Clinically important, potentially hazardous interactions with: acebutolol, alfuzosin, bromocriptine, captopril, cilazapril, cyclopenthiazide, diclofenac, enalapril, ephedrine, fosinopril, irbesartan, levodopa, levomepromazine, linezolid, lisinopril, meloxicam, olmesartan, quinapril, ramipril, risperidone, rotigotine, trandolapril, triamcinolone, zuclopenthixol
Pregnancy category: B
Important contra-indications noted in the prescribing guidelines for: nursing mothers
Note: Aldoril is methyldopa and hydrochlorothiazide. Hydrochlorothiazide is a sulfonamide and can be absorbed systemically. Sulfonamides can produce severe, possibly fatal, reactions such as toxic epidermal necrolysis and Stevens-Johnson syndrome.

Skin
Eczema [3]
Erythema multiforme [2]
Exanthems (3%) [3]
Lichen planus [3]
Lichenoid eruption [9]
Lupus erythematosus [14]
Peripheral edema (>10%)
Photosensitivity [2]
Pigmentation [3]
Seborrheic dermatitis [3]
Stevens-Johnson syndrome [2]
Urticaria [2]

Mucosal
Oral lichenoid eruption [3]
Oral ulceration [6]
Xerostomia (<10%)

Central Nervous System
Anxiety (<10%)
Depression (<10%)
Dyskinesia [2]
Fever (<10%)
Headache (<10%)
Nightmares (<10%)
Parkinsonism [2]

Gastrointestinal/Hepatic
Hepatitis [2]
Hepatotoxicity [8]

Endocrine/Metabolic
Amenorrhea [2]
Galactorrhea [4]

Hematologic
Hemolytic anemia [2]

METHYLPHENIDATE

Trade names: Concerta (Janssen), Metadate CD (Celltech), Methylin (Mallinckrodt), Ritalin (Novartis)
Indications: Attention deficit disorder, narcolepsy
Class: Amphetamine
Half-life: 2–4 hours
Clinically important, potentially hazardous interactions with: amitriptyline, benazepril, bupropion, captopril, citalopram, clevidipine, cyclosporine, enalapril, escitalopram, irbesartan, linezolid, lisinopril, lurasidone, MAO inhibitors, olmesartan, paliperidone, pantoprazole, paroxetine hydrochloride, phenylbutazone, pimozide, quinapril, safinamide, ziprasidone
Pregnancy category: C
Important contra-indications noted in the prescribing guidelines for: the elderly; nursing mothers
Warning: ABUSE AND DEPENDENCE

Skin
Angioedema [2]
Exanthems [2]
Exfoliative dermatitis [2]
Hypersensitivity (<10%)
Leukoderma [2]

Mucosal
Xerostomia [7]

Cardiovascular
Cardiotoxicity [3]
Palpitation [4]
QT prolongation [2]
Tachycardia [5]

Central Nervous System
Agitation [2]
Anorexia [7]
Anxiety [7]
Compulsions [2]
Depression [2]
Fever [2]
Hallucinations [6]
Headache [12]
Insomnia [15]
Irritability [6]
Mood changes [2]
Nervousness [2]
Neurotoxicity [3]
Seizures [3]
Somnolence (drowsiness) [3]
Suicidal ideation [2]
Tic disorder [6]
Tremor [2]
Vertigo (dizziness) [5]

Neuromuscular/Skeletal
Asthenia (fatigue) [2]
Dystonia [2]

Gastrointestinal/Hepatic
Abdominal pain [12]
Nausea [7]
Vomiting [5]

Respiratory
Cough [3]
Nasopharyngitis [4]
Upper respiratory tract infection [3]

Endocrine/Metabolic
Appetite decreased [16]
Weight loss [9]

Genitourinary
Priapism [5]

Ocular
Hallucinations, visual [6]

Other
Adverse effects [7]
Bruxism [2]

METHYL-PREDNISOLONE

Trade names: Advantan (Intendis), Medrol (Pharmacia), Solu-Medrol (Pharmacia)
Indications: Arthralgias, asthma, dermatoses, inflammatory ocular conditions, rhinitis
Class: Corticosteroid, systemic
Half-life: 12–36 hours; 2–4 hours (plasma)
Clinically important, potentially hazardous interactions with: aminophylline, aprepitant, aspirin, carbamazepine, clarithromycin, conivaptan, cyclosporine, daclizumab, darunavir, delavirdine, erythromycin, indinavir, itraconazole, ketoconazole, live vaccines, oral contraceptives, phenobarbital, phenytoin, rifampin, telaprevir, telithromycin, troleandomycin, voriconazole, warfarin
Pregnancy category: C
Important contra-indications noted in the prescribing guidelines for: nursing mothers; pediatric patients

---

Skin
Anaphylactoid reactions/Anaphylaxis [15]
Dermatitis [5]
Flushing [2]
Hypersensitivity [3]
Pruritus [2]
Rash [2]
Urticaria [5]

Cardiovascular
Arrhythmias [2]
Bradycardia [6]
Hypertension [6]
Myocardial infarction [2]
Myocardial toxicity [2]

Central Nervous System
Depression [5]
Dysgeusia (taste perversion) [4]
Headache [2]
Neurotoxicity [2]
Psychosis [3]
Seizures [3]
Vertigo (dizziness) [2]

Neuromuscular/Skeletal
Arthralgia [2]
Myalgia/Myopathy [4]
Osteonecrosis [9]
Osteoporosis [2]
Tendinopathy/Tendon rupture [2]

Gastrointestinal/Hepatic
Abdominal pain [3]
Gastrointestinal bleeding [2]
Hepatotoxicity [8]

Respiratory
Dysphonia [2]

Endocrine/Metabolic
Hyperglycemia [4]

Ocular
Cataract [3]
Glaucoma [2]

Other
Adverse effects [7]
Allergic reactions [3]
Death [2]
Hiccups [2]
Infection [7]

METHYL-TESTOSTERONE

Trade names: Android (Valeant), Estratest (Solvay), Testred (Valeant)
Indications: Hypogonadism, impotence, metastatic breast cancer
Class: Androgen
Half-life: 2.5–3.5 hours
Clinically important, potentially hazardous interactions with: anticoagulants, cyclosporine, warfarin
Pregnancy category: X
Important contra-indications noted in the prescribing guidelines for: nursing mothers; pediatric patients

---

Skin
Acneform eruption (>10%) [12]
Edema (>10%)
Flushing (<5%)

Hair
Alopecia [2]
Hirsutism (in females) (<10%) [9]

Endocrine/Metabolic
Mastodynia (>10%)

Genitourinary
Priapism (>10%)

METHYSERGIDE

Trade name: Sansert (Novartis)
Indications: Vascular (migraine) headaches
Class: Hallucinogen, Psychotomimetic
Half-life: 10 hours
Clinically important, potentially hazardous interactions with: acebutolol, almotriptan, amprenavir, azithromycin, chlortetracycline, clarithromycin, delavirdine, demeclocycline, doxycycline, efavirenz, eletriptan, erythromycin, frovatriptan, indinavir, itraconazole, lymecycline, minocycline, naratriptan, nelfinavir, oxytetracycline, ritonavir, rizatriptan, saquinavir, sibutramine, sumatriptan, telithromycin, tetracycline, tigecycline, troleandomycin, voriconazole, zolmitriptan
Pregnancy category: X
Important contra-indications noted in the prescribing guidelines for: nursing mothers; pediatric patients

---

Skin
Lupus erythematosus [2]
Peripheral edema (<10%)
Rash (<10%)
Scleroderma [4]

Hair
Alopecia [4]

Cardiovascular
Valvulopathy [3]

METOPROLOL

Trade names: Lopressor (Novartis), Toprol XL (AstraZeneca)
Indications: Hypertension, angina pectoris
Class: Adrenergic beta-receptor agonist, Antiarrhythmic class II
Half-life: 3–4 hours
Clinically important, potentially hazardous interactions with: cinacalcet, clonidine, cobicistat/elvitegravir/emtricitabine/tenofovir alafenamide, cobicistat/elvitegravir/emtricitabine/tenofovir disoproxil, dronedarone, epinephrine, mirabegron, paroxetine hydrochloride, propoxyphene, tadalafil, telithromycin, tipranavir, venlafaxine, verapamil
Pregnancy category: C
Important contra-indications noted in the prescribing guidelines for: the elderly; pediatric patients
Note: Cutaneous side effects of beta-receptor blockers are clinically polymorphous. They apparently appear after several months of continuous therapy.

Skin
Eczema [2]
Erythroderma [2]
Lichenoid eruption [4]
Pruritus (<5%)
Psoriasis (induction and aggravation of) [8]
Rash (<5%) [3]
Raynaud's phenomenon [3]

Cardiovascular
Arrhythmias [2]
Bradycardia [8]
Hypotension [4]

Central Nervous System
Delirium [3]
Hallucinations [2]
Sleep disturbances [2]

Neuromuscular/Skeletal
Asthenia (fatigue) [2]

Gastrointestinal/Hepatic
Gastrointestinal disorder [2]

Genitourinary
Peyronie's disease [5]

Ocular
Hallucinations, visual [3]

METRONIDAZOLE

Trade names: Flagyl (Pfizer), Metrocream (Galderma), MetroGel (Galderma), Metrolotion (Galderma), Noritate (Dermik), Vandazole (Upsher-Smith)
Indications: Various infections caused by susceptible organisms, rosacea
Class: Antibacterial, Antibiotic, nitroimidazole
Half-life: 6–12 hours
Clinically important, potentially hazardous interactions with: alcohol, anisindione, anticoagulants, astemizole, barbiturates, busulfan, cimetidine, dicumarol, disulfiram, dronabinol, fluorouracil, lithium, lopinavir, mycophenolate, phenytoin, primidone, thalidomide, tipranavir, uracil/tegafur, warfarin
Pregnancy category: B (in patients with trichomoniasis, metronidazole is contra-indicated during the first trimester of pregnancy)
Important contra-indications noted in the prescribing guidelines for: nursing mothers

---

Skin
AGEP [2]
Dermatitis [2]
Exanthems (<5%) [2]
Fixed eruption [14]
Flushing [2]
Pruritus (<10%) [6]
Stevens-Johnson syndrome [5]
Toxic epidermal necrolysis [2]
Urticaria [4]

Mucosal
Glossitis [2]
Tongue furry [2]
Xerostomia [2]

Cardiovascular
Hypertension [2]
Torsades de pointes [2]

Central Nervous System
Cerebellar syndrome [6]
Dysgeusia (taste perversion) [8]
Encephalopathy [22]
Fever [7]
Headache (7%) [7]
Neurotoxicity [14]
Peripheral neuropathy [2]
Psychosis [3]

Neuromuscular/Skeletal
Ataxia [2]

Gastrointestinal/Hepatic
Abdominal pain (5%) [8]
Diarrhea [15]
Hepatotoxicity [5]
Nausea [19]
Pancreatitis [6]
Vomiting [14]

Endocrine/Metabolic
ALT increased [2]
AST increased [2]

Genitourinary
Vulvovaginal candidiasis [2]

Hematologic
Anemia [2]
Bleeding [2]

Otic
Hearing loss [2]

Ocular
Vision loss [2]

Other
Adverse effects [12]
Death [3]
Infection (fungal) (12%)

MICAFUNGIN

Trade name: Mycamine (Astellas)
Indications: Invasive candidiasis, esophageal candidiasis
Class: Antifungal
Half-life: 11–21 hours
Clinically important, potentially hazardous interactions with: amphotericin B, conivaptan, cyclosporine, itraconazole, nifedipine, sirolimus
Pregnancy category: C
Important contra-indications noted in the prescribing guidelines for: nursing mothers; pediatric patients

---

Skin
Anaphylactoid reactions/Anaphylaxis [2]
Peripheral edema (7%)
Pruritus (6%)
Rash (9%) [6]
Ulcerations (5%)

Mucosal
Epistaxis (nosebleed) (6%) [2]
Mucosal inflammation (14%)

Cardiovascular
Bradycardia (3%)
Hypertension (7%) [2]
Hypotension (9%)
Phlebitis (6%)
Tachycardia (8%)

Central Nervous System
Anorexia (6%)
Anxiety (6%)
Fever (20%) [6]
Headache (16%) [3]
Insomnia (10%)
Rigors (9%)
Shock (8%)

Neuromuscular/Skeletal
Asthenia (fatigue) (6%)
Back pain (5%)

Gastrointestinal/Hepatic
Abdominal pain (10%) [3]
Constipation (11%)
Diarrhea (23%) [8]
Dyspepsia (6%)
Hepatotoxicity [8]
Nausea (22%) [6]
Vomiting (22%) [5]

Respiratory
Cough (8%)
Dyspnea (6%)
Pneumonia (2%)

Endocrine/Metabolic
ALP increased (5%) [2]
ALT increased (5%) [6]
AST increased (6%) [4]

Hyperbilirubinemia [3]
Hyperglycemia (6%)
Hyperkalemia (5%)
Hypernatremia (5%)
Hypocalcemia (7%)
Hypoglycemia (6%)
Hypokalemia (18%) [3]
Hypomagnesemia (13%)

Hematologic
Anemia (10%) [3]
Febrile neutropenia (6%)
Hemolysis [3]
Neutropenia (14%)
Sepsis (5%)
Thrombocytopenia (15%) [2]

Local
Infusion-related reactions [2]

Other
Adverse effects [5]
Infection (40%)

MICONAZOLE

Trade names: Monistat (Janssen), Oravig (Dara)
Indications: Fungal infections, oropharyngeal candidiasis
Class: Antibiotic, imidazole, Antifungal, azole
Half-life: initial: 40 minutes; terminal: 24 hours
Clinically important, potentially hazardous interactions with: anisindione, anticoagulants, astemizole, clopidogrel, dicumarol, gliclazide, simvastatin, thioridazine, tolvaptan, vinblastine, vincristine, warfarin
Pregnancy category: C
Important contra-indications noted in the prescribing guidelines for: nursing mothers; pediatric patients

---

Skin
Angioedema (2%)
Contact dermatitis [2]
Dermatitis [11]
Exanthems (2–87%) [5]
Flushing (<2%) [2]
Pruritus (2–36%) [3]
Purpura (3–8%)
Rash (9%)
Toxicity [2]
Urticaria (2%)

Cardiovascular
Phlebitis (5–79%) [3]

Central Nervous System
Chills (>5%)

Gastrointestinal/Hepatic
Nausea [2]

Local
Injection-site pain (10%)

Other
Adverse effects [2]

MIDAZOLAM

Trade name: Versed (Roche)
Indications: Preoperative sedation
Class: Benzodiazepine
Half-life: 1–4 hours
Clinically important, potentially hazardous interactions with: amprenavir, aprepitant, atazanavir, atorvastatin, boceprevir, carbamazepine, chlorpheniramine, cimetidine, clarithromycin, clorazepate, CNS depressants, cobicistat/elvitegravir/emtricitabine/tenofovir alafenamide, cobicistat/elvitegravir/emtricitabine/tenofovir disoproxil, conivaptan, darunavir, dasabuvir/ombitasvir/paritaprevir/ritonavir, delavirdine, dexamethasone, efavirenz, enzalutamide, erythromycin, esomeprazole, fluconazole, fluoxetine, fosamprenavir, grapefruit juice, griseofulvin, imatinib, indinavir, itraconazole, ivermectin, ketoconazole, letermovir, lopinavir, nelfinavir, nevirapine, nilotinib, ombitasvir/paritaprevir/ritonavir, phenobarbital, phenytoin, posaconazole, primidone, ribociclib, rifabutin, rifampin, ritonavir, roxithromycin, saquinavir, St John's wort, telaprevir, telithromycin, tibolone, tipranavir, voriconazole
Pregnancy category: D

Skin
Edema [2]
Pruritus [3]
Urticaria [2]

Cardiovascular
Bradycardia [2]
Hypotension [10]

Central Nervous System
Agitation [3]
Amnesia [38]
Dysphoria [2]
Hallucinations [2]
Sedation [2]
Vertigo (dizziness) [2]

Gastrointestinal/Hepatic
Vomiting [4]

Respiratory
Apnea [2]
Hypoxia [2]

Local
Injection-site pain (>10%)
Injection-site reactions (>10%)

Other
Adverse effects [7]
Hiccups [3]

MIDOSTAURIN

Trade name: Rydapt (Novartis)
Indications: Aggressive systemic mastocytosis, systemic mastocytosis with associated hematological neoplasm, or mast cell leukemia, acute myeloid leukemia (FLT3 mutation-positive) in combination with cytarabine and daunorubicin induction and cytarabine consolidation
Class: Multikinase inhibitor
Half-life: 21 hours
Clinically important, potentially hazardous interactions with: boceprevir, carbamazepine, clarithromycin, cobicistat, conivaptan, danoprevir, dasabuvir/ombitasvir/paritaprevir/ritonavir, diltiazem, elvitegravir, enzalutamide, grapefruit juice, idelalisib, indinavir, itraconazole, ketoconazole, lopinavir, mitotane, nefazodone, nelfinavir, ombitasvir/paritaprevir/ritonavir, phenytoin, posaconazole, rifampin, ritonavir, saquinavir, St John's wort, stong CYP3A inducers and inhibitors, tipranavir, troleandomycin, voriconazole
Pregnancy category: N/A (May cause fetal toxicity based on findings in animal studies)
Important contra-indications noted in the prescribing guidelines for: the elderly; nursing mothers; pediatric patients

---

Skin
Cellulitis (5%)
Desquamation [2]
Edema (40%)
Erysipelas (5%)
Hematoma (6%)
Herpes zoster (10%)
Hypersensitivity (4%)
Rash (14%) [4]

Mucosal
Epistaxis (nosebleed) (12%)
Mucositis [2]
Oropharyngeal pain (4%)
Stomatitis [2]

Cardiovascular
Cardiac failure (6%)
Cardiotoxicity [2]
Hypotension (9%)
Myocardial infarction (4%)
Myocardial ischemia (4%)
Pulmonary edema (3%)
QT prolongation (11%) [3]

Central Nervous System
Altered mental status (4%)
Chills (5%)
Fever (27%) [2]
Headache (26%) [2]
Impaired concentration (7%)
Insomnia (11%)
Pain [2]
Tremor (6%)
Vertigo (dizziness) (13%)

Neuromuscular/Skeletal
Arthralgia (19%)
Asthenia (fatigue) (34%) [6]
Bone or joint pain (35%)

Gastrointestinal/Hepatic
Abdominal pain (34%)
Constipation (29%) [3]

Diarrhea (54%) [7]
Dyspepsia (6%)
Gastritis (3%)
Gastrointestinal bleeding (14%)
Nausea (82%) [12]
Vomiting (68%) [11]

Respiratory
Bronchitis (6%)
Cough (18%) [2]
Dyspnea (23%)
Pleural effusion (13%)
Pneumonia (10%) [2]
Pneumonitis (2%) [2]
Upper respiratory tract infection (30%)

Endocrine/Metabolic
ALP increased (39%)
ALT increased (31%) [2]
AST increased (32%)
GGT increased (35%)
Hyperamylasemia (20%)
Hyperbilirubinemia (29%) [2]
Hyperglycemia (80%) [3]
Hyperkalemia (23%)
Hyperuricemia (37%)
Hypoalbuminemia (27%)
Hypocalcemia (39%)
Hypokalemia (25%) [4]
Hypomagnesemia (20%)
Hyponatremia (34%) [2]
Hypophosphatemia (22%)
Serum creatinine increased (25%)
Weight gain (6%)

Genitourinary
Urinary tract infection (16%)

Renal
Nephrotoxicity (11%)

Hematologic
Anemia (60%) [4]
Febrile neutropenia (8%) [3]
Hyperlipasemia (37%)
Leukopenia (61%) [2]
Lymphopenia (66%) [2]
Neutropenia (49%) [3]
Sepsis (9%)
Thrombocytopenia (50%) [3]

Other
Infection [3]

MIFEPRISTONE

Trade names: Korlym (Corcept), Mifeprex (Danco)
Indications: Medical termination of intrauterine pregnancy (Mifeprex), Cushing's syndrome in patients with Type II diabetes (Korlym)
Class: Corticosteroid antagonist, CYP3A4 inhibitor, Progestogen antagonist
Half-life: 85 hours
Clinically important, potentially hazardous interactions with: amprenavir, aprepitant, atazanavir, boceprevir, bupropion, carbamazepine, ciclesonide, ciprofloxacin, clarithromycin, conivaptan, cyclosporine, darunavir, dihydroergotamine, diltiazem, efavirenz, ergotamine, erythromycin, fentanyl, fluconazole, fluvastatin, fosamprenavir, grapefruit juice, imatinib, indinavir, itraconazole, lopinavir, lovastatin, mibefradil, nefazodone, nelfinavir, NSAIDs, oral contraceptives, phenobarbital, phenytoin, pimozide, posaconazole, quinidine, repaglinide, rifabutin, rifampin, rifapentine, ritonavir, ritonavir, saquinavir, simvastatin, sirolimus, St John's wort, tacrolimus, telaprevir, telithromycin, tenoxicam, triamcinolone, verapamil, voriconazole, warfarin
Pregnancy category: X
Important contra-indications noted in the prescribing guidelines for: nursing mothers; pediatric patients
Note: Contra-indicated in pregnancy, with concurrent use of simvastatin or lovastatin and CYP3A substrates with narrow therapeutic range or long-term corticosteroid use, and in women with a history of unexplained vaginal bleeding or with endometrial hyperplasia with atypia or endometrial carcinoma.
Warning: TERMINATION OF PREGNANCY

Skin
Edema (5–10%)
Peripheral edema (26%)
Pruritus (4%)
Rash (4%)

Mucosal
Xerostomia (18%)

Cardiovascular
Chest pain (5–10%)
Hypertension (24%)

Central Nervous System
Anorexia (10%)
Anxiety (10%)
Chills (3–38%)
Fever (4%)
Headache (2–44%)
Insomnia (5–10%)
Pain (14%)
Somnolence (drowsiness) (10%)
Vertigo (dizziness) (<22%)

Neuromuscular/Skeletal
Arthralgia (30%)
Asthenia (fatigue) (<48%)
Back pain (9–16%)
Myalgia/Myopathy (14%)
Pain in extremities (12%)

Gastrointestinal/Hepatic
Abdominal pain (5–89%) [2]
Constipation (10%)
Diarrhea (12–20%)
Gastroesophageal reflux (5–10%)
Nausea (43–61%)
Vomiting (16–26%)

Respiratory
Dyspnea (16%)
Nasopharyngitis (12%)
Sinusitis (14%)

Endocrine/Metabolic
Adrenal insufficiency (4%)
Appetite decreased (20%)
Hypoglycemia (5–10%)
Hypokalemia (44%) [2]
Menstrual irregularities [2]

Genitourinary
Metrorrhagia (5–10%)
Uterine pain (83%)
Vaginal bleeding (5–10%)
Vaginitis (3%)

Other
Dipsia (thirst) (5–10%)
Infection [3]

MIGALASTAT HYDROCHLORIDE *

Trade name: Galafold (Amicus Therapeutics US Inc)
Indications: indicated for the treatment of adults with a confirmed diagnosis of Fabry disease and is an amenable galactosidase alpha gene (GLA) variant
Class: Alpha-galactosidase A (alpha-Gal A) pharmacological chaperone
Half-life: ~4 hours
Clinically important, potentially hazardous interactions with: none known
Pregnancy category: N/A (available data are not sufficient to assess drug associated risks)

Mucosal
Epistaxis (nosebleed) (9%)

Central Nervous System
Fever (12%)
Headache (35%)

Neuromuscular/Skeletal
Back pain (9%)

Gastrointestinal/Hepatic
Abdominal pain (9%)
Diarrhea (9%)
Nausea (12%)
Vomiting (>5%)

Respiratory
Cough (9%)
Nasopharyngitis (18%)

Genitourinary
Urinary tract infection (15%)

MILK THISTLE

Family: Asteraceae; Compositae
Scientific names: *Carduus marainum, Silibum marianum*
Indications: Dyspepsia, liver protectant, hepatitis, loss of appetite, spleen diseases, supportive treatment for mushroom poisoning
Class: Immunomodulator
Half-life: N/A
Clinically important, potentially hazardous interactions with: simeprevir
Pregnancy category: N/A
Note: Seed, as opposed to the above-ground parts

Other
Adverse effects [3]

MILNACIPRAN

Trade name: Savella (Forest)
Indications: Fibromyalgia
Class: Antidepressant, Selective norepinepherine reuptake inhibitor
Half-life: 6–8 hours
Clinically important, potentially hazardous interactions with: alcohol, alpha / beta argonists, antipsychotics, aspirin, clomipramine, clonidine, CNS-active drugs, digoxin, droperidol, epinephrine, levomepromazine, lithium, MAO inhibitors, norepinephrine, NSAIDs, serotonergic drugs, sibutramine, St John's wort, tryptophan, vitamin K antagonists
Pregnancy category: C
Important contra-indications noted in the prescribing guidelines for: the elderly; nursing mothers; pediatric patients
Note: Contra-indicated in patients with uncontrolled narrow-angle glaucoma.
Warning: SUICIDALITY AND ANTIDEPRESSANT DRUGS

Skin
- Flushing (4%)
- Hot flashes (12%)
- Hyperhidrosis (9%) [6]
- Pruritus (2%)
- Rash (4%)

Mucosal
- Xerostomia (5%)

Cardiovascular
- Chest pain (2%)
- Hypertension (4%) [4]
- Palpitation (7%)
- Tachycardia (2%) [2]

Central Nervous System
- Anxiety (3%)
- Chills (2%)
- Headache (17%) [7]
- Hypoesthesia (2%)
- Insomnia (12%) [2]
- Migraine (4%)
- Paresthesias (3%)
- Serotonin syndrome [2]
- Tremor (2%)
- Vertigo (dizziness) (10%) [3]

Gastrointestinal/Hepatic
- Abdominal pain (3%)
- Constipation (15%) [6]
- Nausea (39%) [17]
- Vomiting (7%)

Respiratory
- Dyspnea (2%)
- Upper respiratory tract infection (6%)

Endocrine/Metabolic
- Appetite decreased (2%)

Genitourinary
- Dysuria (>2%) [2]
- Ejaculatory dysfunction (>2%) [2]

Ocular
- Vision blurred (2%)

Other
- Adverse effects [3]

MILRINONE

Trade name: Primacor (Sanofi-Aventis)
Indications: Severe congestive heart failure unresponsive to conventional maintenance therapy, acute heart failure, including low output states following cardiac surgery
Class: Phosphodiesterase inhibitor
Half-life: 2.3 hours
Clinically important, potentially hazardous interactions with: anagrelide
Pregnancy category: C
Important contra-indications noted in the prescribing guidelines for: nursing mothers; pediatric patients

---

Cardiovascular
- Arrhythmias [2]
- Hypotension (<10%) [7]
- Supraventricular arrhythmias (<10%)
- Vasodilation [2]
- Ventricular tachycardia (<10%)

Central Nervous System
- Headache (<10%)

MINOCYCLINE

Trade names: Dynacin (Medicis), Minocin (Wyeth), Solodyn (Medicis)
Indications: Various infections caused by susceptible organisms
Class: Antibiotic, tetracycline, Disease-modifying antirheumatic drug (DMARD)
Half-life: 11–23 hours
Clinically important, potentially hazardous interactions with: acitretin, aluminum, amoxicillin, ampicillin, antacids, bacampicillin, BCG vaccine, bismuth, carbenicillin, cloxacillin, coumarins, digoxin, ergotamine, estradiol, estrogens, isotretinoin, kaolin, magnesium salts, methotrexate, methoxyflurane, methysergide, mezlocillin, nafcillin, oral iron, oral typhoid vaccine, oxacillin, penicillin G, penicillin V, penicillins, phenindione, piperacillin, quinapril, retinoids, St John's wort, strontium ranelate, sucralfate, sulfonylureas, ticarcillin, tripotassium dicitratobismuthate, vitamin A, zinc
Pregnancy category: D
Important contra-indications noted in the prescribing guidelines for: nursing mothers; pediatric patients

---

Skin
- Anaphylactoid reactions/Anaphylaxis [3]
- Angioedema [2]
- Candidiasis [2]
- Cellulitis [2]
- DRESS syndrome [14]
- Erythema multiforme [2]
- Erythema nodosum [2]
- Exanthems [5]
- Exfoliative dermatitis [3]
- Fixed eruption [8]
- Folliculitis [2]
- Hypersensitivity [25]
- Livedo reticularis [3]
- Lupus erythematosus [50]
- Photosensitivity (<10%) [9]
- Pigmentation [125]
- Pruritus [7]
- Purpura [4]
- Rash [9]
- Raynaud's phenomenon [2]
- Serum sickness [4]
- Serum sickness-like reaction (3–5%) [6]
- Stevens-Johnson syndrome [3]
- Sweet's syndrome [4]
- Urticaria [9]
- Vasculitis [13]

Hair
- Alopecia [2]

Nails
- Nail pigmentation (<5%) [19]
- Photo-onycholysis [2]

Mucosal
- Black tongue [2]
- Gingival pigmentation (8%) [2]
- Oral pigmentation (7%) [22]

Cardiovascular
- Polyarteritis nodosa [12]

Central Nervous System
- Fever [2]
- Headache [6]
- Intracranial pressure increased [4]
- Pseudotumor cerebri [14]
- Vertigo (dizziness) [8]

Neuromuscular/Skeletal
- Arthralgia [6]
- Asthenia (fatigue) [4]
- Black bone disease [6]
- Myalgia/Myopathy [7]

Gastrointestinal/Hepatic
- Abdominal pain [2]
- Diarrhea [2]
- Hepatitis [11]
- Hepatotoxicity [20]
- Nausea [6]
- Pancreatitis [2]
- Vomiting [3]

Respiratory
- Eosinophilic pneumonia [5]
- Pneumonitis [2]

Endocrine/Metabolic
- Black thyroid syndrome [5]
- Galactorrhea (black) [2]
- Thyroid dysfunction [2]

Otic
- Tinnitus [2]

Ocular
- Conjunctival pigmentation [2]
- Diplopia [2]
- Papilledema [2]
- Scleral pigmentation [5]

Other
- Adverse effects [5]
- Tooth pigmentation (primarily in children) (>10%) [22]

MINOXIDIL

Trade names: Loniten (Par), Rogaine (Pfizer) (topical)
Indications: Hypertension, androgenetic alopecia
Class: Vasodilator
Half-life: 4.2 hours
Clinically important, potentially hazardous interactions with: acebutolol, alcohol, alfuzosin, captopril, cilazapril, diclofenac, enalapril, fosinopril, guanethidine, levodopa, levomepromazine, lisinopril, meloxicam, olmesartan, quinapril, ramipril, trandolapril, triamcinolone, trifluoperazine
Pregnancy category: C
Note: Topical [T].

Skin
Bullous dermatitis [2]
Dermatitis [T] (7%) [18]
Eczema [2]
Edema [T] (>10%) [2]
Exanthems [4]
Irritation [2]
Lupus erythematosus [3]
Peripheral edema (7%)
Pruritus [T] [10]
Stevens-Johnson syndrome [2]
Xerosis [2]

Hair
Alopecia [T] [2]
Hair pigmentation [2]
Hirsutism (in women) (100%) [4]
Hypertrichosis (80–100%) [23]

Cardiovascular
Palpitation [3]
Pericardial effusion [2]

Central Nervous System
Headache [2]
Vertigo (dizziness) [2]

Respiratory
Pleural effusion [2]

MIRABEGRON

Trade name: Myrbetriq (Astellas)
Indications: Overactive bladder
Class: Beta-3 adrenergic agonist
Half-life: 50 hours
Clinically important, potentially hazardous interactions with: antimuscarinics, desipramine, digoxin, flecainide, metoprolol, propafenone, thioridazine
Pregnancy category: C
Important contra-indications noted in the prescribing guidelines for: nursing mothers; pediatric patients

---

Mucosal
Xerostomia (3%) [6]

Cardiovascular
Hypertension (8–11%) [7]
Tachycardia (<2%) [3]

Central Nervous System
Headache (2–4%) [4]
Vertigo (dizziness) (3%) [2]

Neuromuscular/Skeletal
Arthralgia (<2%)
Back pain (3%)

Gastrointestinal/Hepatic
Constipation (2–3%) [4]
Diarrhea (≳2%)
Gastrointestinal disorder [2]

Respiratory
Influenza (3%)
Nasopharyngitis (4%) [2]
Sinusitis (<3%)
Upper respiratory tract infection (2%)

Genitourinary
Cystitis (2%)
Dysuria [2]
Urinary tract infection (3–6%) [4]

Other
Adverse effects [4]

MIRTAZAPINE

Trade name: Remeron (Organon)
Indications: Depression
Class: Adrenergic alpha-receptor agonist, Antidepressant, tetracyclic
Half-life: 20–40 hours
Clinically important, potentially hazardous interactions with: linezolid, tapentadol, venlafaxine
Pregnancy category: C
Warning: SUICIDALITY AND ANTIDEPRESSANT DRUGS

Skin
Diaphoresis [2]
Edema (<10%) [2]
Peripheral edema (<10%)
Pigmentation [2]
Rash (<10%)

Mucosal
Glossitis (<10%)
Xerostomia (25%) [3]

Central Nervous System
Abnormal dreams (4%)
Anorexia (<10%)
Cognitive impairment [2]
Headache [2]
Mania [2]
Neurotoxicity [3]
Nightmares [3]
Restless legs syndrome [9]
Sedation [4]
Seizures [3]
Serotonin syndrome [7]
Somnolence (drowsiness) (54%) [10]
Tremor (<10%) [2]
Vertigo (dizziness) (7%) [2]

Neuromuscular/Skeletal
Arthralgia [4]
Asthenia (fatigue) [7]
Myalgia/Myopathy (<10%)
Rhabdomyolysis [4]

Gastrointestinal/Hepatic
Abdominal pain (<10%)
Constipation (<10%) [2]
Hepatotoxicity [3]
Pancreatitis [3]
Vomiting (<10%)

Respiratory
Flu-like syndrome (<10%)

Endocrine/Metabolic
ALT increased (2%)
Appetite increased (12%) [2]
Galactorrhea [2]
Gynecomastia [2]
Weight gain (12%) [10]

Other
Adverse effects [2]

MISOPROSTOL

Trade names: Arthrotec (Pfizer), Cytotec (Pfizer)
Indications: Prevention of NSAID-induced ulcer
Class: Corticosteroid antagonist, Progestogen antagonist
Half-life: 20–40 minutes
Clinically important, potentially hazardous interactions with: none known
Pregnancy category: X
Important contra-indications noted in the prescribing guidelines for: nursing mothers; pediatric patients
Note: Arthrotec is diclofenac and misoprostol.

Skin
Anaphylactoid reactions/Anaphylaxis [2]

Central Nervous System
Chills [7]
Dysgeusia (taste perversion) [2]
Fever [14]
Headache (2%)
Shivering (17%) [9]

Gastrointestinal/Hepatic
Abdominal pain (7%) [8]
Diarrhea (13%)
Dyspepsia (2%)
Flatulence (3%)
Nausea (3%) [5]
Vomiting [5]

Other
Adverse effects [6]

MISTLETOE

Family: Loranthacae; Viscaceae
Scientific names: *Phoradendron flavescens, Phoradendron leucarpum, Phoradendron macrophyllum, Phoradendron rubrum, Phoradendron serotinum, Phoradendron tomentosum, Viscum album*
Indications: Injected: adjuvant tumor therapy. **Oral:** abortifacient, arteriosclerosis, arthritis, asthma, colds, depression, headache, HIV infection, hypertension, hypotension, hysteria, labor pain, lumbago, metrorrhagia, muscle spasms, otitis, whooping cough, hemorrhoids, internal bleeding, gout, sleep disorders, amenorrhea, liver and gallbladder conditions
Class: Immunomodulator
Half-life: N/A
Clinically important, potentially hazardous interactions with: bepridil, clevidipine, corticosteroids, immunosuppressants, MAO inhibitors, squill
Pregnancy category: N/A
Note: Purified extracts injected intramuscularly, subcutaneously or by intravenous infusion. Unless otherwise indicated, side effects listed are from injected preparations. The FDA considers *Viscum album* unsafe.
The well-known mistletoe is an evergreen parasitic plant, growing on the branches of some tree species. Shakespeare calls it ?the baleful mistletoe,? an illusion to the Scandinavian legend that Balder, the god of Peace, was slain with an arrow made of mistletoe.

Skin
- Anaphylactoid reactions/Anaphylaxis (28%) [3]
- Erythema [3]
- Pruritus [2]

Mucosal
- Gingivitis [2]

Cardiovascular
- Hypertension [2]

Central Nervous System
- Chills [4]
- Fever [6]
- Headache [2]

Gastrointestinal/Hepatic
- Hepatotoxicity [3]
- Nausea [2]

Respiratory
- Flu-like syndrome [3]

Local
- Injection-site edema [2]
- Injection-site inflammation [8]
- Injection-site reactions [5]

Other
- Adverse effects [8]
- Allergic reactions [4]
- Death (low incidence – accidental ingestion) [4]

MITOMYCIN

Synonyms: mitomycin-C; MTC
Trade name: Mutamycin (Bristol-Myers Squibb)
Indications: Carcinomas
Class: Alkylating agent, Antibiotic, anthracycline
Half-life: 23–78 minutes
Clinically important, potentially hazardous interactions with: aldesleukin
Pregnancy category: D
Important contra-indications noted in the prescribing guidelines for: nursing mothers; pediatric patients

---

Skin
- Dermatitis [9]
- Erythema multiforme [2]
- Exanthems [2]
- Exfoliative dermatitis [2]
- Hand–foot syndrome [2]
- Thrombocytopenic purpura [2]

Hair
- Alopecia (<10%) [2]

Nails
- Nail pigmentation (purple) (<10%)

Mucosal
- Oral lesions (2–8%) [4]
- Oral ulceration (<10%)
- Stomatitis (>10%)

Cardiovascular
- Congestive heart failure (3–15%)
- Veno-occlusive disease [2]

Central Nervous System
- Anorexia (14%)
- Fever (14%)
- Paresthesias (<10%)

Neuromuscular/Skeletal
- Asthenia (fatigue) [2]

Gastrointestinal/Hepatic
- Nausea (14%)
- Vomiting (14%)

Respiratory
- Cough (7%)
- Pneumonitis [2]

Renal
- Nephrotoxicity [2]

Hematologic
- Anemia (19–24%)
- Hemolytic uremic syndrome [41]
- Neutropenia [2]

Ocular
- Epiphora [2]
- Keratitis [2]
- Ocular toxicity [3]

Local
- Injection-site cellulitis (>10%)
- Injection-site necrosis (>10%) [3]

MITOXANTRONE

Trade name: Novantrone (OSI)
Indications: Acute myelogenous leukemia, multiple sclerosis, prostate cancer
Class: Antibiotic, anthracycline, Antineoplastic
Half-life: median terminal: 75 hours
Clinically important, potentially hazardous interactions with: aldesleukin, safinamide
Pregnancy category: D
Important contra-indications noted in the prescribing guidelines for: nursing mothers; pediatric patients

---

Skin
- Diaphoresis (<10%)
- Ecchymoses (7%)
- Edema (>10%)
- Fungal dermatitis (>15%)
- Peripheral edema [2]
- Petechiae (>10%)
- Purpura (>10%)

Hair
- Alopecia (20–60%) [7]

Cardiovascular
- Cardiac failure [2]
- Cardiotoxicity [4]
- Congestive heart failure [3]

Central Nervous System
- Chills (<10%)

Gastrointestinal/Hepatic
- Diarrhea [2]
- Nausea [6]
- Vomiting [3]

Endocrine/Metabolic
- Amenorrhea [4]
- Menstrual irregularities [2]

Genitourinary
- Urinary tract infection [2]

Hematologic
- Anemia [2]
- Febrile neutropenia [2]
- Leukemia [4]
- Leukopenia [4]
- Neutropenia [6]
- Thrombocytopenia [2]

Other
- Death [2]
- Infection (>66%) [3]

MODAFINIL

Trade name: Provigil (Cephalon)
Indications: Narcolepsy
Class: Analeptic, CNS stimulant, CYP1A2 inducer, CYP3A4 inducer
Half-life: ~15 hours
Clinically important, potentially hazardous interactions with: elbasvir & grazoprevir, enzalutamide, neratinib, olaparib, oral contraceptives, palbociclib, sonidegib, thalidomide, venetoclax

Pregnancy category: C
Important contra-indications noted in the prescribing guidelines for: the elderly; nursing mothers; pediatric patients

---

Skin
Fixed eruption [2]

Mucosal
Xerostomia (5%)

Cardiovascular
Hypertension [2]
Palpitation [2]

Central Nervous System
Agitation [2]
Chills (2%)
Hallucinations [2]
Headache (28%) [13]
Insomnia (5%) [6]
Nervousness [2]
Paresthesias (3%)
Psychosis [2]
Vertigo (dizziness) (5%) [3]

Neuromuscular/Skeletal
Back pain (6%)

Gastrointestinal/Hepatic
Abdominal pain [2]
Diarrhea (6%) [3]
Nausea (11%) [6]

Respiratory
Rhinitis (7%)

Ocular
Hallucinations, visual [2]

Other
Adverse effects [3]

MONOSODIUM GLUTAMATE

Family: N/A
Scientific name: *Monosodium glutamate*
Indications: Food additive, flavor enhancer
Class: Food additive
Half-life: N/A
Clinically important, potentially hazardous interactions with: BCG vaccine, MAO inhibitors
Pregnancy category: N/A
Note: The US Food & Drug Administration has determined that MSG is a safe food ingredient if used in moderation. Only a very small subset of individuals is allergic to MSG.
The etiologic agent of Chinese Restaurant Syndrome.

Skin
Anaphylactoid reactions/Anaphylaxis [2]
Angioedema [5]
Atopic dermatitis [2]
Churg-Strauss syndrome [2]
Sensitivity [2]
Urticaria [5]

Central Nervous System
Headache [6]
Hypoesthesia [2]
Paresthesias [2]

MONTELUKAST

Trade name: Singulair (Merck)
Indications: Asthma
Class: Leukotriene receptor antagonist
Half-life: 2.7–5.5 hours
Clinically important, potentially hazardous interactions with: prednisone
Pregnancy category: B
Important contra-indications noted in the prescribing guidelines for: nursing mothers

---

Skin
Angioedema [3]
Churg-Strauss syndrome [27]
Rash (2%) [2]
Urticaria (2%)

Central Nervous System
Aggression [3]
Anxiety [2]
Depression [3]
Hallucinations [2]
Headache [4]
Irritability [2]
Neurotoxicity [5]
Nightmares [2]
Sleep disturbances [3]
Suicidal ideation [2]

Gastrointestinal/Hepatic
Abdominal pain [2]
Hepatotoxicity [3]

Respiratory
Cough [2]
Flu-like syndrome (<10%)

Other
Adverse effects [3]

MORPHINE

Trade names: Avinza (Ligand), Duramorph (Baxter) (Elkins-Sinn), Infumorph (Baxter), Kadian (aaiPharma), Morphabond (Inspirion), MS Contin (Purdue), MSIR Oral (Purdue), Roxanol (aaiPharma)
Indications: Severe pain, acute myocardial infarction
Class: Opiate agonist
Half-life: 2–4 hours
Clinically important, potentially hazardous interactions with: buprenorphine, cimetidine, furazolidone, MAO inhibitors, metformin, mianserin, pentazocine, rifapentine, trospium
Pregnancy category: C
Important contra-indications noted in the prescribing guidelines for: nursing mothers; pediatric patients
Warning: ADDICTION, ABUSE, AND MISUSE; LIFETHREATENING RESPIRATORY DEPRESSION; ACCIDENTAL INGESTION; NEONATAL OPIOID WITHDRAWAL SYNDROME; and INTERACTION WITH ALCOHOL

Skin
AGEP [3]
Edema [2]
Pruritus (5–65%) [39]

Mucosal
Xerostomia (>10%) [8]

Cardiovascular
Cardiotoxicity [3]
Hypotension [5]

Central Nervous System
Allodynia [4]
Confusion [2]
Hallucinations [4]
Hyperalgesia [10]
Sedation [2]
Somnolence (drowsiness) [5]
Trembling (<10%)
Vertigo (dizziness) [5]

Neuromuscular/Skeletal
Myoclonus [5]
Rhabdomyolysis [2]

Gastrointestinal/Hepatic
Constipation [7]
Nausea [16]
Vomiting [13]

Respiratory
Respiratory depression [6]

Endocrine/Metabolic
Amenorrhea [2]

Genitourinary
Urinary retention [2]

Local
Injection-site pain (>10%)

Other
Adverse effects [2]
Death [3]
Hiccups [3]

MOXIDECTIN *

Trade name: Moxidectin (Medicines Development for Global Health)
Indications: treatment of onchocerciasis due to Onchocerca volvulus in patients aged 12 years and older
Class: Anthelmintic
Half-life: 23 days
Clinically important, potentially hazardous interactions with: none known
Pregnancy category: N/A (Limited available data is insufficient to establish risk)

Skin
Lymphoma (>10%)
Peripheral edema (>10%)
Pruritus (>10%)
Rash (>10%)
Urticaria (>10%)

Cardiovascular
Hypotension (>10%)
Orthostatic hypotension (>10%)
Tachycardia (>10%)

Central Nervous System
Fever (>10%)
Headache (>10%)
Pain (>10%)
Vertigo (dizziness) (>10%)

Neuromuscular/Skeletal
Arthralgia (>10%)

Back pain (>10%)
Myalgia/Myopathy (>10%)

Gastrointestinal/Hepatic
Abdominal pain (>10%)
Diarrhea (>10%)
Enteritis (>10%)
Gastroenteritis (>10%)

Respiratory
Cough (>10%)
Influenza (>10%)

Endocrine/Metabolic
ALT increased (<5%)
AST increased (<5%)
Hyperbilirubinemia (<5%)
Hyponatremia (>10%)

Hematologic
Eosinophilia (>10%)
Leukocytosis (>10%)
Lymphopenia (>10%)
Neutropenia (>10%)

Ocular
Conjunctival hyperemia (<10%)
Conjunctivitis (<10%)
Eyelid edema (<10%)
Foreign body sensation (<10%)
Lacrimation (<10%)
Ocular hyperemia (<10%)
Ocular pain (<10%)
Ocular pruritus (<10%)
Vision blurred (<10%)
Vision impaired (<10%)

MOXIFLOXACIN

Trade names: Avelox (Bayer), Moxeza (Alcon)
Indications: Various infections caused by susceptible organisms
Class: Antibiotic, fluoroquinolone
Half-life: 12 hours
Clinically important, potentially hazardous interactions with: alfuzosin, aminophylline, amiodarone, amitriptyline, antacids, arsenic, artemether/lumefantrine, asenapine, atomoxetine, BCG vaccine, benperidol, bepridil, bretylium, chloroquine, ciprofloxacin, corticosteroids, cyclosporine, degarelix, didanosine, disopyramide, dronedarone, droperidol, erythromycin, gadobutrol, haloperidol, hydroxychloroquine, insulin, lanthanum, levomepromazine, magnesium salts, mefloquine, mizolastine, mycophenolate, nilotinib, NSAIDs, oral iron, oral typhoid vaccine, pentamidine, phenothiazines, pimavanserin, pimozide, probenecid, procainamide, QT prolonging agents, quinapril, quinidine, quinine, ribociclib, sevelamer, sotalol, strontium ranelate, sucralfate, sulfonylureas, tetrabenazine, thioridazine, tricyclic antidepressants, vandetanib, vitamin K antagonists, warfarin, zinc, ziprasidone, zolmitriptan, zuclopenthixol
Pregnancy category: C
Important contra-indications noted in the prescribing guidelines for: the elderly; nursing mothers; pediatric patients
Note: Fluoroquinolones are associated with an increased risk of tendinitis and tendon rupture in all ages. This risk is further increased in older patients usually over 60 years of age, in patients taking corticosteroid drugs, and in patients with kidney, heart or lung transplants.
Fluoroquinolones may exacerbate muscle weakness in persons with myasthenia gravis.
Moxeza is for topical ophthalmic use only.
Warning: SERIOUS ADVERSE REACTIONS INCLUDING TENDINITIS, TENDON RUPTURE, PERIPHERAL NEUROPATHY, CENTRAL NERVOUS SYSTEM EFFECTS and EXACERBATION OF MYASTHENIA GRAVIS

Skin
AGEP [2]
Anaphylactoid reactions/Anaphylaxis [5]
Bullous dermatitis [2]
Hypersensitivity [6]
Photosensitivity [5]
Pruritus [3]
Rash [4]
Thrombocytopenic purpura [2]
Toxic epidermal necrolysis [2]
Urticaria [3]

Cardiovascular
Phlebitis [2]
QT prolongation [15]
Torsades de pointes [8]

Central Nervous System
Delirium [2]
Dysgeusia (taste perversion) [3]
Hallucinations [2]
Headache (4%) [5]
Somnolence (drowsiness) [2]
Vertigo (dizziness) (3%) [6]

Neuromuscular/Skeletal
Myasthenia gravis (exacerbation) [2]
Tendinopathy/Tendon rupture [3]

Gastrointestinal/Hepatic
Abdominal pain [5]
Diarrhea (6%) [6]
Gastrointestinal disorder [2]
Hepatotoxicity [3]
Nausea (7%) [9]
Vomiting [5]

Otic
Tinnitus [2]

Local
Injection-site reactions [2]

Other
Adverse effects [8]

MYCOPHENOLATE

Synonyms: mycophenolate mofetil, mycophenolate sodium
Trade names: CellCept (Roche), Myfortic (Novartis)
Indications: Prophylaxis of organ rejection
Class: Immunosuppressant
Half-life: 18 hours
Clinically important, potentially hazardous interactions with: antacids, azathioprine, basiliximab, belatacept, cholestyramine, ciprofloxacin, corticosteroids, cyclophosphamide, cyclosporine, daclizumab, gemifloxacin, Hemophilus B vaccine, levofloxacin, mercaptopurine, metronidazole, moxifloxacin, norfloxacin, ofloxacin, pantoprazole, rifapentine, sevelamer, tacrolimus, vaccines
Pregnancy category: D
Important contra-indications noted in the prescribing guidelines for: the elderly; nursing mothers; pediatric patients
Warning: EMBRYOFETAL TOXICITY, MALIGNANCIES AND SERIOUS INFECTIONS

Skin
Acneform eruption (>10%) [3]
Carcinoma (non-melanoma) (4%)
Edema (12%)
Herpes simplex [3]
Herpes zoster [7]
Peripheral edema (29%)
Rash (8%) [2]
Warts [2]

Hair
Alopecia [4]

Mucosal
Gingival hyperplasia/hypertrophy [2]
Oral candidiasis (10%)
Oral ulceration [5]

Cardiovascular
Hypertension [4]
Thrombophlebitis (<10%)

Central Nervous System
Encephalopathy [2]
Fever [3]
Headache (>20%) [5]
Insomnia [3]
Leukoencephalopathy [4]
Neurotoxicity [2]
Pain (>20%)
Tremor (11%)

Neuromuscular/Skeletal
Arthralgia [4]
Asthenia (fatigue) [6]
Back pain (6%)
Myalgia/Myopathy [4]

Gastrointestinal/Hepatic
Abdominal distension [2]
Abdominal pain [6]
Colitis [3]
Diarrhea [14]
Hepatotoxicity [5]
Nausea [5]
Vomiting [5]

Respiratory
Bronchitis [2]
Cough [2]
Upper respiratory tract infection [3]

Endocrine/Metabolic
ALT increased [2]
Hyperglycemia [4]
Hyperlipidemia [3]

Genitourinary
Urinary tract infection [3]

Renal
Nephrotoxicity [3]

Hematologic
Anemia (>20%) [2]
Bone marrow suppression [2]
Dyslipidemia [2]
Leukopenia [5]
Lymphopenia [3]

Myelotoxicity [2]
Neutropenia [4]
Thrombocytopenia [4]

Other
Adverse effects [21]
Death [2]
Infection (12–20%) [18]
Teratogenicity [4]

MYRRH

Family: Burseraceae
Scientific names: *Commiphora abyssinica, Commiphora erythraea, Commiphora habessinica, Commiphora kataf, Commiphora madagascariensis, Commiphora molmol, Commiphora myrrh*
Indications: Fascioliasis, schistosomiasis, ulcers, eczema, catarrh, amenorrhea, gum disease, aphthous stomatitis
Class: Anthelmintic, Anti-inflammatory
Half-life: N/A
Clinically important, potentially hazardous interactions with: none known
Pregnancy category: N/A

Skin
Dermatitis [5]

Neuromuscular/Skeletal
Asthenia (fatigue) (2%)

Gastrointestinal/Hepatic
Abdominal pain (2%)

NABILONE

Trade name: Cesamet (Valeant)
Indications: Nausea and vomiting
Class: Antiemetic, Cannabinoid
Half-life: 2 hours
Clinically important, potentially hazardous interactions with: CNS depressants
Pregnancy category: C

Mucosal
Xerostomia [6]

Cardiovascular
Hypotension [8]

Central Nervous System
Dyskinesia [3]
Euphoria [2]
Somnolence (drowsiness) [3]
Vertigo (dizziness) [15]

Neuromuscular/Skeletal
Asthenia (fatigue) [5]

NABUMETONE

Trade name: Relafen (GSK)
Indications: Arthritis
Class: Non-steroidal anti-inflammatory (NSAID)
Half-life: 22.5–30 hours
Clinically important, potentially hazardous interactions with: methotrexate
Pregnancy category: C
Important contra-indications noted in the prescribing guidelines for: nursing mothers; pediatric patients
Note: NSAIDs may cause an increased risk of serious cardiovascular and gastrointestinal adverse events, which can be fatal. This risk may increase with duration of use.
Warning: CARDIOVASCULAR AND GASTROINTESTINAL RISKS

Skin
Diaphoresis (<3%)
Edema (3–9%)
Erythema [2]
Hypersensitivity [3]
Photosensitivity [2]
Pruritus (3–9%) [2]
Rash (3–9%) [4]

Mucosal
Stomatitis (<3%)
Xerostomia (<3%)

Central Nervous System
Headache (3–9%) [2]
Insomnia (3–9%)
Nervousness (3–9%)
Somnolence (drowsiness) (3–9%)
Vertigo (dizziness) (3–9%)

Gastrointestinal/Hepatic
Abdominal pain (12%) [5]
Constipation (3–9%)
Diarrhea (14%) [5]
Dyspepsia (13%) [4]
Flatulence (3–9%)
Gastrointestinal ulceration [3]
Hepatotoxicity [2]
Nausea (3–9%) [2]
Vomiting (3–9%)

Endocrine/Metabolic
Pseudoporphyria [8]

Renal
Nephrotoxicity [2]

Otic
Tinnitus (<10%)

Other
Adverse effects [6]

NADOLOL

Trade name: Corzide (Monarch)
Indications: Hypertension, angina pectoris
Class: Adrenergic beta-receptor antagonist, Antiarrhythmic class II
Half-life: 10–24 hours
Clinically important, potentially hazardous interactions with: clonidine, epinephrine, verapamil
Pregnancy category: C
Important contra-indications noted in the prescribing guidelines for: nursing mothers; pediatric patients
Note: Corzide is nadolol and bendroflumethiazide. Cutaneous side effects of beta-receptor blockers are clinically polymorphous. They apparently appear after several months of continuous therapy. Contra-indicated in patients with bronchial asthma, sinus bradycardia and greater than first degree conduction block, cardiogenic shock, and overt cardiac failure.

Skin
Edema (<5%)
Psoriasis [4]
Raynaud's phenomenon (2%) [2]

Cardiovascular
Bradycardia (2%)

Central Nervous System
Hypoesthesia (fingers and toes) (>5%)
Paresthesias (>5%)
Vertigo (dizziness) (2%)

Neuromuscular/Skeletal
Asthenia (fatigue) (2%)

Other
Adverse effects [4]

NALBUPHINE

Trade name: Nubain (Endo)
Indications: Moderate to severe pain
Class: Opiate agonist
Half-life: 5 hours
Clinically important, potentially hazardous interactions with: CNS depressants, diazepam, hydrocodone, hydromorphone, oxymorphone, pentobarbital, promethazine, tapentadol
Pregnancy category: B
Note: Nalbuphine contains sulfites.

Skin
Clammy skin (9%)
Diaphoresis (9%)

Mucosal
Xerostomia (4%)

Central Nervous System
Vertigo (dizziness) (5%)

Local
Injection-site pain [4]

NALDEMEDINE

Trade name: Symproic (Shionogi)
Indications: Opioid-induced constipation in adult patients with chronic non-cancer pain
Class: Opioid antagonist
Half-life: 11 hours
Clinically important, potentially hazardous interactions with: amiodarone, aprepitant, atazanavir, captopril, carbamazepine, clarithromycin, cyclosporine, diltiazem, erythromycin, fluconazole, itraconazole, ketoconazole, moderate or strong CYP3A inhibitors, other opioid antagonists, P-gp inhibitors, phenytoin, quercetin, quinidine, rifampin, ritonavir, saquinavir, St John's wort, strong CYP3A inducers, verapamil

Pregnancy category: N/A (Potential for opioid withdrawal in fetus)
Important contra-indications noted in the prescribing guidelines for: nursing mothers; pediatric patients
Note: Contra-indicated in patients with known or suspected gastrointestinal obstruction. Opioid withdrawal symptoms have occurred in patients treated with naldemedine.

Skin
Hypersensitivity (<2%)
Rash (<2%)

Gastrointestinal/Hepatic
Abdominal pain (8–11%)
Diarrhea (7%) [4]
Gastroenteritis (2–3%)
Nausea (4–6%)
Vomiting (3%)

Respiratory
Bronchospasm (<2%)

Other
Adverse effects [3]

NALOXEGOL

Trade name: Movantik (AstraZeneca)
Indications: Opioid-induced constipation
Class: Opioid receptor antagonist
Half-life: 6–11 hours
Clinically important, potentially hazardous interactions with: diltiazem, erythromycin, grapefruit juice, verapamil
Pregnancy category: C
Important contra-indications noted in the prescribing guidelines for: nursing mothers; pediatric patients
Note: Contra-indicated in patients with known or suspected gastrointestinal obstruction, patients at increased risk of recurrent gastrointestinal obstruction, and patients concomitantly using strong CYP3A4 inhibitors.

Skin
Hyperhidrosis (<3%)

Central Nervous System
Headache (4%) [3]

Gastrointestinal/Hepatic
Abdominal pain (12–21%) [5]
Diarrhea (6–9%) [5]
Flatulence (3–6%) [2]
Nausea (7–8%) [5]
Vomiting (3–5%)

Other
Adverse effects [2]

NALOXONE

Trade names: Suboxone (Reckitt Benckiser), Talwin-NX (Sanofi-Aventis), Targiniq (Purdue)
Indications: Narcotic overdose
Class: Opioid antagonist
Half-life: <1.5 hours
Clinically important, potentially hazardous interactions with: cobicistat/elvitegravir/emtricitabine/tenofovir alafenamide, cobicistat/elvitegravir/emtricitabine/tenofovir disoproxil, thioridazine
Pregnancy category: C
Important contra-indications noted in the prescribing guidelines for: nursing mothers
Note: Subuxone contains buprenorphine; Targiniq is naloxone and oxycodone.

Skin
Diaphoresis (<10%)
Pruritus [2]
Rash (<10%)

Mucosal
Xerostomia [2]

Cardiovascular
Arrhythmias [2]
Bradycardia [2]
Hypertension [8]
Hypotension [2]
Pulmonary edema [2]

Central Nervous System
Headache [4]
Seizures [5]
Somnolence (drowsiness) [3]

Neuromuscular/Skeletal
Asthenia (fatigue) [3]
Myoclonus [2]

Gastrointestinal/Hepatic
Constipation [7]
Nausea [4]
Vomiting [2]

Other
Adverse effects [5]
Death [2]

NALTREXONE

Trade names: Contrave (Takeda), Depade (Mallinckrodt), Nalorex (Bristol-Myers Squibb), Opizone (Genus), ReVia (Meda), Troxyca (Pfizer), Vivitrex (Alkermes), Vivitrol (Alkermes)
Indications: Substance abuse, opioid dependence, alcohol dependence
Class: Opioid antagonist
Half-life: 4 hours
Clinically important, potentially hazardous interactions with: lofexidine, opioid analgesics, opioid containing medications
Pregnancy category: C
Important contra-indications noted in the prescribing guidelines for: nursing mothers; pediatric patients
Note: Naltrexone has the capacity to cause hepatocellular injury when given in excessive doses.
Troxyca is naltrexone and oxycodone. Contra-indicated in acute hepatitis or liver failure; patients receiving opioid analgesics, with current physiologic opioid dependence, or in acute opioid withdrawal.

Skin
Pruritus [2]
Rash (<10%)

Cardiovascular
Hypertension [4]

Central Nervous System
Anxiety [2]
Chills (<10%)
Compulsions [2]
Depression [2]
Headache [5]
Insomnia [5]
Seizures [2]
Somnolence (drowsiness) [2]
Vertigo (dizziness) [5]

Neuromuscular/Skeletal
Arthralgia (>10%)
Asthenia (fatigue) [3]

Gastrointestinal/Hepatic
Constipation [6]
Hepatotoxicity [5]
Nausea [10]
Vomiting [6]

Respiratory
Influenza [2]
Nasopharyngitis [2]

Local
Injection-site pain [2]
Injection-site reactions [5]

Other
Adverse effects [3]

NANDROLONE

Trade name: Deca-Durabolin (Organon)
Indications: Anemia of renal insufficiency, control of metastatic breast cancer, osteoporosis in post-menopausal women
Class: Anabolic steroid
Half-life: 6–14 days
Clinically important, potentially hazardous interactions with: acenocoumarol, anisindione, anticoagulants, dabigatran, danaparoid, fondaparinux, heparin, warfarin
Pregnancy category: X
Important contra-indications noted in the prescribing guidelines for: nursing mothers; pediatric patients
Note: Deca Durabolin contains Arachis oil (peanut oil) and should not be taken / applied by patients known to be allergic to peanut.

Hair
Hirsutism [3]

Other
Adverse effects [2]

NAPROXEN

Trade names: Aleve (Bayer), Naprosyn (Roche), Synflex (Roche)
Indications: Pain, arthritis
Class: Non-steroidal anti-inflammatory (NSAID)
Half-life: 15 hours
Clinically important, potentially hazardous interactions with: methotrexate, methyl salicylate, prednisolone
Pregnancy category: C
Important contra-indications noted in the prescribing guidelines for: the elderly; nursing mothers; pediatric patients
Note: NSAIDs may cause an increased risk of serious cardiovascular and gastrointestinal adverse events, which can be fatal. This risk may increase with duration of use.

Skin
Anaphylactoid reactions/Anaphylaxis [2]
Angioedema [5]
Bullous dermatitis [5]
Diaphoresis (<3%) [3]
DRESS syndrome [4]
Ecchymoses (3–9%)
Edema (<9%)
Erythema multiforme [2]
Exanthems (<14%) [9]
Fixed eruption [26]
Hypersensitivity [2]
Lichen planus [3]
Lichenoid eruption [3]
Lupus erythematosus [2]
Photosensitivity [16]
Pruritus (3–17%) [5]
Purpura (<3%) [4]
Pustules [2]
Rash (3–9%) [2]
Toxic epidermal necrolysis [5]
Urticaria (<5%) [6]
Vasculitis [9]

Hair
Alopecia [3]

Mucosal
Stomatitis (<3%)
Xerostomia [2]

Cardiovascular
Chest pain [2]
Myocardial infarction [2]

Central Nervous System
Somnolence (drowsiness) [2]
Vertigo (dizziness) [6]

Neuromuscular/Skeletal
Leg cramps [2]

Gastrointestinal/Hepatic
Abdominal pain [4]
Constipation [2]
Diarrhea [3]
Dyspepsia [9]
Hepatotoxicity [4]
Nausea [10]

Respiratory
Nasopharyngitis [2]

Endocrine/Metabolic
Pseudoporphyria [29]

Renal
Nephrotoxicity [3]

Hematologic
Thrombocytopenia [2]

Otic
Tinnitus [2]

Other
Adverse effects [11]
Death [2]
Side effects (5–9%) [3]

NATALIZUMAB

Synonym: antegren
Trade name: Tysabri (Biogen)
Indications: Multiple sclerosis, Crohn's disease
Class: Immunomodulator, Monoclonal antibody
Half-life: 11 days
Clinically important, potentially hazardous interactions with: abatacept, alefacept, azacitidine, azathioprine, betamethasone, cabazitaxel, certolizumab, cortocosteroids, cyclosporine, denileukin, docetaxel, fingolimod, gefitinib, leflunomide, lenalidomide, mercaptopurine, methotrexate, oxaliplatin, pazopanib, pemetrexed, rilonacept, temsirolimus, triamcinolone, vedolizumab
Pregnancy category: C
Important contra-indications noted in the prescribing guidelines for: nursing mothers; pediatric patients
Note: Contra-indicated in patients who have or have had progressive multifocal leukoencephalopathy.
Warning: PROGRESSIVE MULTIFOCAL LEUKOENCEPHALOPATHY

Skin
Dermatitis (6%)
Herpes simplex [2]
Hypersensitivity [6]
Pruritus (4%)
Rash (9%)

Central Nervous System
Depression (17%)
Headache (35%) [3]
Leukoencephalopathy [77]
Tremor (3%)

Neuromuscular/Skeletal
Asthenia (fatigue) (24%) [4]

Gastrointestinal/Hepatic
Hepatotoxicity [4]

Genitourinary
Vaginitis (8%)

Local
Application-site reactions (22%)
Infusion-related reactions [3]
Infusion-site reactions [2]

Other
Adverse effects [5]
Allergic reactions (7%) [4]
Death [6]
Infection (2%) [3]

NATEGLINIDE

Trade name: Starlix (Novartis)
Indications: Diabetes Type II
Class: Meglitinide
Half-life: 1.5 hours
Clinically important, potentially hazardous interactions with: none known
Pregnancy category: C
Important contra-indications noted in the prescribing guidelines for: nursing mothers; pediatric patients

---

Respiratory
Flu-like syndrome (4%)

NEBIVOLOL

Trade names: Bystolic (Forest), Byvalson (Forest), Nebilet (Menarini)
Indications: Hypertension
Class: Adrenergic beta-receptor antagonist, Beta blocker
Half-life: 8 hours
Clinically important, potentially hazardous interactions with: beta blockers, cinacalcet, clonidine, CYP2D6 inhibitors, delavirdine, digitalis glycosides, duloxetine, terbinafine, tipranavir
Pregnancy category: C
Important contra-indications noted in the prescribing guidelines for: nursing mothers; pediatric patients
Note: Byvalson is nebivolol and valsartan.
Warning: Byvalson: FETAL TOXICITY

Cardiovascular
Bradycardia [3]

Central Nervous System
Headache (6–9%) [9]
Vertigo (dizziness) (2–4%) [5]

Neuromuscular/Skeletal
Asthenia (fatigue) (2–5%) [4]

Gastrointestinal/Hepatic
Diarrhea (<2%)
Nausea (<3%)

Respiratory
Nasopharyngitis [3]
Upper respiratory tract infection [3]

Other
Adverse effects [3]

NECITUMUMAB

Trade name: Portrazza (Lilly)
Indications: Metastatic squamous non-small cell lung cancer (in combination with cisplatin and gemcitabine)
Class: Epidermal growth factor receptor (EGFR) inhibitor, Monoclonal antibody
Half-life: 14 days
Clinically important, potentially hazardous interactions with: none known

Pregnancy category: N/A (Can cause fetal harm)
Important contra-indications noted in the prescribing guidelines for: nursing mothers; pediatric patients
Note: See separate entries for cisplatin and gemcitabine.
Warning: CARDIOPULMONARY ARREST and HYPOMAGNESEMIA

Skin
Acneform eruption (9–15%)
Fissures (5%)
Hypersensitivity (2%)
Pruritus (7%) [2]
Rash (44%) [9]
Toxicity (8%) [2]
Xerosis (7%) [2]

Mucosal
Stomatitis (11%)

Cardiovascular
Cardiac arrest (3%)
Phlebitis (2%)
Venous thromboembolism (9%) [4]

Central Nervous System
Headache (11%) [2]

Neuromuscular/Skeletal
Asthenia (fatigue) [3]
Muscle spasm (2%)

Gastrointestinal/Hepatic
Diarrhea (16%) [2]
Dysphagia (3%)
Vomiting (29%)

Respiratory
Hemoptysis (10%)
Pulmonary embolism (5%)
Pulmonary toxicity [2]

Endocrine/Metabolic
Hypocalcemia (45%)
Hypokalemia (28%)
Hypomagnesemia (83%) [8]
Hypophosphatemia (31%)
Weight loss (13%)

Hematologic
Anemia [2]
Febrile neutropenia [2]
Neutropenia [4]
Thrombocytopenia [3]

Ocular
Conjunctivitis (7%)

Local
Infusion-related reactions (2%) [2]

Other
Adverse effects [2]
Death [2]

NELFINAVIR

Trade name: Viracept (ViiV)
Indications: HIV infection
Class: Antiretroviral, CYP3A4 inhibitor, HIV-1 protease inhibitor
Half-life: 3.5–5 hours
Clinically important, potentially hazardous interactions with: abiraterone, afatinib, alfuzosin, amiodarone, amprenavir, aripiprazole, artemether/lumefantrine, atorvastatin, avanafil, barbiturates, benzodiazepines, brigatinib, cabazitaxel, cabozantinib, calcifediol, carbamazepine, chlordiazepoxide, ciclesonide, cisapride, clonazepam, clorazepate, copanlisib, crizotinib, cyclosporine, darifenacin, dasatinib, delavirdine, diazepam, dihydroergotamine, eletriptan, eplerenone, ergot alkaloids, ergotamine, erlotinib, estrogens, eszopiclone, etravirine, eucalyptus, everolimus, fentanyl, fesoterodine, flibanserin, flurazepam, fluticasone propionate, indinavir, ivabradine, ixabepilone, lapatinib, lomitapide, lopinavir, lorazepam, lovastatin, maraviroc, methadone, methylergonovine, methysergide, midazolam, midostaurin, mifepristone, neratinib, olaparib, omeprazole, oral contraceptives, oxazepam, paclitaxel, palbociclib, pantoprazole, pazopanib, phenytoin, pimozide, ponatinib, primidone, progestogens, quazepam, quinidine, quinine, ranolazine, rifabutin, rifampin, rilpivirine, ritonavir, rivaroxaban, romidepsin, rosuvastatin, ruxolitinib, saquinavir, sildenafil, simeprevir, simvastatin, solifenacin, St John's wort, sunitinib, tacrolimus, tadalafil, telithromycin, temazepam, temsirolimus, ticagrelor, tolterodine, tolvaptan, triazolam, vardenafil, vemurafenib, vorapaxar
Pregnancy category: B
Important contra-indications noted in the prescribing guidelines for: nursing mothers
Note: Protease inhibitors cause dyslipidemia which includes elevated triglycerides and cholesterol and redistribution of body fat centrally to produce the so-called 'protease paunch', breast enlargement, facial atrophy, and 'buffalo hump'.

Skin
Rash (<10%) [4]

Gastrointestinal/Hepatic
Diarrhea [3]
Hepatotoxicity [3]

Genitourinary
Urolithiasis [2]

Hematologic
Lymphopenia [2]

NEOMYCIN

Trade names: Maxitrol (Falcon), Neosporin (Monarch)
Indications: Various infections caused by susceptible organisms
Class: Antibiotic, aminoglycoside
Half-life: 3 hours
Clinically important, potentially hazardous interactions with: acarbose, aldesleukin, aminoglycosides, atracurium, bacitracin, bumetanide, doxacurium, ethacrynic acid, furosemide, methoxyflurane, neostigmine, pancuronium, penicillin V, polypeptide antibiotics, rocuronium, sorafenib, succinylcholine, teicoplanin, torsemide, vecuronium
Pregnancy category: D
Important contra-indications noted in the prescribing guidelines for: nursing mothers; pediatric patients
Note: Aminoglycosides may cause neurotoxicity and/or nephrotoxicity.

Skin
Anaphylactoid reactions/Anaphylaxis [2]
Contact dermatitis (<10%) [70]
Eczema [2]
Exanthems [2]
Rash (<10%)
Toxic epidermal necrolysis [2]
Urticaria (<10%)

Otic
Hearing loss [3]

NEOSTIGMINE

Trade name: Prostigmin (Valeant)
Indications: Myasthenia gravis
Class: Acetylcholinesterase inhibitor, Cholinesterase inhibitor, Parasympathomimetic
Half-life: 52 minutes
Clinically important, potentially hazardous interactions with: aminoglycosides, antiarrhythmics, anticholinergics, chloroquine, clindamycin, hydroxychloroquine, kanamycin, lithium, local and general anesthetics, neomycin, non-depolarising muscle relaxants, polymixins, propafenone, propranolol, streptomycin, succinylcholine
Pregnancy category: C (Anticholinesterase drugs may cause uterine irritability and induce premature labor when given intravenously to pregnant women near term)
Important contra-indications noted in the prescribing guidelines for: nursing mothers; pediatric patients
Note: Neostigmine bromide is given orally; neostigmine methylsulfate is given parenterally. Contra-indicated in patients with a previous history of reaction to bromides, or those with peritonitis or mechanical obstruction of the intestinal or urinary tract.

Skin
Anaphylactoid reactions/Anaphylaxis [3]

Cardiovascular
Atrioventricular block [3]

Bradycardia [4]
Cardiac arrest [3]
Tachycardia [2]

Central Nervous System
Anxiety [2]
Sedation [2]

Gastrointestinal/Hepatic
Abdominal pain [3]
Diarrhea [2]
Nausea [14]
Vomiting [12]

Respiratory
Bronchospasm [3]

NERATINIB

Trade name: Nerlynx (Puma)
Indications: Early stage HER2-overexpressed/amplified breast cancer, to follow adjuvant trastuzumab-based therapy
Class: Kinase inhibitor
Half-life: 7–17 hours
Clinically important, potentially hazardous interactions with: aprepitant, boceprevir, bosentan, carbamazepine, cimetidine, ciprofloxacin, clarithromycin, clotrimazole, cobicistat, conivaptan, crizotinib, cyclosporine, dabigatran, dasabuvir/ombitasvir/paritaprevir/ritonavir, digoxin, diltiazem, dronedarone, efavirenz, enzalutamide, erythromycin, etravirine, fexofenadine, fluconazole, fluvoxamine, grapefruit juice, H2-receptor antagonists, idelalisib, imatinib, indinavir, itraconazole, ketoconazole, lansoprazole, lopinavir, mitotane, modafinil, nefazodone, nelfinavir, ombitasvir/paritaprevir/ritonavir, phenytoin, posaconazole, rifampin, ritonavir, saquinavir, St John's wort, strong or moderate CYP3A4 inhibitors or inducers, tipranavir, tofisopam, troleandomycin, verapamil, voriconazole
Pregnancy category: N/A (Can cause fetal harm)
Important contra-indications noted in the prescribing guidelines for: nursing mothers; pediatric patients

---

Skin
Fissures (2%)
Rash (18%)
Xerosis (6%)

Nails
Nail disorder (8%)

Mucosal
Epistaxis (nosebleed) (5%)
Stomatitis (14%) [2]
Xerostomia (3%)

Cardiovascular
Cardiotoxicity [2]

Central Nervous System
Anorexia [4]
Peripheral neuropathy [2]

Neuromuscular/Skeletal
Asthenia (fatigue) (27%) [5]
Muscle spasm (11%)

Gastrointestinal/Hepatic
Abdominal distension (5%)
Abdominal pain (36%) [2]
Diarrhea (95%) [15]
Dyspepsia (10%)
Hepatotoxicity (<2%)
Nausea (43%) [10]
Vomiting (26%) [7]

Endocrine/Metabolic
ALT increased (9%)
Appetite decreased (12%)
AST increased (7%)
Dehydration (4%)
Weight loss (5%)

Genitourinary
Urinary tract infection (5%)

Hematologic
Anemia [2]
Leukopenia [2]
Neutropenia [3]

NETUPITANT & PALONOSETRON

Synonym: NEPA
Trade name: Akynzeo (Helsinn)
Indications: Acute and delayed nausea and vomiting associated with cancer chemotherapy
Class: Neurokinin 1 receptor antagonist (netupitant), Serotonin type 3 receptor antagonist (palonosetron)
Half-life: 40 hours
Clinically important, potentially hazardous interactions with: rifampin
Pregnancy category: C
Important contra-indications noted in the prescribing guidelines for: nursing mothers; pediatric patients

---

Skin
Erythema (3%)

Central Nervous System
Headache (9%) [7]

Neuromuscular/Skeletal
Asthenia (fatigue) (4–8%)

Gastrointestinal/Hepatic
Constipation (3%) [6]
Dyspepsia (4%) [2]

Other
Adverse effects [2]
Hiccups [2]

NEVIRAPINE

Trade name: Viramune (Boehringer Ingelheim)
Indications: HIV infection
Class: Antiretroviral, CYP3A4 inducer, Non-nucleoside reverse transcriptase inhibitor
Half-life: 45 hours
Clinically important, potentially hazardous interactions with: amiodarone, amprenavir, atazanavir, carbamazepine, caspofungin, clarithromycin, clonazepam, cyclosporine, diltiazem, disopyramide, efavirenz, ethosuximide, etravirine, fentanyl, fluconazole, fosamprenavir, indinavir, itraconazole, ketoconazole, levonorgestrel, lidocaine, lopinavir, midazolam, nifedipine, rifampin, rilpivirine, simeprevir, St John's wort, verapamil
Pregnancy category: B
Important contra-indications noted in the prescribing guidelines for: nursing mothers
Warning: LIFE-THREATENING (INCLUDING FATAL) HEPATOTOXICITY and SKIN REACTIONS

Skin
Angioedema [2]
DRESS syndrome [12]
Exanthems [6]
Hypersensitivity [15]
Lipodystrophy [2]
Rash (<48%) [31]
Stevens-Johnson syndrome [35]
Toxic epidermal necrolysis [17]
Toxicity [3]

Mucosal
Gingivitis (<3%)
Ulcerative stomatitis (4%)

Central Nervous System
Fever [2]
Paresthesias (2%)
Peripheral neuropathy [2]

Neuromuscular/Skeletal
Myalgia/Myopathy (<10%)

Gastrointestinal/Hepatic
Hepatic failure [2]
Hepatotoxicity [31]

Endocrine/Metabolic
Acidosis [2]

Other
Adverse effects [7]
Death [3]

NIACIN

Synonyms: nicotinic acid; vitamin B_3
Trade names: Advicor (Kos), Niacor (Upsher-Smith), Niaspan (Merck), Simcor (AbbVie), Slo-Niacin (Upsher-Smith)
Indications: Hyperlipidemia
Class: Vitamin
Half-life: 45 minutes
Clinically important, potentially hazardous interactions with: antihypertensives, atorvastatin, bile acid sequestrants, insulin aspart, insulin degludec, insulin detemir, insulin glargine, insulin glulisine, pitavastatin, rosuvastatin, selenium
Pregnancy category: C (Where niacin is co-administered with a statin, refer to the pregnancy category for the statin)
Important contra-indications noted in the prescribing guidelines for: nursing mothers; pediatric patients
Note: Contra-indicated in patients with active liver or peptic ulcer disease, or arterial bleeding. Simcor is niacin and simvastatin.

Skin
Acanthosis nigricans (8%) [14]
Exanthems (<3%)
Flushing (<30%) [31]
Pruritus (<5%) [9]

Rash [5]

Central Nervous System
Paresthesias (<10%) [2]

Neuromuscular/Skeletal
Myalgia/Myopathy [5]

Gastrointestinal/Hepatic
Hepatotoxicity [3]

Endocrine/Metabolic
Hyperglycemia [2]

Ocular
Maculopathy [3]

Other
Adverse effects [2]
Side effects [2]

NIACINAMIDE

Synonyms: nicotinamide; vitamin B_3
Indications: Prophylaxis and treatment of pellagra
Class: Vitamin
Half-life: 45 minutes
Clinically important, potentially hazardous interactions with: atorvastatin, primidone, rosuvastatin
Pregnancy category: A (the pregnancy category will be C if used in doses above the RDA)

Skin
Pruritus (<5%) [2]

Central Nervous System
Paresthesias (<10%)

Hematologic
Thrombocytopenia [2]

NICARDIPINE

Trade name: Cardene (Roche)
Indications: Angina, hypertension
Class: Calcium channel blocker
Half-life: 2–4 hours
Clinically important, potentially hazardous interactions with: amprenavir, atazanavir, boceprevir, cobicistat/elvitegravir/emtricitabine/tenofovir alafenamide, cobicistat/elvitegravir/emtricitabine/tenofovir disoproxil, delavirdine, epirubicin, imatinib, indinavir, lopinavir, posaconazole, propranolol, telaprevir
Pregnancy category: C
Important contra-indications noted in the prescribing guidelines for: the elderly; pediatric patients

---

Skin
Flushing (6%) [2]
Peripheral edema (7%) [2]
Rash [3]
Urticaria [3]

Mucosal
Gingival hyperplasia/hypertrophy [2]

Cardiovascular
Erythromelalgia [2]
Pulmonary edema [5]

Endocrine/Metabolic
Gynecomastia [2]

NICOTINE

Trade names: Habitrol Patch (Novartis), Nicoderm (GSK), Nicorette (GSK), Nicotrol (Pfizer)
Indications: Aid to smoking cessation
Class: Alkaloid
Half-life: varies with the delivery system
Clinically important, potentially hazardous interactions with: adenosine, bendamustine, heparin, horsetail
Pregnancy category: D
Important contra-indications noted in the prescribing guidelines for: nursing mothers; pediatric patients
Note: Smoking cessation therapy has various delivery systems. These include: transdermal patches, chewing gum, nasal spray, inhaler, and oral forms.

Skin
Acneform eruption (3%)
Diaphoresis (<3%)
Erythema (>10%)
Pigmentation [3]
Pruritus (>10%)

Mucosal
Sialorrhea (>10%)
Stomatitis (>10%)
Xerostomia (<3%)

Central Nervous System
Headache (18–26%)

Neuromuscular/Skeletal
Arthralgia (5%)
Back pain (6%)
Myalgia/Myopathy (<10%)

Gastrointestinal/Hepatic
Dyspepsia (18%)
Flatulence (4%)
Pancreatitis [2]
Throat irritation/pain (66%)

Respiratory
Cough (32%) [2]
Rhinitis (23%)

Other
Death [2]
Hiccups [2]

NIFEDIPINE

Trade names: Adalat (Bayer), Coracten (UCB), Procardia (Pfizer), Tenif (AstraZeneca), Tensipine MR (Genus), Valni XL (Winthrop)
Indications: Angina, hypertension
Class: Calcium channel blocker
Half-life: 2–5 hours (immediate release products)
Clinically important, potentially hazardous interactions with: acebutolol, amprenavir, atazanavir, beta blockers, boceprevir, carbamazepine, cobicistat/elvitegravir/emtricitabine/tenofovir alafenamide, cobicistat/elvitegravir/emtricitabine/tenofovir disoproxil, cyclosporine, delavirdine, digoxin, diltiazem, dronedarone, efavirenz, epirubicin, fentanyl, fluoxetine, grapefruit juice, imatinib, indinavir, insulin, lopinavir, micafungin, mizolastine, nevirapine, oxcarbazepine, parenteral magnesium, phenytoin, posaconazole, propranolol, rifampin, ritonavir, St John's wort, tacrolimus, vardenafil, vincristine
Pregnancy category: C
Important contra-indications noted in the prescribing guidelines for: the elderly; nursing mothers; pediatric patients
Note: Tenif is atenolol and nifedipine.

Skin
AGEP [3]
Angioedema [2]
Bullous dermatitis [2]
Dermatitis (<2%)
Diaphoresis (<2%) [2]
Edema [3]
Erysipelas [2]
Erythema [2]
Erythema multiforme [5]
Erythema nodosum [2]
Exanthems [9]
Exfoliative dermatitis [5]
Fixed eruption [2]
Flushing (3–25%) [9]
Lichenoid eruption [3]
Lupus erythematosus [3]
Peripheral edema [12]
Photosensitivity [5]
Pruritus (<2%) [3]
Purpura (<2%) [3]
Rash (<3%) [2]
Stevens-Johnson syndrome [3]
Telangiectasia [2]
Toxic epidermal necrolysis [2]
Urticaria [7]
Vasculitis [4]

Hair
Alopecia [4]

Mucosal
Gingival hyperplasia/hypertrophy (6–10%) [75]
Xerostomia (<3%)

Cardiovascular
Erythromelalgia [4]
Hypotension [9]
Pulmonary edema [3]
Tachycardia [4]

Central Nervous System
Chills (2%)
Headache (19%) [7]
Paresthesias (<3%)
Tremor (2–8%)
Vertigo (dizziness) [5]

Neuromuscular/Skeletal
Asthenia (fatigue) (4%)

Gastrointestinal/Hepatic
Hepatotoxicity [3]
Nausea (2%) [2]

Endocrine/Metabolic
Gynecomastia [6]

Other
Adverse effects [4]
Side effects [3]

NILOTINIB

Trade name: Tasigna (Novartis)
Indications: Chronic myelogenous leukemia
Class: Antineoplastic, Epidermal growth factor receptor (EGFR) inhibitor, Tyrosine kinase inhibitor
Half-life: 17 hours
Clinically important, potentially hazardous interactions with: amiodarone, amitriptyline, amoxapine, arsenic, astemizole, bepridil, carbamazepine, chloroquine, cisapride, citalopram, clarithromycin, clozapine, conivaptan, darunavir, dasatinib, degarelix, delavirdine, digoxin, dihydroergotamine, disopyramide, dolasetron, efavirenz, ergotamine, grapefruit juice, halofantrine, haloperidol, indinavir, itraconazole, ketoconazole, lapatinib, levofloxacin, lopinavir, methadone, midazolam, moxifloxacin, oxcarbazepine, pazopanib, phenobarbital, phenytoin, pimozide, procainamide, quinidine, rifampin, rifapentine, ritonavir, sotalol, St John's wort, telavancin, telithromycin, terfenadine, voriconazole, vorinostat, ziprasidone
Pregnancy category: D
Important contra-indications noted in the prescribing guidelines for: nursing mothers; pediatric patients
Note: Contra-indicated in patients with hypokalemia, hypomagnesemia, or long QT syndrome.
Warning: QT PROLONGATION AND SUDDEN DEATHS

Skin
Acneform eruption (<10%)
Dermatitis (<10%)
Eczema (<10%)
Edema [3]
Erythema (<10%) [2]
Exanthems [2]
Flushing (<10%)
Folliculitis (<10%)
Hematoma (<10%)
Hyperhidrosis (<10%)
Peripheral edema (<10%)
Pruritus (<10%) [16]
Rash (<10%) [18]
Sweet's syndrome [3]
Toxicity [8]
Urticaria (<10%)
Xerosis [2]

Hair
Alopecia (<10%) [5]

Cardiovascular
Angina (<10%)
Arrhythmias (<10%) [2]
Arterial occlusion [5]
Atrial fibrillation (<10%) [2]
Atrioventricular block (<10%)
Bradycardia (<10%)
Cardiotoxicity [5]
Chest pain (<10%)
Extrasystoles (<10%)
Hypertension (<10%)
Myocardial infarction [3]
Palpitation (<10%)
QT prolongation (<10%) [8]

Central Nervous System
Anorexia (<10%) [2]
Depression (<10%) [2]
Fever (<10%) [2]
Headache (~10%) [14]
Hypoesthesia (<10%)
Insomnia (<10%)
Pain [2]
Paresthesias (<10%)
Stroke [2]
Vertigo (dizziness) (<10%) [2]

Neuromuscular/Skeletal
Arthralgia (<10%) [3]
Asthenia (fatigue) (<10%) [9]
Bone or joint pain (<10%)
Muscle spasm [3]
Myalgia/Myopathy (<10%) [5]
Neck pain (<10%)

Gastrointestinal/Hepatic
Abdominal distension (<10%)
Abdominal pain (<10%) [2]
Constipation (~10%) [3]
Diarrhea (~10%) [5]
Dyspepsia (<10%)
Flatulence (<10%)
Hepatotoxicity [6]
Nausea (~10%) [8]
Pancreatitis (<10%) [4]
Vomiting (~10%)

Respiratory
Cough (<10%)
Dysphonia (<10%)
Dyspnea (<10%) [2]
Nasopharyngitis [2]
Pleural effusion [2]
Pulmonary hypertension [3]
Upper respiratory tract infection [2]

Endocrine/Metabolic
ALP increased [2]
ALT increased (4%) [5]
AST increased (<3%) [3]
Diabetes mellitus (<10%)
Hyperamylasemia [3]
Hyperbilirubinemia [8]
Hypercalcemia (<10%)
Hypercholesterolemia (<10%) [2]
Hyperglycemia (6–12%) [6]
Hyperkalemia (2–6%)
Hyperlipidemia (<10%)
Hypocalcemia (<10%)
Hypokalemia (<10%) [2]
Hypomagnesemia (<10%)
Hyponatremia (<10%)
Hypophosphatemia (5–17%) [4]
Hypothyroidism [2]
Weight gain (<10%)
Weight loss (<10%)

Genitourinary
Pollakiuria (<10%)

Hematologic
Anemia (4–27%) [9]
Febrile neutropenia (<10%)
Hyperlipasemia [5]
Leukopenia [2]
Lymphopenia (<10%) [2]
Neutropenia (12–42%) [9]
Pancytopenia (<10%)
Thrombocytopenia (10–42%) [11]

Ocular
Conjunctivitis (<10%)
Ocular hemorrhage (<10%)
Periorbital edema (<10%)
Xerophthalmia (<10%)

Other
Adverse effects [3]
Death [3]
Side effects [3]

NINTEDANIB

Trade name: Ofev (Boehringer Ingelheim)
Indications: Idiopathic pulmonary fibrosis
Class: Tyrosine kinase inhibitor
Half-life: 9.5 hours
Clinically important, potentially hazardous interactions with: anticoagulants, carbamazepine, erythromycin, phenytoin, St John's wort
Pregnancy category: D
Important contra-indications noted in the prescribing guidelines for: nursing mothers; pediatric patients

---

Skin
Hand–foot syndrome [2]
Rash [4]

Hair
Alopecia [2]

Mucosal
Epistaxis (nosebleed) [2]

Cardiovascular
Cardiotoxicity [2]
Hypertension (5%) [7]
Myocardial infarction (2%)

Central Nervous System
Anorexia [6]
Headache (8%)
Peripheral neuropathy [2]

Neuromuscular/Skeletal
Asthenia (fatigue) [15]

Gastrointestinal/Hepatic
Abdominal pain (15%) [6]
Diarrhea (62%) [34]
Gastrointestinal disorder [4]
Hepatotoxicity (14%) [10]
Nausea (24%) [25]
Vomiting (12%) [20]

Respiratory
Bronchitis [3]
Cough [3]
Dyspnea [4]
Nasopharyngitis [3]
Pneumonia [3]
Upper respiratory tract infection [2]

Endocrine/Metabolic
ALT increased [12]
Appetite decreased (11%) [6]
AST increased [10]
Weight loss (10%) [3]

Hematologic
Anemia [3]
Bleeding (10%) [3]
Leukopenia [2]
Neutropenia [4]

Thrombocytopenia [2]

Other

Adverse effects [6]
Death [3]

NIRAPARIB

Trade name: Zejula (Tesaro)
Indications: Maintenance treatment of adult patients with recurrent epithelial ovarian, fallopian tube, or primary peritoneal cancer who are in a complete or partial response to platinum-based chemotherapy
Class: Poly (ADP-ribose) polymerase (PARP) inhibitor
Half-life: 36 hours
Clinically important, potentially hazardous interactions with: none known
Pregnancy category: N/A (Can cause fetal harm)
Important contra-indications noted in the prescribing guidelines for: nursing mothers; pediatric patients

---

Skin

Peripheral edema (<10%)
Rash (21%)

Mucosal

Epistaxis (nosebleed) (<10%)
Mucositis (20%)
Stomatitis (20%)
Xerostomia (10%)

Cardiovascular

Hypertension (20%) [2]
Palpitation (10%)
Tachycardia (<10%)

Central Nervous System

Anxiety (11%)
Depression (<10%)
Dysgeusia (taste perversion) (10%)
Headache (26%)
Insomnia (27%)
Vertigo (dizziness) (18%)

Neuromuscular/Skeletal

Arthralgia (13%)
Asthenia (fatigue) (57%) [2]
Back pain (18%)
Myalgia/Myopathy (19%)

Gastrointestinal/Hepatic

Abdominal distension (33%)
Abdominal pain (33%)
Constipation (40%)
Diarrhea (20%)
Dyspepsia (18%)
Nausea (74%) [2]
Vomiting (34%) [2]

Respiratory

Bronchitis (<10%)
Dyspnea (20%)
Nasopharyngitis (23%)

Endocrine/Metabolic

ALT increased (10%)
Appetite decreased (25%) [2]
AST increased (10%)
Creatine phosphokinase increased (<10%)
GGT increased (<10%)
Hypokalemia (<10%)
Serum creatinine increased (<10%)
Weight loss (<10%)

Genitourinary

Urinary tract infection (13%)

Hematologic

Anemia (50%) [3]
Leukopenia (17%)
Neutropenia (30%) [3]
Thrombocytopenia (61%) [3]

Ocular

Conjunctivitis (<10%)

NISOLDIPINE

Trade name: Sular (First Horizon)
Indications: Hypertension
Class: Calcium channel blocker
Half-life: 7–12 hours
Clinically important, potentially hazardous interactions with: amprenavir, conivaptan, cyclosporine, darunavir, delavirdine, efavirenz, epirubicin, grapefruit juice, imatinib, indinavir, itraconazole, ketoconazole, oxcarbazepine, propranolol, telaprevir, telithromycin, voriconazole
Pregnancy category: C

Skin

Peripheral edema (22%) [6]
Rash (2%)

Central Nervous System

Headache [4]

Endocrine/Metabolic

Gynecomastia [2]

NITAZOXANIDE

Trade name: Alinia (Romark)
Indications: Diarrhea caused by *Cryptosporidium parvum* or *Giardia lamblia* (in children)
Class: Antiprotozoal
Half-life: N/A
Clinically important, potentially hazardous interactions with: none known
Pregnancy category: B

Central Nervous System

Headache [2]

Gastrointestinal/Hepatic

Abdominal pain [3]
Diarrhea [2]

NITROFURANTOIN

Trade names: Furadantin (First Horizon), Macrobid (Procter & Gamble), Macrodantin (Procter & Gamble)
Indications: Various urinary tract infections caused by susceptible organisms
Class: Antibiotic
Half-life: 1–2 minutes
Clinically important, potentially hazardous interactions with: norfloxacin
Pregnancy category: B
Important contra-indications noted in the prescribing guidelines for: nursing mothers; pediatric patients

---

Skin

Anaphylactoid reactions/Anaphylaxis [2]
Angioedema [4]
Dermatitis [3]
DRESS syndrome [4]
Eczema [2]
Erythema multiforme [3]
Exanthems (<5%) [9]
Exfoliative dermatitis [3]
Lupus erythematosus [8]
Purpura [2]
Rash [2]
Stevens-Johnson syndrome [2]
Toxic epidermal necrolysis [5]
Urticaria [8]

Hair

Alopecia [5]

Central Nervous System

Neurotoxicity [2]
Paresthesias (<10%)

Gastrointestinal/Hepatic

Hepatitis [2]
Hepatotoxicity [14]

Respiratory

Pneumonitis [3]
Pulmonary toxicity [8]

Other

Adverse effects [3]
Death [3]

NITROGLYCERIN

Synonyms: glyceryl trinitrate; nitroglycerol; NTG
Trade names: Minitran (3M), Nitrodur (Schering) (Key), Nitrolingual (First Horizon), Nitrostat (Pfizer)
Indications: Acute angina
Class: Nitrate, Vasodilator
Half-life: 1–4 minutes
Clinically important, potentially hazardous interactions with: acetylcysteine, alteplase, heparin, sildenafil, tadalafil, vardenafil
Pregnancy category: C
Important contra-indications noted in the prescribing guidelines for: nursing mothers; pediatric patients

---

Skin

Dermatitis (to topical systems) [25]
Eczema [2]
Erythema (to transdermal delivery system) [2]
Exfoliative dermatitis (<10%)
Flushing (>10%)
Purpura [2]
Rash (<10%)
Urticaria [2]

Cardiovascular

Bradycardia [2]
Hypotension [4]

Central Nervous System
- Headache [14]
- Migraine [2]

NIVOLUMAB

Trade name: Opdivo (Bristol-Myers Squibb)
Indications: Metastatic squamous non-small cell lung cancer with progression on or after platinum-based chemotherapy, unresectable or metastatic melanoma and disease progression following ipilimumab and, if BRAF V600 mutation positive, a BRAF inhibitor, advanced renal cell carcinoma with prior anti-angiogenic therapy, Hodgkin lymphoma that has relapsed or progressed after autologous hematopoietic stem cell transplantation and post-transplantation brentuximab vedotin
Class: Monoclonal antibody, Programmed death receptor-1 (PD-1) inhibitor
Half-life: 27 days
Clinically important, potentially hazardous interactions with: none known
Pregnancy category: N/A (Can cause fetal harm)
Important contra-indications noted in the prescribing guidelines for: nursing mothers; pediatric patients

---

Skin
- Bullous pemphigoid [7]
- Dermatitis [3]
- Eczema [2]
- Edema (17%) [3]
- Erythema [4]
- Erythema multiforme (<10%) [2]
- Exanthems [3]
- Exfoliative dermatitis (<10%)
- Granulomatous reaction [2]
- Hypersensitivity [3]
- Lichen planus [2]
- Lichenoid eruption [2]
- Pruritus (11–19%) [27]
- Psoriasis (<10%) [6]
- Rash (16–21%) [36]
- Sarcoidosis [6]
- Stevens-Johnson syndrome [2]
- Thrombocytopenic purpura [2]
- Toxic epidermal necrolysis [2]
- Toxicity [7]
- Urticaria [2]
- Vitiligo (<10%) [12]

Mucosal
- Stomatitis (<10%) [2]
- Xerostomia [3]

Cardiovascular
- Chest pain (13%)
- Myocarditis [7]
- Ventricular arrhythmia (<10%)

Central Nervous System
- Encephalopathy [8]
- Fever (17%) [9]
- Neurotoxicity [5]
- Pain (10%)
- Peripheral neuropathy (<10%)
- Vertigo (dizziness) (<10%)

Neuromuscular/Skeletal
- Arthralgia (13%) [10]
- Asthenia (fatigue) (19–50%) [29]
- Bone or joint pain (36%)
- Myalgia/Myopathy [14]
- Myasthenia gravis [13]
- Polymyositis [2]
- Rhabdomyolysis [3]
- Synovial effusions [3]

Gastrointestinal/Hepatic
- Abdominal pain (16%)
- Colitis [25]
- Constipation (24%)
- Diarrhea (18%) [30]
- Hepatitis [8]
- Hepatotoxicity [14]
- Nausea (29%) [14]
- Pancreatitis [4]
- Vomiting (19%) [2]

Respiratory
- Bronchitis (<10%)
- Cough (17–32%) [2]
- Dyspnea (38%) [3]
- Pneumonia (10%) [4]
- Pneumonitis [30]
- Pulmonary granuloma [2]
- Pulmonary toxicity [3]
- Upper respiratory tract infection (11%)

Endocrine/Metabolic
- Adrenal insufficiency [5]
- ALP increased (14–22%)
- ALT increased (12–16%) [9]
- Appetite decreased (35%) [9]
- AST increased (16–28%) [7]
- Diabetes mellitus [15]
- Diabetic ketoacidosis [3]
- Hyperamylasemia [2]
- Hypercalcemia (20%)
- Hyperkalemia (15–18%)
- Hyperthyroidism [12]
- Hypocalcemia (18%)
- Hypokalemia (20%)
- Hypomagnesemia (20%)
- Hyponatremia (25–38%)
- Hypophosphatemia [2]
- Hypophysitis [13]
- Hypothyroidism [23]
- Serum creatinine increased (22%) [2]
- Thyroid dysfunction [9]
- Thyroiditis [11]
- Weight loss (13%)

Renal
- Glomerulonephritis [2]
- Nephrotoxicity [11]
- Renal failure [4]

Hematologic
- Anemia (28%) [5]
- Cytopenia [2]
- Eosinophilia [2]
- Hemolytic anemia [5]
- Hyperlipasemia [6]
- Lymphopenia (47%) [4]
- Neutropenia [7]
- Thrombocytopenia (14%) [6]

Ocular
- Iridocyclitis (<10%)
- Ocular adverse effects [2]
- Uveitis [5]

Local
- Infusion-related reactions (<10%) [7]

Other
- Adverse effects [33]
- Death [19]
- Side effects [2]

NORFLOXACIN

Trade names: Chibroxin (Merck), Noroxin (Merck)
Indications: Various urinary tract infections caused by susceptible organisms, conjunctivitis
Class: Antibiotic, fluoroquinolone, CYP3A4 inhibitor
Half-life: 3–4 hours
Clinically important, potentially hazardous interactions with: aminophylline, amiodarone, antacids, arsenic, artemether/lumefantrine, bepridil, bretylium, caffeine, ciprofibrate, clozapine, cyclosporine, dairy products, didanosine, disopyramide, erythromycin, glyburide, lanthanum, mycophenolate, nitrofurantoin, NSAIDs, oral iron, oral typhoid vaccine, oxtriphylline, phenothiazines, probenecid, procainamide, quinidine, ropinirole, sotalol, strontium ranelate, sucralfate, tacrine, tamoxifen, tizanidine, tricyclic antidepressants, warfarin, zinc, zolmitriptan
Pregnancy category: C
Important contra-indications noted in the prescribing guidelines for: the elderly; nursing mothers; pediatric patients
Note: Fluoroquinolones are associated with an increased risk of tendinitis and tendon rupture in all ages. This risk is further increased in older patients usually over 60 years of age, in patients taking corticosteroid drugs, and in patients with kidney, heart or lung transplants.
Fluoroquinolones may exacerbate muscle weakness in persons with myasthenia gravis.

Skin
- Erythema [2]
- Exanthems [2]
- Fixed eruption [3]
- Phototoxicity [4]
- Stevens-Johnson syndrome [2]
- Toxic epidermal necrolysis [2]

Nails
- Photo-onycholysis [2]

Neuromuscular/Skeletal
- Rhabdomyolysis [2]
- Tendinopathy/Tendon rupture [4]

Other
- Adverse effects [2]

NORTRIPTYLINE

Trade names: Aventyl (Ranbaxy), Pamelor (Mallinckrodt)
Indications: Depression
Class: Antidepressant, tricyclic
Half-life: 28–31 hours
Clinically important, potentially hazardous interactions with: amprenavir, arbutamine, clonidine, cobicistat/elvitegravir/emtricitabine/tenofovir alafenamide, cobicistat/elvitegravir/emtricitabine/tenofovir disoproxil, epinephrine, fluoxetine, formoterol, guanethidine,

isocarboxazid, linezolid, MAO inhibitors, phenelzine, quinolones, sparfloxacin, tranylcypromine
Pregnancy category: D
Important contra-indications noted in the prescribing guidelines for: pediatric patients
Warning: SUICIDALITY AND ANTIDEPRESSANT DRUGS

Skin
Diaphoresis (<10%)
Photosensitivity [2]

Mucosal
Xerostomia (>10%) [9]

Central Nervous System
Dysgeusia (taste perversion) (>10%)
Parkinsonism (<10%)
Vertigo (dizziness) [2]

Other
Adverse effects [2]

NUSINERSEN

Trade name: Spinraza (Biogen)
Indications: Spinal muscular atrophy
Class: Survival motor neuron-2 (SMN2)-directed antisense oligonucleotide
Half-life: 63–87 days (in plasma)
Clinically important, potentially hazardous interactions with: none known
Pregnancy category: N/A (No data available)
Important contra-indications noted in the prescribing guidelines for: nursing mothers

---

Central Nervous System
Headache (50%) [2]

Neuromuscular/Skeletal
Back pain (41%) [2]
Scoliosis (5%)

Gastrointestinal/Hepatic
Constipation (30%)

Respiratory
Bronchitis (>5%)
Upper respiratory tract infection (39%)

Otic
Ear infection (5%)

NYSTATIN

Trade names: Mycology-II (Bristol-Myers Squibb), Mycostatin (Bristol-Myers Squibb)
Indications: Candidiasis
Class: Antifungal
Half-life: ~2–3 hours
Clinically important, potentially hazardous interactions with: none known
Pregnancy category: C
Important contra-indications noted in the prescribing guidelines for: nursing mothers

---

Skin
AGEP [5]
Dermatitis [12]
Eczema [2]
Fixed eruption [2]

OBETICHOLIC ACID

Trade name: Ocaliva (Intercept)
Indications: Primary biliary cholangitis
Class: Farnesoid X receptor (FXR) agonist
Half-life: N/A
Clinically important, potentially hazardous interactions with: aminophylline, tizanidine, warfarin
Pregnancy category: N/A (Insufficient evidence to inform drug-associated risk)
Important contra-indications noted in the prescribing guidelines for: nursing mothers; pediatric patients
Note: Contra-indicated in patients with complete biliary obstruction.

Skin
Eczema (3–6%)
Peripheral edema (3–7%)
Pruritus (56–70%) [8]
Rash (7–10%)
Urticaria (<10%)

Mucosal
Oropharyngeal pain (7–8%)

Cardiovascular
Palpitation (3–7%)

Central Nervous System
Fever (<7%)
Syncope (<7%)
Vertigo (dizziness) (7%)

Neuromuscular/Skeletal
Arthralgia (6–10%)
Asthenia (fatigue) (19–25%)

Gastrointestinal/Hepatic
Abdominal pain (10–19%)
Constipation (7%)

Endocrine/Metabolic
Thyroid dysfunction (4–6%)

OBINUTUZUMAB

Trade name: Gazyva (Genentech)
Indications: Chronic lymphocytic leukemia (in combination with chlorambucil), follicular lymphoma (firstly with bendamustine then as monotherapy)
Class: CD20-directed cytolytic monoclonal antibody, Monoclonal antibody
Half-life: 28 days
Clinically important, potentially hazardous interactions with: live vaccines
Pregnancy category: N/A (Insufficient evidence to inform drug-associated risk)
Important contra-indications noted in the prescribing guidelines for: nursing mothers; pediatric patients
Warning: HEPATITIS B VIRUS REACTIVATION AND PROGRESSIVE MULTIFOCAL LEUKOENCEPHALOPATHY

Skin
Tumor lysis syndrome [5]

Central Nervous System
Fever (10%) [5]
Headache [2]
Leukoencephalopathy [2]

Gastrointestinal/Hepatic
Nausea [3]

Respiratory
Cough (10%) [2]

Endocrine/Metabolic
ALP increased (16%)
AST increased (25%)
Hyperkalemia (31%)
Hypoalbuminemia (22%)
Hypocalcemia (32%)
Hypokalemia (13%)

Hematologic
Anemia (12%) [6]
Leukopenia (7%)
Neutropenia (40%) [17]
Thrombocytopenia (15%) [9]

Local
Infusion-related reactions (69%) [16]

Other
Death [2]
Infection (38%) [8]

OCRIPLASMIN

Trade name: Jetrea (ThromboGenics)
Indications: Symptomatic vitreomacular adhesion
Class: Enzyme
Half-life: N/A
Clinically important, potentially hazardous interactions with: none known
Pregnancy category: C
Important contra-indications noted in the prescribing guidelines for: nursing mothers; pediatric patients

---

Ocular
Cataract (2–4%)
Conjunctival hemorrhage (5–20%)
Conjunctival hyperemia (2–4%)
Dyschromatopsia (2%)
Intraocular inflammation (7%)
Intraocular pressure increased (4%)
Iritis (2–4%)
Macular edema (2–4%)
Macular hole (5–20%)
Ocular adverse effects [2]
Ocular hemorrhage (2%)
Ocular pain (5–20%) [2]
Photophobia (2–4%)
Photopsia (5–20%) [4]
Reduced visual acuity (5–20%) [2]
Retinal edema (5–20%)
Vision blurred (5–20%)
Vision impaired (5–20%)
Vision loss [3]
Vitreous detachment (2–4%)
Vitreous floaters (5–20%) [4]
Xerophthalmia (2–4%)

OCTREOTIDE

Trade name: Sandostatin (Novartis)
Indications: Diarrhea, sulfonylurea poisoning
Class: Somatostatin analog
Half-life: 1.5 hours
Clinically important, potentially hazardous interactions with: bromocriptine, insulin aspart, insulin degludec, metformin
Pregnancy category: B
Important contra-indications noted in the prescribing guidelines for: the elderly; nursing mothers; pediatric patients

---

Skin
Cellulitis (<4%)
Diaphoresis (5–15%)
Edema (<10%)
Flushing (<4%)
Petechiae (<4%)
Pruritus (18%)
Purpura (<4%)
Rash (5–15%)
Raynaud's phenomenon (<4%)
Urticaria (<4%)

Hair
Alopecia (~13%) [4]

Cardiovascular
Arrhythmias (3–9%)
Bradycardia (19–25%) [4]
Chest pain (20%)
Hypertension (13%) [3]
QT prolongation [2]
Thrombophlebitis (<4%)

Central Nervous System
Anorexia (4–6%)
Headache [3]
Pain (4–6%)
Rigors (5–15%)
Vertigo (dizziness) [2]

Neuromuscular/Skeletal
Arthralgia (5–15%)
Asthenia (fatigue) [5]
Myalgia/Myopathy (5–15%) [2]

Gastrointestinal/Hepatic
Abdominal pain (5–61%) [5]
Diarrhea (34–58%) [5]
Flatulence (38%) [2]
Hepatotoxicity [4]
Loose stools [2]
Nausea (5–61%) [6]
Pancreatitis [2]
Vomiting (4–21%)

Respiratory
Cough (5–15%)
Pharyngitis (5–15%)
Rhinitis (5–15%)
Sinusitis (5–15%)

Endocrine/Metabolic
Galactorrhea (<4%)
Gynecomastia (<4%)
Hyperglycemia [7]
Hypoglycemia [2]
Hypothyroidism (12%)

Genitourinary
Vaginitis (<4%)

Hematologic
Anemia (15%)
Neutropenia [2]
Thrombocytopenia [3]

Otic
Ear pain (5–15%)

Local
Injection-site granuloma [2]
Injection-site pain (8%) [2]

OFATUMUMAB

Trade name: Arzerra (Novartis)
Indications: Chronic lymphocytic leukemia
Class: CD20-directed cytolytic monoclonal antibody, Monoclonal antibody
Half-life: 14 days
Clinically important, potentially hazardous interactions with: live vaccines
Pregnancy category: N/A (May cause fetal B-cell depletion)
Important contra-indications noted in the prescribing guidelines for: nursing mothers; pediatric patients
Warning: HEPATITIS B VIRUS REACTIVATION AND PROGRESSIVE MULTIFOCAL LEUKOENCEPHALOPATHY

Skin
Herpes (6%)
Hyperhidrosis (5%)
Peripheral edema (9%)
Rash (14%) [2]
Toxicity [3]
Urticaria (8%)

Cardiovascular
Angina [2]
Hypertension (5%)
Hypotension (5%)
Tachycardia (5%)

Central Nervous System
Chills (8%)
Fever (20%) [2]
Headache (6%)
Insomnia (7%)
Peripheral neuropathy [2]

Neuromuscular/Skeletal
Asthenia (fatigue) (15%) [4]
Back pain (8%)

Gastrointestinal/Hepatic
Diarrhea (18%) [2]
Nausea (11%) [3]

Respiratory
Bronchitis (11%)
Cough (19%)
Dyspnea (14%)
Nasopharyngitis (8%)
Pneumonia (23%)
Pulmonary toxicity [3]
Upper respiratory tract infection (11%)

Hematologic
Anemia (16%) [4]
Hemolysis [2]
Hemolytic anemia [2]
Leukopenia [2]
Lymphopenia [3]
Neutropenia (>10%) [11]
Sepsis (8%)
Thrombocytopenia [5]

Local
Infusion-related reactions [10]
Infusion-site reactions [2]

Other
Adverse effects [2]
Infection (70%) [10]

OFLOXACIN

Trade names: Floxin (Ortho-McNeil), Ocuflox (Allergan), Taravid (Sanofi-Aventis)
Indications: Various infections caused by susceptible organisms
Class: Antibiotic, fluoroquinolone
Half-life: 4–8 hours
Clinically important, potentially hazardous interactions with: aminophylline, amiodarone, antacids, arsenic, artemether/lumefantrine, BCG vaccine, bendamustine, bepridil, bretylium, calcium salts, clozapine, corticosteroids, cyclosporine, CYP1A2 substrates, didanosine, disopyramide, erythromycin, insulin, lanthanum, magnesiuim salts, mycophenolate, NSAIDs, oral iron, oral typhoid vaccine, oxtriphylline, phenothiazines, probenecid, procainamide, quinapril, quinidine, sevelamer, sotalol, St John's wort, strontium ranelate, sucralfate, sulfonylureas, tricyclic antidepressants, vitamin K antagonists, warfarin, zinc, zolmitriptan
Pregnancy category: C
Important contra-indications noted in the prescribing guidelines for: the elderly; nursing mothers; pediatric patients
Note: Fluoroquinolones are associated with an increased risk of tendinitis and tendon rupture in all ages. This risk is further increased in older patients usually over 60 years of age, in patients taking corticosteroid drugs, and in patients with kidney, heart or lung transplants.
Fluoroquinolones may exacerbate muscle weakness in persons with myasthenia gravis.
Warning: SERIOUS ADVERSE REACTIONS INCLUDING TENDINITIS, TENDON RUPTURE, PERIPHERAL NEUROPATHY, CENTRIAL NERVOUS SYSTEM EFFECTS and EXACERBATION OF MYASTHENIA GRAVIS

Skin
Anaphylactoid reactions/Anaphylaxis [4]
Angioedema [3]
Exanthems [3]
Fixed eruption [4]
Hypersensitivity [2]
Photosensitivity [8]
Phototoxicity [3]
Pruritus (<3%) [5]
Pruritus ani et vulvae (<3%)
Rash (<10%) [5]
Stevens-Johnson syndrome [4]
Toxic epidermal necrolysis [4]
Urticaria [3]
Vasculitis [4]

Nails
Photo-onycholysis [2]

Mucosal
- Oral mucosal eruption [3]
- Xerostomia (<3%)

Cardiovascular
- QT prolongation [3]

Central Nervous System
- Dysgeusia (taste perversion) (<3%) [2]
- Hallucinations [3]
- Headache [3]
- Insomnia [2]
- Peripheral neuropathy [2]
- Psychosis [2]
- Seizures [2]
- Vertigo (dizziness) [3]

Neuromuscular/Skeletal
- Arthralgia [2]
- Arthropathy [2]
- Asthenia (fatigue) [2]
- Myalgia/Myopathy [2]
- Rhabdomyolysis [2]
- Tendinopathy/Tendon rupture [7]

Gastrointestinal/Hepatic
- Abdominal pain [3]
- Diarrhea [2]
- Nausea [4]
- Vomiting [2]

Genitourinary
- Vaginitis (<10%)

Local
- Injection-site pain (<10%)

Other
- Adverse effects [10]
- Death [3]
- Side effects [2]

OLANZAPINE

Trade names: Symbyax (Lilly), Zyprexa (Lilly), Zyprexa Relprevv (Lilly)
Indications: Schizophrenia, bipolar I disorder
Class: Antipsychotic, Muscarinic antagonist
Half-life: 21–54 hours
Clinically important, potentially hazardous interactions with: alcohol, antihypertensive agents, carbamazepine, ciprofloxacin, CNS acting drugs, diazepam, dopamine agonists, eszopiclone, fluoxetine, fluvoxamine, insulin degludec, insulin detemir, insulin glargine, levodopa, lithium, tetrabenazine, valproic acid
Pregnancy category: C
Important contra-indications noted in the prescribing guidelines for: the elderly; nursing mothers; pediatric patients
Note: Can cause DRESS and other serious skin reactions.
Symbyax is olanzapine and fluoxetine; Zypraxa Relprevv is olanzapine pamoate.
Warning: INCREASED MORTALITY IN ELDERLY PATIENTS WITH DEMENTIA-RELATED PSYCHOSIS
POST-INJECTION DELIRIUM/SEDATION SYNDROME (Zyprexa Relprevv)

Skin
- Angioedema [2]
- Edema [3]
- Hypersensitivity [2]
- Peripheral edema (<10%) [5]
- Psoriasis [3]
- Purpura (<10%)
- Rash (>2%) [2]
- Vesiculobullous eruption (2%)
- Xanthomas [2]

Hair
- Alopecia [3]

Mucosal
- Epistaxis (nosebleed) (<10%)
- Sialorrhea [4]
- Xerostomia (13%) [11]

Cardiovascular
- Hypertension (<10%)
- Hypotension (<10%) [4]
- Orthostatic hypotension [2]
- QT prolongation [6]
- Tachycardia (<10%)
- Torsades de pointes [3]
- Venous thromboembolism [4]

Central Nervous System
- Akathisia (<10%) [8]
- Amnesia [2]
- Compulsions [2]
- Confusion [2]
- Delirium [6]
- Extrapyramidal symptoms [4]
- Fever [2]
- Hallucinations [2]
- Headache (17%) [3]
- Insomnia (12%) [3]
- Neuroleptic malignant syndrome [35]
- Parkinsonism (<10%) [6]
- Psychosis [2]
- Restless legs syndrome [7]
- Restlessness [2]
- Sedation [17]
- Seizures [8]
- Serotonin syndrome [2]
- Somnolence (drowsiness) (20–39%) [14]
- Suicidal ideation [2]
- Tardive dyskinesia [5]
- Tremor (<10%) [5]
- Twitching (2%)
- Vertigo (dizziness) [5]

Neuromuscular/Skeletal
- Asthenia (fatigue) (8–20%) [4]
- Back pain (<10%)
- Dystonia [6]
- Myalgia/Myopathy [2]
- Rhabdomyolysis [9]

Gastrointestinal/Hepatic
- Abdominal pain (<10%)
- Constipation (9–11%) [5]
- Diarrhea (<10%) [2]
- Dyspepsia (7–11%)
- Flatulence (<10%)
- Hepatotoxicity [6]
- Nausea (<10%)
- Pancreatitis [7]
- Vomiting (<10%)

Respiratory
- Cough (<10%)
- Nasopharyngitis [2]
- Pharyngitis (<10%)
- Pneumonia [2]
- Pulmonary embolism [3]
- Rhinitis (<10%)
- Sinusitis (<10%)

Endocrine/Metabolic
- Appetite increased [2]
- Diabetes mellitus [7]
- Diabetic ketoacidosis [2]
- Galactorrhea [2]
- Glucose dysregulation [3]
- Gynecomastia [2]
- Hypercholesterolemia [3]
- Hyperglycemia [7]
- Hyperprolactinemia [2]
- Metabolic syndrome [11]
- Weight gain (5–40%) [62]

Genitourinary
- Priapism [19]
- Sexual dysfunction [2]
- Urinary incontinence (<10%)
- Urinary tract infection (<10%)

Hematologic
- Agranulocytosis [2]
- Dyslipidemia [4]
- Eosinophilia [2]
- Leukopenia [2]
- Neutropenia [4]
- Pancytopenia [2]

Ocular
- Amblyopia (<10%)
- Oculogyric crisis [2]
- Vision blurred [2]

Other
- Adverse effects [10]
- Death [7]

OLAPARIB

Trade name: Lynparza (AstraZeneca)
Indications: BRCA-mutated ovarian cancer
Class: Poly (ADP-ribose) polymerase (PARP) inhibitor
Half-life: 7–17 hours
Clinically important, potentially hazardous interactions with: amprenavir, aprepitant, atazanavir, boceprevir, bosentan, carbamazepine, ciprofloxacin, clarithromycin, crizotinib, darunavir, diltiazem, efavirenz, erythromycin, etravirine, fluconazole, fosamprenavir, grapefruit juice, imatinib, indinavir, itraconazole, ketoconazole, lopinavir, modafinil, nafcillin, nefazodone, nelfinavir, phenytoin, posaconazole, rifampin, ritonavir, saquinavir, St John's wort, strong and moderate CYP3A inhibitors, telaprevir, telithromycin, verapamil, voriconazole
Pregnancy category: D
Important contra-indications noted in the prescribing guidelines for: nursing mothers; pediatric patients

---

Skin
- Eczema (<10%)
- Hot flashes (<10%)
- Peripheral edema (10–20%)
- Pruritus (<10%)
- Rash (25%) [2]
- Xerosis (<10%)

Hair
- Alopecia [2]

Mucosal
Stomatitis (<10%)

Cardiovascular
Hypertension (<10%) [2]
Venous thromboembolism (<10%)

Central Nervous System
Anxiety (<10%)
Depression (<10%)
Dysgeusia (taste perversion) (21%) [2]
Fever (<10%)
Headache (25%) [4]
Insomnia (<10%)
Peripheral neuropathy (<10%) [2]

Neuromuscular/Skeletal
Arthralgia (21–32%)
Asthenia (fatigue) (66–68%) [18]
Back pain (25%)
Myalgia/Myopathy (22–25%)

Gastrointestinal/Hepatic
Abdominal pain (43–47%) [3]
Constipation (10–20%) [2]
Diarrhea (28–31%) [8]
Dyspepsia (25%) [3]
Gastric obstruction [2]
Nausea (64–75%) [14]
Vomiting (32–43%) [10]

Respiratory
Cough (21%) [2]
Dyspnea (10–20%)
Nasopharyngitis (26–43%)
Pharyngitis (43%)
Pulmonary embolism (<10%)
Upper respiratory tract infection (26–43%)

Endocrine/Metabolic
ALT increased [2]
Appetite decreased (22–25%) [4]
Creatine phosphokinase increased (26–30%)
Hyperglycemia (<10%)
Hypomagnesemia (<10%)

Genitourinary
Dysuria (<10%)
Urinary incontinence (<10%)
Urinary tract infection (10–20%)

Hematologic
Anemia (25–34%) [18]
Febrile neutropenia [2]
Leukopenia (<10%) [3]
Lymphopenia (56%)
Myelodysplastic syndrome [2]
Myeloid leukemia [2]
Neutropenia (25–32%) [12]
Thrombocytopenia (26–30%) [8]

Other
Adverse effects [5]
Death [3]

OLARATUMAB

Trade name: Lartruvo (Lilly)
Indications: Treatment of adult patients with soft tissue sarcoma (with doxorubicin) with a histologic subtype for which an anthracycline-containing regimen is appropriate and which is not amenable to curative treatment with radiotherapy or surgery
Class: Monoclonal antibody, Platelet-derived growth factor receptor alpha blocking antibody
Half-life: ~11 days
Clinically important, potentially hazardous interactions with: none known
Pregnancy category: N/A (Can cause fetal harm)
Important contra-indications noted in the prescribing guidelines for: the elderly; nursing mothers; pediatric patients
Note: See separate entry for doxorubicin.

Hair
Alopecia (52%)

Mucosal
Mucositis (53%) [3]

Central Nervous System
Anxiety (11%)
Headache (20%)
Neurotoxicity (22%)

Neuromuscular/Skeletal
Asthenia (fatigue) (64%) [2]
Bone or joint pain (64%)

Gastrointestinal/Hepatic
Abdominal pain (23%)
Diarrhea (34%) [4]
Nausea (73%) [3]
Vomiting (45%) [2]

Endocrine/Metabolic
ALP increased (16%)
Appetite decreased (31%)
AST increased [2]
Hyperglycemia (52%) [2]
Hypokalemia (21%)
Hypomagnesemia (16%)

Renal
Proteinuria [2]

Hematologic
Lymphopenia (77%)
Neutropenia (65%) [3]
Prothrombin time increased (33%)
Thrombocytopenia (63%)

Ocular
Xerophthalmia (11%)

Local
Infusion-related reactions (13%) [2]

OLMESARTAN

Trade names: Benicar (Sankyo), Olmetec (Daiichi Sankyo)
Indications: Hypertension
Class: Angiotensin II receptor antagonist (blocker), Antihypertensive
Half-life: ~13 hours
Clinically important, potentially hazardous interactions with: ACE inhibitors, adrenergic neurone blockers, aldesleukin, aliskiren, alprostadil, amifostine, antihypertensives, antipsychotics, anxiolytics and hypnotics, baclofen, beta blockers, calcium channel blockers, clonidine, colesevelam, corticosteroids, cyclosporine, diazoxide, diuretics, eltrombopag, eplerenone, estrogens, general anesthetics, heparins, hydralazine, levodopa, lithium, MAO inhibitors, methyldopa, methylphenidate, minoxidil, moxisylyte, moxonidine, nitrates, nitroprusside, NSAIDs, pentoxifylline, phosphodiesterase 5 inhibitors, potassium salts, quinine, rituximab, tacrolimus, tizanidine, tolvaptan, trimethoprim
Pregnancy category: D (category C in first trimester; category D in second and third trimesters)
Important contra-indications noted in the prescribing guidelines for: nursing mothers; pediatric patients
Note: Contra-indicated in patients with diabetes.
Warning: FETAL TOXICITY

Skin
Angioedema [3]
Edema [2]
Peripheral edema [2]

Cardiovascular
Hypotension [2]

Central Nervous System
Vertigo (dizziness) (3%) [8]

Neuromuscular/Skeletal
Asthenia (fatigue) [2]

Gastrointestinal/Hepatic
Diarrhea [4]
Enteropathy [20]
Gastrointestinal disorder [6]

Respiratory
Upper respiratory tract infection [2]

Endocrine/Metabolic
Hyperkalemia [3]

Other
Adverse effects [6]

OLODATEROL

Trade names: Stiolto Respimat (Boehringer Ingelheim), Striverdi Respimat (Boehringer Ingelheim)
Indications: Chronic obstructive pulmonary disease including chronic bronchitis and emphysema
Class: Beta-2 adrenergic agonist
Half-life: 8 hours
Clinically important, potentially hazardous interactions with: adrenergics, beta blockers, diuretics, MAO inhibitors, QT interval prolonging agents, steroids, tricyclic antidepressants, xanthine derivatives
Pregnancy category: C
Important contra-indications noted in the prescribing guidelines for: nursing mothers; pediatric patients
Note: Stiolto Respimat is olodaterol and tiotropium.
Warning: ASTHMA-RELATED DEATH

Skin
Rash (2%)

Cardiovascular
Extrasystoles [2]
Hypertension [3]

Central Nervous System
Fever (>2%)
Headache [4]
Vertigo (dizziness) (2%) [3]

Neuromuscular/Skeletal
Arthralgia (2%) [3]
Back pain (4%) [4]
Myalgia/Myopathy [2]

Gastrointestinal/Hepatic
Constipation (>2%)
Diarrhea (3%) [3]
Nausea [2]

Respiratory
Bronchitis (5%) [4]
COPD [2]
Cough (4%) [4]
Dyspnea [3]
Nasopharyngitis (11%) [5]
Pneumonia (>2%) [3]
Upper respiratory tract infection (8%) [4]

Genitourinary
Urinary tract infection (3%) [3]

Other
Adverse effects [2]

OMALIZUMAB

Trade name: Xolair (Genentech)
Indications: Asthma
Class: IgE-targeting monoclonal antibody, Monoclonal antibody
Half-life: 26 days
Clinically important, potentially hazardous interactions with: none known
Pregnancy category: B
Important contra-indications noted in the prescribing guidelines for: nursing mothers
Warning: ANAPHYLAXIS

Skin
Anaphylactoid reactions/Anaphylaxis [10]
Angioedema [3]
Churg-Strauss syndrome [13]
Dermatitis (2%)
Hypersensitivity [2]
Pruritus (2%)
Rash [2]
Serum sickness [2]
Serum sickness-like reaction [2]
Urticaria (7%) [4]

Central Nervous System
Headache (15%) [8]
Pain (7%)
Vertigo (dizziness) (3%)

Neuromuscular/Skeletal
Arthralgia (8%) [3]
Asthenia (fatigue) (3%) [3]
Myalgia/Myopathy [3]

Gastrointestinal/Hepatic
Abdominal pain [3]
Diarrhea [2]
Nausea [3]

Respiratory
Cough [2]
Nasopharyngitis [4]
Sinusitis (16%) [4]
Upper respiratory tract infection (20%) [5]

Local
Injection-site pain [2]
Injection-site reactions (45%) [8]

Other
Adverse effects [7]
Infection [2]

OMBITASVIR/ PARITAPREVIR/ RITONAVIR

Trade names: Technivie (AbbVie), Viekira Pak (AbbVie), Viekirax (AbbVie)
Indications: Genotype 4 chronic hepatitis C virus infection in patients without cirrhosis (in combination with ribavirin)
Class: CYP3A4 inhibitor (ritonavir), Direct-acting antiviral, Hepatitis C virus NS3/4A protease inhibitor (paritaprevir), Hepatitis C virus NS5A inhibitor (ombitasvir)
Half-life: 21–25 hours (ombitasvir); 6 hours (paritaprevir); 4 hours (ritonavir)
Clinically important, potentially hazardous interactions with: atazanavir, carbamazepine, cisapride, colchicine, dihydroergotamine, dronedarone, efavirenz, ergotamine, ethinyl estradiol-containing medications, lopinavir, lovastatin, lurasidone, methylergonovine, midazolam, midostaurin, neratinib, phenobarbital, phenytoin, pimozide, ranolazine, rifampin, rilpivirine, salmeterol, sildenafil, simvastatin, St John's wort, triazolam, voriconazole
Pregnancy category: B (pregnancy category will be X when administered with ribavirin)
Important contra-indications noted in the prescribing guidelines for: nursing mothers; pediatric patients
Note: Contra-indicated in patients with moderate or severe hepatic impairment or with known hypersensitivity to ritonavir (see separate entry). See also separate entry for ribavirin. Viekira Pak is ombitasvir/paritaprevir/ritonavir co-packaged with dasabuvir.

Skin
Dermatitis (<5%)
Eczema (<5%)
Erythema (<5%)
Exfoliative dermatitis (<5%)
Photosensitivity (<5%)
Pruritus (5%) [9]
Psoriasis (<5%)
Rash (<5%) [4]
Ulcerations (<5%)
Urticaria (<5%)
Xerosis [2]

Central Nervous System
Headache [19]
Insomnia (5%) [13]
Irritability [3]
Vertigo (dizziness) [2]

Neuromuscular/Skeletal
Arthralgia [2]
Asthenia (fatigue) (7–25%) [19]
Myalgia/Myopathy [2]

Gastrointestinal/Hepatic
Diarrhea [11]
Nausea (9%) [15]
Vomiting [2]

Respiratory
Cough [3]
Dyspnea [3]
Nasopharyngitis [2]

Endocrine/Metabolic
Acidosis [2]
ALT increased [4]
AST increased [4]

Hematologic
Anemia [8]
Hemoglobin decreased [2]

Other
Adverse effects [3]
Death [2]

OMEGA-3 FATTY ACIDS

Family: N/A
Scientific names: *docosahexaenoic acid (DHA), eicosapentaenoic acid (EPA), Lovaza (GSK), Omega-3 fatty acids, Omtryg*
Indications: Albuminuria, anorexia nervosa, hypertension, lupus erythematosus, macular degeneration, osteoarthritis, otitis media, psoriasis
Class: Anti-inflammatory, Lipid regulator
Half-life: N/A
Clinically important, potentially hazardous interactions with: abciximab, clopidogrel

Pregnancy category: C
Important contra-indications noted in the prescribing guidelines for: pediatric patients
Note: More than 25 mL or 3 g per day can increase the risk of bleeding. Fish oils contain a significant amount of vitamins A and D and high doses may be toxic.

Central Nervous System
Dysgeusia (taste perversion) (4%) [4]

Gastrointestinal/Hepatic
Diarrhea [4]
Dyspepsia (3%)
Eructation (belching) (4%)
Nausea [2]

Other
Adverse effects [3]

OMEPRAZOLE

Trade names: Prilosec (AstraZeneca), Yosprala (Aralez)
Indications: Duodenal ulcer, gastric ulcer, gastroesophageal reflux disease (GERD), erosive esophagitis
Class: CYP1A2 inducer, Proton pump inhibitor (PPI)
Half-life: 0.5–1 hour
Clinically important, potentially hazardous interactions with: amoxicillin, atazanavir, bendamustine, benzodiazepines, cilostazol, clarithromycin, clobazam, clopidogrel, clozapine, coumarins, cyclosporine, dasatinib, delavirdine, diazepam, digoxin, disulfiram, enzalutamide, erlotinib, escitalopram, itraconazole, ketoconazole, lapatinib, letermovir, methotrexate, nelfinavir, phenytoin, posaconazole, prednisone, raltegravir, rilpivirine, saquinavir, sofosbuvir & velpatasvir, St John's wort, tacrolimus, tipranavir, ulipristal, voriconazole, warfarin
Pregnancy category: C
Important contra-indications noted in the prescribing guidelines for: nursing mothers; pediatric patients
Note: Yosprala is omeprazole and aspirin.

Skin
AGEP [2]
Anaphylactoid reactions/Anaphylaxis [7]
Angioedema [5]
Baboon syndrome (SDRIFE) [2]
Bullous pemphigoid [2]
Contact dermatitis [2]
Eczema [2]
Edema (<10%) [2]
Erythroderma [2]
Exfoliative dermatitis [3]
Hypersensitivity [2]
Lichen planus [2]
Lichen spinulosus [2]
Lichenoid eruption [2]
Lupus erythematosus [5]
Pemphigus (exacerbation) [2]
Peripheral edema [2]
Pruritus (<10%) [8]
Rash (2%) [6]
Toxic epidermal necrolysis [5]
Urticaria (<10%) [9]
Vasculitis [2]
Xerosis [2]

Hair
Alopecia [2]

Mucosal
Oral candidiasis [3]
Xerostomia (<10%) [2]

Central Nervous System
Anorexia [3]
Dysgeusia (taste perversion) (<10%) [4]
Headache (7%) [2]
Paresthesias [2]
Somnolence (drowsiness) [2]
Vertigo (dizziness) (2%)

Neuromuscular/Skeletal
Asthenia (fatigue) [2]
Myalgia/Myopathy (<10%)
Rhabdomyolysis [2]

Gastrointestinal/Hepatic
Abdominal distension [2]
Abdominal pain (5%) [4]
Constipation [3]
Diarrhea (4%) [9]
Flatulence (3%)
Hepatitis [4]
Hepatotoxicity [3]
Nausea (4%) [7]
Pancreatitis [2]
Vomiting (3%) [6]

Respiratory
Cough [2]
Upper respiratory tract infection (2%)

Endocrine/Metabolic
Gynecomastia [11]
Hypomagnesemia [7]

Renal
Nephrotoxicity [9]

Hematologic
Agranulocytosis [3]
Hemolytic anemia [2]
Leukopenia [3]
Neutropenia [3]

Ocular
Visual disturbances [2]

Other
Adverse effects [9]

ONDANSETRON

Trade names: Zofran (GSK), Zuplenz (Par)
Indications: Nausea and vomiting
Class: 5-HT3 antagonist, Antiemetic, Serotonin type 3 receptor antagonist
Half-life: 3–6 hours
Clinically important, potentially hazardous interactions with: apomorphine, carbamazepine, phenytoin, ribociclib, rifampin, tramadol
Pregnancy category: B
Important contra-indications noted in the prescribing guidelines for: nursing mothers; pediatric patients

---

Skin
Anaphylactoid reactions/Anaphylaxis [5]
Fixed eruption [2]
Flushing [2]
Pruritus (5%)

Mucosal
Sialopenia (<5%)
Xerostomia (<10%) [3]

Cardiovascular
Bradycardia [2]
Hypotension [3]
Myocardial ischemia [2]
QT prolongation [12]
Torsades de pointes [3]
Ventricular tachycardia [2]

Central Nervous System
Anxiety (6%)
Chills (5–10%)
Fever (2–8%)
Headache (17–25%) [15]
Paresthesias (2%)
Seizures [3]
Somnolence (drowsiness) (8%) [5]
Vertigo (dizziness) (4–7%) [9]

Neuromuscular/Skeletal
Asthenia (fatigue) (9–13%)

Gastrointestinal/Hepatic
Abdominal pain [2]
Constipation (6–11%) [7]
Diarrhea (8–16%) [3]

Respiratory
Hypoxia (9%)

Endocrine/Metabolic
ALT increased [2]

Local
Injection-site reactions (4%)

Other
Adverse effects [3]
Death [2]
Hiccups [2]

ORAL CONTRACEPTIVES

Trade names: Alesse (Wyeth), Aviane (Barr), Brevicon (Watson), Demulen (Pfizer), Desogen (Organon), Estrostep (Pfizer), Evra (Johnson & Johnson), Levlen (Bayer), Levlite (Bayer), Levora (Watson), Lo/Ovral (Wyeth), Loestrin (Barr), Lunelle (Pfizer), Mircette (Organon), Modicon (Ortho), Necon (Watson), Nordette (Monarch), Norinyl (Watson), Ortho Tri-Cyclen (Ortho-McNeil), Ortho-Cept (Ortho-McNeil), Ortho-Cyclen (Ortho-McNeil), Ortho-Novum (Ortho-McNeil), Ovcon (Warner Chilcott), Ovral (Wyeth), Tri-Levlen (Bayer), Tri-Norinyl (Watson), Triphasil (Wyeth), Trivora (Watson), Yasmin (Bayer), Yaz (Bayer), Zovia (Watson)
Indications: Prevention of pregnancy
Class: Hormone
Half-life: N/A
Clinically important, potentially hazardous interactions with: aminophylline, amprenavir, anticonvulsants, aprepitant, atazanavir, atorvastatin, beclomethasone, bexarotene,

bosentan, budesonide, cigarette smoking, danazol, doxycycline, efavirenz, eslicarbazepine, exenatide, flucloxacillin, flunisolide, fluticasone propionate, glecaprevir & pibrentasvir, hydrocortisone, insulin aspart, insulin degludec, insulin detemir, insulin glargine, insulin glulisine, isotretinoin, lamotrigine, lomitapide, lymecycline, metformin, methylprednisolone, mifepristone, modafinil, naratriptan, nelfinavir, oxcarbazepine, perampanel, prednisolone, prednisone, rifabutin, rifampin, ritonavir, roflumilast, selegiline, St John's wort, teriflunomide, tigecycline, triamcinolone, troleandomycin, tuberculostatics, ursodiol, zolmitriptan
Warning: CIGARETTE SMOKING AND SERIOUS CARDIOVASCULAR EVENTS

Skin
- Acneform eruption [17]
- Angioedema [4]
- Candidiasis [9]
- Chloasma [13]
- Erythema multiforme [2]
- Erythema nodosum [18]
- Exanthems [2]
- Herpes gestationis [3]
- Lupus erythematosus [29]
- Melanoma [5]
- Melasma [8]
- Perioral dermatitis [8]
- Photosensitivity [12]
- Pigmentation [18]
- Pruritus [5]
- Purpura [3]
- Seborrhea [3]
- Spider angioma [2]
- Sweet's syndrome [2]
- Telangiectasia [6]
- Urticaria [2]

Hair
- Alopecia [19]
- Alopecia areata [4]
- Hirsutism [12]

Mucosal
- Gingival hyperplasia/hypertrophy [2]

Cardiovascular
- Thrombophlebitis [2]
- Venous thromboembolism [6]

Central Nervous System
- Chorea [2]
- Depression [2]
- Headache [3]

Gastrointestinal/Hepatic
- Colitis [3]
- Nausea [4]

Endocrine/Metabolic
- Acute intermittent porphyria [5]
- Galactorrhea [2]
- Mastodynia [3]
- Porphyria cutanea tarda [28]
- Porphyria variegata [2]

Genitourinary
- Vaginal bleeding [4]

Local
- Application-site reactions (92%) [2]

Other
- Adverse effects [3]

ORITAVANCIN

Trade name: Orbactiv (Medicines Co)
Indications: Acute bacterial skin and skin structure infections caused or suspected to be caused by susceptible isolates of designated Gram-positive microorganisms
Class: Antibiotic, lipoglycopeptide
Half-life: 245 hours
Clinically important, potentially hazardous interactions with: warfarin
Pregnancy category: C
Important contra-indications noted in the prescribing guidelines for: nursing mothers; pediatric patients

---

Skin
- Abscess (4%) [3]
- Angioedema (<2%)
- Cellulitis [4]
- Erythema multiforme (<2%)
- Hypersensitivity (<2%)
- Leukocytoclastic vasculitis (<2%)
- Pruritus (<2%) [3]
- Rash (<2%)
- Urticaria (<2%)

Cardiovascular
- Phlebitis [2]
- Tachycardia (3%)

Central Nervous System
- Fever [4]
- Headache (7%) [7]
- Vertigo (dizziness) (3%) [4]

Neuromuscular/Skeletal
- Myalgia/Myopathy (<2%)
- Osteomyelitis (<2%)

Gastrointestinal/Hepatic
- Constipation [5]
- Diarrhea (4%) [6]
- Nausea (10%) [8]
- Vomiting (5%) [6]

Respiratory
- Bronchospasm (<2%)
- Wheezing (<2%)

Endocrine/Metabolic
- ALT increased (3%) [4]
- AST increased (2%) [2]
- Hyperuricemia (<2%)
- Hypoglycemia (<2%)

Hematologic
- Anemia (<2%)
- Eosinophilia (<2%)

Local
- Infusion-site reactions (2%) [3]
- Injection-site extravasation [3]
- Injection-site phlebitis [3]
- Injection-site reactions [2]

ORLISTAT

Trade names: Alli (GSK), Xenical (Roche)
Indications: Obesity, weight reduction
Class: Lipase inhibitor
Half-life: 1–2 hours
Clinically important, potentially hazardous interactions with: acarbose, amiodarone, antiepileptics, coumarins, cyclosporine, ergocalciferol, ethosuximide, lacosamide, levothyroxine, oxcarbazepine, paricalcitol, phytonadione, tiagabine, vigabatrin, vitamin A, vitamin E, warfarin
Pregnancy category: B
Important contra-indications noted in the prescribing guidelines for: nursing mothers; pediatric patients
Note: Contra-indicated in organ transplant recipients. Orlistat interferes with the medicines used to prevent transplant rejection.

Skin
- Lichenoid eruption [2]
- Peripheral edema (3%)
- Rash (4%)
- Xerosis (2%)

Mucosal
- Gingivitis (2–4%)

Central Nervous System
- Anxiety (3–5%)
- Depression (3%)
- Headache (31%) [2]
- Sleep related disorder (4%)
- Vertigo (dizziness) (5%)

Neuromuscular/Skeletal
- Arthralgia (5%)
- Asthenia (fatigue) (3–7%)
- Back pain (14%)
- Bone or joint pain (2%)
- Myalgia/Myopathy (4%)
- Tendinitis (2%)

Gastrointestinal/Hepatic
- Abdominal pain (26%) [4]
- Cholelithiasis (gallstones) (3%)
- Defecation (increased) (3–11%) [3]
- Fecal incontinence (2–8%) [2]
- Fecal urgency (3–23%) [2]
- Flatulence (with discharge) (2–24%) [3]
- Hepatic failure [2]
- Hepatitis [3]
- Hepatotoxicity [5]
- Nausea (4–8%)
- Pancreatitis [5]
- Vomiting (4%)

Respiratory
- Influenza (40%)
- Upper respiratory tract infection (26–38%) [2]

Endocrine/Metabolic
- Hypoglycemia (in diabetic patients) [2]
- Menstrual irregularities (10%)

Genitourinary
- Urinary tract infection (6–8%)
- Vaginitis (3–4%)

Renal
- Nephrotoxicity [11]
- Renal failure [2]

Otic
Otitis media (3–4%)

Other
Adverse effects [7]
Tooth disorder (3–4%)

OSELTAMIVIR

Trade name: Tamiflu (Roche)
Indications: Influenza infection
Class: Antiviral, Neuraminidase inhibitor
Half-life: 6–10 hours
Clinically important, potentially hazardous interactions with: none known
Pregnancy category: C

Skin
Rash [5]
Toxic epidermal necrolysis [2]

Central Nervous System
Delirium [5]
Hallucinations [3]
Headache [2]
Insomnia [2]
Neuropsychiatric disturbances [3]
Neurotoxicity [5]
Seizures [2]
Suicidal ideation [2]

Gastrointestinal/Hepatic
Abdominal pain (2–5%) [2]
Diarrhea (<3%) [9]
Hemorrhagic colitis [5]
Nausea (4–10%) [16]
Vomiting (2–15%) [17]

Respiratory
Respiratory failure [2]
Upper respiratory tract infection [2]

Hematologic
Thrombocytopenia [2]

Other
Adverse effects [7]

OSIMERTINIB

Trade name: Tagrisso (AstraZeneca)
Indications: Metastatic epidermal growth factor receptor T790M mutation-positive non-small cell lung cancer
Class: Kinase inhibitor
Half-life: 48 hours
Clinically important, potentially hazardous interactions with: carbamazepine, cyclosporine, ergot alkaloids, fentanyl, itraconazole, nefazodone, phenytoin, quinidine, rifampin, ritonavir, St John's wort, strong CYP3A inhibitors or inducers, telithromycin
Pregnancy category: N/A (Can cause fetal harm)
Important contra-indications noted in the prescribing guidelines for: nursing mothers; pediatric patients

---

Skin
Rash (41%) [9]
Xerosis (31%) [4]

Nails
Nail toxicity (25%) [2]
Paronychia [4]

Mucosal
Stomatitis (12%)

Cardiovascular
QT prolongation (3%) [2]
Venous thromboembolism (7%)

Central Nervous System
Cerebrovascular accident (3%)
Headache (10%)

Neuromuscular/Skeletal
Asthenia (fatigue) (14%) [3]
Back pain (13%)

Gastrointestinal/Hepatic
Constipation (15%)
Diarrhea (42%) [9]
Nausea (17%) [2]

Respiratory
Cough (14%)
Dyspnea [2]
Pneumonia (4%)
Pneumonitis (3%) [2]
Pulmonary toxicity [5]

Endocrine/Metabolic
Appetite decreased (16%) [2]
Hypermagnesemia (20%)
Hyponatremia (26%)

Hematologic
Anemia (44%)
Lymphopenia (63%)
Neutropenia (33%)
Thrombocytopenia (54%)

Ocular
Ocular adverse effects (18%)

Other
Adverse effects [2]

OSPEMIFENE

Trade name: Osphena (Shionogi)
Indications: Dyspareunia due to menopausal vulvar and vaginal atrophy
Class: Estrogen agonist, Estrogen antagonist, Selective estrogen receptor modulator (SERM)
Half-life: 26 hours
Clinically important, potentially hazardous interactions with: fluconazole, ketoconazole, other estrogen agonists or antagonists, rifampin
Pregnancy category: X
Important contra-indications noted in the prescribing guidelines for: nursing mothers; pediatric patients
Note: Contra-indicated in patients with undiagnosed abnormal genital bleeding, known or suspected estrogen-dependent neoplasia, active DVT or pulmonary embolism, or active arterial thromboembolic disease.
Warning: ENDOMETRIAL CANCER AND CARDIOVASCULAR DISORDERS

Skin
Hot flashes (8%) [8]
Hyperhidrosis (2%)

Neuromuscular/Skeletal
Muscle spasm (3%)

Genitourinary
Urinary tract infection [3]
Vaginal discharge (4%)

OXACILLIN

Indications: Various infections caused by susceptible organisms
Class: Antibiotic, penicillin
Half-life: 23–60 minutes
Clinically important, potentially hazardous interactions with: anticoagulants, cyclosporine, demeclocycline, doxycycline, imipenem/cilastatin, methotrexate, minocycline, oxytetracycline, tetracycline
Pregnancy category: B
Important contra-indications noted in the prescribing guidelines for: the elderly; nursing mothers; pediatric patients

---

Skin
Exanthems [2]
Rash (<22%)

Other
Adverse effects [2]

OXALIPLATIN

Trade name: Eloxatin (Sanofi-Aventis)
Indications: Metastatic carcinoma of the colon or rectum (in combination with fluorouracil/leucovorin (FOLFOX))
Class: Alkylating agent, Antineoplastic
Half-life: 391 hours
Clinically important, potentially hazardous interactions with: aminoglycosides, BCG vaccine, capreomycin, cardiac glycosides, clozapine, denosumab, diuretics, leflunomide, natalizumab, pimecrolimus, polymyxins, sipuleucel-T, tacrolimus, taxanes, topotecan, trastuzumab, vaccines, vitamin K antagonists
Pregnancy category: D
Important contra-indications noted in the prescribing guidelines for: nursing mothers; pediatric patients
Warning: ANAPHYLACTIC REACTIONS

Skin
Anaphylactoid reactions/Anaphylaxis [11]
Diaphoresis (5%) [2]
Edema (13–15%) [2]
Erythema [4]
Exanthems (2–5%)
Flushing (2–7%) [2]
Hand-foot syndrome (7–13%) [14]
Hot flashes (2–5%)
Hypersensitivity (12%) [29]
Peripheral edema (11%)
Pruritus (6%) [5]
Purpura (2–5%)
Radiation recall dermatitis [3]
Rash (5–11%) [11]
Thrombocytopenic purpura [2]
Toxicity [3]
Urticaria [2]

Xerosis (6%)

Hair

Alopecia (3–38%) [4]

Mucosal

Epistaxis (nosebleed) (<16%)
Gingivitis (2–5%)
Mucositis (10%) [5]
Oral mucositis [2]
Stomatitis (32–42%) [4]
Xerostomia (5%)

Cardiovascular

Chest pain (4%) [2]
Extravasation [2]
Hypertension [6]
Hypotension (5%) [2]
Tachycardia [3]
Thromboembolism (4%)
Vascular trauma [2]

Central Nervous System

Anorexia (13–35%) [5]
Anxiety (5%)
Chills [3]
Depression (9%)
Dysesthesia (often cold-induced or cold-exacerbated) (38%) [7]
Dysgeusia (taste perversion) (<14%)
Dysphasia (5%)
Fever (16–27%) [9]
Headache (7–13%)
Hyperalgesia [2]
Hypoesthesia [2]
Insomnia (4–13%)
Leukoencephalopathy [4]
Neurotoxicity (48%) [37]
Pain (5–9%)
Paresthesias (77%) [7]
Peripheral neuropathy (92%) [42]
Rigors (8%)
Sensory disturbances (8%)
Vertigo (dizziness) (7–8%)

Neuromuscular/Skeletal

Arthralgia (5–10%)
Asthenia (fatigue) (44–70%) [22]
Ataxia [2]
Back pain (11–16%)
Myalgia/Myopathy (14%)

Gastrointestinal/Hepatic

Abdominal pain (18–31%) [4]
Constipation (22–32%) [2]
Diarrhea (44–56%) [44]
Dyspepsia (8–12%)
Flatulence (6–9%)
Gastroesophageal reflux (3%)
Hepatotoxicity [8]
Nausea (59–74%) [24]
Sinusoidal obstruction syndrome [2]
Vomiting (27–47%) [19]

Respiratory

Cough (9–35%)
Dyspnea (5–18%) [2]
Pharyngitis (10%)
Pneumonia [2]
Pulmonary embolism [2]
Pulmonary fibrosis [2]
Pulmonary toxicity [2]
Rhinitis (4–10%)
Upper respiratory tract infection (4%)

Endocrine/Metabolic

ALP increased (42%)
ALT increased (57%)
AST increased [2]
Dehydration (9%)
Hyperglycemia (14%)
Hypoalbuminemia (8%)
Hypocalcemia (7%)
Hypokalemia (11%)
Hyponatremia (8%) [2]
Serum creatinine increased (4%) [2]
Weight gain (10%)
Weight loss (11%)

Genitourinary

Urinary frequency (5%)

Renal

Nephrotoxicity [3]
Proteinuria [2]

Hematologic

Anemia (27–76%) [25]
Febrile neutropenia (<4%) [10]
Hemolytic anemia [4]
Leukocytopenia [2]
Leukopenia (34–85%) [14]
Lymphopenia (6%)
Myelosuppression [4]
Neutropenia (25–81%) [59]
Thrombocytopenia (20–77%) [41]
Thrombosis (6%)

Ocular

Abnormal vision (5%)
Conjunctivitis (9%)
Epiphora [3]
Lacrimation (4–9%)
Vision blurred [2]

Local

Injection-site reactions (5–11%) [2]

Other

Adverse effects [3]
Allergic reactions (3%) [4]
Death [4]
Hiccups (5%)
Infection (8–25%) [3]

OXAPROZIN

Trade name: Daypro (Pfizer)
Indications: Arthritis
Class: Non-steroidal anti-inflammatory (NSAID)
Half-life: 42–50 hours
Clinically important, potentially hazardous interactions with: methotrexate
Pregnancy category: C
Important contra-indications noted in the prescribing guidelines for: nursing mothers; pediatric patients
Note: NSAIDs may cause an increased risk of serious cardiovascular and gastrointestinal adverse events, which can be fatal. This risk may increase with duration of use.

Skin

Pruritus (<10%)
Rash (>10%) [2]
Stevens-Johnson syndrome [2]
Toxic epidermal necrolysis [4]

Gastrointestinal/Hepatic

Hepatotoxicity [3]

Endocrine/Metabolic

Pseudoporphyria [3]

Renal

Nephrotoxicity [2]

Other

Adverse effects [3]

OXAZEPAM

Trade name: Serax (Mayne)
Indications: Anxiety, depression
Class: Benzodiazepine
Half-life: 3–6 hours
Clinically important, potentially hazardous interactions with: amprenavir, chlorpheniramine, clarithromycin, efavirenz, esomeprazole, imatinib, nelfinavir
Pregnancy category: D
Important contra-indications noted in the prescribing guidelines for: pediatric patients

---

Skin

Dermatitis (<10%)
Diaphoresis (>10%)
Rash (>10%)

Mucosal

Sialopenia (>10%)
Sialorrhea (<10%)
Xerostomia (>10%)

OXCARBAZEPINE

Trade names: Oxtellar XR (Supernus), Trileptal (Novartis)
Indications: Partial epileptic seizures
Class: Anticonvulsant, CYP3A4 inducer, Mood stabilizer
Half-life: 1–2.5 hours
Clinically important, potentially hazardous interactions with: alcohol, antipsychotics, bictegravir/emtricitabine/tenofovir alafenamide, carbamazepine, chloroquine, clopidogrel, cobicistat/elvitegravir/emtricitabine/tenofovir alafenamide, cobicistat/elvitegravir/emtricitabine/tenofovir disoproxil, cyclosporine, CYP3A4 substrates, dronedarone, emtricitabine/rilpivirine/tenofovir alafenamide, eslicarbazepine, everolimus, exemestane, guanfacine, hydroxychloroquine, imatinib, ixabepilone, ledipasvir & sofosbuvir, levomepromazine, levonorgestrel, MAO inhibitors, maraviroc, mefloquine, nifedipine, nilotinib, nisoldipine, oral contraceptives, orlistat, pazopanib, perampanel, phenobarbital, phenytoin, praziquantel, ranolazine, rilpivirine, risperidone, romidepsin, saxagliptin, selegiline, simeprevir, sofosbuvir, sofosbuvir & velpatasvir, sofosbuvir/velpatasvir/voxilaprevir, sorafenib, SSRIs, St John's wort, tadalafil, tenofovir alafenamide, thiazide diuretics, tolvaptan, tricyclic antidepressants, ulipristal, valproic acid, zuclopenthixol

Pregnancy category: C
Important contra-indications noted in the prescribing guidelines for: nursing mothers; pediatric patients

---

Skin
Acneform eruption (<2%)
Diaphoresis (3%)
DRESS syndrome [6]
Ecchymoses (4%)
Edema (<2%)
Exanthems [4]
Hot flashes (<2%)
Hyperhidrosis (3%)
Hypersensitivity [6]
Lymphadenopathy (2%)
Purpura (2%)
Rash (<6%) [11]
Stevens-Johnson syndrome [11]
Toxic epidermal necrolysis [4]

Mucosal
Epistaxis (nosebleed) (4%)
Rectal hemorrhage (2%)
Xerostomia (3%)

Cardiovascular
Chest pain (2%)
Hypotension (<3%)

Central Nervous System
Agitation (<2%)
Amnesia (4%)
Anorexia (3–5%)
Anxiety (5–7%)
Coma [2]
Confusion (<7%)
Dysgeusia (taste perversion) (5%)
Emotional lability (2–3%)
Fever (3%)
Gait instability (5–17%)
Headache (13–32%) [8]
Hyperesthesia (3%)
Hypoesthesia (<3%)
Incoordination (<4%)
Insomnia (2–6%)
Nervousness (2–4%)
Seizures (2–5%) [5]
Somnolence (drowsiness) (5–36%) [5]
Speech disorder (<3%)
Tremor (3–16%) [2]
Vertigo (dizziness) (3–49%) [12]

Neuromuscular/Skeletal
Asthenia (fatigue) (3–15%) [5]
Ataxia (<31%) [2]
Back pain (4%)
Myoclonus [3]
Osteoporosis [2]

Gastrointestinal/Hepatic
Abdominal pain (3–13%)
Constipation (2–6%)
Diarrhea (5–7%)
Dyspepsia (5–6%)
Gastritis (<2%)
Nausea (15–29%) [8]
Vomiting (13–36%) [4]

Respiratory
Cough (5%)
Pharyngitis (3%)
Pneumonia (2%)
Rhinitis (2–5%)
Sinusitis (4%)
Upper respiratory tract infection (5–10%)

Endocrine/Metabolic
Hyponatremia (<5%) [17]
SIADH [3]
Weight gain (<2%)

Genitourinary
Ejaculatory dysfunction [3]
Urinary frequency (<2%)
Urinary tract infection (<5%)
Vaginitis (2%)

Hematologic
Leukopenia [3]
Thrombocytopenia [2]

Otic
Ear pain (<2%)

Ocular
Abnormal vision (2–14%)
Accommodation disorder (<3%)
Diplopia (<40%) [10]
Nystagmus (2–26%)

Other
Adverse effects [8]
Allergic reactions (2%) [3]
Dipsia (thirst) (2%)
Infection (2–7%)
Teratogenicity [3]
Toothache (2%)

OXYBUTYNIN

Trade names: Cystrin (Sanofi-Aventis), Ditropan (Ortho-McNeil), Lyrinel (Janssen-Cilag)
Indications: Neurogenic bladder, urinary incontinence, palmar and axillary hyperhidrosis
Class: Anticholinergic, Antimuscarinic, Muscarinic antagonist
Half-life: 2–3 hours
Clinically important, potentially hazardous interactions with: alcohol, anticholinergics, antihistamines, arbutamine, cannabinoids, clozapine, conivaptan, diphenoxylate, disopyramide, domperidone, haloperidol, ketoconazole, levodopa, MAO inhibitors, memantine, metoclopramide, nefopam, nitrates, parasympathomimetics, pramlintide, secretin, tricyclic antidepressants
Pregnancy category: B
Important contra-indications noted in the prescribing guidelines for: nursing mothers
Note: Contra-indicated in patients with urinary retention, gastric retention and other severe decreased gastrointestinal motility conditions, uncontrolled narrow-angle glaucoma and in patients who are at risk for these conditions.

Skin
Hot flashes (<10%)
Pruritus [2]
Rash (<10%)

Mucosal
Sialopenia [2]
Xerostomia (71%) [31]

Central Nervous System
Cognitive impairment [4]
Headache (8%) [2]
Insomnia (6%)
Nervousness (7%)
Somnolence (drowsiness) (14%)
Vertigo (dizziness) (17%) [2]

Gastrointestinal/Hepatic
Constipation (15%) [4]
Dyspepsia (6%)
Nausea [3]

Genitourinary
Urinary retention (6%)
Urinary tract infection (7%)

Ocular
Vision blurred (10%)

Other
Adverse effects [4]
Allergic reactions [2]

OXYCODONE

Trade names: OxyContin (Purdue), OxyIR (Purdue), Percocet (Endo), Roxicodone (aaiPharma), Targiniq (Purdue), Troxyca (Pfizer), Tylox (Ortho-McNeil), Xtampza ER (Collegium)
Indications: Pain
Class: Opiate agonist
Half-life: 4.6 hours
Clinically important, potentially hazardous interactions with: cimetidine, clonazepam, telithromycin, voriconazole
Pregnancy category: B
Important contra-indications noted in the prescribing guidelines for: the elderly; nursing mothers; pediatric patients
Note: Oxycodone is often combined with acetaminophen (Percocet, Roxicet, Tylox) or aspirin (Percodan, Roxiprin); Targiniq is oxycodone and naloxone; Troxyca is oxycodone and naltrexone. Contra-indicated in patients with significant respiratory depression, acute or severe bronchial asthma, or with known or suspected gastrointestinal obstruction, including paralytic ileus.
Warning: ADDICTION, ABUSE and MISUSE; LIFETHREATENING RESPIRATORY DEPRESSION; ACCIDENTAL INGESTION; NEONATAL OPIOID WITHDRAWAL SYNDROME; and CYTOCHROME P450 3A4 INTERACTION

Skin
Pruritus [8]

Mucosal
Xerostomia [2]

Cardiovascular
Bradycardia [2]

Central Nervous System
Fever [2]
Headache [6]
Insomnia [3]
Sedation [2]
Serotonin syndrome [2]
Somnolence (drowsiness) [14]
Vertigo (dizziness) [9]

Neuromuscular/Skeletal
Asthenia (fatigue) [9]

Gastrointestinal/Hepatic
- Abdominal pain [3]
- Constipation [14]
- Diarrhea [2]
- Ileus [2]
- Nausea [25]
- Vomiting [20]

Ocular
- Hallucinations, visual [2]

Local
- Injection-site pain (<10%)

Other
- Adverse effects [10]
- Death [3]
- Tooth disorder [2]

OXYMETAZOLINE

Trade name: Rhofade (Allergan)
Indications: Persistant facial erythema associated with rosacea
Class: Alpha adrenoceptor agonist
Half-life: N/A
Clinically important, potentially hazardous interactions with: none known
Pregnancy category: N/A (No available data to inform drug-associated risk)
Important contra-indications noted in the prescribing guidelines for: nursing mothers; pediatric patients
Note: For topical use only. See separate entry for tetracaine & oxymetazoline as intranasal formulation.
Oxymetazoline is also available as an ophthalmic solution and a nasal decongestant in over-the-counter products.

Skin
- Rosacea (exacerbation) (<3%)

Local
- Application-site dermatitis (<3%) [3]
- Application-site erythema [2]
- Application-site pain (<2%) [2]
- Application-site pruritus (<2%) [2]

OXYMORPHONE

Trade name: Opana (Endo)
Indications: Pain (moderate to severe)
Class: Analgesic, Opiate agonist
Half-life: 7–9 hours
Clinically important, potentially hazardous interactions with: anticholinergics, buprenorphine, butorphanol, cimetidine, CNS depressants, MAO inhibitors, nalbuphine, pentazocine
Pregnancy category: C
Important contra-indications noted in the prescribing guidelines for: the elderly; nursing mothers; pediatric patients
Note: Contra-indicated in patients with a known hypersensitivity to morphine analogs such as codeine; in patients with respiratory depression, except in monitored settings and in the presence of resuscitative equipment; in patients with acute or severe bronchial asthma or hypercarbia; in any patient who has or is suspected of having paralytic ileus; and in patients with moderate or severe hepatic impairment.

Skin
- Hyperhidrosis (<10%)
- Pruritus (8%) [2]

Mucosal
- Xerostomia (<10%)

Cardiovascular
- Hypotension (<10%)
- Tachycardia (<10%)

Central Nervous System
- Anxiety (<10%)
- Confusion (3%)
- Fever (14%)
- Headache (7%)
- Sedation (<10%)
- Somnolence (drowsiness) (9%) [2]
- Vertigo (dizziness) (7%)

Gastrointestinal/Hepatic
- Abdominal distension (<10%)
- Constipation (4%) [3]
- Flatulence (<10%)
- Nausea (19%) [4]
- Vomiting (9%) [2]

Respiratory
- Hypoxia (<10%)

Local
- Injection-site reactions (<10%)

OXYTOCIN

Trade name: Pitocin (Par)
Indications: Induction of labor
Class: Oxytocic
Half-life: N/A
Clinically important, potentially hazardous interactions with: cyclopropane, gemeprost, halothane, prostaglandins
Pregnancy category: X

Skin
- Anaphylactoid reactions/Anaphylaxis [7]

Mucosal
- Xerostomia [3]

Cardiovascular
- Bradycardia [2]

Central Nervous System
- Fever [2]
- Shivering [2]

Respiratory
- Hypoxia [2]

Genitourinary
- Urinary frequency [3]
- Uterine hyperstimulation [3]

PACLITAXEL

Trade name: Taxol (Bristol-Myers Squibb)
Indications: Breast cancer and metastatic carcinoma of the ovary
Class: Antineoplastic, Taxane
Half-life: 5–17 hours
Clinically important, potentially hazardous interactions with: atazanavir, bexarotene, buspirone, carbamazepine, cisplatin, clarithromycin, delavirdine, doxorubicin, efavirenz, eletriptan, felodipine, gadobenate, gemfibrozil, indinavir, itraconazole, ketoconazole, lapatinib, lovastatin, nefazodone, nelfinavir, repaglinide, rifampin, ritonavir, rosiglitazone, saquinavir, sildenafil, simvastatin, telithromycin, teriflunomide, thalidomide, trastuzumab, triazolam
Pregnancy category: D
Important contra-indications noted in the prescribing guidelines for: the elderly; nursing mothers; pediatric patients
Note: Studies have shown that elderly patients have an increased risk of severe myelosuppression, severe neuropathy and a higher incidence of cardiovascular events.

Skin
- Acneform eruption [6]
- Acral erythema [4]
- Anaphylactoid reactions/Anaphylaxis [3]
- Dermatitis [2]
- Desquamation (7%)
- Edema (21%) [2]
- Erythema [6]
- Exanthems [2]
- Fixed eruption [2]
- Flushing (28%) [3]
- Folliculitis [2]
- Hand–foot syndrome [18]
- Hypersensitivity (31–45%) [26]
- Lupus erythematosus [5]
- Photosensitivity [4]
- Pigmentation [3]
- Pruritus [6]
- Pustules [2]
- Radiation recall dermatitis [11]
- Rash (12%) [19]
- Recall reaction [2]
- Scleroderma [6]
- Stevens-Johnson syndrome [2]
- Toxicity [10]
- Tumor lysis syndrome [2]
- Urticaria (2–4%) [4]

Hair
- Alopecia (87–100%) [50]

Nails
- Leukonychia (Mees' lines) [2]
- Nail changes (2%) [6]
- Nail pigmentation (2%) [3]
- Onycholysis [9]
- Pyogenic granuloma [2]

Mucosal
- Epistaxis (nosebleed) [2]
- Mucosal inflammation [3]
- Mucositis (17–35%) [15]
- Oral lesions (3–8%)
- Stomatitis (2–39%) [9]

Cardiovascular
Atrial fibrillation [2]
Bradycardia (3%)
Cardiotoxicity [3]
Congestive heart failure [3]
Hypertension [16]
Hypotension (4–12%)
Myocardial infarction [2]
Tachycardia (2%)

Central Nervous System
Anorexia [8]
Dysgeusia (taste perversion) [3]
Fever [4]
Headache [2]
Insomnia [2]
Neurotoxicity [42]
Pain [9]
Paresthesias (>10%) [5]
Peripheral neuropathy (42–70%) [46]
Seizures [2]
Vertigo (dizziness) [7]

Neuromuscular/Skeletal
Arthralgia (60%) [16]
Asthenia (fatigue) (17%) [61]
Bone or joint pain [3]
Myalgia/Myopathy (19–60%) [24]

Gastrointestinal/Hepatic
Abdominal pain (>10%) [2]
Constipation [8]
Diarrhea (38%) [41]
Dyspepsia [2]
Gastrointestinal bleeding [2]
Gastrointestinal disorder [2]
Gastrointestinal perforation [5]
Hepatotoxicity [6]
Nausea (52%) [36]
Pancreatitis [4]
Vomiting [28]

Respiratory
Cough [3]
Dyspnea (2%) [4]
Pneumonia [5]
Pneumonitis [4]
Pulmonary toxicity [6]

Endocrine/Metabolic
ALP increased [2]
ALT increased [11]
Appetite decreased [5]
AST increased [8]
Hyperbilirubinemia [2]
Hyperglycemia [4]
SIADH [3]

Renal
Proteinuria [6]

Hematologic
Anemia (47%) [41]
Bleeding [3]
Febrile neutropenia [27]
Hemotoxicity [11]
Leukocytopenia [2]
Leukopenia (90%) [33]
Lymphopenia [2]
Myelosuppression [4]
Myelotoxicity [3]
Neutropenia (78–98%) [101]
Thrombocytopenia (4–20%) [32]

Ocular
Macular edema [11]
Maculopathy [2]

Local
Injection-site cellulitis (>10%)
Injection-site extravasation (>10%) [4]
Injection-site pain (>10%)
Injection-site reactions (13%) [2]

Other
Adverse effects [9]
Allergic reactions (15%) [8]
Death [14]
Infection (3–22%) [16]
Kounis syndrome [2]

PALBOCICLIB

Trade name: Ibrance (Pfizer)
Indications: Treatment of postmenopausal women with estrogen receptor (ER)-positive, human epidermal growth factor receptor 2 (HER2)-negative advanced breast cancer (in combination with letrozole)
Class: CDK4/6 inhibitor
Half-life: 29 hours
Clinically important, potentially hazardous interactions with: bosentan, carbamazepine, clarithromycin, efavirenz, etravirine, grapefruit juice, indinavir, itraconazole, ketoconazole, lopinavir, modafinil, nafcillin, nefazodone, nelfinavir, phenytoin, posaconazole, rifampin, ritonavir, saquinavir, St John's wort, telaprevir, telithromycin, verapamil, voriconazole
Pregnancy category: N/A (Can cause fetal harm)
Important contra-indications noted in the prescribing guidelines for: nursing mothers; pediatric patients

---

Skin
Peripheral edema [2]
Rash [5]

Hair
Alopecia (22%) [2]

Mucosal
Epistaxis (nosebleed) (11%) [2]
Stomatitis (25%) [5]

Central Nervous System
Fever [2]
Headache [2]
Peripheral neuropathy (13%)

Neuromuscular/Skeletal
Asthenia (fatigue) (13–41%) [12]

Gastrointestinal/Hepatic
Constipation [2]
Diarrhea (21%) [8]
Nausea (25%) [9]
Vomiting (15%) [4]

Respiratory
Dyspnea [2]
Upper respiratory tract infection (31%)

Endocrine/Metabolic
Appetite decreased (16%)

Hematologic
Anemia (35%) [11]
Febrile neutropenia [11]
Leukopenia (43%) [13]
Lymphopenia [2]
Neutropenia (75%) [27]
Thrombocytopenia (17%) [8]

Other
Adverse effects [3]
Infection [4]

PALIFERMIN

Trade name: Kepivance (Amgen)
Indications: Severe oral mucositis in cancer patients
Class: Keratinocyte growth factor
Half-life: 4.5 hours
Clinically important, potentially hazardous interactions with: heparin
Pregnancy category: C
Important contra-indications noted in the prescribing guidelines for: nursing mothers

---

Skin
Acanthosis nigricans [2]
Edema (28%) [2]
Erythema (32%) [3]
Hand–foot syndrome [3]
Pruritus (35%) [3]
Rash (62%) [7]

Mucosal
Tongue edema (17%) [3]
Tongue pigmentation (17%)

Cardiovascular
Hypertension (~12%)

Central Nervous System
Dysesthesia (12%)
Dysgeusia (taste perversion) (16%) [4]
Fever (39%)
Pain (16%)
Paresthesias (12%)

Neuromuscular/Skeletal
Arthralgia (10%)

PALIPERIDONE

Trade name: Invega (Janssen)
Indications: Schizophrenia
Class: Antipsychotic
Half-life: ~23 hours
Clinically important, potentially hazardous interactions with: ACE inhibitors, alcohol, alpha blockers, amphetamines, angiotensin II receptor antagonists, carbamazepine, CNS depressants, dopamine agonists, droperidol, general anesthetics, itraconazole, levodopa, levomepromazine, lithium, methylphenidate, metoclopramide, myleosuppressives, P-glycoprotein inhibitors or inducers, quinagolide, risperidone, tetrabenazine, valproic acid
Pregnancy category: C
Important contra-indications noted in the prescribing guidelines for: the elderly; nursing mothers; pediatric patients
Note: Invega is not recommended for patients with creatinine clearance below 10 mL/min. Paliperidone is the active metabolite of risperidone (see separate entry).

Warning: INCREASED MORTALITY IN ELDERLY PATIENTS WITH DEMENTIA-RELATED PSYCHOSIS

Skin
- Anaphylactoid reactions/Anaphylaxis (<2%)
- Edema (<2%)
- Peripheral edema [4]
- Pruritus (<2%)
- Rash (<2%)

Mucosal
- Nasal congestion (<2%)
- Sialorrhea (<6%) [2]
- Tongue edema (3%)
- Xerostomia (<4%)

Cardiovascular
- Arrhythmias (<2%)
- Atrioventricular block (<2%)
- Bradycardia (<2%)
- Bundle branch block (<3%)
- Hypertension (<2%)
- Palpitation (<2%) [2]
- Tachycardia (<14%) [6]

Central Nervous System
- Agitation (<2%) [6]
- Akathisia (3–17%) [23]
- Anxiety (2–9%) [9]
- Depression [2]
- Dysarthria (<4%) [2]
- Extrapyramidal symptoms (4–23%) [17]
- Headache (4–14%) [17]
- Insomnia (<2%) [23]
- Neuroleptic malignant syndrome [6]
- Nightmares (<2%)
- Parkinsonism [5]
- Psychosis [3]
- Schizophrenia [6]
- Sleep related disorder (2–3%)
- Somnolence (drowsiness) (6–26%) [13]
- Tardive dyskinesia [3]
- Tremor [7]
- Vertigo (dizziness) (2–6%) [3]

Neuromuscular/Skeletal
- Asthenia (fatigue) (<4%) [4]
- Bone or joint pain [2]
- Dystonia [6]
- Hyperkinesia [2]
- Rhabdomyolysis [3]

Gastrointestinal/Hepatic
- Abdominal pain (<3%)
- Constipation (4–5%) [4]
- Dyspepsia (5–6%)
- Flatulence (<2%)
- Nausea [3]
- Vomiting (3–11%)

Respiratory
- Cough (<3%)
- Nasopharyngitis (2–5%) [6]
- Pharyngolaryngeal pain (<2%)
- Pulmonary embolism [2]
- Rhinitis (<3%)

Endocrine/Metabolic
- ALT increased (<2%)
- Amenorrhea (6%) [3]
- Appetite decreased (<2%)
- Appetite increased (2–3%)
- AST increased (<2%)
- Galactorrhea (4%) [5]
- Gynecomastia (3%)
- Hyperprolactinemia [10]
- Hyponatremia [2]
- Menstrual irregularities (<2%)
- Weight gain (2–7%) [19]

Genitourinary
- Ejaculatory dysfunction (<2%)
- Erectile dysfunction [2]
- Sexual dysfunction [3]
- Urinary tract infection (<2%)

Ocular
- Vision blurred (3%)

Local
- Injection-site pain [9]

Other
- Adverse effects [7]
- Death [3]

PALIVIZUMAB

Trade name: Synagis (Medimmune)
Indications: Prophylaxis of serious lower respiratory tract disease caused by respiratory syncytial virus in pediatric patients
Class: Immunomodulator, Monoclonal antibody
Half-life: 18 days
Clinically important, potentially hazardous interactions with: none known
Pregnancy category: C

Skin
- Anaphylactoid reactions/Anaphylaxis [3]
- Rash (26%)

Central Nervous System
- Fever [2]

Local
- Injection-site bruising (<3%)
- Injection-site edema (<3%)
- Injection-site erythema [3]
- Injection-site induration (<3%)
- Injection-site pain (<9%) [2]
- Injection-site reactions [2]

PALONOSETRON

Trade name: Aloxi (MGI)
Indications: Antiemetic (for cancer chemotherapy)
Class: 5-HT3 antagonist, Antiemetic, Serotonin type 3 receptor antagonist
Half-life: 40 hours
Clinically important, potentially hazardous interactions with: none known
Pregnancy category: B
Note: See also the fixed drug combination Netupitant & Palonosetron (separate entry).

Skin
- Hot flashes (<15)
- Pruritus (8–22%)
- Rash (6%)

Central Nervous System
- Anorexia [2]
- Fever [2]
- Headache (9%) [13]
- Vertigo (dizziness) [4]

Neuromuscular/Skeletal
- Asthenia (fatigue) [4]
- Osteonecrosis (jaw) [13]

Gastrointestinal/Hepatic
- Abdominal pain [2]
- Constipation [10]
- Diarrhea [3]

Endocrine/Metabolic
- AST increased [2]

Renal
- Nephrotoxicity [3]

Other
- Hiccups [4]

PAMIDRONATE

Trade name: Aredia (Novartis)
Indications: Hypercalcemia, Paget's disease, osteogenesis imperfecta
Class: Bisphosphonate
Half-life: 1.6 hours
Clinically important, potentially hazardous interactions with: none known
Pregnancy category: D
Important contra-indications noted in the prescribing guidelines for: nursing mothers; pediatric patients

---

Skin
- Candidiasis (6%)

Cardiovascular
- Atrial fibrillation (6%)
- Hypertension (6%)
- Tachycardia (6%)

Central Nervous System
- Anorexia (26%)
- Fever (18–39%) [8]
- Headache (26%)
- Insomnia (22%)
- Somnolence (drowsiness) (6%)

Neuromuscular/Skeletal
- Arthralgia (14%) [2]
- Asthenia (fatigue) (37%) [2]
- Bone or joint pain [3]
- Fractures [3]
- Myalgia/Myopathy [3]
- Osteonecrosis [19]

Gastrointestinal/Hepatic
- Abdominal pain (23%)
- Constipation (6%)
- Dyspepsia (23%)
- Nausea (54%)
- Vomiting (36%) [2]

Respiratory
- Cough (26%)
- Flu-like syndrome [3]
- Rhinitis (6%)
- Sinusitis (16%)

Endocrine/Metabolic
- Hypocalcemia [10]
- Hypophosphatemia [2]
- Hypothyroidism (6%)

Genitourinary
- Azotemia (prerenal) (4%)

Urinary tract infection (19%)

Renal

Nephrotoxicity [11]

Hematologic

Anemia (43%)
Granulocytopenia (20%)

Ocular

Conjunctivitis [5]
Episcleritis [2]
Orbital inflammation [2]
Scleritis [4]
Uveitis [12]
Vision blurred [2]

Local

Injection-site reactions (18%)

PANDEMIC INFLUENZA VACCINE (H1N1)

Trade names: Celvapan (Baxter), Focetria (Novartis), Pandemrix (GSK), Tamiflu (Roche)
Indications: Pandemic influenza vaccine (H1N1)
Class: Vaccine
Half-life: N/A
Clinically important, potentially hazardous interactions with: none known
Pregnancy category: C
Note: This is the vaccine for swine flu.

Skin

Lymphadenopathy (<10%)

Central Nervous System

Fever [3]
Guillain–Barré syndrome [2]
Headache (>10%)
Seizures [2]

Neuromuscular/Skeletal

Asthenia (fatigue) [2]

Other

Adverse effects [4]

PANITUMUMAB

Trade name: Vectibix (Amgen)
Indications: Metastatic colorectal carcinoma progression
Class: Antineoplastic, Biologic, Epidermal growth factor receptor (EGFR) inhibitor, Monoclonal antibody
Half-life: ~7.5 days
Clinically important, potentially hazardous interactions with: none known
Pregnancy category: C
Important contra-indications noted in the prescribing guidelines for: nursing mothers; pediatric patients
Warning: DERMATOLOGIC TOXICITY and INFUSION REACTIONS

Skin

Acneform eruption (57%) [18]
Desquamation [3]
Eczema [2]
Erythema (65%) [5]
Exfoliative dermatitis (25%) [2]
Fissures (20%) [5]
Folliculitis [3]
Hand–foot syndrome [3]
Papulopustular eruption [4]
Peripheral edema (12%)
Pruritus (57%) [10]
Rash (22%) [33]
Toxicity (90%) [26]
Xerosis (10%) [12]

Hair

Alopecia [3]
Hair changes (9%) [2]

Nails

Nail changes (9–29%) [2]
Paronychia (25%) [13]

Mucosal

Mucosal inflammation (6%)
Mucositis [4]
Stomatitis (7%) [4]

Central Nervous System

Anorexia [4]
Fever [2]
Neurotoxicity [2]

Neuromuscular/Skeletal

Asthenia (fatigue) (26%) [17]

Gastrointestinal/Hepatic

Abdominal pain (25%) [3]
Constipation (21%) [4]
Diarrhea (21%) [21]
Nausea (23%) [9]
Vomiting (19%) [9]

Respiratory

Cough (14%)
Dyspnea [3]
Pulmonary embolism [3]
Pulmonary fibrosis [3]
Pulmonary toxicity [7]

Endocrine/Metabolic

Dehydration [3]
Hypocalcemia [3]
Hypokalemia [6]
Hypomagnesemia [20]

Hematologic

Anemia [2]
Febrile neutropenia [2]
Leukopenia [2]
Neutropenia [7]
Thrombocytopenia [3]

Ocular

Conjunctivitis (4%) [2]
Corneal perforation [2]
Eyelashes – hypertrichosis (6%)
Lacrimation (2%)
Ocular toxicity (15%) [2]
Trichomegaly [3]

Local

Infusion-related reactions (3%) [5]
Injection-site reactions (4%)

Other

Adverse effects [5]
Death [2]
Infection [3]

PANOBINOSTAT

Trade name: Farydak (Novartis)
Indications: Multiple myeloma (in combination with bortezomib and dexamethasone)
Class: Histone deacetylase (HDAC) inhibitor
Half-life: 37 hours
Clinically important, potentially hazardous interactions with: antiarrhythmics, QT prolonging agents, sensitive CYP2D6 substrates, strong CYP3A4 inducers
Pregnancy category: N/A (can cause fetal harm)
Important contra-indications noted in the prescribing guidelines for: the elderly; pediatric patients
Warning: FATAL AND SERIOUS TOXICITIES: SEVERE DIARRHEA AND CARDIAC TOXICITIES

Skin

Edema (<10%)
Erythema (<10%)
Lesions (<10%)
Peripheral edema (29%) [3]
Rash (<10%) [5]

Mucosal

Cheilitis (<10%)
Xerostomia (<10%)

Cardiovascular

Arrhythmias (12%)
Hypertension (<10%)
Hypotension (<10%) [2]
Orthostatic hypotension (<10%)
Palpitation (<10%)
QT prolongation [7]

Central Nervous System

Anorexia [5]
Chills (<10%)
Dysgeusia (taste perversion) (<10%) [3]
Fever (26%) [3]
Headache (<10%) [3]
Insomnia (<10%)
Peripheral neuropathy [9]
Syncope (<10%) [2]
Tremor (<10%)
Vertigo (dizziness) (<10%) [2]

Neuromuscular/Skeletal

Asthenia (fatigue) (60%) [31]
Back pain [2]
Joint disorder (<10%)

Gastrointestinal/Hepatic

Abdominal distension (<10%)
Abdominal pain (<10%) [4]
Colitis (<10%)
Constipation [5]
Diarrhea (68%) [29]
Dyspepsia (<10%) [2]
Flatulence (<10%)
Gastritis (<10%)
Nausea (36%) [18]
Vomiting (26%) [12]

Respiratory

Cough (<10%)
Dyspnea (<10%) [5]
Pneumonia [5]
Respiratory failure (<10%)
Wheezing (<10%)

Endocrine/Metabolic
ALP increased (<10%)
Appetite decreased (28%) [4]
Creatine phosphokinase increased (41%) [4]
Dehydration (<10%) [3]
Hyperbilirubinemia (21%) [3]
Hyperglycemia (<10%)
Hypermagnesemia (27%)
Hyperphosphatemia (29%)
Hyperuricemia (<10%)
Hypoalbuminemia (63%)
Hypocalcemia (67%) [2]
Hypokalemia (52%) [7]
Hypomagnesemia (<10%)
Hyponatremia (49%) [2]
Hypophosphatemia (63%) [4]
Hypothyroidism (<10%)
Weight loss (12%) [3]

Genitourinary
Urinary incontinence (<10%)

Renal
Renal failure (<10%)

Hematologic
Anemia (62%) [14]
Febrile neutropenia [2]
Leukopenia (81%) [5]
Lymphopenia (82%) [8]
Myelosuppression [5]
Neutropenia (75%) [21]
Sepsis [2]
Thrombocytopenia (97%) [36]

Other
Adverse effects [2]
Death (8%)

PANTOPRAZOLE

Trade names: Protium (Nycomed), Protonix (Wyeth)
Indications: Esophagitis associated with gastroesophageal reflux disease (GERD), Zollinger-Ellison syndrome, erosive esophagitis
Class: Proton pump inhibitor (PPI)
Half-life: 1 hour
Clinically important, potentially hazardous interactions with: alcohol, allopurinol, atazanavir, cefditoren, clopidogrel, conivaptan, CYP2C19 inducers and substrates, dabigatran, dasatinib, delavirdine, dexmethylphenidate, digoxin, erlotinib, eucalyptus, fluconazole, indinavir, iron salts, itraconazole, ketoconazole, lapatinib, letermovir, mesalamine, methotrexate, methylphenidate, mycophenolate, nelfinavir, PEG-interferon, posaconazole, raltegravir, rilpivirine, saquinavir, tipranavir, topotecan, ulipristal, voriconazole, warfarin
Pregnancy category: B
Important contra-indications noted in the prescribing guidelines for: nursing mothers

Skin
Anaphylactoid reactions/Anaphylaxis [7]
Edema (<2%)
Facial edema (<4%)
Hypersensitivity [2]
Lupus erythematosus (discoid) [3]
Peripheral edema [2]
Photosensitivity (<2%)
Pruritus (<2%)
Rash (<2%) [3]
Urticaria (<4%) [2]

Mucosal
Xerostomia (<2%)

Central Nervous System
Depression (<2%)
Fever (>4%) [3]
Headache (12%) [3]
Vertigo (dizziness) (3%)

Neuromuscular/Skeletal
Arthralgia (<4%)
Myalgia/Myopathy (<4%)

Gastrointestinal/Hepatic
Abdominal pain (6%)
Constipation (<4%) [2]
Diarrhea (9%)
Flatulence (<4%)
Hepatitis (<2%)
Nausea (7%) [2]
Pancreatitis [2]
Vomiting (4%)

Respiratory
Flu-like syndrome (<10%)
Upper respiratory tract infection (>4%)

Endocrine/Metabolic
Creatine phosphokinase increased (<2%)
Hypomagnesemia [3]

Renal
Nephrotoxicity [4]

Hematologic
Leukopenia (<2%)
Thrombocytopenia (<2%) [5]

Ocular
Vision blurred (<2%)

Other
Adverse effects [2]
Allergic reactions (<4%)
Infection (<10%)
Kounis syndrome [2]

PAPAVERINE

Indications: Peripheral and cerebral ischemia
Class: Opium alkaloid, Vasodilator, peripheral
Half-life: 0.5–2 hours
Clinically important, potentially hazardous interactions with: levodopa, reboxetine
Pregnancy category: C
Important contra-indications noted in the prescribing guidelines for: nursing mothers; pediatric patients

Cardiovascular
Hypotension [2]

Genitourinary
Priapism (11%) [16]

PAROMOMYCIN

Trade name: Humatin (Pfizer)
Indications: Intestinal amebiasis
Class: Antibiotic, aminoglycoside
Half-life: N/A
Clinically important, potentially hazardous interactions with: methotrexate, succinylcholine
Pregnancy category: C

Skin
Pruritus [2]

Central Nervous System
Pain [2]

Gastrointestinal/Hepatic
Abdominal pain [2]

Local
Injection-site pain [2]

PAROXETINE HYDROCHLORIDE

Trade names: Paxil (GSK), Paxil CR (GSK), Seroxat (GSK)
Indications: Depression, obsessive-compulsive disorder, panic disorder, social and generalized anxiety disorders, post-traumatic stress disorder
Class: Antidepressant, Selective serotonin reuptake inhibitor (SSRI)
Half-life: 21 hours
Clinically important, potentially hazardous interactions with: alcohol, amitriptyline, amphetamines, antiepileptics, aprepitant, aripiprazole, artemether/lumefantrine, asenapine, aspirin, astemizole, atomoxetine, barbiturates, clarithromycin, clozapine, cobicistat/elvitegravir/emtricitabine/tenofovir alafenamide, cobicistat/elvitegravir/emtricitabine/tenofovir disoproxil, coumarins, cyproheptadine, darifenacin, darunavir, deutetrabenazine, dexibuprofen, dextroamphetamine, diethylpropion, digitalis, digoxin, duloxetine, eluxadoline, entacapone, erythromycin, galantamine, iloperidone, isocarboxazid, linezolid, lithium, MAO inhibitors, mazindol, methadone, methamphetamine, methylene blue, methylphenidate, metoprolol, moclobemide, molindone, NSAIDs, perphenazine, phendimetrazine, phenelzine, phenobarbital, phentermine, phenylpropanolamine, phenytoin, pimozide, primidone, procyclidine, propafenone, propranolol, pseudoephedrine, ranolazine, rasagiline, risperidone, ritonavir, selegiline, sibutramine, St John's wort, sumatriptan, sympathomimetics, tamoxifen, tamsulosin, tetrabenazine, thioridazine, tramadol, tranylcypromine, trazodone, tricyclic antidepressants, troleandomycin, tryptophan, valbenazine, vortioxetine
Pregnancy category: D
Important contra-indications noted in the prescribing guidelines for: nursing mothers; pediatric patients
Note: For menopausal indications see separate entry for paroxetine mesylate.

Warning: SUICIDALITY AND ANTIDEPRESSANT DRUGS

Skin
Diaphoresis (11%) [10]
Ecchymoses [2]
Exanthems [2]
Hyperhidrosis [2]
Photosensitivity [3]
Pruritus [3]
Rash (2%)
Vasculitis [2]

Mucosal
Xerostomia (18%) [17]

Cardiovascular
Venous thromboembolism [2]

Central Nervous System
Abnormal dreams (3–4%)
Agitation (3–6%)
Akathisia [3]
Anxiety (5%) [2]
Chills (2%) [2]
Delirium [3]
Depression [3]
Dysarthria [2]
Dysgeusia (taste perversion) (2%)
Extrapyramidal symptoms [2]
Headache (17–28%) [12]
Insomnia (11–24%) [5]
Irritability [2]
Mania [2]
Nervousness (4–9%)
Neuroleptic malignant syndrome [4]
Paresthesias (4%)
Parkinsonism [3]
Restless legs syndrome [7]
Serotonin syndrome [19]
Sleep disturbances [2]
Somnolence (drowsiness) (15–24%) [5]
Suicidal ideation [4]
Tic disorder [3]
Tremor (4–11%) [5]
Vertigo (dizziness) (6–14%) [7]
Yawning (2–4%)

Neuromuscular/Skeletal
Asthenia (fatigue) [4]
Myalgia/Myopathy (<10%)

Gastrointestinal/Hepatic
Abdominal pain (4%) [2]
Constipation (5–18%) [2]
Diarrhea (9–12%) [3]
Nausea (26%) [8]
Vomiting [3]

Respiratory
Pharyngitis (4%)
Rhinitis (3%)
Sinusitis (4%)

Endocrine/Metabolic
Galactorrhea [4]
Gynecomastia [2]
Libido decreased (3–15%)
SIADH [18]
Weight gain [9]

Genitourinary
Ejaculatory dysfunction (13–28%)
Erectile dysfunction [2]
Priapism [4]
Sexual dysfunction [8]

Otic
Hallucinations, auditory [3]

Ocular
Glaucoma [2]
Hallucinations, visual [2]
Vision impaired [2]

Other
Adverse effects [4]
Bruxism [4]
Congenital malformations [2]
Death [2]
Infection (5–6%)

PAROXETINE MESYLATE

Trade name: Brisdelle (Noven)
Indications: Vasomotor symptoms associated with the menopause
Class: Selective serotonin reuptake inhibitor (SSRI)
Half-life: N/A
Clinically important, potentially hazardous interactions with: eluxadoline, linezolid, MAO inhibitors, methylene blue, pimozide, tamoxifen, thioridazine
Pregnancy category: X
Important contra-indications noted in the prescribing guidelines for: the elderly; nursing mothers; pediatric patients
Note: Brisdelle contains a low dose of paroxetine and is not indicated for psychiatric conditions. Paroxetine mesylate is also available as Pexeva. For psychiatric indications see separate entry for paroxetine hydrochloride.
Warning: SUICIDAL THOUGHTS AND BEHAVIORS

Central Nervous System
Headache (6%)

Neuromuscular/Skeletal
Asthenia (fatigue) (5%)

Gastrointestinal/Hepatic
Nausea (4%) [2]
Vomiting (4%)

Other
Adverse effects [2]

PATIROMER

Trade name: Veltassa (Relypsa)
Indications: Hyperkalemia
Class: Potassium binder
Half-life: N/A
Clinically important, potentially hazardous interactions with: none known
Pregnancy category: N/A (Not expected to cause fetal risk)
Important contra-indications noted in the prescribing guidelines for: pediatric patients
Warning: BINDING TO OTHER ORAL MEDICATIONS

Gastrointestinal/Hepatic
Abdominal pain (2%)
Constipation (7%) [13]
Diarrhea (5%) [6]
Flatulence (2%) [3]
Nausea (2%) [2]
Vomiting (<2%) [3]

Endocrine/Metabolic
Hypokalemia (5%) [5]
Hypomagnesemia (5–9%) [7]

PATISIRAN *

Trade name: Onpattro (Alnylam Pharma Inc)
Indications: indicated for the treatment of the polyneuropathy of hereditary transthyretin-mediated amyloidosis in adults
Class: Transthyretin-directed small interfering RNA
Half-life: 1.8–3.2 days
Clinically important, potentially hazardous interactions with: none known
Pregnancy category: N/A (no available data)

Skin
Erythema (7%)
Facial edema (1–19%)
Facial erythema (1–19%)
Flushing (1–19%)
Rash (1–19%)

Cardiovascular
Atrioventricular block (3%)
Chest pain (1–19%)
Hypertension (1–19%)
Hypotension (1–19%)
Tachycardia (1–19%)

Central Nervous System
Chills (1–19%)
Headache (1–19%)
Pain (1–19%)
Vertigo (dizziness) (5%)

Neuromuscular/Skeletal
Arthralgia (7%)
Asthenia (fatigue) (1–19%)
Back pain (1–19%)
Muscle spasm (8%)
Neck pain (1–19%)

Gastrointestinal/Hepatic
Abdominal pain (1–19%)
Dyspepsia (8%)
Nausea (1–19%)

Respiratory
Bronchitis (7%)
Cough (1–19%)
Dyspnea (8%)
Nasopharyngitis (1–29%)
Pharyngitis (1–29%)
Respiratory tract infection (1–29%)
Rhinitis (1–29%)
Sinusitis (1–29%)
Upper respiratory tract infection (1–29%)

Ocular
Keratoconjunctivitis (5%)
Vision blurred (3%)
Vitreous floaters (2%)

Other
Adverse effects [2]

PEG-INTERFERON

Trade names: PegIntron (Schering), Sylatron (Schering)
Indications: Chronic hepatitis C, melanoma
Class: Immunomodulator, Interferon
Half-life: ~40 hours
Clinically important, potentially hazardous interactions with: ACE inhibitors, acetaminophen, aldesleukin, bupivacaine, cilostazol, cinacalcet, CYP2C9 substrates, CYP2D6 substrates, delavirdine, duloxetine, estradiol, fesoterodine, fingolimod, fluoxetine, indinavir, melphalan, methadone, methylnaltrexone, pantoprazole, pegloticase, ribavirin, sildenafil, tapentadol, telbivudine, theophylline, theophylline derivatives, tiotropium, trimethoprim, voriconazole, warfarin, zidovudine
Pregnancy category: C (pregnancy category will be X when used in combination with ribavirin)
Important contra-indications noted in the prescribing guidelines for: nursing mothers; pediatric patients
Note: PEG-interferon is commonly administered with ribavirin and many of the reactions listed below are in combination therapy with this drug. Contra-indicated in patients with known hypersensitivity reactions, such as urticaria, angioedema, bronchoconstriction, anaphylaxis, Stevens-Johnson syndrome, and toxic epidermal necrolysis to interferon alpha or any other product component; or with autoimmune hepatitis.
Warning: RISK OF SERIOUS DISORDERS AND RIBAVIRIN-ASSOCIATED EFFECTS DEPRESSION AND OTHER NEUROPSYCHIATRIC DISORDERS

Skin
Dermatitis (7%)
Diaphoresis (6%)
DRESS syndrome [2]
Eczema [2]
Exanthems [5]
Fixed eruption [2]
Flushing (6%)
Lupus erythematosus [3]
Nummular eczema [2]
Photosensitivity [4]
Pruritus (12%) [11]
Psoriasis [4]
Rash (6%) [24]
Rosacea fulminans [2]
Sarcoidosis [9]
Stevens-Johnson syndrome [2]
Toxic epidermal necrolysis [2]
Toxicity [3]
Vasculitis [2]
Vitiligo [3]
Xerosis (11%) [2]

Hair
Alopecia (22%) [5]
Alopecia areata [2]

Central Nervous System
Anorexia (17%) [2]
Chills [2]
Cognitive impairment [2]
Depression (16–29%) [10]
Dysgeusia (taste perversion) (<10%) [5]
Fever (37%) [8]
Headache (54%) [16]
Insomnia (19%) [4]
Irritability [2]
Neurotoxicity [2]
Pain (12%)
Parkinsonism [2]
Psychosis [2]
Vertigo (dizziness) (16%) [3]

Neuromuscular/Skeletal
Arthralgia (28%) [2]
Asthenia (fatigue) (56%) [24]
Back pain (9%)
Myalgia/Myopathy (38–42%) [4]

Gastrointestinal/Hepatic
Abdominal pain (15%)
Diarrhea (16%) [4]
Hepatotoxicity [5]
Nausea (24%) [12]
Pancreatitis [4]
Vomiting (24%) [2]

Respiratory
Cough (6%)
Dyspnea (13%) [2]
Flu-like syndrome (46%) [11]
Pneumonitis [2]

Endocrine/Metabolic
ALT increased [3]
Appetite decreased [2]
AST increased [3]
Diabetes mellitus [2]
Thyroid dysfunction [2]
Weight loss (16%) [3]

Genitourinary
Urinary tract infection [2]

Renal
Nephrotoxicity [4]

Hematologic
Anemia (14%) [44]
Hemotoxicity [2]
Leukopenia [6]
Lymphopenia (14%) [3]
Neutropenia (21%) [20]
Sepsis [2]
Thrombocytopenia (5%) [15]

Otic
Hearing loss [2]
Tinnitus [2]

Ocular
Retinopathy [7]
Vision blurred (4%)

Local
Injection-site pain (2%)
Injection-site reactions (22%) [4]

Other
Adverse effects [26]
Death [2]
Infection (3%) [4]

PEGAPTANIB

Trade name: Macugen (Valeant)
Indications: Neovascular (wet) age-related macular degeneration
Class: Vascular endothelial growth factor antagonist
Half-life: 6–14 days
Clinically important, potentially hazardous interactions with: none known
Pregnancy category: B
Important contra-indications noted in the prescribing guidelines for: nursing mothers; pediatric patients
Note: Contra-indicated in patients with ocular or periocular infections.

Skin
Dermatitis (<5%)

Cardiovascular
Arterial occlusion (carotid) (<5%)
Chest pain (<5%)
Hypertension (10–40%)
Myocardial ischemia (transient) (<5%)

Central Nervous System
Cerebrovascular accident (<5%)
Headache (6–10%)
Ischemic injury (transient) (<5%)
Vertigo (dizziness) (<10%)

Neuromuscular/Skeletal
Arthralgia (<5%)

Gastrointestinal/Hepatic
Diarrhea (6–10%)
Nausea (6–10%)
Vomiting (<5%)

Respiratory
Bronchitis (6–10%)
Pleural effusion (<5%)

Endocrine/Metabolic
Diabetes mellitus (<5%)

Genitourinary
Urinary retention (<5%)
Urinary tract infection (6–10%)

Otic
Hearing loss (<5%)
Otitis media (<5%)

Ocular
Blepharitis (6–10%)
Cataract (10–40%) [2]
Conjunctival edema (<5%)
Conjunctival hemorrhage (10–40%)
Conjunctivitis (<10%)
Corneal abnormalities (<5%)
Corneal deposits (<5%)
Corneal edema (10–40%)
Endophthalmitis (<5%) [4]
Eyelid irritation (<5%)
Intraocular pressure increased (10–40%)
Meibomianitis (<5%)
Mydriasis (<5%)
Ocular edema (<5%)
Ocular hypertension (10–40%)
Ocular inflammation (<5%) [2]
Ocular pain (10–40%)
Ocular stinging (10–40%)
Ophthalmitis (<5%)
Periorbital hematoma (<5%)

Photopsia (6–10%)
Punctate keratitis (10–40%)
Reduced visual acuity (10–40%)
Retinal detachment (<10%) [5]
Retinal edema (<5%)
Vision blurred (10–40%)
Visual disturbances (10–40%)
Vitreous floaters (10–40%)

PEGASPARGASE

Trade name: Oncaspar (Enzon)
Indications: Acute lymphoblastic leukemia
Class: Antineoplastic
Half-life: 5.7 days
Clinically important, potentially hazardous interactions with: none known
Pregnancy category: C

Skin
Anaphylactoid reactions/Anaphylaxis (<5%) [2]
Angioedema (<5%)
Edema (>5%)
Rash (<5%)
Urticaria (<5%)

Cardiovascular
Hypotension (>5%)
Tachycardia (>5%)
Venous thromboembolism [2]

Central Nervous System
Chills (<5%)
Fever (>5%)
Headache (<5%)
Paresthesias (<5%)
Seizures (<5%) [2]

Neuromuscular/Skeletal
Arthralgia (<5%)
Myalgia/Myopathy (<5%)

Gastrointestinal/Hepatic
Abdominal pain (<5%)
Hepatotoxicity [3]
Pancreatitis [4]

Endocrine/Metabolic
Hyperglycemia [2]
Hypertriglyceridemia [2]

Hematologic
Leukopenia [2]
Neutropenia [2]
Prothrombin time increased [2]
Thrombocytopenia [2]

Other
Allergic reactions (>5%) [7]

PEGLOTICASE

Trade name: Krystexxa (Savient)
Indications: Chronic gout
Class: Enzyme
Half-life: N/A
Clinically important, potentially hazardous interactions with: PEG-interferon
Pregnancy category: C
Important contra-indications noted in the prescribing guidelines for: nursing mothers; pediatric patients
Note: Contra-indicated for patients at higher risk for G6PD deficiency (e.g. those of African and Mediterranean ancestry) who should be screened due to the risk of hemolysis and methemoglobinemia.
Warning: ANAPHYLAXIS and INFUSION REACTIONS

Skin
Anaphylactoid reactions/Anaphylaxis (5%) [3]
Ecchymoses (11%)

Cardiovascular
Chest pain (6%)

Central Nervous System
Vertigo (dizziness) [3]

Neuromuscular/Skeletal
Arthralgia [3]
Back pain [2]
Gouty tophi (flare) (77%) [7]

Gastrointestinal/Hepatic
Constipation (6%)
Nausea (12%) [3]
Vomiting (5%)

Respiratory
Dyspnea [2]
Nasopharyngitis (7%)

Local
Infusion-related reactions [4]
Infusion-site reactions (26%) [4]

Other
Adverse effects [2]

PEGVISOMANT

Trade name: Somavert (Pfizer)
Indications: Acromegaly
Class: Growth hormone analog
Half-life: 6 days
Clinically important, potentially hazardous interactions with: acarbose, exenatide, hydromorphone, insulin, latex, metformin, opioids, oral hypoglycemics, pioglitazone, saxagliptin, tapentadol
Pregnancy category: B
Important contra-indications noted in the prescribing guidelines for: the elderly; nursing mothers; pediatric patients

---

Skin
Lipohypertrophy (<5%) [2]
Peripheral edema (4–8%)

Cardiovascular
Chest pain (4–8%)
Hypertension (8%)

Central Nervous System
Pain (4–14%)
Paresthesias (7%)
Vertigo (dizziness) (4–8%)

Neuromuscular/Skeletal
Back pain (4–8%)

Gastrointestinal/Hepatic
Diarrhea (4–14%)
Hepatitis [2]
Hepatotoxicity [6]
Nausea (8–14%)

Respiratory
Flu-like syndrome (4–12%)
Sinusitis (4–8%)

Local
Injection-site reactions (8–11%) [4]

Other
Adverse effects [3]
Infection (23%)

PEMBROLIZUMAB

Synonym: lambrolizumab
Trade name: Keytruda (Merck Sharpe & Dohme)
Indications: Unresectable or metastatic melanoma and disease progression following ipilimumab and, if BRAF V600 mutation positive, a BRAF inhibitor
Class: Monoclonal antibody, Programmed death receptor-1 (PD-1) inhibitor
Half-life: 26 days
Clinically important, potentially hazardous interactions with: none known
Pregnancy category: D
Important contra-indications noted in the prescribing guidelines for: nursing mothers; pediatric patients

---

Skin
Bullous pemphigoid [5]
Dermatitis [2]
Erythema [3]
Exanthems [4]
Lichen planus [2]
Lichenoid eruption [3]
Peripheral edema (17%)
Pruritus (30%) [19]
Psoriasis [4]
Rash (29%) [20]
Sarcoidosis [5]
Scleroderma [2]
Toxicity [6]
Vasculitis [2]
Vitiligo (11%) [11]

Hair
Alopecia [2]
Alopecia areata [2]

Mucosal
Oral mucositis [2]
Xerostomia [2]

Cardiovascular
Myocarditis [3]

Central Nervous System
Chills (14%)
Encephalopathy [3]
Fever (11%) [6]
Headache (16%) [3]
Insomnia (14%)
Neurotoxicity [3]
Pain [2]
Peripheral neuropathy [3]
Vertigo (dizziness) (11%)

Neuromuscular/Skeletal
- Arthralgia (20%) [10]
- Asthenia (fatigue) (47%) [25]
- Back pain (12%)
- Myalgia/Myopathy (14%) [9]
- Myasthenia gravis [7]
- Pain in extremities (18%)

Gastrointestinal/Hepatic
- Abdominal pain (12%) [2]
- Colitis [13]
- Constipation (21%)
- Diarrhea (20%) [14]
- Hepatitis [8]
- Hepatotoxicity [6]
- Nausea (30%) [12]
- Pancreatitis [6]
- Vomiting (16%) [3]

Respiratory
- Cough (30%) [5]
- Dyspnea (18%) [4]
- Pneumonia [5]
- Pneumonitis (3%) [19]
- Upper respiratory tract infection (11%)

Endocrine/Metabolic
- ALT increased [6]
- Appetite decreased (26%) [10]
- AST increased (24%) [4]
- Diabetes mellitus [6]
- Hyperthyroidism [7]
- Hypertriglyceridemia (25%)
- Hypoalbuminemia (34%)
- Hypocalcemia (24%)
- Hyponatremia (35%) [4]
- Hypophysitis [9]
- Hypothyroidism (8%) [15]
- Thyroid dysfunction [5]
- Thyroiditis [5]

Renal
- Nephrotoxicity [6]
- Renal failure [3]

Hematologic
- Anemia (14–55%) [8]
- Hemolytic anemia [2]
- Lymphopenia [2]
- Neutropenia [5]
- Sepsis (<10%) [2]
- Thrombocytopenia [4]

Ocular
- Iridocyclitis [2]
- Uveitis [6]

Local
- Infusion-related reactions [2]

Other
- Adverse effects [23]
- Death [6]
- Side effects [3]

PEMETREXED

Trade name: Alimta (Lilly)
Indications: Non-squamous non-small cell lung cancer, mesothelioma (in combination with cisplatin)
Class: Antimetabolite, Folic acid antagonist
Half-life: 3.5 hours
Clinically important, potentially hazardous interactions with: clozapine, digoxin, leflunomide, meloxicam, natalizumab, nephrotoxic drugs, NSAIDs, phenytoin, pimecrolimus, probenecid, pyrimethamine, sipuleucel-T, tacrolimus, trastuzumab, vaccines
Pregnancy category: D
Important contra-indications noted in the prescribing guidelines for: nursing mothers; pediatric patients

---

Skin
- AGEP [4]
- Cellulitis [3]
- Desquamation (10–14%)
- Edema (<5%)
- Erythema multiforme (<5%)
- Hypersensitivity (<5%)
- Peripheral edema [4]
- Pruritus (<7%)
- Radiation recall dermatitis [7]
- Rash (10–14%) [20]
- Toxic epidermal necrolysis [5]
- Toxicity [2]
- Urticaria [3]
- Vasculitis [2]

Hair
- Alopecia (<6%) [5]

Mucosal
- Epistaxis (nosebleed) [2]
- Mucositis (7%) [6]
- Stomatitis (7–15%) [6]

Cardiovascular
- Hypertension [7]
- Venous thromboembolism [2]

Central Nervous System
- Anorexia (19–22%) [9]
- Depression (14%)
- Dysgeusia (taste perversion) [2]
- Fever (<8%) [2]
- Headache [4]
- Insomnia [2]
- Neurotoxicity (<9%)
- Peripheral neuropathy [2]

Neuromuscular/Skeletal
- Asthenia (fatigue) (25–34%) [34]

Gastrointestinal/Hepatic
- Abdominal pain (<5%)
- Constipation (<6%) [4]
- Diarrhea (5–13%) [13]
- Hepatotoxicity [7]
- Nausea (19–31%) [18]
- Vomiting (9–16%) [10]

Respiratory
- Cough [2]
- Dysphonia [2]
- Dyspnea [4]
- Hemoptysis [2]
- Pharyngitis (15%)
- Pneumonitis [2]
- Pulmonary toxicity [2]

Endocrine/Metabolic
- ALT increased (8–10%) [3]
- Appetite decreased [5]
- AST increased (7–8%) [3]
- Creatine phosphokinase increased (<5%) [3]
- Hyperglycemia [2]
- Hyperkalemia [2]
- Hypokalemia [2]
- Hypomagnesemia [3]
- Hyponatremia [3]

Renal
- Nephrotoxicity [3]

Hematologic
- Anemia (15–19%) [23]
- Febrile neutropenia (<5%) [11]
- Hemotoxicity [4]
- Leukocytopenia [2]
- Leukopenia (6–12%) [11]
- Lymphopenia [3]
- Myelosuppression [3]
- Neutropenia (6–11%) [24]
- Sepsis [2]
- Thrombocytopenia (<8%) [15]
- Thrombotic complications [2]

Ocular
- Conjunctivitis (<5%)
- Eyelid edema [3]
- Lacrimation (<5%)

Other
- Adverse effects (53%) [16]
- Allergic reactions (<5%)
- Death [5]
- Hiccups [2]
- Infection (<5%) [7]

PENICILLAMINE

Trade name: Depen (MedPointe)
Indications: Wilson's disease, rheumatoid arthritis
Class: Antidote, Chelator, Disease-modifying antirheumatic drug (DMARD)
Half-life: 1.7–3.2 hours
Clinically important, potentially hazardous interactions with: aluminum, antacids, ascorbic acid, bone marrow suppressants, chloroquine, clozapine, cytotoxic agents, diclofenac, ferrous sulfate, food, gold & gold compounds, hydroxychloroquine, iron, magnesium, meloxicam, primaquine, probenecid, sodium picosulfate
Pregnancy category: D
Important contra-indications noted in the prescribing guidelines for: nursing mothers; pediatric patients
Note: As an antidote, it is difficult to differentiate side effects due to the drug from those due to the effects of the poison.

Skin
- Bullous dermatitis [3]
- Bullous pemphigoid [6]
- Cicatricial pemphigoid [2]
- Cutis laxa [13]

Dermatitis [4]
Dermatomyositis [14]
Edema of lip (<10%)
Ehlers–Danlos syndrome [2]
Elastosis perforans serpiginosa [43]
Epidermolysis bullosa [4]
Epidermolysis bullosa acquisita [2]
Erythema multiforme (<5%)
Exanthems [8]
Fragility [2]
Hypersensitivity [3]
Lichen planus [4]
Lichenoid eruption [7]
Lupus erythematosus [43]
Morphea [2]
Pemphigus [76]
Pemphigus erythematodes (Senear–Usher) [10]
Pemphigus foliaceus [16]
Pemphigus herpetiformis [3]
Pemphigus vulgaris [2]
Peripheral edema (<10%)
Pruritus (44–50%) [2]
Pseudoxanthoma elasticum [16]
Psoriasis [4]
Purpura [5]
Rash (44–50%) [6]
Scleroderma [7]
Toxic epidermal necrolysis [2]
Urticaria (44–50%) [2]
Vasculitis [7]

Hair
Alopecia [3]
Hirsutism [2]

Nails
Nail pigmentation [4]

Mucosal
Aphthous stomatitis [2]
Mucosal lesions (pemphigus-like) [2]
Oral ulceration [5]
Stomatitis [6]

Central Nervous System
Ageusia (taste loss) (12%) [2]
Dysgeusia (taste perversion) (metallic taste) [8]
Hypogeusia (25–33%) [2]

Neuromuscular/Skeletal
Dystonia [4]
Myasthenia gravis [73]
Polymyositis [8]

Respiratory
Pulmonary toxicity [2]

Endocrine/Metabolic
Gynecomastia [5]

Renal
Glomerulonephritis [3]
Nephrotoxicity [5]
Proteinuria [2]

Hematologic
Hemotoxicity [2]

Other
Adverse effects [2]

PENICILLIN G

Trade name: Crystapen (Britannia)
Indications: Anthrax, cellulitis, endocarditis, infections, otitis media, rheumatic fever, respiratory infections, septicemia
Class: Antibiotic, penicillin
Half-life: 4 hours
Clinically important, potentially hazardous interactions with: estrogens, methotrexate, minocycline, phenindione, probenecid, sulfinpyrazone, warfarin
Pregnancy category: B
Important contra-indications noted in the prescribing guidelines for: nursing mothers

---

Skin
Anaphylactoid reactions/Anaphylaxis [5]
Dermatitis [2]
Hypersensitivity [4]
Jarisch–Herxheimer reaction [21]
Nicolau syndrome [2]
Rash [4]
Serum sickness-like reaction [2]

Central Nervous System
Hoigne's syndrome [16]
Seizures [2]

Gastrointestinal/Hepatic
Hepatotoxicity [2]

Genitourinary
Cystitis [3]

Renal
Nephrotoxicity [2]

Hematologic
Thrombosis [2]

PENICILLIN V

Trade name: V-cillin K (Lilly)
Indications: Cellulitis, endocarditis, erysipelas, oral infections, otitis media, rheumatic fever, scarlet fever, tonsillitis
Class: Antibiotic, penicillin
Half-life: 4 hours
Clinically important, potentially hazardous interactions with: estrogens, methotrexate, minocycline, neomycin, phenindione, probenecid, sulfinpyrazone, warfarin
Pregnancy category: B

Skin
Anaphylactoid reactions/Anaphylaxis [2]
DRESS syndrome [2]
Hypersensitivity [3]
Serum sickness [2]
Serum sickness-like reaction [2]
Urticaria [3]

Central Nervous System
Fever [3]

Neuromuscular/Skeletal
Arthralgia [2]

Gastrointestinal/Hepatic
Diarrhea [2]

PENTAMIDINE

Trade names: NebuPent (Astellas), Pentacarinat (Sanofi-Aventis), Pentam 300 (Astellas)
Indications: *Pneumocystis jiroveci* infection, trypanosomiasis, leishmaniasis
Class: Antiprotozoal
Half-life: 9.1–13.2 hours (intramuscular); 6.5 hours (intravenous)
Clinically important, potentially hazardous interactions with: adefovir, aminoglycosides, amiodarone, amisulpride, amitriptyline, amphotericin B, cisplatin, droperidol, erythromycin, foscarnet, insulin aspart, insulin degludec, insulin detemir, insulin glargine, insulin glulisine, ivabradine, levomepromazine, moxifloxacin, phenothiazines, saquinavir, sparfloxacin, sulpiride, tricyclic antidepressants, trifluoperazine, vancomycin
Pregnancy category: C
Important contra-indications noted in the prescribing guidelines for: nursing mothers; pediatric patients
Note: The rate of adverse side effects is increased in patients with AIDS.

Skin
Exanthems (<15%) [10]
Pruritus [2]
Rash (<47%) [4]
Toxic epidermal necrolysis [3]
Urticaria [3]

Cardiovascular
QT prolongation [8]
Torsades de pointes [4]

Central Nervous System
Dysgeusia (taste perversion) (metallic taste) (2%)
Paresthesias [2]
Vertigo (dizziness) [2]

Neuromuscular/Skeletal
Myalgia/Myopathy (<5%)
Rhabdomyolysis [4]

Gastrointestinal/Hepatic
Pancreatitis [6]

Local
Injection-site irritation [2]
Injection-site pain [2]
Injection-site reactions (>10%)

Other
Adverse effects [4]

PENTOXIFYLLINE

Trade names: Pentoxil (Upsher-Smith), Trental (Sanofi-Aventis)
Indications: Peripheral vascular disease, intermittent claudication
Class: Vasodilator, peripheral, Xanthine alkaloid
Half-life: 0.4–0.8 hours
Clinically important, potentially hazardous interactions with: abciximab, benazepril, captopril, ceftobiprole, cilostazol, ciprofloxacin, citalopram, clevidipine, clopidogrel, diclofenac, enalapril, eptifibatide, fosinopril, insulin degludec, insulin glargine, insulin glulisine, irbesartan,

lisinopril, meloxicam, olmesartan, quinapril, ramipril, tinzaparin
Pregnancy category: C

Skin
Flushing (2%) [2]

Mucosal
Xerostomia [2]

PEPPERMINT

Family: Labiatae
Scientific name: *Mentha piperita*
Indications: Dyspepsia, regress pancreatic, mammary, and liver tumors, irritable bowel syndrome, colonic spasm, colic, nausea, vomiting, biliary disorders, common cold, dysmenorrhoea, anxiolytic. **Topical:** pain, itching, inflammations, headaches, toothache, pruritus, urticaria, mosquito repellant. **Vapor:** bronchial catarrh, fever, influenza. Flavoring, cosmetics, toothpaste, mouthwash
Class: Analgesic, Antiemetic, Carminative, Vasodilator, peripheral
Half-life: N/A
Clinically important, potentially hazardous interactions with: cisapride
Pregnancy category: N/A

Skin
Burning (anal) [3]
Contact dermatitis [5]
Dermatitis [5]
Hypersensitivity [2]
Sensitivity [2]

Mucosal
Cheilitis [3]
Oral ulceration [2]
Stomatitis [2]

Gastrointestinal/Hepatic
Dyspepsia [3]
Hepatotoxicity [2]
Nausea [2]
Vomiting [2]

Other
Adverse effects [6]
Allergic reactions [2]
Side effects [3]

PERAMIVIR

Trade name: Rapivab (BioCryst)
Indications: Influenza
Class: Antiviral, Neuraminidase inhibitor
Half-life: ~20 hours
Clinically important, potentially hazardous interactions with: live attenuated influenza vaccine
Pregnancy category: C
Important contra-indications noted in the prescribing guidelines for: nursing mothers; pediatric patients

Skin
Rash [2]

Cardiovascular
Hypertension (2%)

Central Nervous System
Behavioral disturbances [2]
Insomnia (3%)

Gastrointestinal/Hepatic
Constipation (4%)
Diarrhea (8%) [6]
Nausea [4]
Vomiting [4]

Endocrine/Metabolic
ALT increased (3%)
AST increased (3%)
Creatine phosphokinase increased (4%)
Hyperglycemia (5%)

Hematologic
Leukopenia [2]
Neutropenia (8%) [4]
Thrombocytopenia [2]

PERAMPANEL

Trade name: Fycompa (Eisai)
Indications: Partial-onset seizures, primary generalized tonic-clonic seizures
Class: AMPA glutamate receptor antagonist, Anticonvulsant, Antiepileptic
Half-life: ~105 hours
Clinically important, potentially hazardous interactions with: alcohol, carbamazepine, oral contraceptives, oxcarbazepine, phenobarbital, phenytoin, primidone, rifampin, St John's wort
Pregnancy category: C
Important contra-indications noted in the prescribing guidelines for: the elderly; nursing mothers; pediatric patients
Warning: SERIOUS PSYCHIATRIC AND BEHAVIORAL REACTIONS

Skin
Peripheral edema (<2%)

Mucosal
Oropharyngeal pain (2%)

Central Nervous System
Aggression (<3%) [11]
Anxiety (2–4%)
Balance disorder (<5%)
Behavioral disturbances [6]
Confusion (<2%)
Depression [2]
Dysarthria (<4%)
Euphoria (<2%)
Gait instability (<4%) [11]
Headache (11–13%) [15]
Hypersomnia (<3%)
Hypoesthesia (<3%)
Incoordination (<2%)
Irritability (4–12%) [16]
Memory loss (<2%)
Mood changes (<2%)
Neurotoxicity [2]
Paresthesias (<2%)
Sedation [3]
Seizures [3]
Somnolence (drowsiness) (9–18%) [32]
Suicidal ideation [3]
Vertigo (dizziness) (16–43%) [36]

Neuromuscular/Skeletal
Arthralgia (<3%)
Asthenia (fatigue) (<12%) [18]
Ataxia (<8%) [7]
Back pain (2–5%)
Bone or joint pain (<2%)
Myalgia/Myopathy (<3%)
Pain in extremities (<3%)

Gastrointestinal/Hepatic
Constipation (2–3%)
Nausea (3–8%) [6]
Vomiting (2–4%) [2]

Respiratory
Cough (<4%)
Nasopharyngitis [2]
Upper respiratory tract infection (3–4%)

Endocrine/Metabolic
Hyponatremia (<2%)
Weight gain (4%) [8]

Ocular
Diplopia (<3%)
Vision blurred (<4%)

Other
Adverse effects [6]

PERINDOPRIL

Trade names: Aceon (Solvay), Prestalia (Symplmed)
Indications: Hypertension, coronary disease
Class: Angiotensin-converting enzyme (ACE) inhibitor, Antihypertensive
Half-life: 1.5–3 hours
Clinically important, potentially hazardous interactions with: none known
Pregnancy category: D (category C in first trimester; category D in second and third trimesters)
Important contra-indications noted in the prescribing guidelines for: nursing mothers; pediatric patients
Note: Prestalia is perindopril and amlodipine.
Warning: FETAL TOXICITY

Skin
Angioedema [6]
Edema (4%)
Peripheral edema [4]
Pruritus (<10%)
Rash (<10%)

Mucosal
Tongue edema [2]

Central Nervous System
Paresthesias (2%)
Vertigo (dizziness) [3]

Neuromuscular/Skeletal
Back pain (6%)

Respiratory
Cough (12%) [17]

Other
Adverse effects [2]

PERPHENAZINE

Trade names: Decentan (Merck), Fentazin (Goldshield), Trilafon (Schering)
Indications: Psychotic disorders, nausea and vomiting
Class: Antiemetic, Antipsychotic, Phenothiazine
Half-life: 9 hours
Clinically important, potentially hazardous interactions with: cobicistat/elvitegravir/emtricitabine/tenofovir alafenamide, cobicistat/elvitegravir/emtricitabine/tenofovir disoproxil, paroxetine hydrochloride, sparfloxacin
Pregnancy category: C
Note: Perphenazine is also used in combination with amitriptyline.

Skin
Exanthems [2]
Lupus erythematosus [4]
Rash (<10%)

Central Nervous System
Tardive dyskinesia [2]

Neuromuscular/Skeletal
Rhabdomyolysis [2]

Endocrine/Metabolic
Mastodynia (<10%)

Genitourinary
Priapism [2]

PHELLODENDRON

Family: Rutaceae
Scientific names: *Phellodendron amurense, Phellodendron chinense, Phellodendron wilsonii*
Indications: Anti-inflammatory, muscle and joint pain, gastroenteritis, abdominal pain, diarrhea, gastric ulcers, thrush, cholera, night sweats, fever, nocturnal emissions, dysentery, jaundice, leukorrhea, weakness and edema of legs, consumptive fever. **Topical:** sores, skin infection with local redness and swelling, eczema with itching, periodontal disease (in dentifrice)
Class: COX-2 selective inhibitor, Immunosuppressant
Half-life: N/A
Clinically important, potentially hazardous interactions with: aspirin, NSAIDs
Pregnancy category: N/A
Note: Contra-indicated in patients with impaired renal function, impaired heart function, or hypertension.

PHENOBARBITAL

Synonyms: phenobarbitone; phenylethylmalonylurea
Trade name: Luminal (Sanofi-Aventis)
Indications: Insomnia, seizures
Class: Anticonvulsant, Barbiturate, CYP3A4 inducer
Half-life: 2–6 days
Clinically important, potentially hazardous interactions with: abacavir, abiraterone, afatinib, alcohol, amprenavir, anticoagulants, antihistamines, apremilast, aprepitant, betamethasone, bictegravir/emtricitabine/tenofovir alafenamide, boceprevir, brompheniramine, buclizine, buprenorphine, cabazitaxel, cabozantinib, caffeine, calcifediol, chlorpheniramine, cobicistat/elvitegravir/emtricitabine/tenofovir disoproxil, crizotinib, darunavir, dasabuvir/ombitasvir/paritaprevir/ritonavir, dasatinib, deferasirox, delavirdine, dexamethasone, dicumarol, doxercalciferol, dronedarone, eliglustat, emtricitabine/rilpivirine/tenofovir alafenamide, enzalutamide, estradiol, ethanolamine, ethosuximide, etravirine, fesoterodine, flibanserin, fluconazole, flunisolide, fosamprenavir, gefitinib, hydrocortisone, imatinib, indinavir, influenza vaccine, itraconazole, ixabepilone, lacosamide, lapatinib, ledipasvir & sofosbuvir, lisdexamfetamine, lopinavir, meperidine, methsuximide, methylprednisolone, midazolam, mifepristone, nilotinib, ombitasvir/paritaprevir/ritonavir, oxcarbazepine, oxtriphylline, paroxetine hydrochloride, perampanel, piracetam, pizotifen, prednisolone, prednisone, propranolol, ranolazine, regorafenib, rilpivirine, riociguat, rivaroxaban, roflumilast, romidepsin, rufinamide, simeprevir, sodium oxybate, sofosbuvir, sofosbuvir & velpatasvir, sofosbuvir/velpatasvir/voxilaprevir, solifenacin, sonidegib, sorafenib, sunitinib, telaprevir, telithromycin, temsirolimus, teniposide, tenofovir alafenamide, tezacaftor/ivacaftor, tiagabine, ticagrelor, tipranavir, trabectedin, triamcinolone, ulipristal, vandetanib, vemurafenib, voriconazole, warfarin
Pregnancy category: D
Important contra-indications noted in the prescribing guidelines for: the elderly; nursing mothers
Note: Aromatic antiepileptic drugs, phenytoin, phenobarbital, carbamazepine and primidone, are a frequent cause of severe cutaneous adverse reactions. A strong genetic association between HLA-B*1502 and phenobarbital-induced Stevens-Johnson syndrome and toxic epidermal necrolysis has been shown in Han Chinese patients.

Skin
Anticonvulsant hypersensitivity syndrome [10]
Bullous dermatitis [5]
DRESS syndrome [15]
Erythema multiforme [7]
Erythroderma [2]
Exanthems [13]
Exfoliative dermatitis [6]
Fixed eruption [9]
Hypersensitivity [12]
Lupus erythematosus [2]
Purpura [2]
Rash [4]
Stevens-Johnson syndrome [23]
Toxic epidermal necrolysis [28]

Nails
Nail hypoplasia [2]

Mucosal
Gingival hyperplasia/hypertrophy [4]

Central Nervous System
Behavioral disturbances [3]
Somnolence (drowsiness) [2]
Vertigo (dizziness) [2]

Neuromuscular/Skeletal
Asthenia (fatigue) [2]
Hypoplasia of phalanges [2]

Gastrointestinal/Hepatic
Hepatotoxicity [2]

Local
Injection-site pain (>10%)
Injection-site thrombophlebitis (>10%)

Other
Allergic reactions [2]
Death [2]
Side effects [2]
Teratogenicity [5]

PHENTERMINE

Trade names: Adipex-P (Teva), Ionamin (Celltech), Lomaira (Avanthi), Qsymia (Vivus)
Indications: Obesity
Class: Amphetamine
Half-life: 19–24 hours
Clinically important, potentially hazardous interactions with: fluoxetine, fluvoxamine, MAO inhibitors, paroxetine hydrochloride, phenelzine, sertraline, tranylcypromine
Pregnancy category: X
Important contra-indications noted in the prescribing guidelines for: the elderly; nursing mothers; pediatric patients
Note: Qsymia is phentermine and topiramate.

Mucosal
Xerostomia [7]

Cardiovascular
Cardiotoxicity [3]
Hypertension [11]
Palpitation [3]
Tachycardia [5]
Valvulopathy [17]

Central Nervous System
Anxiety [2]
Cognitive impairment [4]
Depression [3]
Dysgeusia (taste perversion) [5]
Headache [2]
Insomnia [8]
Paresthesias [7]
Vertigo (dizziness) [5]

Gastrointestinal/Hepatic
Constipation [6]

Endocrine/Metabolic
Acidosis [3]

Renal
Nephrotoxicity [2]

Other
Death [4]
Teratogenicity [2]

PHENTOLAMINE

Trade name: Regitine (Novartis)
Indications: Hypertensive episodes in pheochromocytoma
Class: Adrenergic alpha-receptor antagonist
Half-life: 19 minutes
Clinically important, potentially hazardous interactions with: none known
Pregnancy category: C
Important contra-indications noted in the prescribing guidelines for: nursing mothers

---

Skin
Flushing (<10%) [2]

Central Nervous System
Headache [2]

Genitourinary
Priapism [4]

PHENYLEPHRINE

Trade names: Rynatan (MedPointe), Tussi-12D (MedPointe)
Indications: Nasal congestion, glaucoma, hypotension
Class: Adrenergic alpha-receptor agonist, Sympathomimetic
Half-life: 2.5 hours
Clinically important, potentially hazardous interactions with: epinephrine, furazolidone, iobenguane, MAO inhibitors, oxprenolol, phenelzine, tranylcypromine
Pregnancy category: C
Important contra-indications noted in the prescribing guidelines for: nursing mothers; pediatric patients

---

Skin
Dermatitis [16]
Hypersensitivity [2]
Stinging (from nasal or ophthalmic preparations) (<10%)

Cardiovascular
Bradycardia [3]
Hypertension [2]

Ocular
Blepharoconjunctivitis [4]
Periorbital dermatitis [4]

Other
Adverse effects [2]

PHENYTOIN

Synonyms: diphenylhydantoin; DPH; phenytoin sodium
Trade name: Dilantin (Pfizer)
Indications: Grand mal seizures
Class: Antiarrhythmic class Ib, Anticonvulsant, Antiepileptic, hydantoin, CYP3A4 inducer
Half-life: 7–42 hours (dose dependent)
Clinically important, potentially hazardous interactions with: abacavir, abiraterone, acitretin, afatinib, amiodarone, amitriptyline, amlodipine, amprenavir, apixaban, apremilast, aprepitant, artemether/lumefantrine, beclomethasone, bictegravir/emtricitabine/tenofovir alafenamide, boceprevir, brigatinib, brivaracetam, buprenorphine, cabazitaxel, cabozantinib, caffeine, calcium, capecitabine, caspofungin, cefazolin, ceritinib, chloramphenicol, cimetidine, ciprofloxacin, citalopram, clobazam, clorazepate, cobicistat/elvitegravir/emtricitabine/tenofovir disoproxil, cobimetinib, colesevelam, copanlisib, crizotinib, cyclosporine, cyproterone, dabigatran, daclatasvir, darunavir, dasabuvir/ombitasvir/paritaprevir/ritonavir, dasatinib, deferasirox, deflazacort, delavirdine, dexamethasone, diazoxide, disulfiram, dopamine, doxycycline, dronedarone, efavirenz, elbasvir & grazoprevir, eliglustat, emtricitabine/rilpivirine/tenofovir alafenamide, enzalutamide, erlotinib, eslicarbazepine, ethosuximide, etravirine, everolimus, ezogabine, fesoterodine, flibanserin, floxuridine, fluconazole, flunisolide, fluoxetine, fosamprenavir, gefitinib, gold & gold compounds, hydrocortisone, ibrutinib, idelalisib, imatinib, indinavir, influenza vaccine, isoniazid, isotretinoin, isradipine, itraconazole, ixabepilone, ixazomib, lacosamide, lapatinib, ledipasvir & sofosbuvir, leflunomide, letermovir, levodopa, levomepromazine, levonorgestrel, lisdexamfetamine, lomustine, lopinavir, meperidine, metformin, methsuximide, methylprednisolone, metronidazole, midazolam, midostaurin, mifepristone, mivacurium, naldemedine, nelfinavir, neratinib, nifedipine, nilotinib, nilutamide, nintedanib, olaparib, ombitasvir/paritaprevir/ritonavir, omeprazole, ondansetron, osimertinib, oxcarbazepine, oxtriphylline, palbociclib, paroxetine hydrochloride, pemetrexed, perampanel, phenylbutazone, pimavanserin, piracetam, ponatinib, posaconazole, prednisolone, prednisone, propranolol, regorafenib, rifapentine, rilpivirine, riociguat, risperidone, ritonavir, rivaroxaban, roflumilast, romidepsin, saquinavir, simeprevir, sofosbuvir, sofosbuvir & velpatasvir, sofosbuvir/velpatasvir/voxilaprevir, solifenacin, sonidegib, sorafenib, St John's wort, sucralfate, sunitinib, tegafur/gimeracil/oteracil, telaprevir, telithromycin, temsirolimus, teniposide, tenofovir alafenamide, tezacaftor/ivacaftor, thalidomide, tiagabine, ticagrelor, ticlopidine, tinidazole, tipranavir, tizanidine, tolvaptan, triamcinolone, trimethoprim, ulipristal, uracil/tegafur, valbenazine, vandetanib, vemurafenib, venetoclax, vigabatrin, vorapaxar, voriconazole, vortioxetine, zidovudine, zuclopenthixol
Pregnancy category: D
Note: Aromatic antiepileptic drugs, phenytoin, phenobarbital, carbamazepine and primidone, are a frequent cause of severe cutaneous adverse reactions. A strong genetic association between HLA-B*1502 and phenytoin-induced Stevens-Johnson syndrome and toxic epidermal necrolysis has been shown in Han Chinese patients. Children whose mothers receive phenytoin during pregnancy are born with fetal hydantoin syndrome. The main features of this syndrome are mental and growth retardation, unusual facies, digital and nail hypoplasia, and coarse scalp hair. Occasionally neonatal acne will be present.

Skin
Acne keloid [2]
Acneform eruption [8]
AGEP [5]
Angioedema [2]
Anticonvulsant hypersensitivity syndrome [10]
Coarse facies [4]
Dermatomyositis [2]
DRESS syndrome [34]
Erythema multiforme [11]
Erythroderma [9]
Exanthems (6–71%) [22]
Exfoliative dermatitis [15]
Fixed eruption [5]
Hypersensitivity [47]
Kaposi's varicelliform eruption [2]
Linear IgA bullous dermatosis [8]
Lupus erythematosus [19]
Lymphoma [6]
Mycosis fungoides [7]
Pemphigus [2]
Pigmentation [4]
Pruritus [5]
Pseudolymphoma [31]
Purple glove syndrome [10]
Purpura [4]
Pustules [3]
Rash (<10%) [13]
Reticular hyperplasia [2]
Serum sickness-like reaction [2]
Stevens-Johnson syndrome (14%) [60]
Toxic epidermal necrolysis (2%) [66]
Urticaria [5]
Vasculitis (2%) [11]

Hair
Alopecia [3]
Hirsutism [8]

Nails
Nail changes [2]
Nail hypoplasia [3]

Mucosal
Gingival hyperplasia/hypertrophy (>10%) [57]
Mucocutaneous eruption [2]

Cardiovascular
Bradycardia [3]
Polyarteritis nodosa [2]

Central Nervous System
Ageusia (taste loss) [2]
Fetal hydantoin syndrome [8]
Hallucinations [2]
Neurotoxicity [2]
Paresthesias [2]
Restless legs syndrome [2]

Neuromuscular/Skeletal
Digital malformations [4]
Myalgia/Myopathy [2]
Myasthenia gravis [2]
Osteoporosis [2]
Rhabdomyolysis [6]

Gastrointestinal/Hepatic
Hepatotoxicity [10]

Respiratory
Cough [2]

Ocular
Hallucinations, visual [2]

Local
- Injection-site extravasation [2]
- Injection-site necrosis [2]

Other
- Adverse effects [3]
- Death [4]
- Hiccups [2]
- Teratogenicity [3]

PHYSOSTIGMINE

Synonym: eserine
Indications: Miotic in glaucoma treatment, reverses toxic CNS effects caused by anticholinergic drugs
Class: Cholinesterase inhibitor
Half-life: 15–40 minutes
Clinically important, potentially hazardous interactions with: bethanechol, corticosteroids, galantamine, methacholine, succinylcholine
Pregnancy category: C
Important contra-indications noted in the prescribing guidelines for: nursing mothers
Note: Antilirium is a derivative of the Calabar bean, and its active moiety, physostigmine, is also known as eserine. Physostigmine is used to reverse the effect upon the nervous system caused by clinical or toxic dosages of drugs and herbs capable of producing the anticholinergic syndrome. Some of the drugs responsible are: amitriptyline, amoxapine, atropine, benztropine, biperiden, clidinium, cyclobenzaprine, desipramine, doxepin, hyoscyamine, imipramine, lorazepam, maprotiline, nortriptyline, protriptyline, propantheline, scopolamine, trimipramine. Some herbals that can elicit the anticholinergic syndrome are black henbane, deadly nightshade, Devil's apple, Jimson weed, Loco seeds or weeds, Matrimony vine, night blooming jessamine, stinkweed.

Skin
- Diaphoresis (>10%)
- Erythema (<10%)

Mucosal
- Sialorrhea (>10%)

Cardiovascular
- Atrial fibrillation [2]
- Bradycardia [3]

Central Nervous System
- Seizures (<10%) [4]
- Twitching (<10%)

Gastrointestinal/Hepatic
- Nausea [4]
- Vomiting [3]

Ocular
- Epiphora (>10%)
- Ocular burning (<10%)
- Ocular stinging (>10%)

PHYTONADIONE

Synonym: vitamin K_1
Trade names: Mephyton (Valeant), Vitamin K (AbbVie)
Indications: Coagulation disorders
Class: Vitamin
Half-life: 2–4 hours
Clinically important, potentially hazardous interactions with: cholestyramine, orlistat, warfarin
Pregnancy category: C
Important contra-indications noted in the prescribing guidelines for: nursing mothers; pediatric patients

---

Skin
- Anaphylactoid reactions/Anaphylaxis [4]
- Dermatitis [9]
- Eczema [2]
- Nicolau syndrome [2]
- Scleroderma [12]
- Urticaria [4]

Local
- Injection-site eczematous eruption [10]
- Injection-site erythema [2]
- Injection-site induration [15]

Other
- Allergic reactions [2]

PILOCARPINE

Trade names: Ocusert Pilo (Akorn), Pilopine (Alcon), Salagen (MGI)
Indications: Glaucoma, miosis induction, xerostomia
Class: Miotic, Muscarinic cholinergic agonist
Half-life: N/A
Clinically important, potentially hazardous interactions with: acebutolol, galantamine
Pregnancy category: C
Important contra-indications noted in the prescribing guidelines for: nursing mothers; pediatric patients

---

Skin
- Burning (<10%)
- Dermatitis [4]
- Diaphoresis [6]
- Edema (4%)
- Hyperhidrosis [2]
- Hypersensitivity (<10%)
- Stinging (<10%)

Central Nervous System
- Dysgeusia (taste perversion) (2%)
- Headache [2]

Ocular
- Cataract [2]

PIMAVANSERIN

Trade name: Nuplazid (Acadia)
Indications: Hallucinations and delusions associated with Parkinson's disease psychosis
Class: Antipsychotic
Half-life: 57 hours
Clinically important, potentially hazardous interactions with: amiodarone, carbamazepine, chlorpromazine, clarithromycin, disopyramide, drugs known to prolong the QT interval, gatifloxacin, indinavir, itraconazole, ketoconazole, moxifloxacin, phenytoin, procainamide, quinidine, rifampin, sotalol, St John's wort, strong CYP3A4 inhibitors and inducers, thioridazine, ziprasidone
Pregnancy category: N/A (No available data to inform drug-associated risk)
Important contra-indications noted in the prescribing guidelines for: the elderly; nursing mothers; pediatric patients
Warning: INCREASED MORTALITY IN ELDERLY PATIENTS WITH DEMENTIA-RELATED PSYCHOSIS

Skin
- Peripheral edema (7%) [5]

Cardiovascular
- QT prolongation [3]

Central Nervous System
- Confusion (6%) [4]
- Gait instability (2%) [6]
- Hallucinations (5%) [3]
- Headache [2]

Gastrointestinal/Hepatic
- Constipation (4%)
- Nausea (7%) [2]

Genitourinary
- Urinary tract infection [5]

PIMECROLIMUS

Trade name: Elidel (Valeant)
Indications: Second-line therapy for the short-term and non-continuous chronic treatment of mild to moderate atopic dermatitis
Class: Immunomodulator, Macrolactam
Half-life: N/A
Clinically important, potentially hazardous interactions with: abatacept, alcohol, alefacept, aprepitant, azacitidine, betamethasone, cabazitaxel, calcium channel blockers, cimetidine, conivaptan, CYP3A4 inhibitors, darunavir, delavirdine, denileukin, docetaxel, efavirenz, erythromycin, fingolimod, fluconazole, gefitinib, immunosuppressants, indinavir, itraconazole, ketoconazole, lapatinib, leflunomide, lenalidomide, oxaliplatin, pazopanib, pemetrexed, telithromycin, temsirolimus, triamcinolone, voriconazole
Pregnancy category: C
Important contra-indications noted in the prescribing guidelines for: nursing mothers; pediatric patients
Warning: LONG-TERM SAFETY OF TOPICAL CALCINEURIN INHIBITORS HAS NOT BEEN ESTABLISHED.

Skin
- Burning [4]
- Dermatitis [2]
- Peripheral edema [3]
- Rosacea [5]
- Tinea [3]

Cardiovascular
- Cardiac arrest [2]

Respiratory
- Upper respiratory tract infection (19%)

Local
- Application-site burning (8–26%)
- Application-site reactions (2%)

Other
- Infection (5%) [2]

PIMOZIDE

Trade name: Orap (Teva)
Indications: Tourette's syndrome, schizophrenia
Class: Antipsychotic
Half-life: 50 hours
Clinically important, potentially hazardous interactions with: amitriptyline, amoxapine, amphetamines, amprenavir, aprepitant, arsenic, artemether/lumefantrine, astemizole, atazanavir, azithromycin, azole antifungals, boceprevir, ceritinib, citalopram, clarithromycin, crizotinib, darunavir, dasabuvir/ombitasvir/paritaprevir/ritonavir, dasatinib, degarelix, delavirdine, dirithromycin, dolasetron, droperidol, efavirenz, eluxadoline, enzalutamide, erythromycin, fluoxetine, fosamprenavir, grapefruit juice, imatinib, indinavir, itraconazole, ketoconazole, lapatinib, letermovir, levofloxacin, levomepromazine, lopinavir, lurasidone, methylphenidate, mifepristone, moxifloxacin, nefazodone, nelfinavir, nilotinib, ombitasvir/paritaprevir/ritonavir, paroxetine hydrochloride, pazopanib, pemoline, phenothiazines, posaconazole, protease inhibitors, quinidine, quinine, ribociclib, ritonavir, saquinavir, sertraline, sotalol, sparfloxacin, sulpiride, telaprevir, telavancin, telithromycin, thioridazine, tipranavir, tricyclic antidepressants, trifluoperazine, troleandomycin, vandetanib, voriconazole, vorinostat, zileuton, ziprasidone
Pregnancy category: C
Important contra-indications noted in the prescribing guidelines for: nursing mothers; pediatric patients

---

Skin
- Facial edema (<10%)
- Rash (8%)

Mucosal
- Sialorrhea (14%)
- Xerostomia (>10%) [3]

Cardiovascular
- QT prolongation [4]

Neuromuscular/Skeletal
- Myalgia/Myopathy (3%)

Endocrine/Metabolic
- Gynecomastia (>10%)

PIOGLITAZONE

Trade name: Actos (Takeda)
Indications: Type II diabetes
Class: Antidiabetic, CYP3A4 inducer, Thiazolidinedione
Half-life: 3–7 hours
Clinically important, potentially hazardous interactions with: alcohol, conivaptan, corticosteroids, CYP2C8 inhibitors and inducers, dapagliflozin, deferasirox, gemfibrozil, insulin, pegvisomant, pregabalin, rifampin, saxagliptin, somatropin, teriflunomide, trimethoprim
Pregnancy category: C
Important contra-indications noted in the prescribing guidelines for: nursing mothers; pediatric patients
Note: Contra-indicated in patients with established NYHA Class III or IV heart failure.
Warning: CONGESTIVE HEART FAILURE

Skin
- Edema (4–11%) [29]
- Peripheral edema [12]

Cardiovascular
- Cardiac failure (<10%) [14]
- Cardiomyopathy [3]
- Cardiotoxicity [2]
- Myocardial infarction [3]

Central Nervous System
- Headache (9%) [4]
- Stroke [2]

Neuromuscular/Skeletal
- Asthenia (fatigue) (4%)
- Bone loss [4]
- Fractures [10]
- Myalgia/Myopathy (5%)

Gastrointestinal/Hepatic
- Diarrhea [4]
- Hepatotoxicity [8]
- Nausea [3]
- Vomiting [2]

Respiratory
- Nasopharyngitis [3]
- Pharyngitis (5%)
- Sinusitis (6%)
- Upper respiratory tract infection (13%)

Endocrine/Metabolic
- Hypoglycemia [10]
- Weight gain [19]

Genitourinary
- Bladder cancer [7]

Hematologic
- Anemia (<2%) [2]
- Pancytopenia [2]

Ocular
- Macular edema [2]

Other
- Adverse effects [4]
- Death [3]
- Tooth disorder (5%)

PIPERACILLIN/ TAZOBACTAM

Trade name: Zosyn (Wyeth)
Indications: Moderate to severe infections
Class: Antibacterial
Half-life: 0.7–1.2 hours
Clinically important, potentially hazardous interactions with: heparin, methotrexate
Pregnancy category: B
Important contra-indications noted in the prescribing guidelines for: nursing mothers

---

Skin
- AGEP [2]
- DRESS syndrome [3]
- Hypersensitivity [2]
- Rash [5]

Central Nervous System
- Fever [3]
- Neurotoxicity [2]

Gastrointestinal/Hepatic
- Diarrhea [4]
- Hepatotoxicity [3]
- Nausea [2]
- Vomiting [2]

Endocrine/Metabolic
- Hypokalemia [3]

Renal
- Nephrotoxicity [5]

Hematologic
- Hemolytic anemia [3]
- Hemotoxicity [2]
- Thrombocytopenia [4]

Other
- Adverse effects [4]

PIRFENIDONE

Trade name: Esbriet (Intermune)
Indications: Idiopathic pulmonary fibrosis
Class: Immunosuppressant, Pyridone
Half-life: 3 hours
Clinically important, potentially hazardous interactions with: ciprofloxacin, fluvoxamine
Pregnancy category: C
Important contra-indications noted in the prescribing guidelines for: nursing mothers; pediatric patients

---

Skin
- Photosensitivity (9%) [22]
- Phototoxicity [2]
- Pruritus (8%) [3]
- Rash (30%) [14]

Cardiovascular
- Chest pain (5%) [3]

Central Nervous System
- Anorexia (13%) [11]
- Dysgeusia (taste perversion) (6%)
- Headache (22%) [3]
- Insomnia (10%)
- Sedation [2]
- Vertigo (dizziness) (18%) [7]

Neuromuscular/Skeletal
Arthralgia (10%)
Asthenia (fatigue) (6–26%) [9]

Gastrointestinal/Hepatic
Abdominal pain (24%) [7]
Diarrhea (26%) [12]
Dyspepsia (19%) [10]
Gastroesophageal reflux (11%) [6]
Gastrointestinal disorder [3]
Hepatotoxicity [5]
Nausea (36%) [20]
Vomiting (13%) [7]

Respiratory
Bronchitis [2]
Cough [3]
Dyspnea [3]
Nasopharyngitis [2]
Sinusitis (11%)
Upper respiratory tract infection (27%) [3]

Endocrine/Metabolic
ALT increased [5]
Appetite decreased (8%) [4]
AST increased [5]
Hyponatremia [3]
Weight loss (10%) [4]

Other
Adverse effects [9]

PIROXICAM

Trade name: Feldene (Pfizer)
Indications: Arthritis
Class: Non-steroidal anti-inflammatory (NSAID)
Half-life: 50 hours
Clinically important, potentially hazardous interactions with: ACE inhibitors, aspirin, furosemide, lithium, methotrexate, ritonavir, warfarin
Pregnancy category: D (pregnancy category C prior to 30 weeks gestation; category D starting at 30 weeks gestation)
Important contra-indications noted in the prescribing guidelines for: the elderly; nursing mothers
Note: NSAIDs may cause an increased risk of serious cardiovascular and gastrointestinal adverse events, which can be fatal. This risk may increase with duration of use.
Elderly patients are at greater risk for serious gastrointestinal events.
Warning: CARDIOVASCULAR AND GASTROINTESTINAL RISKS

Skin
AGEP [2]
Angioedema [3]
Dermatitis [5]
Erythema multiforme [12]
Erythroderma [2]
Exanthems (>5%) [8]
Fixed eruption [15]
Lichenoid eruption [5]
Linear IgA bullous dermatosis [3]
Pemphigus [3]
Photosensitivity [40]
Pruritus (<10%) [6]
Purpura [2]
Rash (>10%)
Stevens-Johnson syndrome [2]
Toxic epidermal necrolysis [12]
Urticaria [7]
Vasculitis [3]
Vesiculation [2]

Hair
Alopecia [3]

Mucosal
Aphthous stomatitis [4]

Central Nervous System
Anorexia (<10%)
Vertigo (dizziness) (<10%)

Gastrointestinal/Hepatic
Abdominal pain (<10%)
Constipation (<10%)
Diarrhea (<10%)
Dyspepsia (<10%)
Flatulence (<10%)
Gastrointestinal ulceration (<10%)
Nausea (<10%)
Vomiting (<10%)

Renal
Renal function abnormal (<10%)

Otic
Hearing loss [2]
Tinnitus [2]

Other
Adverse effects [2]
Side effects (47%)

PITAVASTATIN

Trade name: Livalo (Kowa)
Indications: Primary hyperlipidemia, mixed dyslipidemia
Class: Statin
Half-life: 12 hours
Clinically important, potentially hazardous interactions with: alcohol, cyclosporine, erythromycin, gemfibrozil, letermovir, lopinavir, niacin, rifampin, ritonavir, sofosbuvir/velpatasvir/voxilaprevir
Pregnancy category: X
Important contra-indications noted in the prescribing guidelines for: nursing mothers; pediatric patients
Note: Contra-indicated in patients with active liver disease.

Skin
Hypersensitivity (<2%)
Rash (<2%)
Urticaria (<2%)

Central Nervous System
Headache (<2%)

Neuromuscular/Skeletal
Arthralgia (<2%)
Back pain (2–4%)
Myalgia/Myopathy (2–3%) [5]
Pain in extremities (<2%)

Gastrointestinal/Hepatic
Constipation (2–4%)
Diarrhea (2–3%)

Respiratory
Influenza (<2%)
Nasopharyngitis (<2%) [2]

Endocrine/Metabolic
ALT increased [2]
AST increased [2]
Creatine phosphokinase increased [2]

Other
Adverse effects [4]

PLAZOMICIN *

Trade name: Zemdri (Achaogen Inc)
Indications: treatment of patients 18 years of age or older with Complicated Urinary Tract Infections (cUTI) including Pyelonephritis
Class: Antibiotic, aminoglycoside
Half-life: 3.5 hours
Clinically important, potentially hazardous interactions with: none known
Pregnancy category: N/A (Aminoglycosides can cause fetal harm, however, there are no available data on the use of Plazomicin in pregnant women to inform a drug associated risk of adverse developmental outcomes.)
Warning: NEPHROTOXICITY, OTOTOXICITY, NEUROMUSCULAR BLOCKADE and FETAL HARM

Cardiovascular
Hypertension (2%)

Gastrointestinal/Hepatic
Diarrhea (2%)

Endocrine/Metabolic
Serum creatinine increased (7%)

Renal
Renal function abnormal (4%)

PLECANATIDE

Trade name: Trulance (Synergy)
Indications: Chronic idiopathic constipation
Class: Guanylate cyclase-C agonist
Half-life: N/A
Clinically important, potentially hazardous interactions with: none known
Pregnancy category: N/A (Insufficient data to inform drug-associated risks)
Important contra-indications noted in the prescribing guidelines for: the elderly; nursing mothers; pediatric patients
Warning: RISK OF SERIOUS DEHYDRATION IN PEDIATRIC PATIENTS

Gastrointestinal/Hepatic
Abdominal distension (<2%)
Abdominal pain [2]
Diarrhea (5%) [9]
Flatulence (<2%)
Nausea [3]
Vomiting [2]

Respiratory
Sinusitis (<2%)
Upper respiratory tract infection (<2%)

Endocrine/Metabolic
ALT increased (<2%)
AST increased (<2%)

PNEUMOCOCCAL VACCINE

Trade names: PCV (Lederle), PncOMP (Merck), Pneumovax II (Sanofi-Aventis), Pnu-Immune (Lederle), PPV (Lederle), Prevnar (Wyeth)
Indications: Prevention of bacteremia, meningitis, pneumonia, respiratory tract infections, otitis media, sinusitis
Class: Vaccine
Half-life: N/A
Clinically important, potentially hazardous interactions with: none known
Pregnancy category: C

Skin
Anaphylactoid reactions/Anaphylaxis [2]
Rash [2]
Serum sickness [2]
Sweet's syndrome [2]
Urticaria [5]

Central Nervous System
Fever [21]
Headache [4]
Irritability [3]
Seizures [4]
Sleep disturbances [2]

Neuromuscular/Skeletal
Arthralgia [3]
Asthenia (fatigue) [7]
Myalgia/Myopathy [4]

Respiratory
Respiratory tract infection [2]

Endocrine/Metabolic
Appetite decreased [3]

Local
Injection-site edema [8]
Injection-site erythema [10]
Injection-site induration [3]
Injection-site pain [10]
Injection-site reactions [10]

Other
Adverse effects [3]

POLIDOCANOL

Trade names: Asclera (Chemische Fabrik Kreussler), Varithena (BTG)
Indications: Uncomplicated spider veins and uncomplicated reticular veins in the lower extremity
Class: Sclerosant, local
Half-life: 1.5 hours
Clinically important, potentially hazardous interactions with: none known
Pregnancy category: C
Important contra-indications noted in the prescribing guidelines for: nursing mothers; pediatric patients
Note: Severe allergic reactions have been reported following polidocanol use, including anaphylactic reactions, some of them fatal. Severe reactions are more frequent with use of larger volumes (>3 mL).
Contra-indicated in patients with acute thromboembolic diseases.

Skin
Anaphylactoid reactions/Anaphylaxis [4]
Pigmentation [2]
Urticaria [2]

Cardiovascular
Cardiac arrest [2]
Phlebitis [2]

Central Nervous System
Migraine [2]

Neuromuscular/Skeletal
Leg pain [2]

Hematologic
Thrombosis [2]

Local
Injection-site hematoma (42%)
Injection-site irritation (41%)
Injection-site pain (24%)
Injection-site pigmentation (38%)
Injection-site pruritus (19%)
Injection-site reactions [3]
Injection-site thrombosis (6%)

POLYPODIUM LEUCOTOMOS

Family: Polypodiaceae
Scientific names: *Anapsos, Calagualine, Calagula, Difur, Fernblock, Heliocare, Polypodium leucotomos*
Indications: Oral and topical photoprotection, vitiligo, psoriasis, dermatitis, arthritis
Class: Anti-inflammatory, Antioxidant
Half-life: N/A
Clinically important, potentially hazardous interactions with: none known
Note: It is the first oral agent effective in reducing side effects of PUVA treatment.

POMALIDOMIDE

Trade name: Pomalyst (Celgene)
Indications: Multiple myeloma in patients who have received at least two prior therapies including lenalidomide and bortezomib
Class: Immunomodulator, Thalidomide analog
Half-life: 7.5–9.5 hours
Clinically important, potentially hazardous interactions with: ketoconazole, P-glycoprotein, rifampin
Pregnancy category: X
Important contra-indications noted in the prescribing guidelines for: nursing mothers; pediatric patients
Warning: EMBRYO-FETAL TOXICITY and VENOUS AND ARTERIAL THROMBOEMBOLISM

Skin
Edema [4]
Hyperhidrosis (6%)
Peripheral edema (23%)
Pruritus (15%)
Rash (22%) [2]
Xerosis (9%)

Mucosal
Epistaxis (nosebleed) (15%)

Cardiovascular
Chest pain (22%)
Venous thromboembolism [8]

Central Nervous System
Anorexia [2]
Anxiety (11%)
Chills (9%)
Confusion (10%)
Fever (19%) [3]
Headache (13%)
Insomnia (7%)
Neurotoxicity (18%) [3]
Pain (6%)
Peripheral neuropathy (10%) [3]
Tremor (9%) [2]
Vertigo (dizziness) (20%)

Neuromuscular/Skeletal
Arthralgia (16%)
Asthenia (fatigue) (12–55%) [11]
Back pain (32%) [3]
Bone or joint pain (11–12%) [2]
Muscle spasm (19%)
Myalgia/Myopathy [2]
Pain in extremities (5%)

Gastrointestinal/Hepatic
Constipation (36%) [2]
Diarrhea (34%) [2]
Nausea (36%)
Vomiting (14%)

Respiratory
Cough (14%)
Dyspnea (34%) [5]
Pneumonia (23%) [7]
Upper respiratory tract infection (32%)

Endocrine/Metabolic
Appetite decreased (22%)
Dehydration [2]
Hypercalcemia (21%)
Hyperglycemia (12%) [2]
Hypocalcemia (6%)
Hypokalemia (10%)
Hyponatremia (10%)
Serum creatinine increased (15%)
Weight loss (14%)

Genitourinary
Urinary tract infection (8%)

Renal
Renal failure (15%)

Hematologic
Anemia (38%) [16]
Febrile neutropenia [3]
Leukopenia (11%) [3]
Lymphopenia (4%) [2]
Myelosuppression [4]
Neutropenia (52%) [27]
Sepsis [2]
Thrombocytopenia (25%) [17]

Other
Death [3]
Infection [11]

POSACONAZOLE

Trade name: Noxafil (Schering)
Indications: *Aspergillus* and *Candida* infection prophylaxis in immunocompromised patients
Class: Antibiotic, triazole, Antifungal, azole
Half-life: 35 hours
Clinically important, potentially hazardous interactions with: alprazolam, atazanavir, atorvastatin, boceprevir, brigatinib, cabozantinib, calcium channel blockers, cimetidine, copanlisib, cyclosporine, digoxin, dihydroergotamine, diltiazem, dronedarone, efavirenz, ergotamine, esomeprazole, everolimus, felodipine, flibanserin, fosamprenavir, HMG-CoA reductase inhibitors, ibrutinib, lapatinib, lomitapide, lovastatin, metoclopramide, midazolam, midostaurin, mifepristone, neratinib, nicardipine, nifedipine, olaparib, omeprazole, palbociclib, pantoprazole, phenytoin, pimozide, ponatinib, quinidine, regorafenib, rifabutin, rilpivirine, ritonavir, rivaroxaban, ruxolitinib, simeprevir, simvastatin, sirolimus, sonidegib, tacrolimus, telaprevir, temsirolimus, tezacaftor/ivacaftor, triazolam, venetoclax, verapamil, vinblastine, vincristine, vorapaxar
Pregnancy category: C
Important contra-indications noted in the prescribing guidelines for: nursing mothers; pediatric patients

---

Skin
- Edema (9%)
- Herpes (14%)
- Herpes simplex (3–15%)
- Hyperhidrosis (2–10%)
- Jaundice (<5%)
- Peripheral edema (15%)
- Petechiae (11%)
- Pruritus (11%)
- Rash (3–19%) [3]
- Thrombocytopenic purpura (<5%)

Mucosal
- Epistaxis (nosebleed) (14%)
- Mucositis (17%)
- Oral candidiasis (<12%)

Cardiovascular
- Hypertension (18%)
- Hypotension (14%)
- QT prolongation [3]
- Tachycardia (12%)
- Torsades de pointes (<5%)

Central Nervous System
- Anorexia (2–19%)
- Anxiety (9%)
- Dysgeusia (taste perversion) (~2%)
- Fever (6–45%)
- Headache (8–28%) [6]
- Insomnia (<17%)
- Neurotoxicity [2]
- Paresthesias (<5%)
- Rigors (<20%)
- Tremor (~2%)
- Vertigo (dizziness) (11%) [3]

Neuromuscular/Skeletal
- Arthralgia (11%)
- Asthenia (fatigue) (3–17%) [3]
- Back pain (10%)
- Bone or joint pain (16%)
- Myalgia/Myopathy (16%)

Gastrointestinal/Hepatic
- Abdominal pain (5–27%) [3]
- Constipation (21%)
- Diarrhea (10–42%) [6]
- Dyspepsia (10%)
- Flatulence [2]
- Hepatitis (<5%)
- Hepatomegaly (<5%)
- Hepatotoxicity (<5%) [6]
- Nausea (9–38%) [13]
- Vomiting (7–29%) [6]

Respiratory
- Cough (3–25%)
- Dyspnea (<20%)
- Pharyngitis (12%)
- Pneumonia (3–10%)
- Pulmonary embolism (<5%)
- Upper respiratory tract infection (7%)

Endocrine/Metabolic
- Adrenal insufficiency (<5%)
- ALP increased (3–13%)
- ALT increased (3–11%) [2]
- AST increased (6–17%) [2]
- Dehydration (<11%)
- Hyperbilirubinemia [2]
- Hyperglycemia (11%)
- Hypocalcemia (9%)
- Hypokalemia (30%)
- Hypomagnesemia (18%)
- Weight loss (<14%)

Genitourinary
- Vaginal bleeding (10%)

Renal
- Renal failure (<5%)

Hematologic
- Anemia (2–25%)
- Febrile neutropenia (20%)
- Hemolytic uremic syndrome (<5%)
- Neutropenia (4–23%) [2]
- Thrombocytopenia (29%) [2]

Ocular
- Vision blurred (~2%)

Other
- Adverse effects [11]
- Allergic reactions (<5%)
- Infection (18%)

POTASSIUM IODIDE

Synonyms: KI; Lugol's solution
Trade name: SSKI (Upsher-Smith)
Indications: Hyperthyroidism, erythema nodosum, sporotrichosis
Class: Antihyperthyroid, Antimycobacterial
Half-life: N/A
Clinically important, potentially hazardous interactions with: ACE inhibitors, potassium-sparing diuretics, spironolactone, triamterene
Pregnancy category: D
Important contra-indications noted in the prescribing guidelines for: nursing mothers

---

Skin
- Acneform eruption (<10%) [3]
- Angioedema (<10%)
- Bullous pemphigoid [2]
- Dermatitis herpetiformis [2]
- Iododerma [17]
- Psoriasis [2]
- Urticaria (<10%)
- Vasculitis [3]

Central Nervous System
- Dysgeusia (taste perversion) (<10%) [2]

Gastrointestinal/Hepatic
- Gastrointestinal disorder [2]

Endocrine/Metabolic
- Hypothyroidism [2]

PRALIDOXIME

Trade name: Protopam (Baxter)
Indications: Muscle weakness and respiratory depression caused by organophosphate drugs which have anticholinesterase activity, antidote to overdose of anticholinesterase drugs
Class: Antidote
Half-life: 2.4–5.3 hours
Clinically important, potentially hazardous interactions with: succinylcholine
Pregnancy category: C
Important contra-indications noted in the prescribing guidelines for: the elderly; nursing mothers
Note: Pralidoxime is not effective in the treatment of poisoning due to phosphorus, inorganic phosphates, or organophosphates not having anticholinesterase activity. Pralidoxime is not indicated as an antidote for intoxication by pesticides of the carbamate class since it may increase the toxicity of carbaryl. In therapy it has been difficult to differentiate side effects due to the drug from those due to the effects of the poison.

PRAMIPEXOLE

Trade name: Mirapex (Boehringer Ingelheim)
Indications: Parkinsonism, restless legs syndrome
Class: Dopamine receptor agonist
Half-life: ~8 hours
Clinically important, potentially hazardous interactions with: levomepromazine, risperidone, zuclopenthixol
Pregnancy category: C
Important contra-indications noted in the prescribing guidelines for: nursing mothers; pediatric patients

---

Skin
- Edema (5%)
- Peripheral edema (5%) [4]

Mucosal
- Xerostomia (7%) [3]

Cardiovascular
- Chest pain (3%)
- Hypotension (~53%) [2]
- Orthostatic hypotension [2]

Central Nervous System
- Abnormal dreams (11%)

Akathisia (2–3%)
Amnesia (4–6%)
Anorexia (<5%)
Compulsions [6]
Confusion [2]
Depression (2%)
Dyskinesia (17–47%) [3]
Hallucinations (5–17%) [6]
Headache (4–7%) [3]
Hyperesthesia (3%)
Impulse control disorder [10]
Insomnia (4–27%) [2]
Restless legs syndrome [2]
Somnolence (drowsiness) (9–36%) [9]
Tremor (4%)
Twitching (2%)
Vertigo (dizziness) (2–26%) [6]

Neuromuscular/Skeletal
Antecollis [2]
Arthralgia (4%)
Asthenia (fatigue) (<14%) [2]

Gastrointestinal/Hepatic
Constipation [5]
Nausea [9]
Vomiting (4%) [3]

Respiratory
Cough (3%)
Dyspnea (4%)
Rhinitis (3%)

Genitourinary
Urinary frequency (6%)
Urinary tract infection (4%)

Other
Adverse effects (2%) [5]

PRASUGREL

Trade name: Effient (Lilly)
Indications: Acute coronary syndrome in patients who are to be managed with percutaneous coronary intervention
Class: Antiplatelet, thienopyridine
Half-life: 2–15 hours
Clinically important, potentially hazardous interactions with: cangrelor, clopidogrel, conivaptan, coumarins, darunavir, delavirdine, diclofenac, indinavir, meloxicam, NSAIDs, phenindione, telithromycin, voriconazole, warfarin
Pregnancy category: B
Important contra-indications noted in the prescribing guidelines for: the elderly; nursing mothers; pediatric patients
Note: Contra-indicated in patients with active pathological bleeding, prior transient ischemic attack or stroke.
Warning: BLEEDING RISK

Skin
Hypersensitivity [2]
Peripheral edema (3%)
Rash (3%) [4]

Mucosal
Epistaxis (nosebleed) (6%)

Cardiovascular
Atrial fibrillation (3%)
Bradycardia (3%)
Chest pain (3%)
Hypertension (8%)
Hypotension (4%)

Central Nervous System
Fever (3%)
Headache (6%)
Vertigo (dizziness) (4%)

Neuromuscular/Skeletal
Asthenia (fatigue) (4%)
Back pain (5%)
Pain in extremities (3%)

Gastrointestinal/Hepatic
Diarrhea (3%)
Gastrointestinal bleeding (2%)
Nausea (5%)

Respiratory
Cough (4%)
Dyspnea (5%)
Respiratory distress [2]

Endocrine/Metabolic
Hypercholesterolemia (7%)
Hyperlipidemia (7%)

Hematologic
Anemia (2%)
Bleeding (<14%) [25]
Hemorrhage [2]
Leukopenia (3%)

Other
Adverse effects [2]
Malignant neoplasms (2%)

PRAVASTATIN

Trade names: Lipostat (Bristol-Myers Squibb), Pravachol (Bristol-Myers Squibb)
Indications: Hypercholesterolemia
Class: HMG-CoA reductase inhibitor, Statin
Half-life: ~2–3 hours
Clinically important, potentially hazardous interactions with: azithromycin, ciprofibrate, clarithromycin, colchicine, cyclosporine, darunavir, efavirenz, erythromycin, gemfibrozil, imatinib, letermovir, red rice yeast, telithromycin
Pregnancy category: X
Important contra-indications noted in the prescribing guidelines for: nursing mothers

---

Skin
Dermatomyositis [2]
Eczema (generalized) [2]
Edema (3%)
Lichenoid eruption [2]
Pruritus [2]
Rash (5–7%) [7]

Cardiovascular
Angina (5%)
Chest pain (3–10%)

Central Nervous System
Anxiety (5%)
Fever (2%)
Headache (6%)
Nervousness (5%)
Paresthesias (3%)
Sleep disturbances (3%)
Vertigo (dizziness) (4–7%)

Neuromuscular/Skeletal
Asthenia (fatigue) (3–8%)
Bone or joint pain (25%)
Cramps (5%)
Myalgia/Myopathy (2–3%) [9]
Rhabdomyolysis [24]

Gastrointestinal/Hepatic
Abdominal distension (2%)
Diarrhea (7%)
Dyspepsia (3%)
Flatulence (3%)
Nausea (7%)
Pancreatitis [4]
Vomiting (7%)

Respiratory
Bronchitis (3%)
Cough (3–8%)
Influenza (9%)
Pharyngitis (2%)
Pulmonary toxicity (4%)
Rhinitis (4%)
Upper respiratory tract infection (6–21%)

Endocrine/Metabolic
ALT increased (3%)
Creatine phosphokinase increased (4%) [3]
GGT increased (2%)
Weight gain (4%)
Weight loss (3%)

Genitourinary
Urinary tract infection (3%)

Renal
Renal failure [2]

Ocular
Diplopia (3%)
Vision blurred (3%)

Other
Adverse effects [2]
Infection (3%)

PRAZIQUANTEL

Trade name: Biltricide (Bayer)
Indications: Helmintic infections
Class: Anthelmintic
Half-life: 0.8–1.5 hours
Clinically important, potentially hazardous interactions with: dexamethasone, efavirenz, oxcarbazepine, rifampin, rifapentine
Pregnancy category: B
Important contra-indications noted in the prescribing guidelines for: nursing mothers

---

Skin
Diaphoresis (<10%)
Edema [2]
Pruritus [3]
Rash [2]
Urticaria [5]

Central Nervous System
Fever [2]
Headache [8]
Seizures [2]
Somnolence (drowsiness) [2]
Vertigo (dizziness) [7]

Neuromuscular/Skeletal
Asthenia (fatigue) [3]

Gastrointestinal/Hepatic
- Abdominal pain [10]
- Diarrhea [5]
- Nausea [5]
- Vomiting [7]

Other
- Adverse effects [2]
- Allergic reactions [2]

PREDNISOLONE

Trade names: Blephamide (Allergan), Delta-Cortef (Pharmacia), Hydeltrasol (Merck), Inflamase (Novartis), Pediapred (UCB), Prelone (Teva)
Indications: Arthralgias, asthma, dermatoses, inflammatory ocular conditions
Class: Corticosteroid, systemic
Half-life: 2–4 hours
Clinically important, potentially hazardous interactions with: aluminum, aminophylline, carbamazepine, carbimazole, cyclosporine, daclizumab, diuretics, etoposide, etretinate, grapefruit juice, indomethacin, isoniazid, itraconazole, ketoconazole, live vaccines, methotrexate, naproxen, oral contraceptives, pancuronium, phenobarbital, phenytoin, rifampin, troleandomycin
Pregnancy category: C

Skin
- Acneform eruption [4]
- AGEP [2]
- Candidiasis [2]
- Cushingoid features [2]
- Dermatitis [3]
- Edema [7]
- Erythema [2]
- Erythema multiforme [2]
- Exanthems [3]
- Flushing [2]
- Kaposi's sarcoma [3]
- Pruritus [2]
- Stevens-Johnson syndrome [2]
- Toxicity [3]

Hair
- Alopecia [2]

Cardiovascular
- Atrial fibrillation [2]
- Cardiotoxicity [4]
- Hypertension [13]
- Tachycardia [2]

Central Nervous System
- Behavioral disturbances [2]
- Depression [4]

Neuromuscular/Skeletal
- Arthralgia [4]
- Asthenia (fatigue) [5]
- Back pain [4]
- Bone or joint pain [5]
- Myalgia/Myopathy [2]
- Osteonecrosis [4]
- Osteoporosis [32]

Gastrointestinal/Hepatic
- Constipation [3]
- Diarrhea [2]
- Hepatotoxicity [6]
- Nausea [2]
- Pancreatitis [2]

Respiratory
- Upper respiratory tract infection [2]

Endocrine/Metabolic
- Cushing's syndrome [2]
- Diabetes mellitus [4]
- Hyperglycemia [3]
- Hypokalemia [7]
- Weight gain [2]

Hematologic
- Anemia [3]
- Febrile neutropenia [3]
- Neutropenia [4]
- Thrombocytopenia [2]

Ocular
- Cataract [5]
- Chorioretinopathy [2]
- Glaucoma [2]
- Intraocular pressure increased [4]

Other
- Adverse effects [12]
- Allergic reactions [2]
- Death [2]
- Infection [18]
- Side effects [4]

PREDNISONE

Trade names: Deltasone (Pharmacia), Meticorten (Schering)
Indications: Arthralgias, asthma, dermatoses, inflammatory ocular conditions
Class: Corticosteroid, systemic
Half-life: N/A
Clinically important, potentially hazardous interactions with: aluminum, aminophylline, aspirin, chlorambucil, cimetidine, clarithromycin, cyclophosphamide, cyclosporine, dicumarol, diuretics, docetaxel, estrogens, grapefruit juice, indomethacin, influenza vaccine, itraconazole, ketoconazole, lansoprazole, live vaccines, methotrexate, montelukast, omeprazole, oral contraceptives, pancuronium, phenobarbital, phenytoin, ranitidine, rifampin, timolol, tolbutamide, vitamin A, yellow fever vaccine
Pregnancy category: B
Important contra-indications noted in the prescribing guidelines for: the elderly; nursing mothers

---

Skin
- Dermatitis [4]
- Ecchymoses [2]
- Erythema [3]
- Kaposi's sarcoma [7]
- Squamous cell carcinoma [2]
- Thinning [2]
- Toxicity [2]

Hair
- Alopecia [2]

Mucosal
- Stomatitis [2]

Cardiovascular
- Cardiotoxicity [3]
- Hypertension [8]

Central Nervous System
- Headache [3]
- Leukoencephalopathy [3]
- Peripheral neuropathy [4]
- Psychosis [2]

Neuromuscular/Skeletal
- Arthralgia [2]
- Asthenia (fatigue) [7]
- Bone or joint pain [2]
- Fractures [3]
- Myalgia/Myopathy [4]
- Osteonecrosis [3]
- Osteoporosis [23]

Gastrointestinal/Hepatic
- Constipation [3]
- Diarrhea [4]
- Nausea [4]
- Vomiting [2]

Respiratory
- Cough [2]
- Upper respiratory tract infection [2]

Endocrine/Metabolic
- Diabetes mellitus [2]
- Hyperglycemia [3]
- Hypokalemia [2]
- Weight gain [2]

Hematologic
- Anemia [5]
- Febrile neutropenia [3]
- Leukopenia [3]
- Lymphopenia [3]
- Neutropenia [15]
- Thrombocytopenia [10]

Ocular
- Cataract [3]

Other
- Adverse effects [10]
- Death [3]
- Infection [12]
- Side effects [3]

PREGABALIN

Trade name: Lyrica (Pfizer)
Indications: Neuropathy, post-herpetic neuralgia, partial epilepsy, fibromyalgia
Class: Anticonvulsant, GABA analog
Half-life: 6 hours
Clinically important, potentially hazardous interactions with: lacosamide, pioglitazone
Pregnancy category: C
Important contra-indications noted in the prescribing guidelines for: nursing mothers; pediatric patients

---

Skin
- Edema (2%) [9]
- Peripheral edema (9%) [15]

Mucosal
- Xerostomia (5%) [11]

Cardiovascular
- Cardiac failure [4]
- Chest pain (2%)

Central Nervous System
- Anorgasmia [3]
- Confusion [2]

Depression [2]
Gait instability [4]
Headache (7%) [8]
Impaired concentration [2]
Insomnia [3]
Memory loss [2]
Neurotoxicity [4]
Pain (5%)
Sedation [6]
Somnolence (drowsiness) [47]
Suicidal ideation [4]
Tremor [2]
Vertigo (dizziness) (4%) [60]

Neuromuscular/Skeletal
Asthenia (fatigue) (5%) [8]
Ataxia [8]
Back pain (2%)
Muscle spasm [2]
Myoclonus [4]
Rhabdomyolysis [4]

Gastrointestinal/Hepatic
Constipation [6]
Diarrhea [2]
Hepatotoxicity [2]
Nausea [9]
Vomiting [3]

Endocrine/Metabolic
Appetite increased [2]
Weight gain [22]

Genitourinary
Erectile dysfunction [4]

Ocular
Diplopia (9%) [2]
Ocular edema [2]
Vision blurred (6%) [8]

Other
Adverse effects [6]
Dipsia (thirst) [2]
Infection (7%)
Side effects [2]

PRILOCAINE

Trade name: Citanest (AstraZeneca)
Indications: Local anesthetic
Class: Membrane integrity antagonist, Potassium channel antagonist, Sodium channel antagonist
Half-life: 2 hours
Clinically important, potentially hazardous interactions with: adenosine, amide-type anesthetics, antimalarials, co-trimoxazole, dronedarone, nitric compounds, sulfonamides
Pregnancy category: B
Important contra-indications noted in the prescribing guidelines for: nursing mothers; pediatric patients

---

Skin
Angioedema [3]
Contact dermatitis [3]
Hypersensitivity [2]
Petechiae [3]
Purpura [3]

Central Nervous System
Coma [4]
Paresthesias [3]
Seizures [2]

Hematologic
Methemoglobinemia [12]

Other
Adverse effects [2]

PROBENECID

Indications: Gouty arthritis
Class: Uricosuric
Half-life: 6–12 hours (dose-dependent)
Clinically important, potentially hazardous interactions with: acemetacin, acetaminophen, amphotericin B, ampicillin/sulbactam, benzodiazepines, captopril, cefazolin, cefditoren, cefixime, ceftaroline fosamil, ceftazidime & avibactam, ceftriaxone, ciprofloxacin, deferiprone, doripenem, ertapenem, flucloxacillin, furosemide, gemifloxacin, glibenclamide, ketoprofen, ketorolac, levodopa, levofloxacin, meloxicam, meropenem & vaborbactam, methotrexate, moxifloxacin, norfloxacin, NSAIDs, ofloxacin, pemetrexed, penicillamine, penicillin G, penicillin V, salicylates, sulfamethoxazole, sulfonamides, torsemide, zidovudine
Pregnancy category: C
Important contra-indications noted in the prescribing guidelines for: nursing mothers; pediatric patients

---

Skin
Flushing (<10%)
Pruritus (<10%)
Rash (<10%)
Urticaria (<5%)

Mucosal
Gingivitis (<10%)

Renal
Nephrotoxicity [3]

Hematologic
Thrombocytopenia [2]

PROCAINAMIDE

Trade names: Procan (Pfizer), Procanbid (Pfizer)
Indications: Ventricular arrhythmias
Class: Antiarrhythmic, Antiarrhythmic class Ia
Half-life: 2.5–4.5 hours
Clinically important, potentially hazardous interactions with: abarelix, amiodarone, amisulpride, arsenic, artemether/lumefantrine, asenapine, astemizole, ciprofloxacin, enoxacin, ethoxzolamide, gatifloxacin, glycopyrrolate, glycopyrronium, imidapril, lomefloxacin, lurasidone, metformin, mivacurium, moxifloxacin, nilotinib, norfloxacin, ofloxacin, pimavanserin, quinine, quinolones, ribociclib, rocuronium, sotalol, sparfloxacin, tetrabenazine, trimethoprim, trospium, vandetanib, zofenopril
Pregnancy category: C
Important contra-indications noted in the prescribing guidelines for: nursing mothers; pediatric patients

---

Skin
Dermatitis (6%)
Exanthems (<8%) [5]
Hypersensitivity [2]
Lupus erythematosus (>10%) [176]
Purpura [3]
Urticaria (<5%)
Vasculitis [5]

Mucosal
Oral mucosal eruption (2%)

Cardiovascular
Hypotension [2]
QT prolongation [5]
Torsades de pointes [3]

Central Nervous System
Dysgeusia (taste perversion) (3–4%)
Psychosis [2]

Neuromuscular/Skeletal
Myalgia/Myopathy [2]
Myasthenia gravis [3]

Gastrointestinal/Hepatic
Hepatotoxicity [3]
Nausea [3]

Respiratory
Pulmonary toxicity [2]

Hematologic
Agranulocytosis [4]
Neutropenia [3]
Pancytopenia [2]
Pure red cell aplasia [3]

PROCHLORPERAZINE

Trade name: Compazine (GSK)
Indications: Psychotic disorders, control of severe nausea and vomiting
Class: Antiemetic, Antipsychotic, Muscarinic antagonist, Phenothiazine
Half-life: 23 hours
Clinically important, potentially hazardous interactions with: antihistamines, arsenic, chlorpheniramine, dofetilide, pericyazine, piperazine, quinine, quinolones, sparfloxacin
Pregnancy category: C
Important contra-indications noted in the prescribing guidelines for: the elderly; nursing mothers; pediatric patients

---

Skin
Anaphylactoid reactions/Anaphylaxis (<10%)
Fixed eruption [3]
Photosensitivity (<10%) [3]
Pruritus (<10%)
Rash (<10%)
Toxic epidermal necrolysis [2]

Mucosal
Xerostomia (>10%)

Central Nervous System
Akathisia [14]
Extrapyramidal symptoms [3]
Neuroleptic malignant syndrome [3]
Parkinsonism [4]
Somnolence (drowsiness) [2]

Neuromuscular/Skeletal
Dystonia [6]

Endocrine/Metabolic
Gynecomastia (<10%)

PROGESTINS

Trade names: Aygestin (Barr), Megace (Bristol-Myers Squibb), Micronor (Ortho), Ovrette (Wyeth), Provera (Pfizer)
Indications: Prevention of pregnancy
Class: Progestogen
Half-life: N/A
Clinically important, potentially hazardous interactions with: acitretin, aprepitant, dofetilide, rosuvastatin, voriconazole

---

Skin
Acneform eruption [3]
Dermatitis [4]
Diaphoresis (31%)
Erythema multiforme [2]
Flushing (12%)
Urticaria [2]

Endocrine/Metabolic
Amenorrhea [2]

PROMETHAZINE

Trade name: Phenergan (Wyeth)
Indications: Allergic rhinitis, urticaria
Class: Histamine H1 receptor antagonist
Half-life: 10–14 hours
Clinically important, potentially hazardous interactions with: antihistamines, arsenic, chlorpheniramine, dofetilide, nalbuphine, piperazine, quinolones, sparfloxacin, zaleplon
Pregnancy category: C
Important contra-indications noted in the prescribing guidelines for: the elderly; nursing mothers; pediatric patients
Note: Not for intra-arterial or subcutaneous injection and contra-indicated in comatose states.
Warning: RESPIRATORY DEPRESSION and SEVERE TISSUE INJURY, INCLUDING GANGRENE

Skin
Dermatitis [3]
Erythema multiforme [2]
Lupus erythematosus [2]
Photosensitivity [12]
Purpura [2]
Toxic epidermal necrolysis [2]
Urticaria [3]

Mucosal
Xerostomia (<10%) [2]

Cardiovascular
QT prolongation [2]

Central Nervous System
Neuroleptic malignant syndrome [2]
Seizures [2]
Somnolence (drowsiness) [3]

PROPAFENONE

Trade name: Rythmol (Reliant)
Indications: Ventricular arrhythmias
Class: Antiarrhythmic, Antiarrhythmic class Ic
Half-life: 10–32 hours
Clinically important, potentially hazardous interactions with: amitriptyline, boceprevir, carvedilol, clozapine, cobicistat/elvitegravir/emtricitabine/tenofovir alafenamide, cobicistat/elvitegravir/emtricitabine/tenofovir disoproxil, delavirdine, digoxin, efavirenz, fosamprenavir, grapefruit juice, mirabegron, neostigmine, paroxetine hydrochloride, propranolol, pyridostigmine, rifapentine, ritonavir, telaprevir, tipranavir
Pregnancy category: C
Important contra-indications noted in the prescribing guidelines for: nursing mothers; pediatric patients

---

Skin
Lupus erythematosus [3]
Psoriasis [2]
Rash (<3%)

Mucosal
Oral lesions (>5%)
Xerostomia (2%)

Cardiovascular
Bradycardia [3]
Brugada syndrome [7]
Cardiotoxicity [3]
Congestive heart failure [2]
Hypotension [3]

Central Nervous System
Dysgeusia (taste perversion) (3–23%)
Seizures [3]
Syncope [2]

Gastrointestinal/Hepatic
Hepatotoxicity [8]

Local
Injection-site pain (28–90%) [4]

PROPOFOL

Trade name: Diprivan (AstraZeneca)
Indications: Induction and maintenance of anesthesia
Class: Anesthetic, general
Half-life: initial: 40 minutes; terminal: 3 days
Clinically important, potentially hazardous interactions with: zinc
Pregnancy category: B
Important contra-indications noted in the prescribing guidelines for: nursing mothers; pediatric patients

---

Skin
Anaphylactoid reactions/Anaphylaxis (<10%) [9]
Angioedema [2]
Exanthems (6%) [2]
Rash (5%)
Urticaria [2]

Hair
Hair pigmentation [3]

Cardiovascular
Bradycardia [15]
Brugada syndrome [2]
Cardiac failure [2]
Hypotension [20]
Tachycardia [2]

Central Nervous System
Amnesia [10]
Hallucinations [3]
Seizures [8]
Shivering [2]
Twitching (<10%)

Neuromuscular/Skeletal
Ataxia [2]
Myoclonus [2]
Rhabdomyolysis [10]

Gastrointestinal/Hepatic
Nausea [4]
Pancreatitis [8]
Vomiting [5]

Respiratory
Apnea [4]
Cough [2]
Hypoxia [7]
Respiratory depression [4]

Endocrine/Metabolic
Acidosis [3]
Hypertriglyceridemia [2]

Renal
Green urine [8]

Local
Infusion-related reactions [3]
Injection-site pain (>10%) [35]

Other
Adverse effects [5]
Death [9]
Hiccups [3]

PROPOLIS

Family: None
Scientific name: *Propolis*
Indications: Tuberculosis, bacterial, fungal and protozoal infections, nasopharyngeal carcinoma, duodenal ulcer, *Helicobacter pylori* infection, cold, wound cleansing, mouth rinse, genital herpes. Ingredient in cosmetics
Class: Immunomodulator
Half-life: N/A
Clinically important, potentially hazardous interactions with: none known

---

Skin
Contact dermatitis [3]
Dermatitis [39]
Hypersensitivity [4]
Sensitivity [4]

Mucosal
Cheilitis [2]

Other
Allergic reactions [8]

PROPRANOLOL

Trade names: Hemangeol (Pierre Fabre), Inderal (Wyeth)
Indications: Hypertension, angina pectoris, atrial fibrillation, myocardial infarction, migraine, tremor, infantile hemangioma
Class: Antiarrhythmic, Antiarrhythmic class II, Beta adrenergic blocker, Beta blocker
Half-life: 2–6 hours
Clinically important, potentially hazardous interactions with: alcohol, aluminum hydroxide, aminophylline, amiodarone, barbiturates, bupivacaine, chlorpromazine, cholestyramine, cimetidine, ciprofloxacin, clonidine, colestipol, delavirdine, diazepam, dronedarone, epinephrine, ethanol, fluconazole, fluoxetine, fluvoxamine, haloperidol, imipramine, insulin, insulin detemir, insulin glargine, insulin glulisine, isoniazid, levothyroxine, lidocaine, neostigmine, nicardipine, nifedipine, nilutamide, nisoldipine, oxtriphylline, paroxetine hydrochloride, phenobarbital, phenytoin, propafenone, pyridostigmine, quinidine, rifampin, ritonavir, rizatriptan, sodium iodide I-131, teniposide, terbutaline, tolbutamide, verapamil, warfarin, zileuton, zolmitriptan
Pregnancy category: C
Important contra-indications noted in the prescribing guidelines for: nursing mothers; pediatric patients
Note: Cutaneous side effects of beta-receptor blockers are clinically polymorphous. They apparently appear after several months of continuous therapy.

Skin
Acneform eruption [2]
Angioedema [2]
Cold extremities [6]
Dermatitis [2]
Eczema [2]
Exanthems [4]
Flushing [2]
Lichenoid eruption [3]
Lupus erythematosus [2]
Necrosis [3]
Pemphigus [2]
Psoriasis [21]
Rash (<10%) [2]
Raynaud's phenomenon [3]
Stevens-Johnson syndrome [2]
Urticaria [3]

Hair
Alopecia [6]

Nails
Nail thickening [2]

Cardiovascular
Bradycardia [20]
Cardiac arrest [2]
Hypertension [2]
Hypotension [19]

Central Nervous System
Agitation [2]
Amnesia [2]
Confusion [2]
Delirium [3]
Hallucinations [5]
Headache [2]
Insomnia [2]
Nightmares [2]
Psychosis [3]
Sleep disturbances [9]
Somnolence (drowsiness) [4]
Vertigo (dizziness) [3]

Neuromuscular/Skeletal
Asthenia (fatigue) [4]
Myalgia/Myopathy [3]

Gastrointestinal/Hepatic
Constipation [2]
Diarrhea [6]
Gastroesophageal reflux [2]
Nausea [2]

Respiratory
Bronchospasm [3]
Upper respiratory tract infection [2]
Wheezing [3]

Endocrine/Metabolic
Hyperkalemia [4]
Hypoglycemia [15]
Weight gain [2]

Genitourinary
Peyronie's disease [6]

Ocular
Hallucinations, visual [4]

Other
Adverse effects [10]
Death [3]
Side effects [2]
Tooth decay [2]

PROTAMINE SULFATE

Indications: Heparin overdose
Class: Heparin antagonist
Half-life: 2 hours
Clinically important, potentially hazardous interactions with: none known
Pregnancy category: C

Skin
Anaphylactoid reactions/Anaphylaxis [42]
Angioedema [3]
Hypersensitivity [10]
Rash [2]
Urticaria [5]

Cardiovascular
Hypertension [2]
Hypotension [6]

Respiratory
Pulmonary hypertension [2]

Other
Adverse effects [2]
Allergic reactions [13]
Death [13]

PROTHROMBIN COMPLEX CONCENTRATE (HUMAN)

Synonym: PCC
Trade name: Kcentra (CSL Behring)
Indications: Urgent reversal of acquired coagulation factor deficiency induced by vitamin K antagonist therapy in adult patients with acute major bleeding
Class: Coagulant
Half-life: 4–60 hours
Clinically important, potentially hazardous interactions with: none known
Pregnancy category: C
Important contra-indications noted in the prescribing guidelines for: nursing mothers; pediatric patients
Warning: ARTERIAL AND VENOUS THROMBOEMBOLIC COMPLICATIONS

Skin
Hematoma (3%)

Cardiovascular
Hypertension (3%)
Hypotension (5%)
Orthostatic hypotension (4%)
Tachycardia (3%)

Central Nervous System
Headache (8%)
Intracranial hemorrhage (3%)
Neurotoxicity (3%)

Neuromuscular/Skeletal
Arthralgia (4%)

Gastrointestinal/Hepatic
Constipation (2%)
Nausea (4%)
Vomiting (4%)

Respiratory
Dyspnea (2%)
Hypoxia (2%)
Respiratory distress (2%)

Endocrine/Metabolic
Hypokalemia (2%)

Hematologic
Prothrombin time increased (3%)

PSEUDOEPHEDRINE

Trade names: Allegra-D (Sanofi-Aventis), Benadryl (Pfizer), Bromfed (Muro), Entex (Andrx), Robitussin-CF (Wyeth), Sudafed (Pfizer), Trinalin (Schering)
Indications: Nasal congestion
Class: Adrenergic alpha-receptor agonist
Half-life: 9–16 hours
Clinically important, potentially hazardous interactions with: bromocriptine, fluoxetine, fluvoxamine, furazolidone, iobenguane, MAO inhibitors, paroxetine hydrochloride, phenelzine, rasagiline, sertraline, tranylcypromine
Pregnancy category: C

Skin
AGEP [3]
Baboon syndrome (SDRIFE) [2]

Dermatitis [3]
Diaphoresis (<10%)
Erythroderma [2]
Exanthems [4]
Fixed eruption [14]

Cardiovascular
Myocardial infarction [2]
Palpitation [2]

Central Nervous System
Somnolence (drowsiness) [2]

Ocular
Hallucinations, visual [2]

PSORALENS

Trade names: Oxsoralen (Valeant), Trisoralen (Valeant)
Indications: Psoriasis, eczema, vitiligo, cutaneous T-cell lymphoma
Class: Psoralen
Half-life: 2 hours
Clinically important, potentially hazardous interactions with: none known
Pregnancy category: C

Skin
Anaphylactoid reactions/Anaphylaxis [2]
Basal cell carcinoma [3]
Bullous pemphigoid (with UVA) [14]
Burning (<10%) [3]
Dermatitis [11]
Eczema [2]
Edema (<10%)
Ephelides (<10%) [5]
Erythema [2]
Herpes simplex [2]
Herpes zoster [2]
Hypomelanosis (<10%)
Lupus erythematosus [5]
Melanoma [3]
Photosensitivity [14]
Phototoxicity [15]
Pigmentation [9]
Porokeratosis (actinic) [3]
Pruritus (>10%) [4]
Rash (<10%)
Squamous cell carcinoma [4]
Tumors (for the most part malignant) [18]
Vesiculation [2]
Vitiligo [2]

Hair
Hypertrichosis [4]

Nails
Nail pigmentation [4]
Photo-onycholysis [3]

Mucosal
Cheilitis (<10%)

Central Nervous System
Pain [3]

PYRIDOSTIGMINE

Trade names: Mestinon (Valeant), Regonol (Novartis)
Indications: Myasthenia gravis
Class: Acetylcholinesterase inhibitor
Half-life: ~2 hours
Clinically important, potentially hazardous interactions with: aminoglycosides, bacitracin, clindamycin, colistin, edrophonium, polymyxin B, propafenone, propranolol, quinidine, tetracyclines
Pregnancy category: B
Important contra-indications noted in the prescribing guidelines for: nursing mothers; pediatric patients

---

Central Nervous System
Neurotoxicity [3]
Parkinsonism [2]

Gastrointestinal/Hepatic
Abdominal pain [5]
Diarrhea [2]
Nausea [3]

Other
Adverse effects [2]
Side effects [2]

PYRIMETHAMINE

Trade names: Daraprim (GSK), Fansidar (Roche)
Indications: Malaria
Class: Antimalarial, Antiprotozoal
Half-life: 80–95 hours
Clinically important, potentially hazardous interactions with: dapsone, pemetrexed, trimethoprim, zidovudine
Pregnancy category: C
Important contra-indications noted in the prescribing guidelines for: the elderly; nursing mothers
Note: Fansidar is pyrimethamine and sulfadoxine. Sulfadoxine is a sulfonamide and can be absorbed systemically. Sulfonamides can produce severe, possibly fatal, reactions such as toxic epidermal necrolysis and Stevens-Johnson syndrome.

Skin
Angioedema [2]
Bullous dermatitis [2]
DRESS syndrome [2]
Erythema multiforme [4]
Exanthems [3]
Exfoliative dermatitis [2]
Fixed eruption [3]
Hypersensitivity (>10%)
Lichenoid eruption [2]
Photosensitivity (>10%) [3]
Pigmentation [5]
Pruritus [2]
Stevens-Johnson syndrome (<10%) [25]
Toxic epidermal necrolysis [15]

Central Nervous System
Vertigo (dizziness) [2]

Neuromuscular/Skeletal
Asthenia (fatigue) [2]

Gastrointestinal/Hepatic
Diarrhea [2]
Nausea [2]
Vomiting [2]

Other
Adverse effects [2]
Death [4]

QUETIAPINE

Trade name: Seroquel (AstraZeneca)
Indications: Schizophrenia, bipolar I disorder
Class: Antipsychotic, Mood stabilizer
Half-life: ~6 hours
Clinically important, potentially hazardous interactions with: alcohol, amoxapine, antihypertensive agents, arsenic, atazanavir, azithromycin, CNS acting drugs, darunavir, dolasetron, dopamine, drugs known to cause electrolyte imbalance or increase QT interval, erythromycin, fluconazole, hepatic enzyme inducers, itraconazole, ketoconazole, levodopa, methadone, P4503A inhibitors, pazopanib, telavancin, tipranavir, tricyclic antidepressants, voriconazole
Pregnancy category: C
Important contra-indications noted in the prescribing guidelines for: the elderly; nursing mothers; pediatric patients
Warning: INCREASED MORTALITY IN ELDERLY PATIENTS WITH DEMENTIA-RELATED PSYCHOSIS
SUICIDALITY AND ANTIDEPRESSANT DRUGS

Skin
Diaphoresis (<10%)
Hyperhidrosis (2%)
Peripheral edema [5]
Rash (4%)

Mucosal
Sialorrhea [3]
Xerostomia (9%) [22]

Cardiovascular
Bradycardia [2]
Hypertension (41%)
Hypotension [6]
Postural hypotension [2]
QT prolongation [7]
Tachycardia (6%) [3]

Central Nervous System
Abnormal dreams (2–3%)
Agitation (20%) [3]
Akathisia (8%) [6]
Anxiety (2–4%)
Compulsions [3]
Confusion [2]
Delirium [2]
Depression (3%) [3]
Extrapyramidal symptoms [4]
Headache (21%) [6]
Hypoesthesia (2%)
Hypomania [3]
Impulse control disorder [2]
Insomnia (9%) [2]
Mania [3]
Neuroleptic malignant syndrome [15]
Pain (7%)
Paresthesias (3%)
Parkinsonism (4%) [4]
Psychosis [2]
Restless legs syndrome [7]
Sedation [15]
Seizures [7]
Serotonin syndrome [2]
Sleep related disorder [2]
Somnambulism [2]

Somnolence (drowsiness) (18%) [23]
Suicidal ideation [3]
Tardive dyskinesia (5%) [3]
Tic disorder [3]
Tremor [3]
Vertigo (dizziness) (11%) [14]

Neuromuscular/Skeletal
Asthenia (fatigue) (5%) [5]
Ataxia (2%)
Dystonia [2]
Pisa syndrome [2]
Rhabdomyolysis [4]

Gastrointestinal/Hepatic
Abdominal pain (4–7%)
Colitis [3]
Constipation (8%) [6]
Dyspepsia (5%)
Hepatotoxicity [2]
Nausea (7%)
Pancreatitis [5]
Vomiting (6%)

Respiratory
Pneumonia [2]

Endocrine/Metabolic
ALT increased (5%)
Appetite increased [3]
Diabetes mellitus [2]
Hyperglycemia [3]
Hypertriglyceridemia [4]
Libido decreased (2%)
Metabolic syndrome [2]
SIADH [2]
Weight gain (5%) [23]

Genitourinary
Priapism [14]
Sexual dysfunction [2]
Urinary retention [2]

Hematologic
Leukopenia [3]
Neutropenia [2]
Thrombocytopenia [3]

Ocular
Amblyopia (2–3%)
Vision blurred (<4%)

Other
Adverse effects [11]
Death [8]
Toothache (2–3%)

QUINACRINE

Synonym: mepacrine
Trade name: Atabrine (Winthrop)
Indications: Various infections caused by susceptible helminths
Class: Antibiotic, Antimalarial
Half-life: 4–10 hours
Clinically important, potentially hazardous interactions with: none known
Pregnancy category: N/A

Skin
Exanthems [3]
Exfoliative dermatitis (8%) [3]
Fixed eruption [3]
Lichenoid eruption (12%) [6]
Ochronosis [2]
Pigmentation [9]
Squamous cell carcinoma [2]

Hair
Alopecia (80%) [2]

Nails
Nail pigmentation (ala nasi) (blue-gray) [2]

Mucosal
Oral pigmentation [4]

Gastrointestinal/Hepatic
Nausea [2]
Vomiting [2]

QUINAPRIL

Trade names: Accupril (Pfizer), Accupro (Pfizer), Accuretic (Pfizer)
Indications: Hypertension, heart failure
Class: Angiotensin-converting enzyme (ACE) inhibitor, Antihypertensive, Vasodilator
Half-life: 2 hours
Clinically important, potentially hazardous interactions with: alcohol, aldesleukin, allopurinol, alpha blockers, alprostadil, amifostine, amiloride, angiotensin II receptor antagonists, antacids, antidiabetics, antihypertensives, antipsychotics, anxiolytics and hypnotics, aprotinin, azathioprine, baclofen, beta blockers, calcium channel blockers, chlortetracycline, ciprofloxacin, clonidine, corticosteroids, cyclosporine, demeclocycline, diazoxide, diuretics, doxycycline, eplerenone, estrogens, everolimus, gemifloxacin, general anesthetics, gold & gold compounds, heparins, hydralazine, insulin, levodopa, lithium, lymecycline, MAO inhibitors, metformin, methyldopa, methylphenidate, minocycline, minoxidil, moxifloxacin, moxisylyte, moxonidine, nitrates, nitroprusside, NSAIDs, ofloxacin, oxytetracycline, pentoxifylline, phosphodiesterase 5 inhibitors, potassium salts, prostacyclin analogues, quinine, quinolones, rituximab, salicylates, sirolimus, spironolactone, sulfonylureas, temsirolimus, tetracycline, tetracyclines, tigecycline, tizanidine, tolvaptan, triamterene, trimethoprim
Pregnancy category: D (category C in first trimester; category D in second and third trimesters)
Important contra-indications noted in the prescribing guidelines for: nursing mothers; pediatric patients
Note: Contra-indicated in patients with a history of angioedema related to previous treatment with an ACE inhibitor.
Warning: FETAL TOXICITY

Skin
Angioedema [9]
Diaphoresis [3]
Edema [4]
Peripheral edema [3]
Photosensitivity [2]
Pruritus [7]
Rash [5]

Central Nervous System
Dysgeusia (taste perversion) [3]

Neuromuscular/Skeletal
Myalgia/Myopathy (2%)

Respiratory
Cough [9]

Other
Adverse effects [2]

QUINIDINE

Indications: Tachycardia, atrial fibrillation
Class: Antiarrhythmic, Antiarrhythmic class Ia, Antimalarial, Antiprotozoal
Half-life: 6–8 hours
Clinically important, potentially hazardous interactions with: abarelix, afatinib, amiloride, amiodarone, amisulpride, amitriptyline, amprenavir, anisindione, anticoagulants, aripiprazole, arsenic, artemether/lumefantrine, asenapine, astemizole, atazanavir, boceprevir, celiprolol, ceritinib, ciprofloxacin, clevidipine, clozapine, cobicistat/elvitegravir/emtricitabine/tenofovir alafenamide, cobicistat/elvitegravir/emtricitabine/tenofovir disoproxil, crizotinib, dabigatran, darunavir, dasatinib, degarelix, delavirdine, deutetrabenazine, dicumarol, digoxin, duloxetine, eluxadoline, enoxacin, enzalutamide, ethoxzolamide, fosamprenavir, gatifloxacin, glycopyrrolate, glycopyrronium, indinavir, itraconazole, ketoconazole, letermovir, lomefloxacin, lopinavir, lurasidone, metformin, mifepristone, mivacurium, moxifloxacin, naldemedine, nelfinavir, nilotinib, norfloxacin, ofloxacin, osimertinib, oxprenolol, pimavanserin, pimozide, pipecuronium, posaconazole, pristinamycin, propranolol, pyridostigmine, quinine, quinolones, ranolazine, ribociclib, rifapentine, ritonavir, rocuronium, sertindole, sotalol, sparfloxacin, sulpiride, telaprevir, telithromycin, tetrabenazine, tipranavir, tramadol, valbenazine, vecuronium, venetoclax, verapamil, voriconazole, vortioxetine, warfarin, zuclopenthixol
Pregnancy category: C
Important contra-indications noted in the prescribing guidelines for: nursing mothers; pediatric patients

---

Skin
Acneform eruption [2]
AGEP [2]
Dermatitis [4]
Exanthems [6]
Exfoliative dermatitis [5]
Fixed eruption [2]
Flushing [2]
Lichen planus [7]
Lichenoid eruption [6]
Livedo reticularis [6]
Lupus erythematosus [35]
Photosensitivity [21]
Pigmentation [3]
Pruritus [3]
Psoriasis [5]
Purpura [13]
Rash (<10%)
Toxic epidermal necrolysis [2]
Vasculitis [5]

Mucosal
Oral mucosal eruption [2]

Cardiovascular
Congestive heart failure [2]
QT prolongation [9]
Torsades de pointes [13]

Central Nervous System
Dysgeusia (taste perversion) (>10%)
Headache (<10%) [2]
Syncope [2]
Tremor (2%)
Vertigo (dizziness) [2]

Gastrointestinal/Hepatic
Diarrhea (>10%) [7]

Genitourinary
Urinary tract infection [2]

Hematologic
Thrombocytopenia [2]

QUININE

Trade name: Qualaquin (URL Pharma)
Indications: Malaria
Class: Antimalarial, Antiprotozoal
Half-life: 8–14 hours
Clinically important, potentially hazardous interactions with: amantadine, amiodarone, amitriptyline, amoxapine, anisindione, anticoagulants, arsenic, artemether/lumefantrine, astemizole, atazanavir, atorvastatin, cimetidine, cisapride, citalopram, class Ia or III antiarrhythmics, clevidipine, CYP3A4 and CYP2D6 substrates, CYP3A4 inducers or inhibitors, darunavir, dasatinib, degarelix, dicumarol, digoxin, disopyramide, dofetilide, dolasetron, droperidol, enalapril, flecainide, fosamprenavir, halofantrine, haloperidol, histamine, indinavir, lapatinib, levofloxacin, mefloquine, metformin, moxifloxacin, nelfinavir, neuromuscular blocking agents, olmesartan, oral typhoid vaccine, pazopanib, pimozide, procainamide, prochlorperazine, quinapril, quinidine, ramipril, rifampin, ritonavir, saquinavir, sotalol, succinylcholine, telavancin, telithromycin, terfenadine, tipranavir, voriconazole, vorinostat, warfarin, ziprasidone
Pregnancy category: C
Important contra-indications noted in the prescribing guidelines for: nursing mothers; pediatric patients
Note: Qualaquin (quinine sulfate) is not idicated for the prevention or treatment of nocturnal leg cramps.
Contra-indicated in patients with prolongation of QT interval, G6PD deficiency, myasthenia gravis, or optic neuritis.

Skin
Acneform eruption [2]
Acral necrosis [2]
Dermatitis [6]
Erythema multiforme [2]
Exanthems (<5%) [3]
Exfoliative dermatitis [2]
Fixed eruption [12]
Lichen planus [3]
Lichenoid eruption [3]
Livedo reticularis (photosensitive) [3]
Photosensitivity [19]
Pigmentation [6]
Purpura [13]
Raynaud's phenomenon [2]
Stevens-Johnson syndrome [2]
Thrombocytopenic purpura [8]
Toxic epidermal necrolysis [3]
Urticaria [2]
Vasculitis [5]

Cardiovascular
Cardiotoxicity [2]

Neuromuscular/Skeletal
Leg cramps [2]
Rhabdomyolysis [2]

Endocrine/Metabolic
Hypoglycemia [3]

Renal
Nephrotoxicity [2]

Hematologic
Hemolytic anemia [2]
Hemolytic uremic syndrome [16]
Thrombocytopenia [11]
Thrombotic microangiopathy [2]

Otic
Hearing loss [4]
Ototoxicity [2]
Tinnitus [9]

Ocular
Amblyopia [8]

Other
Adverse effects [3]
Death [2]

RABEPRAZOLE

Trade name: Aciphex (Eisai) (Janssen)
Indications: Gastroesophageal reflux disease (GERD), duodenal ulcers, Zollinger-Ellison syndrome
Class: Proton pump inhibitor (PPI)
Half-life: 1–2 hours
Clinically important, potentially hazardous interactions with: atazanavir, clopidogrel, cyclosporine, digoxin, ketoconazole, rilpivirine, simvastatin, warfarin
Pregnancy category: B
Important contra-indications noted in the prescribing guidelines for: nursing mothers

---

Skin
Pruritus [2]
Rash [3]

Central Nervous System
Dysgeusia (taste perversion) [2]
Headache (2–5%) [4]
Pain (3%)
Vertigo (dizziness) [4]

Neuromuscular/Skeletal
Asthenia (fatigue) [3]

Gastrointestinal/Hepatic
Abdominal pain [6]
Constipation (2%)
Diarrhea (3%) [8]
Dyspepsia [3]
Flatulence [2]
Gastrointestinal bleeding [2]
Nausea [5]
Vomiting [5]

Respiratory
Cough [3]
Upper respiratory tract infection [2]

Endocrine/Metabolic
Hypomagnesemia [2]

Renal
Nephrotoxicity [2]

Other
Adverse effects [4]

RADIUM-223 DICHLORIDE

Synonym: Ra-223 dichloride
Trade name: Xofigo (Bayer)
Indications: Castration-resistant prostate cancer
Class: Radiopharmaceutical, alpha-emitting
Half-life: 11.4 days
Clinically important, potentially hazardous interactions with: none known
Pregnancy category: X
Important contra-indications noted in the prescribing guidelines for: nursing mothers; pediatric patients

---

Skin
Peripheral edema (13%) [3]

Central Nervous System
Anorexia [2]

Neuromuscular/Skeletal
Bone or joint pain [3]

Gastrointestinal/Hepatic
Diarrhea (25%) [6]
Nausea (36%) [5]
Vomiting (19%) [4]

Endocrine/Metabolic
Dehydration (3%)

Renal
Renal failure (3%)
Renal function abnormal (<3%)

Hematologic
Anemia (93%) [7]
Leukopenia (35%) [3]
Lymphopenia (72%) [3]
Myelosuppression [2]
Neutropenia (18%) [6]
Pancytopenia (2%)
Thrombocytopenia (31%) [6]

Other
Adverse effects [2]

RALOXIFENE

Trade name: Evista (Lilly)
Indications: Osteoporosis, reduction in risk of invasive breast cancer in postmenopausal women with osteoporosis or at high risk for invasive breast cancer
Class: Selective estrogen receptor modulator (SERM)
Half-life: 27.7 hours
Clinically important, potentially hazardous interactions with: cholestyramine, levothyroxine
Pregnancy category: X
Important contra-indications noted in the prescribing guidelines for: nursing mothers; pediatric patients
Warning: INCREASED RISK OF VENOUS THROMBOEMBOLISM AND DEATH FROM STROKE

Skin
Diaphoresis (3%)
Hot flashes (8–29%) [14]
Peripheral edema (3–5%) [4]
Rash (6%)

Cardiovascular
Chest pain (3%)
Venous thromboembolism [5]

Central Nervous System
Insomnia (6%)
Stroke [4]

Neuromuscular/Skeletal
Arthralgia (11–16%)
Leg cramps (6–12%) [5]
Myalgia/Myopathy (8%)

Gastrointestinal/Hepatic
Abdominal pain (7%)
Vomiting (5%)

Respiratory
Bronchitis (10%)
Flu-like syndrome (~2%)
Pharyngitis (8%)
Pneumonia (3%)
Sinusitis (10%)

Endocrine/Metabolic
Mastodynia (4%) [2]
Weight gain (9%)

Genitourinary
Vaginal bleeding (6%)
Vaginitis (4%)

Hematologic
Thrombosis [2]

Other
Adverse effects [2]
Infection (11%)

RALTEGRAVIR

Trade name: Isentress (Merck)
Indications: HIV-1 infection
Class: Antiretroviral, Integrase strand transfer inhibitor
Half-life: 9 hours
Clinically important, potentially hazardous interactions with: atazanavir, efavirenz, histamine H_2 antagonists, omeprazole, pantoprazole, proton pump inhibitors, rifampin, St John's wort, strong UGT inducers, tipranavir
Pregnancy category: C
Important contra-indications noted in the prescribing guidelines for: nursing mothers; pediatric patients

---

Skin
DRESS syndrome [4]
Herpes zoster (<2%)
Hypersensitivity (<2%) [7]
Pruritus (4%)
Rash [8]

Central Nervous System
Depression (<2%) [2]
Headache (2%) [10]
Insomnia (4%) [4]
Neurotoxicity [2]
Vertigo (dizziness) (<2%) [2]

Neuromuscular/Skeletal
Asthenia (fatigue) (<2%) [4]
Myalgia/Myopathy [3]
Rhabdomyolysis [8]

Gastrointestinal/Hepatic
Abdominal pain (<2%) [2]
Diarrhea [8]
Dyspepsia (<2%)
Gastritis (<2%)
Hepatitis [2]
Hepatotoxicity (<2%) [3]
Nausea (<2%) [9]
Vomiting (<2%) [2]

Endocrine/Metabolic
ALT increased [3]
Creatine phosphokinase increased [2]
Serum creatinine increased [2]

Renal
Nephrolithiasis (<2%)
Renal failure (<2%)

Other
Adverse effects [6]

RAMELTEON

Trade name: Rozerem (Takeda)
Indications: Insomnia
Class: Hypnotic, Melatonin receptor agonist
Half-life: 1–2.6 hours
Clinically important, potentially hazardous interactions with: alcohol, antifungals, CNS depressants, conivaptan, CYP1A2 inhibitors, donepezil, doxepin, droperidol, fluconazole, fluvoxamine, food, ketoconazole, levomepromazine, rifampin, rifapentine, St John's wort, voriconazole, zolpidem
Pregnancy category: C
Important contra-indications noted in the prescribing guidelines for: nursing mothers; pediatric patients

---

Central Nervous System
Depression (2%)
Dysgeusia (taste perversion) (2%)
Headache (7%) [8]
Insomnia (exacerbation) (3%)
Somnolence (drowsiness) (3%) [9]
Vertigo (dizziness) (4%) [6]

Neuromuscular/Skeletal
Arthralgia (2%)
Asthenia (fatigue) (3%) [4]
Myalgia/Myopathy (2%)

Gastrointestinal/Hepatic
Nausea (3%) [3]

Respiratory
Upper respiratory tract infection (3%)

Genitourinary
Urinary tract infection [2]

Other
Adverse effects [7]

RAMIPRIL

Trade names: Altace (Monarch), Tritace (Sanofi-Aventis)
Indications: Hypertension
Class: Angiotensin-converting enzyme (ACE) inhibitor, Antihypertensive, Vasodilator
Half-life: 2–17 hours
Clinically important, potentially hazardous interactions with: alcohol, aldesleukin, allopurinol, alpha blockers, alprostadil, amifostine, amiloride, angiotensin II receptor antagonists, antacids, antihypertensives, antipsychotics, azathioprine, baclofen, beta blockers, calcium channel blockers, clonidine, corticosteroids, cyclosporine, diazoxide, diuretics, eplerenone, estrogens, everolimus, general anesthetics, gold & gold compounds, heparins, hydralazine, hypotensives, insulin, levodopa, lithium, MAO inhibitors, metformin, methyldopa, minoxidil, moxisylyte, moxonidine, nitrates, nitroprusside, NSAIDs, pentoxifylline, phosphodiesterase 5 inhibitors, potassium salts, prostacyclin analogues, quinine, rituximab, sirolimus, spironolactone, sulfonylureas, telmisartan, temsirolimus, tizanidine, tolvaptan, triamterene, trimethoprim
Pregnancy category: D (category C in first trimester; category D in second and third trimesters)
Important contra-indications noted in the prescribing guidelines for: nursing mothers; pediatric patients
Note: Contra-indicated in patients with a history of angioedema related to previous treatment with an ACE inhibitor, or a history of hereditary or idiopathic angioedema.
Warning: FETAL TOXICITY

Skin
Angioedema [11]
Diaphoresis [2]
Flushing [2]

Lichen planus pemphigoides [3]
Photosensitivity [2]
Pruritus [3]
Rash [4]
Stevens-Johnson syndrome [2]

Hair
Alopecia (<10%)

Cardiovascular
Angina (3%)
Hypotension (11%) [3]
Postural hypotension (2%)

Central Nervous System
Headache (5%) [2]
Syncope (2%)
Vertigo (dizziness) (2–4%) [4]

Neuromuscular/Skeletal
Asthenia (fatigue) (2%)

Gastrointestinal/Hepatic
Hepatotoxicity [2]
Nausea (2%)
Pancreatitis [2]
Vomiting (2%)

Respiratory
Cough (8–12%) [22]

Endocrine/Metabolic
Hyperkalemia [2]

Other
Adverse effects [4]

RAMUCIRUMAB

Trade name: Cyramza (Lilly)
Indications: Gastric cancer
Class: Monoclonal antibody, Vascular endothelial growth factor antagonist
Half-life: N/A
Clinically important, potentially hazardous interactions with: none known
Pregnancy category: C
Important contra-indications noted in the prescribing guidelines for: nursing mothers; pediatric patients
Warning: HEMORRHAGE, GASTROINSTINAL PERFORATION, AND IMPAIRED WOUND HEALING

Skin
Peripheral edema [2]
Rash (4%)

Mucosal
Epistaxis (nosebleed) (5%) [2]
Stomatitis [3]

Cardiovascular
Hypertension (16%) [25]
Thromboembolism (2%) [2]
Venous thromboembolism [2]

Central Nervous System
Anorexia [2]
Headache (9%) [3]

Neuromuscular/Skeletal
Asthenia (fatigue) [14]

Gastrointestinal/Hepatic
Abdominal pain [2]
Ascites [2]
Constipation [3]
Diarrhea (14%) [9]
Gastric obstruction (2%)
Gastrointestinal perforation [5]
Hepatotoxicity [2]
Nausea [4]
Vomiting [4]

Respiratory
Dyspnea [3]

Endocrine/Metabolic
Appetite decreased [4]
Hyponatremia (6%)

Renal
Nephrotoxicity [2]
Proteinuria [13]

Hematologic
Anemia [8]
Bleeding [6]
Febrile neutropenia [10]
Hemorrhage [3]
Leukopenia [7]
Neutropenia (5%) [18]
Thrombocytopenia [5]

Local
Infusion-related reactions [4]

Other
Adverse effects [2]
Death [3]

RANIBIZUMAB

Trade name: Lucentis (Genentech)
Indications: Neovascular (wet) age-related macular degeneration, macular edema (following retinal vein occlusion)
Class: Monoclonal antibody, Vascular endothelial growth factor antagonist
Half-life: 9 days
Clinically important, potentially hazardous interactions with: none known
Pregnancy category: C
Important contra-indications noted in the prescribing guidelines for: nursing mothers; pediatric patients
Note: Contra-indicated in patients with ocular or periocular infections.

Cardiovascular
Atrial fibrillation (<5%)
Hypertension [4]
Myocardial infarction [2]
Thromboembolism [3]

Central Nervous System
Anxiety (<4%)
Headache (3–12%)
Insomnia (<5%)
Stroke [3]

Neuromuscular/Skeletal
Arthralgia (2–11%)
Pain in extremities (<5%)

Gastrointestinal/Hepatic
Gastroenteritis (<4%)
Nausea (<9%)

Respiratory
Bronchitis (<12%)
COPD (<7%)
Cough (2–9%)
Dyspnea (<5%)
Influenza (3–7%)
Nasopharyngitis (5–16%) [2]
Sinusitis (3–8%)
Upper respiratory tract infection (2–9%)

Endocrine/Metabolic
Hypercholesterolemia (<5%)

Genitourinary
Urinary tract infection (<9%)

Hematologic
Anemia (<8%)

Ocular
Blepharitis (<13%)
Cataract (2–17%) [4]
Conjunctival hemorrhage (48–74%) [4]
Conjunctival hyperemia (<8%)
Endophthalmitis [9]
Hallucinations, visual [2]
Intraocular inflammation (<18%) [5]
Intraocular pressure increased (7–24%) [7]
Iridocyclitis [2]
Lacrimation (increased) (2–14%)
Maculopathy (6–11%)
Ocular adverse effects [4]
Ocular hemorrhage [5]
Ocular hyperemia (5–11%)
Ocular pain (17–35%) [3]
Ocular pruritus (<12%)
Ocular stinging (7–15%)
Posterior capsule opacification (<8%)
Retinal atrophy [2]
Retinal detachment [2]
Retinal vein occlusion [2]
Vision blurred (5–18%)
Visual disturbances (5–18%)
Vitreous detachment (4–21%)
Vitreous floaters (7–27%) [2]
Xerophthalmia (3–12%)

Local
Injection-site bleeding (<6%)

Other
Adverse effects [5]
Systemic reactions [2]

RANITIDINE

Trade name: Zantac (Concordia)
Indications: Duodenal ulcer
Class: Histamine H2 receptor antagonist
Half-life: 2.5 hours
Clinically important, potentially hazardous interactions with: acalabrutinib, alfentanil, delavirdine, fentanyl, gefitinib, metformin, prednisone, rilpivirine, risperidone
Pregnancy category: B
Important contra-indications noted in the prescribing guidelines for: nursing mothers

---

Skin
AGEP [2]
Anaphylactoid reactions/Anaphylaxis [18]
Dermatitis [6]
Eczema [2]
Exanthems [5]
Hypersensitivity [2]
Photosensitivity [2]
Pseudolymphoma [2]

Purpura [2]
Rash (<10%)
Toxic epidermal necrolysis [2]
Urticaria [4]

Central Nervous System
Confusion [2]
Somnolence (drowsiness) [2]

Respiratory
Pneumonia [2]

Endocrine/Metabolic
Gynecomastia [3]
Porphyria [3]

Other
Adverse effects [3]

RANOLAZINE

Trade name: Ranexa (CV Therapeutics)
Indications: Angina
Class: Anti-ischemic, Fatty acid oxidation inhibitor
Half-life: 7 hours
Clinically important, potentially hazardous interactions with: aprepitant, atazanavir, clarithromycin, conivaptan, cyclosporine, CYP3A inducers, CYP3A inhibitors, darunavir, dasabuvir/ombitasvir/paritaprevir/ritonavir, delavirdine, diltiazem, dofetilide, efavirenz, erythromycin, grapefruit juice, indinavir, itraconazole, ketoconazole, lopinavir, nelfinavir, ombitasvir/paritaprevir/ritonavir, oxcarbazepine, paroxetine hydrochloride, phenobarbital, quinidine, rifampin, rifapentine, ritonavir, simvastatin, sotalol, telithromycin, thioridazine, tipranavir, venetoclax, verapamil, voriconazole, ziprasidone
Pregnancy category: C
Important contra-indications noted in the prescribing guidelines for: nursing mothers
Note: Contra-indicated in patients with existing QT prolongation, and in patients with liver disease.

Mucosal
Xerostomia (<2%)

Cardiovascular
Palpitation (<2%)
QT prolongation [7]
Torsades de pointes [2]

Central Nervous System
Headache (3%) [4]
Vertigo (dizziness) [10]

Neuromuscular/Skeletal
Asthenia (fatigue) [3]

Gastrointestinal/Hepatic
Abdominal pain (<2%)
Constipation [8]
Nausea [9]
Vomiting [2]

Otic
Tinnitus (<2%)

RASAGILINE

Trade name: Azilect (Teva)
Indications: Parkinsonism
Class: Monoamine oxidase B inhibitor
Half-life: 0.6–2.0 hours
Clinically important, potentially hazardous interactions with: aminophylline, amitriptyline, ciprofloxacin, citalopram, dextromethorphan, entacapone, fluoxetine, fluvoxamine, MAO inhibitors, meperidine, paroxetine hydrochloride, pethidine, pseudoephedrine, SSRIs
Pregnancy category: C
Important contra-indications noted in the prescribing guidelines for: nursing mothers; pediatric patients

---

Skin
Ecchymoses (2%)

Mucosal
Xerostomia (3%)

Cardiovascular
Hypotension (5%)

Central Nervous System
Depression (5%) [2]
Dyskinesia (>10%) [2]
Fever (3%)
Gait instability (5%)
Headache (14%) [2]
Paresthesias (2%)
Somnolence (drowsiness) [3]
Vertigo (dizziness) (2%) [3]

Neuromuscular/Skeletal
Arthralgia (7%) [2]
Asthenia (fatigue) (2%)
Dystonia (2%)
Neck pain (2%)

Gastrointestinal/Hepatic
Dyspepsia (7%)
Gastroenteritis (3%)
Nausea [2]

Respiratory
Flu-like syndrome (5%)
Rhinitis (3%)

Ocular
Conjunctivitis (3%)

RASPBERRY LEAF

Family: Rosaceae
Scientific name: *Rubus idaeus*
Indications: Astringent, stimulant, gargle for sore throat, mouth ulcers, bleeding gums, diarrhea, morning sickness, to shorten labor, menstrual complaints, respiratory tract infections, fever, dysmenorrhea, menorrhagia, rash
Class: Food supplement
Half-life: N/A
Clinically important, potentially hazardous interactions with: aminophylline, atropine
Pregnancy category: N/A

REBOXETINE

Trade name: Edronax (Pfizer)
Indications: Clinical depression, panic disorder
Class: Antidepressant, Noradrenaline reuptake inhibitor
Half-life: 13 hours
Clinically important, potentially hazardous interactions with: azithromycin, bosentan, itraconazole, ketoconazole, MAO inhibitors, papaverine, voriconazole
Pregnancy category: N/A (not recommended in pregnancy)
Important contra-indications noted in the prescribing guidelines for: the elderly; nursing mothers; pediatric patients

---

Skin
Diaphoresis [8]

Mucosal
Xerostomia [12]

Central Nervous System
Headache [5]
Insomnia [9]
Somnolence (drowsiness) [2]

Genitourinary
Ejaculatory dysfunction [2]

RED CLOVER

Family: Leguminosae
Scientific name: *Trifolium pratense*
Indications: Menopausal symptoms, hot flashes, muscle spasms, hypercholesterolemia, breast pain, osteoporosis, diuretic, expectorant, mild antispasmodic, sedative, blood purifier, bladder infections, liver disorders. Ointment for acne, eczema, psoriasis and other rashes
Class: Phytoestrogen
Half-life: N/A
Clinically important, potentially hazardous interactions with: conjugated estrogens
Pregnancy category: N/A
Note: Red clover contains phytoestrogens that bind to estrogen and progesterone receptors, potentially adversely affecting breast tissue.

RED RICE YEAST

Family: Monascaceae
Scientific name: *Monascus purpureus*
Indications: Hypercholesterolemia, indigestion, diarrhea, improved circulation. In foodstuff
Class: HMG-CoA reductase inhibitor
Half-life: N/A
Clinically important, potentially hazardous interactions with: atorvastatin, cerivastatin, fluvastatin, grapefruit juice, levothyroxine, lovastatin, pravastatin, simvastatin, St John's wort
Pregnancy category: N/A
Note: Red yeast rice is the product of fermentation with *Monascus purpureus* yeast. Red yeast that is not fermented correctly may contain the nephrotoxin, citrinin.

Neuromuscular/Skeletal
Myalgia/Myopathy [5]
Rhabdomyolysis [3]

Gastrointestinal/Hepatic
Hepatitis [2]

RESLIZUMAB

Trade name: Cinqair (Teva)
Indications: Adjunctive treatment for severe eosinophilic asthma
Class: Interleukin-5 antagonist, Monoclonal antibody
Half-life: 24 days
Clinically important, potentially hazardous interactions with: none known
Pregnancy category: N/A (Insufficient evidence to inform drug-associated risk)
Important contra-indications noted in the prescribing guidelines for: nursing mothers; pediatric patients
Warning: ANAPHYLAXIS

Skin
Anaphylactoid reactions/Anaphylaxis [2]

Mucosal
Oropharyngeal pain (3%)

Central Nervous System
Headache [5]

Neuromuscular/Skeletal
Asthenia (fatigue) [2]

Respiratory
Asthma (exacerbation) [5]
Bronchitis [2]
Cough [2]
Nasopharyngitis [7]
Sinusitis [2]
Upper respiratory tract infection [5]

Endocrine/Metabolic
Creatine phosphokinase increased (14%)

RESVERATROL

Family: N/A
Scientific names: *3,4',5-trihydroxystilbene, trans-resveratrol-3-O-glucuronide, trans-resveratrol-3-sulfate*
Indications: Cancers, dermal wound healing, atherosclerosis, herpes simplex, cholesterol-lowering, heart disease, skin cancers
Class: Immunomodulator, Phytoestrogen
Half-life: N/A
Clinically important, potentially hazardous interactions with: aspirin, warfarin
Note: Resveratrol is extracted from: *Vitis vinifera* ?grape seed and skin?, *Polygonium cuspidatum*, and nuts. Red wine is associated with the so-called French paradox – low incidence of heart disease among French people who drink moderate quantities of red wine. A glass of red wine contains approximately 640 micrograms of resveratrol.

RIBAVIRIN

Trade names: Copegus (Roche), Rebetol (Schering-Plough), Rebetron (Schering), Virazole (Valeant)
Indications: Respiratory syncytial viral infections
Class: Antiviral, nucleoside analog
Half-life: 24 hours
Clinically important, potentially hazardous interactions with: abacavir, azathioprine, didanosine, emtricitabine, interferon alfa, PEG-interferon, stavudine, zidovudine
Pregnancy category: X
Important contra-indications noted in the prescribing guidelines for: nursing mothers
Note: [INH] = Inhalation; [O] = Oral. Rebetron is ribavirin and interferon.
Warning: RISK OF SERIOUS DISORDERS AND RIBAVIRIN-ASSOCIATED EFFECTS

Skin
Dermatitis [O] (16%)
DRESS syndrome [2]
Eczema [O] (4–5%) [3]
Exanthems [5]
Flushing [O] (4%)
Lichenoid eruption [2]
Nummular eczema [2]
Peripheral edema [2]
Photosensitivity [7]
Pruritus [O] (13–29%) [28]
Psoriasis [2]
Rash [O] (5–28%) [39]
Sarcoidosis [16]
Stevens-Johnson syndrome [2]
Toxic epidermal necrolysis [2]
Toxicity [2]
Vasculitis [2]
Vitiligo [2]
Xerosis [O] (10–24%) [2]

Hair
Alopecia [O] (27–36%) [5]
Alopecia areata [2]

Central Nervous System
Depression [O] (20–36%) [10]
Dysgeusia (taste perversion) [O] (4–9%) [4]
Fever [O] (32–55%) [8]
Headache [INH] (<10%) [O] (43–66%) [57]
Insomnia [O] (25–41%) [29]
Irritability [10]
Neurotoxicity [2]
Pain [O] (10%)
Rigors [O] (25–48%)
Suicidal ideation [O] (2%) [2]
Vertigo (dizziness) [O] (14–26%) [7]

Neuromuscular/Skeletal
Arthralgia [INH] (22–34%) [7]
Asthenia (fatigue) [63]
Muscle spasm [3]
Myalgia/Myopathy [INH] (40–64%) [4]

Gastrointestinal/Hepatic
Diarrhea [16]
Dyspepsia [2]
Hepatotoxicity [6]
Nausea [INH] (<10%) [39]
Pancreatitis [4]
Vomiting [O] (9–25%) [3]

Respiratory
Cough [O] (7–23%) [9]
Dyspnea [O] (13–26%) [7]
Flu-like syndrome [O] (13–18%) [9]
Nasopharyngitis [3]
Pneumonitis [2]
Rhinitis [O] (8%)
Upper respiratory tract infection [3]

Endocrine/Metabolic
ALT increased [6]
Appetite decreased [2]
AST increased [5]
Diabetes mellitus [2]
Hyperbilirubinemia [3]
Hyperuricemia [O] (33–38%)
Thyroid dysfunction [2]
Weight loss [O] (10–29%) [2]

Genitourinary
Erectile dysfunction [2]

Renal
Nephrotoxicity [5]

Hematologic
Anemia [INH] (<10%) [80]
Hemoglobin decreased [3]
Hemolytic anemia [2]
Hemotoxicity [2]
Leukopenia [O] (6–45%) [3]
Lymphopenia [O] (12–14%) [2]
Neutropenia [O] (8–42%) [18]
Thrombocytopenia [INH] (<15%) [10]

Otic
Hearing loss [2]
Tinnitus [2]

Ocular
Retinopathy [6]

Local
Injection-site reactions [2]

Other
Adverse effects [25]
Death [4]
Infection [INH] [4]
Vogt-Koyanagi-Harada syndrome [6]

RIBOCICLIB

Trade name: Kisqali (Novartis)
Indications: Treatment of postmenopausal women with hormone receptor (HR)-positive, human epidermal growth factor receptor 2 (HER2)-negative advanced or metastatic breast cancer (in combination with an aromatase inhibitor)
Class: CDK4/6 inhibitor
Half-life: 30–55 hours
Clinically important, potentially hazardous interactions with: alfentanil, amiodarone, bepridil, boceprevir, chloroquine, clarithromycin, conivaptan, cyclosporine, CYP3A4 substrates, dihydroergotamine, disopyramide, ergotamine, everolimus, fentanyl, grapefruit juice, halofantrine, haloperidol, indinavir, itraconazole, ketoconazole, lopinavir, methadone, midazolam, moxifloxacin, ondansetron, pimozide, procainamide, QT prolonging drugs, quinidine, rifampin, ritonavir, saquinavir, sirolimus, sotalol, strong CYP3A4 inducers and inhibitors, tacrolimus, voriconazole

Pregnancy category: N/A (Can cause fetal harm)
Important contra-indications noted in the prescribing guidelines for: nursing mothers; pediatric patients

---

Skin
Peripheral edema (12%)
Pruritus (14%)
Rash (17%) [2]

Hair
Alopecia (33%) [2]

Mucosal
Stomatitis (12%)

Cardiovascular
Hypertension [2]

Central Nervous System
Fever (13%)
Headache (22%) [2]
Insomnia (12%)

Neuromuscular/Skeletal
Asthenia (fatigue) (37%) [5]
Back pain (20%) [2]

Gastrointestinal/Hepatic
Abdominal pain (11%)
Constipation (25%) [2]
Diarrhea (35%) [2]
Nausea (52%) [7]
Vomiting (29%) [4]

Respiratory
Dyspnea (12%)

Endocrine/Metabolic
ALT increased (46%) [2]
Appetite decreased (19%)
AST increased (44%) [3]
Hyperbilirubinemia (18%)
Serum creatinine increased (20%)

Genitourinary
Urinary tract infection (11%)

Hematologic
Anemia (18%) [2]
Leukopenia (33%) [8]
Lymphopenia (11%) [3]
Neutropenia (75%) [11]
Thrombocytopenia [2]

Other
Infection [2]

RIFABUTIN

Trade name: Mycobutin (Pfizer)
Indications: Disseminated *Mycobacterium avium* infection
Class: Antibiotic, rifamycin, CYP3A4 inducer
Half-life: 45 hours
Clinically important, potentially hazardous interactions with: abiraterone, amiodarone, amprenavir, anisindione, anticoagulants, atazanavir, atovaquone, atovaquone/proguanil, azithromycin, bedaquiline, bictegravir/emtricitabine/tenofovir alafenamide, boceprevir, cabazitaxel, cabozantinib, cobicistat/elvitegravir/emtricitabine/tenofovir alafenamide, cobicistat/elvitegravir/emtricitabine/tenofovir disoproxil, corticosteroids, crizotinib, cyclosporine, dapsone, darunavir, delavirdine, dicumarol, efavirenz, enzalutamide, etravirine, flibanserin, fosamprenavir, indinavir, itraconazole, ixabepilone, lapatinib, ledipasvir & sofosbuvir, levonorgestrel, lopinavir, midazolam, mifepristone, nelfinavir, oral contraceptives, posaconazole, rilpivirine, ritonavir, romidepsin, simeprevir, sofosbuvir, sofosbuvir & velpatasvir, sofosbuvir/velpatasvir/voxilaprevir, solifenacin, sonidegib, sorafenib, sunitinib, tacrolimus, temsirolimus, tenofovir alafenamide, tezacaftor/ivacaftor, thalidomide, tipranavir, tolvaptan, vandetanib, vemurafenib, voriconazole
Pregnancy category: B
Important contra-indications noted in the prescribing guidelines for: the elderly; nursing mothers; pediatric patients

---

Skin
Lupus erythematosus [2]
Pigmentation [2]
Rash (11%) [2]

Central Nervous System
Anorexia (2%)
Dysgeusia (taste perversion) (3%)
Fever (2%)
Headache (3%)

Neuromuscular/Skeletal
Arthralgia [6]
Myalgia/Myopathy (2%)

Gastrointestinal/Hepatic
Abdominal pain (4%)
Diarrhea (3%)
Dyspepsia (3%)
Eructation (belching) (3%)
Flatulence (2%)
Hepatotoxicity [2]
Nausea (6%)

Ocular
Intraocular inflammation [2]
Ocular toxicity [2]
Uveitis [31]
Visual disturbances [2]

RIFAMPIN

Synonym: rifampicin
Trade names: Rifadin (Sanofi-Aventis), Rimactane (Novartis)
Indications: Tuberculosis
Class: Antibiotic, rifamycin, CYP1A2 inducer, CYP3A4 inducer
Half-life: 3–5 hours
Clinically important, potentially hazardous interactions with: abacavir, abiraterone, acalabrutinib, afatinib, amiodarone, amprenavir, anisindione, antacids, anticoagulants, apixaban, apremilast, aprepitant, artemether/lumefantrine, atazanavir, atorvastatin, atovaquone, atovaquone/proguanil, beclomethasone, bedaquiline, betamethasone, bictegravir/emtricitabine/tenofovir alafenamide, bisoprolol, boceprevir, bosentan, brentuximab vedotin, brigatinib, brivaracetam, buprenorphine, cabazitaxel, cabozantinib, canagliflozin, caspofungin, ceritinib, clobazam, clozapine, cobimetinib, copanlisib, corticosteroids, cortisone, crizotinib, cyclosporine, cyproterone, dabigatran, daclatasvir, dapsone, darunavir, dasabuvir/ombitasvir/paritaprevir/ritonavir, dasatinib, deferasirox, deflazacort, delavirdine, dexamethasone, diclofenac, dicumarol, digoxin, doxycycline, dronedarone, edoxaban, efavirenz, elbasvir & grazoprevir, eliglustat, eluxadoline, emtricitabine/rilpivirine/tenofovir alafenamide, enzalutamide, estradiol, eszopiclone, etoricoxib, etravirine, everolimus, fesoterodine, flibanserin, fludrocortisone, flunisolide, fosamprenavir, gadoxetate, gefitinib, gestrinone, glecaprevir & pibrentasvir, halothane, hydrocortisone, ibrutinib, idelalisib, imatinib, indinavir, isavuconazonium sulfate, isoniazid, itraconazole, ixabepilone, ixazomib, ketoconazole, lapatinib, ledipasvir & sofosbuvir, leflunomide, lesinurad, letermovir, levodopa, levonorgestrel, linagliptin, linezolid, lopinavir, lorcainide, losartan, lumacaftor/ivacaftor, lurasidone, macitentan, maraviroc, methylprednisolone, midazolam, midostaurin, mifepristone, naldemedine, nelfinavir, neratinib, netupitant & palonosetron, nevirapine, nifedipine, nilotinib, olaparib, ombitasvir/paritaprevir/ritonavir, ondansetron, oral contraceptives, osimertinib, ospemifene, oxtriphylline, paclitaxel, palbociclib, pazopanib, perampanel, phenylbutazone, pimavanserin, pioglitazone, pitavastatin, pomalidomide, ponatinib, praziquantel, prednisolone, prednisone, propranolol, propyphenazone, protease inhibitors, pyrazinamide, quinine, raltegravir, ramelteon, ranolazine, regorafenib, ribociclib, rilpivirine, riociguat, ritonavir, rivaroxaban, roflumilast, romidepsin, rosiglitazone, saquinavir, simeprevir, simvastatin, sofosbuvir, sofosbuvir & velpatasvir, sofosbuvir/velpatasvir/voxilaprevir, solifenacin, sonidegib, sorafenib, sunitinib, tacrolimus, tadalafil, tasimelteon, telaprevir, telithromycin, temsirolimus, tenofovir alafenamide, terbinafine, tezacaftor/ivacaftor, thalidomide, ticagrelor, tipranavir, tofacitinib, tolvaptan, trabectedin, treprostinil, triamcinolone, triazolam, trimethoprim, troleandomycin, ulipristal, valbenazine, vandetanib, vemurafenib, venetoclax, vorapaxar, voriconazole, vortioxetine, warfarin, zaleplon, zidovudine, zolpidem
Pregnancy category: C

Skin
Acneform eruption [3]
AGEP [2]
Anaphylactoid reactions/Anaphylaxis [8]
Dermatitis [3]
Diaphoresis (<10%)
DRESS syndrome [5]
Erythema multiforme [4]
Exanthems (<5%) [6]
Fixed eruption [6]
Flushing (7%) [8]
Hypersensitivity [5]
Linear IgA bullous dermatosis [3]
Pemphigus [9]
Pruritus (<62%) [9]
Purpura [6]
Rash (<5%) [5]
Red man syndrome [7]
Serum sickness-like reaction [2]
Stevens-Johnson syndrome [5]
Thrombocytopenic purpura [2]
Toxic epidermal necrolysis [6]

Urticaria [8]
Vasculitis [5]

Central Nervous System
Fever [2]
Seizures [3]
Vertigo (dizziness) [2]

Neuromuscular/Skeletal
Asthenia (fatigue) [3]

Gastrointestinal/Hepatic
Abdominal pain [3]
Diarrhea [2]
Hepatitis [3]
Hepatotoxicity [18]
Nausea [4]
Vomiting [2]

Respiratory
Pneumonitis [2]

Endocrine/Metabolic
Amenorrhea [2]
Porphyria [2]

Renal
Nephrotoxicity [10]

Hematologic
Agranulocytosis [2]
Anemia [3]
Thrombocytopenia [11]

Other
Adverse effects [13]
Death [7]
Side effects (5%)

RIFAXIMIN

Trade names: Xifaxan (Salix), Xifaxanta (Norgine)
Indications: Diarrhea in travelers (caused by non-invasive strains of *E. coli*), reduction in risk of overt hepatic encephalopathy recurrence (in adults)
Class: Antibiotic, rifamycin
Half-life: 2–5 hours
Clinically important, potentially hazardous interactions with: BCG vaccine
Pregnancy category: C
Important contra-indications noted in the prescribing guidelines for: nursing mothers; pediatric patients

---

Skin
Cellulitis (2–5%)
Clammy skin (<2%)
Diaphoresis (<2%)
Edema (2–5%)
Hot flashes (<2%)
Hyperhidrosis (<2%)
Peripheral edema (15%) [2]
Pruritus (9%)
Rash (<5%)
Sunburn (<2%)

Mucosal
Epistaxis (nosebleed) (2–5%)
Gingival lesions (<2%)
Rhinorrhea (<2%)
Xerostomia (2–5%)

Cardiovascular
Chest pain (<5%) [2]
Hypotension (2–5%)

Central Nervous System
Abnormal dreams (<2%)
Ageusia (taste loss) (<2%)
Amnesia (2–5%)
Anorexia (<5%)
Confusion (2–5%)
Depression (7%)
Dysgeusia (taste perversion) (<2%) [2]
Fever (3–6%)
Headache (10%) [8]
Hypoesthesia (2–5%)
Impaired concentration (2–5%)
Insomnia (<7%)
Migraine (<2%)
Pain (<5%)
Syncope (<2%)
Tremor (2–5%)
Vertigo (dizziness) (<13%) [3]

Neuromuscular/Skeletal
Arthralgia (<6%)
Asthenia (fatigue) (<12%) [3]
Back pain (6%)
Muscle spasm (<9%)
Myalgia/Myopathy (<5%)
Neck pain (<2%)
Pain in extremities (2–5%)

Gastrointestinal/Hepatic
Abdominal distension (<8%)
Abdominal pain (2–9%) [10]
Ascites (11%)
Black stools (<2%)
Constipation (4–6%)
Diarrhea (<2%) [6]
Fecal urgency (6%)
Flatulence (11%) [2]
Hernia (<2%)
Nausea (5–14%) [8]
Tenesmus (7%)
Vomiting (2%) [3]

Respiratory
Cough (7%)
Dyspnea (<6%)
Flu-like syndrome (2–5%)
Nasopharyngitis (<7%) [4]
Pharyngitis (<2%)
Pharyngolaryngeal pain (<2%)
Pneumonia (2–5%)
Rhinitis (<5%)
Sinusitis [2]
Upper respiratory tract infection (2–5%) [6]

Endocrine/Metabolic
AST increased (<2%)
Dehydration (<5%)
Hyperglycemia (2–5%)
Hyperkalemia (2–5%)
Hypoglycemia (2–5%)
Hyponatremia (2–5%)
Weight gain (2–5%)

Genitourinary
Dysuria (<2%)
Hematuria (<2%)
Polyuria (<2%)
Urinary frequency (<2%)

Renal
Proteinuria (<2%)

Hematologic
Anemia (8%)
Lymphocytosis (<2%)
Monocytosis (<2%)
Neutropenia (<2%)

Otic
Ear pain (<2%)
Tinnitus (<2%)

Other
Adverse effects [2]
Breast cancer [2]

RIOCIGUAT

Trade name: Adempas (Bayer)
Indications: Pulmonary hypertension
Class: Soluble guanylate cyclase (sGC) stimulator
Half-life: 7–12 hours
Clinically important, potentially hazardous interactions with: antacids, carbamazepine, dipyridamole, nitrates or nitric oxide donors, nitroprusside, phenobarbital, phenytoin, rifampin, sildenafil, St John's wort, tadalafil, theophylline, vardenafil
Pregnancy category: X
Important contra-indications noted in the prescribing guidelines for: nursing mothers; pediatric patients
Warning: EMBRYO-FETAL TOXICITY

Skin
Peripheral edema [2]

Cardiovascular
Hypotension (10%) [6]

Central Nervous System
Headache (27%) [3]
Syncope [2]
Vertigo (dizziness) (20%)

Gastrointestinal/Hepatic
Constipation (5%)
Diarrhea (12%)
Dyspepsia (21%) [2]
Gastroesophageal reflux (5%)
Nausea (14%)
Vomiting (10%)

Hematologic
Anemia (7%)
Bleeding (2%) [2]

Other
Adverse effects [5]

RISEDRONATE

Trade names: Actonel (Procter & Gamble), Atelvia (Warner Chilcott)
Indications: Paget's disease of bone, osteoporosis
Class: Bisphosphonate
Half-life: terminal: 220 hours
Clinically important, potentially hazardous interactions with: antacids, calcium supplements, iron preparations, laxatives, magnesium-based supplements

Pregnancy category: C
Important contra-indications noted in the prescribing guidelines for: nursing mothers; pediatric patients

---

Skin
Ecchymoses (4%)
Peripheral edema (8%)
Pruritus (3%)
Rash (8%)

Cardiovascular
Chest pain (5%)
Hypertension (11%)

Central Nervous System
Depression (7%)
Fever [2]
Headache (10%) [3]
Insomnia (5%)
Pain (14%)
Paresthesias (2%)
Vertigo (dizziness) (7%)

Neuromuscular/Skeletal
Arthralgia (10–24%) [7]
Asthenia (fatigue) (5%)
Back pain (28%) [5]
Bone or joint pain (7%) [5]
Fractures (9%) [9]
Myalgia/Myopathy (7%) [3]
Neck pain (5%) [3]
Osteonecrosis [5]
Tendinopathy/Tendon rupture (3%)

Gastrointestinal/Hepatic
Abdominal pain (12%) [3]
Constipation (13%) [3]
Diarrhea (11%) [4]
Dyspepsia (11%) [2]
Esophagitis [2]
Gastrointestinal disorder [3]
Hepatotoxicity [6]
Nausea (11%) [2]

Respiratory
Bronchitis (10%)
Cough (6%)
Flu-like syndrome (11%) [2]
Influenza [3]
Nasopharyngitis [3]
Pharyngitis (6%)
Rhinitis (6%)
Sinusitis (9%)

Genitourinary
Urinary tract infection (11%)

Ocular
Cataract (7%)
Ocular adverse effects [3]
Scleritis [2]

Other
Adverse effects [5]
Allergic reactions (4%)
Infection (31%) [3]
Tooth disorder (2%)

RISPERIDONE

Trade names: Risperdal (Ortho-McNeil) (Janssen), Risperdal Consta (Ortho-McNeil) (Janssen)
Indications: Schizophrenia, bipolar mania, irritability associated with autistic disorder
Class: Antipsychotic, Mood stabilizer
Half-life: 3–30 hours
Clinically important, potentially hazardous interactions with: ACE inhibitors, alcohol, alpha blockers, amantadine, angiotensin II receptor antagonists, anxiolytics and hypnotics, apomorphine, artemether/lumefantrine, barbiturates, bromocriptine, cabergoline, calcium channel blockers, carbamazepine, cimetidine, citalopram, clozapine, cobicistat/elvitegravir/emtricitabine/tenofovir alafenamide, cobicistat/elvitegravir/emtricitabine/tenofovir disoproxil, ethosuximide, fluoxetine, general anesthetics, histamine, levodopa, memantine, methyldopa, metoclopramide, opioid analgesics, oxcarbazepine, paliperidone, paroxetine hydrochloride, pergolide, phenytoin, pramipexole, primidone, ranitidine, ritonavir, ropinirole, rotigotine, sodium oxybate, sympathomimetics, tetrabenazine, tramadol, tricyclics, valproic acid
Pregnancy category: C
Important contra-indications noted in the prescribing guidelines for: nursing mothers; pediatric patients
Note: Safety and effectiveness have not been established for pediatric patients with schizophrenia <13 years of age, for bipolar mania <10 years of age, and for autistic disorder <5 years of age. [C] = in children.
Warning: INCREASED MORTALITY IN ELDERLY PATIENTS WITH DEMENTIA-RELATED PSYCHOSIS

Skin
Angioedema [6]
Edema [3]
Peripheral edema (16%) [4]
Photosensitivity (<10%) [2]
Rash [C] (11%) (2–4%)
Seborrhea (2%)
Urticaria [2]
Xerosis (2%)

Hair
Alopecia [2]

Mucosal
Sialopenia (5%)
Sialorrhea [C] (22%) (<3%) [11]
Xerostomia [C] (13%) (4%) [7]

Cardiovascular
Bradycardia [2]
Cardiotoxicity [2]
Hypotension [2]
QT prolongation [4]
Tachycardia [C] (7%) (<5%)
Venous thromboembolism [6]
Ventricular arrhythmia [2]

Central Nervous System
Agitation [2]
Akathisia [C] (16%) (5–9%) [18]
Anorexia [C] (8%) (2%)
Anxiety [C] (16%) (2–16%) [5]
Catatonia [2]
Compulsions [3]
Depression (14%) [7]
Extrapyramidal symptoms [18]
Fever [C] (20%) (<2%)
Headache [9]
Insomnia [9]
Neuroleptic malignant syndrome [25]
Neurotoxicity [2]
Parkinsonism [C] (2–16%) (12–20%) [7]
Psychosis [3]
Rabbit syndrome [3]
Restless legs syndrome [2]
Schizophrenia [2]
Sedation [4]
Seizures [3]
Serotonin syndrome [3]
Somnolence (drowsiness) [C] (12–67%) (5–14%) [16]
Stuttering [2]
Suicidal ideation [3]
Tardive dyskinesia [5]
Tremor [C] (10–12%) (6%) [6]
Vertigo (dizziness) [C] (7–16%) (4–10%) [5]

Neuromuscular/Skeletal
Arthralgia (2–3%)
Asthenia (fatigue) [C] (18–42%) (<3%) [4]
Back pain (2–3%)
Dystonia [C] (9–18%) (5–11%) [5]
Pisa syndrome [3]
Rhabdomyolysis [7]

Gastrointestinal/Hepatic
Abdominal pain [C] (15–18%) (3–4%)
Constipation [C] (21%) (8–9%) [5]
Diarrhea [C] (7%) (73%)
Dyspepsia [C] (5–16%) (4–10%)
Dysphagia [2]
Nausea [C] (8–16%) (4–9%) [4]
Pancreatitis [2]
Vomiting [C] (10–25%)

Respiratory
Cough [C] (34%) (3%)
Dyspnea [C] (2–5%) (2%)
Pneumonia [2]
Pulmonary embolism [3]
Rhinitis [C] (13–36%) (7–11%)
Upper respiratory tract infection [C] (34%) (2–3%)

Endocrine/Metabolic
Amenorrhea [6]
Appetite decreased [2]
Appetite increased [C] (49%) [3]
Diabetes mellitus [2]
Galactorrhea (<10%) [14]
Gynecomastia (<10%) [6]
Hyperprolactinemia [23]
Metabolic syndrome [5]
Weight gain [C] (5%) [33]

Genitourinary
Priapism (<10%) [27]
Sexual dysfunction [3]
Urinary incontinence [C] (5–22%) (2%)
Urinary tract infection (3%)

Renal
Enuresis [4]

Hematologic
Leukopenia [2]

Neutropenia [2]

Ocular

Abnormal vision [C] (4–7%) (<3%)
Periorbital edema [2]
Vision blurred [3]

Local

Injection-site pain [3]

Other

Adverse effects [11]
Death [3]
Tooth disorder (<3%)

RITODRINE

Indications: Preterm labor
Class: Beta-2 adrenergic agonist, Tocolytic
Half-life: 1.3–12 hours
Clinically important, potentially hazardous interactions with: glycopyrrolate
Pregnancy category: B

Skin

Anaphylactoid reactions/Anaphylaxis (<3%)
Diaphoresis (<14%)
Erythema (10–15%) [2]
Pustules [2]
Rash (<3%)
Toxic epidermal necrolysis [2]
Vasculitis [2]

Cardiovascular

Chest pain [2]
Myocardial ischemia [2]
Pulmonary edema [3]

Central Nervous System

Chills (3–10%)
Tremor (>10%)

Neuromuscular/Skeletal

Rhabdomyolysis [4]

Gastrointestinal/Hepatic

Hepatotoxicity [3]

Endocrine/Metabolic

Hypokalemia [2]

Ocular

Glaucoma [2]

Other

Adverse effects [2]

RITONAVIR

Trade names: Kaletra (AbbVie), Norvir (AbbVie)
Indications: HIV infection
Class: Antiretroviral, CYP3A4 inhibitor, HIV-1 protease inhibitor
Half-life: 3–5 hours
Clinically important, potentially hazardous interactions with: abiraterone, afatinib, alfentanil, alfuzosin, alprazolam, amiodarone, amitriptyline, amprenavir, aprepitant, astemizole, atazanavir, atorvastatin, atovaquone, atovaquone/proguanil, avanafil, azithromycin, bepridil, boceprevir, bosentan, brigatinib, buprenorphine, bupropion, buspirone, cabazitaxel, cabozantinib, calcifediol, carbamazepine, ceritinib, chlordiazepoxide, ciclesonide, citalopram, clozapine, cobicistat/elvitegravir/emtricitabine/tenofovir disoproxil, colchicine, conivaptan, copanlisib, crizotinib, cyclosporine, cyproterone, darifenacin, dasatinib, deferasirox, delavirdine, diazepam, diclofenac, dihydroergotamine, docetaxel, dronedarone, dutasteride, efavirenz, eletriptan, eluxadoline, ergot alkaloids, ergotamine, erlotinib, estazolam, estradiol, eszopiclone, etravirine, everolimus, ezetimibe, fentanyl, fesoterodine, flecainide, flibanserin, flurazepam, fluticasone propionate, glecaprevir & pibrentasvir, halazepam, indacaterol, isavuconazonium sulfate, itraconazole, ivabradine, ixabepilone, ketoconazole, lapatinib, ledipasvir & sofosbuvir, levomepromazine, levothyroxine, lomitapide, macitentan, maraviroc, meloxicam, meperidine, meptazinol, methylergonovine, methysergide, midazolam, midostaurin, mifepristone, naldemedine, nelfinavir, neratinib, nifedipine, nilotinib, olaparib, oral contraceptives, osimertinib, paclitaxel, palbociclib, paroxetine hydrochloride, pazopanib, phenytoin, pimozide, piroxicam, pitavastatin, ponatinib, posaconazole, propafenone, propoxyphene, propranolol, quazepam, quinidine, quinine, ranolazine, ribociclib, rifabutin, rifampin, rifapentine, rilpivirine, rimonabant, risperidone, rivaroxaban, romidepsin, rosuvastatin, ruxolitinib, saquinavir, sildenafil, silodosin, simeprevir, simvastatin, sofosbuvir, sofosbuvir/velpatasvir/voxilaprevir, solifenacin, St John's wort, sunitinib, tadalafil, telaprevir, telithromycin, temsirolimus, tenofovir disoproxil, ticagrelor, tolvaptan, trabectedin, triazolam, ulipristal, vardenafil, vemurafenib, venetoclax, vorapaxar, voriconazole, zolpidem, zuclopenthixol
Pregnancy category: B
Important contra-indications noted in the prescribing guidelines for: nursing mothers
Note: Protease inhibitors cause dyslipidemia which includes elevated triglycerides and cholesterol and redistribution of body fat centrally to produce the so-called 'protease paunch', breast enlargement, facial atrophy, and 'buffalo hump'. Kaletra is ritonavir and lopinavir. See also separate entry for ombitasvir/paritaprevir/ritonavir.
Warning: DRUG-DRUG INTERACTIONS LEADING TO POTENTIALLY SERIOUS AND/OR LIFE THREATENING REACTIONS

Skin

Acneform eruption (4%)
Bullous dermatitis (<2%)
Dermatitis (<2%)
Diaphoresis (<10%)
Ecchymoses (<2%)
Eczema (<2%)
Edema (6%)
Exanthems (<2%) [2]
Facial edema (8%)
Flushing (13%)
Folliculitis (<2%)
Hypersensitivity (8%)
Jaundice [3]
Lipodystrophy [4]
Peripheral edema (6%)
Photosensitivity (<2%)
Pruritus (12%)
Psoriasis (<2%)
Rash (27%) [12]
Seborrhea (<2%)
Toxicity [2]
Urticaria (8%)
Xanthomas [2]
Xerosis (<2%)

Hair

Alopecia [2]

Mucosal

Cheilitis (<2%)
Gingivitis (<2%)
Oral candidiasis (<2%)
Oral ulceration (<2%)
Oropharyngeal pain (16%)
Xerostomia (<2%)

Cardiovascular

Cardiotoxicity [2]
Hypertension (3%)
Hypotension (2%)
Orthostatic hypotension (2%)

Central Nervous System

Ageusia (taste loss) (<2%)
Confusion (3%)
Dysgeusia (taste perversion) (16%)
Headache [8]
Hyperesthesia (<2%)
Impaired concentration (3%)
Insomnia [2]
Neurotoxicity [2]
Paresthesias (51%)
Parosmia (<2%)
Peripheral neuropathy (10%)
Syncope (3%)
Vertigo (dizziness) (16%) [2]

Neuromuscular/Skeletal

Arthralgia (19%)
Asthenia (fatigue) (46%) [3]
Back pain (19%)
Myalgia/Myopathy (4–9%)
Rhabdomyolysis [2]

Gastrointestinal/Hepatic

Abdominal pain (26%) [2]
Diarrhea (68%) [14]
Dyspepsia (12%)
Flatulence (8%)
Gastrointestinal bleeding (2%)
Gastrointestinal disorder [4]
Hepatotoxicity (9%) [5]
Nausea (57%) [12]
Vomiting (32%) [7]

Respiratory

Cough (22%)
Nasopharyngitis [2]
Upper respiratory tract infection [2]

Endocrine/Metabolic

ALT increased [3]
Cushing's syndrome [7]
Gynecomastia [2]
Hyperbilirubinemia [6]
Hypercholesterolemia (3%) [2]
Hyperlipidemia [2]
Hypertriglyceridemia (9%) [3]

Genitourinary

Urinary frequency (4%)

Renal

Fanconi syndrome [4]
Nephrolithiasis [3]

Nephrotoxicity [3]
Renal failure [2]

Ocular
Vision blurred (6%)

Other
Adverse effects [9]
Allergic reactions (<2%)

RITUXIMAB

Trade names: MabThera (Roche), Rituxan (Genentech)
Indications: Non-Hodgkin's lymphoma, chronic lymphocytic leukemia, rhematoid arthritis (in combination with methotrexate), granulomatosis with polyangiitis and mycroscopic polyangiitis (in combination with glucocorticoids)
Class: Biologic, CD20-directed cytolytic monoclonal antibody, Disease-modifying antirheumatic drug (DMARD), Immunosuppressant, Monoclonal antibody
Half-life: 60 hours (after first infusion)
Clinically important, potentially hazardous interactions with: benazepril, captopril, certolizumab, cisplatin, clevidipine, enalapril, fosinopril, irbesartan, lisinopril, olmesartan, quinapril, ramipril
Pregnancy category: C
Important contra-indications noted in the prescribing guidelines for: nursing mothers; pediatric patients
Warning: FATAL INFUSION REACTIONS, SEVERE MUCOCUTANEOUS REACTIONS, HEPATITIS B VIRUS REACTIVATION and PROGRESSIVE MULTIFOCAL LEUKOENCEPHALOPATHY

Skin
Anaphylactoid reactions/Anaphylaxis [7]
Angioedema (11%) [4]
Dermatitis [2]
Diaphoresis (15%) [2]
Erythema [2]
Flushing (5%)
Herpes simplex [2]
Herpes zoster [7]
Hypersensitivity [5]
Kaposi's sarcoma [3]
Paraneoplastic pemphigus [2]
Peripheral edema (8%)
Pruritus (14%) [8]
Psoriasis [4]
Pyoderma gangrenosum [3]
Rash (15%) [12]
Sarcoidosis [3]
Serum sickness [22]
Serum sickness-like reaction [5]
Stevens-Johnson syndrome [6]
Toxic epidermal necrolysis [4]
Toxicity [3]
Tumor lysis syndrome [4]
Urticaria (8%) [5]
Vasculitis [4]

Mucosal
Mucocutaneous reactions [2]
Stomatitis [2]

Cardiovascular
Atrial fibrillation [2]
Cardiotoxicity [5]
Hypertension (6%) [3]
Hypotension (10%) [10]
Myocardial infarction [2]

Central Nervous System
Anxiety (5%)
Chills (33%) [15]
Encephalitis [3]
Fever (53%) [23]
Headache (19%) [4]
Leukoencephalopathy [27]
Neurotoxicity [4]
Pain (12%)
Peripheral neuropathy [6]
Rigors [4]
Vertigo (dizziness) (10%)

Neuromuscular/Skeletal
Arthralgia (10%) [3]
Asthenia (fatigue) (26%) [18]
Back pain (10%)
Myalgia/Myopathy (10%) [2]

Gastrointestinal/Hepatic
Abdominal pain (14%)
Colitis [4]
Constipation [2]
Diarrhea (10%) [10]
Hepatitis [4]
Hepatotoxicity [7]
Nausea (23%) [13]
Pancreatitis [2]
Vomiting (10%) [8]

Respiratory
Acute respiratory distress syndrome [3]
Bronchospasm (8%) [6]
Cough (increased) (13%) [6]
Dyspnea (7%) [7]
Flu-like syndrome [3]
Nasopharyngitis [3]
Pneumonia [21]
Pneumonitis [2]
Pulmonary toxicity [15]
Rhinitis (12%) [2]
Sinusitis (6%) [5]
Upper respiratory tract infection [9]

Endocrine/Metabolic
ALT increased [3]
AST increased [3]
Hyperglycemia (9%)
Hypokalemia [2]
Hyponatremia [2]

Genitourinary
Urinary tract infection [8]

Renal
Nephrotoxicity [3]

Hematologic
Anemia (8%) [14]
Cytopenia [3]
Febrile neutropenia [17]
Hemotoxicity [3]
Hypogammaglobulinemia [6]
Leukopenia (14%) [15]
Lymphopenia (48%) [13]
Myelosuppression [5]
Myelotoxicity [2]
Neutropenia (14%) [55]
Sepsis [4]
Thrombocytopenia (12%) [42]
Thrombosis [2]

Local
Application-site reactions [4]
Infusion-related reactions [28]
Infusion-site reactions [11]
Injection-site pain [2]
Injection-site reactions [4]

Other
Adverse effects [30]
Allergic reactions [4]
Death [28]
Infection (31%) [55]

RIVAROXABAN

Trade name: Xarelto (Janssen)
Indications: Prevention of venous thromboembolism in patients undergoing knee or hip replacement surgery, treatment of deep vein thrombosis and pulmonary embolism
Class: Anticoagulant, Direct factor Xa inhibitor
Half-life: 5–9 hours
Clinically important, potentially hazardous interactions with: anticoagulants, aspirin, atazanavir, atorvastatin, carbamazepine, clarithromycin, clopidogrel, combined P-glycoprotein and strong CYP3A4 inhibitors and inducers, conivaptan, dabigatran, darunavir, delavirdine, diclofenac, efavirenz, enoxaparin, erythromycin, fosamprenavir, HIV protease inhibitors, indinavir, itraconazole, ketoconazole, ketorolac, lapatinib, lopinavir, nelfinavir, phenobarbital, phenytoin, posaconazole, rifampin, ritonavir, saquinavir, St John's wort, telithromycin, tipranavir, voriconazole
Pregnancy category: C
Important contra-indications noted in the prescribing guidelines for: nursing mothers; pediatric patients
Note: Contra-indicated in patients with active pathological bleeding.
Warning: PREMATURE DISCONTINUATION OF XARELTO INCREASES THE RISK OF THROMBOTIC EVENTS
SPINAL/EPIDURAL HEMATOMA

Skin
Hematoma [3]
Hypersensitivity [2]
Pruritus (2%)
Rash [3]

Mucosal
Epistaxis (nosebleed) [7]
Gingival bleeding [2]

Cardiovascular
Cardiac tamponade [2]
Congestive heart failure [2]
Hypertension [2]
Myocardial infarction [2]

Central Nervous System
Stroke [2]

Gastrointestinal/Hepatic
Abdominal pain [2]
Black stools [2]
Diarrhea [2]
Gastrointestinal bleeding [3]
Hepatotoxicity [6]

Genitourinary
Hematuria [5]

Hematologic
Anemia (3%)
Bleeding [15]
Hemorrhage [5]

Other
Adverse effects [4]

RIVASTIGMINE

Trade name: Exelon (Novartis)
Indications: Alzheimer's disease and dementia
Class: Acetylcholinesterase inhibitor, Cholinesterase inhibitor
Half-life: 1–2 hours
Clinically important, potentially hazardous interactions with: galantamine
Pregnancy category: B
Important contra-indications noted in the prescribing guidelines for: nursing mothers; pediatric patients

---

Skin
Dermatitis [2]
Diaphoresis (10%)
Exanthems [2]
Hyperhidrosis (4%)
Peripheral edema (>2%)
Rash (>2%) [2]

Cardiovascular
Bradycardia [5]
Chest pain (>2%)
Hypertension (3%) [2]
QT prolongation [2]
Thrombophlebitis (<2%)

Central Nervous System
Aggression (3%)
Agitation (>2%)
Anorexia (6–17%) [3]
Anxiety (4–5%)
Confusion (8%) [2]
Delusions of parasitosis (>2%)
Depression (6%)
Hallucinations (4%)
Headache (4–17%) [3]
Insomnia (3–9%)
Nervousness (>2%)
Pain (>2%)
Parkinsonism (2%)
Restlessness [2]
Somnolence (drowsiness) (3–5%)
Syncope (3%) [4]
Tremor (4–10%) [3]
Vertigo (dizziness) (6–21%) [5]

Neuromuscular/Skeletal
Arthralgia (>2%)
Asthenia (fatigue) (2–9%)
Back pain (>2%)
Dystonia [2]
Fractures (>2%)
Myalgia/Myopathy (20%)
Pisa syndrome [3]

Gastrointestinal/Hepatic
Abdominal pain (4–13%) [2]
Constipation (5%) [2]
Diarrhea (7–19%) [6]
Dyspepsia (9%)
Eructation (belching) (2%)
Flatulence (4%)
Nausea (29–47%) [14]
Vomiting (17–31%) [14]

Respiratory
Bronchitis (>2%)
Cough (>2%)
Flu-like syndrome (3%)
Pharyngitis (>2%)
Rhinitis (4%)

Endocrine/Metabolic
Dehydration (2%)
Weight loss (3%) [3]

Genitourinary
Urinary incontinence (>2%)
Urinary tract infection (7%)

Local
Application-site erythema [2]
Application-site pruritus [3]
Application-site reactions [3]

Other
Adverse effects [5]
Death [2]
Infection (>2%)

RIZATRIPTAN

Trade name: Maxalt (Merck)
Indications: Migraine
Class: 5-HT1 agonist, Serotonin receptor agonist, Triptan
Half-life: 2–3 hours
Clinically important, potentially hazardous interactions with: dihydroergotamine, ergot-containing drugs, isocarboxazid, MAO inhibitors, methysergide, naratriptan, phenelzine, propranolol, sibutramine, SSRIs, St John's wort, sumatriptan, tranylcypromine, zolmitriptan
Pregnancy category: C
Important contra-indications noted in the prescribing guidelines for: nursing mothers

---

Mucosal
Xerostomia (3%)

Cardiovascular
Chest pain (<3%) [2]

Central Nervous System
Headache (<2%)
Neurotoxicity [2]
Pain (3%)
Paresthesias (3–4%)
Somnolence (drowsiness) (4–6%)
Vertigo (dizziness) (4–9%) [10]

Neuromuscular/Skeletal
Asthenia (fatigue) (4–7%) [9]
Jaw pain (<2%)
Neck pain (<2%)

Gastrointestinal/Hepatic
Nausea (4–6%)

Other
Adverse effects [4]

ROFLUMILAST

Trade names: Daliresp (Takeda), Daxas (Takeda)
Indications: To reduce the risk of COPD exacerbations in patients with severe COPD associated with chronic bronchitis and a history of exacerbations
Class: Anti-inflammatory, Phosphodiesterase inhibitor, Phosphodiesterase type 4 (PDE4) inhibitor
Half-life: 17 hours
Clinically important, potentially hazardous interactions with: aminophylline, carbamazepine, cimetidine, denileukin, efavirenz, enoxacin, erythromycin, fingolimod, fluvoxamine, ketoconazole, oral contraceptives, pazopanib, phenobarbital, phenytoin, rifampin
Pregnancy category: C
Important contra-indications noted in the prescribing guidelines for: nursing mothers; pediatric patients
Note: Contra-indicated in patients with moderate to severe liver impairment (Child-Pugh B or C class).

Cardiovascular
Cardiotoxicity [2]
Hypertension [3]

Central Nervous System
Anorexia [3]
Anxiety (<2%) [2]
Depression (<2%)
Headache (4%) [21]
Insomnia (2%) [6]
Neurotoxicity [3]
Suicidal ideation [2]
Tremor (<2%)
Vertigo (dizziness) [4]

Neuromuscular/Skeletal
Back pain (3%) [4]
Muscle spasm (<2%)

Gastrointestinal/Hepatic
Abdominal pain (<2%) [2]
Diarrhea (10%) [26]
Dyspepsia (<2%)
Gastritis (<2%) [2]
Nausea (5%) [24]
Vomiting (<2%) [2]

Respiratory
Bronchitis [3]
COPD [4]
Dyspnea [3]
Influenza (3%) [3]
Nasopharyngitis [4]
Pneumonia [3]
Rhinitis (<2%)
Sinusitis (<2%)
Upper respiratory tract infection [5]

Endocrine/Metabolic
Appetite decreased (2%) [5]
Weight loss (8%) [25]

Genitourinary
Urinary tract infection (<2%)

Other
Adverse effects [6]

ROLAPITANT

Trade name: Varubi (Tesaro)
Indications: Delayed nausea and vomiting from chemotherapy, in combination with dexamethasone and a 5HT3-receptor antagonist
Class: Antiemetic, Neurokinin 1 receptor antagonist
Half-life: ~7 days
Clinically important, potentially hazardous interactions with: thioridazine
Pregnancy category: N/A (No data available)
Important contra-indications noted in the prescribing guidelines for: nursing mothers; pediatric patients

---

Mucosal
Stomatitis (4%)

Central Nervous System
Headache [6]
Vertigo (dizziness) (6%) [2]

Neuromuscular/Skeletal
Asthenia (fatigue) [5]

Gastrointestinal/Hepatic
Abdominal pain (3%)
Constipation [6]
Dyspepsia (4%) [3]

Endocrine/Metabolic
Appetite decreased (9%)

Genitourinary
Urinary tract infection (4%)

Hematologic
Anemia (3%)
Neutropenia (7–9%) [2]

Other
Hiccups (5%) [3]

ROMIDEPSIN

Trade name: Istodax (Celgene)
Indications: Cutaneous T-cell lymphoma (CTCL)
Class: Histone deacetylase (HDAC) inhibitor
Half-life: 3 hours
Clinically important, potentially hazardous interactions with: atazanavir, carbamazepine, clarithromycin, conivaptan, coumadin derivatives, CYP3A4 inhibitors and inducers, darunavir, delavirdine, dexamethasone, efavirenz, indinavir, itraconazole, ketoconazole, nefazodone, nelfinavir, oxcarbazepine, phenobarbital, phenytoin, rifabutin, rifampin, rifapentine, ritonavir, saquinavir, St John's wort, telithromycin, voriconazole, warfarin
Pregnancy category: D
Important contra-indications noted in the prescribing guidelines for: nursing mothers; pediatric patients

---

Skin
Dermatitis (4–27%)
Edema (>2%)
Exfoliative dermatitis (4–27%)
Peripheral edema (6–10%)
Pruritus (7–31%)

Mucosal
Stomatitis (6–10%)

Cardiovascular
Hypotension (7–23%)
Supraventricular arrhythmias (>2%)
Tachycardia (10%)
Ventricular arrhythmia (>2%)

Central Nervous System
Anorexia (23–54%) [5]
Chills (11–17%)
Dysgeusia (taste perversion) (15–40%)
Fever (20–47%)
Headache (15–34%)

Neuromuscular/Skeletal
Asthenia (fatigue) (53–77%) [10]

Gastrointestinal/Hepatic
Abdominal pain (13–14%)
Constipation (12–40%)
Diarrhea (20–36%)
Nausea (56–86%) [9]
Vomiting (34–52%) [5]

Respiratory
Cough (18–21%)
Dyspnea (13–21%)

Endocrine/Metabolic
ALT increased (3–22%)
AST increased (3–28%)
Hyperglycemia (2–51%)
Hypermagnesemia (27%)
Hyperuricemia (33%)
Hypoalbuminemia (3–48%)
Hypocalcemia (4–52%)
Hypokalemia (6–20%)
Hypomagnesemia (22–28%)
Hyponatremia (<20%)
Hypophosphatemia (27%)
Weight loss (10–15%)

Hematologic
Anemia (19–72%) [3]
Leukopenia (4–55%) [2]
Lymphopenia (4–57%) [2]
Neutropenia (11–66%) [5]
Sepsis (>2%)
Thrombocytopenia (17–72%) [8]

Other
Adverse effects [2]
Infection (46–54%) [2]

ROPINIROLE

Trade name: Requip (GSK)
Indications: Parkinsonism
Class: Dopamine receptor agonist
Half-life: ~6 hours
Clinically important, potentially hazardous interactions with: ciprofloxacin, estradiol, levomepromazine, norfloxacin, risperidone, warfarin, zuclopenthixol
Pregnancy category: C
Important contra-indications noted in the prescribing guidelines for: nursing mothers; pediatric patients

---

Skin
Diaphoresis (3–6%)
Flushing (3%)
Herpes simplex (5%)
Hyperhidrosis (3%)
Peripheral edema (2–7%) [2]
Rash [2]

Mucosal
Xerostomia (5%)

Cardiovascular
Cardiotoxicity [2]
Chest pain (4%)
Hypotension [2]
Orthostatic hypotension [4]

Central Nervous System
Amnesia (3%)
Dyskinesia [9]
Hallucinations (<5%) [7]
Headache (6%) [5]
Hyperesthesia (4%)
Impulse control disorder [3]
Insomnia [2]
Pain (3–8%)
Paresthesias (5%)
Psychosis [5]
Sleep related disorder [2]
Somnolence (drowsiness) (11–40%) [13]
Syncope (<12%) [3]
Tremor (6%)
Vertigo (dizziness) (6–40%) [16]
Yawning (3%)

Neuromuscular/Skeletal
Arthralgia (4%)
Asthenia (fatigue) (8–11%) [4]
Back pain [2]
Myalgia/Myopathy (3%)

Gastrointestinal/Hepatic
Abdominal pain (3–7%) [2]
Constipation [2]
Diarrhea (5%)
Dyspepsia (4–10%) [3]
Nausea (40–60%) [19]
Vomiting (11%) [4]

Respiratory
Cough (3%)
Dyspnea (3%)
Flu-like syndrome (3%)
Pharyngitis (6–9%)
Rhinitis (4%)
Sinusitis (4%)

Genitourinary
Impotence (3%)
Urinary tract infection (5%)

Ocular
Abnormal vision (6%)
Xerophthalmia (2%)

Other
Adverse effects [5]
Infection (viral) (11%)

ROSEMARY

Family: Lamiaceae; Labiatae
Scientific name: *Rosmarinus officinalis*
Indications: Oral: dyspepsia, flatulence, gout, cough, headache, loss of appetite, high blood pressure. **Topical:** alopecia areata, circulatory disturbances, toothache, eczema, musculoskeletal pain. Culinary spice, fragrance component, insect repellent
Class: Antibacterial, Antifungal
Half-life: N/A
Clinically important, potentially hazardous interactions with: none known
Pregnancy category: N/A
Note: Oils from rosemary, thyme, lavender and cedarwood, used to treat alopecia areata, improved hair growth by 44% in 7 months (1998 *Arch Dermatol* 134:1349).

Skin
Dermatitis [5]

ROSIGLITAZONE

Trade names: Avandamet (GSK), Avandaryl (GSK), Avandia (GSK)
Indications: Type II diabetes
Class: Antidiabetic, Thiazolidinedione
Half-life: 3–4 hours
Clinically important, potentially hazardous interactions with: CYP2C8 inhibitors and inducers, gemfibrozil, grapefruit juice, letermovir, paclitaxel, rifampin, teriflunomide
Pregnancy category: C
Important contra-indications noted in the prescribing guidelines for: nursing mothers
Note: Thiazolidinediones, including rosiglitazone, cause or exacerbate congestive heart failure in some patients.
Contra-indicated in patients with established NYHA Class III or IV heart failure. Avandaryl is rosiglitazone and glimepiride; Avandamet is rosiglitazone and metformin.
Warning: CONGESTIVE HEART FAILURE

Skin
Edema (5%) [12]
Peripheral edema [11]

Cardiovascular
Cardiac failure [13]
Congestive heart failure [2]
Myocardial infarction [9]
Myocardial ischemia [3]

Central Nervous System
Headache (6%)
Stroke [2]

Neuromuscular/Skeletal
Arthralgia (5%)
Back pain (4%)
Fractures [5]

Gastrointestinal/Hepatic
Hepatotoxicity [9]
Nausea [2]

Respiratory
Dyspnea [2]
Nasopharyngitis (6%)
Respiratory tract infection (10%)

Endocrine/Metabolic
Weight gain [4]

Genitourinary
Bladder disorder [2]

Hematologic
Anemia [2]

Ocular
Macular edema [8]
Proptosis [2]

Other
Adverse effects [3]
Death [6]

ROSUVASTATIN

Trade name: Crestor (AstraZeneca)
Indications: Hypercholesterolemia, mixed dyslipidemia
Class: HMG-CoA reductase inhibitor, Statin
Half-life: ~19 hours
Clinically important, potentially hazardous interactions with: alcohol, amiodarone, antacids, atazanavir, ciprofibrate, colchicine, conivaptan, coumarins, cyclosporine, daptomycin, darunavir, dronedarone, elbasvir & grazoprevir, eltrombopag, eluxadoline, erythromycin, ethinylestradiol, fenofibrate, fibrates, fosamprenavir, fusidic acid, gemfibrozil, indinavir, ledipasvir & sofosbuvir, letermovir, lopinavir, nelfinavir, niacin, niacinamide, phenindione, progestins, protease inhibitors, ritonavir, safinamide, saquinavir, sofosbuvir/velpatasvir/voxilaprevir, tipranavir, trabectedin, vitamin K antagonists, warfarin
Pregnancy category: X
Important contra-indications noted in the prescribing guidelines for: nursing mothers

---

Skin
Peripheral edema (>2%)
Rash (>2%)

Central Nervous System
Depression (>2%)
Headache (6%)
Insomnia [2]
Pain (>2%)
Paresthesias (>2%)
Vertigo (dizziness) (4%) [3]

Neuromuscular/Skeletal
Arthralgia (>2%)
Asthenia (fatigue) (3%) [2]
Back pain (3%)
Myalgia/Myopathy (3%) [19]
Rhabdomyolysis [18]

Gastrointestinal/Hepatic
Abdominal pain (>2%)
Constipation (2%)
Hepatitis [2]
Hepatotoxicity [5]
Nausea (3%)

Respiratory
Cough (>2%)
Flu-like syndrome (2%)
Rhinitis (2%)
Sinusitis (2%)

Endocrine/Metabolic
Creatine phosphokinase increased [2]
Diabetes mellitus [3]

Renal
Nephrotoxicity [4]
Renal failure [3]

Other
Adverse effects [8]

ROTAVIRUS VACCINE

Trade names: Rotarix (GSK), RotaTeq (Merck)
Indications: Prevention of rotavirus gastroenteritis
Half-life: N/A
Clinically important, potentially hazardous interactions with: none known
Pregnancy category: C

Central Nervous System
Fever [3]

Gastrointestinal/Hepatic
Intussusception [2]

ROTIGOTINE

Trade name: Neupro (Schwarz)
Indications: Parkinsonism, restless legs syndrome
Class: Dopamine receptor agonist
Half-life: 5–7 hours
Clinically important, potentially hazardous interactions with: antipsychotics, levomepromazine, memantine, methyldopa, metoclopramide, risperidone, zuclopenthixol
Pregnancy category: C
Important contra-indications noted in the prescribing guidelines for: nursing mothers; pediatric patients
Note: Neupro contains sodium metabisulfite which is capable of causing anaphylactoid reactions in patients with sulfite allergy.

Skin
Diaphoresis (4%)
Erythema (2%)
Peripheral edema (7%) [3]
Rash (2%) [3]

Mucosal
Xerostomia (3%) [3]

Cardiovascular
Chest pain (>2%)
Hypertension (3%)
Hypotension [2]

Central Nervous System
Abnormal dreams (3%)
Anorexia (3%)
Anxiety (>2%)
Depression (>2%)
Dyskinesia [4]
Gait instability [2]
Hallucinations (2%) [3]
Headache (14%) [8]
Impulse control disorder [4]
Insomnia (10%) [3]

Somnolence (drowsiness) (25%) [16]
Tremor (>2%) [2]
Vertigo (dizziness) (3–18%) [7]

Neuromuscular/Skeletal
Arthralgia (4%)
Asthenia (fatigue) (8%) [10]
Back pain (6%)
Myalgia/Myopathy (2%)

Gastrointestinal/Hepatic
Abdominal pain (>2%)
Constipation (5%)
Diarrhea (>2%)
Dyspepsia (4%)
Gastrointestinal disorder [2]
Nausea (38%) [24]
Vomiting (13%) [6]

Respiratory
Cough (>2%)
Flu-like syndrome (>2%)
Rhinitis (>2%)
Sinusitis (3%)
Upper respiratory tract infection (>2%)

Genitourinary
Urinary frequency (>2%)
Urinary tract infection (3%)

Ocular
Abnormal vision (3%)
Hallucinations, visual (2%) [2]
Visual disturbances (3%)

Local
Application-site erythema [4]
Application-site pruritus [4]
Application-site reactions (37%) [31]

Other
Adverse effects [6]

RUCAPARIB

Trade name: Rubraca (Clovis)
Indications: Advanced BRCA-mutated ovarian cancer
Class: Poly (ADP-ribose) polymerase (PARP) inhibitor
Half-life: 17 hours
Clinically important, potentially hazardous interactions with: none known
Pregnancy category: N/A (Can cause fetal harm)
Important contra-indications noted in the prescribing guidelines for: nursing mothers; pediatric patients

---

Skin
Dermatitis (13%)
Erythema (13%)
Exanthems (13%)
Hand–foot syndrome (2%)
Photosensitivity (10%)
Pruritus (9%)
Rash (13%)

Central Nervous System
Dysgeusia (taste perversion) (39%) [3]
Fever (11%)
Headache [2]
Vertigo (dizziness) (17%)

Neuromuscular/Skeletal
Asthenia (fatigue) (77%) [6]

Gastrointestinal/Hepatic
Abdominal pain (32%) [3]
Constipation (40%) [3]
Diarrhea (34%) [3]
Nausea (77%) [6]
Vomiting (46%) [5]

Respiratory
Dyspnea (21%) [2]

Endocrine/Metabolic
ALT increased (74%) [4]
Appetite decreased (39%) [2]
AST increased (73%) [5]
Hypercholesterolemia (40%)
Serum creatinine increased (92%)

Hematologic
Anemia (44%) [8]
Lymphopenia (45%)
Neutropenia (15%) [3]
Thrombocytopenia (21%) [3]

RUE

Family: Rutaceae
Scientific names: *Ruta chalepensis, Ruta corsica, Ruta graveolens, Ruta montana*
Indications: Hysteria, coughs, croup, colic, flatulence, mild stomachic, insomnia, abdominal cramps, nervous headache, giddiness, hysteria, palpitation, abortifacient, cysticide, vermifuge, insecticide. **Topical:** irritant, rubefacient for eczemas, psoriasis and rheumatic pain, sciatica, headache, chronic bronchitis. Flavoring in alcoholic beverages, salads, meats and cheeses
Class: Antispasmodic
Half-life: N/A
Clinically important, potentially hazardous interactions with: none known
Pregnancy category: N/A

Skin
Bullous dermatitis [2]
Erythema [2]
Photosensitivity [11]
Vesiculation [2]

SACCHARIN

Indications: Sugar substitute
Class: Sweetening agent
Half-life: N/A
Clinically important, potentially hazardous interactions with: none known
Pregnancy category: N/A
Note: Saccharin is a sulfonamide and can be absorbed systemically. Sulfonamides can produce severe, possibly fatal, reactions such as toxic epidermal necrolysis and Stevens-Johnson syndrome.

Skin
Dermatitis [3]
Exanthems [2]
Photosensitivity [3]
Pruritus [3]
Urticaria [5]

SACUBITRIL/ VALSARTAN

Trade name: Entresto (Novartis)
Indications: To reduce risk of cardiovascular death and hospitalization for heart failure in chronic heart failure
Class: Angiotensin receptor neprilysin inhibitor (ARNI)
Half-life: <12 hours
Clinically important, potentially hazardous interactions with: ACE inhibitors, aliskiren, lithium, NSAIDs, potassium-sparing diuretics
Pregnancy category: N/A (Can cause fetal harm)
Important contra-indications noted in the prescribing guidelines for: nursing mothers; pediatric patients
Note: Contra-indicated in patients with a history of angioedema related to previous therapy with angiotensin-converting enzyme inhibitor or angiotensin II receptor blocker. See also separate profile for valsartan.
Warning: FETAL TOXICITY

Skin
Angioedema (<2%) [2]
Peripheral edema [2]

Cardiovascular
Hypotension (18%) [4]
Orthostatic hypotension (2%)

Central Nervous System
Gait instability (2%)
Vertigo (dizziness) (6%) [2]

Neuromuscular/Skeletal
Arthralgia [2]

Gastrointestinal/Hepatic
Constipation [2]

Respiratory
Cough (9%) [4]
Nasopharyngitis [2]

Endocrine/Metabolic
Hyperkalemia (12%) [4]
Serum creatinine increased [2]

Renal
Nephrotoxicity [3]
Renal failure (5%)

Other
Adverse effects [3]

SAFINAMIDE

Trade name: Xadago (Newron)
Indications: Adjunctive treatment to levodopa/carbidopa in patients with Parkinson's disease experiencing 'off' episodes
Class: Monoamine oxidase B inhibitor
Half-life: 20–26 hours
Clinically important, potentially hazardous interactions with: cyclobenzaprine, dextromethorphan, dopaminergic antagonists,

imatinib, irinotecan, isoniazid, lapatinib, linezolid, meperidine, methadone, methylphenidate, metoclopramide, mitoxantrone, other MAO inhibitors, propoxyphene, rosuvastatin, serotonergic drugs, St John's wort, sulfasalazine, sympathomimetics, topotecan, tramadol, tricyclic or tetracyclic antidepressants
Pregnancy category: C
Important contra-indications noted in the prescribing guidelines for: nursing mothers; pediatric patients

---

Skin
Peripheral edema [2]

Cardiovascular
Hypertension [3]
Orthostatic hypotension (2%)

Central Nervous System
Anxiety (2%)
Dyskinesia (17–21%) [5]
Fever [3]
Gait instability (4–6%) [2]
Headache [3]
Insomnia (<4%) [2]
Parkinsonism (exacerbation) [2]
Tremor [2]
Vertigo (dizziness) [2]

Neuromuscular/Skeletal
Asthenia (fatigue) [2]
Back pain [3]

Gastrointestinal/Hepatic
Abdominal pain [2]
Constipation [2]
Dyspepsia (<2%)
Nausea (3–6%) [2]
Vomiting [2]

Respiratory
Cough (2%) [2]
Nasopharyngitis [2]

Endocrine/Metabolic
ALT increased (3–7%)
AST increased (6–7%)
Weight loss [2]

Ocular
Cataract [3]
Vision blurred [2]

SALSALATE

Trade name: Mono-Gesic (Schwarz)
Indications: Arthritis
Class: Non-steroidal anti-inflammatory (NSAID), Salicylate
Half-life: 7–8 hours
Clinically important, potentially hazardous interactions with: dichlorphenamide, methotrexate
Pregnancy category: C
Important contra-indications noted in the prescribing guidelines for: nursing mothers; pediatric patients
Note: NSAIDs may cause an increased risk of serious cardiovascular and gastrointestinal adverse events, which can be fatal. This risk may increase with duration of use.

Skin
Anaphylactoid reactions/Anaphylaxis (<10%)
Rash (<10%)

SAQUINAVIR

Trade name: Invirase (Roche)
Indications: Advanced HIV infection
Class: Antiretroviral, CYP3A4 inhibitor, HIV-1 protease inhibitor
Half-life: 12 hours
Clinically important, potentially hazardous interactions with: abiraterone, afatinib, alprazolam, amitriptyline, amprenavir, astemizole, atazanavir, atorvastatin, avanafil, brigatinib, cabazitaxel, cabozantinib, calcifediol, clindamycin, clozapine, copanlisib, crizotinib, darifenacin, darunavir, dasatinib, delavirdine, dihydroergotamine, dronedarone, efavirenz, elbasvir & grazoprevir, eluxadoline, eplerenone, ergot derivatives, everolimus, fentanyl, fesoterodine, flibanserin, fluticasone propionate, itraconazole, ixabepilone, ketoconazole, lapatinib, levomepromazine, lomitapide, lopinavir, maraviroc, methysergide, midazolam, midostaurin, mifepristone, naldemedine, nelfinavir, neratinib, olaparib, omeprazole, paclitaxel, palbociclib, pantoprazole, pazopanib, pentamidine, phenytoin, pimozide, ponatinib, quinine, ribociclib, rifampin, rilpivirine, ritonavir, rivaroxaban, romidepsin, rosuvastatin, ruxolitinib, sildenafil, simeprevir, simvastatin, solifenacin, sonidegib, St John's wort, sunitinib, tadalafil, telithromycin, temsirolimus, ticagrelor, tipranavir, tolvaptan, vardenafil, vemurafenib, vorapaxar, voriconazole
Pregnancy category: B
Important contra-indications noted in the prescribing guidelines for: nursing mothers
Note: Protease inhibitors cause dyslipidemia which includes elevated triglycerides and cholesterol and redistribution of body fat centrally to produce the so-called 'protease paunch', breast enlargement, facial atrophy, and 'buffalo hump'.

Skin
Acneform eruption (<2%)
Candidiasis (<2%)
Dermatitis (<2%)
Diaphoresis (<2%)
Eczema (<2%)
Erythema (<2%)
Exanthems (<2%)
Folliculitis (<2%)
Herpes simplex (<2%)
Herpes zoster (<2%)
Photosensitivity (<2%)
Pigmentation (<2%)
Seborrheic dermatitis (<2%)
Ulcerations (<2%)
Urticaria (<2%)
Verrucae (<2%)
Xerosis (<2%)

Hair
Hair changes (<2%)

Mucosal
Cheilitis (<2%)
Gingivitis (<2%)
Glossitis (<2%)
Oral ulceration (2%)
Stomatitis (<2%)
Xerostomia (<2%)

Cardiovascular
QT prolongation [3]

Central Nervous System
Dysesthesia (<2%)
Dysgeusia (taste perversion) (<2%)
Hyperesthesia (<2%)
Paresthesias (3%)

Gastrointestinal/Hepatic
Hepatotoxicity [2]

Endocrine/Metabolic
Gynecomastia [2]

SARSAPARILLA

Family: Smilacaceae
Scientific names: *Smilax aristolochiaefolia, Smilax febrifuga, Smilax glabra, Smilax japicanga, Smilax officinalis, Smilax ornata, Smilax regelii, Smilax rotundifolia*
Indications: Blood purifier, general tonic, gout, syphilis, gonorrhea, rheumatism, wounds, arthritis, fever, cough, scrofula, hypertension, digestive disorders, psoriasis, skin diseases, cancer
Class: Anti-inflammatory, Immunomodulator
Half-life: N/A
Clinically important, potentially hazardous interactions with: none known
Pregnancy category: N/A
Note: Sarsaparilla vine should not be confused with sasparilla and sassafras (the root and bark of which were once used to flavor root beer). Sarsaparilla is only used in root beer and other beverages for its foaming properties.

SAW PALMETTO

Family: Arecaceae; Palmae
Scientific names: *Sabal serrulata, Serenoa repens, Serenoa serrulata*
Indications: Benign prostatic hyperplasia, diuretic, sedative, prostate cancer (with other herbs), aphrodisiac, hair growth, colds, coughs, sore throat, asthma, chronic bronchitis, migraine
Class: 5-alpha reductase inhibitor, Anti-inflammatory, Hormone modulator
Half-life: N/A
Clinically important, potentially hazardous interactions with: none known
Pregnancy category: N/A

Central Nervous System
Headache [2]

Neuromuscular/Skeletal
Asthenia (fatigue) [2]

Gastrointestinal/Hepatic
Abdominal pain [3]
Diarrhea [2]
Hepatotoxicity [2]

Nausea [3]
Pancreatitis [2]
Vomiting [2]

Respiratory
Rhinitis [2]

Other
Adverse effects [10]

SAXAGLIPTIN

Trade names: Onglyza (Bristol-Myers Squibb), Qtern (AstraZeneca)
Indications: Type II diabetes mellitus
Class: Antidiabetic, Dipeptidyl peptidase-4 (DPP-4) inhibitor
Half-life: 2.5–3.1 hours
Clinically important, potentially hazardous interactions with: ACE inhibitors, alcohol, aprepitant, beta blockers, bexarotene, colchicine, conivaptan, corticosteroids, CYP3A4 inducers, darunavir, dasatinib, delavirdine, diazoxide, diuretics, efavirenz, estradiol, estrogens, hypoglycemic agents, indinavir, ketoconazole, lapatinib, MAO inhibitors, oxcarbazepine, P-glycoprotein inhibitors and inducers, pegvisomant, pioglitazone, rifapentine, somatropin, strong CYP3A4/5 inhibitors, telithromycin, terbinafine, testosterone, voriconazole
Pregnancy category: B
Important contra-indications noted in the prescribing guidelines for: nursing mothers; pediatric patients
Note: Qtern is saxagliptin and dapagliflozin.

Skin
Hypersensitivity (<2%)
Peripheral edema (2–3%)

Cardiovascular
Cardiac disorder [2]
Cardiac failure [2]
Myocardial infarction [2]

Central Nervous System
Headache (7%) [7]
Stroke [2]

Gastrointestinal/Hepatic
Abdominal pain (2%)
Diarrhea [5]
Gastroenteritis (2%)
Vomiting (2%)

Respiratory
Nasopharyngitis [4]
Sinusitis (3%) [2]
Upper respiratory tract infection (8%) [8]

Endocrine/Metabolic
Hypoglycemia [10]

Genitourinary
Urinary tract infection (7%) [7]

Other
Adverse effects [7]
Death [2]
Infection [2]

SEBELIPASE ALFA

Trade name: Kanuma (Alexion)
Indications: Lysosomal acid lipase deficiency
Class: Enzyme replacement
Half-life: 5–7 minutes
Clinically important, potentially hazardous interactions with: none known
Pregnancy category: N/A (No available data)
Important contra-indications noted in the prescribing guidelines for: nursing mothers

Skin
Hypersensitivity (20%)
Urticaria (33%)

Mucosal
Oropharyngeal pain (17%)

Cardiovascular
Chest pain (<8%)
Tachycardia (<30%)

Central Nervous System
Anxiety (<8%)
Fever (25–56%)
Headache (28%)

Neuromuscular/Skeletal
Asthenia (fatigue) (8%)
Hypotonia (<30%)

Gastrointestinal/Hepatic
Constipation (8%)
Diarrhea (67%)
Nausea (8%)
Vomiting (67%)

Respiratory
Cough (33%)
Nasopharyngitis (11–33%)
Rhinitis (56%)

Hematologic
Anemia (44%)

Other
Sneezing (<30%)

SECUKINUMAB

Trade name: Cosentyx (Novartis)
Indications: Moderate-to-severe plaque psoriasis, psoriatic arthritis, ankylosing spondylitis
Class: Interleukin-17A (IL-17A) antagonist, Monoclonal antibody
Half-life: 22–31 days
Clinically important, potentially hazardous interactions with: live vaccines
Pregnancy category: B
Important contra-indications noted in the prescribing guidelines for: nursing mothers; pediatric patients
Note: Use with caution in patients with inflammatory bowel disease.

Skin
Candidiasis [7]
Malignancies [2]
Neoplasms [2]
Pruritus [4]
Psoriasis (exacerbation) [2]

Cardiovascular
Cardiac disorder [2]
Hypertension [3]

Central Nervous System
Headache [15]

Neuromuscular/Skeletal
Arthralgia [4]
Back pain [2]

Gastrointestinal/Hepatic
Colitis [3]
Crohn's disease [3]
Diarrhea (3–4%) [7]

Respiratory
Nasopharyngitis (11–12%) [22]
Upper respiratory tract infection (3%) [14]

Hematologic
Neutropenia [6]

Local
Injection-site reactions [3]

Other
Adverse effects [5]
Infection (29%) [15]

SEGESTERONE ACETATE *

Synonym: Ethinyl Estradiol
Trade name: Annovera (The Population Council Inc)
Indications: indicated for use by females of reproductive potential to prevent pregnancy
Class: Progestin/estrogen CHC
Half-life: 4.5 hours
Clinically important, potentially hazardous interactions with: none known
Pregnancy category: N/A (no increased risk of genital or nongenital birth defects.)
Warning: CIGARETTE SMOKING AND SERIOUS CARDIOVASCULAR EVENTS

Central Nervous System
Headache (39%) [4]
Pain (breast) (10%)

Gastrointestinal/Hepatic
Abdominal pain (13%)
Diarrhea (7%)
Nausea (25%) [3]
Vomiting (25%)

Endocrine/Metabolic
Menstrual irregularities (8%)

Genitourinary
Cystitis (10%)
Dysmenorrhea (13%)
Genital pruritus (6%)
Metrorrhagia (8%)
Urinary tract infection (10%)
Vaginal discharge (12%)
Vulvovaginal candidiasis (15%)
Vulvovaginalmycotic infection (15%)

Renal
Pyelonephritis (10%)

Other
Adverse effects [3]

SELEGILINE

Synonyms: deprenyl; L-deprenyl
Trade names: Eldepryl (Somerset), Emsam (Mylan Specialty), Zelapar (Valeant)
Indications: Parkinsonism
Class: Antidepressant, Monoamine oxidase B inhibitor
Half-life: 9 minutes
Clinically important, potentially hazardous interactions with: amitriptyline, carbidopa, citalopram, doxepin, ephedra, ephedrine, escitalopram, fluoxetine, fluvoxamine, levodopa, meperidine, methadone, moclobemide, naratriptan, nefazodone, oral contraceptives, oxcarbazepine, paroxetine hydrochloride, propoxyphene, sertraline, tramadol, valbenazine, venlafaxine
Pregnancy category: C
Important contra-indications noted in the prescribing guidelines for: nursing mothers; pediatric patients
Warning: SUICIDALITY IN CHILDREN AND ADOLESCENTS

Mucosal
Xerostomia (>10%) [2]

Cardiovascular
Hypertension [2]

Central Nervous System
Hallucinations [2]
Headache [2]
Serotonin syndrome [2]

Gastrointestinal/Hepatic
Nausea [2]

Local
Application-site reactions [5]

Other
Bruxism (<10%)

SELEXIPAG

Trade name: Uptravi (Actelion)
Indications: Pulmonary arterial hypertension
Class: Prostacyclin receptor agonist
Half-life: <3 hours
Clinically important, potentially hazardous interactions with: gemfibrozil, strong CYP2C8 inhibitors
Pregnancy category: N/A (No data available)
Important contra-indications noted in the prescribing guidelines for: nursing mothers

---

Skin
Flushing (12%)
Rash (11%)

Central Nervous System
Headache (65%) [7]

Neuromuscular/Skeletal
Arthralgia (11%)
Jaw pain (26%) [5]
Myalgia/Myopathy (16%)
Pain in extremities (17%)

Gastrointestinal/Hepatic
Diarrhea (42%) [3]
Nausea (33%) [5]
Vomiting (18%)

Endocrine/Metabolic
Appetite decreased (6%)

Hematologic
Anemia (8%)

SENNA

Family: Caesalpiniaceae; Fabaceae
Scientific names: *Cassia acutifolia, Cassia angustifolia, Cassia obtusifloia, Cassia senna, Cassia tora, Senna alexandrina, Senna obtusifolia, Senna tora*
Indications: Laxative, cathartic, cholagogue, purgative
Class: Stimulant laxative
Half-life: N/A
Clinically important, potentially hazardous interactions with: squill
Note: Part used: Leaves and/or seed pods. Prolonged or excessive laxative use can lead to electrolyte and fluid disturbances, development of carthartic colon, and possible increased risk of colorectal cancer. Treatment should be limited to 8 to 10 days.

Skin
AGEP [2]

Neuromuscular/Skeletal
Arthralgia (from abuse) [2]
Finger clubbing (from abuse) (reversible) [3]

Gastrointestinal/Hepatic
Hepatotoxicity [2]

Other
Adverse effects [4]

SERTRALINE

Trade name: Zoloft (Pfizer)
Indications: Depression, panic disorders, obsessive compulsive disorders
Class: Antidepressant, Selective serotonin reuptake inhibitor (SSRI)
Half-life: 24–26 hours
Clinically important, potentially hazardous interactions with: amphetamines, astemizole, clarithromycin, clozapine, darunavir, dextroamphetamine, diethylpropion, droperidol, efavirenz, erythromycin, isocarboxazid, linezolid, MAO inhibitors, mazindol, methamphetamine, metoclopramide, phendimetrazine, phenelzine, phentermine, phenylpropanolamine, pimozide, pseudoephedrine, selegiline, sibutramine, St John's wort, sumatriptan, sympathomimetics, tranylcypromine, trazodone, troleandomycin, zolmitriptan
Pregnancy category: C

Skin
Angioedema [3]
Diaphoresis (8%) [6]
Flushing (2%)
Rash (<10%)
Stevens-Johnson syndrome [2]

Hair
Alopecia [3]

Mucosal
Xerostomia (16%) [7]

Cardiovascular
Chest pain (<10%)
Palpitation (<10%)
QT prolongation [3]
Torsades de pointes [2]

Central Nervous System
Akathisia [6]
Anxiety (<10%)
Coma [2]
Headache (>10%)
Hypoesthesia (5%)
Insomnia (>10%)
Mania [4]
Pain (<10%)
Paresthesias (<10%)
Restless legs syndrome [3]
Seizures [2]
Serotonin syndrome [10]
Somnolence (drowsiness) (>10%)
Tremor (<10%) [3]
Vertigo (dizziness) (>10%) [3]
Yawning (<10%)

Neuromuscular/Skeletal
Asthenia (fatigue) (>10%)
Back pain (<10%)
Rhabdomyolysis [2]

Gastrointestinal/Hepatic
Constipation (<10%)
Diarrhea (>10%) [3]
Hepatotoxicity [5]
Nausea (10%) [3]
Vomiting (>10%)

Respiratory
Eosinophilic pneumonia [2]
Rhinitis (<10%)

Endocrine/Metabolic
Galactorrhea [4]
Gynecomastia [2]
Hyponatremia [4]
Libido decreased (>10%)
SIADH [14]
Weight gain (<10%)

Genitourinary
Impotence (<10%)
Priapism [5]
Sexual dysfunction (10%) [5]

Otic
Tinnitus (<10%)

Ocular
Abnormal vision (<10%)
Hallucinations, visual [3]

Other
Adverse effects [5]
Allergic reactions [2]
Bruxism [3]
Death [5]

SIBERIAN GINSENG

Family: Araliaceae
Scientific names: *Acanthopanax senticosus, Eleutherococcus senticosus*
Indications: Alzheimer's disease, anaphylaxis, arthritis, colds, depression, fatigue, flu, impotence, infertility, menopause, multiple sclerosis, osteoporosis, perimenopause, PMS, stress
Class: Immunomodulator
Half-life: N/A
Clinically important, potentially hazardous interactions with: antihypertensives
Pregnancy category: N/A
Note: Eleutherococcus may prevent biotransformation of some drugs to less toxic compounds.

SILDENAFIL

Trade names: Revatio (Pfizer), Viagra (Pfizer)
Indications: Erectile dysfunction, hypertension
Class: Phosphodiesterase type 5 (PDE5) inhibitor
Half-life: 4 hours
Clinically important, potentially hazardous interactions with: alfuzosin, alpha blockers, amlodipine, amprenavir, amyl nitrite, antifungals, antihypertensives, atazanavir, boceprevir, bosentan, cimetidine, clarithromycin, cobicistat/elvitegravir/emtricitabine/tenofovir alafenamide, cobicistat/elvitegravir/emtricitabine/tenofovir disoproxil, conivaptan, CYP3A4 inhibitors and inducers, darunavir, dasabuvir/ombitasvir/paritaprevir/ritonavir, dasatinib, deferasirox, delavirdine, disopyramide, erythromycin, etravirine, fosamprenavir, grapefruit juice, high-fat foods, HMG-CoA reductase inhibitors, indinavir, isosorbide, isosorbide dinitrate, isosorbide mononitrate, itraconazole, ketoconazole, lopinavir, macrolide antibiotics, nelfinavir, nicorandil, nitrates, nitroglycerin, ombitasvir/paritaprevir/ritonavir, other phosphodiesterase 5 inhibitors, paclitaxel, PEG-interferon, riociguat, ritonavir, sapropterin, saquinavir, St John's wort, telaprevir, telithromycin, tipranavir
Pregnancy category: B
Important contra-indications noted in the prescribing guidelines for: nursing mothers; pediatric patients

---

Skin
Dermatitis (<2%)
Diaphoresis (<2%)
Edema (<2%)
Erythema (6%)
Exfoliative dermatitis (<2%)
Facial edema (<2%)
Flushing (10–25%) [34]
Genital edema (<2%)
Herpes simplex (<2%)
Lichenoid eruption [2]
Peripheral edema (<2%)
Photosensitivity (<2%)
Pruritus (<2%)
Rash (2%)
Ulcerations (<2%)
Urticaria (<2%)

Mucosal
Epistaxis (nosebleed) (9–13%) [2]
Gingivitis (<2%)
Glossitis (<2%)
Nasal congestion [7]
Rectal hemorrhage (<2%)
Stomatitis (<2%)
Xerostomia (<2%)

Cardiovascular
Angina (<2%)
Atrial fibrillation [2]
Atrioventricular block (<2%)
Cardiac arrest (<2%) [2]
Cardiac failure (<2%)
Cardiomyopathy (<2%)
Chest pain (<2%) [2]
Congestive heart failure [2]
Hypotension (<2%) [5]
Myocardial infarction [4]
Myocardial ischemia (<2%)
Palpitation (<2%)
Postural hypotension (<2%)
Tachycardia (<2%)
Vasodilation [3]
Ventricular arrhythmia [2]

Central Nervous System
Abnormal dreams (<2%)
Amnesia [3]
Anorgasmia (<2%)
Chills (<2%)
Depression (<2%)
Fever (6%)
Headache (16–46%) [40]
Hyperesthesia (<2%)
Insomnia (7%)
Migraine (<2%)
Neurotoxicity (<2%)
Pain (<2%)
Paresthesias (3%)
Seizures [3]
Somnolence (drowsiness) (<2%)
Stroke [2]
Subarachnoid hemorrhage [2]
Syncope (<2%)
Tremor (<2%)
Vertigo (dizziness) (2%) [7]

Neuromuscular/Skeletal
Arthralgia (<2%)
Asthenia (fatigue) (<2%) [2]
Ataxia (<2%)
Back pain [3]
Bone or joint pain (<2%)
Gouty tophi (<2%)
Hypertonia (<2%)
Myalgia/Myopathy (7%) [4]
Tendinopathy/Tendon rupture (<2%)

Gastrointestinal/Hepatic
Abdominal pain (<2%) [3]
Colitis (<2%)
Diarrhea (3–9%) [4]
Dyspepsia (7–17%) [15]
Dysphagia (<2%)
Esophagitis (<2%)
Gastritis (<2%)
Gastroenteritis (<2%)
Hepatotoxicity [2]
Nausea [4]
Vomiting (<2%)

Respiratory
Asthma (<2%)
Bronchitis (<2%)
Cough (<2%)
Dyspnea (7%) [4]
Hemoptysis [2]
Hypoxia [3]
Laryngitis (<2%)
Pharyngitis (<2%)
Pneumonia [2]
Respiratory failure [3]
Rhinitis (4%) [6]
Sinusitis (<2%)
Stridor [2]
Upper respiratory tract infection [2]

Endocrine/Metabolic
Gynecomastia (<2%)
Hyperglycemia (<2%)
Hypernatremia (<2%)
Hyperuricemia (<2%)

Genitourinary
Cystitis (<2%)
Ejaculatory dysfunction (<2%)
Nocturia (<2%)
Priapism [6]
Urinary frequency (<2%)
Urinary incontinence (<2%)
Urinary tract infection (3%)

Hematologic
Anemia (<2%)
Leukopenia (<2%)

Otic
Ear pain (<2%)
Hearing loss (<2%) [4]
Tinnitus (<2%) [2]

Ocular
Abnormal vision [3]
Cataract (<2%)
Conjunctivitis (<2%)
Dyschromatopsia (blue-green vision) (3–11%) [5]
Mydriasis (<2%)
Ocular hemorrhage (<2%)
Ocular pain (<2%)
Ocular pigmentation (<2%)
Optic neuropathy [18]
Photophobia (<2%)
Retinal vein occlusion [2]
Vision blurred [4]
Visual disturbances [5]
Xerophthalmia (<2%)

Other
Adverse effects [6]
Allergic reactions (<2%)
Death [3]
Dipsia (thirst) (<2%)

SILODOSIN

Trade names: Rapaflo (Watson), Urief (Kissei)
Indications: Benign prostatic hyperplasia
Class: Adrenergic alpha-receptor antagonist
Half-life: 4.7–6 hours
Clinically important, potentially hazardous interactions with: alpha blockers, antihypertensives, atorvastatin, clarithromycin, conivaptan, cyclosporine, darunavir, delavirdine,

diltiazem, erythromycin, indinavir, itraconazole, ketoconazole, lapatinib, ritonavir, stong CYP3A4 inhibitors, telithromycin, vasodilators, verapamil, voriconazole
Pregnancy category: B (Not indicated for use in women)
Important contra-indications noted in the prescribing guidelines for: pediatric patients
Note: Contra-indicated in patients with severe hepatic or renal impairment.

Mucosal
Nasal congestion (2%) [3]
Rhinorrhea (<2%)
Cardiovascular
Orthostatic hypotension (3%) [9]
Postural hypotension [2]
Central Nervous System
Headache (2%) [3]
Insomnia (<2%)
Vertigo (dizziness) (3%) [8]
Neuromuscular/Skeletal
Asthenia (fatigue) (<2%)
Gastrointestinal/Hepatic
Abdominal pain (<2%)
Diarrhea (3%) [2]
Respiratory
Nasopharyngitis (2%)
Sinusitis (<2%)
Genitourinary
Ejaculatory dysfunction (25%) [29]
Retrograde ejaculation (28%) [5]
Other
Adverse effects [2]
Dipsia (thirst) (7%) [2]

SIMEPREVIR

Trade name: Olysio (Janssen)
Indications: Hepatitis C
Class: Direct-acting antiviral, Hepatitis C virus NS3/4A protease inhibitor
Half-life: 10–13 hours
Clinically important, potentially hazardous interactions with: atazanavir, carbamazepine, cisapride, clarithromycin, cobicistat/elvitegravir/emtricitabine/tenofovir disoproxil, darunavir, delavirdine, dexamethasone, efavirenz, erythromycin, etravirine, fluconazole, fosamprenavir, indinavir, itraconazole, ketoconazole, ledipasvir & sofosbuvir, lopinavir, milk thistle, nelfinavir, nevirapine, oxcarbazepine, phenobarbital, phenytoin, posaconazole, rifabutin, rifampin, rifapentine, ritonavir, saquinavir, St John's wort, telithromycin, tipranavir, voriconazole
Pregnancy category: X (simeprevir is pregnancy category C but must not be used in monotherapy)
Important contra-indications noted in the prescribing guidelines for: nursing mothers; pediatric patients
Note: Must be used in combination with PEG-interferon and ribavirin (see separate entries).
Warning: RISK OF HEPATITIS B VIRUS REACTIVATION IN PATIENTS COINFECTED WITH HCV AND HBV

Skin
Photosensitivity (28%) [5]
Pruritus (22%) [8]
Rash (28%) [10]
Central Nervous System
Fever [2]
Headache [13]
Insomnia [3]
Neuromuscular/Skeletal
Asthenia (fatigue) [10]
Myalgia/Myopathy (16%)
Gastrointestinal/Hepatic
Nausea (22%) [9]
Vomiting [2]
Respiratory
Dyspnea (12%)
Flu-like syndrome [3]
Endocrine/Metabolic
Hyperbilirubinemia [9]
Hematologic
Anemia [11]
Neutropenia [3]
Other
Adverse effects [7]

SIMVASTATIN

Trade names: Inegy (MSD), Simcor (AbbVie), Vytorin (MSD), Zocor (Merck)
Indications: Hypercholesterolemia
Class: HMG-CoA reductase inhibitor, Statin
Half-life: 1.9 hours
Clinically important, potentially hazardous interactions with: alitretinoin, amiodarone, amlodipine, amprenavir, atazanavir, azithromycin, boceprevir, bosentan, carbamazepine, ciprofibrate, clarithromycin, clopidogrel, colchicine, conivaptan, coumarins, cyclosporine, danazol, darunavir, dasabuvir/ombitasvir/paritaprevir/ritonavir, dasatinib, delavirdine, diltiazem, dronedarone, efavirenz, elbasvir & grazoprevir, erythromycin, fosamprenavir, fusidic acid, gemfibrozil, glecaprevir & pibrentasvir, grapefruit juice, HIV protease inhibitors, imatinib, imidazoles, indinavir, itraconazole, ketoconazole, letermovir, lomitapide, lopinavir, miconazole, mifepristone, nefazodone, nelfinavir, ombitasvir/paritaprevir/ritonavir, paclitaxel, pazopanib, posaconazole, rabeprazole, ranolazine, red rice yeast, rifampin, ritonavir, roxithromycin, saquinavir, selenium, St John's wort, tacrolimus, telaprevir, telithromycin, ticagrelor, tipranavir, triazoles, verapamil, voriconazole, warfarin
Pregnancy category: X
Important contra-indications noted in the prescribing guidelines for: nursing mothers; pediatric patients
Note: Simcor is simvastatin and niacin; Vytorin is simvastatin and ezetimibe.

Skin
Dermatomyositis [5]
Eczema (5%) [4]
Edema (3%)
Eosinophilic fasciitis [2]
Erythema multiforme [2]
Lichen planus pemphigoides [2]
Lupus erythematosus [5]
Peripheral edema [2]
Photosensitivity [7]
Pruritus [3]
Purpura [3]
Rash (<10%) [4]
Vasculitis [2]
Mucosal
Stomatitis [2]
Cardiovascular
Atrial fibrillation (6%)
Central Nervous System
Cognitive impairment [3]
Headache (3–7%)
Memory loss [2]
Vertigo (dizziness) (5%)
Neuromuscular/Skeletal
Asthenia (fatigue) (9%) [3]
Compartment syndrome [2]
Myalgia/Myopathy (<10%) [37]
Rhabdomyolysis [88]
Tendinopathy/Tendon rupture [3]
Gastrointestinal/Hepatic
Abdominal pain (7%)
Constipation (2–7%)
Diarrhea [5]
Gastritis (5%)
Hepatitis [4]
Hepatotoxicity [7]
Nausea (5%)
Pancreatitis [7]
Respiratory
Bronchitis (7%)
Upper respiratory tract infection (9%)
Endocrine/Metabolic
Creatine phosphokinase increased [2]
Diabetes mellitus [4]
Renal
Nephrotoxicity [2]
Renal failure [9]
Hematologic
Leukopenia [2]
Other
Adverse effects [9]
Death [5]

SIROLIMUS

Synonym: rapamycin
Trade name: Rapamune (Wyeth)
Indications: Prophylaxis of organ rejection in renal transplants, lymphangioleiomyomatosis
Class: Immunosuppressant, Macrolactam, Non-calcineurin inhibitor
Half-life: 62 hours
Clinically important, potentially hazardous interactions with: atazanavir, benazepril, boceprevir, captopril, ceritinib, cobicistat/elvitegravir/emtricitabine/tenofovir disoproxil, crizotinib, cyclosporine, darunavir, dasatinib, delavirdine, dronedarone, efavirenz, eluxadoline,

enalapril, enzalutamide, fosinopril, Hemophilus B vaccine, indinavir, itraconazole, letermovir, lisinopril, lopinavir, micafungin, mifepristone, posaconazole, quinapril, ramipril, ribociclib, St John's wort, tacrolimus, telaprevir, telithromycin, tipranavir, venetoclax, voriconazole, zotarolimus
Pregnancy category: C
Important contra-indications noted in the prescribing guidelines for: the elderly; nursing mothers; pediatric patients
Warning: IMMUNOSUPPRESSION, USE IS NOT RECOMMENDED IN LIVER OR LUNG TRANSPLANT PATIENTS

Skin
Abscess (3–20%)
Acneform eruption (20–31%) [9]
Angioedema [6]
Cellulitis (3–20%)
Dermatitis [3]
Diaphoresis (3–20%)
Ecchymoses (3–20%)
Edema (16–24%) [6]
Facial edema (3–20%) [2]
Folliculitis [3]
Fungal dermatitis (3–20%)
Hypertrophy (3–20%)
Lymphedema [2]
Peripheral edema (54–64%) [3]
Pruritus (3–20%)
Purpura (3–20%)
Rash (10–20%) [5]
Toxicity [3]
Ulcerations (3–20%)
Vasculitis [2]

Hair
Hirsutism (3–20%)

Nails
Onychopathy [2]

Mucosal
Aphthous stomatitis (9%) [8]
Gingival hyperplasia/hypertrophy (3–20%) [2]
Gingivitis (3–20%)
Mucositis [2]
Oral candidiasis (3–20%)
Oral ulceration (3–20%) [8]
Stomatitis (3–20%) [7]

Cardiovascular
Thrombophlebitis (3–20%)

Central Nervous System
Chills (3–20%)
Depression (3–20%)
Fever [2]
Hyperesthesia (3–20%)
Paresthesias (3–20%)
Tremor (21–31%)

Neuromuscular/Skeletal
Arthralgia (25–31%) [3]
Asthenia (fatigue) [4]
Myalgia/Myopathy [2]

Gastrointestinal/Hepatic
Diarrhea [4]
Hepatitis [3]
Hepatotoxicity [3]

Respiratory
Cough [2]
Flu-like syndrome (3–20%)
Pneumonitis [7]
Pulmonary toxicity [3]
Upper respiratory tract infection (20–26%) [2]

Endocrine/Metabolic
Hypercholesterolemia [2]
Hyperlipidemia [2]
Hypertriglyceridemia [2]

Renal
Nephrotoxicity [2]
Proteinuria [5]

Hematologic
Anemia [4]
Dyslipidemia [5]
Hemolytic uremic syndrome [2]
Leukopenia [2]
Neutropenia [3]
Thrombocytopenia [2]
Thrombosis [2]

Otic
Tinnitus (3–20%)

Ocular
Eyelid edema (40%) [2]

Local
Application-site pruritus [2]

Other
Adverse effects [5]
Death [3]
Infection [5]

SITAGLIPTIN

Trade names: Janumet (Merck Sharpe & Dohme), Januvia (Merck Sharpe & Dohme)
Indications: Type II diabetes mellitus
Class: Antidiabetic, Dipeptidyl peptidase-4 (DPP-4) inhibitor
Half-life: 12 hours
Clinically important, potentially hazardous interactions with: alcohol, anabolic steroids, beta blockers, corticosteroids, diazoxide, digoxin, estrogens, loop diuretics, MAO inhibitors, progestogens, testosterone, thiazides
Pregnancy category: B
Important contra-indications noted in the prescribing guidelines for: the elderly; nursing mothers; pediatric patients
Note: Janumet is sitagliptin and metformin.

Skin
Angioedema [3]
Bullous pemphigoid [2]
Edema [3]
Rash [2]

Central Nervous System
Headache [6]
Stroke [2]

Neuromuscular/Skeletal
Arthralgia [2]
Bone or joint pain [2]
Rhabdomyolysis [4]

Gastrointestinal/Hepatic
Abdominal pain (2%)
Constipation [3]
Diarrhea [9]
Hepatotoxicity [2]
Nausea [11]
Pancreatitis [9]
Vomiting [6]

Respiratory
Nasopharyngitis [5]
Upper respiratory tract infection [2]

Endocrine/Metabolic
Creatine phosphokinase increased [2]
Hypoglycemia [13]
Weight gain [4]
Weight loss [2]

Renal
Renal failure [2]

Other
Adverse effects [7]
Cancer [3]
Death [2]

SMALLPOX VACCINE

Trade name: Dryvax (Wyeth)
Indications: Prevention of smallpox (variola)
Class: Vaccine
Half-life: ~5 years
Clinically important, potentially hazardous interactions with: corticosteroids
Pregnancy category: C

Skin
Basal cell carcinoma [4]
Bullous dermatitis [2]
Carcinoma [2]
Dermatitis [2]
Eczema vaccinatum [13]
Erythema multiforme [8]
Exanthems [7]
Folliculitis [2]
Herpes simplex [2]
Herpes zoster [2]
Melanoma [2]
Papulovesicular eruption [2]
Photosensitivity [2]
Purpura [11]
Rash [3]
Scar [2]
Stevens-Johnson syndrome [3]
Toxic epidermal necrolysis [5]
Tumors [3]
Urticaria [5]
Vaccinia [25]
Vaccinia gangrenosum [3]
Vaccinia necrosum [6]

Central Nervous System
Headache [2]

Other
Allergic reactions [2]
Death [8]

SODIUM ZIRCONIUM CYCLOSILICATE *

Trade name: Lokelma (AstraZeneca)
Indications: hyperkalemia
Class: Potassium binder
Clinically important, potentially hazardous interactions with: none known
Pregnancy category: N/A (maternal use is not expected to result in fetal exposure to the drug)

Skin
Edema (8–11%) [4]

Endocrine/Metabolic
Hypokalemia (4%) [3]

Genitourinary
Urinary tract infection [2]

SOFOSBUVIR

Trade name: Sovaldi (Gilead)
Indications: Hepatitis C
Class: Direct-acting antiviral, Hepatitis C virus nucleotide analog NS5B polymerase inhibitor
Half-life: <27 hours
Clinically important, potentially hazardous interactions with: carbamazepine, oxcarbazepine, phenobarbital, phenytoin, rifabutin, rifampin, rifapentine, ritonavir, St John's wort, tipranavir
Pregnancy category: N/A (May cause fetal harm)
Important contra-indications noted in the prescribing guidelines for: nursing mothers; pediatric patients
Note: Used in combination with daclatasvir, ledipasvir, ribavirin, velpatasvir or with PEG-interferon and ribavirin (see separate entries).

Skin
Pruritus (11–27%) [13]
Rash (8–18%) [10]

Cardiovascular
Bradyarrhythmia [2]
Bradycardia [2]

Central Nervous System
Chills (2–18%) [2]
Fever (4–18%) [3]
Headache (24–44%) [55]
Insomnia (15–29%) [22]
Irritability (10–16%) [6]
Vertigo (dizziness) [4]

Neuromuscular/Skeletal
Arthralgia [3]
Asthenia (fatigue) (30–59%) [53]
Back pain [2]
Myalgia/Myopathy (6–16%) [4]

Gastrointestinal/Hepatic
Abdominal pain [2]
Diarrhea (9–17%) [7]
Dyspepsia [2]
Hepatotoxicity [2]
Nausea (13–34%) [41]
Vomiting [4]

Respiratory
Cough [4]
Dyspnea [3]
Flu-like syndrome (3–18%) [4]
Nasopharyngitis [2]
Upper respiratory tract infection [4]

Endocrine/Metabolic
Appetite decreased (6–18%)

Renal
Renal failure [2]

Hematologic
Anemia (6–21%) [37]
Lymphopenia [2]
Neutropenia (<17%) [5]

Other
Adverse effects [8]
Infection [2]

SOFOSBUVIR & VELPATASVIR

Trade name: Epclusa (Gilead)
Indications: Hepatitis C
Class: Direct-acting antiviral, Hepatitis C virus NS5A inhibitor (velpatasvir), Hepatitis C virus nucleotide analog NS5B polymerase inhibitor (sofosbuvir)
Half-life: <27 hours (sofosbuvir); 15 hours (velpatasvir)
Clinically important, potentially hazardous interactions with: amiodarone, carbamazepine, efavirenz, omeprazole, oxcarbazepine, phenobarbital, phenytoin, rifabutin, rifampin, rifapentine, St John's wort, topotecan
Pregnancy category: N/A (Insufficient evidence to inform drug-associated risk; contra-indicated in pregnancy when given with ribavirin)
Important contra-indications noted in the prescribing guidelines for: nursing mothers; pediatric patients
Note: See also separate entry for sofosbuvir.

Skin
Rash (2%)

Central Nervous System
Headache (22%) [13]
Insomnia (5%) [6]

Neuromuscular/Skeletal
Arthralgia [2]
Asthenia (fatigue) (5–15%) [13]

Gastrointestinal/Hepatic
Hepatotoxicity (2–6%)
Nausea (9%) [11]

Respiratory
Nasopharyngitis [4]

Endocrine/Metabolic
Creatine phosphokinase increased (<2%)

Hematologic
Anemia [3]
Lymphopenia [2]
Thrombocytopenia [2]

SOLIFENACIN

Trade name: Vesicare (Astellas)
Indications: Overactive bladder
Class: Antimuscarinic, Muscarinic antagonist
Half-life: 45–68 hours
Clinically important, potentially hazardous interactions with: atazanavir, carbamazepine, clarithromycin, indinavir, itraconazole, ketoconazole, nefazodone, nelfinavir, phenobarbital, phenytoin, rifabutin, rifampin, rifapentine, ritonavir, saquinavir, St John's wort, troleandomycin, voriconazole
Pregnancy category: C
Important contra-indications noted in the prescribing guidelines for: nursing mothers; pediatric patients

Mucosal
Xerostomia (11–27%) [22]

Cardiovascular
QT prolongation [3]

Central Nervous System
Vertigo (dizziness) (2%) [3]

Neuromuscular/Skeletal
Asthenia (fatigue) (<2%)

Gastrointestinal/Hepatic
Abdominal pain (2%)
Constipation [11]

Ocular
Vision blurred (4–5%) [5]
Xerophthalmia (2%)

Other
Adverse effects [5]

SONIDEGIB

Trade name: Odomzo (Novartis)
Indications: Basal cell carcinoma
Class: Hedgehog (Hh) signaling pathway inhibitor
Half-life: 28 days
Clinically important, potentially hazardous interactions with: atazanavir, carbamazepine, diltiazem, efavirenz, fluconazole, itraconazole, ketoconazole, modafinil, nefazodone, phenobarbital, phenytoin, posaconazole, rifabutin, rifampin, saquinavir, St John's wort, telithromycin, voriconazole
Pregnancy category: N/A (Can cause fetal harm)
Important contra-indications noted in the prescribing guidelines for: nursing mothers; pediatric patients
Note: Patients should not donate blood or blood products while receiving sonidegib and for at least 20 months after the last dose.
Warning: EMBRYO-FETAL TOXICITY

Skin
Pruritus (10%)

Hair
Alopecia (53%) [6]

Central Nervous System
Anorexia [2]
Dysgeusia (taste perversion) (46%) [6]

Headache (15%)
Pain (14%)
Vertigo (dizziness) [2]

Neuromuscular/Skeletal
Asthenia (fatigue) (41%) [5]
Bone or joint pain (32%)
Muscle spasm (54%) [6]
Myalgia/Myopathy (19%) [5]

Gastrointestinal/Hepatic
Abdominal pain (18%)
Diarrhea (32%)
Hepatotoxicity [2]
Nausea (39%) [4]
Vomiting (11%) [3]

Endocrine/Metabolic
ALT increased (19%)
Appetite decreased (30%)
AST increased (19%)
Creatine phosphokinase increased (61%) [8]
Hyperbilirubinemia [2]
Hyperglycemia (51%)
Weight loss (30%) [3]

Hematologic
Anemia (32%)
Lymphopenia (28%)

SORAFENIB

Trade name: Nexavar (Bayer)
Indications: Advanced renal cell carcinoma
Class: Antineoplastic, Epidermal growth factor receptor (EGFR) inhibitor, Tyrosine kinase inhibitor
Half-life: 25–48 hours
Clinically important, potentially hazardous interactions with: bevacizumab, carbamazepine, clozapine, conivaptan, coumarins, CYP3A4 inducers, darunavir, delavirdine, dexamethasone, digoxin, docetaxel, doxorubicin, efavirenz, indinavir, irinotecan, neomycin, oxcarbazepine, phenobarbital, phenytoin, rifabutin, rifampin, rifapentine, St John's wort, telithromycin, voriconazole, warfarin
Pregnancy category: D
Important contra-indications noted in the prescribing guidelines for: nursing mothers; pediatric patients
Note: In combination with carboplatin and paclitaxel, Nexavar is contra-indicated in patients with squamous cell lung cancer.

Skin
Acneform eruption (<10%) [6]
Actinic keratoses [4]
AGEP [2]
Desquamation (19–40%) [8]
Eczema [2]
Edema [3]
Erythema (>10%) [4]
Erythema multiforme [11]
Exanthems [3]
Exfoliative dermatitis (<10%)
Facial erythema [3]
Flushing (<10%)
Folliculitis [3]
Hand–foot syndrome (21–30%) [126]
Hyperkeratosis [4]
Hypersensitivity [2]
Keratoacanthoma [4]
Keratosis pilaris [2]
Milia [2]
Nevi [3]
Palmar–plantar toxicity [2]
Pigmentation [2]
Pruritus (14–19%) [10]
Psoriasis [3]
Radiation recall dermatitis [3]
Rash (19–40%) [54]
Recall reaction [2]
Seborrheic dermatitis [2]
Squamous cell carcinoma [8]
Stevens-Johnson syndrome [2]
Toxicity [19]
Xerosis (10–11%) [6]

Hair
Alopecia (14–27%) [28]
Hair pigmentation [2]

Nails
Splinter hemorrhage [4]
Subungual hemorrhage [2]

Mucosal
Epistaxis (nosebleed) [2]
Glossodynia (<10%)
Mucositis (<10%) [13]
Stomatitis (<10%) [13]
Xerostomia (<10%)

Cardiovascular
Cardiac failure [2]
Cardiotoxicity (3%) [3]
Congestive heart failure (<10%)
Hypertension (9–17%) [58]
Myocardial infarction (<10%)

Central Nervous System
Anorexia (16–29%) [15]
Depression (<10%)
Dysgeusia (taste perversion) [2]
Encephalopathy [2]
Fever (<10%) [7]
Headache (10%) [5]
Neurotoxicity (2–40%) [4]
Pain (>10%) [4]

Neuromuscular/Skeletal
Arthralgia (<10%)
Asthenia (fatigue) (37–46%) [57]
Back pain [3]
Bone or joint pain (>10%) [3]
Myalgia/Myopathy (<10%) [2]

Gastrointestinal/Hepatic
Abdominal pain (11–31%) [10]
Ascites [2]
Constipation (14–15%) [4]
Diarrhea (43–55%) [71]
Dyspepsia (<10%)
Dysphagia (<10%)
Gastrointestinal bleeding [5]
Hepatotoxicity (11%) [25]
Nausea (23–24%) [15]
Pancreatitis [8]
Pneumatosis intestinalis [2]
Vomiting (15–16%) [9]

Respiratory
Cough (13%) [2]
Dysphonia [6]
Dyspnea (14%) [4]
Flu-like syndrome (<10%)
Hoarseness (<10%) [2]
Pulmonary toxicity [2]

Endocrine/Metabolic
ALT increased [11]
Appetite decreased (<10%) [7]
AST increased [10]
Creatine phosphokinase increased [2]
Hyperbilirubinemia [5]
Hypoalbuminemia (56%)
Hypocalcemia [2]
Hypokalemia [2]
Hyponatremia [2]
Hypophosphatemia (35–45%) [10]
Hypothyroidism [8]
Thyroid dysfunction [4]
Weight loss (10–30%) [13]

Genitourinary
Erectile dysfunction (<10%)

Renal
Nephrotoxicity [2]
Proteinuria [4]
Renal failure (<10%) [3]

Hematologic
Anemia (44%) [10]
Bleeding [3]
Cytopenia [2]
Hemorrhage (15–18%) [4]
Hemotoxicity [2]
Hyperlipasemia [2]
Leukopenia (>10%) [4]
Lymphopenia (23–47%) [5]
Myelosuppression [2]
Neutropenia (<10%) [7]
Thrombocytopenia (12–46%) [19]
Thrombosis [2]

Other
Adverse effects [18]
Death [9]
Infection [2]
Side effects (71%) [4]

SOTALOL

Trade name: Betapace (Bayer)
Indications: Ventricular arrhythmias
Class: Antiarrhythmic, Antiarrhythmic class II, Antiarrhythmic class III, Beta adrenergic blocker, Beta blocker
Half-life: 7–18 hours
Clinically important, potentially hazardous interactions with: abarelix, amiodarone, amisulpride, amitriptyline, arsenic, artemether/lumefantrine, asenapine, astemizole, atomoxetine, bepridil, ciprofloxacin, class I and class III antiarrhythmics, clonidine, degarelix, disopyramide, dronedarone, droperidol, enoxacin, gatifloxacin, guanethidine, haloperidol, insulin, isoprenaline, ivabradine, levomepromazine, lomefloxacin, loop diuretics, mizolastine, moxifloxacin, nilotinib, norfloxacin, ofloxacin, oral macrolides, phenothiazines, pimavanserin, pimozide, procainamide, quinidine, quinine, quinolones, ranolazine, reserpine, ribociclib, salbutamol, sertindole, sparfloxacin, sulpiride, terbutaline, tetrabenazine, thiazides and related diruetics, tolterodine, tricyclic antidepressants, trifluoperazine, vandetanib, zuclopenthixol

Pregnancy category: B
Important contra-indications noted in the prescribing guidelines for: nursing mothers; pediatric patients
Note: Contra-indicated in patients with bronchial asthma, sinus bradycardia, second and third degree AV block, unless a functioning pacemaker is present, congenital or acquired long QT syndromes, cardiogenic shock, or uncontrolled congestive heart failure.

Skin
Edema (5%)
Pruritus (<10%)
Psoriasis [3]
Rash (3%)
Scleroderma [3]

Cardiovascular
Arrhythmias [2]
Atrioventricular block [2]
Bradycardia [10]
Cardiac failure [2]
Cardiogenic shock [2]
Cardiotoxicity [3]
Hypotension [3]
QT prolongation [19]
Torsades de pointes [25]

Central Nervous System
Depression [2]
Paresthesias (3%)

Neuromuscular/Skeletal
Asthenia (fatigue) (6%) [2]

Other
Adverse effects [2]

SPIRONOLACTONE

Trade names: Aldactazide (Pfizer), Aldactone (Pfizer)
Indications: Hyperaldosteronism, hirsutism, hypertension, edema for patients with congestive heart failure, cirrhosis of the liver or nephrotic syndrome
Class: Aldosterone antagonist, Diuretic
Half-life: 78–84 minutes
Clinically important, potentially hazardous interactions with: ACE inhibitors, alcohol, amiloride, barbiturates, benazepril, captopril, cyclosporine, enalapril, fosinopril, lisinopril, mitotane, moexipril, narcotics, NSAIDs, potassium chloride, potassium iodide, quinapril, ramipril, trandolapril, triamterene, zofenopril
Pregnancy category: C
Important contra-indications noted in the prescribing guidelines for: nursing mothers; pediatric patients
Note: Aldactazide is spironolactone and hydrochlorothiazide. Hydrochlorothiazide is a sulfonamide and can be absorbed systemically. Sulfonamides can produce severe, possibly fatal, reactions such as toxic epidermal necrolysis and Stevens-Johnson syndrome.
Warning: Spironolactone has been shown to be a tumorigen in chronic toxicity studies in rats

---

Skin
Bullous pemphigoid [2]
Dermatitis [6]
Eczema [2]
Exanthems (<5%) [6]
Lichenoid eruption [2]
Melasma [2]
Pigmentation [3]
Pruritus [3]
Rash (<10%) [2]
Urticaria [2]
Xerosis (40%) [2]

Hair
Alopecia [2]

Endocrine/Metabolic
Amenorrhea [2]
Gynecomastia [30]
Hyperkalemia [9]

Renal
Renal function abnormal [2]

SQUILL

Family: Liliaceae
Scientific names: *Drimia indica, Drimia maritima, Scilla indica, Scilla maritima, Urginea indica, Urginea maritima, Urginea scilla*
Indications: Arrhythmias, asthma, edema, bronchitis, whooping cough, abortifacient. Also used as a rodenticide
Class: Diuretic
Half-life: N/A
Clinically important, potentially hazardous interactions with: ginger, ginseng, hawthorn (fruit, leaf, flower extract), licorice, mistletoe, senna
Pregnancy category: N/A
Note: Squill is unsafe for self-medication.

ST JOHN'S WORT

Family: Hypericaceae
Scientific names: *Hypericum perforatum, Kira (Lichtwer), Quanterra Emotional Balance (Warner Lambert)*
Indications: Depression, dysthymic disorder, fatigue, insomnia, loss of appetite, anxiety, obsessive-compulsive disorders, mood disturbances, migraine headaches, neuralgia, fibrositis, sciatica, palpitations, exhaustion, headache, muscle pain, vitiligo, diuretic, bruises, abrasions, first-degree burns, hemorrhoids
Class: Anxyolytic, CYP3A4 inducer
Half-life: 24–48 hours
Clinically important, potentially hazardous interactions with: acetaminophen, acitretin, afatinib, alfuzosin, alitretinoin, alprazolam, ambrisentan, aminophylline, amiodarone, amitriptyline, amlodipine, amprenavir, apixaban, aprepitant, artemether/lumefantrine, atazanavir, atorvastatin, bexarotene, bictegravir/emtricitabine/tenofovir alafenamide, boceprevir, bosentan, brigatinib, buspirone, cabazitaxel, cabozantinib, carbamazepine, ceritinib, cilostazol, ciprofloxacin, citalopram, cobimetinib, conivaptan, copanlisib, crizotinib, cyclosporine, cyproterone, dabigatran, daclatasvir, darunavir, dasabuvir/ombitasvir/paritaprevir/ritonavir, dasatinib, delavirdine, demeclocycline, digoxin, doxycycline, dronedarone, duloxetine, efavirenz, eliglustat, enzalutamide, eplerenone, escitalopram, estradiol, eszopiclone, ethosuximide, etoposide, etravirine, everolimus, fenfluramine, fesoterodine, fexofenadine, flibanserin, fluoxetine, fluvoxamine, fosamprenavir, gefitinib, gemifloxacin, ginkgo biloba, glecaprevir & pibrentasvir, hydromorphone, ibrutinib, idelalisib, imatinib, indinavir, irinotecan, isavuconazonium sulfate, isotretinoin, ixabepilone, ixazomib, lacosamide, lapatinib, ledipasvir & sofosbuvir, levonorgestrel, loperamide, lopinavir, lorcaserin, lumacaftor/ivacaftor, maraviroc, metaxalone, methadone, midazolam, midostaurin, mifepristone, milnacipran, naldemedine, naratriptan, nefazodone, nelfinavir, neratinib, nevirapine, nifedipine, nilotinib, nintedanib, ofloxacin, olaparib, ombitasvir/paritaprevir/ritonavir, omeprazole, oral contraceptives, osimertinib, oxcarbazepine, palbociclib, paroxetine hydrochloride, pazopanib, perampanel, phenobarbitone, phenprocoumon, phenytoin, pimavanserin, ponatinib, quinolones, raltegravir, ramelteon, regorafenib, reserpine, rilpivirine, riociguat, ritonavir, rivaroxaban, rizatriptan, romidepsin, safinamide, saquinavir, sertraline, sildenafil, simeprevir, simvastatin, sirolimus, sofosbuvir, sofosbuvir & velpatasvir, sofosbuvir/velpatasvir/voxilaprevir, solifenacin, sonidegib, sorafenib, SSRIs, sumatriptan, sunitinib, tacrolimus, tadalafil, tapentadol, telaprevir, telithromycin, temsirolimus, tenofovir alafenamide, tetracyclines, tezacaftor/ivacaftor, thalidomide, tiagabine, tipranavir, tolvaptan, trabectedin, tricyclic antidepressants, ulipristal, valbenazine, vandetanib, venetoclax, venlafaxine, vigabatrin, vorapaxar, voriconazole, warfarin, ziprasidone, zolmitriptan
Pregnancy category: N/A
Note: St John's wort is a natural source of flavoring in Europe. Although not indigenous to Australia, and long considered a weed, St John's wort is now grown there as a cash crop and produces 20% of the world's supply.

Skin
Hyperhidrosis [2]
Photosensitivity [11]
Pruritus [2]
Rash [2]

Mucosal
Xerostomia [5]

Cardiovascular
Hypertension [3]

Central Nervous System
Headache [5]
Insomnia [3]
Irritability [2]
Mania [2]
Neurotoxicity [2]
Psychosis [2]
Restlessness [4]
Serotonin syndrome [8]
Sleep disturbances [3]
Somnolence (drowsiness) [3]
Vertigo (dizziness) [4]

Neuromuscular/Skeletal
Asthenia (fatigue) [6]

Gastrointestinal/Hepatic
Abdominal pain [2]
Constipation [2]
Diarrhea [2]
Hepatotoxicity [6]
Nausea [4]

Other
Adverse effects [20]
Allergic reactions [2]

STANOZOLOL

Trade name: Winstrol (Ovation)
Indications: Hereditary angioedema
Class: Anabolic steroid
Half-life: N/A
Clinically important, potentially hazardous interactions with: anticoagulants, warfarin
Pregnancy category: X
Important contra-indications noted in the prescribing guidelines for: nursing mothers

---

Skin
Acneform eruption (>10%) [2]
Pigmentation (<10%)

Hair
Hirsutism (in women) [3]

Cardiovascular
Cardiomyopathy [2]
Hypertension [2]
Myocardial infarction [2]
Myocardial ischemia [2]

Central Nervous System
Chills (<10%)

Gastrointestinal/Hepatic
Hepatotoxicity [3]

Endocrine/Metabolic
Gynecomastia (>10%)

Genitourinary
Priapism (>10%)

Renal
Nephrotoxicity [3]

Other
Death [3]

STAR ANISE (CHINESE)

Family: Illiciaceae
Scientific name: *Illicium verum*
Indications: Bronchitis, colic, cough, flatulence, menstrual complaints, respiratory tract inflammation. Culinary spice, fragrance component in cosmetics
Class: Antimycobacterial, Insecticide
Half-life: N/A
Clinically important, potentially hazardous interactions with: none known
Pregnancy category: N/A
Note: Star anise preparations are sometimes contaminated with highly poisonous Japanese star anise (*Illicium anisatum*). Star anise contains a compound used in the manufacture of Tamiflu.

Central Nervous System
Seizures [2]

STAVUDINE

Synonym: D4T
Trade name: Zerit (Bristol-Myers Squibb)
Indications: HIV infection
Class: Antiretroviral, Nucleoside analog reverse transcriptase inhibitor
Half-life: 1.44 hours
Clinically important, potentially hazardous interactions with: doxorubicin, ribavirin, zidovudine
Pregnancy category: C
Important contra-indications noted in the prescribing guidelines for: nursing mothers
Warning: LACTIC ACIDOSIS and HEPATOMEGALY with STEATOSIS; PANCREATITIS

Skin
Diaphoresis (19%)
Lipoatrophy [7]
Lipodystrophy [8]
Rash (40%)
Toxic epidermal necrolysis [2]
Toxicity [2]

Central Nervous System
Chills (50%)
Neurotoxicity [4]
Peripheral neuropathy (52%) [11]

Neuromuscular/Skeletal
Myalgia/Myopathy (32%) [2]

Gastrointestinal/Hepatic
Diarrhea (50%)
Hepatotoxicity [2]
Nausea (39%)
Pancreatitis [6]
Vomiting (39%)

Endocrine/Metabolic
Acidosis [11]
Diabetes mellitus [2]
Fat distribution abnormality [4]
Gynecomastia [4]

Renal
Fanconi syndrome [2]

Other
Adverse effects [3]
Allergic reactions (9%)

STIRIPENTOL *

Trade name: Diacomit (Biocodex SA)
Indications: treatment of seizures associated with Dravet syndrome in patients 2 years of age and older taking clobazam
Half-life: 4.5–13 hours
Clinically important, potentially hazardous interactions with: clobazam
Pregnancy category: N/A (Based on animal data, may cause fetal harm)

Mucosal
Salivary hypersecretion (6%)

Central Nervous System
Aggression (9%)
Agitation (27%)
Anorexia [5]
Dysarthria (12%)
Fever (6%)
Insomnia (12%)
Sedation [2]
Somnolence (drowsiness) (67%) [4]
Tremor (15%)

Neuromuscular/Skeletal
Asthenia (fatigue) (9%)
Ataxia (27%) [3]
Hypotonia (18%)

Gastrointestinal/Hepatic
Nausea (15%)
Vomiting (9%)

Respiratory
Bronchitis (6%)
Nasopharyngitis (6%)

Endocrine/Metabolic
Appetite decreased (46%) [6]
Weight gain (6%)
Weight loss (27%) [4]

Hematologic
Neutropenia (13%)
Platelets decreased (13%)

Other
Adverse effects [3]

STREPTOKINASE

Trade names: Kabikinase (Pfizer), Streptase (AstraZeneca)
Indications: Pulmonary embolism, acute myocardial infarction
Class: Fibrinolytic
Half-life: 83 minutes
Clinically important, potentially hazardous interactions with: bivalirudin, lepirudin
Pregnancy category: C

Skin
Anaphylactoid reactions/Anaphylaxis [2]
Angioedema (>10%) [2]
Diaphoresis (<10%)
Exanthems (<5%) [2]
Pruritus (<10%)
Purpura [2]
Rash (<10%)
Serum sickness [4]
Serum sickness-like reaction [3]
Urticaria (<5%)
Vasculitis [7]

Neuromuscular/Skeletal
Rhabdomyolysis [2]

Ocular
Periorbital edema (>10%)

Other
Allergic reactions (4%) [4]

STREPTOMYCIN

Trade name: Streptomycin (Pfizer)
Indications: Tuberculosis
Class: Antibiotic, aminoglycoside
Half-life: 2–5 hours
Clinically important, potentially hazardous interactions with: aldesleukin, aminoglycosides, atracurium, bacitracin, bumetanide, doxacurium, ethacrynic acid, furosemide, methoxyflurane, neostigmine, non-depolarizing muscle relaxants, pancuronium, polypeptide antibiotics, rocuronium, succinylcholine, teicoplanin, torsemide, vecuronium
Pregnancy category: D
Important contra-indications noted in the prescribing guidelines for: nursing mothers
Note: Aminoglycosides may cause neurotoxicity and/or nephrotoxicity.

Skin
Anaphylactoid reactions/Anaphylaxis [3]
Dermatitis [2]
DRESS syndrome [3]
Erythema multiforme [4]
Exanthems (>5%) [8]
Exfoliative dermatitis [11]
Lupus erythematosus [5]
Nicolau syndrome [2]
Photosensitivity [2]
Pruritus [2]
Purpura [3]
Stevens-Johnson syndrome [3]
Toxic epidermal necrolysis [9]
Urticaria [3]

Mucosal
Cheilitis (2%)
Glossitis (2%)
Oral mucosal eruption [2]
Stomatitis [2]

Renal
Nephrotoxicity [2]

Otic
Ototoxicity [6]

Ocular
Optic neuropathy [2]

Other
Adverse effects [2]
Allergic reactions [2]

STREPTOZOCIN

Trade name: Zanosar (Gensia)
Indications: Carcinoma of the pancreas, carcinoid tumor, Hodgkin's disease
Class: Alkylating agent, Antineoplastic
Half-life: 35 minutes
Clinically important, potentially hazardous interactions with: aldesleukin
Pregnancy category: D
Important contra-indications noted in the prescribing guidelines for: nursing mothers

---

Neuromuscular/Skeletal
Asthenia (fatigue) [2]

Gastrointestinal/Hepatic
Abdominal pain [2]
Nausea [2]
Vomiting [2]

Renal
Nephrotoxicity [2]

Hematologic
Neutropenia [2]

Local
Injection-site pain (<10%)

SUCCIMER

Synonym: DMSA
Trade name: Chemet (Sanofi-Aventis)
Indications: Heavy metal poisoning
Class: Chelator
Half-life: 2 days
Clinically important, potentially hazardous interactions with: other chelating agents
Pregnancy category: C
Important contra-indications noted in the prescribing guidelines for: nursing mothers; pediatric patients

---

Skin
Candidiasis (16%)
Exanthems (11%)
Pruritus (11%)
Rash (<11%) [2]

Mucosal
Mucocutaneous eruption (11%)

Central Nervous System
Chills (16%)
Dysgeusia (taste perversion) (metallic) (21%)
Fever (16%)
Headache (16%)
Pain (3%)
Paresthesias (13%)

Neuromuscular/Skeletal
Back pain (16%)

Gastrointestinal/Hepatic
Abdominal pain (16%)

Respiratory
Flu-like syndrome (16%)

SUCCINYLCHOLINE

Synonym: suxamethonium
Trade name: Anectine (Sabex)
Indications: Skeletal muscle relaxation during general anesthesia
Class: Cholinesterase inhibitor, Depolarizing muscle relaxant
Half-life: N/A
Clinically important, potentially hazardous interactions with: amikacin, aminoglycosides, donepezil, galantamine, gentamicin, hydromorphone, kanamycin, levomepromazine, neomycin, neostigmine, paromomycin, physostigmine, pipecuronium, pralidoxime, quinine, streptomycin, tapentadol, thalidomide, tobramycin, vancomycin, vecuronium
Pregnancy category: C
Important contra-indications noted in the prescribing guidelines for: the elderly; nursing mothers
Warning: RISK OF CARDIAC ARREST FROM HYPERKALEMIC RHABDOMYOLYSIS

Skin
Anaphylactoid reactions/Anaphylaxis [13]

Mucosal
Sialorrhea (<10%)

Cardiovascular
Bradycardia [2]

Central Nervous System
Malignant hyperthermia [7]
Paralysis [3]
Twitching [5]

Neuromuscular/Skeletal
Myalgia/Myopathy [11]
Rhabdomyolysis [27]

Endocrine/Metabolic
Hyperkalemia [8]

Other
Death [3]

SUCRALFATE

Trade name: Carafate (Aptalis)
Indications: Duodenal ulcer
Class: Chelator
Half-life: N/A
Clinically important, potentially hazardous interactions with: anagrelide, chlortetracycline, ciprofloxacin, clorazepate, demeclocycline, doxycycline, gemifloxacin, ketoconazole, lansoprazole, levofloxacin, lomefloxacin, lymecycline, minocycline, moxifloxacin, norfloxacin, ofloxacin, oxtriphylline, oxytetracycline, paricalcitol, phenytoin, sparfloxacin, tetracycline, tigecycline, voriconazole
Pregnancy category: B
Important contra-indications noted in the prescribing guidelines for: the elderly; nursing mothers; pediatric patients
Note: Sucralfate use can lead to symptoms of aluminum toxicity.

Mucosal
Xerostomia [2]

Gastrointestinal/Hepatic
Constipation (2%)

SUCRALOSE

Trade name: Splenda (McNeil)
Indications: Weight reduction
Class: Sweetening agent
Half-life: 2–5 hours
Clinically important, potentially hazardous interactions with: none known
Pregnancy category: N/A

Central Nervous System
Migraine [3]

SUGAMMADEX

Trade name: Bridion (Organon)
Indications: Reversal of neuromuscular blockade induced by rocuronium bromide and vecuronium bromide in adults undergoing surgery
Class: Cyclodextrin, Selective relaxant binding agent
Half-life: ~2 hours
Clinically important, potentially hazardous interactions with: toremifene
Pregnancy category: N/A (No data available)
Important contra-indications noted in the prescribing guidelines for: the elderly; nursing mothers; pediatric patients

---

Skin
Anaphylactoid reactions/Anaphylaxis [10]
Erythema (<2%)
Hypersensitivity [7]
Pruritus (2–3%)

Mucosal
Oropharyngeal pain (3–5%)
Xerostomia (<2%) [2]

Cardiovascular
Bradycardia (<5%)
Hypotension [2]
QT prolongation (<6%) [2]
Tachycardia (2–5%)

Central Nervous System
Anxiety (<3%)
Chills (3–7%)
Depression (<2%)
Dysgeusia (taste perversion) [3]
Fever (5–9%)
Headache (5–10%) [2]
Hypoesthesia (<3%)
Insomnia (2–5%)
Pain (36–52%)
Restlessness (<2%)
Somnolence (drowsiness) [2]
Vertigo (dizziness) (3–6%)

Neuromuscular/Skeletal
Bone or joint pain (<2%)
Myalgia/Myopathy (<2%)
Pain in extremities (<6%)

Gastrointestinal/Hepatic
Abdominal pain (4–6%)
Diarrhea [2]
Flatulence (<3%)
Nausea (23–26%) [3]
Vomiting (11–15%) [2]

Respiratory
Bronchospasm [2]
Cough (<8%)

Endocrine/Metabolic
Creatine phosphokinase increased (<2%)
Hypocalcemia (<2%)

Hematologic
Anemia (<2%)

Local
Injection-site pain (4–6%)

Other
Allergic reactions [2]

SULFADOXINE

Trade name: Fansidar (Roche)
Indications: Malaria
Class: Antibiotic, sulfonamide, Antimalarial
Half-life: 5–8 days
Clinically important, potentially hazardous interactions with: none known
Pregnancy category: C
Important contra-indications noted in the prescribing guidelines for: the elderly; nursing mothers; pediatric patients
Note: Sulfadoxine is a sulfonamide and can be absorbed systemically. Sulfonamides can produce severe, possibly fatal, reactions such as toxic epidermal necrolysis and Stevens-Johnson syndrome.
Fansidar is sulfadoxine and pyrimethamine (this combination is almost always prescribed).

Skin
Erythema multiforme [3]
Exfoliative dermatitis [3]
Fixed eruption [2]
Hypersensitivity (>10%)
Photosensitivity (>10%) [2]
Pruritus [2]
Stevens-Johnson syndrome (<10%) [24]
Toxic epidermal necrolysis [17]

Mucosal
Glossitis (>10%)

Central Nervous System
Tremor (>10%)
Vertigo (dizziness) [2]

Neuromuscular/Skeletal
Asthenia (fatigue) [2]

Gastrointestinal/Hepatic
Diarrhea [2]

Other
Death [7]

SULFA-METHOXAZOLE

Trade names: Bactrim (Women First), Septra (Monarch)
Indications: Various infections caused by susceptible organisms
Class: Antibiotic, sulfonamide, Folic acid antagonist
Half-life: 7–12 hours
Clinically important, potentially hazardous interactions with: anticoagulants, azathioprine, cyclosporine, methotrexate, pralatrexate, probenecid, warfarin
Pregnancy category: C
Note: Sulfamethoxazole is a sulfonamide and can be absorbed systemically. Sulfonamides can produce severe, possibly fatal, reactions such as toxic epidermal necrolysis and Stevens-Johnson syndrome.
Sulfamethoxazole is commonly used in conjunction with trimethoprim (see separate entry for co-trimoxazole).

Skin
AGEP [3]
Anaphylactoid reactions/Anaphylaxis [4]
Angioedema (<5%)
Dermatitis [4]
DRESS syndrome [4]
Erythema multiforme [15]
Erythema nodosum [2]
Exanthems (<5%) [30]
Exfoliative dermatitis [3]
Fixed eruption [29]
Hypersensitivity [6]
Linear IgA bullous dermatosis [3]
Lupus erythematosus [3]
Photosensitivity (>10%) [3]
Pruritus (10%) [7]
Purpura [3]
Pustules [6]
Radiation recall dermatitis [3]
Rash (>10%) [3]
Stevens-Johnson syndrome (<10%) [22]
Sweet's syndrome [3]
Toxic epidermal necrolysis (<10%) [32]
Urticaria [9]
Vasculitis [6]

Mucosal
Oral mucosal eruption [2]
Oral ulceration [2]

Neuromuscular/Skeletal
Rhabdomyolysis [4]

Renal
Nephrotoxicity [2]

Hematologic
Thrombocytopenia [2]

Other
Allergic reactions [2]
Side effects (2%) [2]

SULFASALAZINE

Synonyms: salicylazosulfapyridine; salazopyrin
Trade name: Azulfidine (Pfizer)
Indications: Inflammatory bowel disease, ulcerative colitis, rheumatoid arthritis
Class: Aminosalicylate, Disease-modifying antirheumatic drug (DMARD), Sulfonamide
Half-life: 5–10 hours
Clinically important, potentially hazardous interactions with: cholestyramine, methotrexate, safinamide
Pregnancy category: B
Important contra-indications noted in the prescribing guidelines for: nursing mothers; pediatric patients
Note: Sulfasalazine is a sulfonamide and can be absorbed systemically. Sulfonamides can produce severe, possibly fatal, reactions such as toxic epidermal necrolysis and Stevens-Johnson syndrome.
Contra-indicated in patients with intestinal or urinary obstruction, or with porphyria.

Skin
AGEP [3]
Anaphylactoid reactions/Anaphylaxis [4]
Angioedema [3]
Bullous pemphigoid [3]

Cyanosis (<10%)
Dermatitis [2]
DRESS syndrome [31]
Erythema multiforme [8]
Erythema nodosum [2]
Exanthems (2–23%) [23]
Exfoliative dermatitis [5]
Fixed eruption [7]
Flushing [2]
Hypersensitivity (<5%) [21]
Lichen planus [3]
Lupus erythematosus [34]
Photosensitivity (10%) [4]
Pigmentation [3]
Pruritus (10%) [8]
Pseudolymphoma [2]
Pustules [2]
Rash (>10%) [19]
Raynaud's phenomenon [3]
Stevens-Johnson syndrome [9]
Toxic epidermal necrolysis (<10%) [13]
Urticaria (<5%) [11]
Vasculitis [4]

Hair

Alopecia [6]

Mucosal

Mucocutaneous reactions (6%) [2]
Oral mucosal eruption [4]
Oral ulceration [3]
Stomatitis (<10%)

Central Nervous System

Anorexia (10%)
Aseptic meningitis [3]
Fever [4]
Headache (10%) [7]
Vertigo (dizziness) (<10%)

Neuromuscular/Skeletal

Arthralgia [2]
Asthenia (fatigue) [5]

Gastrointestinal/Hepatic

Abdominal pain (<10%)
Dyspepsia (10%) [3]
Hepatotoxicity [14]
Nausea (10%) [7]
Pancreatitis [6]
Vomiting (10%) [2]

Respiratory

Pulmonary toxicity [3]
Upper respiratory tract infection [3]

Renal

Nephrotoxicity [4]
Renal failure [2]

Hematologic

Agranulocytosis [6]
Anemia (<10%)
Leukopenia (<10%) [4]
Neutropenia [2]
Thrombocytopenia (<10%)

Ocular

Conjunctival pigmentation [2]

Other

Adverse effects [9]
Death [4]
Side effects (5%)

SULFITES

Family: N/A
Scientific names: *Ammonium bisulfite [AB], potassium bisulfite [PB], potassium metabisulfite [PM], sodium bisulfite [SB], sodium metabisulfite [SM], sodium sulfite [SS], sulfur dioxide [SD]*
Indications: Food additive, drug additive, sanitary agent
Class: Trace element
Half-life: N/A
Clinically important, potentially hazardous interactions with: aspirin, NSAIDs

---

Skin

Anaphylactoid reactions/Anaphylaxis [11]
Angioedema [2]
Dermatitis [15]
Edema [2]
Hypersensitivity [6]
Rash [2]
Sensitivity [4]
Urticaria [6]

Respiratory

Pulmonary toxicity [2]
Rhinitis [3]

Other

Adverse effects [5]
Allergic reactions [6]
Death [2]

SULINDAC

Trade name: Clinoril (Merck)
Indications: Arthritis
Class: Non-steroidal anti-inflammatory (NSAID)
Half-life: 7.8–16.4 hours
Clinically important, potentially hazardous interactions with: methotrexate, warfarin
Pregnancy category: C (category C in first and second trimesters; category D in third trimester)
Important contra-indications noted in the prescribing guidelines for: nursing mothers; pediatric patients
Note: NSAIDs may cause an increased risk of serious cardiovascular and gastrointestinal adverse events, which can be fatal. This risk may increase with duration of use.

Skin

Anaphylactoid reactions/Anaphylaxis [4]
Erythema multiforme [8]
Exanthems (<5%) [9]
Fixed eruption [5]
Photosensitivity [2]
Pruritus (<10%) [5]
Purpura [2]
Rash (>10%)
Stevens-Johnson syndrome [5]
Toxic epidermal necrolysis [13]
Urticaria [4]

Mucosal

Oral mucosal eruption (3%) [2]
Stomatitis [2]
Xerostomia [2]

Gastrointestinal/Hepatic

Hepatotoxicity [4]
Pancreatitis [3]

SUMATRIPTAN

Trade names: Alsuma (King), Imigran (GSK), Imitrex (GSK), Onzetra Xsail (Avanir), Sumavel DosePro (Endo), Zecuity (Teva)
Indications: Migraine attacks, cluster headaches
Class: 5-HT1 agonist, Serotonin receptor agonist, Triptan
Half-life: 2.5 hours
Clinically important, potentially hazardous interactions with: citalopram, dihydroergotamine, ergot-containing drugs, escitalopram, fluoxetine, fluvoxamine, isocarboxazid, MAO inhibitors, methysergide, naratriptan, nefazodone, paroxetine hydrochloride, phenelzine, rizatriptan, sertraline, sibutramine, SNRIs, SSRIs, St John's wort, tranylcypromine, venlafaxine, zolmitriptan
Pregnancy category: C
Important contra-indications noted in the prescribing guidelines for: the elderly; nursing mothers; pediatric patients
Note: Contra-indicated in patients with Wolff-Parkinson-White syndrome, peripheral vascular disease, ischemic bowel disease, uncontrolled hypertension, severe hepatic impairment or a history of coronary artery disease, coronary vasospasm, stroke, transient ischemic attack, or hemiplegic or basilar migraine; or with recent (within 24 hours) use of another 5-HT1 agonist (e.g. another triptan) or an ergotamine-containing medication, or current or recent (past 2 weeks) use of a monoamine oxidase-A inhibitor.

Skin

Burning (<10%)
Diaphoresis (2%)
Flushing (7%) [4]
Hot flashes (>10%)
Hypersensitivity [2]

Mucosal

Nasal discomfort [3]
Rhinorrhea [2]
Xerostomia [2]

Cardiovascular

Chest pain (<2%) [7]
Hypertension [2]
Myocardial infarction [5]

Central Nervous System

Dysgeusia (taste perversion) [11]
Headache [2]
Neurotoxicity [3]
Pain (<2%) [4]
Paresthesias (3–5%) [11]
Somnolence (drowsiness) [3]
Stroke [2]
Vertigo (dizziness) (<2%) [10]
Warm feeling (2–3%)

Neuromuscular/Skeletal

Asthenia (fatigue) (2–3%) [5]
Jaw pain (<3%)
Muscle spasm [2]
Myalgia/Myopathy (2%) [2]
Neck pain (<3%)

Gastrointestinal/Hepatic
Colitis [2]
Nausea [13]

Respiratory
Nasopharyngitis [2]
Rhinitis [2]
Upper respiratory tract infection [2]

Local
Application-site erythema [2]
Injection-site edema [2]
Injection-site reactions (10–58%) [2]

Other
Adverse effects [10]

SUNITINIB

Trade name: Sutent (Pfizer)
Indications: Gastrointestinal stromal tumor, advanced renal cell carcinoma, advanced pancreatic neuroendocrine tumor
Class: Antineoplastic, Epidermal growth factor receptor (EGFR) inhibitor, Tyrosine kinase inhibitor
Half-life: 40–60 hours
Clinically important, potentially hazardous interactions with: atazanavir, bevacizumab, carbamazepine, clarithromycin, clozapine, dexamethasone, digoxin, efavirenz, grapefruit juice, indinavir, itraconazole, ketoconazole, nefazodone, nelfinavir, phenobarbital, phenytoin, rifabutin, rifampin, rifapentine, ritonavir, saquinavir, St John's wort, telithromycin, temsirolimus, voriconazole
Pregnancy category: D
Important contra-indications noted in the prescribing guidelines for: nursing mothers; pediatric patients
Note: [G] = treated for gastrointestinal tumor; [R] = treated for renal cell carcinoma; [P] treated for pancreatic neuroendocrine tumor.
Warning: HEPATOTOXICITY

Skin
Acral erythema [2]
Edema [6]
Erythema [6]
Facial edema [3]
Hand–foot syndrome (12–14%) [75]
Lesions [2]
Nevi [2]
Peripheral edema [R] (17%)
Pigmentation [15]
Pruritus [R] [3]
Pyoderma gangrenosum [8]
Rash (14–38%) [17]
Thrombocytopenic purpura [4]
Toxicity [24]
Xerosis (17%) [3]

Hair
Alopecia (5–12%) [6]
Hair pigmentation [G] [8]

Nails
Splinter hemorrhage [2]
Subungual hemorrhage [4]

Mucosal
Epistaxis (nosebleed) [2]
Glossodynia [R] [P] (15%)
Mucosal inflammation [4]
Mucositis (29–53%) [19]
Stomatitis [19]
Xerostomia [R] [P] [2]

Cardiovascular
Aortic dissection [3]
Cardiac failure [2]
Cardiomyopathy [2]
Cardiotoxicity [8]
Congestive heart failure [2]
Hypertension [60]
QT prolongation [2]
Ventricular arrhythmia [2]

Central Nervous System
Anorexia [8]
Dysgeusia (taste perversion) (21–43%) [6]
Fever [R] (15–18%) [2]
Headache (13–25%) [4]
Leukoencephalopathy [3]
Neurotoxicity [R] (10%)
Pain [R] (18%)
Vertigo (dizziness) [R] (16%)

Neuromuscular/Skeletal
Arthralgia [R] (12–28%)
Asthenia (fatigue) (22%) [74]
Back pain [R] (11–17%)
Myalgia/Myopathy [G] (14–17%)
Osteonecrosis [4]

Gastrointestinal/Hepatic
Abdominal pain (20–33%) [2]
Constipation [3]
Diarrhea [39]
Dyspepsia [R] [P] [3]
Esophagitis [2]
Gastrointestinal bleeding [4]
Gastrointestinal disorder [2]
Hepatotoxicity [8]
Nausea [18]
Pneumatosis intestinalis [3]
Vomiting [16]

Respiratory
Cough [R] (8–17%) [2]
Dyspnea [5]
Pulmonary toxicity [3]
Radiation recall pneumonitis [2]

Endocrine/Metabolic
ALT increased [4]
Appetite decreased [2]
AST increased [2]
Hypothyroidism [R] [30]
Serum creatinine increased [2]
Thyroid dysfunction [8]

Renal
Nephrotoxicity [5]
Proteinuria [5]

Hematologic
Anemia [21]
Bleeding [5]
Bone marrow suppression [2]
Cytopenia [2]
Hemorrhage [2]
Hemotoxicity [3]
Hyperlipasemia [2]
Leukopenia [20]
Lymphopenia [10]
Myelosuppression [3]
Neutropenia [48]
Thrombocytopenia [44]
Thrombotic microangiopathy [2]

Ocular
Epiphora [R] (6%)
Periorbital edema [R] (7%)

Other
Adverse effects [17]
Death [7]
Side effects [3]

SUVOREXANT

Trade name: Belsomra (Merck Sharpe & Dohme)
Indications: Insomnia
Class: Orexin receptor antagonist
Half-life: 10–22 hours
Clinically important, potentially hazardous interactions with: none known
Pregnancy category: C
Important contra-indications noted in the prescribing guidelines for: nursing mothers; pediatric patients
Note: Contra-indicated in patients with narcolepsy.

Mucosal
Xerostomia (2%)

Central Nervous System
Abnormal dreams (2%) [2]
Headache (7%) [2]
Sedation [2]
Somnolence (drowsiness) (7%) [6]
Vertigo (dizziness) (3%)

Gastrointestinal/Hepatic
Diarrhea (2%)

Respiratory
Cough (2%)
Upper respiratory tract infection (2%)

TACROLIMUS

Trade names: Envarsus XR (Veloxis), Prograf (Astellas), Protopic (Astellas)
Indications: Prophylaxis of organ rejection, atopic dermatitis (topical)
Class: Calcineurin inhibitor, Immunosuppressant, Macrolactam
Half-life: ~8.7 hours
Clinically important, potentially hazardous interactions with: abatacept, afatinib, alefacept, amiodarone, amprenavir, atazanavir, azacitidine, beta blockers, betamethasone, boceprevir, bosentan, cabazitaxel, caspofungin, ceritinib, cinacalcet, cobicistat/elvitegravir/emtricitabine/tenofovir disoproxil, crizotinib, cyclosporine, CYP3A4 inhibitors and inducers, dabigatran, dairy products, danazol, darunavir, dasatinib, delavirdine, denileukin, dexlansoprazole, diclofenac, docetaxel, dronedarone, efavirenz, elbasvir & grazoprevir, eluxadoline, enzalutamide, erythromycin, etoricoxib, fingolimod, gefitinib, grapefruit juice, Hemophilus B vaccine, HMG-CoA reductase inhibitors, ibuprofen, immunosuppressants, indinavir, irbesartan, itraconazole, ketoconazole, leflunomide, lenalidomide, letermovir, lopinavir, lovastatin,

meloxicam, mifepristone, mycophenolate, nelfinavir, nifedipine, olmesartan, omeprazole, oxaliplatin, pazopanib, pemetrexed, posaconazole, potassium, potassium-sparing diuretics, pralatrexate, ribociclib, rifabutin, rifampin, rifapentine, sevelamer, simvastatin, sirolimus, St John's wort, telaprevir, telithromycin, temsirolimus, tinidazole, tipranavir, tofacitinib, triamcinolone, vaccines, voriconazole
Pregnancy category: C
Important contra-indications noted in the prescribing guidelines for: the elderly; nursing mothers; pediatric patients
Warning: MALIGNANCIES AND SERIOUS INFECTIONS

Skin
- Anaphylactoid reactions/Anaphylaxis [3]
- Burning (46%) [13]
- Dermatitis [2]
- Diaphoresis (>3%)
- Ecchymoses (>3%)
- Edema (>10%)
- Erythema (12%) [3]
- Exanthems (4%) [2]
- Flushing [4]
- Folliculitis (10%) [2]
- Graft-versus-host reaction [2]
- Herpes simplex (13%) [4]
- Herpes zoster [2]
- Kaposi's sarcoma [2]
- Kaposi's varicelliform eruption [2]
- Lymphoma [2]
- Neoplasms [2]
- Peripheral edema (26%)
- Photosensitivity (>3%)
- Pigmentation [2]
- Pruritus (25–36%) [12]
- Pustules (6%)
- Rash (24%) [2]
- Rosacea [5]
- Thrombocytopenic purpura [2]
- Toxicity [3]

Hair
- Alopecia (>3%) [6]
- Hypertrichosis [2]

Mucosal
- Gingival hyperplasia/hypertrophy [6]
- Oral candidiasis (>3%)
- Oral pigmentation [2]
- Oral ulceration [2]

Cardiovascular
- Cardiomyopathy [3]
- Hypertension (49%) [9]
- QT prolongation [2]

Central Nervous System
- Encephalopathy [10]
- Fever (>10%) [2]
- Headache [10]
- Insomnia [2]
- Leukoencephalopathy [14]
- Neurotoxicity [12]
- Pain [3]
- Paresthesias (40%) [5]
- Parkinsonism [2]
- Seizures (<10%) [5]
- Tremor (>10%) [11]
- Vertigo (dizziness) [3]

Neuromuscular/Skeletal
- Arthralgia (>10%) [2]
- Asthenia (fatigue) (>10%) [4]
- Back pain (>10%)
- Bone or joint pain [2]
- Myalgia/Myopathy (>3%)

Gastrointestinal/Hepatic
- Abdominal pain [3]
- Constipation (>10%)
- Diarrhea (>10%) [6]
- Dyspepsia (>10%)
- Dysphagia (>3%)
- Hepatotoxicity [11]
- Nausea (>10%) [3]
- Pancreatitis [3]
- Vomiting (>10%)

Respiratory
- Cough (>10%)
- Dyspnea (>10%)
- Pneumonia [2]
- Pulmonary toxicity [2]

Endocrine/Metabolic
- Diabetes mellitus [6]
- Diabetic ketoacidosis [6]
- Gynecomastia [3]
- Hyperglycemia [11]
- Hyperkalemia [4]
- Hyperlipidemia [2]
- Hypomagnesemia (>10%) [2]
- Hypophosphatemia (>10%)
- Serum creatinine increased [4]
- SIADH [2]

Genitourinary
- Urinary tract infection [3]

Renal
- Nephrotoxicity [45]
- Renal failure [2]
- Renal function abnormal [4]

Hematologic
- Anemia (>10%) [2]
- Angiopathy [4]
- Dyslipidemia [3]
- Hemolytic anemia [2]
- Hemolytic uremic syndrome [18]
- Leukopenia (>10%) [5]
- Neutropenia [4]
- Thrombotic microangiopathy [5]

Otic
- Tinnitus [2]

Ocular
- Diplopia [2]
- Ocular burning [3]
- Optic neuropathy [2]
- Vision blurred [2]
- Vision loss [3]

Local
- Application-site burning [7]
- Application-site erythema [3]
- Application-site infection [2]
- Application-site irritation [2]
- Application-site pain [2]
- Application-site pruritus [9]

Other
- Adverse effects [18]
- Cancer [2]
- Infection (>10%) [16]

TADALAFIL

Trade names: Adcirca (Lilly), Cialis (Lilly)
Indications: Erectile dysfunction, pulmonary arterial hypertension
Class: Phosphodiesterase type 5 (PDE5) inhibitor
Half-life: 15–18 hours
Clinically important, potentially hazardous interactions with: alcohol, alfuzosin, alpha blockers, amlodipine, amyl nitrite, angiotensin II receptor blockers, antifungals, antihypertensives, atazanavir, bendroflumethiazide, boceprevir, bosentan, clarithromycin, cobicistat/elvitegravir/emtricitabine/tenofovir alafenamide, cobicistat/elvitegravir/emtricitabine/tenofovir disoproxil, conivaptan, CYP3A4 inhibitors or inducers, darunavir, dasatinib, delavirdine, disopyramide, doxazosin, efavirenz, enalapril, erythromycin, etravirine, fosamprenavir, grapefruit juice, indinavir, itraconazole, ketoconazole, lopinavir, macrolide antibiotics, metoprolol, nelfinavir, nicorandil, nitrates, nitroglycerin, nitroprusside, oxcarbazepine, phosphodiesterase 5 inhibitors, rifampin, rifapentine, riociguat, ritonavir, sapropterin, saquinavir, St John's wort, tamsulosin, telaprevir, telithromycin, voriconazole
Pregnancy category: B (Cialis is not indicated for use in women)
Important contra-indications noted in the prescribing guidelines for: pediatric patients

---

Skin
- Diaphoresis (<2%)
- Facial edema (<2%)
- Flushing (2–3%) [16]
- Peripheral edema [2]
- Pruritus (<2%)
- Rash (<2%)

Mucosal
- Epistaxis (nosebleed) (<2%) [2]
- Nasal congestion [4]
- Rectal hemorrhage (<2%)
- Xerostomia (<2%)

Cardiovascular
- Angina (<2%)
- Chest pain (<2%)
- Hypotension (<2%)
- Myocardial infarction (<2%)
- Palpitation (<2%)
- Postural hypotension (<2%)
- Tachycardia (<2%)

Central Nervous System
- Amnesia [3]
- Headache (4–15%) [38]
- Hyperesthesia (<2%)
- Hypoesthesia (<2%)
- Insomnia (<2%)
- Pain (<3%)
- Paresthesias (<2%)
- Somnolence (drowsiness) (<2%)
- Syncope (<2%)
- Vertigo (dizziness) (<2%) [8]

Neuromuscular/Skeletal
- Arthralgia (<2%)
- Asthenia (fatigue) (<2%)
- Back pain (2–6%) [22]
- Myalgia/Myopathy (<4%) [15]
- Neck pain (<2%)

Gastrointestinal/Hepatic
Diarrhea [2]
Dyspepsia [8]
Dysphagia (<2%)
Esophagitis (<2%)
Gastritis (<2%)
Gastroesophageal reflux (<2%)
Hepatotoxicity [2]
Loose stools (<2%)
Nausea (<2%) [3]
Vomiting (<2%)

Respiratory
Dyspnea (<2%)
Nasopharyngitis [2]
Pharyngitis (<2%)

Endocrine/Metabolic
GGT increased (<2%)

Genitourinary
Erection (<2%)
Priapism (spontaneous) (<2%) [2]

Hematologic
Anemia [2]
Platelets decreased [2]

Otic
Hearing loss (<2%) [4]
Tinnitus (<2%)

Ocular
Chorioretinopathy [2]
Conjunctival hyperemia (<2%)
Conjunctivitis (<2%)
Dyschromatopsia (<2%)
Eyelid edema (<2%)
Eyelid pain (<2%)
Lacrimation (<2%)
Optic neuropathy [7]
Vision blurred (<2%)

Other
Adverse effects [4]

TAFENOQUINE *

Trade name: Krintafel (GSK)
Indications: indicated for the radical cure (prevention of relapse) of *Plasmodium vivax* malaria in patients aged 16 years and older who are receiving appropriate antimalarial therapy for acute *P. vivax* infection
Class: Antimalarial
Half-life: ~15 days
Clinically important, potentially hazardous interactions with: none known
Pregnancy category: N/A (May cause hemolytic anemia in a fetus who is G6PD deficient. Treatment during pregnancy is not recommended)
Important contra-indications noted in the prescribing guidelines for: nursing mothers

---

Skin
Hypersensitivity (<3%)

Central Nervous System
Abnormal dreams (<3%)
Anxiety (<3%)
Headache (5%)
Insomnia (<3%)
Somnolence (drowsiness) (<3%)
Vertigo (dizziness) (8%)

Gastrointestinal/Hepatic
Abdominal pain [2]
Diarrhea [2]
Nausea (6%) [3]
Vomiting (6%)

Endocrine/Metabolic
ALT increased (<3%)
Creatine phosphokinase increased (<3%)

Hematologic
Hemoglobin decreased (5%)
Methemoglobinemia (<3%)

Ocular
Keratopathy (<3%)
Photophobia (<3%)

TAFLUPROST

Trade names: Saflutan (Merck Sharpe & Dohme), Zioptan (Merck Sharpe & Dohme)
Indications: Reduction of elevated intraocular pressure in open angle glaucoma or ocular hypertension
Class: Antiglaucoma, Prostaglandin analog
Half-life: 0.5 hours
Clinically important, potentially hazardous interactions with: none known
Pregnancy category: C
Important contra-indications noted in the prescribing guidelines for: nursing mothers; pediatric patients

---

Central Nervous System
Headache (6%)

Respiratory
Cough (3%)

Genitourinary
Urinary tract infection (2%)

Ocular
Cataract (3%)
Conjunctival hyperemia (4–20%) [7]
Conjunctivitis (5%)
Deepening of upper lid sulcus [4]
Eyelashes – hypertrichosis (2%)
Eyelashes – pigmentation (2%) [2]
Eyelid erythema (<10%)
Eyelid pigmentation [3]
Keratoconjunctivitis (<10%)
Lacrimation (<10%)
Ocular burning [3]
Ocular hyperemia [2]
Ocular itching [6]
Ocular pain (3%)
Ocular pigmentation (<10%)
Ocular pruritus (5%) [2]
Ocular stinging (7%) [4]
Photophobia (<10%)
Vision blurred (2%)
Visual disturbances (<10%)
Xerophthalmia (3%)

Other
Adverse effects [5]

TALIMOGENE LAHERPAREPVEC

Synonym: T-VEC
Trade name: Imlygic (Amgen)
Indications: Unresectable cutaneous, subcutaneous, and nodal lesions in patients with melanoma recurrent after initial surgery
Class: Oncolytic virus immunotherapy
Half-life: N/A
Clinically important, potentially hazardous interactions with: none known
Pregnancy category: N/A (Contraception advised to prevent pregnancy during treatment)
Important contra-indications noted in the prescribing guidelines for: nursing mothers; pediatric patients

---

Skin
Cellulitis (<5%) [3]
Herpes (oral) (<5%)
Vitiligo (<5%)

Mucosal
Oropharyngeal pain (6%)

Central Nervous System
Chills (49%) [5]
Fever (43%) [4]
Headache (19%)
Vertigo (dizziness) (10%)

Neuromuscular/Skeletal
Arthralgia (17%)
Asthenia (fatigue) (50%) [4]
Myalgia/Myopathy (18%)
Pain in extremities (16%)

Gastrointestinal/Hepatic
Abdominal pain (9%)
Constipation (12%)
Diarrhea (19%)
Nausea (36%) [2]
Vomiting (21%)

Respiratory
Flu-like syndrome (31%) [2]

Endocrine/Metabolic
Weight loss (6%)

Renal
Glomerulonephritis (<5%)

Local
Injection-site pain (28%)

TAMOXIFEN

Trade name: Nolvadex (AstraZeneca)
Indications: Advanced breast cancer
Class: Selective estrogen receptor modulator (SERM)
Half-life: 5–7 days
Clinically important, potentially hazardous interactions with: anastrozole, bexarotene, cinacalcet, delavirdine, droperidol, duloxetine, gadobenate, paroxetine hydrochloride, rifapentine, terbinafine, tipranavir

Pregnancy category: D
Important contra-indications noted in the prescribing guidelines for: nursing mothers; pediatric patients

---

Skin
- Carcinosarcoma [2]
- Diaphoresis [4]
- Edema (2–6%) [3]
- Exanthems (3%) [3]
- Flushing (>10%) [9]
- Hot flashes [18]
- Lupus erythematosus [2]
- Pruritus ani et vulvae [2]
- Radiation recall dermatitis [6]
- Rash (<10%) [2]
- Sarcoma [9]
- Toxicity [3]
- Tumors [3]
- Vasculitis [5]
- Xerosis (7%)

Hair
- Alopecia [7]
- Hirsutism [2]

Mucosal
- Stomatitis [2]
- Xerostomia (7%) [2]

Cardiovascular
- Myocardial ischemia [2]
- QT prolongation [3]
- Thromboembolism [6]
- Thrombophlebitis [3]
- Venous thromboembolism [6]

Central Nervous System
- Depression [5]
- Headache [3]
- Insomnia [4]
- Mood changes [3]
- Parkinsonism [2]
- Stroke [4]
- Vertigo (dizziness) [3]

Neuromuscular/Skeletal
- Asthenia (fatigue) [5]
- Bone or joint pain [3]
- Fractures [2]
- Leg cramps [2]
- Myalgia/Myopathy [4]

Gastrointestinal/Hepatic
- Hepatic steatosis [2]
- Hepatotoxicity [10]
- Nausea [4]
- Pancreatitis [4]
- Vomiting [3]

Respiratory
- Pulmonary embolism [7]

Endocrine/Metabolic
- ALP increased [2]
- Amenorrhea [8]
- Galactorrhea (<10%)
- Hypercholesterolemia [2]
- Hypertriglyceridemia [7]
- Libido decreased [4]
- Weight gain [4]

Genitourinary
- Dyspareunia [4]
- Endometrial cancer [5]
- Ovarian hyperstimulation syndrome [2]
- Sexual dysfunction [2]
- Vaginal bleeding [4]
- Vaginal discharge [5]
- Vaginal dryness [5]

Hematologic
- Hemolytic uremic syndrome [2]
- Thrombosis [9]

Ocular
- Cataract [9]
- Keratopathy [4]
- Macular edema [2]
- Maculopathy [5]
- Ocular adverse effects [6]
- Ocular toxicity [5]
- Retinopathy [5]
- Vision impaired [3]

TAMSULOSIN

Trade names: Flomax (Boehringer Ingelheim), Jalyn (GSK)
Indications: Benign prostatic hypertrophy
Class: Adrenergic alpha-receptor antagonist
Half-life: 9–13 hours
Clinically important, potentially hazardous interactions with: alpha adrenergic blockers, cimetidine, conivaptan, darunavir, delavirdine, erythromycin, indinavir, ketoconazole, paroxetine hydrochloride, phosphodiesterase 5 inhibitors, tadalafil, telithromycin, terbinafine, vardenafil, voriconazole, warfarin
Pregnancy category: B (not indicated for use in women; Jalyn is pregnancy category X)
Important contra-indications noted in the prescribing guidelines for: nursing mothers; pediatric patients
Note: Jalyn is tamsulosin and dutasteride.

Mucosal
- Xerostomia [5]

Cardiovascular
- Chest pain (4%)
- Hypotension (6–19%) [3]
- Orthostatic hypotension [3]
- Postural hypotension [3]

Central Nervous System
- Headache (19–21%) [9]
- Insomnia (<2%)
- Somnolence (drowsiness) (3–4%)
- Vertigo (dizziness) (15–17%) [19]

Neuromuscular/Skeletal
- Asthenia (fatigue) (8–9%) [3]
- Back pain (7–8%) [2]

Gastrointestinal/Hepatic
- Constipation [3]
- Diarrhea (4–6%)
- Dyspepsia [2]
- Nausea (3–4%)

Respiratory
- Cough (3–5%)
- Pharyngitis (5–6%)
- Rhinitis (13–18%) [2]
- Sinusitis (2–4%)

Endocrine/Metabolic
- Libido decreased (<2%)

Genitourinary
- Ejaculatory dysfunction (8–18%) [9]
- Erectile dysfunction [2]
- Priapism [4]
- Urinary incontinence [2]
- Urinary retention [3]

Ocular
- Floppy iris syndrome [34]
- Vision blurred (<2%)

Other
- Adverse effects [3]
- Infection (9–11%)
- Tooth disorder (<2%)

TAPENTADOL

Trade names: Nucynta (Janssen), Nucynta ER (Janssen), Palexia (Grunenthal)
Indications: Immediate release formulation: moderate to severe acute pain, extended release formulation: moderate to severe chronic pain and neuropathic pain associated with diabetic peripheral neuropathy when a continuous analgesic is needed for an extended period of time
Class: Analgesic, opioid
Half-life: 5 hours
Clinically important, potentially hazardous interactions with: alcohol, alvimopan, amphetamines, anesthetics, anitemetics, anticholinergics, buprenorphine, butorphanol, CNS depressants, desmopressin, droperidol, hypnotics, linezolid, MAO inhibitors, mirtazapine, nalbuphine, PEG-interferon, pegvisomant, pentazocine, phenothiazines, sedatives, sibutramine, SNRIs, SSRIs, St John's wort, succinylcholine, thiazide diuretics, tramadol, tranquilizers, trazodone, tricyclic antidepressants, triptans
Pregnancy category: C
Important contra-indications noted in the prescribing guidelines for: the elderly; nursing mothers; pediatric patients
Note: Contra-indicated in patients with impaired pulmonary function or paralytic ileus. Should not be used in patients currently using or within 14 days of using a monoamine oxidase inhibitor.
Warning: For extended release oral tablets: ABUSE POTENTIAL, LIFE-THREATENING RESPIRATORY DEPRESSION, ACCIDENTAL EXPOSURE, and INTERACTION WITH ALCOHOL

Mucosal
- Xerostomia [4]

Central Nervous System
- Headache [4]
- Neurotoxicity [2]
- Somnolence (drowsiness) [8]
- Vertigo (dizziness) (4%) [9]

Neuromuscular/Skeletal
- Asthenia (fatigue) [3]

Gastrointestinal/Hepatic
- Constipation [15]
- Diarrhea [2]
- Gastrointestinal disorder [2]
- Nausea (4%) [21]

Vomiting (3%) [14]

Other

Adverse effects [5]

TARTRAZINE

Class: Food additive
Half-life: N/A
Clinically important, potentially hazardous interactions with: none known
Note: Tartrazine intolerance has been estimated to affect between 0.01% and 0.1% of the population. Adverse reactions are most common in people who are sensitive to aspirin.
Banned in Austria and Norway.

Skin

Anaphylactoid reactions/Anaphylaxis [8]
Angioedema [11]
Atopic dermatitis [2]
Hypersensitivity [9]
Pruritus [2]
Purpura [5]
Urticaria (often related to aspirin intolerance) [33]
Vasculitis [3]

Other

Adverse effects [3]
Allergic reactions [9]

TASIMELTEON

Trade name: Hetlioz (Vanda)
Indications: Non-24-hour sleep-wake disorder
Class: Melatonin receptor agonist
Half-life: 2–3 hours
Clinically important, potentially hazardous interactions with: fluvoxamine, ketoconazole, rifampin
Pregnancy category: C
Important contra-indications noted in the prescribing guidelines for: the elderly; nursing mothers; pediatric patients

Central Nervous System

Abnormal dreams (10%) [3]
Headache (17%) [3]
Nightmares (10%) [3]

Respiratory

Upper respiratory tract infection (7%) [2]

Endocrine/Metabolic

ALT increased (10%) [2]

Genitourinary

Urinary tract infection (7%) [3]

TAVABOROLE

Indications: Onychomycosis
Class: Antifungal, oxaborole
Half-life: N/A
Clinically important, potentially hazardous interactions with: none known
Pregnancy category: C
Important contra-indications noted in the prescribing guidelines for: nursing mothers; pediatric patients

Nails

Onychocryptosis (3%)

Local

Application-site erythema (2%) [2]
Application-site exfoliation (3%)

TAZAROTENE

Trade names: Avage (Allergan), Fabior (GSK), Tazorac (Allergan), Zorac (Allergan)
Indications: Acne vulgaris, mild to moderate plaque psoriasis involving up to 10% body surface area
Half-life: 18 hours
Clinically important, potentially hazardous interactions with: none known
Pregnancy category: X
Important contra-indications noted in the prescribing guidelines for: the elderly; nursing mothers; pediatric patients

Skin

Burning (10–20%) [5]
Contact dermatitis (5–10%)
Desquamation (5–10%)
Erythema (10–20%) [5]
Pruritus (10–25%) [11]
Psoriasis (5–10%)
Rash (5–10%)
Scaling [2]
Stinging (<3%) [2]
Xerosis (<3%) [5]

Local

Application-site reactions [2]

Other

Adverse effects [2]
Side effects [2]

TEA TREE

Family: Myrtaceae
Scientific names: *Melaleuca alternifolia, Melaleuca cajeputi, Melaleuca dissitifolia, Melaleuca linafolia*
Indications: Gram-negative and Gram-positive bacteria, acne, vaginal infection, burns, onychomycosis, tinea pedis, bruises, insect bites, skin infections, mouthwash, genital herpes, antiperspirant, gingivitis, disinfectant, scabies
Class: Antiseptic
Half-life: N/A
Clinically important, potentially hazardous interactions with: colophony, turpentine
Pregnancy category: N/A
Note: Tea tree oil in bottles may undergo photooxidation, and degradation products are moderate to strong sensitizers.
The plant was discovered and named by Captain James Cook of the Royal Navy in 1770, who found groves of trees with sticky, aromatic leaves that, when boiled, made a spicy tea.

Skin

Burning [2]
Dermatitis [22]
Hypersensitivity [3]
Pruritus [2]

Endocrine/Metabolic

Gynecomastia [3]

Other

Adverse effects [4]
Allergic reactions [8]

TECOVIRIMAT *

Trade name: Tpoxx (Siga Technologies Inc)
Indications: treatment of human smallpox disease in adults and pediatric patients weighing at least 13 kg
Class: Orthopoxvirus VP37 envelope wrapping protein inhibitor
Half-life: 20 hours
Clinically important, potentially hazardous interactions with: none known
Pregnancy category: N/A (no human data to establish the presence or absence of associated risk)

Mucosal

Oropharyngeal pain (<2%)

Cardiovascular

Tachycardia (<2%)

Central Nervous System

Dysgeusia (taste perversion) (<2%)
Headache (12%)
Irritability (<2%)
Migraine (<2%)
Pain (<2%)
Panic attack (<2%)
Paresthesias (<2%)

Neuromuscular/Skeletal

Arthralgia (<2%)

Gastrointestinal/Hepatic

Abdominal pain (2%)
Dyspepsia (<2%)
Eructation (belching) (<2%)
Nausea (5%)
Vomiting (2%)

Hematologic

Hemoglobin decreased (<2%)

Other

Dipsia (thirst) (<2%)

TEDIZOLID

Trade name: Sivextro (Cubist)
Indications: Acute bacterial skin and skin structure infections caused by susceptible bacteria
Class: Antibiotic, oxazolidinone
Half-life: 12 hours
Clinically important, potentially hazardous interactions with: none known
Pregnancy category: C
Important contra-indications noted in the prescribing guidelines for: nursing mothers; pediatric patients

Skin
- Dermatitis (<2%)
- Flushing (<2%)
- Hypersensitivity (<2%)
- Pruritus (<2%) [2]
- Urticaria (<2%)

Cardiovascular
- Hypertension (<2%)
- Palpitation (<2%)
- Tachycardia (<2%)

Central Nervous System
- Headache (6%) [5]
- Hypoesthesia (<2%)
- Insomnia (<2%) [2]
- Vertigo (dizziness) (2%) [4]

Neuromuscular/Skeletal
- Asthenia (fatigue) [2]

Gastrointestinal/Hepatic
- Constipation [2]
- Diarrhea (4%) [6]
- Nausea (8%) [7]
- Vomiting (3%) [5]

Hematologic
- Anemia (<2%)

Ocular
- Asthenopia (<2%)
- Vision blurred (<2%)
- Vision impaired (<2%)
- Vitreous floaters (<2%)

Local
- Infusion-related reactions (<2%)

Other
- Adverse effects [3]
- Infection (<2%)

TEDUGLUTIDE

Trade name: Gattex (Hospira)
Indications: Treatment of short bowel syndrome in adult patients dependent on parenteral support
Class: Glucagon-like peptide-2 (GLP-2) analog
Half-life: 1–2 hours
Clinically important, potentially hazardous interactions with: none known
Pregnancy category: B
Important contra-indications noted in the prescribing guidelines for: nursing mothers; pediatric patients

---

Skin
- Edema [4]
- Hypersensitivity (<10%)

Cardiovascular
- Congestive heart failure [2]

Central Nervous System
- Headache (16%) [6]
- Sleep disturbances (<10%)

Gastrointestinal/Hepatic
- Abdominal distension (14%) [5]
- Abdominal pain (30%) [8]
- Constipation [3]
- Flatulence (<10%)
- Gastric obstruction [2]
- Gastrointestinal disorder [2]
- Hepatotoxicity [3]
- Nausea (18%) [7]
- Vomiting (<10%) [2]

Respiratory
- Cough (<10%)
- Nasopharyngitis [2]
- Upper respiratory tract infection (12%)

Local
- Injection-site erythema [2]
- Injection-site reactions (22%)

Other
- Adverse effects [10]

TEGAFUR/GIMERACIL/OTERACIL

Synonyms: TS-1; S-1
Trade name: Teysuno (Taiho Pharma)
Indications: Gastric, colorectal, head and neck cancers, non-small cell lung cancer, inoperable or recurrent breast cancer, pancreatic cancer
Class: Antineoplastic
Half-life: N/A
Clinically important, potentially hazardous interactions with: capecitabine, flucytosine, fluorouracil, other fluoropyrimidine-group antineoplastics, phenytoin, uracil/tegafur, warfarin
Pregnancy category: N/A (Contra-indicated in pregnancy)
Important contra-indications noted in the prescribing guidelines for: the elderly; nursing mothers; pediatric patients
Note: Contra-indicated in patients with severe bone marrow depression, hepatic or renal impairment.
Not available in the USA.

Skin
- Dermatitis (<5%)
- Desquamation (<5%)
- Edema (<5%) [3]
- Erythema (<5%)
- Flushing (<5%)
- Hand–foot syndrome (<5%) [12]
- Herpes simplex (<5%)
- Jaundice (<5%)
- Pigmentation (21%) [9]
- Pruritus (<5%)
- Rash (12%) [6]
- Raynaud's phenomenon (<5%)
- Stevens-Johnson syndrome [2]
- Ulcerations (<5%)
- Xerosis (<5%) [2]

Hair
- Alopecia (<5%) [4]

Nails
- Nail disorder (<5%)
- Paronychia (<5%) [2]

Mucosal
- Mucositis [7]
- Stomatitis (17%) [10]

Cardiovascular
- Hypertension (<5%)
- Hypotension (<5%)

Central Nervous System
- Anorexia (34%) [26]
- Fever (<5%) [2]
- Headache (<5%)
- Neurotoxicity [4]
- Paresthesias (<5%)
- Peripheral neuropathy [3]
- Vertigo (dizziness) (<5%)
- Warm feeling (<5%)

Neuromuscular/Skeletal
- Arthralgia (<5%)
- Asthenia (fatigue) (22%) [16]
- Myalgia/Myopathy (<5%)

Gastrointestinal/Hepatic
- Diarrhea (19%) [40]
- Hepatotoxicity [6]
- Nausea (23%) [20]
- Vomiting (8%) [13]

Respiratory
- Pharyngitis (<5%)
- Pneumonitis [4]
- Rhinitis (<5%)

Endocrine/Metabolic
- ALT increased (12%) [6]
- Appetite decreased [6]
- AST increased (12%) [4]
- Hyperbilirubinemia [4]
- Hyponatremia [4]
- Weight loss (<5%)

Genitourinary
- Glycosuria (<5%)
- Hematuria (<5%)

Renal
- Nephrotoxicity [2]
- Proteinuria (<5%)

Hematologic
- Anemia [27]
- Bleeding (<5%)
- Bone marrow suppression [2]
- Febrile neutropenia [13]
- Hemotoxicity [5]
- Leukocytopenia [2]
- Leukopenia (87%) [25]
- Myelosuppression [6]
- Neutropenia (44%) [52]
- Thrombocytopenia (11%) [20]

Ocular
- Conjunctivitis (<5%)
- Keratitis (<5%)
- Lacrimation (<5%) [3]
- Ocular adverse effects [2]
- Ocular pain (<5%)
- Reduced visual acuity (<5%)

Other
- Adverse effects [21]
- Death [3]

TEICOPLANIN

Trade name: Targocid (Sanofi-Aventis)
Indications: Staphylococcal infections
Class: Antibiotic, glycopeptide
Half-life: 150 hours
Clinically important, potentially hazardous interactions with: amikacin, cephaloridine, colistin, gentamicin, kanamycin, neomycin, streptomycin, tobramycin, vancomycin

Pregnancy category: N/A (Not recommended in pregnancy)
Important contra-indications noted in the prescribing guidelines for: nursing mothers

Skin
DRESS syndrome [3]
Erythema (<10%)
Exanthems [2]
Hypersensitivity [3]
Pruritus (<10%)
Rash (<10%) [4]
Red man syndrome [3]
Urticaria [2]

Central Nervous System
Fever (<10%)

Gastrointestinal/Hepatic
Hepatotoxicity (2%) [2]

Renal
Nephrotoxicity [2]

Hematologic
Neutropenia [2]

Otic
Ototoxicity [2]

Other
Adverse effects [2]

TELAPREVIR

Trade name: Incivek (Vertex)
Indications: Hepatitis C (must only be used in combination with PEG-interferon alfa and ribavirin)
Class: CYP3A4 inhibitor, Direct-acting antiviral, Hepatitis C virus NS3/4A protease inhibitor
Half-life: 4–11 hours
Clinically important, potentially hazardous interactions with: alfuzosin, alprazolam, amiodarone, amlodipine, atazanavir, atorvastatin, bepridil, bosentan, budesonide, carbamazepine, cisapride, dabigatran, darunavir, desipramine, dexamethasone, digoxin, dihydroergotamine, diltiazem, efavirenz, ergotamine, escitalopram, estradiol, felodipine, flecainide, flibanserin, fluticasone propionate, fosamprenavir, itraconazole, ketoconazole, lidocaine, lomitapide, lovastatin, methylergonovine, methylprednisolone, midazolam, mifepristone, nicardipine, nisoldipine, olaparib, palbociclib, phenobarbital, phenytoin, pimozide, ponatinib, posaconazole, propafenone, quinidine, rifampin, ritonavir, ruxolitinib, salmeterol, sildenafil, simvastatin, sirolimus, St John's wort, tacrolimus, tadalafil, telithromycin, tenofovir disoproxil, trazodone, triazolam, vardenafil, venetoclax, verapamil, vorapaxar, voriconazole, warfarin, zolpidem
Pregnancy category: X
Important contra-indications noted in the prescribing guidelines for: the elderly; nursing mothers; pediatric patients
Note: Must be used in combination with PEG-interferon alfa and ribavirin (see separate entries).
Warning: SERIOUS SKIN REACTIONS

Skin
Dermatitis [2]
DRESS syndrome [6]
Exanthems [6]
Pruritus (including anal pruritus) (53%) [14]
Rash (56%) [38]
Stevens-Johnson syndrome [3]
Toxic epidermal necrolysis [2]
Toxicity [2]

Central Nervous System
Dysgeusia (taste perversion) (10%)

Neuromuscular/Skeletal
Asthenia (fatigue) (56%) [4]

Gastrointestinal/Hepatic
Anorectal discomfort (11%)
Diarrhea (26%) [2]
Hemorrhoids (12%)
Hepatotoxicity [5]
Nausea (39%) [4]
Vomiting (13%)

Renal
Nephrotoxicity [3]

Hematologic
Anemia [36]
Neutropenia [6]
Thrombocytopenia [6]

Other
Adverse effects [19]
Infection [4]

TELBIVUDINE

Trade names: Sebvio (Novartis), Tyzeka (Novartis)
Indications: Hepatitis B (chronic)
Class: Nucleoside analog reverse transcriptase inhibitor
Half-life: ~15 hours
Clinically important, potentially hazardous interactions with: interferon alfa, PEG-interferon
Pregnancy category: B
Important contra-indications noted in the prescribing guidelines for: the elderly; nursing mothers; pediatric patients

Skin
Pruritus (2%)
Rash (4%)

Cardiovascular
Arrhythmias [2]

Central Nervous System
Fever (4%)
Headache (11%)
Insomnia (3%)
Neurotoxicity [2]
Peripheral neuropathy [2]
Vertigo (dizziness) (4%)

Neuromuscular/Skeletal
Arthralgia (4%)
Asthenia (fatigue) (>5%) [2]
Back pain (4%)
Myalgia/Myopathy (3%) [8]

Gastrointestinal/Hepatic
Abdominal distension (3%)
Abdominal pain (12%)
Diarrhea [2]
Dyspepsia (3%)
Hepatitis (exacerbation) (2%)

Respiratory
Cough (7%)
Flu-like syndrome (7%)
Pharyngolaryngeal pain (5%)
Upper respiratory tract infection (>5%)

Endocrine/Metabolic
Acidosis [2]
ALT increased (3%)
Creatine phosphokinase increased [5]

Hematologic
Neutropenia (2%)

TELMISARTAN

Trade name: Micardis (Boehringer Ingelheim)
Indications: Hypertension
Class: Angiotensin II receptor antagonist (blocker), Antihypertensive
Half-life: 24 hours
Clinically important, potentially hazardous interactions with: ramipril
Pregnancy category: D (category C in first trimester; category D in second and third trimesters)
Important contra-indications noted in the prescribing guidelines for: nursing mothers; pediatric patients
Warning: FETAL TOXICITY

Skin
Angioedema [2]
Peripheral edema [2]

Cardiovascular
Hypotension [2]

Central Nervous System
Headache [4]
Vertigo (dizziness) [5]

Neuromuscular/Skeletal
Asthenia (fatigue) [4]

Gastrointestinal/Hepatic
Enteropathy [2]

Respiratory
Cough [9]

Endocrine/Metabolic
Hyperkalemia [2]

TEMAZEPAM

Trade name: Restoril (Mallinckrodt)
Indications: Insomnia, anxiety
Class: Benzodiazepine
Half-life: 8–15 hours
Clinically important, potentially hazardous interactions with: amprenavir, chlorpheniramine, clarithromycin, efavirenz, esomeprazole, imatinib, mianserin, nelfinavir
Pregnancy category: X
Important contra-indications noted in the prescribing guidelines for: the elderly; nursing mothers; pediatric patients

Skin
Dermatitis (<10%)

Diaphoresis (>10%)
Rash (>10%)

Mucosal
Sialopenia (>10%)
Sialorrhea (<10%)
Xerostomia (2%)

Other
Adverse effects [2]

TEMOZOLOMIDE

Trade name: Temodar (MSD)
Indications: Anaplastic astrocytoma, newly diagnosed glioblastoma multiforme concomitantly with radiotherapy and then as maintenance treatment
Class: Alkylating agent, Antineoplastic
Half-life: 1.8 hours
Clinically important, potentially hazardous interactions with: clozapine, digoxin, valproic acid
Pregnancy category: D
Important contra-indications noted in the prescribing guidelines for: the elderly; nursing mothers; pediatric patients

---

Skin
Peripheral edema (11%)
Pruritus (8%)
Rash (8%) [7]
Toxicity [3]

Hair
Alopecia [3]

Cardiovascular
Thromboembolism [2]
Venous thromboembolism [2]

Central Nervous System
Anorexia [3]
Cerebral hemorrhage [2]
Fever [2]
Headache [3]
Paresthesias (9%)

Neuromuscular/Skeletal
Asthenia (fatigue) [14]
Myalgia/Myopathy (5%)

Gastrointestinal/Hepatic
Constipation [2]
Diarrhea [7]
Gastrointestinal perforation [2]
Hepatotoxicity [6]
Nausea [10]
Vomiting [4]

Endocrine/Metabolic
Mastodynia (6%)

Hematologic
Anemia [3]
Febrile neutropenia [2]
Hemotoxicity [6]
Leukopenia [6]
Lymphopenia [7]
Myelosuppression [3]
Neutropenia [11]
Thrombocytopenia [12]

Other
Death [7]
Infection [5]

TEMSIROLIMUS

Trade name: Torisel (Wyeth)
Indications: Renal cell carcinoma, other cancers
Class: Analog of sirolimus, Antineoplastic, mTOR inhibitor
Half-life: 17 hours
Clinically important, potentially hazardous interactions with: ACE inhibitors, atazanavir, BCG vaccine, benazepril, captopril, carbamazepine, clarithromycin, clozapine, conivaptan, cyclosporine, darunavir, dasatinib, denosumab, dexamethasone, digoxin, enalapril, fluconazole, fosinopril, grapefruit juice, hypoglycemic agents, indinavir, itraconazole, ketoconazole, leflunomide, lisinopril, live and inactive vaccines, macolide antibiotics, natalizumab, nefazodone, nelfinavir, P-glycoprotein inhibitors, phenobarbital, phenytoin, pimecrolimus, posaconazole, protease inhibitors, quinapril, ramipril, rifabutin, rifampin, rifapentine, ritonavir, saquinavir, St John's wort, sunitinib, tacrolimus, telithromycin, tipranavir, trastuzumab, voriconazole
Pregnancy category: D
Important contra-indications noted in the prescribing guidelines for: the elderly; nursing mothers; pediatric patients
Note: Contra-indicated in patients with bilirubin >1.5xULN.

Skin
Acneform eruption (10%) [4]
Edema [2]
Exanthems [3]
Hypersensitivity (9%) [3]
Pruritus (19%) [3]
Rash (47%) [14]
Toxicity [4]
Xerosis (11%)

Nails
Nail disorder (14%)
Paronychia [2]

Mucosal
Mucositis (30%) [12]
Oral mucositis [2]
Stomatitis [17]

Cardiovascular
Chest pain (16%)
Hypertension (7%) [3]

Central Nervous System
Anorexia (30%) [3]
Chills (8%)
Depression (4%)
Dysgeusia (taste perversion) (20%) [2]
Fever (24%)
Headache (15%)
Insomnia (12%) [2]
Neurotoxicity [2]
Pain (28%)

Neuromuscular/Skeletal
Arthralgia (18%)
Asthenia (fatigue) (30%) [21]
Back pain (20%)
Myalgia/Myopathy (8%)

Gastrointestinal/Hepatic
Abdominal pain (21%)
Diarrhea [7]
Nausea [7]
Vomiting [2]

Respiratory
Cough (26%) [3]
Dyspnea [7]
Pharyngitis (12%)
Pneumonia [2]
Pneumonitis (36%) [11]
Rhinitis (10%)
Upper respiratory tract infection (7%)

Endocrine/Metabolic
ALT increased [4]
AST increased [2]
Dehydration [2]
Hypercholesterolemia [4]
Hyperglycemia [14]
Hyperlipidemia [2]
Hypertriglyceridemia [5]
Hypokalemia [3]
Hypophosphatemia [4]
Serum creatinine increased [2]

Genitourinary
Urinary tract infection (15%)

Hematologic
Anemia [10]
Febrile neutropenia [3]
Hemorrhage [2]
Hemotoxicity [3]
Immunosupression [2]
Leukopenia [4]
Lymphopenia [4]
Neutropenia [5]
Thrombocytopenia [16]

Ocular
Conjunctivitis (7%)

Other
Adverse effects [10]
Death [2]
Infection (20%) [5]

TENOFOVIR ALAFENAMIDE

Trade names: Descovy (Gilead), Vemlidy (Gilead)
Indications: Hepatitis B
Class: Antiviral, Hepatitis B virus necleoside analog reverse transcriptase inhibitor
Half-life: <1 hour
Clinically important, potentially hazardous interactions with: carbamazepine, oxcarbazepine, phenobarbital, phenytoin, rifabutin, rifampin, rifapentine, St John's wort
Pregnancy category: N/A (No available data to inform drug-associated risk)
Important contra-indications noted in the prescribing guidelines for: nursing mothers; pediatric patients
Note: Descovy is tenofovir alafenamide and emtricitabine. See also separate profile for tenofovir alafenamide in combination with cobicistat, elvitegravir and emtricitabine.
Warning: LACTIC ACIDOSIS/SEVERE HEPATOMEGALY WITH STEATOSIS and POST TREATMENT SEVERE ACUTE EXACERBATION OF HEPATITIS B

Central Nervous System
Headache (9%) [5]

Neuromuscular/Skeletal
Asthenia (fatigue) (6%)
Back pain (5%)

Gastrointestinal/Hepatic
Abdominal pain (7%)
Nausea (5%)

Respiratory
Cough (6%)
Nasopharyngitis [4]
Upper respiratory tract infection [4]

Endocrine/Metabolic
ALT increased (8%) [2]
AST increased (3%)
Creatine phosphokinase increased (3%)
Hyperamylasemia (3%)
Hypercholesterolemia (4%)

Genitourinary
Glycosuria (5%)

Other
Adverse effects [2]

TENOFOVIR DISOPROXIL

Trade names: Atripla (Gilead), Complera (Gilead), Truvada (Gilead), Viread (Gilead)
Indications: HIV infection in combination with at least two other antiretroviral agents
Class: Antiretroviral, Nucleoside analog reverse transcriptase inhibitor
Half-life: 12–18 hours
Clinically important, potentially hazardous interactions with: acyclovir, adefovir, atazanavir, cidofovir, cobicistat/elvitegravir/emtricitabine/tenofovir disoproxil, darunavir, didanosine, ganciclovir, high-fat foods, indinavir, ledipasvir & sofosbuvir, lopinavir, protease inhibitors, ritonavir, telaprevir, tipranavir, trospium, valacyclovir, valganciclovir
Pregnancy category: B
Important contra-indications noted in the prescribing guidelines for: nursing mothers; pediatric patients
Note: Atripla is tenofovir disoproxil, efavirenz and emtricitabine; Complera is tenofovir disoproxil, emtricitabine and rilpivirine; Truvada is tenofovir disoproxil and emtricitabine. See also separate profile for tenofovir disoproxil in combination with cobicistat, elvitegravir and emtricitabine.
Warning: LACTIC ACIDOSIS/SEVERE HEPATOMEGALY WITH STEATOSIS and POST TREATMENT EXACERBATION OF HEPATITIS

Skin
Diaphoresis (3%)
Lichenoid eruption [2]
Rash (5–18%) [4]
Stevens-Johnson syndrome [2]

Cardiovascular
Chest pain (3%)

Central Nervous System
Abnormal dreams [3]
Anorexia (3%)
Anxiety (6%) [2]
Depression (4–11%)
Fever (2–8%)
Headache (5–14%) [10]
Insomnia (3–5%) [2]
Neurotoxicity (3%) [6]
Pain (7–13%)
Peripheral neuropathy (<3%)
Somnolence (drowsiness) [2]
Vertigo (dizziness) (<3%) [4]

Neuromuscular/Skeletal
Arthralgia (5%)
Asthenia (fatigue) (6–7%) [6]
Back pain (3–9%)
Bone or joint pain [4]
Fractures [2]
Myalgia/Myopathy (3%) [2]
Osteomalacia [5]

Gastrointestinal/Hepatic
Abdominal pain (4–7%) [2]
Diarrhea (11%) [7]
Dyspepsia (3–4%)
Flatulence (3%)
Hepatic failure [2]
Hepatotoxicity [3]
Nausea (8%) [10]
Pancreatitis [5]
Vomiting (4–5%) [5]

Respiratory
Nasopharyngitis [3]
Pneumonia (2–5%)
Upper respiratory tract infection [2]

Endocrine/Metabolic
Acidosis [3]
ALT increased [3]
Creatine phosphokinase increased [3]
Hypokalemia [2]
Hypophosphatemia [3]
Weight loss (2%)

Renal
Fanconi syndrome [26]
Nephrotoxicity [42]
Proteinuria [4]
Renal failure [10]
Renal tubular necrosis [2]

Other
Adverse effects [11]

TERAZOSIN

Trade name: Hytrin (AbbVie)
Indications: Hypertension, benign prostatic hypertrophy
Class: Adrenergic alpha-receptor antagonist
Half-life: 12 hours
Clinically important, potentially hazardous interactions with: vardenafil
Pregnancy category: C

Skin
Edema (<10%)
Lichenoid eruption [2]
Peripheral edema (6%)

Mucosal
Xerostomia (<10%)

Cardiovascular
Postural hypotension [2]

Central Nervous System
Paresthesias (3%)
Vertigo (dizziness) [3]

Genitourinary
Priapism [2]

Ocular
Floppy iris syndrome [2]

TERBINAFINE

Trade name: Lamisil (Novartis)
Indications: Fungal infections of the skin and nails
Class: Antifungal
Half-life: ~36 hours
Clinically important, potentially hazardous interactions with: amitriptyline, amphotericin B, atomoxetine, caffeine, carbamazepine, cimetidine, codeine, conivaptan, cyclosporine, CYP2D6 substrates, desipramine, estrogens, fesoterodine, fluconazole, nebivolol, progestogens, rifampin, rifapentine, saxagliptin, tamoxifen, tamsulosin, tetrabenazine, thioridazine, tramadol, tricyclic antidepressants
Pregnancy category: B
Important contra-indications noted in the prescribing guidelines for: nursing mothers; pediatric patients

---

Skin
AGEP [24]
Baboon syndrome (SDRIFE) [2]
Dermatitis (<10%)
Eczema [2]
Erythema multiforme [9]
Erythroderma [2]
Exanthems [5]
Fixed eruption [3]
Hypersensitivity [3]
Lichenoid eruption [2]
Lupus erythematosus [30]
Pityriasis rosea [2]
Pruritus (3%) [6]
Psoriasis [15]
Pustules [3]
Rash (6%) [3]
Stevens-Johnson syndrome [2]
Toxic epidermal necrolysis [3]
Urticaria [7]

Hair
Alopecia (<10%)

Nails
Onychocryptosis [2]

Central Nervous System
Ageusia (taste loss) [17]
Dysgeusia (taste perversion) (3%) [8]
Headache (13%)

Gastrointestinal/Hepatic
Abdominal pain (2%)
Diarrhea (6%)
Dyspepsia (4%)
Flatulence (2%)
Hepatotoxicity [11]
Nausea (3%)

Other
Adverse effects [3]
Allergic reactions (<10%)
Side effects (3%)

TERBUTALINE

Trade names: Brethine (aaiPharma), Bricanyl (AstraZeneca)
Indications: Bronchospasm
Class: Beta-2 adrenergic agonist, Bronchodilator, Tocolytic
Half-life: 11–16 hours
Clinically important, potentially hazardous interactions with: alpha blockers, atomoxetine, beta blockers, betahistine, cannabinoids, epinephrine, insulin aspart, insulin degludec, insulin detemir, insulin glargine, insulin glulisine, iobenguane, loop diuretics, MAO inhibitors, propranolol, sotalol, sympathomimetics, tricyclic antidepressants, yohimbine
Pregnancy category: C
Important contra-indications noted in the prescribing guidelines for: nursing mothers; pediatric patients
Warning: PROLONGED TOCOLYSIS

Skin
Diaphoresis (<10%)

Mucosal
Xerostomia (<10%)

Cardiovascular
Arrhythmias [2]

Central Nervous System
Dysgeusia (taste perversion) (<10%)
Tremor [2]

Gastrointestinal/Hepatic
Nausea [2]

Other
Side effects [2]

TERIFLUNOMIDE

Trade name: Aubagio (Sanofi-Aventis)
Indications: Relapsing forms of multiple sclerosis
Class: Pyrimidine synthesis inhibitor
Half-life: N/A
Clinically important, potentially hazardous interactions with: alosetron, caffeine, duloxetine, ethinylestradiol, leflunomide, live vaccines, oral contraceptives, paclitaxel, pioglitazone, repaglinide, rosiglitazone, theophylline, tizanidine, warfarin
Pregnancy category: X
Important contra-indications noted in the prescribing guidelines for: the elderly; nursing mothers; pediatric patients
Warning: HEPATOTOXICITY and RISK OF TERATOGENICITY

Skin
Acneform eruption (<3%)
Burning (2–3%)
Herpes (oral) (2–4%)
Pruritus (3–4%)

Hair
Alopecia (10–13%) [15]

Cardiovascular
Hypertension (4%) [3]
Palpitation (2–3%)

Central Nervous System
Anxiety (3–4%)
Carpal tunnel syndrome (<3%)
Headache (19–22%) [4]
Paresthesias (9–10%) [3]
Peripheral neuropathy (<2%) [2]

Neuromuscular/Skeletal
Asthenia (fatigue) [2]
Back pain (<3%) [2]
Bone or joint pain (4–5%)
Myalgia/Myopathy (3–4%)

Gastrointestinal/Hepatic
Abdominal distension (<2%)
Abdominal pain (5–6%)
Diarrhea (15–18%) [11]
Gastroenteritis (2–4%)
Hepatotoxicity [4]
Nausea (9–14%) [9]

Respiratory
Bronchitis (5–8%)
Influenza (9–12%) [2]
Nasopharyngitis [2]
Sinusitis (4–6%)
Upper respiratory tract infection (9%)

Endocrine/Metabolic
ALT increased (12–14%) [11]
AST increased (2–3%)
GGT increased (3–5%)
Hypophosphatemia (mild) (18%)
Weight loss (2–3%)

Genitourinary
Cystitis (2–4%)

Renal
Renal failure [2]

Hematologic
Immunosupression (10–15%)
Leukopenia (<2%) [2]
Lymphopenia [3]
Neutropenia (2–4%) [4]

Ocular
Conjunctivitis (<3%)
Vision blurred (3%)

Other
Adverse effects [4]
Allergic reactions (2–3%)
Infection [5]
Side effects [2]
Toothache (4%)

TERIPARATIDE

Trade name: Forteo (Lilly)
Indications: Osteoporosis in postmenopausal women and men at increased risk of fractures
Class: Parathyroid hormone analog
Half-life: 1 hour
Clinically important, potentially hazardous interactions with: alcohol, digoxin
Pregnancy category: C
Important contra-indications noted in the prescribing guidelines for: nursing mothers; pediatric patients
Warning: POTENTIAL RISK OF OSTEOSARCOMA

Skin
Diaphoresis (2%)
Herpes zoster (3%)
Rash (5%)

Cardiovascular
Angina (3%)
Hypertension (7%)

Central Nervous System
Anxiety (4%)
Depression (4%)
Dysgeusia (taste perversion) (<2%)
Headache (8%) [8]
Insomnia (4–5%)
Pain (21%)
Paresthesias (<2%)
Syncope (3%)
Vertigo (dizziness) (4–8%) [7]

Neuromuscular/Skeletal
Arthralgia (10%) [3]
Asthenia (fatigue) (9%)
Bone tumor [2]
Leg cramps (3%) [4]
Myalgia/Myopathy [2]
Neck pain (3%)
Pain in extremities [3]

Gastrointestinal/Hepatic
Constipation (5%)
Diarrhea (5%)
Dyspepsia (5%)
Gastritis (2–7%)
Nausea (9–14%) [8]
Vomiting (3%)

Respiratory
Cough (6%)
Dyspnea (4–6%)
Pharyngitis (6%)
Pneumonia (4–6%)
Rhinitis (10%)

Endocrine/Metabolic
Hypercalcemia [6]

Local
Injection-site pain (<2%)

Other
Adverse effects [4]
Tooth disorder (2%)

TERLIPRESSIN

Trade names: Glypressin (IS Pharma), Terlipressin (Ferring) (Bissendorf Peptide)
Indications: Esophageal variceal hemorrhage
Class: Vasopressin agonist
Half-life: 50–70 minutes
Clinically important, potentially hazardous interactions with: none known
Pregnancy category: N/A (Contra-indicated in pregnancy)

Skin
Gangrene [2]
Necrosis [12]

Cardiovascular
Myocardial infarction [3]
QT prolongation [2]
Torsades de pointes [2]

Central Nervous System
Seizures [3]

Neuromuscular/Skeletal
Rhabdomyolysis [3]

Endocrine/Metabolic
Hyponatremia [8]

Other
Adverse effects [2]

TESTOSTERONE

Trade names: Androderm (Actavis), AndroGel (AbbVie), Delatestryl (Endo), Fortesta (Endo), Natesto (Endo), Testim (Auxilium)
Indications: Androgen replacement, hypogonadism, postpartum breast pain
Class: Androgen
Half-life: 10–100 minutes
Clinically important, potentially hazardous interactions with: acarbose, anisindione, anticoagulants, cyclosporine, dicumarol, metformin, saxagliptin, sitagliptin, warfarin
Pregnancy category: N/A (Contra-indicated in pregnancy)
Important contra-indications noted in the prescribing guidelines for: nursing mothers; pediatric patients
Note: Contra-indicated in men with carcinoma of the breast or known or suspected carcinoma of the prostate.
Warning: SECONDARY EXPOSURE TO TESTOSTERONE

Skin
Acneform eruption (>10%) [20]
Carcinoma [2]
Dermatitis (4%) [2]
Edema (<10%)
Flushing (<10%)
Rash (2%)

Hair
Alopecia [3]
Hirsutism (<10%) [12]

Cardiovascular
Cardiotoxicity [2]
Myocardial infarction [3]

Endocrine/Metabolic
Gynecomastia [2]
Mastodynia (>10%)

Genitourinary
Priapism (>10%) [10]

Hematologic
Thrombosis [2]

Local
Application-site bullae (12%)
Application-site burning (3%)
Application-site erythema (7%)
Application-site induration (3%)
Application-site pruritus (37%)
Application-site vesicles (6%)
Injection-site pain [2]

Other
Adverse effects [3]

TETRACAINE & OXYMETAZOLINE

Trade name: Kovanaze (St Renatus)
Indications: Regional anesthesia in restorative dentistry
Class: Alpha adrenoceptor agonist (oxymetazoline), Anesthetic, local (tetracaine)
Half-life: <2 hours
Clinically important, potentially hazardous interactions with: beta blockers, MAO inhibitors, other intranasal products, tricyclic antidepressants
Pregnancy category: N/A (Insufficient evidence to inform drug-associated risk)
Important contra-indications noted in the prescribing guidelines for: the elderly; nursing mothers; pediatric patients
Note: For intranasal use only. See separate entry for oxymetazoline as topical formulation.

Mucosal
Epistaxis (nosebleed) (2%)
Mucosal ulceration (2–3%)
Nasal congestion (32%) [3]
Nasal discomfort (26%)
Nasal dryness (2%)
Oropharyngeal pain (14%)
Rhinorrhea (52%) [3]

Cardiovascular
Blood pressure variations (3–5%)
Bradycardia (3%)
Hypertension (3%)

Central Nervous System
Dysgeusia (taste perversion) (8%)
Headache (10%)
Hypoesthesia (intranasal and pharyngeal) (10%)
Sensory disturbances (2%)
Vertigo (dizziness) (3%)

Ocular
Lacrimation (13%)

Other
Sneezing (4%)

TETRACYCLINE

Trade names: Helidac (Prometheus), Sumycin (Par)
Indications: Various infections caused by susceptible organisms
Class: Antibiotic, tetracycline
Half-life: 6–11 hours
Clinically important, potentially hazardous interactions with: ACE inhibitors, acitretin, aluminum, amoxicillin, ampicillin, antacids, atovaquone, atovaquone/proguanil, bacampicillin, betamethasone, bismuth, bromelain, calcium salts, carbenicillin, cholestyramine, cloxacillin, colestipol, corticosteroids, coumarins, dairy products, dicloxacillin, didanosine, digoxin, ergotamine, food, gliclazide, isotretinoin, kaolin, methicillin, methotrexate, methoxyflurane, methysergide, mezlocillin, nafcillin, oral iron, oral typhoid vaccine, oxacillin, penicillins, phenindione, piperacillin, quinapril, retinoids, rocuronium, sodium picosulfate, strontium ranelate, sucralfate, sulfonylureas, ticarcillin, tripotassium dicitratobismuthate, vitamin A, zinc
Pregnancy category: D

Skin
Acneform eruption [2]
Angioedema [2]
Candidiasis [2]
Erythema multiforme [7]
Exanthems [3]
Exfoliative dermatitis [2]
Fixed eruption (15%) [43]
Hypersensitivity [2]
Jarisch–Herxheimer reaction [3]
Lichenoid eruption [3]
Lupus erythematosus [6]
Photosensitivity (<10%) [12]
Phototoxicity [4]
Pigmentation [4]
Psoriasis (exacerbation) [2]
Stevens-Johnson syndrome [4]
Toxic epidermal necrolysis [13]
Urticaria [5]

Nails
Onycholysis [5]
Photo-onycholysis [9]

Central Nervous System
Pseudotumor cerebri [6]

Gastrointestinal/Hepatic
Diarrhea [2]
Hepatotoxicity [2]
Pancreatitis [3]

Genitourinary
Vaginitis [3]

Other
Adverse effects [4]
Tooth pigmentation (commonly in under 8-year-olds) (>10%) [13]

THALIDOMIDE

Trade name: Thalomid (Celgene)
Indications: Graft-versus-host reactions, recalcitrant aphthous stomatitis
Class: Immunosuppressant, TNF modulator
Half-life: 5–7 hours
Clinically important, potentially hazardous interactions with: alcohol, amiodarone, antihistamines, antipsychotics, bortezomib, calcium channel blockers, carbamazepine, cimetidine, cisplatin, CNS depressants, digoxin, disulfiram, docetaxel, famotidine, griseofulvin, lithium, metronidazole, modafinil, opioids, paclitaxel, penicillins, phenytoin, rifabutin, rifampin, St John's wort, succinylcholine, vincristine

Pregnancy category: X
Important contra-indications noted in the prescribing guidelines for: nursing mothers; pediatric patients
Note: Thalidomide is a potent teratogen, an agent that causes congenital malformations and developmental abnormalities if introduced during gestation. Some of these teratogenic side effects of thalidomide include fetal limb growth retardation (arms, legs, hands, feet), ingrown genitalia, absence of lung, partial/total loss of hearing or sight, malformed digestive tract, heart, kidney, and stillborn infant.
Warning: FETAL RISK AND VENOUS THROMBOEMBOLIC EVENTS

Skin
Bullous dermatitis (5%)
Dermatitis [2]
Diaphoresis (13%)
Edema (57%) [11]
Erythema [2]
Erythema nodosum [2]
Erythroderma [2]
Exanthems [2]
Exfoliative dermatitis [4]
Facial erythema (<5%) [2]
Hypersensitivity [3]
Peripheral edema (3–8%) [4]
Pruritus (3–8%) [3]
Psoriasis [2]
Purpura [2]
Rash (11–50%) [25]
Stevens-Johnson syndrome [3]
Toxic epidermal necrolysis [4]
Urticaria (3%) [2]
Vasculitis [2]
Xerosis (21%) [5]

Mucosal
Oral candidiasis (4–11%)
Xerostomia (8%) [9]

Cardiovascular
Bradycardia [5]
Cardiotoxicity [2]
Hypotension (16%)
Thromboembolism [2]
Venous thromboembolism [5]

Central Nervous System
Agitation (9–26%)
Fever (19–23%) [2]
Hyperesthesia [2]
Insomnia (9%)
Neurotoxicity (22%) [24]
Paresthesias (6–16%) [8]
Parkinsonism [2]
Peripheral neuropathy [28]
Somnolence (drowsiness) (36%) [13]
Tremor (4–26%) [6]
Vertigo (dizziness) (4–20%) [16]

Neuromuscular/Skeletal
Arthralgia (13%)
Asthenia (fatigue) (79%) [17]
Myalgia/Myopathy (7%)

Gastrointestinal/Hepatic
Abdominal pain (3%)
Constipation [13]
Diarrhea (4–19%)
Flatulence (8%)
Hepatotoxicity [4]
Pancreatitis [2]

Respiratory
Dyspnea (42%)
Pharyngitis (4–8%)
Pneumonia [2]
Rhinitis (4%)
Sinusitis (3–8%)

Endocrine/Metabolic
Amenorrhea [6]
Gynecomastia [2]
Weight gain (22%)
Weight loss (23%)

Genitourinary
Erectile dysfunction [2]
Impotence (38%)
Leukorrhea (17–35%)

Hematologic
Anemia (6–13%) [5]
Neutropenia (31%) [9]
Thrombocytopenia [6]
Thrombosis [13]

Other
Adverse effects [8]
Death [2]
Infection (6–8%) [6]
Teratogenicity [6]
Toothache (4%)

THALLIUM

Indications: For diagnostic use in myocardial perfusion imaging
Class: Radioactive element
Half-life: 73.1 hours
Clinically important, potentially hazardous interactions with: none known
Pregnancy category: C

Hair
Alopecia [11]

Nails
Leukonychia (Mees' lines) [2]

Cardiovascular
Tachycardia [3]

Central Nervous System
Encephalopathy [5]
Peripheral neuropathy [5]

Gastrointestinal/Hepatic
Abdominal pain [5]

Other
Death [2]

THIABENDAZOLE

Synonym: tiabendazole
Indications: Various infections caused by susceptible helminths
Class: Anthelmintic, Antibiotic, imidazole
Half-life: 1.2 hours
Clinically important, potentially hazardous interactions with: none known
Pregnancy category: C

Skin
Dermatitis [3]
Erythema multiforme [3]
Exanthems (>5%) [4]
Fixed eruption [2]
Rash (<10%)
Sjögren's syndrome [3]
Stevens-Johnson syndrome (<10%)
Toxic epidermal necrolysis [2]
Urticaria (<5%)

Central Nervous System
Vertigo (dizziness) [3]

Gastrointestinal/Hepatic
Abdominal pain [2]
Nausea [2]

TIAGABINE

Trade name: Gabitril (Cephalon)
Indications: Partial seizures
Class: Anticonvulsant, Mood stabilizer
Half-life: 7–9 hours
Clinically important, potentially hazardous interactions with: alcohol, antipsychotics, carbamazepine, chloroquine, conivaptan, CYP3A4 inhibitors and inducers, dasatinib, deferasirox, droperidol, hydroxychloroquine, ketorolac, levomepromazine, MAO inhibitors, mefloquine, orlistat, phenobarbital, phenytoin, SSRIs, St John's wort, tricyclic antidepressants
Pregnancy category: C
Important contra-indications noted in the prescribing guidelines for: the elderly; nursing mothers; pediatric patients

---

Skin
Ecchymoses (<6%)
Pruritus (2%)
Rash (5%) [2]

Cardiovascular
Vasodilation (2%)

Central Nervous System
Confusion (5%)
Depression (<7%) [4]
Emotional lability (3%)
Gait instability (3–5%)
Headache [8]
Hostility (2–5%)
Impaired concentration (6–14%) [2]
Insomnia (5–6%)
Nervousness (10–14%) [10]
Pain (2–7%)
Paresthesias (4%)
Seizures [4]
Somnolence (drowsiness) (18–21%) [9]
Speech disorder (4%)
Status epilepticus (non-convulsive) [17]
Syncope [2]
Tremor (9–21%) [7]
Vertigo (dizziness) (27–31%) [22]

Neuromuscular/Skeletal
Asthenia (fatigue) (18–23%) [16]
Ataxia (5–9%)
Dystonia [5]
Myalgia/Myopathy (2–5%)

Gastrointestinal/Hepatic
Abdominal pain (5–7%)

Diarrhea (2–10%)
Nausea (11%) [7]
Vomiting (7%)

Respiratory
Cough (4%)
Flu-like syndrome (6–9%)
Pharyngitis (7–8%)

Endocrine/Metabolic
Appetite increased (2%)

Genitourinary
Urinary tract infection (<5%)

Ocular
Amblyopia (4–9%)
Nystagmus (2%)

Other
Adverse effects [6]
Infection (10–19%) [3]

TICAGRELOR

Trade name: Brilinta (AstraZeneca)
Indications: Thrombotic cardiovascular events
Class: Antiplatelet, Antiplatelet, cyclopentyl triazolo-pyrimidine (CPTP)
Half-life: 7 hours
Clinically important, potentially hazardous interactions with: atazanavir, carbamazepine, clarithromycin, dexamethasone, digoxin, efavirenz, indinavir, itraconazole, ketoconazole, lovastatin, nefazodone, nelfinavir, phenobarbital, phenytoin, rifampin, ritonavir, saquinavir, simvastatin, telithromycin, venetoclax, voriconazole
Pregnancy category: C
Important contra-indications noted in the prescribing guidelines for: nursing mothers; pediatric patients
Note: Maintenance doses of aspirin above 100 mg reduce the effectiveness of ticagrelor and should be avoided. Contra-indicated in patients with a history of intracranial hemorrhage, or active pathological bleeding, and in patients with severe hepatic impairment.
Warning: BLEEDING RISK

Cardiovascular
Atrial fibrillation (4%)
Bradycardia [2]
Chest pain (3–4%)
Hypertension (4%)
Hypotension (3%)
Ventricular arrhythmia [7]

Central Nervous System
Headache (7%)
Vertigo (dizziness) (5%)

Neuromuscular/Skeletal
Asthenia (fatigue) (3%)
Back pain (4%)
Rhabdomyolysis [4]

Gastrointestinal/Hepatic
Diarrhea (4%)
Nausea (4%)

Respiratory
Cough (5%)
Dyspnea (14%) [19]
Pneumonitis [2]

Hematologic
Bleeding (12%) [14]

Other
Adverse effects [2]

TINZAPARIN

Trade name: Innohep (Leo Pharma)
Indications: Acute symptomatic deep vein thrombosis
Class: Anticoagulant, Heparin, low molecular weight
Half-life: 3–4 hours
Clinically important, potentially hazardous interactions with: aliskiren, angiotensin II recepton antagonists, aspirin, butabarbital, clopidogrel, collagenase, dasatinib, dextran, diclofenac, dipyridamole, drotrecogin alfa, glyceryl trinitrate, ibritumomab, iloprost, ketorolac, NSAIDs, oral anticoagulants, pentosan, pentoxifylline, platelet inhibitors, prostacyclin analogues, salicylates, sulfinpyrazone, throbolytics, ticlopidine, tositumomab & iodine[131]
Pregnancy category: B
Important contra-indications noted in the prescribing guidelines for: the elderly; nursing mothers; pediatric patients
Warning: SPINAL / EPIDURAL HEMATOMAS

Skin
Bullous dermatitis (<10%)
Pruritus (<10%)

Mucosal
Epistaxis (nosebleed) (2%)

Cardiovascular
Chest pain (2%)

Central Nervous System
Fever (2%)
Headache (2%)
Pain (2%)

Neuromuscular/Skeletal
Back pain (2%)

Respiratory
Pulmonary embolism (2%)

Endocrine/Metabolic
ALT increased (13%)
AST increased (9%)

Genitourinary
Urinary tract infection (4%)

Hematologic
Bleeding [4]
Hemorrhage (2%)

Local
Injection-site hematoma (16%)

TIOTROPIUM

Trade names: Spiriva (Boehringer Ingelheim), Stiolto Respimat (Boehringer Ingelheim)
Indications: Bronchospasm (associated with COPD)
Class: Anticholinergic, Muscarinic antagonist
Half-life: 5–6 days
Clinically important, potentially hazardous interactions with: acetylcholinesterase inhibitors, anticholinergics, antihistamines, botulinum toxin (A & B), cannabinoids, conivaptan, disopyramide, domperidone, haloperidol, ketoconazole, levodopa, MAO inhibitors, memantine, metoclopramide, nefopam, parasympathomimetics, PEG-interferon, phenothiazines, potassium chloride, pramlintide, secretin, sublingual nitrates, tricyclic antidepressants
Pregnancy category: C
Important contra-indications noted in the prescribing guidelines for: nursing mothers; pediatric patients
Note: Stiolto Respimat is tiotropium and olodaterol.

Skin
Candidiasis (4%)
Edema (5%)
Herpes zoster (<3%)
Rash (4%)

Mucosal
Epistaxis (nosebleed) (4%)
Oral candidiasis [2]
Stomatitis (<3%)
Xerostomia (10–16%) [22]

Cardiovascular
Angina (<3%)
Cardiotoxicity [2]
Chest pain (7%) [2]
Hypertension [2]

Central Nervous System
Depression (<3%)
Headache [6]
Paresthesias (<3%)
Vertigo (dizziness) [2]

Neuromuscular/Skeletal
Arthralgia (>3%)
Back pain [4]
Bone or joint pain (<3%)
Leg pain (<3%)
Myalgia/Myopathy (4%)

Gastrointestinal/Hepatic
Abdominal pain (5%)
Constipation (4%) [2]
Diarrhea [3]
Dyspepsia (6%)
Gastroesophageal reflux (<3%)
Vomiting (4%)

Respiratory
Asthma [4]
Bronchitis [4]
COPD (exacerbation) [5]
Cough (>3%) [8]
Dysphonia (<3%)
Dyspnea [4]
Flu-like syndrome (>3%)
Influenza [3]

Laryngitis (<3%)
Nasopharyngitis [11]
Pharyngitis (9%)
Pneumonia [3]
Rhinitis (6%) [3]
Sinusitis (11%)
Upper respiratory tract infection (41%) [4]

Endocrine/Metabolic
Hypercholesterolemia (<3%)
Hyperglycemia (<3%)

Genitourinary
Urinary tract infection (7%)

Ocular
Cataract (<3%)

Other
Adverse effects [13]
Allergic reactions (<3%)
Death [7]
Infection (4%)

TIPRANAVIR

Trade name: Aptivus (Boehringer Ingelheim)
Indications: Antiretroviral treatment of HIV-1
Class: HIV-1 protease inhibitor, Sulfonamide
Half-life: 4.8–6.0 hours
Clinically important, potentially hazardous interactions with: abacavir, alcohol, alfuzosin, alprazolam, amiodarone, antacids, antifungals, apixaban, artemether/lumefantrine, atazanavir, atomoxetine, atorvastatin, bepridil, bosentan, buprenorphine, calcium channel blockers, carbamazepine, cisapride, clarithromycin, codeine, conivaptan, copanlisib, corticosteroids, cyclosporine, CYP2D6 substrates, CYP3A4 inducers, dabigatran, darifenacin, deferasirox, delavirdine, didanosine, digoxin, dihydroergotamine, disulfiram, efavirenz, elbasvir & grazoprevir, eluxadoline, enfuvirtide, eplerenone, ergotamine, esomeprazole, estradiol, estrogens, etravirine, fesoterodine, flecainide, fluconazole, fosamprenavir, fusidic acid, garlic, HMG-CoA reductase inhibitors, lopinavir, lovastatin, meperidine, methadone, metoprolol, metronidazole, midazolam, midostaurin, nebivolol, nefazodone, neratinib, omeprazole, P-glycoprotein substrates, pantoprazole, phenobarbital, phenytoin, pimozide, propafenone, protease inhibitors, proton pump inhibitors, quetiapine, quinidine, quinine, raltegravir, ranolazine, rifabutin, rifampin, rilpivirine, rivaroxaban, rosuvastatin, salmeterol, saquinavir, sildenafil, simeprevir, simvastatin, sirolimus, sofosbuvir, sofosbuvir/velpatasvir/voxilaprevir, St John's wort, tacrolimus, tamoxifen, telithromycin, temsirolimus, tenofovir disoproxil, tetrabenazine, theophylline, thioridazine, tramadol, trazodone, triazolam, tricyclic antidepressants, valproic acid, vardenafil, vitamin E, zidovudine
Pregnancy category: C
Important contra-indications noted in the prescribing guidelines for: the elderly; nursing mothers; pediatric patients
Note: Tipranavir is a sulfonamide and can be absorbed systemically. Sulfonamides can produce severe, possibly fatal, reactions such as toxic epidermal necrolysis and Stevens-Johnson syndrome.
Tipranavir is co-administered with ritonavir.
Contra-indicated in patients with moderate or severe (Child-Pugh Class B or C) hepatic impairment.
Warning: HEPATOTOXICITY and INTRACRANIAL HEMORRHAGE

Skin
Exanthems (<2%)
Herpes simplex (<2%)
Herpes zoster (<2%)
Hypersensitivity (<2%)
Lipoatrophy (<2%)
Lipodystrophy (<2%)
Lipohypertrophy (<2%)
Pruritus (<2%)
Rash (3%) [2]

Central Nervous System
Anorexia (<2%)
Depression (2%)
Fever (14%)
Headache (5%)
Insomnia (2%)
Intracranial hemorrhage (<2%) [3]
Neurotoxicity (<2%)
Peripheral neuropathy (2%)
Sleep related disorder (<2%)
Somnolence (drowsiness) (<2%)
Vertigo (dizziness) (<2%)

Neuromuscular/Skeletal
Asthenia (fatigue) (2%)
Cramps (<2%)
Myalgia/Myopathy (2%)

Gastrointestinal/Hepatic
Abdominal distension (<2%)
Abdominal pain (6%)
Dyspepsia (<2%)
Flatulence (<2%)
Gastroesophageal reflux (<2%)
Hepatic failure (<2%)
Hepatitis (<2%)
Hepatotoxicity [4]
Nausea (9%)
Pancreatitis (<2%)
Vomiting (6%)

Respiratory
Dyspnea (2%)
Flu-like syndrome (<2%)

Endocrine/Metabolic
ALT increased (2%) [2]
Appetite decreased (<2%)
Dehydration (2%)
Diabetes mellitus (<2%)
GGT increased (2%)
Hyperamylasemia (<2%)
Hypercholesterolemia (<2%)
Hyperglycemia (<2%)
Hyperlipidemia (3%)
Hypertriglyceridemia (4%) [2]
Weight loss (3%)

Hematologic
Anemia (3%)
Neutropenia (2%)
Thrombocytopenia (<2%)

Other
Adverse effects [3]

TIZANIDINE

Trade name: Zanaflex (Acorda)
Indications: Muscle spasticity, multiple sclerosis
Class: Adrenergic alpha2-receptor agonist
Half-life: 2.5 hours
Clinically important, potentially hazardous interactions with: acebutolol, alfuzosin, benazepril, captopril, cilazapril, ciprofloxacin, enalapril, fluvoxamine, fosinopril, irbesartan, lisinopril, norfloxacin, obeticholic acid, olmesartan, phenytoin, quinapril, ramipril, rofecoxib, teriflunomide, trandolapril
Pregnancy category: C
Important contra-indications noted in the prescribing guidelines for: the elderly; pediatric patients

---

Skin
Pallor [2]
Pruritus (<10%)
Rash (<10%)

Mucosal
Xerostomia (49–88%) [14]

Cardiovascular
Bradycardia (<10%) [5]
Hypotension (16–33%) [3]

Central Nervous System
Dyskinesia (3%)
Nervousness (3%)
Somnolence (drowsiness) (48–92%) [4]
Speech disorder (3%)
Tremor (<10%)
Vertigo (dizziness) (41–45%) [3]

Neuromuscular/Skeletal
Asthenia (fatigue) (41–78%) [5]

Gastrointestinal/Hepatic
Constipation (4%)
Hepatotoxicity (6%) [4]
Vomiting (3%)

Respiratory
Flu-like syndrome (3%)
Pharyngitis (3%)
Rhinitis (3%)

Genitourinary
Urinary frequency (3%)
Urinary tract infection (10%)

Ocular
Amblyopia (3%)

Other
Infection (6%)

TOBRAMYCIN

Trade names: TOBI (Chiron), TobraDex (Alcon)
Indications: Various serious infections caused by susceptible organisms, superficial ocular infections
Class: Antibiotic, aminoglycoside
Half-life: 2–3 hours
Clinically important, potentially hazardous interactions with: adefovir, aldesleukin, aminoglycosides, atracurium, bumetanide, daptomycin, doxacurium, ethacrynic acid, furosemide, neuromuscular blockers, pancuronium, polypeptide antibiotics,

rocuronium, succinylcholine, teicoplanin, torsemide, vecuronium
Pregnancy category: D (Category D for injection and inhalation; category B for ophthalmic use)
Important contra-indications noted in the prescribing guidelines for: the elderly; nursing mothers; pediatric patients
Note: Aminoglycosides may cause neurotoxicity and/or nephrotoxicity.
TobraDex is tobramycin and dexamethasone.

Skin
Exanthems [4]
Hypersensitivity [3]
Rash [2]

Central Nervous System
Dysgeusia (taste perversion) [2]
Fever [2]

Respiratory
Cough [3]

Renal
Nephrotoxicity [6]

Ocular
Conjunctivitis [2]
Eyelid dermatitis [2]
Intraocular pressure increased [2]

TOCILIZUMAB

Trade name: Actemra (Roche)
Indications: Rheumatoid arthritis, juvenile idiopathic arthritis, Castleman's disease
Class: Anti-interleukin-6 receptor monoclonal antibody, Disease-modifying antirheumatic drug (DMARD), Monoclonal antibody
Half-life: 8–14 days
Clinically important, potentially hazardous interactions with: efavirenz, fesoterodine, fingolimod, infliximab, lurasidone, paricalcitol, pazopanib, typhoid vaccine, yellow fever vaccine
Pregnancy category: N/A (Based on animal data, may cause fetal harm)
Important contra-indications noted in the prescribing guidelines for: nursing mothers; pediatric patients
Warning: RISK OF SERIOUS INFECTIONS

Skin
Anaphylactoid reactions/Anaphylaxis [5]
Cellulitis [9]
Herpes zoster [8]
Hypersensitivity [6]
Malignancies [2]
Peripheral edema (<2%)
Psoriasis [3]
Rash (2%) [7]
Urticaria [2]

Mucosal
Mucosal ulceration [2]
Oral ulceration (2%)
Stomatitis (<2%)

Cardiovascular
Cardiotoxicity [3]
Hypertension (6%) [3]

Central Nervous System
Headache (7%) [7]
Neurotoxicity [2]
Vertigo (dizziness) (3%)

Neuromuscular/Skeletal
Arthralgia [4]
Fractures [2]

Gastrointestinal/Hepatic
Abdominal pain (2%)
Diarrhea [2]
Gastroenteritis [6]
Gastrointestinal bleeding [3]
Gastrointestinal perforation [8]
Gastrointestinal ulceration (<2%)
Hepatotoxicity [16]
Nausea [3]
Pancreatitis [2]

Respiratory
Bronchitis (3%) [6]
Cough (<2%)
Dyspnea (<2%)
Influenza [3]
Nasopharyngitis (7%) [7]
Pharyngitis [4]
Pneumonia [12]
Pneumothorax [2]
Pulmonary toxicity [5]
Upper respiratory tract infection (7%) [11]

Endocrine/Metabolic
ALT increased (6%) [10]
AST increased [4]
Hypercholesterolemia [4]
Hyperlipidemia [5]
Hypertriglyceridemia [2]
Hypothyroidism (<2%)
Weight gain (<2%)

Genitourinary
Urinary tract infection [3]

Renal
Nephrolithiasis (<2%)
Pyelonephritis [3]

Hematologic
Hemotoxicity [2]
Leukopenia (<2%) [5]
Lymphopenia [2]
Neutropenia [20]
Sepsis [2]

Ocular
Conjunctivitis (<2%)

Local
Infusion-related reactions [3]
Infusion-site reactions [2]

Other
Adverse effects [12]
Death [5]
Infection [39]

TOFACITINIB

Trade name: Xeljanz (Pfizer)
Indications: Rheumatoid arthritis
Class: Janus kinase (JAK) inhibitor
Half-life: ~3 hours
Clinically important, potentially hazardous interactions with: azathioprine, biologic disease-modifying antirheumatics, cyclosporine, CYP3A4 inhibitors, fluconazole, ketoconazole, live vaccines, potent immunosuppressives, rifampin, strong CYP inducers, strong CYP2C19 inhibitors, tacrolimus
Pregnancy category: C
Important contra-indications noted in the prescribing guidelines for: the elderly; nursing mothers; pediatric patients
Warning: SERIOUS INFECTIONS AND MALIGNANCY

Skin
Erythema (<2%)
Herpes zoster [10]
Peripheral edema (<2%)
Pruritus (<2%)
Psoriasis [2]
Rash (<2%) [3]

Mucosal
Nasal congestion (<2%)

Cardiovascular
Cardiotoxicity [2]
Hypertension (2%)

Central Nervous System
Fever (<2%)
Headache (3–4%) [10]
Insomnia (<2%)
Paresthesias (<2%)

Neuromuscular/Skeletal
Arthralgia (<2%)
Bone or joint pain (<2%)
Tendinitis (<2%)

Gastrointestinal/Hepatic
Abdominal pain (<2%) [2]
Diarrhea (3–4%) [9]
Dyspepsia (<2%) [2]
Gastritis (<2%)
Nausea (<2%) [4]
Vomiting (<2%)

Respiratory
Bronchitis [4]
Cough (<2%)
Dyspnea (<2%)
Influenza [3]
Nasopharyngitis (3–4%) [11]
Tuberculosis [4]
Upper respiratory tract infection (4–5%) [12]

Endocrine/Metabolic
ALT increased [3]
AST increased [3]
Creatine phosphokinase increased [2]
Dehydration (<2%)
Hypercholesterolemia [2]
Hyperlipidemia [2]

Genitourinary
Urinary tract infection (2%) [5]

Hematologic
Anemia (<2%)
Neutropenia [3]

Other
Adverse effects [8]
Death [2]
Infection (20–22%) [14]

TOLTERODINE

Trade name: Detrol (Pharmacia & Upjohn)
Indications: Urinary incontinence
Class: Muscarinic antagonist
Half-life: 2–4 hours
Clinically important, potentially hazardous interactions with: itraconazole, ketoconazole, lopinavir, nelfinavir, sotalol, voriconazole, warfarin
Pregnancy category: C
Important contra-indications noted in the prescribing guidelines for: nursing mothers; pediatric patients

---

Skin
Erythema (2%)
Rash (2%)

Mucosal
Xerostomia (35%) [38]

Cardiovascular
Chest pain (2%)

Central Nervous System
Headache (7%) [4]
Somnolence (drowsiness) (3%)
Vertigo (dizziness) (5%) [4]

Neuromuscular/Skeletal
Arthralgia (2%)
Asthenia (fatigue) (4%)

Gastrointestinal/Hepatic
Abdominal pain (5%) [2]
Constipation (7%) [13]
Diarrhea (4%)
Dyspepsia (4%)

Respiratory
Flu-like syndrome (3%)
Upper respiratory tract infection (6%)

Genitourinary
Dysuria (2%)

Ocular
Vision blurred [3]
Xerophthalmia (3%) [2]

Other
Adverse effects [6]

TOPIRAMATE

Trade names: Qsymia (Vivus), Qudexy (Upsher-Smith), Topamax (Janssen), Trokendi XR (Supernus)
Indications: Partial onset seizures, migraine
Class: Anticonvulsant, Mood stabilizer
Half-life: 21 hours
Clinically important, potentially hazardous interactions with: eslicarbazepine, levonorgestrel, metformin, rufinamide, ulipristal, valproic acid
Pregnancy category: D
Important contra-indications noted in the prescribing guidelines for: nursing mothers; pediatric patients
Note: Qsymia is topiramate and phentermine.

Skin
Anhidrosis [2]
Bromhidrosis (2%)
Diaphoresis (2%)
Edema (2%)
Fixed eruption [2]
Flushing (>5%)
Hot flashes (<10%)
Hypohidrosis [2]
Palmar erythema [2]
Pruritus (2%) [3]
Rash (4%) [3]

Hair
Alopecia [2]

Mucosal
Gingival hyperplasia/hypertrophy [2]
Gingivitis (2%)
Xerostomia (3%) [6]

Cardiovascular
Tachycardia [4]

Central Nervous System
Anorexia (>5%) [4]
Anxiety [3]
Cognitive impairment (>5%) [17]
Confusion (>5%)
Depression [11]
Dysgeusia (taste perversion) (>5%) [10]
Encephalopathy [4]
Fever (>5%)
Headache [2]
Hyperthermia [3]
Impaired concentration [4]
Insomnia [8]
Irritability [2]
Nervousness (>5%)
Neurotoxicity [6]
Palinopsia [3]
Paresthesias (>5%) [36]
Peripheral neuropathy [2]
Psychosis [3]
Seizures [3]
Somnambulism [2]
Somnolence (drowsiness) (>5%) [7]
Suicidal ideation [2]
Tremor (>10%)
Vertigo (dizziness) (>5%) [14]

Neuromuscular/Skeletal
Asthenia (fatigue) (>5%) [10]
Ataxia [2]

Gastrointestinal/Hepatic
Constipation [6]
Diarrhea [3]
Nausea [5]

Respiratory
Flu-like syndrome (<2%)

Endocrine/Metabolic
Acidosis [4]
Appetite decreased [5]
Gynecomastia (8%)
Hyperammonemia [3]
Mastodynia (3–9%)
Weight gain [2]
Weight loss (>5%) [16]

Genitourinary
Erectile dysfunction [2]

Renal
Nephrolithiasis [5]

Ocular
Diplopia [2]
Glaucoma [16]
Myopia [9]
Uveitis [5]
Vision loss [3]

Other
Adverse effects [11]
Death [2]
Infection (>5%)
Side effects [3]
Teratogenicity [8]

TOPOTECAN

Trade name: Hycamtin (GSK)
Indications: Metastatic ovarian carcinoma
Class: Antineoplastic, Topoisomerase I inhibitor
Half-life: 3–6 hours
Clinically important, potentially hazardous interactions with: atorvastatin, darunavir, gefitinib, lapatinib, oxaliplatin, pantoprazole, safinamide, sofosbuvir & velpatasvir
Pregnancy category: D
Important contra-indications noted in the prescribing guidelines for: nursing mothers; pediatric patients
Warning: BONE MARROW SUPPRESSION

Hair
Alopecia (59%) [7]

Mucosal
Mucositis [2]
Stomatitis (24%) [4]

Central Nervous System
Fever [2]
Paresthesias (9%)

Neuromuscular/Skeletal
Asthenia (fatigue) [9]

Gastrointestinal/Hepatic
Abdominal pain [2]
Diarrhea [5]
Hepatotoxicity [3]
Nausea [3]
Vomiting [4]

Respiratory
Dyspnea [3]

Renal
Nephrotoxicity [2]

Hematologic
Anemia [11]
Febrile neutropenia [5]
Granulocytopenia [2]
Myelosuppression [2]
Neutropenia [16]
Thrombocytopenia [15]

Other
Adverse effects [2]
Death [5]
Infection [2]

TOREMIFENE

Trade name: Fareston (ProStrakan)
Indications: Metastatic breast cancer
Class: Selective estrogen receptor modulator (SERM)
Half-life: ~5 days
Clinically important, potentially hazardous interactions with: amoxapine, arsenic, dolasetron, efavirenz, pazopanib, sugammadex, telavancin
Pregnancy category: D
Important contra-indications noted in the prescribing guidelines for: nursing mothers; pediatric patients
Warning: QT PROLONGATION

Skin
Diaphoresis (20%) [6]
Edema (5%) [2]
Flushing [3]
Hot flashes (35%) [4]

Cardiovascular
Thromboembolism [3]
Venous thromboembolism [2]

Central Nervous System
Headache [2]
Vertigo (dizziness) [2]

Gastrointestinal/Hepatic
Hepatotoxicity [3]
Nausea [2]
Vomiting [2]

Endocrine/Metabolic
ALP increased [2]
Galactorrhea (<10%)

Genitourinary
Priapism (<10%)
Vaginal bleeding [2]
Vaginal discharge [2]

Ocular
Cataract [3]

TORSEMIDE

Trade names: Demadex (Roche), Torem (Roche)
Indications: Essential hypertension, edema due to congestive heart failure, hepatic, pulmonary or renal edema
Class: Diuretic, loop
Half-life: 2–4 hours
Clinically important, potentially hazardous interactions with: ACE inhibitors, amikacin, aminoglycosides, aminophylline, anti-diabetics, antihypertensives, cephalosporins, cisplatin, gentamicin, indomethacin, kanamycin, neomycin, probenecid, salicylates, streptomycin, tobramycin
Pregnancy category: B
Important contra-indications noted in the prescribing guidelines for: nursing mothers; pediatric patients
Note: Torsemide is a sulfonamide and can be absorbed systemically. Sulfonamides can produce severe, possibly fatal, reactions such as toxic epidermal necrolysis and Stevens-Johnson syndrome.

Skin
Photosensitivity (<10%)
Urticaria (<10%)
Vasculitis [2]

Central Nervous System
Headache (7%)
Vertigo (dizziness) (3%)

Neuromuscular/Skeletal
Arthralgia (2%)
Asthenia (fatigue) (2%)
Myalgia/Myopathy (2%)

Gastrointestinal/Hepatic
Constipation (2%)
Diarrhea (2%)
Dyspepsia (2%)
Nausea (2%)

Respiratory
Cough (2%)
Pharyngolaryngeal pain (2%)
Rhinitis (3%)

Endocrine/Metabolic
Pseudoporphyria [2]

TRAGACANTH GUM

Family: Fabaceae; Leguminosae
Scientific names: *Astragalus gossypinus, Astragalus gummifer*
Indications: Diarrhea. Ingredient in pharmaceuticals, foods, toothpaste, denture adhesives, emulsifier, binding agent, demulcent, stabilizer
Class: Food additive, Laxative
Half-life: N/A
Clinically important, potentially hazardous interactions with: none known
Pregnancy category: N/A
Note: See also Astragalus root.

TRAMADOL

Trade names: Rybix ODT (Victory Pharma), Ultracet (Ortho-McNeil), Ultram (Ortho-McNeil)
Indications: Pain
Class: Opiate agonist
Half-life: 6–7 hours
Clinically important, potentially hazardous interactions with: alcohol, amitriptyline, carbamazepine, cinacalcet, citalopram, delavirdine, desflurane, desvenlafaxine, duloxetine, erythromycin, fluoxetine, fluvoxamine, ketoconazole, levomepromazine, linezolid, lorcaserin, MAO inhibitors, nefazodone, ondansetron, paroxetine hydrochloride, phenelzine, quinidine, risperidone, safinamide, tapentadol, terbinafine, tianeptine, tipranavir, tranylcypromine, venlafaxine, vilazodone, zuclopenthixol
Pregnancy category: C
Important contra-indications noted in the prescribing guidelines for: the elderly; nursing mothers; pediatric patients

Skin
Anaphylactoid reactions/Anaphylaxis [2]
Angioedema [2]
Contact dermatitis [2]
Diaphoresis (9%) [3]
Flushing [2]
Hypersensitivity [2]
Peripheral edema [2]
Pruritus (<10%) [4]
Rash (<5%) [2]
Urticaria (<18%)

Mucosal
Xerostomia (10%) [5]

Cardiovascular
Vasodilation (<5%)

Central Nervous System
Anorexia (<5%)
Anxiety (<5%)
Catatonia [2]
Confusion (<5%)
Euphoria (<5%)
Fever [2]
Headache [8]
Insomnia [3]
Nervousness (<5%)
Restless legs syndrome [5]
Seizures [16]
Serotonin syndrome [17]
Sleep related disorder (<5%)
Somnolence (drowsiness) [7]
Tremor (5–10%)
Vertigo (dizziness) [18]

Neuromuscular/Skeletal
Asthenia (fatigue) (<5%) [3]
Hypertonia (<5%)

Gastrointestinal/Hepatic
Abdominal pain (<5%) [3]
Constipation [8]
Diarrhea [2]
Flatulence (<5%)
Nausea [25]
Vomiting [23]

Respiratory
Apnea [2]
Respiratory depression [2]

Endocrine/Metabolic
Adrenal insufficiency [2]
Hypoglycemia [8]
Hyponatremia [3]

Genitourinary
Urinary frequency (<5%)
Urinary retention (<5%)

Otic
Hallucinations, auditory [2]

Ocular
Hallucinations, visual [3]
Mydriasis [2]
Visual disturbances (<5%)

Other
Adverse effects [8]
Death [2]

TRAMETINIB

Trade name: Mekinist (Novartis)
Indications: Melanoma (unresectable or metastatic) in patients with BRAF V600E or V600K mutations
Class: MEK inhibitor
Half-life: 4–5 days
Clinically important, potentially hazardous interactions with: none known
Pregnancy category: D
Important contra-indications noted in the prescribing guidelines for: nursing mothers; pediatric patients

---

Skin
Acneform eruption (19%) [8]
Actinic keratoses [2]
Cellulitis (<10%)
Dermatitis (19%) [2]
Edema (32%)
Erythema [2]
Exanthems [2]
Folliculitis (<10%)
Hand–foot syndrome [2]
Hyperkeratosis [3]
Keratosis pilaris [2]
Lymphedema (32%)
Panniculitis [4]
Papillomas [2]
Papulopustular eruption [2]
Peripheral edema (32%) [9]
Pruritus (10%) [4]
Pustules (<10%)
Rash (57%) [18]
Squamous cell carcinoma [4]
Toxicity (87%) [5]
Xerosis (11%) [3]

Hair
Alopecia [4]

Nails
Paronychia (10%)

Mucosal
Aphthous stomatitis (15%)
Epistaxis (nosebleed) (13%)
Gingival bleeding (13%)
Mucosal inflammation (15%)
Oral ulceration (15%)
Rectal hemorrhage (13%)
Stomatitis (15%) [2]
Xerostomia (<10%)

Cardiovascular
Bradycardia (<10%)
Cardiomyopathy (7%)
Cardiotoxicity [6]
Hypertension (15%) [7]

Central Nervous System
Chills [4]
Dysgeusia (taste perversion) (<10%)
Fever [13]
Headache [5]
Vertigo (dizziness) (<10%)

Neuromuscular/Skeletal
Arthralgia [6]
Asthenia (fatigue) [16]
Rhabdomyolysis (<10%)

Gastrointestinal/Hepatic
Abdominal pain (13%)
Black stools (13%)
Constipation [3]
Diarrhea (43%) [19]
Hepatotoxicity [2]
Nausea [14]
Vomiting [8]

Respiratory
Cough [2]
Pneumonitis (2%)

Endocrine/Metabolic
ALP increased (24%)
ALT increased (39%) [4]
Appetite decreased [2]
AST increased (60%) [5]
Hypoalbuminemia (42%)

Genitourinary
Hematuria (13%)
Vaginal bleeding (13%)

Hematologic
Anemia (38%) [3]
Hemorrhage (13%)
Neutropenia [2]
Thrombocytopenia [3]

Ocular
Chorioretinopathy [3]
Conjunctival hemorrhage (13%)
Retinopathy [2]
Uveitis [2]
Vision blurred (<10%) [4]
Xerophthalmia (<10%)

Other
Adverse effects [6]

TRANDOLAPRIL

Trade names: Mavik (AbbVie), Tarka (AbbVie)
Indications: Hypertension
Class: Angiotensin-converting enzyme (ACE) inhibitor, Antihypertensive, Vasodilator
Half-life: 6 hours
Clinically important, potentially hazardous interactions with: alcohol, aldesleukin, aliskiren, allopurinol, alpha blockers, amiloride, angiotensin II receptor antagonists, antacids, antidiabetics, antipsychotics, anxiolytics and hypnotics, baclofen, beta blockers, calcium channel blockers, clonidine, corticosteroids, cyclosporine, diazoxide, diuretics, estrogens, general anesthetics, gold & gold compounds, heparins, hydralazine, insulin, levodopa, lithium, MAO inhibitors, metformin, methyldopa, minoxidil, moxisylyte, moxonidine, nitrates, nitroprusside, NSAIDs, potassium salts, spironolactone, sulfonylureas, tizanidine, triamterene, trimethoprim
Pregnancy category: D (category C in first trimester; category D in second and third trimesters)
Important contra-indications noted in the prescribing guidelines for: nursing mothers; pediatric patients
Note: Contra-indicated in patients with hereditary/idiopathic angioedema and in patients with a history of angioedema related to previous treatment with an ACE inhibitor. Tarka is trandolapril and verapamil.
Warning: FETAL TOXICITY

Skin
Angioedema [3]
Edema (>3%)

Mucosal
Xerostomia (>3%)

Cardiovascular
Bradycardia (5%)
Cardiogenic shock (4%)
Hypotension (11%)

Central Nervous System
Hyperesthesia (>3%)
Stroke (3%)
Syncope (6%)
Vertigo (dizziness) (23%)

Neuromuscular/Skeletal
Asthenia (fatigue) (3%)
Myalgia/Myopathy (5%)

Gastrointestinal/Hepatic
Dyspepsia (6%)
Gastritis (4%)

Respiratory
Cough (35%) [5]

Endocrine/Metabolic
Creatine phosphokinase increased (5%)
Hyperkalemia (5%)
Hypocalcemia (5%)

TRANEXAMIC ACID

Trade name: Cyklokapron (Pharmacia)
Indications: Fibrinolysis
Class: Antifibrinolytic
Half-life: 2 hours
Clinically important, potentially hazardous interactions with: none known
Pregnancy category: B

Skin
Fixed eruption [2]

Central Nervous System
Headache [3]
Seizures [11]

Gastrointestinal/Hepatic
Abdominal pain [2]

Endocrine/Metabolic
Menstrual irregularities [3]

Renal
Nephrotoxicity [3]

Other
Adverse effects [2]

TRASTUZUMAB

Trade name: Herceptin (Genentech)
Indications: Metastatic breast cancer
Class: Antineoplastic, HER2/neu receptor antagonist, Monoclonal antibody
Half-life: 2–16 days (dose dependent)
Clinically important, potentially hazardous interactions with: abatacept, abciximab, alefacept, antineoplastics, azacitidine, betamethasone, cabazitaxel, denileukin, docetaxel, doxorubicin, fingolimod, gefitinib, immunosuppressants, leflunomide, lenalidomide, oxaliplatin, paclitaxel, pazopanib, pemetrexed, temsirolimus
Pregnancy category: D
Important contra-indications noted in the prescribing guidelines for: nursing mothers; pediatric patients
Warning: CARDIOMYOPATHY, INFUSION REACTIONS, EMBRYO-FETAL TOXICITY, and PULMONARY TOXICITY

Skin
Acneform eruption (2%) [4]
Edema (8%)
Erythema [2]
Hand–foot syndrome [10]
Herpes simplex (2%)
Hypersensitivity [3]
Peripheral edema (5–10%)
Photosensitivity [2]
Pruritus (2%)
Radiation recall dermatitis [2]
Rash (4–18%) [12]
Toxicity [3]

Hair
Alopecia [6]

Nails
Nail disorder (2%)

Mucosal
Epistaxis (nosebleed) (2%)
Mucositis [3]
Stomatitis [5]

Cardiovascular
Arrhythmias (3%)
Cardiac disorder [4]
Cardiac failure [4]
Cardiomyopathy [2]
Cardiotoxicity [28]
Congestive heart failure (2–7%) [7]
Hypertension (4%) [3]
Myocardial toxicity [3]
Palpitation (3%)
Tachycardia (5%)

Central Nervous System
Anorexia (14%) [4]
Chills (5–32%) [8]
Depression (6%)
Fever (6–36%) [7]
Headache (10–26%) [2]
Insomnia (14%)
Neurotoxicity [4]
Pain (47%) [2]
Paresthesias (2–9%)
Peripheral neuropathy [6]
Vertigo (dizziness) (4–13%)

Neuromuscular/Skeletal
Arthralgia (6–8%) [4]
Asthenia (fatigue) (5–47%) [19]
Back pain (5–22%)
Bone or joint pain (3–7%)
Muscle spasm (3%)
Myalgia/Myopathy (4%) [3]

Gastrointestinal/Hepatic
Abdominal pain (2–22%)
Constipation (2%)
Diarrhea (7–25%) [32]
Dyspepsia (2%)
Hepatotoxicity [8]
Nausea (6–33%) [9]
Vomiting (4–23%) [4]

Respiratory
Cough (5–26%)
Dyspnea (3–22%)
Flu-like syndrome (10%) [3]
Influenza (4%)
Nasopharyngitis (8%)
Pharyngitis (12%)
Pharyngolaryngeal pain (2%)
Pneumonia [3]
Pneumonitis [2]
Pulmonary toxicity [4]
Rhinitis (2–14%)
Sinusitis (2–9%)
Upper respiratory tract infection (3%)

Endocrine/Metabolic
ALT increased [7]
Appetite decreased [2]
AST increased [3]
Hyperbilirubinemia [2]
Hyperglycemia [4]

Genitourinary
Urinary tract infection (3–5%)

Hematologic
Anemia (4%) [7]
Febrile neutropenia [16]
Leukopenia (3%) [11]
Neutropenia [33]
Thrombocytopenia [6]

Local
Infusion-related reactions [4]
Injection-site reactions (21–40%) [6]

Other
Adverse effects [6]
Allergic reactions (3%) [2]
Death [5]
Infection (20%) [3]

TRASTUZUMAB EMTANSINE

Synonym: T-DM1
Trade name: Kadcyla (Genentech)
Indications: HER2-positive, metastatic breast cancer in patients who previously received trastuzumab and a taxane, separately or in combination
Class: Antibody drug conjugate (ADC), HER2-targeted antibody-drug conjugate
Half-life: 4 days
Clinically important, potentially hazardous interactions with: none known
Pregnancy category: D
Important contra-indications noted in the prescribing guidelines for: nursing mothers; pediatric patients
Warning: HEPATOTOXICITY, CARDIAC TOXICITY, EMBRYO-FETAL TOXICITY

Skin
Hypersensitivity (2%)
Peripheral edema (7%)
Pruritus (6%)
Rash (12%)
Telangiectasia [2]

Mucosal
Epistaxis (nosebleed) (23%) [2]
Stomatitis (14%)
Xerostomia (17%)

Cardiovascular
Cardiotoxicity [2]
Hypertension (5%)

Central Nervous System
Chills (8%)
Dysgeusia (taste perversion) (8%)
Fever (19%) [2]
Headache (28%) [4]
Insomnia (12%)
Peripheral neuropathy (21%) [2]
Vertigo (dizziness) (10%)

Neuromuscular/Skeletal
Arthralgia (19%) [3]
Asthenia (fatigue) (18–36%) [13]
Bone or joint pain (36%)
Myalgia/Myopathy (14%)

Gastrointestinal/Hepatic
Abdominal pain (19%)
Constipation (27%) [3]
Diarrhea (24%) [6]
Dyspepsia (9%)
Hepatotoxicity [15]
Nausea (40%) [10]
Vomiting (19%)

Respiratory
Cough (18%)
Dyspnea (12%)
Pneumonia [3]

Endocrine/Metabolic
ALP increased (5%)
ALT increased (82%) [4]
AST increased (98%) [7]
Hypokalemia (10%) [3]

Genitourinary
Urinary tract infection (9%)

Hematologic
Anemia (14%) [7]
Febrile neutropenia [3]
Hemorrhage (32%) [2]
Neutropenia (7%) [5]
Thrombocytopenia (31%) [25]

Ocular
Conjunctivitis (4%)
Lacrimation (3%)
Vision blurred (5%)
Xerophthalmia (4%)

Other
Adverse effects [5]
Death [3]

TRAVOPROST

Trade names: Izba (Alcon), Travatan (Alcon), Travatan Z (Alcon)
Indications: Reduction of elevated intraocular pressure in open-angle glaucoma or ocular hypertension
Class: Prostaglandin analog
Half-life: N/A
Clinically important, potentially hazardous interactions with: none known
Pregnancy category: C
Important contra-indications noted in the prescribing guidelines for: nursing mothers; pediatric patients

---

Cardiovascular
Angina (<5%)
Bradycardia (<5%)
Chest pain (<5%)
Hypertension (<5%) [2]
Hypotension (<5%)

Central Nervous System
Anxiety (<5%)
Depression (<5%)
Dysgeusia (taste perversion) [3]
Headache (<5%)
Pain (<5%)

Neuromuscular/Skeletal
Arthralgia (<5%)
Back pain (<5%)

Gastrointestinal/Hepatic
Dyspepsia (<5%)
Gastrointestinal disorder (<5%)
Nausea [2]

Respiratory
Bronchitis (<5%)
Flu-like syndrome (<5%)
Sinusitis (<5%)

Endocrine/Metabolic
Hypercholesterolemia (<5%)

Genitourinary
Prostatitis (<5%)
Urinary incontinence (<5%)
Urinary tract infection (<5%)

Ocular
Abnormal vision (<4%)
Blepharitis (<4%)
Cataract (<4%)
Conjunctival hyperemia [10]
Conjunctivitis (<4%)
Corneal staining (<4%)
Deepening of upper lid sulcus [7]
Eyelashes – hypertrichosis [3]
Eyelid crusting (<4%)
Foreign body sensation (5–10%)
Iris pigmentation (<4%) [2]
Keratitis (<4%)
Lacrimation (<4%)
Ocular adverse effects [4]
Ocular hemorrhage (35–50%)
Ocular hyperemia [7]
Ocular inflammation (<4%)
Ocular pain (5–10%)
Ocular pigmentation (<5%) [4]
Ocular pruritus (5–10%) [6]
Ocular stinging (5–10%)
Photophobia (<4%)
Reduced visual acuity (5–10%)
Subconjunctival hemorrhage (<4%)
Uveitis [5]
Vision blurred [2]
Xerophthalmia (<4%)

Other
Allergic reactions (<5%)
Infection (<5%)

TRAZODONE

Trade names: Desyrel (Bristol-Myers Squibb), Oleptro (Angelini)
Indications: Depression
Class: Antidepressant, tricyclic, Serotonin reuptake inhibitor
Half-life: 3–6 hours
Clinically important, potentially hazardous interactions with: amiodarone, amprenavir, atazanavir, boceprevir, citalopram, cobicistat/elvitegravir/emtricitabine/tenofovir alafenamide, cobicistat/elvitegravir/emtricitabine/tenofovir disoproxil, darunavir, delavirdine, fluoxetine, fluvoxamine, ginkgo biloba, indinavir, linezolid, lopinavir, MAO inhibitors, nefazodone, paroxetine hydrochloride, sertraline, tapentadol, telaprevir, tipranavir, venlafaxine
Pregnancy category: C
Important contra-indications noted in the prescribing guidelines for: nursing mothers; pediatric patients
Warning: SUICIDALITY IN CHILDREN AND ADOLESCENTS

Skin
Edema (<10%)
Exanthems [6]
Photosensitivity [2]
Psoriasis (exacerbation) [2]
Urticaria [3]

Hair
Alopecia [2]

Mucosal
Xerostomia (>10%) [6]

Cardiovascular
Arrhythmias [2]
QT prolongation [2]

Central Nervous System
Dysgeusia (taste perversion) (>10%)
Headache [3]
Sedation (>5%)
Serotonin syndrome [7]
Somnolence (drowsiness) (>5%) [3]
Tremor (<10%)
Vertigo (dizziness) (>5%) [4]

Neuromuscular/Skeletal
Myalgia/Myopathy (<10%)

Gastrointestinal/Hepatic
Constipation (>5%)
Nausea [2]

Genitourinary
Priapism (12%) [23]
Sexual dysfunction [2]

Ocular
Vision blurred (>5%)

TRETINOIN

Synonyms: all-trans-retinoic acid; ATRA
Trade names: Aknemycin Plus (EM Industries), Renova (Ortho), Retin-A Micro (Ortho), Solage (Galderma), Vesanoid (Roche)
Indications: Acne vulgaris, skin aging, facial roughness, fine wrinkles, hyperpigmentation [T], acute promyelocytic leukemia [O]
Class: Antineoplastic, Retinoid
Half-life: 0.5–2 hours
Clinically important, potentially hazardous interactions with: aldesleukin, bexarotene
Pregnancy category: D (category B (topical), category C (oral), category D in third trimester)
Important contra-indications noted in the prescribing guidelines for: nursing mothers; pediatric patients
Note: Oral retinoids can cause birth defects, and women should avoid tretinoin when pregnant or trying to conceive. Avoid prolonged exposure to sunlight.
[T] = Topical; [O] = Oral.

Skin
Bullous dermatitis [2]
Burning [O][T] (10–40%) [20]
Cellulitis [O] (<10%)
Crusting [2]
Dermatitis [7]
Desquamation (14%)
Diaphoresis (20%)
Differentiation syndrome [O] (25%) [19]
Edema (29%) [8]
Erythema [O][T] (<49%) [19]
Erythema nodosum [4]
Exfoliative dermatitis [O] (8%) [3]
Facial edema [O] (<10%)
Flaking [O] (23%)
Hyperkeratosis [O] (78%)
Hypomelanosis (5%) [2]
Pallor [O] (<10%)
Palmar–plantar desquamation [O] (<10%)
Peeling [4]
Photosensitivity [O][T] (10%) [3]
Pigmentation (5%) [3]
Pruritus [O][T] (5–40%) [14]
Rash [O][T] (54%) [3]
Scaling (10–40%) [16]
Stinging (<26%) [8]
Sweet's syndrome [21]
Ulcerations (scrotal) [9]
Vasculitis [2]
Xerosis [O] (49–100%) [19]

Hair
Alopecia areata [O] (14%)

Nails
Pyogenic granuloma [3]

Mucosal
Cheilitis [O] (10%)
Xerostomia [O] (10%)

Cardiovascular
Phlebitis (11%)

Central Nervous System
Depression [O] (14%)
Fever [O] [6]
Headache [3]
Intracranial pressure increased [2]

Pain [O] (37%)
Paresthesias [O] (17%)
Pseudotumor cerebri [O] [11]
Shivering [O] (63%)
Tremor [O] (<10%)

Neuromuscular/Skeletal
Arthralgia [O] (10%) [3]
Bone or joint pain [O] (77%) [3]
Myalgia/Myopathy (14%) [3]

Gastrointestinal/Hepatic
Hepatotoxicity [3]
Pancreatitis [2]

Hematologic
Hemorrhage [2]

Ocular
Diplopia [2]
Ocular pigmentation [O] (<10%)
Ocular pruritus [O] (10%)
Xerophthalmia [O] (<10%) [2]

Local
Injection-site reactions (17%)

Other
Death [O] [2]
Infection [O] (58%)

TRIAMTERENE

Trade names: Dyazide (GSK), Dyrenium (Concordia)
Indications: Edema
Class: Diuretic, potassium-sparing
Half-life: 1–2 hours
Clinically important, potentially hazardous interactions with: ACE inhibitors, acemetacin, benazepril, captopril, cyclosporine, enalapril, fosinopril, indomethacin, lisinopril, metformin, moexipril, potassium iodide, potassium salts, quinapril, ramipril, spironolactone, trandolapril, zofenopril
Pregnancy category: C
Important contra-indications noted in the prescribing guidelines for: nursing mothers; pediatric patients
Note: Dyazide and Maxzide are triamterene and hydrochlorothiazide. Hydrochlorothiazide is a sulfonamide and can be absorbed systemically. Sulfonamides can produce severe, possibly fatal, reactions such as toxic epidermal necrolysis and Stevens-Johnson syndrome.

Skin
Edema (<10%)
Lupus erythematosus (with hydrochlorothiazide) [2]
Photosensitivity [2]
Rash (<10%)

TRIFLURIDINE & TIPIRACIL

Trade name: Lonsurf (Monarch)
Indications: Metastatic colorectal cancer in patients who have been previously treated with fluoropyrimidine-, oxaliplatin-and irinotecan-based chemotherapy, an anti-VEGF biological therapy, and if RAS wild-type, an anti-EGFR therapy
Class: Antineoplastic, Thymidine phosphorylase inhibitor, Thymidine-based nucleoside analogue
Half-life: 2 hours
Clinically important, potentially hazardous interactions with: none known
Pregnancy category: N/A (Can cause fetal harm)
Important contra-indications noted in the prescribing guidelines for: nursing mothers; pediatric patients
Note: See also separate entry for trifluridine.

Hair
Alopecia (7%)

Mucosal
Stomatitis (8%)

Central Nervous System
Dysgeusia (taste perversion) (7%)
Fever (19%)

Neuromuscular/Skeletal
Asthenia (fatigue) (52%) [3]

Gastrointestinal/Hepatic
Abdominal pain (21%) [2]
Diarrhea (32%) [2]
Nausea (48%) [3]
Vomiting (28%)

Respiratory
Nasopharyngitis (4%)
Pulmonary embolism (2%)

Endocrine/Metabolic
Appetite decreased (39%)

Genitourinary
Urinary tract infection (4%)

Hematologic
Anemia (77%) [7]
Febrile neutropenia [3]
Granulocytopenia [3]
Leukopenia [7]
Neutropenia (67%) [9]
Thrombocytopenia (42%) [3]

Other
Adverse effects [2]
Infection (27%)

TRIMETHOPRIM

Trade names: Bactrim (Women First), Septra (Monarch)
Indications: Various urinary tract infections caused by susceptible organisms, acute otitis media in children, acute and chronic bronchitis
Class: Antibiotic
Half-life: 8–10 hours
Clinically important, potentially hazardous interactions with: ACE inhibitors, amantadine, angiotensin II receptor antagonists, antidiabetics, azathioprine, benazepril, captopril, carvedilol, cilazapril, conivaptan, coumarins, cyclosporine, CYP2C8 substrates, CYP2C9 inhibitors, CYP3A4 inducers, dapsone, deferasirox, digoxin, dofetilide, enalapril, eplerenone, fosinopril, irbesartan, lamivudine, leucovorin, levoleucovorin, lisinopril, memantine, mercaptopurine, metformin, methotrexate, olmesartan, oral typhoid vaccine, PEG-interferon, phenytoin, pioglitazone, pralatrexate, procainamide, pyrimethamine, quinapril, ramipril, repaglinide, rifampin, sulfonylureas, trandolapril
Pregnancy category: C
Important contra-indications noted in the prescribing guidelines for: nursing mothers
Note: Although trimethoprim has been known to elicit occasional adverse reactions by itself, it is most commonly used in conjunction with sulfamethoxazole (co-trimoxazole - see separate entry).

Skin
DRESS syndrome [2]
Fixed eruption [6]
Pruritus (<10%)
Rash (3–7%)
Stevens-Johnson syndrome [6]
Toxic epidermal necrolysis [3]

Central Nervous System
Aseptic meningitis [3]

Neuromuscular/Skeletal
Rhabdomyolysis [3]

Gastrointestinal/Hepatic
Hepatotoxicity [2]

Endocrine/Metabolic
Hyperkalemia [3]
Hyponatremia [2]

Hematologic
Anemia [2]
Thrombocytopenia [2]

TRIMIPRAMINE

Trade name: Surmontil (Odyssey)
Indications: Major depression
Class: Antidepressant, tricyclic
Half-life: 20–26 hours
Clinically important, potentially hazardous interactions with: amprenavir, arbutamine, bupropion, clonidine, epinephrine, formoterol, guanethidine, isocarboxazid, linezolid, MAO inhibitors, phenelzine, quinolones, sparfloxacin, tranylcypromine, venlafaxine

Pregnancy category: C
Important contra-indications noted in the prescribing guidelines for: pediatric patients
Warning: SUICIDALITY AND ANTIDEPRESSANT DRUGS

Skin
Diaphoresis (<10%)
Mucosal
Xerostomia (>10%) [2]
Cardiovascular
QT prolongation [2]
Central Nervous System
Dysgeusia (taste perversion) (>10%)
Parkinsonism (<10%)
Seizures [4]

TURMERIC

Family: Zingiberaceae
Scientific names: *Curcuma aromatica, Curcuma domestica, Curcuma longa, Curcuma xanthorrhiza*
Indications: Arthritis, anticarcinogen, stimulant, carminative, amenorrhea, angina, asthma, colorectal cancer, delirium, diarrhea, dyspepsia, flatulence, hemorrhage, hepatitis, hypercholesterolemia, hypertension, jaundice, mania, menstrual disorders, ophthalmia, tendonitis. **Topical:** conjuctivitis, skin cancer, smallpox, chickenpox, leg ulcers. Food coloring in cheese, margarine, sweets, snack foods, cosmetics, essential oil in perfumes, culinary spice
Class: Anti-inflammatory, TNF inhibitor
Half-life: N/A
Clinically important, potentially hazardous interactions with: none known
Pregnancy category: N/A
Note: Persons with symptoms of gallstones or obstruction of bile passages should avoid turmeric.

Skin
Dermatitis [6]
Rash [3]
Central Nervous System
Headache [2]
Gastrointestinal/Hepatic
Abdominal pain [2]
Diarrhea [6]
Nausea [2]
Other
Adverse effects [4]

TYPHOID VACCINE

Trade names: Typherix (GSK), Typhim Vi (Sanofi Pasteur), Vivotif (Berna Biotech)
Indications: Immunization against typhoid fever
Class: Vaccine
Half-life: N/A
Clinically important, potentially hazardous interactions with: alcohol, antibiotics, antimalarials, atovaquone/proguanil, azathioprine, belimumab, cefixime, ceftaroline fosamil, ceftobiprole, chloroquine, ciprofloxacin, corticosteroids, daptomycin, fingolimod, gemifloxacin, hydroxychloroquine, immunosuppressants, interferon gamma, leflunomide, mefloquine, mercaptopurine, sulfonamides, telavancin, tigecycline, tinidazole, tocilizumab, ustekinumab
Pregnancy category: C
Important contra-indications noted in the prescribing guidelines for: nursing mothers; pediatric patients
Note: Vivotif is a live oral vaccine.

Skin
Anaphylactoid reactions/Anaphylaxis [2]
Central Nervous System
Fever (<3%) [5]
Headache (5–20%) [3]
Myelitis [2]
Neuromuscular/Skeletal
Asthenia (fatigue) (4–24%) [3]
Myalgia/Myopathy (3–7%) [3]
Gastrointestinal/Hepatic
Abdominal pain (6%) [2]
Diarrhea (<3%)
Nausea (2–8%)
Vomiting (2%)
Local
Injection-site edema [3]
Injection-site erythema (4–5%) [2]
Injection-site induration (5–15%)
Injection-site pain (27–41%) [5]
Other
Adverse effects [4]
Death [2]

UMECLIDINIUM

Trade name: Incruse (GSK)
Indications: Chronic obstructive pulmonary disease (COPD)
Class: Anticholinergic, Muscarinic antagonist
Half-life: 11 hours
Clinically important, potentially hazardous interactions with: anticholinergics
Pregnancy category: C
Important contra-indications noted in the prescribing guidelines for: nursing mothers; pediatric patients

---

Mucosal
Oropharyngeal pain [2]
Cardiovascular
Angina [2]
Arrhythmias [2]
Extrasystoles [3]
Hypertension [3]
Supraventricular tachycardia [2]
Tachycardia [2]
Central Nervous System
Dysgeusia (taste perversion) [3]
Headache [12]
Neuromuscular/Skeletal
Arthralgia (2%) [2]
Back pain [5]
Gastrointestinal/Hepatic
Constipation [2]
Respiratory
Bronchitis [2]
COPD (exacerbation) [5]
Cough (3%) [6]
Dysphonia [4]
Influenza [2]
Nasopharyngitis (8%) [12]
Pharyngitis [2]
Pneumonia [4]
Sinusitis [3]
Upper respiratory tract infection [5]
Genitourinary
Urinary tract infection [2]
Other
Adverse effects [4]

URSODIOL

Synonyms: ursodeoxycholic acid; UDCA
Trade names: Actigall (Watson), Destolit (Norgine), Urdox (Wockhardt), Urso 250 (Aptalis), Urso Forte (Aptalis), Ursogal (Galen)
Indications: The dissolution of radiolucent (i.e. non-radio opaque) cholesterol gallstones in patients with a functioning gallbladder, primary biliary cirrhosis, biliary calculus, cholelithiasis
Class: Cholesterol antagonist, Urolithic
Half-life: 100 hours
Clinically important, potentially hazardous interactions with: aluminum based antacids, aluminum hydroxide, charcoal, cholestyramine, clofibrate, colestimide, colestipol, cyclosporine, dapsone, estradiol, estrogens, nitrendipine, oral contraceptives, P4503A substrates
Pregnancy category: B
Important contra-indications noted in the prescribing guidelines for: the elderly; nursing mothers; pediatric patients

---

Skin
Lichenoid eruption [3]
Pruritus [3]
Rash (3%)
Hair
Alopecia (<5%)
Cardiovascular
Chest pain (3%)
Central Nervous System
Headache (18–25%)
Insomnia (2%)
Vertigo (dizziness) (17%)
Neuromuscular/Skeletal
Arthralgia (7%)
Asthenia (fatigue) (3–7%)
Back pain (7–12%)
Bone or joint pain (6%)
Myalgia/Myopathy (5%)
Gastrointestinal/Hepatic
Abdominal pain (43%)
Cholecystitis (5%)
Constipation (26%)
Diarrhea (27%) [4]
Dyspepsia (16%) [2]
Flatulence (7%)
Nausea (14%) [4]
Vomiting (9–14%) [3]

Respiratory
Bronchitis (6%)
Cough (7%)
Flu-like syndrome (6%)
Pharyngitis (8%)
Rhinitis (5%)
Sinusitis (5–11%)
Upper respiratory tract infection (12–15%)

Endocrine/Metabolic
Weight gain [2]

Genitourinary
Dysmenorrhea (5%)
Urinary tract infection (6%)

Hematologic
Leukopenia (3%)

Other
Adverse effects [3]
Allergic reactions (5%)
Infection (viral) (9–19%)

USTEKINUMAB

Trade name: Stelara (Centocor)
Indications: Plaque psoriasis (moderate to severe), active psoriatic arthritis, active Crohn's disease (moderate to severe)
Class: Interleukin-12/23 antagonist, Monoclonal antibody
Half-life: 15–32 days
Clinically important, potentially hazardous interactions with: live vaccines
Pregnancy category: B
Important contra-indications noted in the prescribing guidelines for: nursing mothers; pediatric patients

---

Skin
Cellulitis (<10%)
Herpes zoster [2]
Malignancies [2]
Pruritus (<10%)
Psoriasis [3]

Mucosal
Nasal congestion (<10%)

Cardiovascular
Cardiotoxicity [3]

Central Nervous System
Depression (<10%)
Headache (<10%) [9]
Leukoencephalopathy [3]
Vertigo (dizziness) (<10%)

Neuromuscular/Skeletal
Arthralgia [3]
Asthenia (fatigue) (<10%) [3]
Back pain (<10%)
Myalgia/Myopathy (<10%)
Psoriatic arthralgia [2]

Gastrointestinal/Hepatic
Diarrhea (<10%)
Hepatotoxicity [3]

Respiratory
Nasopharyngitis (10%) [12]
Pharyngolaryngeal pain (<10%)
Tuberculosis [2]
Upper respiratory tract infection (10%) [9]

Local
Injection-site reactions [7]

Other
Adverse effects [11]
Infection [12]

VALACYCLOVIR

Trade name: Valtrex (GSK)
Indications: Genital herpes, herpes simplex, herpes zoster
Class: Antiviral, Guanine nucleoside analog
Half-life: 3 hours
Clinically important, potentially hazardous interactions with: cobicistat/elvitegravir/emtricitabine/tenofovir alafenamide, cobicistat/elvitegravir/emtricitabine/tenofovir disoproxil, immunosuppressants, meperidine, tenofovir disoproxil
Pregnancy category: B
Important contra-indications noted in the prescribing guidelines for: the elderly; pediatric patients

---

Central Nervous System
Hallucinations [2]
Headache [5]
Neurotoxicity [4]

Gastrointestinal/Hepatic
Abdominal pain [2]
Nausea [4]
Vomiting [3]

Renal
Nephrotoxicity [3]

VALBENAZINE

Trade name: Ingrezza (Neurocrine Biosciences)
Indications: Tardive dyskinesia
Class: Vesicular monoamine transporter 2 inhibitor
Half-life: 15–22 hours
Clinically important, potentially hazardous interactions with: carbamazepine, clarithromycin, digoxin, fluoxetine, isocarboxazid, itraconazole, ketoconazole, MAO inhibitors, paroxetine hydrochloride, phenelzine, phenytoin, quinidine, rifampin, selegiline, St John's wort, strong CYP2D6 inducers, strong CYP3A4 inducers or inhibitors
Pregnancy category: N/A (May cause fetal harm)
Important contra-indications noted in the prescribing guidelines for: nursing mothers; pediatric patients

---

Mucosal
Xerostomia (<5%) [2]

Central Nervous System
Akathisia (<3%)
Depression [2]
Gait instability (<4%)
Headache (3%) [6]
Impaired concentration (<5%)
Restlessness (<3%)
Sedation (<11%)
Somnolence (drowsiness) (<11%) [5]
Suicidal ideation [2]
Vertigo (dizziness) (<4%) [2]

Neuromuscular/Skeletal
Arthralgia (2%)
Asthenia (fatigue) (<11%) [6]

Gastrointestinal/Hepatic
Constipation (<5%) [2]
Diarrhea [2]
Nausea (2%) [3]
Vomiting (3%)

Endocrine/Metabolic
Appetite decreased [2]

Genitourinary
Urinary retention (<5%)
Urinary tract infection [3]

Ocular
Vision blurred (<5%)

VALERIAN

Family: Valerianaceae
Scientific names: *Valeriana edulis, Valeriana jatamansii, Valeriana officinalis, Valeriana sitchensis, Valeriana wallichii*
Indications: Depression, tremors, epilepsy, attention deficit hyperactivity disorder, rheumatism, nervous asthma, gastric spasms, colic, menstrual cramps, hot flashes. Flavoring in foods and beverages
Class: Anxiolytic
Half-life: N/A
Clinically important, potentially hazardous interactions with: amitriptyline, escitalopram, eszopiclone
Pregnancy category: N/A

Central Nervous System
Somnolence (drowsiness) [2]
Tremor [2]

Gastrointestinal/Hepatic
Hepatotoxicity [2]

Other
Adverse effects [2]

VALGANCICLOVIR

Trade name: Valcyte (Roche)
Indications: Cytomegalovirus retinitis (CMV) in patients with AIDS, prevention of CMV disease in high-risk transplant patients
Class: Antiviral, Guanine nucleoside analog
Half-life: 4 hours (in severe renal impairment up to 68%)
Clinically important, potentially hazardous interactions with: abacavir, cobicistat/elvitegravir/emtricitabine/tenofovir alafenamide, cobicistat/elvitegravir/emtricitabine/tenofovir disoproxil, emtricitabine, tenofovir disoproxil
Pregnancy category: N/A (May cause fetal toxicity based on findings in animal studies)
Important contra-indications noted in the prescribing guidelines for: nursing mothers
Note: Valganciclovir is rapidly converted to ganciclovir in the body.

Warning: HEMATOLOGIC TOXICITY, IMPAIRMENT OF FERTILITY, FETAL TOXICITY, MUTAGENESIS AND CARCINOGENESIS

Mucosal
Oral candidiasis [2]

Central Nervous System
Fever [3]
Headache [2]
Neurotoxicity [2]
Paresthesias (8%)

Hematologic
Neutropenia [9]

Other
Allergic reactions (<5%)
Infection (<5%)

VALPROIC ACID

Synonyms: valproate sodium; divalproex
Trade names: Depacon (AbbVie), Depakene (AbbVie), Depakote (AbbVie)
Indications: Seizures, migraine
Class: Anticonvulsant, Antipsychotic
Half-life: 6–16 hours
Clinically important, potentially hazardous interactions with: amitriptyline, aspirin, ceftobiprole, cholestyramine, clobazam, clozapine, doripenem, eslicarbazepine, ethosuximide, indinavir, ivermectin, lesinurad, levomepromazine, meropenem & vaborbactam, olanzapine, oxcarbazepine, paliperidone, risperidone, rufinamide, temozolomide, tipranavir, vorinostat, zidovudine, zinc, zuclopenthixol
Pregnancy category: D
Warning: LIFE THREATENING ADVERSE REACTIONS

Skin
Anticonvulsant hypersensitivity syndrome [6]
DRESS syndrome [10]
Ecchymoses (<5%) [4]
Edema [3]
Erythema multiforme [3]
Erythroderma [3]
Exanthems (5%) [3]
Facial edema (>5%)
Furunculosis (<5%)
Hypersensitivity [5]
Lupus erythematosus [5]
Peripheral edema (<5%)
Petechiae (<5%)
Pruritus (>5%)
Pseudolymphoma [2]
Purpura [2]
Rash (>5%) [7]
Stevens-Johnson syndrome [12]
Toxic epidermal necrolysis [9]
Vasculitis [3]

Hair
Alopecia (7%) [23]
Curly hair [6]
Hirsutism [2]

Nails
Nail pigmentation [2]

Mucosal
Gingival hyperplasia/hypertrophy [8]
Glossitis (<5%)
Stomatitis (<5%)
Xerostomia (<5%) [2]

Central Nervous System
Brain atrophy [2]
Cerebral edema [2]
Cognitive impairment [2]
Coma [3]
Confusion [2]
Delirium [2]
Dysgeusia (taste perversion) (<5%)
Encephalopathy [21]
Gait instability [2]
Headache [2]
Neurotoxicity [4]
Paresthesias (<5%)
Parkinsonism [15]
Sedation [3]
Seizures [10]
Somnolence (drowsiness) [11]
Tremor [15]
Vertigo (dizziness) [7]

Neuromuscular/Skeletal
Asthenia (fatigue) [4]
Osteoporosis [3]
Rhabdomyolysis [3]

Gastrointestinal/Hepatic
Constipation [2]
Dyspepsia [2]
Hepatic steatosis [2]
Hepatotoxicity [19]
Nausea [5]
Pancreatitis [32]
Vomiting [3]

Respiratory
Pleural effusion [3]
Pneumonitis [2]

Endocrine/Metabolic
Acute intermittent porphyria [2]
Appetite increased [2]
Hyperammonemia [22]
Hyponatremia [2]
Metabolic syndrome [3]
Porphyria [2]
SIADH [6]
Weight gain [23]

Genitourinary
Vaginitis (<5%)

Renal
Enuresis [2]
Fanconi syndrome [4]

Hematologic
Bone marrow suppression [4]
Coagulopathy [2]
Eosinophilia [2]
Hemotoxicity [3]
Neutropenia [3]
Thrombocytopenia [4]

Otic
Hearing loss [2]

Ocular
Ocular adverse effects [2]

Other
Adverse effects [8]
Allergic reactions (<5%)
Congenital malformations [4]
Death [8]
Teratogenicity [31]

VALSARTAN

Trade names: Byvalson (Forest), Diovan (Novartis), Diovan HCT (Novartis), Exforge (Novartis), Valturna (Novartis)
Indications: Hypertension
Class: Angiotensin II receptor antagonist (blocker), Antihypertensive
Half-life: 9 hours
Clinically important, potentially hazardous interactions with: none known
Pregnancy category: D
Important contra-indications noted in the prescribing guidelines for: nursing mothers; pediatric patients
Note: Byvalson is valsartan and nebivolol; Exforge is valsartan and amlodipine; Valturna is valsartan and aliskiren; Diovan HCT is valsartan and hydrochlorothiazide. Hydrochlorothiazide is a sulfonamide and can be absorbed systemically. Sulfonamides can produce severe, possibly fatal, reactions such as toxic epidermal necrolysis and Stevens-Johnson syndrome.
See also separate profile for Sacubitril/Valsartan.
Warning: FETAL TOXICITY

Skin
Angioedema (>2%) [9]
Edema [5]
Peripheral edema [3]
Photosensitivity [3]
Pruritus (>2%)
Pseudolymphoma [2]
Rash (>2%)

Mucosal
Aphthous stomatitis (<10%)
Xerostomia (>10%)

Cardiovascular
Hypotension [2]

Central Nervous System
Dysgeusia (taste perversion) (>10%)
Headache [7]
Paresthesias (>2%)
Vertigo (dizziness) [9]

Neuromuscular/Skeletal
Arthralgia (<10%)
Myalgia/Myopathy (10–29%)

Gastrointestinal/Hepatic
Enteropathy [2]

Respiratory
Cough [2]
Nasopharyngitis [3]
Upper respiratory tract infection [2]

Endocrine/Metabolic
Hyperkalemia [3]

Other
Adverse effects [5]
Allergic reactions (>2%)

VANCOMYCIN

Trade name: Vancocin (Lilly)
Indications: Various infections caused by susceptible organisms
Class: Antibiotic, glycopeptide
Half-life: 5–11 hours
Clinically important, potentially hazardous interactions with: meloxicam, metformin, pentamidine, rocuronium, succinylcholine, teicoplanin, trospium
Pregnancy category: C

Skin
- Abscess [2]
- AGEP [8]
- Anaphylactoid reactions/Anaphylaxis [14]
- Angioedema [3]
- Bullous dermatitis [5]
- Cellulitis [3]
- DRESS syndrome [20]
- Erythema multiforme [5]
- Exanthems [16]
- Exfoliative dermatitis [4]
- Fixed eruption [2]
- Flushing (<10%)
- Hypersensitivity [8]
- Leukocytoclastic vasculitis [4]
- Linear IgA bullous dermatosis [50]
- Lupus erythematosus [2]
- Pruritus [12]
- Rash [20]
- Red man syndrome (<14%) [52]
- Red neck syndrome [2]
- Stevens-Johnson syndrome [10]
- Toxic epidermal necrolysis [10]
- Urticaria [8]
- Vasculitis [2]

Cardiovascular
- Cardiac arrest [2]
- Extravasation [2]
- Hypotension [3]
- Phlebitis (14–23%) [6]

Central Nervous System
- Chills (>10%) [2]
- Dysgeusia (taste perversion) (>10%)
- Fever [8]
- Headache [5]
- Vertigo (dizziness) [2]

Gastrointestinal/Hepatic
- Constipation [3]
- Diarrhea [7]
- Gastrointestinal disorder [2]
- Nausea [12]
- Vomiting [6]

Endocrine/Metabolic
- ALT increased [2]
- AST increased [3]

Renal
- Nephrotoxicity [34]
- Renal failure [4]

Hematologic
- Agranulocytosis [2]
- Anemia [2]
- Eosinophilia [3]
- Leukopenia [2]
- Neutropenia [9]
- Thrombocytopenia [17]

Otic
- Ototoxicity [5]
- Tinnitus [2]

Local
- Infusion-related reactions [2]
- Injection-site extravasation [2]

Other
- Adverse effects [7]
- Allergic reactions (<5%) [5]
- Death [6]

VANDETANIB

Trade name: Caprelsa (AstraZeneca)
Indications: Medullary thyroid cancer
Class: Tyrosine kinase inhibitor
Half-life: 19 days
Clinically important, potentially hazardous interactions with: amiodarone, amoxapine, antiarrhythmics, arsenic, carbamazepine, chloroquine, clarithromycin, CYP3A4 inducers, dexamethasone, disopyramide, dofetilide, dolasetron, efavirenz, granisetron, haloperidol, methadone, moxifloxacin, pazopanib, phenobarbital, phenytoin, pimozide, procainamide, QT prolonging agents, rifabutin, rifampin, rifapentine, sotalol, St John's wort, telavancin
Pregnancy category: D
Important contra-indications noted in the prescribing guidelines for: nursing mothers; pediatric patients
Note: Contra-indicated in patients with congenital long QT syndrome.
Warning: QT PROLONGATION, TORSADES DE POINTES, AND SUDDEN DEATH

Skin
- Acneform eruption (35%) [4]
- Folliculitis [5]
- Hand–foot syndrome [4]
- Photosensitivity (13%) [8]
- Phototoxicity [3]
- Pigmentation [6]
- Pruritus (11%) [2]
- Rash (53%) [34]
- Stevens-Johnson syndrome [4]
- Toxicity [9]
- Xerosis (15%) [3]

Hair
- Hair changes [2]

Nails
- Paronychia [5]
- Splinter hemorrhage [2]

Mucosal
- Mucositis [2]
- Stomatitis [2]

Cardiovascular
- Hypertension (33%) [24]
- QT prolongation (14%) [25]

Central Nervous System
- Anorexia [3]
- Depression (10%)
- Headache (26%) [4]
- Insomnia (13%)
- Neurotoxicity [2]

Neuromuscular/Skeletal
- Asthenia (fatigue) (15–24%) [17]

Gastrointestinal/Hepatic
- Abdominal pain (21%)
- Constipation [2]
- Diarrhea (57%) [44]
- Dyspepsia (11%)
- Hepatotoxicity [4]
- Nausea (33%) [14]
- Vomiting (15%) [6]

Respiratory
- Cough (11%)
- Dyspnea [3]
- Nasopharyngitis (11%)

Endocrine/Metabolic
- ALT increased (51%) [2]
- Appetite decreased (21%) [3]
- Hypocalcemia (11%)
- Hypothyroidism [2]
- Thyroid dysfunction [2]
- Weight loss (10%) [2]

Renal
- Proteinuria (10%) [2]

Hematologic
- Anemia [3]
- Hemorrhage [2]
- Hemotoxicity [2]
- Myelosuppression [2]
- Neutropenia [5]
- Platelets decreased (9%)

Other
- Adverse effects [6]
- Death [3]

VARDENAFIL

Trade name: Levitra (Bayer)
Indications: Erectile dysfunction
Class: Phosphodiesterase type 5 (PDE5) inhibitor
Half-life: 4–5 hours
Clinically important, potentially hazardous interactions with: alfuzosin, alpha blockers, amyl nitrite, antifungals, antihypertensives, atazanavir, boceprevir, bosentan, cobicistat/elvitegravir/emtricitabine/tenofovir alafenamide, cobicistat/elvitegravir/emtricitabine/tenofovir disoproxil, conivaptan, CYP3A4 inhibitors, darunavir, dasatinib, disopyramide, doxazosin, erythromycin, etravirine, fosamprenavir, grapefruit juice, high-fat foods, indinavir, itraconazole, ketoconazole, lopinavir, macrolide antibiotics, nelfinavir, nicorandil, nifedipine, nitrates, nitroglycerin, nitroprusside, phosphodiesterase 5 inhibitors, protease inhibitors, riociguat, ritonavir, sapropterin, saquinavir, tamsulosin, telaprevir, terazosin, tipranavir
Pregnancy category: B (not indicated for use in women)
Important contra-indications noted in the prescribing guidelines for: pediatric patients

---

Skin
- Anaphylactoid reactions/Anaphylaxis (<2%)
- Angioedema (<2%)
- Diaphoresis (<2%)
- Erythema (<2%)

Facial edema (<2%)
Flushing (11%) [14]
Photosensitivity (<2%)
Pruritus (<2%)
Rash (<2%)

Mucosal
Nasal congestion [4]
Xerostomia (<2%)

Cardiovascular
Angina (<2%)
Chest pain (<2%)
Hypotension (<2%)
Myocardial infarction (<2%)
Palpitation (<2%)
QT prolongation [2]
Tachycardia (<2%)
Ventricular arrhythmia (<2%)

Central Nervous System
Amnesia (<2%)
Dysesthesia (<2%)
Headache (7–15%) [16]
Pain (<2%)
Paresthesias (<2%)
Seizures (<2%)
Sleep related disorder (<2%)
Somnolence (drowsiness) (<2%)
Syncope (<2%)
Vertigo (dizziness) (2%) [3]

Neuromuscular/Skeletal
Arthralgia (<2%)
Back pain (<2%)
Cramps (<2%)
Myalgia/Myopathy (<2%)

Gastrointestinal/Hepatic
Abdominal pain (<2%)
Diarrhea (<2%)
Dyspepsia [3]
Gastritis (<2%)
Gastroesophageal reflux (<2%)
Nausea (<2%)
Vomiting (<2%)

Respiratory
Dyspnea (<2%)
Flu-like syndrome (3%)
Rhinitis (9%) [10]
Sinusitis (3%)

Endocrine/Metabolic
ALT increased (<2%)
Creatine phosphokinase increased (<2%)

Genitourinary
Erection (<2%)
Priapism (<2%)

Otic
Hearing loss [2]
Tinnitus (<2%)

Ocular
Conjunctivitis (<2%)
Dyschromatopsia (<2%)
Intraocular pressure increased (<2%)
Ocular hyperemia (<2%)
Ocular pain (<2%)
Photophobia (<2%)
Visual disturbances (<2%)

Other
Allergic reactions (<2%)

VARENICLINE

Trade names: Champix (Pfizer), Chantix (Pfizer)
Indications: Smoking deterrent
Class: Nicotinic antagonist
Half-life: 24 hours
Clinically important, potentially hazardous interactions with: none known
Pregnancy category: C
Important contra-indications noted in the prescribing guidelines for: nursing mothers; pediatric patients
Warning: SERIOUS NEUROPSYCHIATRIC EVENTS

Skin
AGEP [3]
Rash (<3%)

Mucosal
Xerostomia (4–6%)

Cardiovascular
Cardiotoxicity [5]

Central Nervous System
Abnormal dreams (9–13%) [17]
Aggression [3]
Anorexia (<2%)
Anxiety [5]
Depression [9]
Dysgeusia (taste perversion) (5–8%)
Hallucinations [2]
Headache (15–19%) [13]
Insomnia (18–19%) [16]
Mania [5]
Mood changes [4]
Neuropsychiatric disturbances [2]
Nightmares (<2%)
Psychosis [7]
Sleep disturbances [7]
Sleep related disorder (2–5%) [3]
Somnolence (drowsiness) (3%) [2]
Suicidal ideation [7]

Neuromuscular/Skeletal
Asthenia (fatigue) (<7%) [5]

Gastrointestinal/Hepatic
Abdominal pain (5–7%) [4]
Constipation (5–8%) [4]
Dyspepsia (5%) [2]
Flatulence (6–9%)
Hepatotoxicity [2]
Nausea (16–30%) [30]
Vomiting (<5%) [3]

Respiratory
Dyspnea (<2%)
Upper respiratory tract infection (5–7%)

Endocrine/Metabolic
Appetite decreased (<2%)
Appetite increased (3–4%)

Ocular
Hallucinations, visual [2]

Other
Adverse effects [10]
Death [3]

VARICELLA VACCINE

Trade names: Varilrix (GSK), Varivax (Merck)
Indications: Immunization, varicella
Class: Vaccine
Half-life: N/A
Clinically important, potentially hazardous interactions with: none known
Pregnancy category: C

Skin
Herpes zoster [10]
Rash [10]
Stevens-Johnson syndrome [2]

Central Nervous System
Fever (15%) [3]

Ocular
Keratitis [2]
Uveitis [2]

Local
Injection-site edema (19%)
Injection-site erythema (19%)
Injection-site hematoma (19%)
Injection-site induration (19%)
Injection-site pain (19%)
Injection-site pruritus (19%)
Injection-site reactions [5]

VEDOLIZUMAB

Trade name: Entyvio (Takeda)
Indications: Ulcerative colitis, Crohn's disease
Class: Integrin receptor antagonist, Monoclonal antibody
Half-life: 25 days
Clinically important, potentially hazardous interactions with: live vaccines, natalizumab, TNF blockers
Pregnancy category: B
Important contra-indications noted in the prescribing guidelines for: nursing mothers; pediatric patients

---

Skin
Pruritus (3%)
Rash (3%) [2]

Mucosal
Oropharyngeal pain (3%)

Central Nervous System
Fever (9%) [5]
Headache (12%) [11]

Neuromuscular/Skeletal
Arthralgia (12%) [8]
Asthenia (fatigue) (6%) [6]
Back pain (4%) [3]
Pain in extremities (3%)

Gastrointestinal/Hepatic
Abdominal pain [7]
Colitis [5]
Crohn's disease (exacerbation) [2]
Nausea (9%) [9]
Vomiting [4]

Respiratory
Bronchitis (4%)
Cough (5%) [3]

Influenza (4%)
Nasopharyngitis (13%) [11]
Sinusitis (3%)
Upper respiratory tract infection (7%) [7]

Hematologic

Anemia [4]

Local

Infusion-related reactions (4%) [4]

Other

Adverse effects [9]
Cancer [2]
Infection [5]

VEMURAFENIB

Trade name: Zelboraf (Roche)
Indications: Melanoma (metastatic or unresectable)
Class: BRAF inhibitor
Half-life: 57 hours
Clinically important, potentially hazardous interactions with: amoxapine, arsenic, atazanavir, carbamazepine, clarithromycin, CYP substrates, dolasetron, efavirenz, indinavir, itraconazole, ketoconazole, nefazodone, nelfinavir, pazopanib, phenobarbital, phenytoin, rifabutin, rifampin, rifapentine, ritonavir, saquinavir, telavancin, telithromycin, voriconazole, warfarin
Pregnancy category: D
Important contra-indications noted in the prescribing guidelines for: nursing mothers; pediatric patients

---

Skin

Acneform eruption [6]
Actinic keratoses [4]
Basal cell carcinoma [2]
DRESS syndrome [4]
Eccrine squamous syringometaplasia [2]
Erythema (14%) [2]
Exanthems [9]
Granulomas [2]
Hand–foot syndrome [8]
Hyperkeratosis (24%) [18]
Keratoacanthoma [28]
Keratoses [4]
Keratosis pilaris [10]
Lymphoma [2]
Melanoma [2]
Milia [2]
Neoplasms [2]
Nevi [6]
Panniculitis [9]
Papillomas (21%) [2]
Papular lesions (5%)
Peripheral edema (17%)
Photosensitivity (33%) [29]
Pruritus (23%) [10]
Radiation recall dermatitis [2]
Rash (37%) [26]
Squamous cell carcinoma (24%) [36]
Stevens-Johnson syndrome [5]
Sunburn (10%)
Toxic epidermal necrolysis [6]
Toxicity [10]
Transient acantholytic dermatosis [4]
Vasculitis [2]
Verruca vulgaris [2]
Verrucous lesions [3]
Vitiligo [2]
Warts [2]
Xerosis [5]

Hair

Alopecia (45%) [19]
Hair changes [2]

Nails

Paronychia [3]
Pyogenic granuloma [2]

Mucosal

Gingival hyperplasia/hypertrophy [2]

Cardiovascular

QT prolongation [3]

Central Nervous System

Dysgeusia (taste perversion) (14%)
Fever (19%) [6]
Headache (23%) [3]
Paralysis [2]

Neuromuscular/Skeletal

Arthralgia (53%) [22]
Asthenia (fatigue) (38%) [20]
Back pain (8%)
Bone or joint pain (8%)
Myalgia/Myopathy (8–13%) [2]
Pain in extremities (18%)

Gastrointestinal/Hepatic

Constipation (12%)
Diarrhea (28%) [9]
Hepatotoxicity [4]
Nausea (35%) [10]
Vomiting (18%) [4]

Respiratory

Cough (8%)

Endocrine/Metabolic

ALT increased [6]
Appetite decreased (18%) [2]
AST increased [5]
GGT increased [2]

Ocular

Chorioretinopathy [2]
Uveitis [3]
Vision blurred [2]

Other

Adverse effects [11]

VENETOCLAX

Trade name: Venclexta (AbbVie)
Indications: Chronic lymphocytic leukemia in patients with 17p deletion, as detected by an FDA approved test, who have received at least one prior therapy
Class: BCL-2 inhibitor
Half-life: 26 hours
Clinically important, potentially hazardous interactions with: amiodarone, azithromycin, bosentan, captopril, carbamazepine, carvedilol, ciprofloxacin, clarithromycin, conivaptan, cyclosporine, digoxin, diltiazem, dronedarone, efavirenz, erythromycin, etravirine, everolimus, felodipine, fluconazole, grapefruit juice, indinavir, itraconazole, ketoconazole, live vaccines, lopinavir, modafinil, nafcillin, phenytoin, posaconazole, quercetin, quinidine, ranolazine, rifampin, ritonavir, sirolimus, St John's wort, stong or moderate P-gp inhibitors or substrates, strong or moderate CYP3A inducers or inhibitors, telaprevir, ticagrelor, verapamil, voriconazole
Pregnancy category: N/A (May cause fetal harm)
Important contra-indications noted in the prescribing guidelines for: nursing mothers; pediatric patients
Note: Concomitant use of strong CYP3A inhibitors during initiation and ramp-up phase is contra-indicated.

Skin

Peripheral edema (11%)
Tumor lysis syndrome (6%) [13]

Central Nervous System

Fever (16%) [4]
Headache (15%) [2]

Neuromuscular/Skeletal

Asthenia (fatigue) (21%) [8]
Back pain (10%)

Gastrointestinal/Hepatic

Constipation (14%)
Diarrhea (35%) [11]
Nausea (33%) [13]
Vomiting (15%) [4]

Respiratory

Cough (13%)
Pneumonia (8%) [4]
Upper respiratory tract infection (22%) [6]

Endocrine/Metabolic

Hyperkalemia (20%)
Hyperphosphatemia (15%)
Hyperuricemia (6%)
Hypocalcemia (9%)
Hypokalemia (12%)

Hematologic

Anemia (29%) [11]
Febrile neutropenia [6]
Leukopenia [4]
Neutropenia (45%) [16]
Thrombocytopenia (22%) [12]

Other

Death [5]
Infection [2]

VENLAFAXINE

Trade names: Effexor (Wyeth), Effexor XL (Wyeth)
Indications: Major depressive disorder
Class: Antidepressant, Serotonin-norepinephrine reuptake inhibitor
Half-life: 3–7 hours
Clinically important, potentially hazardous interactions with: 5HT1 agonists, artemether/lumefantrine, aspirin, atomoxetine, clozapine, desvenlafaxine, dexibuprofen, diclofenac, duloxetine, entacapone, haloperidol, indinavir, isocarboxazid, ketoconazole, linezolid, lithium, MAO inhibitors, meloxicam, metoclopramide, metoprolol, mirtazapine, moclobemide, naratriptan, NSAIDs, phenelzine, selegiline, sibutramine, SNRIs, SSRIs, St John's wort,

sumatriptan, tramadol, tranylcypromine, trazodone, trimipramine, triptans, voriconazole, warfarin
Pregnancy category: C
Important contra-indications noted in the prescribing guidelines for: the elderly; nursing mothers; pediatric patients
Warning: SUICIDALITY AND ANTIDEPRESSANT DRUGS

Skin
- Diaphoresis [7]
- Ecchymoses [2]
- Hyperhidrosis [2]
- Pruritus (<10%)
- Rash (3%)

Hair
- Alopecia [2]

Mucosal
- Xerostomia (22%) [10]

Cardiovascular
- Cardiac failure [2]
- Cardiomyopathy [3]
- Hypertension [7]
- Myocardial infarction [2]
- Orthostatic hypotension [2]
- Preeclampsia [2]
- QT prolongation [6]
- Tachycardia [2]

Central Nervous System
- Akathisia [2]
- Delirium [2]
- Dysgeusia (taste perversion) (2%)
- Headache [8]
- Insomnia [5]
- Mania [10]
- Paresthesias (3%)
- Psychosis [3]
- Restless legs syndrome [3]
- Seizures [8]
- Serotonin syndrome [24]
- Somnolence (drowsiness) [9]
- Tremor (<10%) [3]
- Vertigo (dizziness) [10]
- Yawning [2]

Neuromuscular/Skeletal
- Asthenia (fatigue) [5]
- Dystonia [2]
- Rhabdomyolysis [3]

Gastrointestinal/Hepatic
- Constipation [6]
- Hepatotoxicity [8]
- Nausea [16]
- Vomiting [3]

Respiratory
- Pneumonitis [3]

Endocrine/Metabolic
- Appetite decreased [2]
- Galactorrhea [4]
- Hyponatremia [4]
- Libido increased [2]
- Mastodynia [2]
- SIADH [6]
- Weight gain [2]

Genitourinary
- Ejaculatory dysfunction [2]
- Sexual dysfunction [8]
- Urinary incontinence [2]

Ocular
- Glaucoma [2]
- Hallucinations, visual [3]

Other
- Adverse effects [3]
- Bruxism [7]

VERAPAMIL

Trade names: Calan (Pfizer), Covera-HS (Pfizer), Isoptin (AbbVie), Tarka (AbbVie), Verelan (Schwarz)
Indications: Angina, arrhythmias, hypertension
Class: Antiarrhythmic class IV, Calcium channel blocker, CYP3A4 inhibitor
Half-life: 2–8 hours
Clinically important, potentially hazardous interactions with: acebutolol, afatinib, aliskiren, amiodarone, amitriptyline, amprenavir, aspirin, atazanavir, atenolol, atorvastatin, avanafil, betaxolol, betrixaban, bisoprolol, carbamazepine, carteolol, celiprolol, clonidine, cobicistat/elvitegravir/emtricitabine/tenofovir alafenamide, cobicistat/elvitegravir/emtricitabine/tenofovir disoproxil, colchicine, dabigatran, dantrolene, darifenacin, deflazacort, delavirdine, digoxin, dofetilide, dronedarone, dutasteride, epirubicin, eplerenone, erythromycin, esmolol, everolimus, fingolimod, flibanserin, indacaterol, lovastatin, metoprolol, mifepristone, nadolol, naldemedine, naloxegol, neratinib, nevirapine, olaparib, oxprenolol, oxtriphylline, palbociclib, penbutolol, pindolol, posaconazole, propranolol, quinidine, ranolazine, sibutramine, silodosin, simvastatin, telaprevir, telithromycin, timolol, trabectedin, venetoclax
Pregnancy category: C
Important contra-indications noted in the prescribing guidelines for: nursing mothers; pediatric patients
Note: Tarka is verapamil and trandolapril.

Skin
- Angioedema [3]
- Diaphoresis [2]
- Edema (2%)
- Erythema multiforme [4]
- Exanthems [8]
- Exfoliative dermatitis [2]
- Flushing (<7%) [4]
- Hyperkeratosis (palms) [2]
- Lupus erythematosus [2]
- Peripheral edema (<10%)
- Photosensitivity [4]
- Pruritus [6]
- Rash [2]
- Stevens-Johnson syndrome [5]
- Urticaria [5]
- Vasculitis [2]

Hair
- Alopecia [5]

Mucosal
- Gingival hyperplasia/hypertrophy (19%) [10]

Cardiovascular
- Atrial fibrillation [2]
- Atrioventricular block [2]
- Bradycardia [11]
- Congestive heart failure [2]
- Hypotension [3]
- QT prolongation [2]
- Torsades de pointes [2]

Central Nervous System
- Parkinsonism [2]
- Seizures [3]

Neuromuscular/Skeletal
- Rhabdomyolysis [2]

Gastrointestinal/Hepatic
- Hepatotoxicity [2]

Endocrine/Metabolic
- Gynecomastia [8]

Other
- Death [2]
- Side effects [2]

VERTEPORFIN

Trade name: Visudyne (Novartis)
Indications: Neovascular (wet) age-related macular degeneration
Class: Photosensitizer
Half-life: 5–6 hours
Clinically important, potentially hazardous interactions with: none known
Pregnancy category: C
Important contra-indications noted in the prescribing guidelines for: nursing mothers; pediatric patients

---

Skin
- Eczema (<10%)
- Photosensitivity (<10%) [2]

Mucosal
- Burning mouth syndrome (<10%)

Cardiovascular
- Atrial fibrillation (<10%)
- Chest pain [2]
- Hypertension (<10%)

Central Nervous System
- Fever (<10%)
- Hypoesthesia (<10%)
- Sleep related disorder (<10%)
- Vertigo (dizziness) (<10%)

Neuromuscular/Skeletal
- Arthralgia (<10%)
- Asthenia (fatigue) (<10%)
- Back pain (<10%)
- Myasthenia gravis (<10%)

Gastrointestinal/Hepatic
- Constipation (<10%)
- Nausea (<10%)

Respiratory
- Flu-like syndrome (<10%)
- Pharyngitis (<10%)

Endocrine/Metabolic
- Creatine phosphokinase increased (<10%)

Genitourinary
- Albuminuria (<10%)

Hematologic
- Anemia (<10%)
- Leukocytosis (<10%)

Leukopenia (<10%)

Otic

Hearing loss (<10%)

Ocular

Blepharitis (<10%)
Cataract (<10%)
Conjunctivitis (<10%)
Diplopia (<10%)
Endophthalmitis [2]
Intraocular inflammation [2]
Lacrimation (<10%)
Ocular itching (<10%)
Vision loss (severe) (<5%)
Visual disturbances (10–30%)
Xerophthalmia (<10%)

Local

Infusion-site pain (<10%)
Injection-site reactions (10–30%)

Other

Cancer (gastrointestinal) (<10%)

VIGABATRIN

Trade name: Sabril (Lundbeck)
Indications: Epilepsy, infantile spasms (West's syndrome)
Class: Anticonvulsant, Antiepileptic
Half-life: 7.5 hours
Clinically important, potentially hazardous interactions with: antipsychotics, chloroquine, hydroxychloroquine, MAO inhibitors, mefloquine, orlistat, phenytoin, rufinamide, SSRIs, St John's wort, tricyclic antidepressants
Pregnancy category: C
Important contra-indications noted in the prescribing guidelines for: nursing mothers; pediatric patients
Warning: VISION LOSS

Skin

Peripheral edema (5–7%)
Rash (6%) [2]

Cardiovascular

Chest pain (<5%)

Central Nervous System

Abnormal dreams (<5%)
Anxiety (4%)
Confusion (4–14%)
Depression (8%) [4]
Dysarthria (2%)
Encephalopathy [4]
Fever (4–7%)
Gait instability (6–12%)
Headache (18%)
Hypoesthesia (4–5%)
Hyporeflexia (4–5%)
Impaired concentration (9%)
Incoordination (7%)
Insomnia (7%)
Irritability (7%)
Memory loss (7%)
Nervousness (2–5%)
Peripheral neuropathy (4%)
Psychosis [2]
Sedation (4%)
Seizures (11%) [4]
Somnolence (drowsiness) (17%) [3]
Status epilepticus (2–5%)
Tremor (7%)
Vertigo (dizziness) (15%)

Neuromuscular/Skeletal

Arthralgia (5–10%)
Asthenia (fatigue) (16%) [2]
Back pain (4–7%)
Muscle spasm (3%)
Myalgia/Myopathy (3–5%)
Pain in extremities (2–6%)

Gastrointestinal/Hepatic

Abdominal distension (2%)
Abdominal pain (2–3%)
Constipation (5–8%)
Diarrhea (7%)
Dyspepsia (4–5%)
Nausea (7%)
Vomiting (6%)

Respiratory

Bronchitis (5%)
Cough (2–14%)
Influenza (5–7%)
Nasopharyngitis (10%)
Pharyngolaryngeal pain (7–14%)
Upper respiratory tract infection (10%)

Endocrine/Metabolic

Appetite increased (<5%)
Weight gain (10%) [4]

Genitourinary

Dysmenorrhea (5–9%)
Erectile dysfunction (5%)
Urinary tract infection (4–5%)

Hematologic

Anemia (6%)

Otic

Tinnitus (2%)

Ocular

Diplopia (6%)
Nystagmus (7%)
Ocular pain (5%)
Optic atrophy [2]
Retinopathy [12]
Vision blurred (6%)
Vision impaired [20]

Other

Adverse effects [3]
Dipsia (thirst) (2%)
Toothache (2–5%)

VILAZODONE

Trade name: Viibryd (Merck KGaA)
Indications: Major depressive disorder
Class: Antidepressant, Serotonin-norepinephrine reuptake inhibitor
Half-life: 25 hours
Clinically important, potentially hazardous interactions with: anticoagulants, aspirin, buspirone, CNS-active agents, CYP3A4 inhibitors or inducers, efavirenz, erythromycin, ketoconazole, MAO inhibitors, NSAIDs, SNRIs, SSRIs, tramadol, triptans, tryptophan, warfarin
Pregnancy category: C
Important contra-indications noted in the prescribing guidelines for: nursing mothers; pediatric patients
Warning: SUICIDALITY AND ANTIDEPRESSANT DRUGS

Mucosal

Xerostomia (8%) [2]

Cardiovascular

Palpitation (2%)

Central Nervous System

Abnormal dreams (4%)
Headache [4]
Insomnia (6%) [5]
Paresthesias (3%)
Restlessness (3%)
Somnolence (drowsiness) (3%) [3]
Tremor (2%)
Vertigo (dizziness) (9%) [2]

Neuromuscular/Skeletal

Arthralgia (3%)
Asthenia (fatigue) (4%)

Gastrointestinal/Hepatic

Diarrhea (28%) [15]
Dyspepsia (3%)
Flatulence (3%)
Gastroenteritis (3%)
Nausea (23%) [15]
Vomiting (5%) [5]

Endocrine/Metabolic

Appetite increased (2%)
Libido decreased (4–5%)

Genitourinary

Ejaculatory dysfunction (2%)
Erectile dysfunction (2%)
Sexual dysfunction (3%) [2]

Other

Adverse effects [3]

VINBLASTINE

Trade names: Velban (Lilly), Velbe (Lilly), Velsar (Lilly)
Indications: Lymphomas, melanoma, carcinomas
Class: Antimitotic, Vinca alkaloid
Half-life: initial: 3.7 minutes; terminal: 24.8 hours
Clinically important, potentially hazardous interactions with: aldesleukin, aprepitant, erythromycin, fluconazole, itraconazole, ketoconazole, lopinavir, miconazole, posaconazole
Pregnancy category: D
Important contra-indications noted in the prescribing guidelines for: nursing mothers

---

Skin

Acral necrosis [2]
Dermatitis (<10%)
Photosensitivity (<10%) [2]
Pigmentation [3]
Radiation recall dermatitis [2]
Rash (<10%)
Raynaud's phenomenon (<10%) [17]

Hair

Alopecia (>10%)

Mucosal
Mucositis [2]
Oral lesions (<5%)
Stomatitis (>10%)

Central Nervous System
Dysgeusia (taste perversion) (metallic taste) (>10%)
Paresthesias (<10%)
Peripheral neuropathy [2]

Neuromuscular/Skeletal
Myalgia/Myopathy (<10%)

Gastrointestinal/Hepatic
Diarrhea [2]

Endocrine/Metabolic
SIADH [4]

Renal
Nephrotoxicity [2]

Hematologic
Hemolytic uremic syndrome [2]
Neutropenia [3]

Otic
Tinnitus [2]

Local
Injection-site necrosis [2]

Other
Adverse effects [2]

VINCRISTINE

Synonym: oncovin
Trade name: Vincasar (Teva)
Indications: Leukemias, lymphomas, neuroblastoma, Wilm's tumor
Class: Antimitotic, Vinca alkaloid
Half-life: 24 hours
Clinically important, potentially hazardous interactions with: aldesleukin, aprepitant, bromelain, fluconazole, gadobenate, influenza vaccine, itraconazole, ketoconazole, lopinavir, miconazole, nifedipine, posaconazole, thalidomide
Pregnancy category: D
Important contra-indications noted in the prescribing guidelines for: nursing mothers

---

Skin
Erythroderma [2]
Exanthems [3]
Hand–foot syndrome [2]
Rash (<10%)
Raynaud's phenomenon [2]

Hair
Alopecia (20–70%) [9]

Nails
Beau's lines (transverse nail bands) [2]
Leukonychia (Mees' lines) [5]

Mucosal
Oral lesions (<10%) [2]
Oral ulceration (<10%)

Cardiovascular
Hypertension [2]
Phlebitis (<10%)

Central Nervous System
Anorexia [2]
Dysgeusia (taste perversion) (<10%)
Neurotoxicity [16]
Paresthesias (<10%)
Peripheral neuropathy [11]
Seizures [6]

Neuromuscular/Skeletal
Asthenia (fatigue) [2]
Myalgia/Myopathy (<10%)

Gastrointestinal/Hepatic
Abdominal pain [2]

Respiratory
Pneumonia [2]

Endocrine/Metabolic
Hyponatremia [2]
SIADH [10]

Hematologic
Anemia [2]
Febrile neutropenia [5]
Hemolytic uremic syndrome [4]
Hemotoxicity [2]
Leukopenia [3]
Neutropenia [10]
Thrombocytopenia [10]

Ocular
Ptosis [4]

Local
Injection-site cellulitis (>10%)
Injection-site necrosis (>10%)

Other
Adverse effects [7]
Death [6]
Infection [3]

VINORELBINE

Trade name: Navelbine (Kyowa)
Indications: Non-small cell lung cancer
Class: Antimitotic, Vinca alkaloid
Half-life: 28–44 hours
Clinically important, potentially hazardous interactions with: aldesleukin, itraconazole
Pregnancy category: D
Important contra-indications noted in the prescribing guidelines for: nursing mothers; pediatric patients
Warning: MYELOSUPPRESSION

Skin
Acneform eruption [3]
Hand–foot syndrome [8]
Rash (<5%) [2]
Recall reaction [2]

Hair
Alopecia (12%) [5]

Mucosal
Mucositis [2]
Stomatitis (>10%) [6]

Cardiovascular
Extravasation [2]
Hypertension [2]
Phlebitis (7%)

Central Nervous System
Anorexia [7]
Dysgeusia (taste perversion) (metallic taste) (>10%)
Hyperesthesia (<10%)
Neurotoxicity [4]
Paresthesias (<10%)

Neuromuscular/Skeletal
Asthenia (fatigue) [14]
Bone or joint pain [3]
Myalgia/Myopathy (<5%)

Gastrointestinal/Hepatic
Constipation [4]
Diarrhea [13]
Esophagitis [2]
Hepatotoxicity [2]
Nausea [11]
Vomiting [8]

Endocrine/Metabolic
ALT increased [2]
AST increased [2]
SIADH [3]

Hematologic
Anemia [8]
Febrile neutropenia [5]
Leukopenia [9]
Myelotoxicity [2]
Neutropenia [28]
Thrombocytopenia [4]

Local
Injection-site irritation (<10%)
Injection-site necrosis (<10%)
Injection-site phlebitis (12%) [2]

Other
Adverse effects [2]
Death [2]
Infection [4]

VISMODEGIB

Trade name: Erivedge (Genentech)
Indications: Basal cell carcinoma
Class: Hedgehog (Hh) signaling pathway inhibitor
Half-life: 4–12 days
Clinically important, potentially hazardous interactions with: none known
Pregnancy category: D
Important contra-indications noted in the prescribing guidelines for: nursing mothers; pediatric patients
Note: Patients should not donate blood or blood products while receiving vismodegib and for at least 7 months after the last dose.
Warning: EMBRYO-FETAL TOXICITY

Skin
Squamous cell carcinoma [2]
Toxicity [2]

Hair
Alopecia (64%) [23]

Central Nervous System
Ageusia (taste loss) (11%) [6]
Anorexia [2]
Dysgeusia (taste perversion) (55%) [20]

Neuromuscular/Skeletal
Arthralgia (16%) [2]
Asthenia (fatigue) (40%) [15]
Muscle spasm (72%) [19]
Myalgia/Myopathy [5]

Gastrointestinal/Hepatic
Constipation (21%)
Diarrhea (29%) [7]
Hepatotoxicity [3]
Nausea (30%) [7]
Vomiting (14%) [2]

Endocrine/Metabolic
Amenorrhea [3]
Appetite decreased (25%) [6]
Hyperglycemia [2]
Hyponatremia (4%) [3]
Hypophosphatemia [2]
Weight loss (45%) [15]

Genitourinary
Azotemia (2%)

Other
Adverse effects [9]
Death [3]

VITAMIN A

Trade name: Aquasol A (aaiPharma)
Indications: Vitamin A deficiency
Class: Vitamin
Half-life: N/A
Clinically important, potentially hazardous interactions with: acitretin, alitretinoin, bexarotene, cholestyramine, fish oil supplements, isotretinoin, minocycline, orlistat, prednisone, tetracycline, warfarin
Pregnancy category: A (the pregnancy category will be X if used in doses above the RDA)

Skin
Dermatitis [7]
Pruritus [2]
Xerosis (<10%)

Hair
Alopecia [11]

Mucosal
Oral mucosal eruption [2]

VITAMIN E

Synonym: alpha tocopherol
Trade name: Aquasol E (aaiPharma)
Indications: Vitamin E deficiency
Class: Vitamin
Half-life: N/A
Clinically important, potentially hazardous interactions with: amprenavir, cholestyramine, orlistat, tipranavir, warfarin
Pregnancy category: A (the pregnancy category will be C if used in doses above the RDA)

Skin
Dermatitis [13]
Erythema multiforme [3]
Sclerosing lipogranuloma [2]

Genitourinary
Prostate cancer (increased risk) [4]

VORAPAXAR

Trade name: Zontivity (Merck)
Indications: Reduction of thrombotic cardiovascular events in patients with a history of myocardial infarction or with peripheral arterial disease
Class: Protease-activated receptor-1 (PAR-1) antagonist
Half-life: 3–4 days
Clinically important, potentially hazardous interactions with: boceprevir, carbamazepine, clarithromycin, conivaptan, indinavir, itraconazole, ketoconazole, nefazodone, nelfinavir, phenytoin, posaconazole, rifampin, ritonavir, saquinavir, St John's wort, strong CYP3A inhibitors or inducers, telaprevir, telithromycin
Pregnancy category: B
Important contra-indications noted in the prescribing guidelines for: nursing mothers; pediatric patients
Note: Contra-indicated in patients with a history of stroke, transient ischemic attack, or intracranial hemorrhage, or with active pathological bleeding.
Warning: BLEEDING RISK

Skin
Exanthems (2%)
Rash (2%)

Cardiovascular
Cardiotoxicity [2]

Central Nervous System
Depression (2%)
Intracranial hemorrhage [5]

Hematologic
Anemia (5%)
Bleeding (25%) [10]

Ocular
Diplopia (<2%)
Retinopathy (<2%)

Other
Adverse effects [3]

VORICONAZOLE

Trade name: Vfend (Pfizer)
Indications: Invasive aspergillosis
Class: Antibiotic, triazole, Antifungal, azole, CYP3A4 inhibitor
Half-life: 6–24 hours (dose dependent)
Clinically important, potentially hazardous interactions with: abiraterone, alfentanil, alfuzosin, almotriptan, alosetron, amphotericin B, antineoplastics, apixaban, aprepitant, artemether/lumefantrine, astemizole, atazanavir, atorvastatin, barbiturates, benzodiazepines, boceprevir, bortezomib, bosentan, brigatinib, brinzolamide, buspirone, busulfan, cabazitaxel, cabozantinib, calcifediol, calcium channel blockers, carbamazepine, carvedilol, chloramphenicol, chloroquine, ciclesonide, cilostazol, cinacalcet, ciprofloxacin, cisapride, clopidogrel, cobicistat/elvitegravir/emtricitabine/tenofovir alafenamide, cobicistat/elvitegravir/emtricitabine/tenofovir disoproxil, colchicine, conivaptan, copanlisib, coumarins, crizotinib, cyclosporine, CYP2C19 inhibitors and inducers, CYP2C9 inhibitors and substrates, CYP3A4 substrates, darunavir, diazepam, diclofenac, didanosine, dienogest, docetaxel, dofetilide, dronedarone, dutasteride, efavirenz, eletriptan, eplerenone, ergot alkaloids, ergotamine, erlotinib, esomeprazole, estrogens, eszopiclone, etravirine, everolimus, fentanyl, fesoterodine, food, gadobutrol, gefitinib, grapefruit juice, guanfacine, halofantrine, HMG-CoA reductase inhibitors, ibrutinib, ibuprofen, imatinib, irinotecan, ixabepilone, lapatinib, letermovir, lomitapide, lopinavir, losartan, macrolide antibiotics, maraviroc, meloxicam, methadone, methylergonovine, methylprednisolone, methysergide, midazolam, midostaurin, mifepristone, mometasone, neratinib, nilotinib, nisoldipine, olaparib, ombitasvir/paritaprevir/ritonavir, omeprazole, oxycodone, palbociclib, pantoprazole, paricalcitol, pazopanib, PEG-interferon, phenobarbital, phenytoin, phosphodiesterase 5 inhibitors, pimecrolimus, pimozide, ponatinib, prasugrel, progestins, progestogens, protease inhibitors, proton pump inhibitors, QT prolonging agents, quetiapine, quinidine, quinine, ramelteon, ranolazine, reboxetine, regorafenib, repaglinide, ribociclib, rifabutin, rifampin, rifapentine, rilpivirine, ritonavir, rivaroxaban, romidepsin, ruxolitinib, salmeterol, saquinavir, saxagliptin, silodosin, simeprevir, simvastatin, sirolimus, solifenacin, sonidegib, sorafenib, St John's wort, sucralfate, sulfonylureas, sunitinib, tacrolimus, tadalafil, tamsulosin, telaprevir, temsirolimus, tetrabenazine, tezacaftor/ivacaftor, thioridazine, ticagrelor, tolterodine, tolvaptan, vemurafenib, venetoclax, venlafaxine, vitamin K antagonists, ziprasidone, zolpidem
Pregnancy category: D
Important contra-indications noted in the prescribing guidelines for: nursing mothers; pediatric patients

---

Skin
Actinic keratoses [2]
Anaphylactoid reactions/Anaphylaxis (<2%)
Angioedema (<2%)
Cellulitis (<2%)
Contact dermatitis (<2%)
Cyanosis (<2%)
Dermatitis (<2%)
Diaphoresis (<2%) [2]
Ecchymoses (<2%)
Eczema (<2%)
Edema (<2%)
Erythema [5]
Erythema multiforme (<2%)
Exfoliative dermatitis (<2%)
Facial edema (<2%)
Fixed eruption (<2%)
Furunculosis (<2%)
Graft-versus-host reaction (<2%)
Granulomas (<2%)
Herpes simplex (<2%)
Lentigo [2]
Lupus erythematosus (<2%) [5]
Lymphadenopathy (<2%)
Malignancies [2]
Melanoma (<2%)
Melanosis (<2%)
Peripheral edema (<2%)
Petechiae (<2%)

Photosensitivity (8%) [18]
Phototoxicity [13]
Pigmentation (<2%)
Pruritus (8%)
Psoriasis (<2%)
Purpura (<2%)
Rash (5%) [7]
Squamous cell carcinoma (<2%) [8]
Stevens-Johnson syndrome (<2%) [4]
Toxic epidermal necrolysis (<2%) [4]
Urticaria (<2%)
Xerosis (<2%) [2]

Hair

Alopecia (<2%) [4]

Nails

Nail changes [3]

Mucosal

Cheilitis (<2%) [4]
Gingival bleeding (<2%)
Gingival hyperplasia/hypertrophy (<2%)
Gingivitis (<2%)
Glossitis (<2%)
Rectal hemorrhage (<2%)
Stomatitis (<2%)
Tongue edema (<2%)
Xerostomia (<2%)

Cardiovascular

Arrhythmias (<2%)
Atrial fibrillation (<2%)
Atrioventricular block (<2%)
Bradycardia (<2%)
Bundle branch block (<2%)
Cardiac arrest (<2%)
Cardiomyopathy (<2%)
Chest pain (<2%)
Congestive heart failure (<2%)
Extrasystoles (<2%)
Hypertension (<2%)
Hypotension (<2%)
Myocardial infarction (<2%)
Palpitation (<2%)
Phlebitis (<2%)
Postural hypotension (<2%)
QT prolongation (<2%) [11]
Supraventricular tachycardia (<2%)
Tachycardia (2%) [2]
Thrombophlebitis (<2%)
Torsades de pointes [7]
Vasodilation (<2%)
Ventricular arrhythmia (<2%)
Ventricular fibrillation (<2%)
Ventricular tachycardia (<2%)

Central Nervous System

Abnormal dreams (<2%)
Ageusia (taste loss) (<2%)
Agitation (<2%)
Akathisia (<2%)
Amnesia (<2%)
Anorexia (<2%)
Anxiety (<2%)
Cerebral edema (<2%)
Cerebral hemorrhage (<2%)
Cerebral ischemia (<2%)
Cerebrovascular accident (<2%)
Chills (4%)
Coma (<2%)
Confusion (<2%) [2]
Delirium (<2%) [2]
Dementia (<2%)
Depersonalization (<2%)
Depression (<2%)
Dysgeusia (taste perversion) (<2%)
Encephalitis (<2%)
Encephalopathy (<2%) [3]
Euphoria (<2%)
Extrapyramidal symptoms (<2%)
Fever (6%)
Guillain–Barré syndrome (<2%)
Hallucinations (2%) [8]
Headache (3%) [3]
Hypoesthesia (<2%)
Insomnia (<2%)
Intracranial pressure increased (<2%)
Neurotoxicity [6]
Paresthesias (<2%)
Peripheral neuropathy [4]
Psychosis (<2%) [2]
Seizures (<2%)
Somnolence (drowsiness) (<2%)
Status epilepticus (<2%)
Suicidal ideation (<2%)
Syncope (<2%)
Tremor (<2%)
Vertigo (dizziness) (<2%)

Neuromuscular/Skeletal

Arthralgia (<2%) [2]
Asthenia (fatigue) (<2%) [2]
Ataxia (<2%)
Back pain (<2%)
Bone or joint pain (<2%)
Hypertonia (<2%)
Leg cramps (<2%)
Myalgia/Myopathy (<2%)
Osteomalacia (<2%)
Osteoporosis (<2%)
Periostitis deformans [23]
Skeletal fluorosis [2]

Gastrointestinal/Hepatic

Abdominal pain (<2%)
Ascites (<2%)
Black stools (<2%)
Cholecystitis (<2%)
Cholelithiasis (gallstones) (<2%)
Constipation (<2%)
Diarrhea (<2%) [2]
Duodentitis (<2%)
Dyspepsia (<2%)
Dysphagia (<2%)
Esophagitis (<2%)
Flatulence (<2%)
Gastroenteritis (<2%)
Gastrointestinal bleeding (<2%)
Gastrointestinal perforation (<2%)
Gastrointestinal ulceration (<2%)
Hematemesis (<2%)
Hepatic failure (<2%)
Hepatotoxicity [19]
Nausea (5%) [3]
Pancreatitis (<2%)
Peritonitis (<2%)
Pseudomembranous colitis (<2%)
Vomiting (4%) [2]

Respiratory

Cough (<2%)
Dysphonia (<2%)
Dyspnea (<2%)
Flu-like syndrome (<2%)
Hemoptysis (<2%)
Hypoxia (<2%)
Pharyngitis (<2%)
Pleural effusion (<2%)
Pneumonia (<2%)
Pneumonitis [2]
Pulmonary embolism (<2%)
Respiratory distress (<2%)
Rhinitis (<2%)
Sinusitis (<2%)
Upper respiratory tract infection (<2%)

Endocrine/Metabolic

ALP increased (4%)
ALT increased [2]
AST increased [2]
Creatine phosphokinase increased (<2%)
Diabetes insipidus (<2%)
GGT increased (<2%)
Hypercalcemia (<2%)
Hypercholesterolemia (<2%)
Hyperglycemia (<2%)
Hyperkalemia (<2%)
Hypermagnesemia (<2%)
Hypernatremia (<2%)
Hyperthyroidism (<2%)
Hyperuricemia (<2%)
Hypervolemia (<2%)
Hypocalcemia (<2%)
Hypoglycemia (<2%)
Hypokalemia (2%) [3]
Hypomagnesemia (<2%)
Hyponatremia (<2%)
Hypophosphatemia (<2%)
Hypothyroidism (<2%)
Libido decreased (<2%)
Pseudoporphyria [6]

Genitourinary

Anuria (<2%)
Cystitis (<2%)
Dysmenorrhea (<2%)
Dysuria (<2%)
Epididymitis (<2%)
Glycosuria (<2%)
Hematuria (<2%)
Impotence (<2%)
Oliguria (<2%)
Urinary incontinence (<2%)
Urinary retention (<2%)
Urinary tract infection (<2%)
Uterine bleeding (<2%)
Vaginal bleeding (<2%)

Renal

Nephrotoxicity (<2%) [5]
Renal tubular necrosis (<2%)

Hematologic

Agranulocytosis (<2%)
Anemia (<2%)
Bone marrow suppression (<2%)
Eosinophilia (<2%)
Hemolytic anemia (<2%)
Leukopenia (<2%)
Pancytopenia (<2%)
Prothrombin time increased (<2%)
Sepsis (<2%)
Thrombocytopenia (<2%)

Otic

Ear pain (<2%)
Hearing loss (<2%)
Hypoacusis (<2%)
Tinnitus (<2%)

Ocular
Abnormal vision (19%)
Accommodation disorder (<2%)
Blepharitis (<2%)
Conjunctivitis (<2%)
Corneal opacity (<2%)
Diplopia (<2%)
Hallucinations, visual [5]
Keratitis (<2%)
Keratoconjunctivitis (<2%)
Mydriasis (<2%)
Night blindness (<2%)
Nystagmus (<2%)
Ocular adverse effects [2]
Ocular hemorrhage (<2%)
Ocular pain (<2%)
Oculogyric crisis (<2%)
Optic atrophy (<2%)
Optic neuritis (<2%)
Papilledema (<2%)
Photophobia (2%)
Retinitis (<2%)
Scleritis (<2%)
Uveitis (<2%)
Visual disturbances (19%) [15]
Xerophthalmia (<2%)

Local
Injection-site infection (<2%)
Injection-site inflammation (<2%)
Injection-site pain (<2%)

Other
Adverse effects (20%) [12]
Infection (<2%)
Multiorgan failure (<2%)
Periodontal infection (<2%)

VORINOSTAT

Trade name: Zolinza (Merck)
Indications: Cutaneous T-cell lymphoma
Class: Antineoplastic, Histone deacetylase (HDAC) inhibitor
Half-life: ~2 hours
Clinically important, potentially hazardous interactions with: alfuzosin, artemether/lumefantrine, chloroquine, ciprofloxacin, coumarins, dronedarone, gadobutrol, nilotinib, pimozide, QT prolonging agents, quinine, tetrabenazine, thioridazine, valproic acid, vitamin K antagonists, ziprasidone
Pregnancy category: D
Important contra-indications noted in the prescribing guidelines for: nursing mothers; pediatric patients

---

Skin
Exanthems [2]
Peripheral edema (13%)
Pruritus (12%)

Hair
Alopecia (19%) [2]

Mucosal
Mucositis [2]
Xerostomia (16%)

Cardiovascular
QT prolongation [3]

Central Nervous System
Anorexia [5]
Chills (16%)
Dysgeusia (taste perversion) (28%)
Fever (10%)
Headache (12%)
Vertigo (dizziness) (15%)

Neuromuscular/Skeletal
Asthenia (fatigue) (52%) [11]

Gastrointestinal/Hepatic
Abdominal pain [2]
Constipation [2]
Diarrhea [7]
Nausea [10]
Vomiting [4]

Respiratory
Cough (11%)
Upper respiratory tract infection (10%)

Endocrine/Metabolic
Creatine phosphokinase increased [2]
Dehydration [2]
Hyperglycemia [3]
Weight loss [4]

Renal
Renal failure [2]

Hematologic
Anemia (14%) [7]
Febrile neutropenia [2]
Hemotoxicity [2]
Leukopenia [3]
Lymphopenia [6]
Neutropenia [10]
Thrombocytopenia [15]

Other
Adverse effects [2]

VORTIOXETINE

Trade name: Trintellix (formerly Brintellix) (Takeda)
Indications: Major depressive disorder
Class: Antidepressant, Serotonin receptor agonist, Serotonin receptor antagonist, Serotonin reuptake inhibitor
Half-life: ~66 hours
Clinically important, potentially hazardous interactions with: bupropion, carbamazepine, fluoxetine, MAO inhibitors, paroxetine hydrochloride, phenytoin, quinidine, rifampin
Pregnancy category: C
Important contra-indications noted in the prescribing guidelines for: nursing mothers; pediatric patients
Warning: SUICIDAL THOUGHTS AND BEHAVIORS

Skin
Hyperhidrosis [6]
Pruritus (<3%)

Mucosal
Xerostomia (6–8%) [18]

Central Nervous System
Abnormal dreams (<3%) [2]
Agitation [2]
Anxiety [2]
Headache [25]
Insomnia [7]
Somnolence (drowsiness) [4]
Vertigo (dizziness) (6–9%) [18]

Neuromuscular/Skeletal
Asthenia (fatigue) [7]

Gastrointestinal/Hepatic
Constipation (3–6%) [13]
Diarrhea (7–10%) [16]
Flatulence (<3%)
Nausea (21–32%) [38]
Vomiting (3–6%) [17]

Respiratory
Nasopharyngitis [6]
Upper respiratory tract infection [2]

Endocrine/Metabolic
Weight gain [2]

Genitourinary
Sexual dysfunction (<5%) [10]

Other
Adverse effects [2]

WARFARIN

Trade name: Coumadin (Bristol-Myers Squibb)
Indications: Thromboembolic disease, pulmonary embolism
Class: Anticoagulant, Coumarin
Half-life: 1.5–2.5 days (highly variable)
Clinically important, potentially hazardous interactions with: acemetacin, amiodarone, amobarbital, amprenavir, antithyroid agents, aprepitant, aprobarbital, aspirin, atazanavir, atorvastatin, azathioprine, azithromycin, barbiturates, beclomethasone, betamethasone, bezafibrate, bismuth, bivalirudin, boceprevir, bosentan, butabarbital, capecitabine, cefixime, celecoxib, ceritinib, chondroitin, cimetidine, ciprofloxacin, clarithromycin, clofibrate, clopidogrel, clorazepate, co-trimoxazole, cobicistat/elvitegravir/emtricitabine/tenofovir alafenamide, cobicistat/elvitegravir/emtricitabine/tenofovir disoproxil, colesevelam, cyclosporine, danazol, daptomycin, darunavir, delavirdine, desvenlafaxine, dexamethasone, dexibuprofen, dexlansoprazole, diclofenac, dicloxacillin, dirithromycin, disulfiram, dronedarone, duloxetine, econazole, efavirenz, enzalutamide, ergotamine, erlotinib, erythromycin, eslicarbazepine, etoricoxib, exenatide, fenofibrate, fluconazole, flunisolide, fluoxymesterone, fosamprenavir, gefitinib, gemfibrozil, glucagon, grapefruit juice, heparin, imatinib, influenza vaccine, itraconazole, ketoconazole, leflunomide, lepirudin, letermovir, levofloxacin, levothyroxine, liothyronine, liraglutide, lomitapide, lopinavir, menadione, mephobarbital, methimazole, methyl salicylate, methylprednisolone, methyltestosterone, metronidazole, miconazole, mifepristone, moricizine, moxifloxacin, nafcillin, nalidixic acid, nandrolone, nilutamide, norfloxacin, obeticholic acid, ofloxacin, omeprazole, oritavancin, orlistat, pantoprazole, PEG-interferon, penicillin G, penicillin V, penicillins, pentobarbital, phenobarbital, phenylbutazones, phytonadione, piperacillin, piroxicam, prasugrel, primidone, propoxyphene, propranolol, propylthiouracil,

quinidine, quinine, rabeprazole, resveratrol, rifampin, rifapentine, rofecoxib, romidepsin, ropinirole, rosuvastatin, roxithromycin, salicylates, secobarbital, simvastatin, sitaxentan, sorafenib, St John's wort, stanozolol, sulfamethoxazole, sulfinpyrazone, sulfisoxazole, sulfonamides, sulindac, tamsulosin, tegafur/gimeracil/oteracil, telaprevir, telithromycin, teriflunomide, testosterone, tibolone, tigecycline, tinidazole, tolmetin, tolterodine, triamcinolone, troleandomycin, uracil/tegafur, valdecoxib, vemurafenib, venlafaxine, vilazodone, vitamin A, vitamin E, zafirlukast, zileuton
Pregnancy category: X (category D for women with mechanical heart valves)
Note: Alternative remedies, including herbals, may potentially increase the risk of bleeding or potentiate the effects of warfarin therapy. Some of these include the following: angelica root, arnica flower, anise, asafetida, bogbean, borage seed oil, bromelain, dan-shen, devil's claw, fenugreek, feverfew, garlic, ginger, ginkgo biloba, ginseng, horse chestnut, lovage root, meadowsweet, onion, parsley, passionflower herb, poplar, quassia, red clover, rue, turmeric and willow bark.
Warning: BLEEDING RISK

Skin
Bullous dermatitis [2]
Calcification [3]
Dermatitis [2]
Ecchymoses [2]
Exanthems [7]
Gangrene [6]
Hematoma [3]
Hypersensitivity [3]
Necrosis (>10%) [117]
Pruritus [2]
Purplish erythema (feet and toes) [8]
Purpura [3]
Rash [2]
Urticaria [3]
Vasculitis [7]

Hair
Alopecia (>10%) [6]

Cardiovascular
Myocardial infarction [2]

Central Nervous System
Headache [2]
Intracranial hemorrhage [2]
Vertigo (dizziness) [2]

Neuromuscular/Skeletal
Rhabdomyolysis [2]

Gastrointestinal/Hepatic
Black stools [2]
Gastrointestinal bleeding [5]
Hematemesis [2]

Genitourinary
Priapism [4]

Renal
Nephrotoxicity [4]

Hematologic
Anticoagulation [3]
Bleeding [18]
Hemorrhage [8]
Prothrombin time increased [5]
Thrombosis [2]

Other
Adverse effects [9]
Death [3]

WILLOW BARK

Family: Salicaceae
Scientific names: *Salix alba, Salix fragilis, Salix purpurea*
Indications: Colds, infections, headaches, pain, muscle and joint aches, influenza, gouty arthritis, ankylosing spondylitis, rheumatoid arthritis, osteoarthritis
Class: Anti-inflammatory
Half-life: N/A
Clinically important, potentially hazardous interactions with: NSAIDs, salicylates
Pregnancy category: N/A

XYLOMETAZOLINE

Trade name: Otrivine (Novartis)
Indications: Nasal congestion, perennial and allergic rhinitis, sinusitis
Class: Alpha adrenoceptor agonist
Half-life: N/A
Clinically important, potentially hazardous interactions with: none known
Pregnancy category: C
Important contra-indications noted in the prescribing guidelines for: nursing mothers

---

Mucosal
Epistaxis (nosebleed) [2]
Mucosal bleeding [2]

YARROW

Family: Compositae
Scientific name: *Achillea millefolium*
Indications: Fevers, common cold, essential hypertension, digestive complaints, loss of appetite, amenorrhea, dysentery, diarrhea, cerebral and coronary thromboses, menstrual pain, bleeding piles, toothache, muscle spasms, gastrointestinal disorders. **Topical:** slow-healing wounds, skin inflammations, cosmetics
Class: Anti-inflammatory
Half-life: N/A
Clinically important, potentially hazardous interactions with: anticoagulants, antiepileptics, hypertensives, hypotensives
Pregnancy category: N/A

Skin
Dermatitis [4]

YELLOW FEVER VACCINE

Trade names: Stamaril (Sanofi Pasteur), YF-VAX (Sanofi Pasteur)
Indications: Immunization against yellow fever
Class: Vaccine
Half-life: N/A
Clinically important, potentially hazardous interactions with: azathioprine, belimumab, corticosteroids, fingolimod, hydroxychloroquine, immunosuppressants, interferon-gamma, leflunomide, mercaptopurine, prednisone, tocilizumab, ustekinumab
Pregnancy category: C
Important contra-indications noted in the prescribing guidelines for: the elderly; nursing mothers; pediatric patients
Note: Contra-indicated in patients with hypersensitivity to egg or chick embryo protein.

Skin
Anaphylactoid reactions/Anaphylaxis [8]
Hypersensitivity [2]
Rash (3%)
Urticaria [2]

Central Nervous System
Encephalopathy [4]
Fever (low-grade) (<5%) [3]
Headache (<30%) [2]
Myelitis [2]
Neurotoxicity [11]

Neuromuscular/Skeletal
Asthenia (fatigue) (10–30%) [2]
Myalgia/Myopathy (10–30%) [2]

Gastrointestinal/Hepatic
Diarrhea (<10%) [2]
Hepatitis [2]
Nausea (<10%)
Vomiting (<10%) [2]

Respiratory
Influenza [2]

Local
Infusion-site erythema (<5%)
Infusion-site pain (<5%)

Other
Adverse effects [14]
Death [13]
Multiorgan failure [3]
Viscerotropic disease [20]

YOHIMBINE

Family: Rubiaceae
Scientific name: *Pausinystalia yohimbe*
Indications: Impotence, alpha2-adrenergic blocker, orthostatic hypertension
Class: Rauwolfia alkaloid
Half-life: 36 minutes
Clinically important, potentially hazardous interactions with: amitriptyline, benazepril, captopril, clevidipine, lisinopril, terbutaline, tricyclic antidepressants
Pregnancy category: N/A

Skin
Flushing [2]

Mucosal
Sialorrhea [2]

Cardiovascular
Hypertension [5]
Tachycardia [4]

Central Nervous System
Agitation [2]
Anxiety [6]
Headache [3]

Gastrointestinal/Hepatic
Hepatotoxicity [4]

Genitourinary
Urinary frequency [2]

ZAFIRLUKAST

Trade name: Accolate (AstraZeneca)
Indications: Asthma
Class: Leukotriene receptor antagonist
Half-life: 10 hours
Clinically important, potentially hazardous interactions with: aminophylline, aspirin, carvedilol, CYP2C9 substrates, CYP3A4 substrates, erythromycin, high protein foods, interferon alfa, primidone, vitamin K antagonists, warfarin
Pregnancy category: B
Important contra-indications noted in the prescribing guidelines for: nursing mothers; pediatric patients
Note: Contra-indicated in patients with hepatic impairment including hepatic cirrhosis.

Skin
Churg-Strauss syndrome [6]

Central Nervous System
Fever (2%)
Headache (13%)
Pain (generalized) (2%)
Vertigo (dizziness) (2%)

Neuromuscular/Skeletal
Asthenia (fatigue) (2%)
Back pain (2%)
Myalgia/Myopathy (2%)

Gastrointestinal/Hepatic
Abdominal pain (2%)
Diarrhea (3%)
Nausea (3%)
Vomiting (2%)

Respiratory
Cough [2]

Other
Infection (4%)

ZALCITABINE

Synonyms: dideoxycytidine; ddC
Trade name: Hivid (Roche)
Indications: Advanced HIV infection
Class: Antiretroviral, Nucleoside analog reverse transcriptase inhibitor
Half-life: 2.9 hours
Clinically important, potentially hazardous interactions with: none known
Pregnancy category: C
Important contra-indications noted in the prescribing guidelines for: the elderly; nursing mothers; pediatric patients

---

Skin
Edema [3]
Exanthems [9]
Pruritus (3–5%)
Rash (2–11%) [2]
Urticaria (3%)

Mucosal
Aphthous stomatitis [6]
Oral lesions (40–73%) [3]
Oral ulceration (3–64%) [4]
Stomatitis (3%)

Central Nervous System
Neurotoxicity [2]

Neuromuscular/Skeletal
Myalgia/Myopathy (<6%)

Other
Side effects [2]

ZALEPLON

Trade name: Sonata (Wyeth)
Indications: Insomnia
Class: Hypnotic, non-benzodiazepine
Half-life: 1 hour
Clinically important, potentially hazardous interactions with: alcohol, cimetidine, erythromycin, imipramine, ketoconazole, promethazine, rifampin, rifapentine, thioridazine
Pregnancy category: C
Important contra-indications noted in the prescribing guidelines for: nursing mothers; pediatric patients

---

Cardiovascular
Tachycardia [2]

Central Nervous System
Amnesia (2–4%)
Anorexia (<2%)
Confusion [2]
Depersonalization (<2%)
Hallucinations [3]
Headache (30–42%) [3]
Hypoesthesia (<2%)
Paresthesias (3%)
Parosmia (<2%)
Slurred speech [2]
Somnambulism [2]
Somnolence (drowsiness) (5–6%) [4]
Tremor (2%)
Vertigo (dizziness) (7–9%) [4]

Neuromuscular/Skeletal
Asthenia (fatigue) (5–7%)
Ataxia [2]

Gastrointestinal/Hepatic
Abdominal pain (6%)
Nausea (6–8%)
Vomiting [2]

Genitourinary
Dysmenorrhea (3–4%)

Otic
Hyperacusis (<2%)

Ocular
Ocular pain (3–4%)

Other
Adverse effects [2]
Viscerotropic disease [2]

ZANAMIVIR

Trade name: Relenza (GSK)
Indications: Influenza A and B
Class: Antiviral, Neuraminidase inhibitor
Half-life: 2.5–5.1 hours
Clinically important, potentially hazardous interactions with: live attenuated influenza vaccine
Pregnancy category: C
Important contra-indications noted in the prescribing guidelines for: nursing mothers

---

Skin
Urticaria (<2%)

Mucosal
Nasal discomfort (12%)

Central Nervous System
Anorexia (4%)
Chills (5–9%)
Fever (5–9%)
Headache (13–24%) [2]
Vertigo (dizziness) (<2%)

Neuromuscular/Skeletal
Arthralgia (<2%)
Asthenia (fatigue) (5–8%)
Bone or joint pain (6%)
Myalgia/Myopathy (<8%)

Gastrointestinal/Hepatic
Abdominal pain (<2%)
Diarrhea (3%) [2]
Nausea (3%) [2]

Respiratory
Bronchitis (2%)
Bronchospasm [3]
Cough (7–17%)
Respiratory failure [2]
Sinusitis (2%)
Upper respiratory tract infection (3–13%) [2]

Endocrine/Metabolic
Appetite decreased (4%)
Appetite increased (4%)

Other
Infection (2%)

ZIDOVUDINE

Synonyms: azidothymidine; AZT
Trade names: Combivir (ViiV), Retrovir (ViiV), Trizivir (ViiV)
Indications: HIV infection
Class: Antiretroviral, Nucleoside analog reverse transcriptase inhibitor
Half-life: 0.5–3 hours
Clinically important, potentially hazardous interactions with: atovaquone, bone marrow suppressives, clarithromycin, darunavir, diclofenac, doxorubicin, fluconazole, ganciclovir, indinavir, interferon alfa, interferon beta, lopinavir, meloxicam, methadone, NSAIDs, PEG-interferon, phenytoin, probenecid, pyrimethamine, ribavirin, rifampin, rifapentine, stavudine, tipranavir, valproic acid
Pregnancy category: C
Important contra-indications noted in the prescribing guidelines for: the elderly; nursing mothers
Note: Combivir is zidovudine and lamivudine; Trizivir is zidovudine, abacavir and lamivudine.
Warning: HEMATOLOGICAL TOXICITY, MYOPATHY, LACTIC ACIDOSIS AND SEVERE HEPATOMEGALY, and EXACERBATIONS OF HEPATITIS B

Skin
Acneform eruption (<5%)
Bromhidrosis (<5%)
Diaphoresis (5–19%)
Edema of lip (<5%)
Erythema multiforme [2]
Exanthems (<5%) [6]
Lipoatrophy [2]
Lipodystrophy [2]
Pigmentation [10]
Pruritus [4]
Rash (17%) [8]
Stevens-Johnson syndrome [4]
Toxic epidermal necrolysis [3]
Urticaria (<5%) [2]
Vasculitis [2]

Hair
Alopecia [2]
Hypertrichosis (eyelashes) [2]

Nails
Nail pigmentation [27]

Mucosal
Oral lichenoid eruption [2]
Oral pigmentation [7]
Oral ulceration (<5%)
Tongue edema (<5%)
Tongue pigmentation [4]

Central Nervous System
Dysgeusia (taste perversion) (5–19%) [2]
Headache [3]
Paresthesias (<8%)

Neuromuscular/Skeletal
Asthenia (fatigue) [3]
Myalgia/Myopathy [5]

Gastrointestinal/Hepatic
Abdominal pain [3]
Diarrhea [2]
Hepatotoxicity [2]
Nausea [3]
Pancreatitis [3]
Vomiting [2]

Endocrine/Metabolic
Acidosis [6]

Hematologic
Anemia [14]
Neutropenia [3]

Other
Adverse effects [9]
Teratogenicity [2]

ZILEUTON

Trade name: Zyflo (AbbVie)
Indications: Asthma
Class: Leukotriene receptor antagonist
Half-life: 2.5 hours
Clinically important, potentially hazardous interactions with: anisindione, anticoagulants, astemizole, dicumarol, methylergonovine, pimozide, propranolol, warfarin
Pregnancy category: C
Important contra-indications noted in the prescribing guidelines for: nursing mothers; pediatric patients

---

Neuromuscular/Skeletal
Myalgia/Myopathy (3%)

ZINC

Trade name: Cold-Eeze (The Quigley Corp)
Indications: Supplement to intravenous solutions given for total parenteral nutrition (TPN)
Class: Food supplement, Trace element
Half-life: N/A
Clinically important, potentially hazardous interactions with: chlorothiazide, chlortetracycline, chlorthalidone, ciprofloxacin, cisplatin, deferoxamine, demeclocycline, doxycycline, eltrombopag, ethambutol, ferrous sulfate, gatifloxacin, gemifloxacin, hydrochlorothiazide, indapamide, levofloxacin, lymecycline, metolozone, minocycline, moxifloxacin, norfloxacin, ofloxacin, oxytetracycline, propofol, tetracycline, valproic acid
Pregnancy category: C
Note: Zinc is found in meats, seafood, dairy products, legumes, nuts, whole grains. Zinc oxide and zinc sulfate are used to fortify wheat products.

Skin
Churg-Strauss syndrome [2]
Dermatitis [4]

Mucosal
Oral mucosal irritation [2]

Central Nervous System
Anosmia [2]
Dysgeusia (taste perversion) [5]

ZIPRASIDONE

Trade name: Geodon (Pfizer)
Indications: Schizophrenia, bipolar I disorder
Class: Antipsychotic
Half-life: 7 hours
Clinically important, potentially hazardous interactions with: acetylcholinesterase inhibitors, alcohol, alfuzosin, amitriptyline, amoxapine, amphetamines, antifungals, arsenic, artemether/lumefantrine, asenapine, astemizole, carbamazepine, chloroquine, ciprofloxacin, citalopram, CNS depressants, conivaptan, dasatinib, degarelix, dolasetron, dopamine agonists, dopamine agonists, dronedarone, food, gadobutrol, ketoconazole, lapatinib, levodopa, levofloxacin, lithium, methylphenidate, metoclopramide, moxifloxacin, nilotinib, pazopanib, pimavanserin, pimozide, QT prolonging agents, quinagolide, quinine, ranolazine, St John's wort, telavancin, telithromycin, tetrabenazine, thioridazine, voriconazole, vorinostat
Pregnancy category: C
Important contra-indications noted in the prescribing guidelines for: the elderly; nursing mothers; pediatric patients
Note: ZIprasidone should be avoided in patients with congenital long QT syndrome or a history of cardiac arrhythmias.
Warning: INCREASED MORTALITY IN ELDERLY PATIENTS WITH DEMENTIA-RELATED PSYCHOSIS

Skin
Angioedema [2]
Diaphoresis (2%)
DRESS syndrome [2]
Fungal dermatitis (2%)
Furunculosis (2%)
Lupus erythematosus [2]
Rash (4%)
Urticaria (5%)

Mucosal
Rectal hemorrhage (2%)
Sialorrhea (4%)
Tongue edema (3%)
Xerostomia (<5%)

Cardiovascular
Bradycardia (2%)
Chest pain (3%)
Hypertension (2–3%)
Postural hypotension (5%)
QT prolongation [22]
Tachycardia (2%) [2]
Torsades de pointes [6]

Central Nervous System
Agitation (2%) [3]
Akathisia (2–10%) [5]
Anorexia (2%)
Anxiety (2–5%) [2]
Depression [2]
Dyskinesia (<10%) [2]
Extrapyramidal symptoms (2–31%) [6]
Headache (3–18%) [3]
Hyperesthesia (<2%)
Hypokinesia (<5%)
Insomnia (3%) [5]
Mania [2]

Neuroleptic malignant syndrome [6]
Paralysis (<10%)
Paresthesias (<2%)
Sedation [4]
Somnolence (drowsiness) (8–31%) [10]
Speech disorder (2%)
Tardive dyskinesia [5]
Tremor (<10%) [2]
Twitching (<10%)
Vertigo (dizziness) (3–16%) [2]

Neuromuscular/Skeletal
Asthenia (fatigue) (2–6%) [2]
Dystonia (<10%) [6]
Hypertonia (<10%)
Myalgia/Myopathy (2%)
Rhabdomyolysis [2]

Gastrointestinal/Hepatic
Abdominal pain (<2%)
Constipation (2–9%)
Diarrhea (3–5%)
Dyspepsia (<8%)
Dysphagia (2%)
Nausea (4–12%) [2]
Vomiting (3–5%)

Respiratory
Cough (increased) (3%)
Dyspnea (2%)
Pharyngitis (3%)
Respiratory tract infection (8%)
Rhinitis (<4%)
Upper respiratory tract infection (8%)

Endocrine/Metabolic
Diabetes mellitus [2]
Galactorrhea [3]
Weight gain [7]

Genitourinary
Dysmenorrhea (2%)
Priapism [4]

Ocular
Abnormal vision (3–6%)

Local
Infusion-site pain (7–9%)

Other
Adverse effects [8]
Death [2]

ZOLEDRONATE

Synonym: zoledronic acid
Trade names: Aclasta (Novartis), Reclast (Novartis), Zometa (Novartis)
Indications: Hypercalcemia of malignancy, Paget's disease, osteoporosis
Class: Bisphosphonate
Half-life: 7 days
Clinically important, potentially hazardous interactions with: aminoglycosides, bisphosphonates, loop diuretics, nephrotoxics
Pregnancy category: D
Important contra-indications noted in the prescribing guidelines for: the elderly; nursing mothers; pediatric patients

---

Skin
Candidiasis (12%)
Dermatitis (11%)
Dermatomyositis [3]
Edema [3]
Neoplasms (malignant / aggrevated) (20%)
Peripheral edema (5–21%)
Rash [3]

Hair
Alopecia (12%)

Mucosal
Mucositis (5–10%)
Stomatitis (8%)

Cardiovascular
Atrial fibrillation [3]
Chest pain (5–10%)
Hypotension (11%)

Central Nervous System
Agitation (13%)
Anorexia (9–22%)
Anxiety (11–14%)
Chills [2]
Confusion (7–13%)
Depression (14%)
Fever (32–44%) [20]
Headache (5–19%) [4]
Hypoesthesia (12%)
Insomnia (15–16%)
Paresthesias (15%)
Rigors (11%)
Seizures [2]
Somnolence (drowsiness) (5–10%)
Vertigo (dizziness) (18%)

Neuromuscular/Skeletal
Arthralgia (5–10%) [9]
Asthenia (fatigue) (5–39%) [11]
Back pain (15%)
Bone or joint pain (12–55%) [15]
Fractures [4]
Myalgia/Myopathy (23%) [7]
Osteonecrosis [53]
Pain in extremities (14%)

Gastrointestinal/Hepatic
Abdominal pain (14–16%)
Constipation (27–31%) [3]
Diarrhea (17–24%) [2]
Dyspepsia (10%)
Dysphagia (5–10%)
Hepatotoxicity [3]
Nausea (29–46%) [12]
Vomiting (14–32%) [2]

Respiratory
Cough (12–22%)
Dyspnea (22–27%)
Flu-like syndrome [9]
Pharyngolaryngeal pain (8%)
Upper respiratory tract infection (10%)

Endocrine/Metabolic
Appetite decreased (13%)
Creatine phosphokinase increased [2]
Dehydration (5–14%)
Hyperparathyroidism [2]
Hypocalcemia (5–10%) [26]
Hypokalemia (12%)
Hypomagnesemia (11%)
Hypophosphatemia (13%) [4]
Weight loss (16%)

Genitourinary
Urinary tract infection (12–14%)

Renal
Fanconi syndrome [2]
Nephrotoxicity [15]
Renal failure [4]
Renal function abnormal [2]

Hematologic
Anemia (22–33%) [8]
Granulocytopenia (5–10%)
Neutropenia (12%)
Pancytopenia (5–10%)
Thrombocytopenia (5–10%)

Ocular
Ocular adverse effects [2]
Ocular inflammation [3]
Scleritis [2]
Uveitis [10]

Other
Adverse effects [6]
Infection (5–10%)

ZOLMITRIPTAN

Trade name: Zomig (AstraZeneca)
Indications: Migraine attacks
Class: 5-HT1 agonist, Serotonin receptor agonist, Triptan
Half-life: 3 hours
Clinically important, potentially hazardous interactions with: cimetidine, ciprofloxacin, dihydroergotamine, ergot-containing drugs, fluoxetine, fluvoxamine, isocarboxazid, levofloxacin, MAO inhibitors, methysergide, moclobemide, moxifloxacin, naratriptan, norfloxacin, ofloxacin, oral contraceptives, phenelzine, propranolol, rizatriptan, sertraline, sibutramine, SNRIs, SSRIs, St John's wort, sumatriptan, tranylcypromine
Pregnancy category: C
Important contra-indications noted in the prescribing guidelines for: nursing mothers; pediatric patients

---

Skin
Diaphoresis (2–3%)
Hot flashes (>10%)

Mucosal
Xerostomia (3–5%)

Cardiovascular
Chest pain (2–4%)
Myocardial infarction [4]

Central Nervous System
Dysgeusia (taste perversion) [4]
Headache [2]
Neurotoxicity [2]
Paresthesias (5–9%) [6]
Somnolence (drowsiness) (5–8%)
Vertigo (dizziness) (2–10%) [3]
Warm feeling (5–7%)

Neuromuscular/Skeletal
Jaw pain (4–10%)
Myalgia/Myopathy (2%) [2]
Neck pain (4–10%)

Gastrointestinal/Hepatic
Dyspepsia (<3%)
Dysphagia (<2%)
Nausea (4–9%) [2]

Renal
Nephrotoxicity [2]

Other
Adverse effects [6]

ZOLPIDEM

Trade name: Ambien (Sanofi-Aventis)
Indications: Insomnia
Class: Hypnotic, non-benzodiazepine
Half-life: 2.6 hours
Clinically important, potentially hazardous interactions with: alcohol, antihistamines, azatadine, azelastine, brompheniramine, buclizine, chlorpheniramine, chlorpromazine, cimetidine, clemastine, cobicistat/elvitegravir/emtricitabine/tenofovir alafenamide, cobicistat/elvitegravir/emtricitabine/tenofovir disoproxil, dexchlorpheniramine, erythromycin, imipramine, ketoconazole, meclizine, pizotifen, ramelteon, rifampin, rifapentine, ritonavir, telaprevir, voriconazole
Pregnancy category: C
Important contra-indications noted in the prescribing guidelines for: nursing mothers; pediatric patients

---

Skin
Rash (2%)

Mucosal
Xerostomia (3%) [3]

Cardiovascular
Palpitation (2%)
Tachycardia [2]
Torsades de pointes [2]

Central Nervous System
Amnesia [16]
Anxiety [2]
Compulsions [2]
Confusion [3]
Delirium [5]
Depression (2%)
Dysgeusia (taste perversion) [4]
Gait instability [3]
Hallucinations [13]
Headache (7%) [11]
Nightmares [2]
Seizures [7]
Sleep related disorder [19]
Slurred speech [2]
Somnambulism [16]
Somnolence (drowsiness) (2–8%) [10]
Vertigo (dizziness) (<5%) [12]

Neuromuscular/Skeletal
Asthenia (fatigue) (3%) [4]
Ataxia [3]
Back pain (3%)
Fractures [2]
Myalgia/Myopathy (7%)

Gastrointestinal/Hepatic
Abdominal pain (2%)
Constipation (2%)
Diarrhea (<3%)
Hepatotoxicity [2]
Nausea [5]
Vomiting [2]

Respiratory
Flu-like syndrome (2%)
Pharyngitis (3%)
Sinusitis (4%)

Ocular
Hallucinations, visual [8]

Other
Adverse effects [8]
Allergic reactions (4%)

ZONISAMIDE

Trade name: Zonegran (Concordia)
Indications: Epilepsy
Class: Anticonvulsant, Antiepileptic, sulfonamide
Half-life: 63 hours
Clinically important, potentially hazardous interactions with: caffeine, metformin
Pregnancy category: C
Important contra-indications noted in the prescribing guidelines for: nursing mothers; pediatric patients
Note: Zonisamide is a sulfonamide and can be absorbed systemically. Sulfonamides can produce severe, possibly fatal, reactions such as toxic epidermal necrolysis and Stevens-Johnson syndrome.

Skin
DRESS syndrome [3]
Ecchymoses (2%)
Hypersensitivity [4]
Oligohydrosis [8]
Purpura (2%)
Rash (3%) [6]
Stevens-Johnson syndrome [3]

Mucosal
Xerostomia (2%)

Central Nervous System
Agitation (9%) [4]
Anorexia (13%) [9]
Anxiety (3%)
Cognitive impairment (6%) [4]
Confusion (6%)
Depression (6%) [4]
Dysgeusia (taste perversion) (2%)
Fever [2]
Headache (10%) [7]
Insomnia (6%)
Irritability (9%) [4]
Mania [2]
Nervousness (2%)
Neuroleptic malignant syndrome [2]
Paresthesias (4%)
Psychosis [3]
Restless legs syndrome [3]
Schizophrenia (2%)
Somnolence (drowsiness) (17%) [22]
Speech disorder (2–5%)
Suicidal ideation [2]
Vertigo (dizziness) (13%) [18]

Neuromuscular/Skeletal
Asthenia (fatigue) (7–8%) [9]
Ataxia (6%) [3]

Gastrointestinal/Hepatic
Abdominal pain (6%)
Constipation (2%)
Diarrhea (5%)
Dyspepsia (3%)
Nausea (9%) [2]
Vomiting [2]

Respiratory
Flu-like syndrome (4%)
Pneumonitis [2]
Rhinitis (2%)

Endocrine/Metabolic
Appetite decreased [7]
Weight loss (3%) [20]

Renal
Nephrolithiasis [4]
Nephrotoxicity [2]

Ocular
Diplopia (6%) [2]
Nystagmus (4%)

Other
Adverse effects [12]
Side effects [4]
Teratogenicity [2]

ZOSTER VACCINE

Trade name: Zostavax (Oka/Merck)
Indications: To reduce the risk of developing herpes zoster (in people over 60)
Class: Vaccine
Half-life: N/A
Clinically important, potentially hazardous interactions with: none known
Pregnancy category: C

Skin
Herpes zoster [7]
Rash [2]

Central Nervous System
Fever (<2%)
Headache [4]

Respiratory
Flu-like syndrome (<2%)

Local
Injection-site edema [3]
Injection-site erythema [3]
Injection-site pain [4]
Injection-site reactions [11]

Other
Adverse effects [2]
Death [2]

ZOTAROLIMUS

Trade names: Endeavor (Medtronic), ZoMaxx Drug-Eluting Coronary Stent (AbbVie)
Indications: Ischemic heart disease, restenosis
Class: Angiogenesis inhibitor, Macrolide immunosuppressant (derivative of sirolimus), mTOR inhibitor
Half-life: 33–36 hours
Clinically important, potentially hazardous interactions with: ketoconazole, sirolimus
Pregnancy category: C
Important contra-indications noted in the prescribing guidelines for: nursing mothers; pediatric patients

---

Skin
Rash (<6%)
Xerosis (<13%)

Cardiovascular
Cardiotoxicity [4]
Myocardial infarction [3]
Subacute thrombosis [2]

Central Nervous System
Headache (4–13%)
Pain (13–63%)

Gastrointestinal/Hepatic
Abdominal pain (<6%)
Diarrhea (<6%)

Genitourinary
Hematuria (<13%)

Local
Application-site reactions (13–63%)
Injection-site reactions (13–38%)

Descriptions of important reactions

Acanthosis nigricans

Acanthosis nigricans (AN) is a process characterized by a soft, velvety, brown or grayish-black thickening of the skin that is symmetrically distributed over the axillae, neck, inguinal areas and other body folds.

While most cases of AN are seen in obese and prepubertal children, it can occur as a marker for various endocrinopathies as well as in female patients with elevated testosterone levels, irregular menses, and hirsutism.

It is frequently a concomitant of an underlying malignant condition, principally an adenocarcinoma of the intestinal tract.

Acneform lesions

Acneform eruptions are inflammatory follicular reactions that resemble acne vulgaris and that are manifested clinically as papules or pustules. They are monomorphic reactions, have a monomorphic appearance, and are found primarily on the upper parts of the body. Unlike acne vulgaris, there are rarely comedones present. Consider a drug-induced acneform eruption if:

- The onset is sudden
- There is a worsening of existing acne lesions
- The extent is considerable from the outset
- The appearance is monomorphic
- The localization is unusual for acne as, for example, when the distal extremities are involved
- The patient's age is unusual for regular acne
- There is an exposure to a potentially responsible drug.

The most common drugs responsible for acneform eruptions are: ACTH, androgenic hormones, anticonvulsants (hydantoin derivatives, phenobarbital, trimethadione), corticosteroids, danazol, disulfiram, halogens (bromides, chlorides, iodides), lithium, oral contraceptives, tuberculostatics (ethionamide, isoniazid, rifampin), vitamins B_2, B_6 and B_{12}.

Acute febrile neutrophilic dermatosis

Acute febrile neutrophilic dermatosis is a disorder that appears more frequently in females and has several characteristic features.

The lesions - tender, erythematous or purple, annular plaques or nodules - appear suddenly and are most prominent on the face, neck and upper extremities. Pain and fever often accompany the eruption.

While the cause is unknown, about 15% of the patients have some type of myeloproliferative disorder, primarily leukemias.

Drugs commonly reported to cause Sweet's syndrome are clofazimine, co-trimoxazole, furosemide, granulocyte-colony stimulating factor and minocycline.

Acute generalized exanthematous pustulosis

Arising on the face or intertriginous areas, acute generalized exanthematous pustulosis (AGEP) is characterized by a rapidly evolving, widespread, scarlatiniform eruption covered with hundreds of small superficial pustules.

Often accompanied by a high fever, AGEP is most frequently associated with acetaminophen, carbamazepine, penicillin and macrolide antibiotics, and usually occurs within 24 hours of the drug exposure.

Ageusia

Ageusia is the loss of taste functions of the tongue, essentially the inability to detect sweet, sour, bitter, or salty substances, and umami (the taste of monosodium glutamate).

Atorvastatin, captopril, enalapril, indomethacin, and paroxetine are some of the drugs that can occasion ageusia.

Alopecia

Many drugs have been reported to occasion hair loss. Commonly appearing as a diffuse alopecia, it affects women more frequently than men and is limited in most instances to the scalp. Axillary and pubic hairs are rarely affected except with anticoagulants.

The hair loss from cytostatic agents, which is dose-dependent and begins about 2 weeks after the onset of therapy, is a result of the interruption of the anagen (growing) cycle of hair. With other drugs the hair loss does not begin until 2–5 months after the medication has been begun. With cholesterol-lowering drugs, diffuse alopecia is a result of interference with normal keratinization.

The scalp is normal and the drug-induced alopecia is almost always reversible within 1–3 months after the therapy has been discontinued. The regrown hair is frequently depigmented and occasionally more curly

The most frequent offenders are cytostatic agents and anticoagulants, but hair loss can occur with a variety of common drugs, including hormones, anticonvulsants, amantadine, amiodarone, captopril, cholesterol-lowering drugs, cimetidine, colchicine, etretinate, isotretinoin, ketoconazole, heavy metals, lithium, penicillamine, valproic acid, and propranolol.

Angioedema

Angioedema is a term applied to a variant of urticaria in which the subcutaneous tissues, rather than the dermis, are mainly involved.

Also known as Quincke's edema, giant urticaria, and angioneurotic edema, this acute, evanescent, skin-colored, circumscribed edema usually affects the most distensible tissues: the lips, eyelids, earlobes, and genitalia. It can also affect the mucous membranes of the tongue, mouth, and larynx.

Symptoms of angioedema, frequently unilateral, asymmetrical and non-pruritic, last for an hour or two but can persist for 2–5 days.

The etiological factors associated with angioedema are as varied as that of urticaria (see separate entry).

Anosmia

Anosmia, or odor blindness, is the total absence of the sense of smell. It can be either temporary or permanent.

Some of the drugs that can cause anosmia are ciprofloxacin, doxycycline, enalapril, paroxetine and sparfloxacin.

Aphthous stomatitis

Aphthous stomatitis – also known as canker sores – is a common disease of the oral mucous membranes.

Arising as tiny, discrete or grouped, papules or vesicles, these painful lesions develop into small (2–5 mm in diameter), round, shallow ulcerations having a grayish, yellow base surrounded by a thin red border.

Located predominantly over the labial and buccal mucosae, these aphthae heal without scarring in 10–14 days. Recurrences are common.

Baboon syndrome (SDRIFE)

Baboon syndrome or symmetric drug-related intertriginous and flexural exanthema (SDRIFE) is an unusual presentation of a drug eruption with a characteristic intertriginous distribution pattern. Several drugs have been implicated, notably mercury, nickel, heparin, aminophylline, pseudoephedrine, terbinafine, IVIG, various antibiotics (amoxicillin, ampicillin), and food additives.

Originally described as a type of systemic contact dermatitis characterized by a pruritic exanthems involving the buttocks and major flexures – groins and axillae, some investigators believe that this entity is a form of recall phenomenon. In children, it is important in the differential diagnosis of viral exanthems.

Black tongue (lingua villosa nigra)

Black hairy tongue (BHT) represents a benign hyperplasia of the filiform papillae of the anterior two-thirds of the tongue.

These papillary elongations, usually associated with black, brown, or yellow pigmentation attributed to the overgrowth of pigment-producing bacteria, may be as long as 2 cm.

Occurring only in adults, BHT has been associated with the administration of oral antibiotics, poor dental hygiene, and excessive smoking.

Bullous dermatitis

Bullous and vesicular drug eruptions are diseases in which blisters and vesicles occur as a complication of the administration of drugs. Blisters are a well-known manifestation of cutaneous reactions to drugs.

In many types of drug reactions, bullae and vesicles may be found in addition to other manifestations. Bullae are usually noted in: erythema multiforme; Stevens–Johnson syndrome; toxic epidermal necrolysis; fixed eruptions when very intense; urticaria; vasculitis; porphyria cutanea tarda; and phototoxic reactions (from furosemide and nalidixic acid). Tense, thick-walled bullae can be seen in bromoderma and iododerma as well as in barbiturate overdosage.

Common drugs that cause bullous eruptions and bullous pemphigoid are: nadalol, penicillamine, piroxicam, psoralens, rifampin, clonidine, furosemide, diclofenac, mefenamic acid, and bleomycin.

DRESS syndrome

The DRESS syndrome is an acronym for Drug Rash with Eosinophilia and Systemic Symptoms. It is also known as the Drug-Induced Pseudolymphoma and Drug Hypersensitivity Syndrome.

The symptoms of DRESS syndrome usually begin 1 to 8 weeks after exposure to the offending drug. Common causes include carbamazepine, phenobarbital, phenytoin, terbinafine, and valproic acid.

Erythema multiforme

Erythema multiforme is a relatively common, acute, self-limited, inflammatory reaction pattern that is often associated with a preceding herpes simplex or mycoplasma infection. Other causes are associated with connective tissue disease, physical agents, X-ray therapy, pregnancy and internal malignancies, to mention a few. In 50% of the cases, no cause can be found. In a recent prospective study of erythema multiforme, only 10% were drug related.

The eruption rapidly occurs over a period of 12 to 24 hours. In about half the cases there are prodromal symptoms of an upper respiratory infection accompanied by fever, malaise, and varying degrees of muscular and joint pains.

Clinically, bluish-red, well-demarcated, macular, papular, or urticarial lesions, as well as the classical 'iris' or 'target lesions', sometimes with central vesicles, bullae, or purpura, are distributed preferentially over the distal extremities, especially over the dorsa of the hands and extensor aspects of the forearms. Lesions tend to spread peripherally and may involve the palms and trunk as well as the mucous membranes of the mouth and genitalia. Central healing and overlapping lesions often lead to arciform, annular and gyrate patterns. Lesions appear over the course of a week or 10 days and resolve over the next two weeks.

The following drugs have been most often associated with erythema multiforme: allopurinol, barbiturates, carbamazepine, estrogens/progestins, gold, lamotrigine, NSAIDs, penicillamine, phenytoin, sulfonamides, tetracycline, tolbutamide and valproic acid.

Erythema nodosum

Erythema nodosum is a cutaneous reaction pattern characterized by erythematous, tender or painful subcutaneous nodules commonly distributed over the anterior aspect of the lower legs, and occasionally elsewhere.

More common in young women, erythema nodosum is often associated with increased estrogen levels as occurs during pregnancy and with the ingestion of oral contraceptives. It is also an occasional manifestation of streptococcal infection, sarcoidosis, secondary syphilis, tuberculosis, certain deep fungal infections, Hodgkin's disease, leukemia, ulcerative colitis, and radiation therapy and is often preceded by fever, fatigue, arthralgia, vomiting, and diarrhea.

The incidence of erythema nodosum due to drugs is low and it is impossible to distinguish clinically between erythema nodosum due to drugs and that caused by other factors.

Some of the drugs that are known to occasion erythema nodosum are: antibiotics, estrogens, amiodarone, gold, NSAIDs, oral contraceptives, sulfonamides, and opiates.

Exanthems

Exanthems, commonly resembling viral rashes, represent the most common type of cutaneous drug eruption. Described as maculopapular or morbilliform eruptions, these flat, barely raised, erythematous patches, from one to several millimeters in diameter, are usually bilateral and symmetrical. They commonly begin on the head and neck or upper torso and progress downward to the limbs. They may present or develop into confluent areas and may be accompanied by pruritus and a mild fever.

The exanthems caused by drugs can be classified as:

- Morbilliform eruptions: fingernail-sized erythematous patches
- Scarlatiniform eruptions: punctate, pinpoint, or pinhead-sized lesions in erythematous areas that have a tendency to coalesce. Circumoral pallor and the subsequent appearance of scaling may also be noted.

Maculopapular drug eruptions usually fade with desquamation and, occasionally, postinflammatory hyperpigmentation, in about 2 weeks. They invariably recur on rechallenge.

Exanthems often have a sudden onset during the first 2 weeks of administration, except in cases of semisynthetic penicillin administration, when the exanthems frequently develop after the first 2 weeks following the initial dose.

The drugs most commonly associated with exanthems are: amoxicillin, ampicillin, bleomycin, captopril, carbamazepine, chlorpromazine, co-trimoxazole, gold, nalidixic acid, naproxen, phenytoin, penicillamine, and piroxicam.

Exfoliative dermatitis

Exfoliative dermatitis is a rare but serious reaction pattern that is characterized by erythema, pruritus and scaling over the entire body (erythroderma).

Drug-induced exfoliative dermatitis usually begins a few weeks or longer following the administration of a culpable drug. Beginning as erythematous, edematous patches, often on the face, it spreads to involve the entire integument. The skin becomes swollen and scarlet and may ooze a straw-colored fluid; this is followed in a few days by desquamation.

High fever, severe malaise and chills, along with enlargement of lymph nodes, often coexist with the cutaneous changes.

One of the most dangerous of all reaction patterns, exfoliative dermatitis can be accompanied by any or all of the following: hypothermia, fluid and electrolyte loss, cardiac failure, and gastrointestinal hemorrhage. Death may supervene if the drug is continued after the onset of the eruption. Secondary infection often complicates the course of the disease. Once the active dermatitis has receded, hyperpigmentation as well as loss of hair and nails may ensue.

The following drugs, among others, can bring about exfoliative dermatitis: barbiturates, captopril, carbamazepine, cimetidine, furosemide, gold, isoniazid, lithium, nitrofurantoin, NSAIDs, penicillamine, phenytoin, pyrazolons, quinidine, streptomycin, sulfonamides, and thiazides.

Fixed eruption

A fixed eruption is an unusual hypersensitivity reaction characterized by one or more well-demarcated erythematous plaques that recur at the same cutaneous (or mucosal) site or sites each time exposure to the offending agent occurs. The sizes of the lesions vary from a few millimeters to as much as 20 centimeters in diameter. Almost any drug that is ingested, injected, inhaled, or inserted into the body can trigger this skin reaction.

The eruption typically begins as a sharply marginated, solitary edematous papule or plaque – occasionally surmounted by a large bulla – which usually develops 30 minutes to 8 hours following the administration of a drug. If the offending agent is not promptly eliminated, the inflammation intensifies, producing a dusky red, violaceous or brown patch that may crust, desquamate, or blister within 7 to 10 days. The lesions are rarely pruritic. Favored sites are the hands, feet, face, and genitalia – especially the glans penis.

The reason for the specific localization of the skin lesions in a fixed drug eruption is unknown. The offending drug cannot be detected at the skin site. Certain drugs cause a fixed eruption at specific sites, for example, tetracycline and ampicillin often elicit a fixed eruption on the penis, whereas aspirin usually causes skin lesions on the face, limbs and trunk.

Common causes of fixed eruptions are: ampicillin, aspirin, barbiturates, dapsone, metronidazole, NSAIDs, oral contraceptives, phenolphthalein, phenytoin, quinine, sulfonamides, and tetracyclines.

Gingival hyperplasia/hypertrophy

Gingival hyperplasia, a common, undesirable, non-allergic drug reaction begins as a diffuse swelling of the interdental papillae.

Particularly prevalent with phenytoin therapy, gingival hyperplasia begins about 3 months after the onset of therapy, and occurs in 30 to 70% of patients receiving it. The severity of the reaction is dose-dependent and children and young adults are more frequently affected. The most severe cases are noted in young women.

In many cases, gingival hyperplasia is accompanied by painful and bleeding gums. There is often superimposed secondary bacterial gingivitis. This can be so extensive that the teeth of the maxilla and mandible are completely overgrown.

While it is characteristically a side effect of hydantoin derivatives, it may occur during the administration of phenobarbital, nifedipine, diltiazem and other medications.

Hand-foot syndrome

Hand-foot syndrome (also known as acral erythema, palmar-plantar erythrodysesthesia, palmoplantar erythrodysesthesia, palmar-plantar erythema, and Bergdorf's reaction) is a syndrome that is characterized by well-demarcated painful erythema, edema, numbness and desquamation over the palms and soles that may develop following treatment with a variety of chemotherapeutic agents including bleomycin, cisplatin, cyclophosphamide, hydroxyurea, idarubicin, methotrexate, sorafenib, sunitinib, and others. Tenderness involving the skin overlying the fingers and toes, followed by bulla formation and subsequent desquamation, often supervenes.

This side effect results when a small amount of the culpable drug leaks out of the blood vessels, damaging tissues. This reaction predominates over the palms and soles, where eccrine glands are more numerous, and also as a result of the increased friction and heat that extremities are exposed to through daily activities.

Lichenoid (lichen planus-like) eruptions

Lichenoid eruptions are so called because of their resemblance to lichen planus, a papulosquamous disorder that characteristically presents as multiple, discrete, violaceous, flat-topped papules, often polygonal in shape and which are extremely pruritic.

Not infrequently, lichenoid lesions appear weeks or months following exposure to the responsible drug. As a rule, the symptoms begin to recede a few weeks following the discontinuation of the drug.

Common drug causes of lichenoid eruptions are: antimalarials, beta-blockers, chlorpropamide, furosemide, gold, methyldopa, phenothiazines, quinidine, thiazides, and tolazamide.

Lupus erythematosus

A reaction, clinically and pathologically resembling idiopathic systemic lupus erythematosus (SLE), has been reported in association with a large variety of drugs. There is some evidence that drug-induced SLE, invariably accompanied by a positive ANA reaction with 90% having antihistone antibodies, may have a genetically determined basis. These symptoms of SLE, a relatively benign form of lupus, recede within days or weeks following the discontinuation of the responsible drug. Skin lesions occur in about 20% of cases. Drugs cause fewer than 8% of all cases of SLE.

The following drugs have been commonly associated with inducing, aggravating or unmasking SLE: beta-blockers, carbamazepine, chlorpromazine, estrogens, griseofulvin, hydralazine, isoniazid (INH), lithium, methyldopa, minoxidil, oral contraceptives, penicillamine, phenytoin (diphenylhydantoin), procainamide, propylthiouracil, quinidine, and testosterone.

Onycholysis

Onycholysis, the painless separation of the nail plate from the nail bed, is one of the most common nail disorders.

The unattached portion, which is white and opaque, usually begins at the free margin and proceeds proximally, causing part or most of the nail plate to become separated. The attached, healthy portion of the nail, by contrast, is pink and translucent.

Paresthesias

Paresthesias are abnormal neurological sensations such as burning, prickling, numbness, pruritus, formication, or tingling, often described as 'pins and needles' or of a limb being 'asleep'. It is a symptom of partial damage to a peripheral nerve, as occurs from a head or spinal injury, lack of blood supply to a nerve, or in many cases medications.

Paresthesias can affect various parts of the body; hands, fingers, and feet are common sites but all areas are possibilities.

Scores of generic drugs have been reported to occasion paresthesias including alprazolam, allopurinol, buspirone, celecoxib, ciprofloxacin, cyclosporine, enalapril, glipizine and many others.

Pemphigus vulgaris

Pemphigus vulgaris (PV) is a rare, serious, acute or chronic, blistering disease involving the skin and mucous membranes.

Characterized by thin-walled, easily ruptured, flaccid bullae that are seen to arise on normal or erythematous skin and over mucous membranes, the lesions of PV appear initially in the mouth (in about 60% of the cases) and then spread, after weeks or months, to involve the axillae and groin, scalp, face and neck. The lesions may become generalized.

Because of their fragile roofs, the bullae rupture leaving painful erosions and crusts may develop principally over the scalp.

Peyronie's disease

First described in 1743 by the French surgeon, François de la Peyronie, Peyronie's disease is a rare, benign connective tissue disorder involving the growth of fibrous plaques in the soft tissue of the penis. Beginning as a localized inflammation, it often develops into a hardened scar. Affecting as many as 1% of men, it may cause deformity, pain, cord-like lesions, or abnormal curvature of the penis when erect.

It has been associated with several drugs, including all the adrenergic blocking agents (beta-blockers), methotrexate, colchicine and others.

Photosensitivity

A photosensitive reaction is a chemically induced change in the skin that makes an individual unusually sensitive to electromagnetic radiation (light). On absorbing light of a specific wavelength, an oral, injected or topical drug may be chemically altered to produce a reaction ranging from macules and papules, vesicles and bullae, edema, urticaria, or an acute eczematous reaction.

Any eruption that is prominent on the face, the dorsa of the hands, the 'V' of the neck, and the presternal area should suggest an adverse reaction to light. The distribution is the key to the diagnosis.

Initially the eruption, which consists of erythema, edema, blisters, weeping and desquamation, involves the forehead, rims of the ears, the nose, the malar eminences and cheeks, the sides and back of the neck, the extensor surfaces of the forearms and the dorsa of the hands. These reactions commonly spare the shaded areas: those under the chin, under the nose, behind the ears and inside the fold of the upper eyelids. There is usually a sharp cut-off at the site of jewelry and at clothing margins. All light-exposed areas need not be affected equally.

There are two main types of photosensitive reactions: the phototoxic and the photoallergic reaction.

Phototoxic reactions, the most common type of drug-induced photosensitivity, resemble an exaggerated sunburn and occur within 5 to 20 hours after the skin has been exposed to a photosensitizing substance and light of the proper wavelength and intensity. It is not a form of allergy – prior sensitization is not required – and, theoretically, could occur in anyone given enough drug and light. Phototoxic reactions are dose-dependent both for drug and sunlight. Patients with phototoxicity reactions are commonly sensitive to ultraviolet A (UVA radiation), the so-called 'tanning rays' at 320–400 nm. Phototoxic reactions may cause onycholysis, as the nailbed is particularly susceptible because of its lack of melanin protection.

Patients with a true photoallergy (the interaction of drug, light and the immune system), a less common form of drug-induced photosensitivity, are often sensitive to UVB radiation, the so-called 'burning rays' at 290–320 nm. Photoallergic reactions, unlike phototoxic responses, represent an immunologic change and require a latent period of from 24 to 48 hours during which sensitization occurs. They are not dose-related.

If the photosensitizer acts internally, it is a photodrug reaction; if it acts externally, it is photocontact dermatitis.

Drugs that are likely to cause phototoxic reactions are: amiodarone, nalidixic acid, various NSAIDs, phenothiazines (especially chlorpromazine), and tetracyclines (particularly demeclocycline).

Photoallergic reactions may occur as a result of exposure to systemically-administered drugs such as griseofulvin, NSAIDs, phenothiazines, quinidine, sulfonamides, sulfonylureas, and thiazide diuretics as well as to external agents such as para-aminobenzoic acid (found in sunscreens), bithionol (used in soaps and cosmetics), paraphenylenediamine, and others.

Pigmentation

Drug-induced pigmentation on the skin, hair, nails, and mucous membranes is a result of either melanin synthesis, increased lipofuscin synthesis, or post-inflammatory pigmentation.

Color changes, which can be localized or widespread, can also be a result of a deposition of bile pigments (jaundice), exogenous metal compounds, and direct deposition of elements such as carotene or quinacrine.

Post-inflammatory pigmentation can follow a variety of drug-induced inflammatory cutaneous reactions; fixed eruptions are known to leave a residual pigmentation that can persist for months.

The following is a partial list of those drugs that can cause various pigmentary changes: anticonvulsants, antimalarials, cytostatics, hormones, metals, tetracyclines, phenothiazine tranquilizers, psoralens and amiodarone.

Pityriasis rosea-like eruption

Pityriasis rosea, commonly mistaken for ringworm, is a unique disorder that usually begins as a single, large, round or oval pinkish patch known as the 'mother' or 'herald' patch. The most common sites for this solitary lesion are the chest, the back, or the abdomen. This is followed in about 2 weeks by a blossoming of small, flat, round or oval, scaly patches of similar color, each with a central collarette scale, usually distributed in a Christmas tree pattern over the trunk and, to a lesser degree, the extremities. This eruption seldom itches and usually limits itself to areas from the neck to the knees.

While the etiology of idiopathic pityriasis rosea is unknown, various medications have been reported to give rise to this disorder. These include: barbiturates, beta-blockers, bismuth, captopril, clonidine, gold, griseofulvin, isotretinoin, labetalol, meprobamate, metronidazole, penicillin, and tripelennamine.

In drug-induced pityriasis rosea, the 'herald patch' is usually absent, and the eruption will often not follow the classic pattern.

Pruritus

Generalized itching, without any visible signs, is one of the least common adverse reactions to drugs. More frequently than not, drug-induced itching – moderate or severe – is fairly generalized.

For most drugs it is not known in what way they elicit pruritus; some drugs can cause itching directly or indirectly through cholestasis. Pruritus may develop by different pathogenetic mechanisms: allergic, pseudoallergic (histamine release), neurogenic, by vasodilatation, cholestatic effect, and others.

A partial list of those drugs that can cause pruritus are as follows: aspirin, NSAIDs, penicillins, sulfonamides, chloroquine, ACE-inhibitors, amiodarone, nicotinic acid derivatives, lithium, bleomycin, tamoxifen, interferons, gold, penicillamine, methoxsalen and isotretinoin.

Pseudolymphoma

Pseudolymphoma is not a specific disease. It is an inflammatory response to various stimuli – known or unknown – that results in a lymphomatous-appearing, but benign, accumulation of inflammatory cells. It may resemble true lymphoma clinically and histologically. Localized, nodular pseudolymphomas typically mimic B-cell lymphoma.

The following drugs, among others, are known to occasion pseudolymphoma: alprazolam, carbamazepine, co-trimoxazole, gold, lamotrigine, lithium, methotrexate, etc.

Pseudoporphyria

Pseudoporphyria is an uncommon, reversible, photoinduced, cutaneous bullous disorder with clinical, histologic and immunofluorescent similarities to porphyria cutanea tarda but without the accompanying biochemical porphyrin abnormalities.

It is commonly seen as localized bullae and skin fragility on sun-exposed skin, often on the dorsum of the hands and fingers. While pseudoporphyria has been linked with numerous causes, including chronic renal failure, dialysis, and ultraviolet radiation, several medications, primarily naproxen and other nonsteroidal inflammatory drugs, have been reported to trigger this reaction pattern. Blue/gray eye color appears to be an independent risk factor for the development of pseudoporphyria.

Psoriasis

Many drugs, as a result of their pharmacological action, have been implicated in the precipitation or exacerbation of psoriasis or psoriasiform eruptions.

Psoriasis is a common, chronic, papulosquamous disorder of unknown etiology with characteristic histopathological features and many biochemical, physiological, and immunological abnormalities.

Drugs that can precipitate psoriasis are, among others, beta-blockers and lithium. Drugs that are reported to aggravate psoriasis are antimalarials, beta-blockers, lithium, NSAIDs, quinidine, and photosensitizing drugs. The effect and extent of these drug-induced psoriatic eruptions are dose-dependent.

Purpura

Purpura, a result of hemorrhage into the skin, can be divided into thrombocytopenic purpura and non-thrombocytopenic purpura (vascular purpura). Both thrombocytopenic and vascular purpura may be due to drugs, and most of the drugs producing purpura may do so by giving rise to vascular damage and thrombocytopenia. In both types of purpura, allergic or toxic (nonallergic) mechanisms may be involved.

Some drugs combine with platelets to form an antigen, stimulating formation of antibody to the platelet–drug combination. Thus, the drug appears to act as a hapten; subsequent antigen–antibody reaction causes platelet destruction leading to thrombocytopenia.

The purpuric lesions are usually more marked over the lower portions of the body, notably the legs and dorsal aspects of the feet in ambulatory patients.

Other drug-induced cutaneous reactions – erythema multiforme, erythema nodosum, fixed eruption, necrotizing vasculitis, and others – can have a prominent purpuric component.

A whole host of drugs can give rise to purpura, the most common being: NSAIDs, thiazide diuretics, phenothiazines, cytostatics, gold, penicillamine, hydantoins, thiouracils, and sulfonamides.

Raynaud's phenomenon

Raynaud's phenomenon is the paroxysmal, cold-induced constriction of small arteries and arterioles of the fingers and, less often, the toes.

Although estimates vary, recent surveys show that Raynaud's phenomenon may affect 5 to 10 percent of the general population in the United States. Occurring more frequently in women, Raynaud's phenomenon is characterized by blanching, pallor, and cyanosis. In severe cases, secondary changes may occur: thinning and ridging of the nails, telangiectases of the nail folds, and, in the later stages, sclerosis and atrophy of the digits.

Rhabdomyolysis

Rhabdomyolysis is the breakdown of muscle fibers, the result of skeletal muscle injury, that leads to the release of potentially toxic intracellular contents into the plasma. The causes are diverse: muscle trauma from vigorous exercise, electrolyte imbalance, extensive thermal burns, crush injuries, infections, various toxins and drugs, and a host of other factors.

Rhabdomyolysis can result from direct muscle injury by myotoxic drugs such as cocaine, heroin and alcohol. About 10–40% of patients with rhabdomyolysis develop acute renal failure.

The classic triad of symptoms of rhabdomyolysis is muscle pain, weakness and dark urine. Most frequently, the involved muscle groups are those of the back and lower calves. The primary diagnostic indicator of this syndrome is significantly elevated serum creatine phosphokinase.

Some of the drugs that have been reported to cause rhabdomyolysis are salicylates, amphotericin, quinine, statin drugs, SSRIs, theophylline, and amphetamines.

Stevens-Johnson syndrome

The Stevens-Johnson syndrome (erythema multiforme major), a severe and occasionally fatal variety of erythema multiforme, has an abrupt onset and is accompanied by any or all of the following: fever, myalgia, malaise, headache, arthralgia, ocular involvement, with occasional bullae and erosions covering less than 10% of the body surface. Painful stomatitis is an early and conspicuous symptom. Hemorrhagic bullae may appear over the lips, mouth and genital mucous membranes. Patients are often acutely ill with high fever. The course from eruption to the healing of the lesions may extend up to six weeks.

The following drugs have been most often associated with Stevens-Johnson syndrome: allopurinol, barbiturates, carbamazepine, estrogens/progestins, gold, lamotrigine, NSAIDs, penicillamine, phenytoin, sulfonamides, tetracycline, tolbutamide, and valproic acid.

Tinnitus

Tinnitus (from the Latin word to tinkle or ring like a bell) is the perception of sound—ringing, buzzing, hissing, humming, whistling, whining, roaring, or ticking, clicking, banging, beeping, pulsating—in the human ear, when none exists. It has also been described as a 'whooshing' sound, like wind or waves, 'crickets' or 'tree frogs' or 'locusts.' To some it's a chirping, clanging, sizzling, rumbling, or a dreadful shrieking noise. And it can be like rushing water, breaking glass or chain saws running. Nearly 40 million Americans suffer from this disorder.

There are more than 200 drugs listed in the Litt's Drug Eruption & Reaction Database that have been reported to trigger tinnitus, the more common being aspirin, quinine, aminoglycoside antibiotics, cytotoxic drugs, diuretics, and NSAIDs.

Toxic epidermal necrolysis (TEN)

Also known as Lyell's syndrome, toxic epidermal necrolysis is a rare, serious, acute exfoliative, bullous eruption of the skin and mucous membranes that usually develops as a reaction to diverse drugs. TEN can also be a result of a bacterial or viral infection and can develop after radiation therapy or vaccinations.

In the drug-induced form of TEN, a morbilliform eruption accompanied by large red, tender areas of the skin will develop shortly after the drug has been administered. This progresses rapidly to blistering, and a widespread exfoliation of the epidermis develops dramatically over a very short period accompanied by high fever. The hairy parts of the body are usually spared. The mucous membranes and eyes are often involved.

The clinical picture resembles an extensive second-degree burn; the patient is acutely ill. Fatigue, vomiting, diarrhea and angina are prodromal symptoms. In a few hours the condition becomes grave.

TEN is a medical emergency and unless the offending agent is discontinued immediately, the outcome may be fatal in the course of a few days.

Drugs that are the most common cause of TEN are: allopurinol, ampicillin, amoxicillin, carbamazepine, NSAIDs, phenobarbital, pentamidine, phenytoin (diphenylhydantoin), pyrazolons, and sulfonamides.

Urticaria

Urticaria induced by drugs is, after exanthems, the second most common type of drug reaction. Urticaria, or hives, is a vascular reaction of the skin characterized by pruritic, erythematous wheals. These welts – or wheals – caused by localized edema, can vary in size from one millimeter in diameter to large palm-sized swellings, favor the covered areas (trunk, buttocks, chest), and are, more often than not, generalized. Urticaria usually develops within 36 hours following the administration of the responsible drug. Individual lesions rarely persist for more than 24 hours.

Urticaria may be the only symptom of drug sensitivity, or it may be a concomitant or followed by the manifestations of serum sickness. Urticaria may be accompanied by angioedema of the lips or eyelids. It may, on rare occasions, progress to anaphylactoid reactions or to anaphylaxis.

The following are the most common causes of drug-induced urticaria: antibiotics, notably penicillin (more commonly following parenteral administration than by ingestion), barbiturates, captopril, levamisole, NSAIDs, quinine, rifampin, sulfonamides, thiopental, and vancomycin.

Vasculitis

Drug-induced cutaneous necrotizing vasculitis, a clinicopathologic process characterized by inflammation and necrosis of blood vessels, often presents with a variety of small, palpable purpuric lesions most frequently distributed over the lower extremities: urticaria-like lesions, small ulcerations, and occasional hemorrhagic vesicles and pustules. The basic process involves an immunologically mediated response to antigens that result in vessel wall damage.

Beginning as small macules and papules, they ultimately eventuate into purpuric lesions and, in the more severe cases, into hemorrhagic blisters and frank ulcerations. A polymorphonuclear infiltrate and fibrinoid changes in the small dermal vessels characterize the vasculitic reaction.

Drugs that are commonly associated with vasculitis are: ACE-inhibitors, amiodarone, ampicillin, cimetidine, coumadin, furosemide, hydantoins, hydralazine, NSAIDs, pyrazolons, quinidine, sulfonamides, thiazides, and thiouracils.

Vertigo

Vertigo, a specific type of dizziness, is a feeling of unsteadiness. It is the sensation of spinning or swaying while actually remaining stationary with respect to the surroundings. It is a result of either motion sickness, a viral infection of the organs of balance, low blood sugar, or medications. It is a symptom of multiple sclerosis, carbon monoxide poisoning, and Ménière's disease.

Vertigo is one of the most common health problems in adults. According to the National Institutes of Health, about 40% of people in the United States experience vertigo at least once during their lifetime. Prevalence is higher in women and increases with age.

Classes of drugs that have been reported to trigger vertigo include, aminoglycoside antibiotics, antihypertensives, diuretics, vasodilators, phenothiazines, tranquilizers, antidepressants, anticonvulsants, hypnotics, analgesics, alcohol, caffeine, and tobacco.

Xerostomia

Xerostomia is a dryness of the oral cavity that makes speaking, chewing and swallowing difficult. Some people also experience changes in taste and salivary gland enlargement. Lack of saliva may predispose one to oral infection, such as candidiasis, and increase the risk of dental caries.

Resulting from a partial or complete absence of saliva production, xerostomia can be caused by more than 400 generic drugs.

Class Reactions*

ACE INHIBITORS

	B	C	E	F	L	P	Q	R	T	Z	=
SKIN											
Anaphylaxis		[1]	[1]		•	[1]		•			✓
Angioedema	[8]	[45] (15%)	[73]	[3]	[43] (70%)	[6]	[9]	[11]	[3]	[1]	✓✓
Bullous dermatitis		[1]			[1]						
Bullous pemphigoid		[2]	[2]		[1]						
Dermatitis		[3]		[1]				[1]			
Diaphoresis	[1]		[1]	•	•	•	[3]	[2]			✓
DRESS syndrome		[2]				[1]		[1]			
Edema			[1]	•		•	[4]	[1]	•		✓
Erythema		[1]	[1]		•	•		[1]			✓
Erythema multiforme			•					•			
Erythroderma		[2]	[1]	[1]							
Exanthems	[1]	[19] (10%)	[9]		[4]		[1]	[1]			✓
Exfoliative dermatitis		[4]	•		[2]		•				
Facial edema					[1]	•	[1]				
Flushing	[1]	[2]	[4]		[2]		•	[2]	•		✓
Jaundice		[1]						[1]			
Kaposi's sarcoma		[2]			[2]		[1]				
Lichen planus pemphigoides		[2]						[3]			
Lichenoid eruption		[12]	[2]		[2]						
Linear IgA	[1]	[5]									
Lupus erythematosus		[8]	[2]		[1]						
Mycosis fungoides		[2]	[1]								
Palmar–plantar pustulosis		[1]				[1]					

B Benazepril; **C** Captopril; **E** Enalapril; **F** Fosinopril; **L** Lisinopril; **P** Perindopril; **Q** Quinapril; **R** Ramipril; **T** Trandolapril; **Z** Zofenopril

These tables concentrate on skin, hair, nails and mucosal reactions.

* The following conventions are followed in these tables:

•	reaction noted (package inserts)
[3]	number of published reports of a reaction
(8%)	highest incidence that has ever been noted or reported
?	20 reports or over or an incidence of 20% or over recorded for this reaction for a minority of drugs in the class
✓	at least half the drugs in the class selection have this reaction noted or reported
✓✓	all drugs in the class selection have this reaction noted or reported
Note:	reactions noted or reported for only one drug in a class selection have been excluded

	B	C	E	F	L	P	Q	R	T	Z	=
Pemphigus	[1]	[24]	[11]	[1]			[1]	[1]	•		✓
Pemphigus foliaceus	[1]	[2]	[2]	[1]	[2]	[1]	[1]	[1]	[1]		✓
Peripheral edema	[3]		[2]		[1]	[4]	[3]				✓
Photosensitivity	•	[3]	[2]	•	•		[2]	[2]			✓
Pityriasis rosea		[6]			[2]						
Pruritus	[1]	[8] (10%)	[3]	[1]	•	(<10%)	[7]	[3]	•		✓
Pseudolymphoma		[2]		[1]	[1]						
Psoriasis		[8]	[3]		[1]	•		[1]			✓
Purpura		[1]	[1]		[2]	•		•			✓
Rash	[1]	[12] (4–7%)	[5]	[1]	[5]	[1] (<10%)	[5]	[4]	•	•	✓✓
Stevens-Johnson syndrome		[1]	[1] (5%)					[2]			
Toxic epidermal necrolysis		[3]	[1] (5%)								
Urticaria	[1]	[9] (7%)	[5]	•	[2]		•	•			✓
Vasculitis		[7]	[2]		[1]		•	[1]			✓
Xerosis		[1]				•					
HAIR											
Alopecia		[4]	[1]		[1]		•	(<10%)			✓
NAILS											
Nail dystrophy		[2]	[1]								
MUCOSAL											
Burning mouth syndrome		[1]	[1]		[1]						
Gingival bleeding			[1]					[1]			
Glossitis		[3]	•								
Glossopyrosis		[1]	[1]								
Oral burn		[1]	[1]								
Oral ulceration		[4]	[2]								
Sialorrhea		[1]						•			
Tongue edema			[2]		[2]	[2]					
Xerostomia		[1]	•	•	•	•	•	•	•		✓

B Benazepril; **C** Captopril; **E** Enalapril; **F** Fosinopril; **L** Lisinopril; **P** Perindopril; **Q** Quinapril; **R** Ramipril; **T** Trandolapril; **Z** Zofenopril

ANTIARRHYTHMICS

	A	Di	Dr	F	I	L	Pn	Pf	Pr	Q	S	=
SKIN												
Acneform eruption								•	[2]	[2]		
AGEP								[1]		[2]		
Anaphylaxis	[2]		[2]			[7]			[1]			
Angioedema	[2]		[1]			[3]	[1]	[1]	[2]	•		✓
Bullous dermatitis					[1]				[1]			
Dermatitis		•	[1] (<10%)			[27]	[1] (6%)		[2]	[4]		✓
Diaphoresis	[2]			•	[1]	[1]		•				
Eczema			[1] (<10%)			[3]			[2]			
Edema	(<10%)	•		•		[2]		•			(5%)	✓
Erythema			(5%)			[3]		[1]	[1]			
Erythema multiforme	[1]					[2]			[1]	[1]		
Erythema nodosum	[2]	[1]				[1]						
Exanthems	[5]	[1] (<5%)	[1]	[1]		[2]	[5] (8%)	[1]	[4]	[6] (17%)		✓
Exfoliative dermatitis	[1]			•		[2]			[1]	[5]		
Fixed eruption				[1]		[2]			[1]	[2]		
Flushing	(<10%)			•			•	•	[2]	[2]		✓
Hypersensitivity	[1]		[1]			[9]	[2]			[1]		
Leukocytoclastic vasculitis									[1]		[1]	
Lichen planus							[1]			[7]		
Lichenoid eruption									[3]	[6]	[1]	
Lupus erythematosus	[5] (5%)	[3]				[1]	[176] (15–20%)	[3]	[2]	[35]		✓
Necrosis	[1]								[3]			
Photosensitivity	[42] (10–75%)	[1]	[1]				[1]		[1]	[21]	•	✓
Phototoxicity	[3]		[1]						[1]	[1]		
Pigmentation	[68] (<10%)					[1]				[3]		?
Pruritus	[2] (<5%)	•	[1] (<10%)	•		[3]	•	•	[1]	[3]	(<10%)	✓
Psoriasis	[2]			[2]				[2]	[21]	[5]	[3]	✓
Purpura	[1]	[1]				[1]	[3]	•	[1]	[13]		✓

A Amiodarone; **Di** Disopyramide; **Dr** Dronedarone; **F** Flecainide; **I** Ibutilide; **L** Lidocaine; **Pn** Procainamide; **Pf** Propafenone; **Pr** Propranolol; **Q** Quinidine; **S** Sotalol

	A	Di	Dr	F	I	L	Pn	Pf	Pr	Q	S	=
Rash	[1]	•	[8] (<10%)	•		•	•	•	[2] (<10%)	(<10%)	•	✓
Raynaud's phenomenon									[3] (59%)		•	?
Sjögren's syndrome							[1]			[1]		
Stevens-Johnson syndrome	•					[1]			[2]			
Toxic epidermal necrolysis	[2]		[1]						[1]	[2]		
Toxicity	[5]	[1]	[1]	[1]		[3]		[1]				✓
Urticaria	[1]			•		[5]	[1] (<5%)	[1]	[3]	[1]		✓
Vasculitis	[6]		[1]				[5]			[5]	[1]	
HAIR												
Alopecia	[5]			•				•	[6]	[1]	•	✓
MUCOSAL												
Oral lesions		[1] (40%)						[1]				?
Oral mucosal eruption							[1]			[2]		
Oral ulceration		[1]				[1]			[1]			
Sialorrhea	(<10%)							[1]				
Xerostomia		[2] (40%)		•				•	[1]		•	?

A Amiodarone; **Di** Disopyramide; **Dr** Dronedarone; **F** Flecainide; **I** Ibutilide; **L** Lidocaine; **Pn** Procainamide; **Pf** Propafenone; **Pr** Propranolol; **Q** Quinidine; **S** Sotalol

ANTIBIOTICS, MACROLIDE

	A	C	E	=
SKIN				
AGEP	[3]		[2]	✓
Anaphylaxis	[2]	[2]	[2]	✓✓
Angioedema	[1]	[1]	[1]	✓✓
Dermatitis	[1]		[4]	✓
Exanthems	[3]	[3]	[4] (<5%)	✓✓
Fixed eruption		[3]	[6]	✓
Hypersensitivity	[3]	[3]	[3] (<10%)	✓✓
Jarisch–Herxheimer reaction	[2]		[1]	✓
Pruritus	[3]	[1]		✓
Pustules	[1]		[1]	✓
Rash	[6] (2–10%)	[2]	[3]	✓✓
SDRIFE		[1]	[2]	✓
Stevens-Johnson syndrome	[9] (5%)	[1]	[8] (10%)	✓✓
Toxic epidermal necrolysis	[1] (5%)	[4]	[8] (10%)	✓✓
Toxicity	[1]	[1]		✓
Urticaria	[2]	[1]	[4]	✓✓
Vasculitis	[1]	[3]	[1]	✓✓
HAIR				
Alopecia		[1]	[1]	✓
MUCOSAL				
Gingival hyperplasia/hypertrophy		[1]	[1]	✓

A Azithromycin; **C** Clarithromycin; **E** Erythromycin

ANTICONVULSANTS

	B	C	G	La	Le	O	Phb	Phy	Ti	To	V	Z	=
SKIN													
Acne keloid		[1]						[2]					
Acneform eruption		[1]	•	[1]		•	[1]	[8]	•	•		•	✓
AGEP		[5]		[1]	[1]		[1]	[5]			[1]		✓
Angioedema	•	[5]		[1] (<10%)			•	[2]					
Anticonvulsant hypersensitivity syndrome		[19]	[2]	[17]		[1]	[10]	[10]			[6]		✓
Bullae		[1]					[1]						
Bullous dermatitis		[4]		[1]			[5]	[1]			[1]		
Bullous pemphigoid			[2]		[1]								
Dermatitis		[7]					[1]		•	•			
Diaphoresis		(<10%)		•		•	[1]		•	•	[1]	•	✓
DRESS syndrome		[51] (77%)		[18] (11%)	[7]	[6]	[15] (6%)	[34] (68%)			[10]	[3]	✓
Ecchymoses				•	•	•			(<6%)		[4] (<5%)	•	✓
Eczema		[2]		•					•	•		•	
Edema			[5]		[1]	•	[1]		•	•	[3]	•	✓
Epidermolysis bullosa		[1]						[1]					
Erythema		[1]		[2] (~10%)	[2]								
Erythema multiforme		[16]		[4]	[2]		[7]	[11]			[3]		✓
Erythroderma		[12]			[1]		[2] (16%)	[9] (6%)			[3]		
Exanthems		[36] (17%)	[2]	[19] (20%)	[1]	[4]	[13] (70%)	[22] (71%)	•	[1]	[3] (14%)	•	✓
Exfoliative dermatitis		[24]				[1]	[6]	[15]	•				?
Facial edema		[2]	•	•					•	[1]	•	•	✓
Fixed eruption		[10]		[1]		[1]	[9]	[5]		[2]	[1]		✓
Flushing				•						[1] (27%)			?
Furunculosis									•		(<5%)		
Granuloma annulare					[1]					[1]			
Hand–foot syndrome								[1]			[1]		
Hot flashes			[1]	(<10%)		•				(<10%)			
Hyperhidrosis				[1]		•							

B Brivaracetam; **C** Carbamazepine; **G** Gabapentin; **La** Lamotrigine; **Le** Levetiracetam; **O** Oxcarbazepine; **Phb** Phenobarbital; **Phy** Phenytoin; **Ti** Tiagabine; **To** Topiramate; **V** Valproic Acid; **Z** Zonisamide

	B	C	G	La	Le	O	Phb	Phy	Ti	To	V	Z	=
Hypersensitivity	•	[71]	[1]	[29] (<10%)	[1]	[6]	[12]	[47] (23%)			[5]	[4]	✓
Leukocytoclastic vasculitis			[1]		[1]								
Lichen planus		[2]						[1]					
Lichenoid eruption		[8]						[1]					
Linear IgA		[1]						[8]					
Lupus erythematosus		[35]		[4]			[2]	[19]			[5]	[1]	✓
Lymphadenopathy		[1]		[1]		•			•			•	
Lymphoma		[2]						[6]					
Lymphoproliferative disease		[5]						[1]					
Mycosis fungoides		[3]			[1]	[1]		[7]					
Neoplasms								[1]	•				
Oligohydrosis										[1]		[8]	
Pemphigus		[3]					[1]	[2]					
Peripheral edema		[1]	[13] (8%)				[1]	[1]	•		[1] (<5%)	•	✓
Petechiae		[1]		•					•		[1] (<5%)	•	
Photosensitivity		[9]		[2]			[1]	[1]	•	•	[1]		✓
Pigmentation					[1]		[1]	[4]	•	•			
Pruritus		[7]	[1]	[3]	[1]		[1]	[5]	•	[3]	[1]	[1] (2–6%)	✓
Pseudolymphoma		[17]		[1]			[1]	[31]			[2]		?
Psoriasis		[1]			[1]				•				
Purpura		[8]	[1]	[1]		•	[2]	[4]		•	[2]	•	✓
Pustules		[5]					[1]	[3]				•	
Rash		[31] (12%)	[2]	[54] (12–22%)	[5]	[11] (9%)	[4]	[13] (17%)	[2] (5%)	[3] (6%)	[7]	[6] (7%)	✓
Scleroderma								[1]			[1]		
Sjögren's syndrome				[1]			[1]	[1]			[1]		
Stevens-Johnson syndrome		[103] (68%)	[2]	[53] (30%)	[4]	[11]	[23] (29%)	[60] (68%)			[12]	[3]	✓
Toxic epidermal necrolysis		[93] (68%)		[54] (13%)	[2]	[4]	[28] (29%)	[66] (68%)			[9]	[1]	✓
Toxicity		[2]	[1]					[1]					
Toxicoderma		[1]					[1]						
Urticaria		[14] (7%)		[1]	[2]		[1]	[5]	•	[1]		[1]	✓
Vasculitis		[7]	[1]		[1]		[1]	[11]			[3]		✓

B Brivaracetam; **C** Carbamazepine; **G** Gabapentin; **La** Lamotrigine; **Le** Levetiracetam; **O** Oxcarbazepine; **Phb** Phenobarbital; **Phy** Phenytoin; **Ti** Tiagabine; **To** Topiramate; **V** Valproic Acid; **Z** Zonisamide

	B	C	G	La	Le	O	Phb	Phy	Ti	To	V	Z	=
Vesiculobullous eruption									•			•	
Xerosis				•					•	[1]		[1]	
HAIR													
Alopecia		[7] (~6%)	[2]	[2]				[3]	•	[2]	[23] (<10%)	•	✓
Hirsutism		[1] (25%)		•				[8] (13%)	•		[2] (60%)	•	✓
Poliosis							[1]				[1]		
NAILS													
Nail changes								[2]		•			
Nail hypoplasia		[1]					[2]	[3]					
Nail pigmentation								[1]			[2]		
Onychomadesis		[1]									[1]		
MUCOSAL													
Epistaxis						•			•				
Gingival hyperplasia/hypertrophy		[1]		•	[1]		[4] (16%)	[57] (16–94%)	•	[2]	[8] (42%)	•	✓
Gingivitis			•	•	•				•	•		•	✓
Glossitis									•		(<5%)	•	
Halitosis									•		[1]		
Mucocutaneous eruption		[4]						[2]					
Mucocutaneous lymph node syndrome		[2]						[1]					
Oral ulceration		[2]		[1]		[1]		[1]	•			•	✓
Rectal hemorrhage						•			•			•	
Sialorrhea				•						[1] (4–5%)			
Stomatitis				•					•	•	(<5%)	•	
Ulcerative stomatitis									•			•	
Xerostomia			[1] (5%)	(6%)		•	[1]		[1]	[6] (16%)	[2] (<5%)	•	✓

B Brivaracetam; **C** Carbamazepine; **G** Gabapentin; **La** Lamotrigine; **Le** Levetiracetam; **O** Oxcarbazepine; **Phb** Phenobarbital; **Phy** Phenytoin; **Ti** Tiagabine; **To** Topiramate; **V** Valproic Acid; **Z** Zonisamide

ANTIDEPRESSANTS, TRICYCLIC

	Ami	Amo	C	I	N	T	=
SKIN							
Angioedema	[1]			[1]			
Bullous dermatitis	[1]			[1]			
Dermatitis	[1]		[1]				
Diaphoresis	[1] (<10%)	(<10%)	[2] (43%)	[8] (25%)	(<10%)	[1] (<10%)	✓
DRESS syndrome	[2]		[1]				
Edema	[1]	(<10%)	•	[1]			✓
Exanthems		[2]		[6] (6%)			
Fixed eruption	[1]			[1]			
Flushing			(8%)	[1]			
Hypersensitivity	[1]		[2]				
Lichen planus	[1]			[1]			
Lupus erythematosus	[1]			[1]			
Photosensitivity	[3]	•	[3]	[3]	[2]	•	✓✓
Pigmentation	[4]		[1]	[13]			✓
Pruritus	[3]	[1]	[1] (6%)	[6]			✓
Purpura	[2]		•	[3]			✓
Rash		(<10%)	(8%)				
Toxic epidermal necrolysis	[1] (5%)	[2]					
Urticaria		•	[1]	[6]			✓
Vasculitis	[1]	[1]		[1]			✓
HAIR							
Alopecia	[1]	•	•	[2]	•	•	✓✓
Alopecia areata			[1]	[1]			
MUCOSAL							
Stomatitis	[1]			[2]			
Xerostomia	[17] (79%)	[1] (14%)	[6] (84%)	[16] (21%)	[9]	[2]	✓✓

Ami Amitriptyline; **Amo** Amoxapine; **C** Clomipramine; **I** Imipramine; **N** Nortriptyline; **T** Trimipramine

ANTIHISTAMINES (HI)

	Ce	Chl	Des	Dy	Fex	H	Lev	Lor	O	P	=
SKIN											
AGEP	[1]			[1]	[1]	[3]					
Anaphylaxis	[2]	[1]		[4]		[2]		•		[1]	✓
Angioedema	•	(<10%)		[1]		[3]		[1]		•	✓
Bullous dermatitis	•									•	
Dermatitis	•	[4] (<10%)		[4]		[1]	[1]	•		[3]	✓
Desquamation	[1]					[1]					
Diaphoresis	•							•			
Eczema				[2]						[1]	
Edema				•		•					
Erythema multiforme						[2]		•		[2]	
Exanthems	[1]			[1]		[3]				[1]	
Fixed eruption	[7]			[4]		[3]	[3]	[3]	[1]	[1]	✓
Flushing	[1] (60%)					[1]		•			?
Hypersensitivity						[1]				[1]	
Palmar erythema	[1]					[1]					
Photosensitivity	•	(<10%)		[3]		•		•		[12]	✓
Phototoxicity	•			[1]		[1]				[1]	
Pruritus	[1]	[1]		[2]				[1]			
Purpura	•			[1]		[1]		•		[2]	✓
Rash	•			•		•		[1]		[1]	✓
Stevens-Johnson syndrome					[2]					[1]	
Toxic epidermal necrolysis				[3]	[1]					[2]	
Toxicity				[2]		[1]					
Urticaria	[9]		[2]		[3]	[4]	[1]	[4]		[3]	✓
Xerosis	•							•			
HAIR											
Alopecia	•							•			
MUCOSAL											
Oral ulceration			[1]							[1]	
Sialorrhea	•							•			
Stomatitis	•							•			
Xerostomia	[2] (6%)	(<10%)	[5]	[1] (<10%)		[4] (12%)	•	[9]		[2] (<10%)	✓

Ce Cetirizine; **Chl** Chlorpheniramine; **Des** Desloratadine; **Dy** Diphenhydramine; **Fex** Fexofenadine; **H** Hydroxyzine; **Lev** Levocetirizine; **Lor** Loratadine; **O** Olopatadine; **P** Promethazine

ANTIMALARIALS

	Amo	A/L	Art	A/P	C	H	M	P	Quc	Qud	Qun	S	T	=
SKIN														
Acneform eruption										[2]	[2]			
AGEP				[1]	[1]	[23] (25%)		[1]		[2]				?
Anaphylaxis						[1]	[2]	•						
Angioedema	[1]				[1]	•		[2]		•	•	[1]		✓
Bullous dermatitis						[2]		[2]				[1]		
Dermatitis		[1]			[2]	[1]		•		[4]	[6]			✓
DRESS syndrome						[3]		[2]			[1]			
Erythema							[2]	[1]				[1]		
Erythema annulare centrifugum					[2]	[3]								
Erythema multiforme				[2]	•	[2]		[4]		[1]	[2]	[3]		✓
Erythema nodosum						[1]			[1]					
Erythroderma					[3]	[3]								
Exanthems				[1]	[3] (<5%)	[4] (<5%)	[1] (30%)	[3]	[3] (80%)	[6] (17%)	[3] (<5%)	[1]		✓
Exfoliative dermatitis					[4]	[3]	[1]	[2]	[3] (8%)	[5]	[2]	[3]		✓
Fixed eruption	[1]				•	•		[3]	[3]	[2]	[12]	[2]		✓
Flushing										[2]	•			
Hypersensitivity		[1]						[1]		[1]	[1]	•	•	
Lesions						[1]	[1]							
Lichen planus						[1]				[7]	[3]			
Lichenoid eruption					[6]	[4]		[2]	[6] (12%)	[6]	[3]			
Livedo reticularis										[6]	[3]			
Lupus erythematosus										[35]	[1]			?
Lymphoproliferative disease						[1]		[1]		[1]				
Ochronosis									[2]		[1]			
Pemphigus					[1]	[1]								
Photosensitivity					[8]	[6]		[3]	[1]	[21]	[19]	[2]		✓
Phototoxicity				[1]	[1]	[3]				[1]				
Pigmentation					[15]	[19] (<10%)		[5]	[9]	[3]	[6]			

Amo Amodiaquine; **A/L** Artemether/Lumefantrine; **Art** Artesunate; **A/P** Atovaquone/Proguanil; **C** Chloroquine; **H** Hydroxychloroquine; **M** Mefloquine; **P** Pyrimethamine; **Quc** Quinacrine; **Qud** Quinidine; **Qun** Quinine; **S** Sulfadoxine; **T** Tafenoquine

	Amo	A/L	Art	A/P	C	H	M	P	Quc	Qud	Qun	S	T	=
Pruritus	[4]	[2]	[4]	(<10%)	[36] (47%)	[13] (47%)	[2] (4–10%)	[2]	•	[3]	[1]	[2]		✓
Psoriasis					[19]	[14]	[2]		[1]	[5]				
Purpura		[1]					[1]	[1]		[13]	[13]	[1]		
Pustules		[1]			[1]	[1]		[1]		[1]				
Rash		[6] (11%)			[1]	[4] (<10%)	[1] (<10%)	•	[1]	(<10%)	[1]	•		✓
Stevens-Johnson syndrome				[1]	[4]	[1]	[2]	[25] (<10%)			[2]	[24] (<10%)		✓
Thrombocytopenic purpura						[2]					[8]			
Toxic epidermal necrolysis					[5]	[3]	[2]	[15]		[2]	[3]	[17]		✓
Toxicity					[2]	[1]								
Urticaria	[1]	[2]	[1]	[1]	[4]	[2]	[1]		[1]	[1]	[2]			✓
Vasculitis						[1]	[3]			[5]	[5]			
HAIR														
Alopecia				[1]		[2]	•		[2] (80%)	[1]				?
Hair pigmentation					[10]	[8] (<10%)								
NAILS														
Discoloration					[1]	[1]								
Nail pigmentation					[2]	[3]			[2]					
MUCOSAL														
Aphthous stomatitis	[1]		[1]					[1]				[1]		
Gingival pigmentation					[1]	[1]								
Glossitis								•				•		
Oral edema			[1]					[1]				[1]		
Oral mucosal eruption										[2]	[1]			
Oral pigmentation					[13]	[7]			[4]	[1]				
Oral ulceration				[3] (6%)	[1]							[1]		
Stomatitis					•	[2]						[1]		

Amo Amodiaquine; **A/L** Artemether/Lumefantrine; **Art** Artesunate; **A/P** Atovaquone/Proguanil; **C** Chloroquine; **H** Hydroxychloroquine; **M** Mefloquine; **P** Pyrimethamine; **Quc** Quinacrine; **Qud** Quinidine; **Qun** Quinine; **S** Sulfadoxine; **T** Tafenoquine

ANTIPSYCHOTICS

	Ap	As	Chl	Clo	H	Lo	Lu	O	Pal	Per	Q	R	Z	=
SKIN														
Acneform eruption	[1]											•		
AGEP				[1]				[1]			[1]			
Anaphylaxis			[1]					[1]	•					
Angioedema		[1]	[1]	[2]	[1]		•	[2]				[6]	[2]	✓
Bullous dermatitis			[1]									•		
Candidiasis								•			•			
Dermatitis			[1]	•	•	[1]		[1]						
Diaphoresis				[4] (31%)	[2]			•			(<10%)	•	[1]	?
DRESS syndrome				[1]				[1]					[2]	
Ecchymoses								•					•	
Eczema				•				•	[1]			[1]	•	
Edema				•				[3]	•		[1]	[3]		
Erythema multiforme			•	•							[1]	[1]		
Exanthems			[8] (13%)	[2]				•	[1]	[2]			•	
Exfoliative dermatitis												•	•	
Facial edema			[1]					•			•		•	
Fixed eruption			•					[1]						
Flushing			[1]									[1]		
Furunculosis												•	•	
Hyperhidrosis	[1]										•			
Hypersensitivity		[1]						[2]						
Lichenoid eruption			[1]					[1]				•		
Lupus erythematosus			[12]	[4]						[4]			[2]	
Peripheral edema		[1]						[5] (<10%)	[4]		[5]	[4] (16%)	•	
Photosensitivity			[23] (<10%)	[1]	[3]	[1]		•			•	[2] (<10%)	•	✓
Pigmentation			[16]		•	•		[1]		•		•		
Pityriasis rosea		[1]		[2]										
Pruritus			[2] (<10%)	•	•	[1]	•	•	[1]			•		✓
Pseudolymphoma			[1]							[1]				
Psoriasis								[3]				•		
Purpura			[6]	•				(<10%)				•		

Ap Aripiprazole; **As** Asenapine; **Chl** Chlorpromazine; **Clo** Clozapine; **H** Haloperidol; **Lo** Loxapine; **Lu** Lurasidone; **O** Olanzapine; **Pal** Paliperidone; **Per** Perphenazine; **Q** Quetiapine; **R** Risperidone; **Z** Ziprasidone

	Ap	As	Chl	Clo	H	Lo	Lu	O	Pal	Per	Q	R	Z	=
Pustules			[1]					[1]						
Rash	[2] (7%)		(<10%)	[2]	•	(<10%)	•	[2]	[1]	(<10%)	•	[1]	•	✓
SDRIFE				[1]								[1]		
Seborrhea						[1]		•				•		
Seborrheic dermatitis			[4]		[2]									
Stevens-Johnson syndrome	[1]			[1]										
Sweet's syndrome				[1]	[1]					[1]				
Ulcerations								•				•		
Urticaria			[4]	•				•		[1]		[2]	[1] (5%)	
Vasculitis			[3]	•				[1]						
Vesiculobullous eruption								•					•	
Xerosis								•			•	•		
HAIR														
Alopecia					[1]			[3]			[1]	[2]	•	
Alopecia areata				[1]	[2]									
NAILS														
MUCOSAL														
Epistaxis								(<10%)				[1]	•	
Gingival bleeding												[1]	•	
Gingivitis								•			[1]	•	[1]	
Glossitis								•			•			
Glossodynia		[1]		•										
Nasal congestion									•			[1]		
Oral ulceration								•			•			
Sialorrhea	[5] (4–11%)	[1]		[77] (30–80%)	[1]		•	[4]	[2] (<6%)		[3]	[11] (13%)	•	✓
Stomatitis								•			•	•		
Tongue edema								•	•		•	•	•	
Tongue pigmentation								•				•		
Xerostomia	[7] (15%)	[1]	[1] (<10%)	[3] (6%)	[4] (21%)	•		[11] (19%)	[1]		[22] (31%)	[7] (18%)	[1] (<5%)	✓

Ap Aripiprazole; **As** Asenapine; **Chl** Chlorpromazine; **Clo** Clozapine; **H** Haloperidol; **Lo** Loxapine; **Lu** Lurasidone; **O** Olanzapine; **Pal** Paliperidone; **Per** Perphenazine; **Q** Quetiapine; **R** Risperidone; **Z** Ziprasidone

ANTIRETROVIRALS

	Amp	Ata	C	Ef	Em	H	I	L	R	=
SKIN										
Acneform eruption								(<10%)	•	
Dermatitis						[3]	•	[1]	[1]	
Diaphoresis				[1]			•		(<10%)	
DRESS syndrome				[2]	[1]				[1]	
Eczema				•					•	
Edema					[1]				(6%)	
Exanthems	[1]	[1]		[3] (27%)	(17%)	[1] (<10%)	[1]		[2]	✓
Flushing				•			•		(13%)	
Folliculitis				•			•		•	
Hypersensitivity		[1]		[5]	[1]			[1]	(8%)	✓
Jaundice		[11] (13%)					[1]	[1]	[3] (13%)	
Lesions		[1]							[1]	
Lichenoid eruption				[1]		[3]				
Lipodystrophy				[2]			[8] (14%)	(<10%)	[4]	
Lupus erythematosus					[1]	[3]				
Peripheral edema				•		[1]			(6%)	
Photosensitivity				[4]		[1]			•	
Pigmentation					[3] (32%)	[18] (59%)				?
Pruritus		[1]		(11%)	(17–30%)	[3]	[2] (86%)		(12%)	✓
Psoriasis						[1]			•	
Rash	[6] (20–27%)	[7] (3–20%)	[3] (22%)	[16] (31%)	[5] (17–30%)		[2] (67%)	[5] (69%)	[12] (69%)	✓
Seborrhea							•		•	
Stevens-Johnson syndrome	[1]			[4] (8%)			[2]			
Toxicity		[1] (21%)		[2] (39%)		[1] (5%)	[1]	[1] (6%)	[2]	✓
Urticaria				[1]	[1] (17–30%)		•		(8%)	?
Vasculitis				[1]		[6]	[1]			
Xerosis						[7] (<10%)	[2] (12%)		•	

Amp Amprenavir; **Ata** Atazanavir; **C** Cobicistat/Elvitegravir/Emtricitabine/Tenofovir Disoproxil; **Ef** Efavirenz; **Em** Emtricitabine; **H** Hydroxyurea; **I** Indinavir; **L** Lopinavir; **R** Ritonavir

	Amp	Ata	C	Ef	Em	H	I	L	R	=
HAIR										
Alopecia				•		[8] (<10%)	[5] (12%)	[3]	[2]	✓
Alopecia areata		[1]					[1]	[1]	[1]	✓
NAILS										
Nail pigmentation						[18]		[1]	[1]	
Onychocryptosis							[2]		[1]	
MUCOSAL										
Cheilitis							[4] (52%)		[1]	?
Gingivitis							•		•	
Oral ulceration						[8]			•	
Oropharyngeal pain								[1]	(16%)	
Sialolithiasis		[1]							[1]	
Sialorrhea								[1]	[1]	
Xerostomia				•			•		•	

Amp Amprenavir; **Ata** Atazanavir; **C** Cobicistat/Elvitegravir/Emtricitabine/Tenofovir Disoproxil; **Ef** Efavirenz; **Em** Emtricitabine; **H** Hydroxyurea; **I** Indinavir; **L** Lopinavir; **R** Ritonavir

BENZODIAZEPINES

	A	Cln	Clo	D	L	M	O	=
SKIN								
Acneform eruption	[1]			[1]				
Anaphylaxis				[1]		[1]		
Angioedema	[1]	[1]		[1]		[1]		✓
Bullous dermatitis		[2]		[1]				
Dermatitis	[5]	(<10%)	(<10%)	[3] (<10%)	(<10%)		(<10%)	✓
Diaphoresis	(16%)	[1]	•	•	•		•	✓
DRESS syndrome		[1]					[1]	
Edema	(5%)					[2]		
Erythema multiforme		[1]			[1]		[1]	
Exanthems	[1]	[1]	[1]	[6]				✓
Exfoliative dermatitis		[1]		[2]				
Fixed eruption				[2]	[1]		[1]	
Flushing				[1]		[1]		
Peripheral edema				[1]		•		
Photosensitivity	[4]		[1]					
Pruritus	[2] (<10%)			[1]		[3]		
Pseudolymphoma	[1]	[2]			[2]			
Purpura		[1]		[4]				
Rash	[4] (11%)	•	•	[2]	•	•	•	✓✓
Urticaria			[1]	[1]		[2]		
Vasculitis			[1]	[1]				
MUCOSAL								
Sialopenia	(33%)	•	•		•		•	✓
Sialorrhea	•	(<10%)	(<10%)		[1]	•	(<10%)	✓
Xerostomia	[6] (15%)	[1]	•	[1]	•		•	✓

A Alprazolam; **Cln** Clonazepam; **Clo** Clorazepate; **D** Diazepam; **L** Lorazepam; **M** Midazolam; **O** Oxazepam

BETA BLOCKERS

	A	B	C	N	P	S	=
SKIN							
Anaphylaxis	[2]				[1]		
Cold extremities		[1]			[6] (36%)		?
Dermatitis	[1]			[1]	[2]		✓
Diaphoresis		•	[1]				
Edema		[1]				(5%)	
Fixed eruption	[1]	[1]			[1]		✓
Leukocytoclastic vasculitis					[1]	[1]	
Lichenoid eruption	[1]			[1]	[3]	[1]	✓
Lupus erythematosus	[2]		[1]		[2]		✓
Necrosis	[3]				[3]		
Peripheral edema		(<10%)		•			
Photosensitivity					[1]	•	
Pruritus	(<5%)				[1]	(<10%)	✓
Psoriasis	[7]	[1]			[21]	[3]	✓
Rash	[1]	(<10%)		•	[2] (<10%)	•	✓
Raynaud's phenomenon	[2]	(<10%)			[3] (59%)	•	✓
Urticaria	[2]				[3]		
Vasculitis	[1]					[1]	
HAIR							
Alopecia	[1]				[6]	•	✓
MUCOSAL							
Xerostomia		•			[1]	•	✓

A Atenolol; **B** Bisoprolol; **C** Celiprolol; **N** Nebivolol; **P** Propranolol; **S** Sotalol

BIOLOGICS

	Ald	Alm	Be	Bo	C	D	E	G	Ib	In	Ip	L	P	R	=
SKIN															
Abscess			[1]		[1]										
Acne keloid			[1]		[1]		[2]								
Acneform eruption			[6] (83%)		[66] (97%)	[2] (<10%)	[29] (73–80%)	[34] (66–85%)	[3]	•	[1]	[1]	[18] (81%)		✓
AGEP	[1]						[2]	[1]	[7]						
Anaphylaxis		•			[5] (13%)		[1] (30%)	[1]				[1]	[1]	[7]	✓
Angioedema	[2]	•	[1]							[3]			[1]	[4] (11%)	
Bullae	[1]					[1]									
Bullous dermatitis	[1]	•					[1]			[4]				[1]	
Bullous pemphigoid	[1]						[1]								
Burning				[1]	[1]										
Carcinoma		[2]							[1]						
Cellulitis		•	[1]									(5%)		[1]	
Dermatitis	[2]		[1]	[1]	[4] (80%)	[1] (<10%)	[4] (30%)			[1] (6%)	[14] (12%)	[1]		[2]	✓
Dermatomyositis									[1]	[1]	[2]				
Desquamation	[1]		[1] (8%)		[3] (89%)		[1]	[2] (39%)					[3] (13%)		?
Diaphoresis									(13%)	[1]		(8%)		[2] (15%)	
DRESS syndrome							[2]		[3]		[1]	[3]			
Ecchymoses				[1] (16%)								[1] (16%)			
Eczema					[1]	(<10%)	[1]	[1]		[6] (39%)	[1]		[2]		✓
Edema	[3] (47%)		[1] (15%)	(23%)		[6] (38%)	[1]		[36] (80%)	[2] (15%)		[1] (10%)	[1] (15%)	[1]	✓
Embolia cutis medicamentosa (Nicolau syndrome)				[1]						[1]					
Erythema	[5] (41%)	[1]	[1]	[2]	[3] (14%)	[2]	(18%)	[1]	[5] (<10%)	[2]	[5]	(5%)	[5] (65%)	[2] (16%)	✓✓
Erythema multiforme	[1]			[1] (16%)					[2]		[2]	[1] (16%)			
Erythema nodosum	[3]					•			[1]	[1]					
Erythroderma	[4]								[3]						

Ald Aldesleukin; **Alm** Alemtuzumab; **Be** Bevacizumab; **Bo** Bortezomib; **C** Cetuximab; **D** Dasatinib; **E** Erlotinib; **G** Gefitinib; **Ib** Imatinib; **In** Interferon Alfa; **Ip** Ipilimumab; **L** Lenalidomide; **P** Panitumumab; **R** Rituximab

	Ald	Alm	Be	Bo	C	D	E	G	Ib	In	Ip	L	P	R	=
Exanthems	[5]		[1]	[1] (16%)	[5]		[3] (8%)	[3] (21%)	[9]	[3]	[6] (20%)	[3] (16%)		[1]	✓
Exfoliative dermatitis	[1] (18%)					[1]		[1]	[4]			[1]	[2] (25%)		?
Facial edema		•					[1]		[3] (<10%)					[1]	
Fissures					[4] (14%)		[1]						[5] (21%)		?
Flushing		[2]			[2]	[1] (<10%)								(5%)	
Folliculitis				[2]	[13] (83%)		[9] (11%)	[4]	[1]		[1] (7%)	[2]	[3]		✓
Graft-versus-host reaction	[1]					[1]			[1]		[1] (14%)	[2] (43%)			?
Granulomas		[1]								[1]	[5]				
Hand–foot syndrome			[13] (57%)		[5] (6%)	[1]	[3] (30–60%)	[2]	[3]	[1] (10%)	[1]		[3] (23%)		✓
Hematoma		•	[1]		[1]										
Herpes		[2]				(<10%)									
Herpes simplex		[2] (6%)								[2]				[2]	
Herpes zoster		[3] (9%)		[13] (10–15%)										[7]	
Hyperhidrosis			[1] (8%)			[1] (<10%)			[1]			[2] (11%)			
Hypersensitivity				[1] (7%)	[9]	•				[1]	[1]			[5]	
Kaposi's sarcoma	[1]									[2]				[3]	
Keratoses									[1]	[1]					
Lesions									[1]	[1] (8%)					
Lichen planus									[5]	[8]					
Linear IgA	[4]									[3]					
Livedo reticularis								[1]		[2]					
Lupus erythematosus	[1]		[1]	[1]		[1]				[17]				[1]	
Lupus syndrome			[1]							[2]	[1]			[1]	
Lymphoma		[2]												[1]	
Malignancies										[1]		[6]			
Malignant lymphoma		•								[1]					
Necrolysis								[1]	[1]						

Ald Aldesleukin; **Alm** Alemtuzumab; **Be** Bevacizumab; **Bo** Bortezomib; **C** Cetuximab; **D** Dasatinib; **E** Erlotinib; **G** Gefitinib; **Ib** Imatinib; **In** Interferon Alfa; **Ip** Ipilimumab; **L** Lenalidomide; **P** Panitumumab; **R** Rituximab

	Ald	Alm	Be	Bo	C	D	E	G	Ib	In	Ip	L	P	R	=
Necrosis	[2]		[2]				[1]			[6]				[1]	
Neutrophilic eccrine hidradenitis					[1]				[3]						
Panniculitis						[4]			[3]						
Papulopustular eruption					[7] (83%)		[9] (29%)	[3] (21%)					[4] (21–41%)		?
Pemphigus	[2]									[2]				[1]	
Peripheral edema	(28%)	(13%)	[1] (8%)	[5] (83%)	[1] (40%)	[3] (44%)		[1] (22%)	[5] (75%)			[5] (83%)	[1] (12%)	[1] (14%)	✓
Petechiae	•								[1] (<10%)						
Photosensitivity	[1]					[1]	[1]		[3] (<10%)	[2]					
Pigmentation			[1]	[1] (16%)		[1]		[1]	[14] (60%)	[3] (21%)	[1] (23%)	[2] (16%)	[1]		✓
Pityriasis rubra pilaris			[1]						[1]						
Pruritus	[7] (24%)	(14–24%)	[1] (91%)	[1] (11%)	[9] (40%)	[4] (14%)	[9] (21%)	[6] (61%)	[3] (10%)	[4] (30%)	[22] (65%)	[3] (42%)	[10] (91%)	[8] (14%)	✓✓
Pseudolymphoma	[1]								[3]	[1]					
Psoriasis	[4]				[1]				[3]	[24]	[1]			[4]	?
Purpura	[1]	(8%)	[1]	[2]			[3]	[1]	[1]	[2]		[1]		[1]	✓
Pustules					[1]			[1]					[1]		
Pyoderma gangrenosum								[1]	[1]	[1]		[1]		[3]	
Radiation recall dermatitis			[1]		[2]		[1]			[1]					
Rash	[2] (42%)	[5] (13–40%)	[17] (91%)	[11] (67%)	[52] (89%)	[10] (34%)	[116] (80%)	[67] (66–85%)	[26] (69%)	[5] (11%)	[29] (83%)	[18] (36%)	[33] (91%)	[12] (58%)	✓✓
Rosacea					[1]		[2]		[1]	[1]	[1]				
Sarcoidosis	[1]									[47]	[4]			[3]	?
Scleroderma	[2]									[1]					
Sclerosis	[1]									[1]					
Seborrheic dermatitis	[1]						[1]			[2]					
Serum sickness												[1] (8%)		[22] (<20%)	?
Sjögren's syndrome										[4]	[1]				
Squamous cell carcinoma		[1]						[1]	[2]		[1] (7%)				
Stevens-Johnson syndrome	[1]				[2]				[15]		[3]	[6]	[1]	[6]	✓

Ald Aldesleukin; **Alm** Alemtuzumab; **Be** Bevacizumab; **Bo** Bortezomib; **C** Cetuximab; **D** Dasatinib; **E** Erlotinib; **G** Gefitinib; **Ib** Imatinib; **In** Interferon Alfa; **Ip** Ipilimumab; **L** Lenalidomide; **P** Panitumumab; **R** Rituximab

	Ald	Alm	Be	Bo	C	D	E	G	Ib	In	Ip	L	P	R	=
Sweet's syndrome	[1]			[7]		[1]			[4]		[1]	[3]			
Telangiectasia			[1]		[1]		[1]		[1]	[1]			[1]		
Thrombocytopenic purpura		[11]	[1]							[2]	[1]				
Toxic epidermal necrolysis	[2]			[1]	[4]			[2]	[2]		[3]	[1]		[4]	✓
Toxicity	[6]	[1]	[9] (16%)	[4] (38%)	[20] (63%)	[8] (36%)	[10] (84%)	[10] (68%)	[9] (30–44%)	[4]	[4] (35%)	[6] (75%)	[26] (95%)	[3] (12%)	✓✓
Transient acantholytic dermatosis					[1]						[2]				
Tumor lysis syndrome				[2] (17%)		[1] (<5%)					[1]	[3] (<5%)		[4] (21%)	
Tumors												[5] (11%)		[1] (11%)	
Ulcerations			[3]	[1]	[1]	[1]		[2]		[1]	[1]				✓
Urticaria	[3]	[2] (16–30%)				[1] (<10%)		[1]	[3]	[3]	[3]	[1]		[5] (8%)	✓
Vasculitis	[1]	[1]	[1]	[4]			[1]	[1]	[2]	[7]	[3]			[4]	✓
Vitiligo	[3]									[9]	[3]				
Xerosis	(15%)		[1]	[1] (16%)	[15] (49%)	[1] (<10%)	[13] (56%)	[13] (53%)	[2] (<10%)	[1]	[1] (13%)	[2] (16%)	[12] (62%)		✓
HAIR															
Abnormal hair growth					[2]							[1]			
Alopecia	[2] (10%)		[5] (43%)		(5%)	[3] (<10%)	[10] (14%)	[6]	[2] (10–15%)	[16] (48%)	[3] (19%)		[3] (54%)	[1]	✓
Alopecia areata		[1]								[1]					
Alopecia universalis		[1]									[1]				
Hair changes					[3]		[4] (20%)						[2] (9%)		?
Hair pigmentation						[2]				[3] (18%)					
Hirsutism							[1]			[1]					
Hypertrichosis					[3]		[4]	[2]		[3]					
NAILS															
Nail changes					[1] (21%)		[3] (25%)	[1] (17%)					[2] (9–29%)		?
Nail disorder					[3]	[1]			[1]				[1]		
Nail pigmentation								[1]	[2]						?

Ald Aldesleukin; **Alm** Alemtuzumab; **Be** Bevacizumab; **Bo** Bortezomib; **C** Cetuximab; **D** Dasatinib; **E** Erlotinib; **G** Gefitinib; **Ib** Imatinib; **In** Interferon Alfa; **Ip** Ipilimumab; **L** Lenalidomide; **P** Panitumumab; **R** Rituximab

	Ald	Alm	Be	Bo	C	D	E	G	Ib	In	Ip	L	P	R	=
Paronychia			[2] (25%)		[17] (39%)		[14] (23%)	[14] (14–32%)					[13] (85%)		?
Pyogenic granuloma					[1]		[1]	[2]					[1]		
MUCOSAL															
Aphthous stomatitis	[1] (5%)				[1]		[1]		[1]	[2]	[1]				
Epistaxis			[5] (17%)					[1]		[1] (17%)		(15%)	[1]		
Mucocutaneous eruption						[1]			[1]						
Mucosal inflammation			[2] (59%)				[1] (18%)			[1]			(6%)		?
Mucositis			[13] (75%)	[2] (45%)	[10]	[1] (16%)	[10] (21%)	[4] (6–17%)	[2] (15%)		[1]		[4] (75%)		✓
Oral lichenoid eruption									[3]	[1]					
Oral mucositis					[2] (82%)			[1] (33%)					(6%)		?
Oral pigmentation									[4]	[1]					
Oral ulceration	[1]		[2] (18%)	[1]	[1]		[1]	[1]	[3] (15%)						✓
Oropharyngeal pain									[1]					[1]	
Perianal fistula			[1] (67%)								[1]				?
Rectal hemorrhage				[1]		[1]									
Stomatitis	[1] (22%)	[1] (14%)	[8] (75%)	[1] (43%)	[4] (25%)	[1]	[12] (26%)	[8] (6–17%)		[1] (30%)			[4] (100%)	[2] (69%)	✓
Xerostomia	[1]				(11%)	[1] (33%)			[1] (44%)	[4] (41%)	[1]	(7%)			✓

Ald Aldesleukin; **Alm** Alemtuzumab; **Be** Bevacizumab; **Bo** Bortezomib; **C** Cetuximab; **D** Dasatinib; **E** Erlotinib; **G** Gefitinib; **Ib** Imatinib; **In** Interferon Alfa; **Ip** Ipilimumab; **L** Lenalidomide; **P** Panitumumab; **R** Rituximab

BISPHOSPHONATES

	A	E	I	P	R	Z	=
SKIN							
Angioedema	[2]	•		•			✓
Candidiasis				(6%)		(12%)	
Eczema	[1] (13%)				[1]		
Edema				•		[3]	
Erythema multiforme	[2]				[1]		
Exanthems				[1]		[1]	
Hypersensitivity	[3] (19%)	•		•	[1]		✓
Peripheral edema	[1]				(8%)	(5–21%)	✓
Pruritus	[1]	[1]	[1] (4–5%)		•		✓
Rash	[5]	•	[1]	[1]	[1] (8%)	[3] (6%)	✓✓
Stevens-Johnson syndrome					[1]	[1]	
Toxic epidermal necrolysis		[1]	[1]				
Urticaria	[1]				[1]		
HAIR							
Alopecia			[1]			[1] (12%)	
MUCOSAL							
Stomatitis	[1]			•		(8%)	✓

A Alendronate; **E** Etidronate; **I** Ibandronate; **P** Pamidronate; **R** Risedronate; **Z** Zoledronate

CALCIUM CHANNEL BLOCKERS

	A	D	F	I	Nic	Nif	Nis	V	=
SKIN									
Acneform eruption		[1]					•	[1]	
AGEP		[21]				[3]			?
Anaphylaxis					[1]	[1]			
Angioedema	[6] (6%)	[3]	[1]		[1]	[2]		[3]	✓
Dermatitis	(<10%)	[1]				[1]			
Diaphoresis	•	[2]	[1]	•		[2]	•	[2]	✓
Ecchymoses		•					•	[1]	
Eczema	[2]	[1]							
Edema	[20] (5–14%)	[4] (<10%)	[1]	[6] (7%)	•	[3]	[1]	[1]	✓✓
Erythema		[2]	•			[2]			
Erythema multiforme	[2]	[11] (31%)				[5]		[4]	✓
Erythema nodosum						[2]		[1]	
Exanthems	[2]	[17] (31%)	[2]	[1]		[9]	[1]	[8]	✓
Exfoliative dermatitis		[6]				[5]	•	[2]	✓
Facial edema	[1]		•			•	•		✓
Flushing	[5] (<10%)	[6] (<10%)	[10] (44%)	[9] (10%)	[2] (6%)	[9] (44%)	[1] (13%)	[4] (<7%)	✓✓
Hyperkeratosis		[1]						[2]	
Hypersensitivity	[1]	[2]							
Lichenoid eruption		[1]				[3]			
Linear IgA	[1]							[1]	
Lupus erythematosus		[5]				[3]		[2]	
Peripheral edema	[45] (34%)	[1] (5–8%)	[6] (22%)		[2] (7%)	[12] (6%)	[6] (22%)	[1] (<10%)	✓
Petechiae	[1]	•					•		
Photosensitivity	[1]	[11]				[5]		[4]	✓
Pigmentation	[2]	[10]					•		
Pruritus	[3]	[6]	•	[1] (6%)		[3]	•	[6]	✓
Pseudolymphoma	[1]	[1]							
Purpura	[2]	[3]	[1]			[3]		[1]	✓
Pustules		[2]					•		
Rash	(<10%)	[4]	•	•	[3]	[2]	•	[2]	✓✓

A Amlodipine; **D** Diltiazem; **F** Felodipine; **I** Isradipine; **Nic** Nicardipine; **Nif** Nifedipine; **Nis** Nisoldipine; **V** Verapamil

	A	D	F	I	Nic	Nif	Nis	V	=
Stevens-Johnson syndrome	[1]	[4]				[3]		[5]	✓
Telangiectasia	[5]		[2]			[2]			
Toxic epidermal necrolysis	[2]	[4]				[2]			
Toxicity	[2]	[2]						[1]	
Ulcerations						[1]	•		
Urticaria	[1]	[5]	[1]	•	[3]	[7]	•	[5]	✓✓
Vasculitis	[2]	[6]				[4]		[2]	✓
Xerosis	•						•		
HAIR									
Alopecia	•	[2]				[4]	•	[5]	✓
Hair pigmentation						[1]		[1]	
NAILS									
Nail dystrophy		[1]				[1]		[1]	
MUCOSAL									
Gingival hyperplasia/hypertrophy	[31] (31%)	[10] (21%)	[5] (2–10%)	[1]	[2]	[75] (75%)	•	[10] (19%)	✓✓
Oral ulceration		[1]					•	[1]	
Xerostomia	[1]	[2]	[1]	•	•	•	•	•	✓✓

A Amlodipine; **D** Diltiazem; **F** Felodipine; **I** Isradipine; **Nic** Nicardipine; **Nif** Nifedipine; **Nis** Nisoldipine; **V** Verapamil

CEPHALOSPORINS

	Cclor	Cdxl	Cnir	Cpm	Cixm	Ctxm	Ctan	CF	Czim	Cple	Caxn	Coxm	=
SKIN													
AGEP	[2]			[1]		[1]			[1]		[4]	[2]	✓
Anaphylaxis	[5] (65%)	[1]			[1]	[1]	[3]	•	[3]		[15]	[7]	✓
Angioedema	•	[1]			•				•		[3]	•	✓
Candidiasis			•	•			•		•		[3] (5%)		
Dermatitis	[1]										[2]		
DRESS syndrome		[1]			[1]	[4]					[2]		
Erythema		[1]								(9%)		[1]	
Erythema multiforme	[6]	•			[1] (13%)	[2]			[1]		[1]	•	✓
Exanthems	[9]	[1]	•	•		[3]			[1]		[7] (6%)	[2] (6%)	✓
Fixed eruption	[2]				[1]				[1]		[1]		
Hypersensitivity				[2]	[1]	[2]	[1]	[2]	[1]	[1]	[4]	[4]	✓
Jarisch–Herxheimer reaction											[1]	[1]	
Lupus erythematosus				[2]								[1]	
Pemphigus		[1]			[1]						[1]	[1]	
Pemphigus erythematodes									[2]			[1]	
Pruritus	[4]	[1]	•	[3]	[1]	[3]	•	[7]	[3]	[1] (9%)	[2]	•	✓✓
Pseudolymphoma					[1]							[1]	
Pustules	[1]											[1]	
Rash	[2] (12%)	•	•	[12] (51%)	[2]	[3]	[2]	[9] (10%)	[5]	[1]	[5]	[1]	✓✓
SDRIFE		[1]										[1]	
Serum sickness	[7]	•											
Serum sickness-like reaction	[23]	•	•		[1]		•				[2]	[2]	✓
Stevens-Johnson syndrome	[1]	•	•	[2]	[1]	[2]	•		•		[1]	•	✓
Toxic epidermal necrolysis	[1]				•	[1]			[1]		[1]	[2]	✓
Urticaria	[5]	[2]	•	[1]	[2] (13%)	•	•	•	•		[4]	[2]	✓
MUCOSAL													
Glossitis		[1]									[2]		
Oral candidiasis				•							[1]	[1]	
Oral mucosal eruption		[1]									[1]		

Cclor Cefaclor; **Cdxl** Cefadroxil; **Cnir** Cefdinir; **Cpm** Cefepime; **Cixm** Cefixime; **Ctxm** Cefotaxime; **Ctan** Cefotetan; **CF** Ceftaroline Fosamil; **Czim** Ceftazidime; **Cple** Ceftobiprole; **Caxn** Ceftriaxone; **Coxm** Cefuroxime

DISEASE-MODIFYING ANTIRHEUMATIC DRUG (DMARDS)

	Ab	Ad	Az	Ce	Cy	E	G	H	I	M	P	R	S	=
SKIN														
Abscess		[1]				[2]			[4]	[2]				
Acneform eruption		[3]	[2]		[7] (13%)	[1]			[6]	[1] (67%)				?
AGEP			[2]			[1]		[23] (25%)	[2]				[3]	?
Anaphylaxis		[2]	[1]		[8]	[2]		[1]	[11]	[9] (<10%)		[7]	[4]	✓
Angioedema		[4]	[2]	•	[1]	[1]		•	[2] (11%)	[1]		[4] (11%)	[3]	✓
Angioma					[1]					[1]				
Atrophy								[1]			[1]			
Basal cell carcinoma	[3]		[2]		[4]		[1]		[1]	[1]				
Bullous dermatitis					[1]			[2]	[1]	[4]	[3]	[1]		
Bullous pemphigoid		[1]				[1]					[6]		[3]	
Burning					[1]					[1]				
Candidiasis		[1]			[2] (16%)				[4] (5%)	[1]	[1]			
Carcinoma		[2]	[3]			[2]				[2]				
Cellulitis	[1]	[2] (<5%)				[2]			[5]	[1]		[1]		
Churg-Strauss syndrome			[1]		[1]									
Cicatricial pemphigoid			[1]								[2]			
Cyst					[5]						[1]			
Dermatitis		[1]	[4]	•		[3]		[1]	[4]	[2]	[4]	[2]	[2]	✓
Dermatomyositis		[5]				[4]		[1]			[14]			?
Diaphoresis												[2] (15%)	[1]	
DRESS syndrome								[3]					[31] (7%)	?
Ecchymoses								[1]	[1]	[1]				
Eccrine squamous syringometaplasia					[1]					[1]				
Eczema	[2] (15%)	[2]							[5] (19–30%)				[1]	?
Edema					[1] (5–14%)				[3]	[2]		[1]	[1]	
Erysipelas	[1]	[1] (<5%)												

Ab Abatacept; **Ad** Adalimumab; **Az** Azathioprine; **Ce** Certolizumab; **Cy** Cyclosporine; **E** Etanercept; **G** Golimumab; **H** Hydroxychloroquine; **I** Infliximab; **M** Methotrexate; **P** Penicillamine; **R** Rituximab; **S** Sulfasalazine

	Ab	Ad	Az	Ce	Cy	E	G	H	I	M	P	R	S	=
Erythema		[1]	[1]		[1]				[1]	[1] (7%)		[2] (16%)		
Erythema annulare centrifugum								[3]				[1]		
Erythema multiforme		[1]	[2]					[2]	[2]	[4]	(<5%)		[8]	✓
Erythema nodosum	[1]		[4]	[1]		[1]		[1]			[1]		[2]	✓
Erythroderma								[3]		[2]			[1]	
Exanthems			[10] (5%)		[1]	[2]		[4] (<5%)	[4]	[5] (15%)	[8]	[1]	[23] (23%)	✓
Exfoliative dermatitis			[1]					[3]		[1]			[5]	
Facial edema	[1]				[1]				[1]	[1]	[1]	[1]	[1]	✓
Fixed eruption		[1]	[1]			[1]		•	[1]				[7]	
Flushing	[1]				[5] (2–5%)				[2] (39%)		[1]	(5%)	[2]	✓
Folliculitis				[1]	[8]	[1]			[2]	[2]				
Fungal dermatitis			[1] (42%)		[1]									?
Furunculosis	[1]	[1]								[1]				
Granuloma annulare						[1]			[1]					
Granulomas		[1]				[2]			[1]					
Granulomatous reaction		[5]				[5]			[1]		[1]			
Hand–foot syndrome									[2] (31%)	[3]				?
Henoch–Schönlein purpura		[2]				[3]			[1]					
Herpes		[1]			[1]				[2]					
Herpes simplex	[3] (<5%)	[1]	[3] (35%)		[4]	[1]			[4] (10%)	[2]		[2]		✓
Herpes zoster	[3]	[10]	[8] (27%)	[3]	[2]	[6]			[11]	[7]		[7]		✓
Hidradenitis		[2]			[1]	[2]			[1]			[1]		
Hyperkeratosis					[1]		[1]							
Hypersensitivity	[2]	[3]	[29]	•	[2]	[1]			[11] (11%)	[4]	[3]	[5]	[21] (9%)	✓
Ichthyosis					[1]					[1]				
Kaposi's sarcoma		[1]	[14]		[5]				[1]			[3]		
Keratoacanthoma			[1]		[1]				[1]					
Leprosy		[1]				[2]			[1]					
Lesions		[2]						[1]	[1]					
Leukocytoclastic vasculitis		[1]		[1]			[1]		[2]					
Lichen planus						[2]		[1]	[2]		[4]		[3]	

Ab Abatacept; **Ad** Adalimumab; **Az** Azathioprine; **Ce** Certolizumab; **Cy** Cyclosporine; **E** Etanercept; **G** Golimumab; **H** Hydroxychloroquine; **I** Infliximab; **M** Methotrexate; **P** Penicillamine; **R** Rituximab; **S** Sulfasalazine

	Ab	Ad	Az	Ce	Cy	E	G	H	I	M	P	R	S	=
Lichenoid eruption		[5]	[1]		[1]	[3]		[4]	[3]		[7]			✓
Linear IgA					[2]				[1]					
Lupus erythematosus		[16]			[1]	[25]	[3]		[35] (59%)		[43]	[1]	[34]	✓
Lupus syndrome		[3]		[1]		[4]			[12]		[1]	[1]		
Lymphadenopathy		[1]							[1]	[1]				
Lymphoma		[8]	[1]		[12]	[3]	[1]		[9]	[5]		[1]		✓
Lymphomatoid papulosis		[1]			[1]									
Lymphoproliferative disease			[4]		[2]	[1]		[1]	[1]				[1]	
Malignancies	[10] (23%)	[6]	[2]		[2] (8%)	[4]	[5]		[2]	[2]				✓
Melanoma		[6]			[1]	[2]	[1]		[1]	[1]				
Molluscum contagiosum		[1]							[2]	[2]				
Morphea		[1]				[1]					[2]			
Necrosis										[6]		[1]	[1]	
Necrotizing fasciitis					[1]	[1]			[1]	[1]				
Neoplasms		[2]	[2]	[2]	[1]	[2]			[2]	[2]		[1]		✓
Neutrophilic dermatosis	[1]	[1]	[4] (76%)			[1]								?
Nevi			[3]			[1]			[2]					
Nodular eruption					[1]	[3]				[15]				
Non-Hodgkin's lymphoma		[1]	[1]			[1]				[2]				
Palmar–plantar pustulosis									[3]			[1]		
Pemphigus								[1]			[76]	[1]		?
Pemphigus foliaceus			[1]								[16]			
Peripheral edema	[1]	(<5%)			[3] (10%)	[1]			[1]		(<10%)	[1] (14%)		✓
Photoallergic reaction								[1]					[1]	
Photosensitivity			[1]					[6]		[9] (5%)			[4] (10%)	
Phototoxicity								[3]		[1]				
Pigmentation			[1] (37%)					[19] (<10%)		(<10%)			[3]	?
Pityriasis lichenoides chronica		[1]				[1]			[2]					
Porokeratosis			[4]		[1]	[1]								
Pruritus	•	[6]	[1]	[1]	[2] (12%)	[2] (14%)		[13] (47%)	[8] (20%)	[1] (<5%)	[2] (44–50%)	[8] (14%)	[8] (10%)	✓
Pseudolymphoma		[1]			[6]	[1]			[2]	[10]			[2]	

Ab Abatacept; **Ad** Adalimumab; **Az** Azathioprine; **Ce** Certolizumab; **Cy** Cyclosporine; **E** Etanercept; **G** Golimumab; **H** Hydroxychloroquine; **I** Infliximab; **M** Methotrexate; **P** Penicillamine; **R** Rituximab; **S** Sulfasalazine

	Ab	Ad	Az	Ce	Cy	E	G	H	I	M	P	R	S	=
Psoriasis	[13]	[40]		[6]	[2]	[20]	[2]	[14]	[57] (19%)	[1]	[4]	[4]	[1]	✓
Purpura					[4]						[5]	[1]	[1]	
Pustules		[1]				[2]		[1]	[5]				[2]	
Pyoderma gangrenosum		[1]	[1]			[1]			[1]			[3]		
Rash	[6] (23%)	[6] (12%)	[10] (<10%)	[2] (5%)	[1] (7–12%)	[8] (15%)	[3]	[4] (<10%)	[13] (25%)	[13] (5%)	[6] (44–50%)	[12] (58%)	[19] (6%)	✓✓
Raynaud's phenomenon					[2]					[1]			[3]	
Rosacea		[1]				[1]			[1]					
Sarcoidosis		[9]		[1]		[10]			[5]	[1]		[3]	[1]	✓
Scabies			[5]			[1]				[1]				
Scleroderma		[1]	[1]								[7]			
Serum sickness				•					[2]			[22] (<20%)	[1]	?
Serum sickness-like reaction				•					[5]		[1]	[5] (<17%)		
Sjögren's syndrome	[4]										[1]			
Skin cancer		[1]							[1]					
Squamous cell carcinoma	[5]	[5]	[11]		[12]	[4]	[1]		[1]	[2]				✓
Stevens-Johnson syndrome		[2]	[1]					[1]	[1]	[4]		[6]	[9]	✓
Striae					[1]					[1] (9%)				
Sweet's syndrome			[12]						[1]				[1]	
Thrombocytopenic purpura		[1]			[5]			[2]						
Tinea		[1]	[3]											
Toxic epidermal necrolysis			[1]		[1]			[3]	[2]	[8]	[2]	[4]	[13] (<10%)	✓
Toxicity		[1]	[3] (6%)	[1]	[2]		[1]	[1]	[2] (75%)	[9] (10%)		[3] (12%)		✓
Tumors		[1]	[8] (14%)	[1]	[1]							[1] (11%)		
Ulcerations			[1]		•				[1]	[12]				
Urticaria	[1]	[4]	[5]	•	[2]	[2]		[2]	[6] (17%)	[4]	[2] (44–50%)	[5] (8%)	[11] (<5%)	✓
Vasculitis	[2]	[9] (13%)	[5]	•	[3]	[23] (25%)	[1]	[1]	[18] (63%)	[9]	[7]	[4]	[4]	✓✓
Vesiculation		[1]								[1]	[1]			
Vitiligo		[2]			[1]				[4]					
Xerosis	[1]										[1]		[1]	

Ab Abatacept; **Ad** Adalimumab; **Az** Azathioprine; **Ce** Certolizumab; **Cy** Cyclosporine; **E** Etanercept; **G** Golimumab; **H** Hydroxychloroquine; **I** Infliximab; **M** Methotrexate; **P** Penicillamine; **R** Rituximab; **S** Sulfasalazine

	Ab	Ad	Az	Ce	Cy	E	G	H	I	M	P	R	S	=
HAIR														
Alopecia		[5]	[10] (54%)	[1]	[2]	[5] (20%)		[2]	[6]	[28] (10%)	[3]	[1]	[6]	✓
Alopecia areata		[7]			[6]	[1]	[1]		[3]					
Follicular mucinosis		[1]							[1]					
Hair pigmentation								[8] (<10%)		[1]				
Hirsutism					[10]						[2]			
NAILS														
Discoloration			[1]					[1]						
Leukonychia (Mees' lines)					[2]					[1]	[1]			
Nail pigmentation								[3]		[2]	[4]			
Onychocryptosis		[1]			[1]			[1]						?
Onycholysis		[1]								[1]				
Onychomycosis			[2] (5%)						[1] (33%)	[1]				?
Pyogenic granuloma					[1]	[1]								
MUCOSAL														
Aphthous stomatitis			•	•	[2] (9%)					[2]	[2]		[1]	
Cheilitis						[1] (10%)				[1]			[1]	
Gingival hyperplasia/hypertrophy					[160] (86%)						[1]			?
Gingivitis					•	[1] (7%)				•			[1]	
Glossitis					[1]					•	[1]			
Mucocutaneous reactions						[1]				[2]	[1]	[2]	[2] (6%)	
Mucosal ulceration			[1]								[1]			
Oral candidiasis									[1]	[1] (11%)	[1]			
Oral mucositis			[1]						[1]	[8]				
Oral ulceration			[2]		[2]	[1]				[11] (61%)	[5]		[3]	✓
Oropharyngeal pain						[1] (9%)						[1]		
Stomatitis	[3] (24%)		[1]		(5–7%)			[2]		[19] (43%)	[6]	[2] (69%)	[1] (<10%)	✓
Tonsillitis		[1]							[1]					

Ab Abatacept; **Ad** Adalimumab; **Az** Azathioprine; **Ce** Certolizumab; **Cy** Cyclosporine; **E** Etanercept; **G** Golimumab; **H** Hydroxychloroquine; **I** Infliximab; **M** Methotrexate; **P** Penicillamine; **R** Rituximab; **S** Sulfasalazine

DPP-4 INHIBITORS

	Alog	Lina	Saxa	Sita	=
SKIN					
Anaphylaxis	[1]			[1]	✓
Angioedema	[1]		[1]	[3]	✓
Edema			[1]	[3]	✓
Hypersensitivity	[2]	[1]	[1]		✓
Peripheral edema	[1]	[1] (10%)	•		✓
Pruritus	[2]	[1]	[1]		✓
Rash	[1]		[1]	[2]	✓
Stevens-Johnson syndrome	[1]			[1]	✓

Alog Alogliptin; **Lina** Linagliptin; **Saxa** Saxagliptin; **Sita** Sitagliptin

EGFR INHIBITORS

	C	E	G	L	Nec	Nil	P	Sor	Sun	=
SKIN										
Acneform eruption	[66] (97%)	[29] (73–80%)	[34] (66–85%)	[8] (90%)	[1] (23–43%)	[1] (<10%)	[18] (81%)	[6] (<10%)	[1] (<10%)	✓✓
AGEP		[2]	[1]					[2]		
Anaphylaxis	[5] (13%)	[1] (30%)	[1]				[1]			?
Angioedema							[1]	[1]		
Bullous dermatitis		[1]							[1] (7%)	
Dermatitis	[4] (80%)	[4] (30%)				(<10%)				?
Desquamation	[3] (89%)	[1]	[2] (39%)				[3] (13%)	[8] (50%)		✓
DRESS syndrome		[2]						[1]		
Eczema	[1]	[1]	[1]			(<10%)	[2]	[2]		✓
Edema		[1]		[2] (29%)		[3]	[1] (15%)	[3] (11%)	[6] (32%)	✓
Erythema	[3] (14%)	(18%)	[1]	[2]		[2] (<10%)	[5] (65%)	[4] (19%)	[6] (7%)	✓
Erythema multiforme						[1]		[11] (17%)		
Exanthems	[5]	[3] (8%)	[3] (21%)	[2]		[2]		[3]		✓
Exfoliative dermatitis			[1]	[2] (14%)		[1]	[2] (25%)	[1] (<10%)	[1] (10%)	✓
Facial edema		[1]				•		[1]	[3] (24%)	?
Fissures	[4] (14%)	[1]			[1] (22%)		[5] (21%)			?
Flushing	[2]					(<10%)		(<10%)		
Folliculitis	[13] (83%)	[9] (11%)	[4]	[2]		[1] (<10%)	[3]	[3]		✓
Hand–foot syndrome	[5] (6%)	[3] (30–60%)	[2]	[20] (76%)			[3] (23%)	[126] (89%)	[75] (45–65%)	✓
Hematoma	[1]					(<10%)				
Hypersensitivity	[9]				[1]			[2]		
Jaundice				[2] (35%)		•		[1]	[1]	?
Keratosis pilaris		[1]				[1]		[2]		
Necrosis		[1]							[1]	
Nevi						[1]		[3]	[2]	

C Cetuximab; **E** Erlotinib; **G** Gefitinib; **L** Lapatinib; **Nec** Necitumumab; **Nil** Nilotinib; **P** Panitumumab; **Sor** Sorafenib; **Sun** Sunitinib

	C	E	G	L	Nec	Nil	P	Sor	Sun	=
Papulopustular eruption	[7] (83%)	[9] (29%)	[3] (21%)				[4] (21–41%)			✓
Peripheral edema	[1] (40%)		[1] (22%)			[1] (44%)	[1] (12%)		[1] (17%)	✓
Pigmentation			[1]	[2] (18%)			[1]	[2]	[15] (91%)	✓
Pruritus	[9] (40%)	[9] (21%)	[6] (61%)	[6] (33%)	[2] (60%)	[16] (9–21%)	[10] (91%)	[10] (21%)	[3] (<10%)	✓✓
Psoriasis	[1]			[2]		[1]		[3]		
Purpura		[3]	[1]							
Pustules	[1]		[1]				[1]			
Pyoderma gangrenosum			[1]						[8]	
Radiation recall dermatitis	[2]	[1]						[3]	[1]	
Rash	[52] (89%)	[116] (80%)	[67] (66–85%)	[52] (55%)	[9] (76–81%)	[18] (56%)	[33] (91%)	[54] (30–75%)	[17] (14–38%)	✓✓
Rosacea	[1]	[2]				[1]				
Seborrheic dermatitis		[1]						[2]	[1]	
Squamous cell carcinoma			[1]			[1]		[8]		
Stevens-Johnson syndrome	[2]						[1]	[2]	[1]	
Telangiectasia	[1]	[1]					[1]			
Toxic epidermal necrolysis	[4]		[2]					[1]		
Toxicity	[20] (63%)	[10] (84%)	[10] (68%)	[14] (46%)	[2] (8%)	[8]	[26] (95%)	[19] (75%)	[24] (67%)	✓✓
Ulcerations	[1]		[2]						[1]	
Urticaria			[1]			(<10%)		•		
Vasculitis		[1]	[1]					[1]		
Xerosis	[15] (49%)	[13] (56%)	[13] (53%)	[2] (29%)	[2] (67%)	[2] (13–17%)	[12] (62%)	[6] (14%)	[3] (17%)	✓✓
HAIR										
Alopecia	(5%)	[10] (14%)	[6]	[4] (33%)		[5] (<10%)	[3] (54%)	[28] (67%)	[6] (5–12%)	✓
Hair changes	[3]	[4] (20%)					[2] (9%)	[1] (26%)		?
Hair pigmentation								[2]	[8] (38%)	?
Hypertrichosis	[3]	[4]	[2]							
NAILS										
Nail changes	[1] (21%)	[3] (25%)	[1] (17%)				[2] (9–29%)			?

C Cetuximab; **E** Erlotinib; **G** Gefitinib; **L** Lapatinib; **Nec** Necitumumab; **Nil** Nilotinib; **P** Panitumumab; **Sor** Sorafenib; **Sun** Sunitinib

	C	E	G	L	Nec	Nil	P	Sor	Sun	=
Nail disorder	[3]			[2] (10%)			[1]		[1] (<10%)	
Paronychia	[17] (39%)	[14] (23%)	[14] (14–32%)	[8] (27%)			[13] (85%)			✓
Pyogenic granuloma	[1]	[1]	[2]				[1]			
Splinter hemorrhage								[4] (70%)	[2]	?
Subungual hemorrhage								[2]	[4]	
MUCOSAL										
Aphthous stomatitis	[1]	[1]						[1]		
Cheilitis				[2] (14%)				[1]		
Epistaxis			[1]				[1]	[2] (11%)	[2] (13%)	
Glossodynia								(<10%)	[1] (15%)	
Mucosal inflammation		[1] (18%)		[2] (15%)			(6%)		[4] (54%)	?
Mucositis	[10]	[10] (21%)	[4] (6–17%)	[4] (11–35%)			[4] (75%)	[13] (28%)	[19] (~60%)	✓
Oral mucositis	[2] (82%)		[1] (33%)				(6%)		[1] (20%)	?
Oral ulceration	[1]	[1]	[1]	[2] (13%)		•		[1] (5%)		✓
Oropharyngeal pain					•			[1] (10%)		
Stomatitis	[4] (25%)	[12] (26%)	[8] (6–17%)	[2] (41%)	(11%)	•	[4] (100%)	[13] (28%)	[19] (60%)	✓✓
Xerostomia	(11%)					[1] (11%)		[1] (<10%)	[2] (~60%)	

C Cetuximab; **E** Erlotinib; **G** Gefitinib; **L** Lapatinib; **Nec** Necitumumab; **Nil** Nilotinib; **P** Panitumumab; **Sor** Sorafenib; **Sun** Sunitinib

FLUOROQUINOLONES

	B	C	L	M	N	=
SKIN						
AGEP		[4]	[1]	[2]		✓
Anaphylaxis		[15]	[6]	[5]		✓
Angioedema		[8]	[1]			
Bullous dermatitis		[1]		[2]	[1]	✓
Candidiasis		[2]	•	•		✓
Diaphoresis		[5]	[1]	•	•	✓
DRESS syndrome		[1]		[1]		
Edema		•	[1]			
Erythema			[2]		[2]	
Erythema multiforme		[5]	[1]			
Erythema nodosum		[1]	[1]			
Exanthems		[4]	[2]		[2]	✓
Fixed eruption		[14]			[3]	
Flushing		[1]		[1]		
Hypersensitivity	[1]	[5]	[5]	[6]		✓
Peripheral edema		[1]		[1]		
Photosensitivity		[20]	[3]	[5]	[1]	✓
Phototoxicity		[5]	[5]		[4]	✓
Pigmentation		[1]	[1]			
Pruritus		[11]	[3]	[3]	[1]	✓
Purpura		[4]	[3]			
Radiation recall dermatitis		[1]	[2]			
Rash		[14] (<10%)	[2]	[4]	•	✓
Stevens-Johnson syndrome		[10]	[3] (5%)		[2]	✓
Sweet's syndrome		[1]			[1]	
Thrombocytopenic purpura		[1]		[2]		
Toxic epidermal necrolysis		[11]	[6] (5%)	[2]	[2]	✓
Toxicity		[3]	[1]			
Urticaria		[10]	[1]	[3]	[1]	✓
Vasculitis		[11]	[3]			
Xerosis		[1]	[1]	•		✓

B Besifloxacin; **C** Ciprofloxacin; **L** Levofloxacin; **M** Moxifloxacin; **N** Norfloxacin

	B	C	L	M	N	=
MUCOSAL						
Stomatitis		[4]		[1]		
Xerostomia		[3]	[1]	[1]	•	✓

B Besifloxacin; **C** Ciprofloxacin; **L** Levofloxacin; **M** Moxifloxacin; **N** Norfloxacin

NON-STEROIDAL ANTI-INFLAMMATORY (NSAIDS)

	A	C	D	E	F	Ib	In	Ktp	Ktl	Mx	Np	O	P	S	=
SKIN															
AGEP	[2]	[7]		[1]		[5] (50%)				[1]			[2]		?
Anaphylaxis	[16] (<10%)	[8]	[16] (48%)		[1]	[5] (25%)	•	[4]	[3]	[1]	[2]	•	•	[4]	✓
Angioedema	[64] (22%)	[9]	[2]	[1]	[1]	[8]	[2]	[1]	[1]	[3]	[5]	•	[3]	•	✓✓
Bullous dermatitis	[8]	[1]	[2]			[3]	[2]	[1] (29%)		•	[5]		[1]		✓
Bullous pemphigoid	[2]	[1]	[1]			[2]									
Churg-Strauss syndrome	[2]						[1]								
Dermatitis		[2]	[10]		[1]	[5]	[5]	[29]	(3–9%)				[5]	[1]	✓
Dermatitis herpetiformis	[2]		[2]		[1]	[1]	[2]								
Dermatomyositis	[2]		[1]												
Diaphoresis		•	•			[1]	•	[1]	[2] (<10%)		[3]	•	[1]		✓
DRESS syndrome	[2]	[1]	[1]			[4]					[4]		[1]		
Ecchymoses						[1]	•		•	[1]	(3–9%)	•	•	•	✓
Eczema			•		(3–9%)	[1]	[1]	[3]		[1]					
Edema		[5] (6%)			(3–9%)	[1]	[1] (3–9%)		(<10%)	[1] (6%)	[1] (<9%)	•	•		✓
Embolia cutis medicamentosa (Nicolau syndrome)			[16]			[2]		[1]					[1]		
Erythema		[2] (14%)	[4]					[4] (21%)	[1]	[2]	[1]		[1]	[1]	✓
Erythema multiforme	[18]	[3]	[6]	•	•	[11] (13%)	[1]	[1]		[1]	[2]	[1]	[12]	[8]	✓
Erythema nodosum	[18]		•			[1] (<5%)	[1]				[1]				
Erythroderma	[4]												[2]		
Exanthems	[22] (18%)	[7] (49%)	[6] (<5%)	[2]	[3]	[9]	[7] (11%)	[3]	[1] (3–9%)	[1]	[9] (14%)	[1]	[8]	[9] (<5%)	✓✓
Excoriations						[1] (6%)			[1]						
Exfoliative dermatitis	[2]	[1]	[1]		•	[1]	[1]	•	•			•	[1]	•	✓
Facial edema		[1]	[1]	[2]				•		[1]					
Fixed eruption	[44]	[2]	[4] (18%)	[2]	[2]	[15]	[3]			[1]	[26] (24%)		[15]	[5]	✓
Flushing	[2]		•	[1]			•		•						

A Aspirin; **C** Celecoxib; **D** Diclofenac; **E** Etodolac; **F** Flurbiprofen; **Ib** Ibuprofen; **In** Indomethacin; **Ktp** Ketoprofen; **Ktl** Ketorolac; **Mx** Meloxicam; **Np** Naproxen; **O** Oxaprozin; **P** Piroxicam; **S** Sulindac

	A	C	D	E	F	Ib	In	Ktp	Ktl	Mx	Np	O	P	S	=
Hematoma	[2]								[2]	[3]					
Henoch–Schönlein purpura						[1]				[1]					
Herpes simplex	[2]	•									[1]				
Herpes zoster		•				[1]									
Hot flashes		[1]			•	•	•	•		•	[1]		•	•	✓
Hypersensitivity	[10]	[8]	[5]		[4]	[5]	[1]		[2]	[2] (5%)	[2]		[1]	•	✓
Jaundice		[1]			[1]				•					[1]	
Lichen planus							[1]				[3]			[1]	
Lichenoid eruption	[4]										[3]		[5]		
Linear IgA			[6]					[1]			[1]	[1]	[3]		
Lupus erythematosus		[1]				[5]					[2]		[1]		
Pemphigus	[2]		[1]			[1]		[1]					[3]		
Peripheral edema	[2]	[2]	[1]	[1]		[2] (5%)		•		[1]	[1]		[1]		✓
Petechiae							•						•		
Photoallergic reaction		[1]	[1]					[2]							
Photosensitivity		•	[4]	[1]	•	[6]	[1]	[36] (11%)	•	•	[16]	•	[40]	[2]	✓
Phototoxicity											[1]	[1]			
Pityriasis rosea	[6]										[1]				
Pruritus	[12]	[6]	[6] (<10%)	[7] (<10%)	[1] (<5%)	[6] (<5%)	[3] (<10%)	[4] (<10%)	[1] (<10%)	[3]	[5] (17%)	(<10%)	[6] (<10%)	[5] (<10%)	✓✓
Pseudolymphoma	[2]		[1]			[1]	[1]	[1]			[1]	[1]		[1]	✓
Psoriasis	[6]		[1]			[2]	[7]	[1]		[1]					
Purpura	[16]	[1]	[2]			[1]	[5]	[1]	[1] (<10%)	•	[4]		[2]	[2]	✓
Purpura fulminans			[2]						[1]						
Pustules		[1]									[2]				
Rash	(<10%)	[11] (40%)	[4] (6%)	[5]	•	[3]	[1]	[1]	[1] (<10%)	[3]	[2] (3–9%)	[2]	[1]	•	✓✓
SDRIFE	[2]	[1]									[1]				
Serum sickness												•	•	[1]	
Serum sickness-like reaction						[1]	[1]				[1]	•	•		
Stevens-Johnson syndrome	[12]	[2]	[7] (5%)	•	•	[12] (17%)	•	•	•	[1]	[1]	[2]	[2]	[5]	✓✓
Toxic epidermal necrolysis	[18]	[5]	[5] (5%)	•	[1]	[9] (6%)	[6]	[1]	•	[1]	[5]	[4]	[12]	[13]	✓✓
Urticaria	[144] (83%)	[11]	[7]	•	•	[10]	[7]	[6]	[1]	[4]	[6] (<5%)	•	[7]	[4]	✓✓

A Aspirin; **C** Celecoxib; **D** Diclofenac; **E** Etodolac; **F** Flurbiprofen; **Ib** Ibuprofen; **In** Indomethacin; **Ktp** Ketoprofen; **Ktl** Ketorolac; **Mx** Meloxicam; **Np** Naproxen; **O** Oxaprozin; **P** Piroxicam; **S** Sulindac

	A	C	D	E	F	Ib	In	Ktp	Ktl	Mx	Np	O	P	S	=
Vasculitis	[4]	[4]	[3]	[2]	[1]	[8]	[5]		[1]	•	[9]		[3]	•	✓
Vesiculobullous eruption						[2]					[1]				
Wound complications						[1]			[1]						
Xerosis		•	[3]					[1]					[1]		
HAIR															
Alopecia	[2]	[3]	•		•	[2]	•	[1]	•	•	[3]		[3]	•	✓
NAILS															
Nail changes		•			•	[1]									
Onycholysis						[1]		[1]							
MUCOSAL															
Aphthous stomatitis	[6]		[1]						[1]		[1]		[4]		
Epistaxis	[4]								•	[1]					
Glossitis									•					•	
Oral lesions						[1]	[2] (7%)	[1]							
Oral lichenoid eruption					[2]	[1]	[1]							[1]	
Oral mucosal eruption	[6]													[2]	
Oral mucosal fixed eruption											[1]		[1]		
Oral ulceration	[8]		[1]			[1]	[4]				[1]		[1]		
Rectal hemorrhage									•	[1]					
Rectal mucosal ulceration	[2]													[1]	
Stomatitis		[4] (8%)	•					•	(<10%)		•	•	•	[2]	✓
Tongue edema			[1]				[1]		•						
Ulcerative stomatitis							[1]			•					
Xerostomia		•	[2] (26%)		•	•		[1]	[2]	•	[2]		[1]	[2]	✓

A Aspirin; **C** Celecoxib; **D** Diclofenac; **E** Etodolac; **F** Flurbiprofen; **Ib** Ibuprofen; **In** Indomethacin; **Ktp** Ketoprofen; **Ktl** Ketorolac; **Mx** Meloxicam; **Np** Naproxen; **O** Oxaprozin; **P** Piroxicam; **S** Sulindac

PROTON PUMP INHIBITOR (PPI)

	D	E	L	O	P	R	=
SKIN							
Acneform eruption		•	•		•		✓
AGEP			[1]	[2]			
Anaphylaxis		[1]	[6]	[7]	[7]		✓
Angioedema		•		[5]	•		✓
Candidiasis		•	•				
Dermatitis		•	[1]	[1]	•		✓
Diaphoresis		•	[1]	[1]	[1]	•	✓
Ecchymoses					•	•	
Eczema		[1]		[2]	[1] (9%)		✓
Edema		•	[1]	[2] (<10%)	•		✓
Erythema				[1]			
Erythema multiforme			[2]	[1]	•		✓
Erythroderma			[1]	[2]			
Exanthems		•		[1]	•		✓
Exfoliative dermatitis		[1]	[1]	[3]			✓
Facial edema			[2]	[1]	[1]	•	✓
Fixed eruption		[2]		[1]			
Flushing		•	[1]				
Fungal dermatitis		•			•		
Herpes zoster					•	•	
Hypersensitivity			[3]	[2]	[2]	[1]	✓
Lichenoid eruption			[1]	[2]	[1]		✓
Lupus erythematosus		[3]	[3]	[5]	[3]		✓
Peripheral edema		•	[2]	[2]	[2]	•	✓
Photosensitivity		[1]			[1]	•	✓
Pigmentation				[1]		•	
Pruritus		•	[1] (3–10%)	[8] (<10%)	[1]	[2]	✓
Pruritus ani et vulvae		•	[1]				
Psoriasis				[1]		•	
Rash		[1]	(3–10%)	[6]	[3] (9%)	[3]	✓
Stevens-Johnson syndrome			[1]	•	•		✓

D Dexlansoprazole; **E** Esomeprazole; **L** Lansoprazole; **O** Omeprazole; **P** Pantoprazole; **R** Rabeprazole

	D	E	L	O	P	R	=
Sweet's syndrome		[1]		[1]			
Toxic epidermal necrolysis			[4]	[5]	•		✓
Urticaria		[1]	[3]	[9] (<10%)	[2]	•	✓
Vasculitis				[2]	[1]		
Xerosis		[1]		[2]	•	•	✓
HAIR							
Alopecia			[1]	[2]	•	•	✓
MUCOSAL							
Gingivitis					•	•	
Glossitis			[1]		•	•	✓
Oral candidiasis	•			[3]	•		✓
Stomatitis			[2]	[1]	•	•	✓
Tongue edema		•			[1]		
Xerostomia	•		•	[2] (<10%)	•	•	✓

D Dexlansoprazole; **E** Esomeprazole; **L** Lansoprazole; **O** Omeprazole; **P** Pantoprazole; **R** Rabeprazole

STATINS

	A	F	L	Pi	Pr	R	S	=
SKIN								
Acneform eruption	•						[1] (36%)	?
Dermatomyositis	[4]	[1]	[1]		[2]		[5]	✓
Diaphoresis	•						[1]	
Ecchymoses	•					•		
Eczema	•				[2]		[4] (5%)	
Edema	•		[1] (6%)		•		[1]	✓
Eosinophilic fasciitis	[1]						[2]	
Erythema multiforme					[1]		[2]	
Exanthems			[3] (5%)				[1]	
Flushing			[1] (10%)		[1]		[1] (30%)	?
Herpes zoster	[1]	[1]	[1]		[1]	[1]	[1]	✓
Hypersensitivity			[1]				[1]	
Jaundice	[2]						[1]	
Lichenoid eruption	[1]	[1]	[1]		[2]		[1]	✓
Lupus erythematosus	[2]	[2]	[4]		[1]		[5]	✓
Peripheral edema						•	[2] (50%)	?
Petechiae	•						[1]	
Photosensitivity	•				[1]		[7]	
Pruritus	[1]		[2] (5%)		[2]	•	[3]	✓
Purpura			[1]		[1]		[3]	
Radiation recall dermatitis						[1]	[1]	
Rash	[2]	•	[3] (5%)		[7] (5–7%)	•	[4] (<10%)	✓
Toxicity	[2]					[1]	[1]	
Urticaria	[1]						[1]	
Vasculitis	[1]						[2]	
HAIR								
Alopecia	[1]		•					
MUCOSAL								
Cheilitis	•						[1]	
Stomatitis	•						[2] (64%)	?

A Atorvastatin; **F** Fluvastatin; **L** Lovastatin; **Pi** Pitavastatin; **Pr** Pravastatin; **R** Rosuvastatin; **S** Simvastatin

TNF INHIBITORS

	A	C	E	G	I	M	=
SKIN							
Abscess	[1]		[2]		[4]		✓
Acneform eruption	[3]		[1]		[6]	[3]	✓
AGEP			[1]		[2]		
Anaphylaxis	[2]		[2]		[11]		✓
Angioedema	[4]	•	[1]		[2] (11%)		✓
Basal cell carcinoma				[1]	[1]	[1]	✓
Bullous pemphigoid	[1]		[1]				
Candidiasis	[1]				[4] (5%)		
Carcinoma	[2]		[2]			•	✓
Cellulitis	[2] (<5%)		[2]		[5]		✓
Dermatitis	[1]	•	[3]		[4]	[1] (3–15%)	✓
Dermatomyositis	[5]		[4]				
Eczema	[2]				[5] (19–30%)		?
Erythema	[1]				[1]		
Erythema multiforme	[1]				[2]		
Erythema nodosum		[1]	[1]				
Exanthems			[2]		[4]		
Fixed eruption	[1]		[1]		[1]		✓
Folliculitis		[1]	[1]		[2]	[1]	✓
Granuloma annulare			[1]		[1]		
Granulomas	[1]		[2]		[1]		✓
Granulomatous reaction	[5]		[5]		[1]		✓
Henoch-Schönlein purpura	[2]		[3]		[1]		✓
Herpes	[1]				[2]	[1]	✓
Herpes simplex	[1]		[1]		[4] (10%)	[3] (15%)	✓
Herpes zoster	[10]	[3]	[6]		[11]	[7] (14%)	✓
Hidradenitis	[2]		[2]		[1]		✓
Hypersensitivity	[3]	•	[1]		[11] (11%)	[1]	✓

A Adalimumab; **C** Certolizumab; **E** Etanercept; **G** Golimumab; **I** Infliximab; **M** Mycophenolate

	A	C	E	G	I	M	=
Kaposi's sarcoma	[1]				[1]	[1]	✓
Leprosy	[1]		[2]		[1]		✓
Lesions	[2]				[1]		
Leukocytoclastic vasculitis	[1]	[1]		[1]	[2]		✓
Lichen planus			[2]		[2]		
Lichenoid eruption	[5]		[3]		[3]		✓
Lupus erythematosus	[16]		[25]	[3]	[35] (59%)		✓
Lupus syndrome	[3]	[1]	[4]		[12]		✓
Lymphadenopathy	[1]				[1]		
Lymphoma	[8]		[3]	[1]	[9]		✓
Lymphoproliferative disease			[1]		[1]		
Malignancies	[6]		[4]	[5]	[2]	[1] (9–15%)	✓
Melanoma	[6]		[2]	[1]	[1]		✓
Molluscum contagiosum	[1]				[2]		
Morphea	[1]		[1]				
Necrotizing fasciitis			[1]		[1]		
Neoplasms	[2]	[2]	[2]		[2]		✓
Neutrophilic dermatosis	[1]		[1]				
Nevi			[1]		[2]		
Non-Hodgkin's lymphoma	[1]		[1]				
Peripheral edema	(<5%)		[1]		[1]	[1] (29%)	✓
Pityriasis lichenoides chronica	[1]		[1]		[2]		✓
Pruritus	[6]	[1]	[2] (14%)		[8] (20%)	[1] (30%)	✓
Pseudolymphoma	[1]		[1]		[2]		✓
Psoriasis	[40]	[6]	[20]	[2]	[57] (19%)	[1]	✓✓
Pustules	[1]		[2]		[5]		✓
Pyoderma gangrenosum	[1]		[1]		[1]		✓
Rash	[6] (12%)	[2] (5%)	[8] (15%)	[3]	[13] (25%)	[2] (8%)	✓✓
Rosacea	[1]		[1]		[1]		✓
Sarcoidosis	[9]	[1]	[10]		[5]		✓

A Adalimumab; **C** Certolizumab; **E** Etanercept; **G** Golimumab; **I** Infliximab; **M** Mycophenolate

	A	C	E	G	I	M	=
Serum sickness		•			[2]		
Skin cancer	[1]				[1]		
Squamous cell carcinoma	[5]		[4]	[1]	[1]	[1]	✓
Stevens-Johnson syndrome	[2]				[1]		
Toxicity	[1]	[1]		[1]	[2] (75%)	[1]	✓
Tumors	[1]	[1]					
Urticaria	[4]	•	[2]		[6] (17%)	[1]	✓
Vasculitis	[9] (13%)	•	[23] (25%)	[1]	[18] (63%)		✓
Vitiligo	[2]				[4]		
HAIR							
Alopecia	[5]	[1]	[5] (20%)		[6]	[4]	✓
Alopecia areata	[7]		[1]	[1]	[3]		✓
Follicular mucinosis	[1]				[1]		
MUCOSAL							
Tonsillitis	[1]				[1]		

A Adalimumab; **C** Certolizumab; **E** Etanercept; **G** Golimumab; **I** Infliximab

TYROSINE-KINASE INHIBITORS

	Aft	Axt	Cbo	Crz	Dsa	Erl	Gft	Imt	Lpt	Lnv	Nlo	Nnt	Srf	Snt	Vnd	=
SKIN																
Acneform eruption	[27] (92%)				[2] (<10%)	[29] (73–80%)	[34] (66–85%)	[3]	[4] (90%)		[1] (<10%)		[6] (<10%)	[1] (<10%)	[4] (35%)	✓
AGEP						[2]	[1]	[7]					[2]			
Anaphylaxis						[1] (30%)	[1]									?
Bullous dermatitis	•					[1]								[1] (7%)		
Cyst				[1]									[1]			
Dermatitis	[1] (21%)				[1] (<10%)	[4] (30%)					(<10%)				[1]	?
Desquamation						[1]	[2] (39%)						[8] (50%)			?
Diaphoresis								(13%)					[1] (6%)			
DRESS syndrome						[2]		[3]					[1]			
Eczema					(<10%)	[1]	[1]				(<10%)		[2]			
Edema				[13] (23–55%)	[6] (38%)	[1]		[36] (80%)	[1] (29%)		[3]		[3] (11%)	[6] (32%)		✓
Erythema		[1]	(11%)		[2]	(18%)	[1]	[5] (<10%)	[1]		[2] (<10%)		[4] (19%)	[6] (7%)		✓
Erythema multiforme				[1]				[2]			[1]		[11] (17%)		[1]	
Erythema nodosum					•			[1]								
Exanthems						[3] (8%)	[3] (21%)	[9]	[1]	(21%)	[2]		[3]			✓
Exfoliative dermatitis	•				[1]		[1]	[4]	[1] (14%)		[1]		[1] (<10%)	[1] (10%)		✓
Facial edema						[1]		[3] (<10%)			•		[1]	[3] (24%)		?
Fissures	[2] (12%)					[1]										
Flushing					[1] (<10%)						(<10%)	[1] (19%)	(<10%)			
Folliculitis	[1]					[9] (11%)	[4]	[1]	[1]		[1] (<10%)		[3]		[5] (49%)	✓
Graft-versus-host reaction					[1]			[1]								
Hand–foot syndrome	[2] (10%)	[18] (64%)	[20] (50%)		[1]	[3] (30–60%)	[2]	[3]	[10] (76%)	[3] (47%)		[2]	[126] (89%)	[75] (45–65%)	[4] (36%)	✓
Hematoma											(<10%)	[1]				

Aft Afatinib; **Axt** Axitinib; **Cbo** Cabozantinib; **Crz** Crizotinib; **Dsa** Dasatinib; **Erl** Erlotinib; **Gft** Gefitinib; **Imt** Imatinib; **Lpt** Lapatinib; **Lnv** Lenvatinib; **Nlo** Nilotinib; **Nnt** Nintedanib; **Srf** Sorafenib; **Snt** Sunitinib; **Vnd** Vandetanib

	Aft	Axt	Cbo	Crz	Dsa	Erl	Gft	Imt	Lpt	Lnv	Nlo	Nnt	Srf	Snt	Vnd	=
Herpes					(<10%)						•					
Hyperhidrosis					[1] (<10%)			[1]			(<10%)	[1] (12%)				
Hyperkeratosis			(7%)							(7%)			[4]			
Hypersensitivity					•								[2]			
Hypomelanosis								[5]						[1]		
Jaundice			(25%)						[1] (35%)		•		[1]	[1]		?
Keratosis pilaris						[1]					[1]		[2]			
Lesions								[1]						[2] (38%)		?
Leukocytoclastic vasculitis	[1]							[1]								
Lichen planus								[5]			[1]					
Necrolysis							[1]	[1]								
Necrosis						[1]								[1]		
Nevi											[1]		[3]	[2]		
Palmar–plantar hyperkeratosis								[1]						[1]		
Panniculitis					[4]			[3]								
Papulopustular eruption						[9] (29%)	[3] (21%)								[1]	?
Peripheral edema				[6] (28%)	[3] (44%)		[1] (22%)	[5] (75%)		[3] (37%)	[1] (44%)			[1] (17%)		?
Photosensitivity				[2]	[1]	[1]		[3] (<10%)							[8] (23%)	?
Phototoxicity													[1]		[3]	
Pigmentation					[1]		[1]	[14] (60%)	[1] (18%)				[2]	[15] (91%)	[6]	?
Pityriasis rubra pilaris								[1]					[1]			
Pruritus	[3] (13%)	[1] (8%)			[4] (14%)	[9] (21%)	[6] (61%)	[3] (10%)	[3] (33%)		[16] (9–21%)	[1] (19%)	[10] (21%)	[3] (<10%)	[2] (11%)	✓
Psoriasis								[3]	[1]		[1]		[3]			
Purpura						[3]	[1]	[1]								
Pyoderma gangrenosum							[1]	[1]						[8]		
Radiation recall dermatitis						[1]							[3]	[1]		
Rash	[52] (92%)	[3] (14%)	[1] (30%)	[4] (16%)	[10] (34%)	[116] (80%)	[67] (66–85%)	[26] (69%)	[26] (55%)	[1] (23%)	[18] (56%)	[4] (41%)	[54] (30–75%)	[17] (14–38%)	[34] (67%)	✓✓
Rosacea						[2]		[1]			[1]					

Aft Afatinib; **Axt** Axitinib; **Cbo** Cabozantinib; **Crz** Crizotinib; **Dsa** Dasatinib; **Erl** Erlotinib; **Gft** Gefitinib; **Imt** Imatinib; **Lpt** Lapatinib; **Lnv** Lenvatinib; **Nlo** Nilotinib; **Nnt** Nintedanib; **Srf** Sorafenib; **Snt** Sunitinib; **Vnd** Vandetanib

	Aft	Axt	Cbo	Crz	Dsa	Erl	Gft	Imt	Lpt	Lnv	Nlo	Nnt	Srf	Snt	Vnd	=
Seborrheic dermatitis						[1]							[2]	[1]		
Squamous cell carcinoma							[1]	[2]			[1]		[8]			
Stevens-Johnson syndrome	[4]							[15]					[2]	[1]	[4]	
Sweet's syndrome					[1]			[4]			[3]					
Telangiectasia						[1]		[1]								
Toxic epidermal necrolysis							[2]	[2]					[1]			
Toxicity	[3]		[3]	[1]	[8] (36%)	[10] (84%)	[10] (68%)	[9] (30–44%)	[7] (46%)	[3]	[8]		[19] (75%)	[24] (67%)	[9] (48–50%)	✓
Ulcerations					[1]		[2]							[1]		
Urticaria					[1] (<10%)		[1]	[3]			(<10%)		•			
Vasculitis						[1]	[1]	[2]					[1]			
Wound complications			[2]										[1]		[1]	
Xerosis	[8] (36%)	(10%)	[1] (23%)		[1] (<10%)	[13] (56%)	[13] (53%)	[2] (<10%)	[1] (29%)	[1] (20%)	[2] (13–17%)		[6] (14%)	[3] (17%)	[3] (15%)	✓
HAIR																
Alopecia	[1] (7%)	[2] (6%)	(16%)	[1] (7%)	[3] (<10%)	[10] (14%)	[6]	[2] (10–15%)	[2] (33%)	(12%)	[5] (<10%)	[2] (71%)	[28] (67%)	[6] (5–12%)	[1]	✓✓
Hair changes			(34%)			[4] (20%)							[1] (26%)		[2]	?
Hair pigmentation			[2] (34%)		[2]								[2]	[8] (38%)		?
Hypertrichosis						[4]	[2]									
NAILS																
Nail changes	[2] (16%)					[3] (25%)	[1] (17%)									?
Nail disorder					[1]			[1]	[1] (10%)					[1] (<10%)		
Nail pigmentation							[1]	[2]								
Paronychia	[17] (33–85%)					[14] (23%)	[14] (14–32%)		[4] (27%)						[5] (7%)	?
Pyogenic granuloma						[1]	[2]									
Splinter hemorrhage													[4] (70%)	[2]	[2]	?

Aft Afatinib; **Axt** Axitinib; **Cbo** Cabozantinib; **Crz** Crizotinib; **Dsa** Dasatinib; **Erl** Erlotinib; **Gft** Gefitinib; **Imt** Imatinib; **Lpt** Lapatinib; **Lnv** Lenvatinib; **Nlo** Nilotinib; **Nnt** Nintedanib; **Srf** Sorafenib; **Snt** Sunitinib; **Vnd** Vandetanib

	Aft	Axt	Cbo	Crz	Dsa	Erl	Gft	Imt	Lpt	Lnv	Nlo	Nnt	Srf	Snt	Vnd	=
Subungual hemorrhage													[2]	[4]		
MUCOSAL																
Aphthous stomatitis	•					[1]		[1]		(41%)			[1]			
Cheilitis	[1] (7%)							[1]	[1] (14%)				[1]			
Epistaxis	[3] (17%)	[1] (8%)					[1]			[1] (24%)		[2]	[2] (11%)	[2] (13%)		?
Glossodynia		[1]								(25%)			(<10%)	[1] (15%)		?
Mucocutaneous eruption					[1]			[1]			[1]					
Mucosal inflammation	[7] (69%)	[2] (15%)	[3] (35%)			[1] (18%)			[1] (15%)	[1] (50%)				[4] (54%)	[1] (27%)	✓
Mucositis	[10] (50–90%)	[1] (30%)	[1]		[1] (16%)	[10] (21%)	[4] (6–17%)	[2] (15%)	[2] (11–35%)				[13] (28%)	[19] (~60%)	[2] (14%)	✓
Oral mucositis		[1]					[1] (33%)							[1] (20%)		?
Oral ulceration						[1]	[1]	[3] (15%)	[1] (13%)	(41%)	•		[1] (5%)			?
Oropharyngeal pain								[1]		(25%)			[1] (10%)			?
Rhinorrhea	(11%)												•			
Stomatitis	[21] (50–90%)	[1] (15%)	[1] (51%)	[1] (11%)	[1]	[12] (26%)	[8] (6–17%)		[1] (41%)	[3] (47%)	•	[1]	[13] (28%)	[19] (60%)	[2] (33%)	✓
Xerostomia	[1] (20%)				[1] (33%)			[1] (44%)		(17%)	[1] (11%)		[1] (<10%)	[2] (~60%)		?

Aft Afatinib; **Axt** Axitinib; **Cbo** Cabozantinib; **Crz** Crizotinib; **Dsa** Dasatinib; **Erl** Erlotinib; **Gft** Gefitinib; **Imt** Imatinib; **Lpt** Lapatinib; **Lnv** Lenvatinib; **Nlo** Nilotinib; **Nnt** Nintedanib; **Srf** Sorafenib; **Snt** Sunitinib; **Vnd** Vandetanib

MAIN CLASSES OF DRUGS

5-HT1 agonist
- Almotriptan
- Eletriptan
- Frovatriptan
- Naratriptan
- Rizatriptan
- Sumatriptan
- Zolmitriptan

5-HT3 antagonist
- Alosetron
- Dolasetron
- Granisetron
- Ondansetron
- Palonosetron

ACE inhibitor
- Benazepril
- Captopril
- Cilazapril
- Enalapril
- Fosinopril
- Imidapril
- Lisinopril
- Moexipril
- Perindopril
- Quinapril
- Ramipril
- Trandolapril
- Zofenopril

Adrenergic alpha-receptor agonist
- Clonidine
- Dexmedetomidine
- Dopamine
- Ephedrine
- Guanabenz
- Guanadrel
- Guanethidine
- Guanfacine
- Methyldopa
- Midodrine
- Mirtazapine
- Phenylephrine
- Phenylpropanolamine
- Polythiazide
- Pseudoephedrine

Adrenergic alpha-receptor antagonist
- Alfuzosin
- Doxazosin
- Phenoxybenzamine
- Phentolamine
- Prazosin
- Silodosin
- Tamsulosin
- Terazosin
- Urapidil

Adrenergic alpha2-receptor agonist
- Apraclonidine
- Brimonidine
- Lofexidine
- Tizanidine

Adrenergic beta-receptor agonist
- Arbutamine
- Dobutamine
- Isoetharine
- Isoproterenol
- Isoxsuprine
- Metoprolol

Adrenergic beta-receptor antagonist
- Betaxolol
- Carteolol
- Carvedilol
- Esmolol
- Labetalol
- Levobetaxolol
- Levobunolol
- Metipranolol
- Nadolol
- Nebivolol
- Penbutolol
- Pindolol
- Timolol

Alkylating agent
- Altretamine
- Bendamustine
- Busulfan
- Carboplatin
- Carmustine
- Chlorambucil
- Cisplatin
- Cyclophosphamide
- Dacarbazine
- Estramustine
- Ifosfamide
- Lomustine
- Mechlorethamine
- Melphalan
- Mitomycin
- Oxaliplatin
- Procarbazine
- Streptozocin
- Temozolomide
- Thiotepa

Amphetamine
- Benzphetamine
- Dextroamphetamine
- Diethylpropion
- MDMA
- Methamphetamine
- Methylphenidate
- Pemoline
- Phendimetrazine
- Phentermine
- Prenylamine

Analeptic
- Doxapram
- Modafinil

Analgesic
- **narcotic**
  - Dextromethorphan
- **non-narcotic**
  - Acetaminophen
- **non-opioid**
  - Ketorolac
- **opioid**
  - Alfentanil
  - Dihydrocodeine
  - Fentanyl
  - Meptazinol
  - Tapentadol
- **urinary**
  - Pentosan
  - Phenazopyridine

Anesthetic
- Alfentanil
- Edrophonium
- Fentanyl
- Ketamine
- **general**
  - Chloral Hydrate
  - Propofol
  - Sodium Oxybate
  - Sufentanil
- **inhalation**
  - Desflurane
  - Enflurane
  - Halothane
  - Isoflurane
  - Methoxyflurane
  - Sevoflurane
- **local**
  - Articaine
  - Bupivacaine
  - Cocaine
  - Levobupivacaine
  - Lidocaine
  - Mepivacaine
  - Ropivacaine
  - Tetracaine & Oxymetazoline

Angiotensin II receptor antagonist (blocker)
- Azilsartan
- Candesartan
- Eprosartan
- Irbesartan
- Losartan
- Olmesartan
- Telmisartan
- Valsartan

Anti-inflammatory
- Aloe Vera (Gel, Juice, Leaf)
- Amlexanox
- Amodiaquine
- Bloodroot
- Boswellia
- Bromelain
- Butterbur
- Caraway
- Clofazimine
- Colchicine
- Devil's Claw
- Eucalyptus
- Evening Primrose
- Fish Oils
- Fluprednisolone
- Henna
- Horsetail
- Juniper
- Licorice
- Linseed
- Meadowsweet
- Myrrh
- Omega-3 Fatty Acids
- Polypodium Leucotomos
- Roflumilast
- Sarsaparilla
- Saw Palmetto
- Turmeric
- Willow Bark
- Yarrow

Antiarrhythmic
- **class Ia**
  - Disopyramide
  - Procainamide
  - Quinidine
- **class Ib**
  - Lidocaine
  - Mexiletine
  - Phenytoin
  - Tocainide
- **class Ic**
  - Flecainide
  - Lorcainide
  - Moricizine
  - Propafenone
- **class II**
  - Acebutolol
  - Atenolol
  - Esmolol
  - Labetalol
  - Metoprolol
  - Nadolol
  - Propranolol
  - Sotalol
- **class III**
  - Amiodarone
  - Bretylium
  - Dofetilide
  - Dronedarone
  - Ibutilide
  - Sotalol
  - Vernakalant
- **class IV**
  - Adenosine
  - Amlodipine
  - Bepridil
  - Digoxin
  - Diltiazem
  - Verapamil

Antibiotic
- Doripenem
- Ertapenem

Imipenem/Cilastatin
Meropenem
Meropenem & Vaborbactam
aminoglycoside
Amikacin
Gentamicin
Kanamycin
Neomycin
Paromomycin
Plazomicin
Streptomycin
Tobramycin
anthracycline
Bleomycin
Dactinomycin
Daunorubicin
Doxorubicin
Epirubicin
Idarubicin
Mitomycin
Mitoxantrone
Peplomycin
Valrubicin
beta-lactam
Ampicillin/Sulbactam
Aztreonam
Ceftazidime & Avibactam
Ceftolozane & Tazobactam
Flucloxacillin
fluoroquinolone
Besifloxacin
Ciprofloxacin
Delafloxacin
Enoxacin
Finafloxacin
Gatifloxacin
Gemifloxacin
Levofloxacin
Lomefloxacin
Moxifloxacin
Norfloxacin
Ofloxacin
Sparfloxacin
Tosufloxacin
glycopeptide
Daptomycin
Teicoplanin
Vancomycin
imidazole
Clotrimazole
Ketoconazole
Mebendazole
Miconazole
Sertaconazole
Thiabendazole
lincosamide
Clindamycin
Clindamycin/Tretinoin
Lincomycin
macrolide
Azithromycin
Clarithromycin
Dirithromycin
Erythromycin
Fidaxomicin
Roxithromycin
Telithromycin
Troleandomycin
nitrofuran
Furazolidone
Nitrofurazone
nitroimidazole
Benznidazole
Metronidazole
Secnidazole
Tinidazole
oxazolidinone
Linezolid
Tedizolid
penicillin
Amoxicillin
Ampicillin
Ampicillin/Sulbactam
Bacampicillin
Carbenicillin
Cloxacillin
Dicloxacillin
Methicillin
Mezlocillin
Nafcillin
Oxacillin
Penicillin G
Penicillin V
Piperacillin
Ticarcillin
quinolone
Cinoxacin
Grepafloxacin
Nalidixic Acid
Ozenoxacin
Trovafloxacin
rifamycin
Rifabutin
Rifampin
Rifapentine
Rifaximin
streptogramin
Pristinamycin
Quinupristin/Dalfopristin
sulfonamide
Co-Trimoxazole
Sulfacetamide
Sulfadiazine
Sulfadoxine
Sulfamethoxazole
Sulfisoxazole
tetracycline
Chlortetracycline
Demeclocycline
Doxycycline
Lymecycline
Minocycline
Oxytetracycline
Tetracycline
Tigecycline
topical
Mupirocin
Retapamulin
triazole
Fluconazole
Itraconazole
Posaconazole
Terconazole
Voriconazole
miscellaneous
Aminosalicylate Sodium
Bacitracin
Capreomycin
Ceftriaxone
Chloramphenicol
Cycloserine
Dapsone
Ethionamide
Fosfomycin
Isoniazid
Methenamine
Nitrofurantoin
Plicamycin
Pyrazinamide
Quinacrine
Spectinomycin
Tigecycline
Trimethoprim

Anticonvulsant
Brivaracetam
Carbamazepine
Ezogabine
Felbamate
Gabapentin
Lacosamide
Lamotrigine
Levetiracetam
Mephenytoin
Oxcarbazepine
Perampanel
Phenacemide
Phenobarbital
Phensuximide
Phenytoin
Pregabalin
Primidone
Tetrazepam
Tiagabine
Topiramate
Valproic Acid
Vigabatrin
Zonisamide
antiepileptic
Brivaracetam
Clobazam
Eslicarbazepine
Lacosamide
Lamotrigine
Perampanel
Rufinamide
Vigabatrin
hydantoin
Ethotoin
Fosphenytoin
Mephenytoin
Phenytoin
oxazolidinedione
Paramethadione
Trimethadione
succinimide
Ethosuximide
Methsuximide

Antidepressant
Bupropion
Citalopram
Desvenlafaxine
Duloxetine
Escitalopram
Fluoxetine
Fluvoxamine
Isocarboxazid
Levomilnacipran
Milnacipran
Moclobemide
Nefazodone
Paroxetine Hydrochloride
Phenelzine
Reboxetine
Selegiline
Sertraline
Tianeptine
Tranylcypromine
Tryptophan
Venlafaxine
Vilazodone
Vortioxetine
tetracyclic
Maprotiline
Mianserin
Mirtazapine
tricyclic
Amitriptyline
Amoxapine
Clomipramine
Desipramine
Doxepin
Imipramine
Nortriptyline
Protriptyline
Trazodone
Trimipramine

Antiemetic
Aprepitant
Artichoke
Chlorpromazine
Dexamethasone
Dimenhydrinate
Diphenhydramine
Domperidone
Dronabinol
Droperidol
Granisetron
Haloperidol
Marihuana
Meclizine
Metoclopramide
Nabilone
Ondansetron
Palonosetron
Peppermint
Perphenazine
Prochlorperazine
Rolapitant
Scopolamine
Trimethobenzamide

Antifungal
Amphotericin B
Caspofungin
Ciclopirox
Clioquinol
Econazole
Efinaconazole
Griseofulvin
Micafungin
Nystatin
Rosemary
Terbinafine
azole
Clotrimazole
Fluconazole
Isavuconazonium Sulfate
Itraconazole
Ketoconazole
Luliconazole
Miconazole
Posaconazole
Voriconazole

oxaborole
Tavaborole

Antimalarial
Amodiaquine
Artemether/Lumefantrine
Artemisia
Artesunate
Atovaquone
Atovaquone/Proguanil
Chloroquine
Halofantrine
Hydroxychloroquine
Mefloquine
Primaquine
Pyrimethamine
Quinacrine
Quinidine
Quinine
Sulfadoxine
Tafenoquine

Antimycobacterial
Bedaquiline
Clofazimine
Dapsone
Ethambutol
Flucytosine
Isoniazid
Potassium Iodide
Star Anise (Chinese)
echinocandin
Anidulafungin

Antineoplastic
Anastrozole
Arsenic
Asparaginase
Asparaginase *Erwinia chrysanthemi*
Azacitidine
Bexarotene
Cabazitaxel
Capecitabine
Carboplatin
Cetuximab
Cisplatin
Cladribine
Cytarabine
Dacarbazine
Dasatinib
Decitabine
Denileukin
Docetaxel
Eribulin
Erlotinib
Everolimus
Floxuridine
Fludarabine
Fluorouracil
Gefitinib
Gemcitabine
Gemtuzumab
Hydroxyurea
Ibritumomab
Imatinib
Irinotecan
Ixabepilone
Lapatinib
Levamisole
Mercaptopurine
Mitotane
Mitoxantrone
Nelarabine
Nilotinib
Nilutamide
Oxaliplatin
Paclitaxel
Panitumumab
Pazopanib
Pegaspargase
Pentostatin
Porfimer
Raltitrexed
Sorafenib
Streptozocin
Sunitinib
Tegafur/Gimeracil/Oteracil
Temozolomide
Temsirolimus
Teniposide
Testolactone
Thioguanine
Topotecan
Tositumomab & Iodine[131]
Trabectedin
Trastuzumab
Tretinoin
Trifluridine & Tipiracil
Vorinostat

Antiplatelet
Abciximab
Aspirin
Cangrelor
Cilostazol
Clopidogrel
Dipyridamole
Eptifibatide
Ticagrelor
Tirofiban
CPTP
Cangrelor
Ticagrelor
thienopyridine
Clopidogrel
Prasugrel
Ticlopidine

Antiprotozoal
Atovaquone
Chloroquine
Hydroxychloroquine
Mefloquine
Nitazoxanide
Pentamidine
Primaquine
Pyrimethamine
Quinidine
Quinine

Antipsychotic
Amisulpride
Aripiprazole
Asenapine
Brexpiprazole
Carbamazepine
Cariprazine
Chlorpromazine
Clozapine
Droperidol
Fluphenazine
Haloperidol
Iloperidone
Levomepromazine
Lithium
Loxapine
Lurasidone
Mesoridazine
Molindone
Olanzapine
Paliperidone
Perphenazine
Pimavanserin
Pimozide
Prochlorperazine
Promazine
Quetiapine
Risperidone
Sertindole
Thioridazine
Thiothixene
Trifluoperazine
Trimeprazine
Valproic Acid
Ziprasidone
Zuclopenthixol
Zuclopenthixol Acetate
Zuclopenthixol Decanoate
Zuclopenthixol Dihydrochloride

Antiretroviral
Adefovir
Amprenavir
Atazanavir
Bictegravir/Emtricitabine/Tenofovir Alafenamide
Cobicistat/Elvitegravir/Emtricitabine/Tenofovir Alafenamide
Cobicistat/Elvitegravir/Emtricitabine/Tenofovir Disoproxil
Darunavir
Delavirdine
Didanosine
Dolutegravir
Efavirenz
Emtricitabine
Enfuvirtide
Fosamprenavir
Hydroxyurea
Ibalizumab
Indinavir
Lamivudine
Lopinavir
Maraviroc
Nelfinavir
Nevirapine
Raltegravir
Rilpivirine
Ritonavir
Saquinavir
Stavudine
Tenofovir Disoproxil
Zalcitabine
Zidovudine

Antiviral
Acyclovir
Amantadine
Cytarabine
Entecavir
Famciclovir
Foscarnet
Ganciclovir
Imiquimod
Letermovir
Oseltamivir
Penciclovir
Peramivir
Podophyllotoxin
Rimantadine
Tenofovir Alafenamide
Trifluridine
Valacyclovir
Valganciclovir
Zanamivir
nucleoside analog
Ribavirin
Vidarabine
nucleotide analog
Cidofovir
topical
Acyclovir
Docosanol

Anxiolytic
Buspirone
Chlormezanone
Kava
Lavender
Meprobamate
Tetrazepam
Valerian

Barbiturate
Amobarbital
Aprobarbital
Butabarbital
Butalbital
Mephobarbital
Methohexital
Pentobarbital
Phenobarbital
Primidone
Secobarbital
Thiopental

Benzodiazepine
Alprazolam
Chlordiazepoxide
Clobazam
Clonazepam
Clorazepate
Diazepam
Estazolam
Flurazepam
Lorazepam
Midazolam
Nitrazepam
Oxazepam
Prazepam
Quazepam
Temazepam
Tetrazepam
Triazolam

Bisphosphonate
Alendronate
Etidronate
Ibandronate
Pamidronate
Risedronate
Tiludronate
Zoledronate

Calcium channel blocker
- Amlodipine
- Bepridil
- Clevidipine
- Diltiazem
- Felodipine
- Isradipine
- Nicardipine
- Nifedipine
- Nimodipine
- Nisoldipine
- Prenylamine
- Verapamil

Carbonic anhydrase inhibitor
- Acetazolamide
- Brinzolamide
- Dichlorphenamide
- Dorzolamide
- Ethoxzolamide
- Methazolamide

CB1 Cannabinoid receptor antagonist
- Rimonabant

Central muscle relaxant
- Carisoprodol
- Chlormezanone
- Chlorzoxazone
- Cyclobenzaprine
- Meprobamate
- Metaxalone
- Methocarbamol
- Orphenadrine

Cephalosporin

1st generation
- Cefadroxil
- Cefazolin
- Cephalexin
- Cephalothin
- Cephapirin
- Cephradine

2nd generation
- Cefaclor
- Cefamandole
- Cefmetazole
- Cefonicid
- Cefotetan
- Cefoxitin
- Cefprozil
- Cefuroxime
- Loracarbef

3rd generation
- Cefdinir
- Cefditoren
- Cefixime
- Cefoperazone
- Cefotaxime
- Cefpodoxime
- Ceftazidime
- Ceftazidime & Avibactam
- Ceftibuten
- Ceftizoxime
- Ceftriaxone

4th generation
- Cefepime

5th generation
- Ceftaroline Fosamil
- Ceftobiprole
- Ceftolozane & Tazobactam

Cholinesterase inhibitor
- Donepezil
- Edrophonium
- Galantamine
- Neostigmine
- Physostigmine
- Rivastigmine
- Succinylcholine
- Tacrine

CNS stimulant
- Cocaine
- Dexmethylphenidate
- Dextroamphetamine
- Lisdexamfetamine
- Modafinil

Corticosteroid
- Alclometasone
- Amcinonide
- Beclomethasone
- Betamethasone
- Budesonide
- Ciclesonide
- Clobetasol
- Cortisone
- Deflazacort
- Desonide
- Desoximetasone
- Dexamethasone
- Difluprednate
- Fludrocortisone
- Flumetasone
- Flunisolide
- Fluocinolone
- Fluocinonide
- Fluprednisolone
- Fluticasone Furoate
- Fluticasone Propionate
- Halcinonide
- Halobetasol
- Halometasone
- Hydrocortisone
- Loteprednol
- Methylprednisolone
- Mometasone
- Prednicarbate
- Prednisolone
- Prednisone
- Tixocortol
- Triamcinolone

antagonist
- Mifepristone
- Misoprostol

COX-2 inhibitor
- Celecoxib
- Etodolac
- Etoricoxib
- Meloxicam
- Nimesulide
- Rofecoxib
- Valdecoxib

CYP3A4 inhibitor
- Amiodarone
- Aprepitant
- Boceprevir
- Chloramphenicol
- Cimetidine
- Ciprofloxacin
- Clarithromycin
- Conivaptan
- Dasabuvir/Ombitasvir/Paritaprevir/Ritonavir
- Delavirdine
- Diltiazem
- Erythromycin
- Fluconazole
- Fluvoxamine
- Grapefruit Juice
- Imatinib
- Indinavir
- Itraconazole
- Ketoconazole
- Mifepristone
- Nefazodone
- Nelfinavir
- Norfloxacin
- Ombitasvir/Paritaprevir/Ritonavir
- Ritonavir
- Saquinavir
- Telaprevir
- Telithromycin
- Verapamil
- Voriconazole

Dermal filler
- Azficel-T
- Calcium Hydroxylapatite

Disease-modifying antirheumatic drug (DMARD)
- Abatacept
- Adalimumab
- Azathioprine
- Bucillamine
- Certolizumab
- Chloroquine
- Cyclosporine
- Etanercept
- Gold & Gold Compounds
- Golimumab
- Hydroxychloroquine
- Infliximab
- Leflunomide
- Methotrexate
- Minocycline
- Penicillamine
- Rituximab
- Sulfasalazine
- Tocilizumab

Diuretic
- Acetazolamide
- Blue Cohosh
- Boswellia
- Brinzolamide
- Caffeine
- Chicory
- Cranberry
- Dorzolamide
- Eplerenone
- Eucalyptus
- Horse Chestnut (Bark, Flower, Leaf, Seed)
- Horsetail
- Isosorbide
- Meadowsweet
- Methazolamide
- Spironolactone
- Squill

loop
- Bumetanide
- Ethacrynic Acid
- Furosemide
- Torsemide

potassium-sparing
- Amiloride
- Triamterene

thiazide
- Bendroflumethiazide
- Benzthiazide
- Chlorothiazide
- Chlorthalidone
- Cyclothiazide
- Hydrochlorothiazide
- Hydroflumethiazide
- Indapamide
- Methyclothiazide
- Metolazone
- Polythiazide
- Quinethazone
- Trichlormethiazide

Dopamine receptor agonist
- Apomorphine
- Bromocriptine
- Cabergoline
- Dopexamine
- Fenoldopam
- Pergolide
- Pramipexole
- Quinagolide
- Ropinirole
- Rotigotine

Dopamine receptor antagonist
- Amisulpride
- Domperidone
- Metoclopramide
- Sulpiride

Endothelin receptor (ETR) antagonist
- Ambrisentan
- Bosentan
- Macitentan
- Sitaxentan

Epidermal growth factor receptor (EGFR) inhibitor
- Cetuximab
- Erlotinib
- Gefitinib
- Lapatinib
- Necitumumab
- Nilotinib
- Panitumumab
- Pazopanib
- Sorafenib
- Sunitinib

Eugeroic
- Armodafinil

Fibrinolytic
- Alteplase
- Anistreplase
- Reteplase
- Streptokinase
- Tenecteplase
- Urokinase

Gonadotropin-releasing hormone (GnRH)
agonist
Buserelin
Goserelin
Histrelin
Leuprolide
Nafarelin
Triptorelin
antagonist
Abarelix
Cetrorelix
Degarelix
Elagolix Sodium
Ganirelix

Histamine
H1 receptor antagonist
Alcaftadine
Astemizole
Azatadine
Azelastine
Bepotastine
Brompheniramine
Buclizine
Carbinoxamine
Cetirizine
Chlorpheniramine
Cinnarizine
Clemastine
Cyproheptadine
Desloratadine
Dexchlorpheniramine
Diphenhydramine
Epinastine
Fexofenadine
Hydroxyzine
Ketotifen
Levocetirizine
Loratadine
Meclizine
Mizolastine
Olopatadine
Phenindamine
Promethazine
Pyrilamine
Rupatadine
Terfenadine
Trimeprazine
Tripelennamine
Triprolidine
H2 receptor antagonist
Cimetidine
Famotidine
Nizatidine
Ranitidine
Roxatidine

Histone deacetylase (HDAC) inhibitor
Belinostat
Panobinostat
Romidepsin
Vorinostat

HMG-CoA reductase inhibitor
Atorvastatin
Fluvastatin
Lovastatin
Pravastatin
Red Rice Yeast
Rosuvastatin
Simvastatin

Hormone
Estradiol
Levonorgestrel
Melatonin
Oral Contraceptives
Sincalide
polypeptide
Glucagon
Insulin
Insulin Aspart
Mecasermin
Nesiritide
Secretin

Immunomodulator
Aldesleukin
Aristolochia
Arnica
Bifidobacteria
Brewer's Yeast
Cordyceps
Dong Quai
Echinacea
Efalizumab
Garlic
Ginseng
Glatiramer
Goldenseal
Imiquimod
Immune Globulin IV
Immune Globulin SC
Interferon Alfa
Interferon Beta
Interferon Gamma
Lactobacillus
Lemon Balm
Lenalidomide
Levamisole
Milk Thistle
Mistletoe
Natalizumab
Palivizumab
PEG-Interferon
Pimecrolimus
Pomalidomide
Propolis
Resveratrol
Sarsaparilla
Siberian Ginseng
Sinecatechins

Immunosuppressant
Alefacept
Alemtuzumab
Anti-Thymocyte Globulin (Equine)
Anti-Thymocyte Immunoglobulin (Rabbit)
Azathioprine
Belatacept
Belimumab
Cyclosporine
Daclizumab
Everolimus
Fingolimod
Mizoribine
Muromonab-CD3
Mycophenolate
Phellodendron
Pirfenidone
Rituximab
Sirolimus
Tacrolimus
Thalidomide

Mast cell stabilizer
Cromolyn
Lodoxamide
Nedocromil
Pemirolast

Monoamine oxidase (MAO) inhibitor
Isocarboxazid
Phenelzine
Tranylcypromine

mTOR inhibitor
Everolimus
Temsirolimus
Zotarolimus

Muscarinic antagonist
Amitriptyline
Amoxapine
Atropine Sulfate
Benactyzine
Benztropine
Biperiden
Chlorpheniramine
Chlorpromazine
Cinnarizine
Clidinium
Clomipramine
Darifenacin
Dicyclomine
Diphenhydramine
Disopyramide
Doxepin
Fesoterodine
Flavoxate
Glycopyrrolate
Hydroxyzine
Hyoscyamine
Imipramine
Ipratropium
Maprotiline
Mepenzolate
Olanzapine
Orphenadrine
Oxybutynin
Phenelzine
Prochlorperazine
Procyclidine
Propantheline
Scopolamine
Solifenacin
Tiotropium
Tolterodine
Trihexyphenidyl
Trospium
Umeclidinium

Muscarinic cholinergic agonist
Bethanechol
Carbachol
Cevimeline
Methantheline
Pilocarpine

Non-depolarizing neuromuscular blocker
Atracurium
Cisatracurium
Doxacurium
Pancuronium
Pipecuronium
Rapacuronium
Rocuronium
Vecuronium

Non-nucleoside reverse transcriptase inhibitor
Delavirdine
Doravirine
Efavirenz
Emtricitabine/Rilpivirine/Tenofovir Alafenamide
Etravirine
Nevirapine
Rilpivirine

Non-steroidal anti-inflammatory (NSAID)
Aceclofenac
Acemetacin
Aspirin
Benzydamine
Bromfenac
Celecoxib
Dexibuprofen
Dexketoprofen
Diclofenac
Diflunisal
Etodolac
Etoricoxib
Fenbufen
Fenoprofen
Flurbiprofen
Ibuprofen
Indomethacin
Ketoprofen
Ketorolac
Meclofenamate
Mefenamic Acid
Meloxicam
Metamizole
Methyl salicylate
Nabumetone
Naproxen
Nepafenac
Nimesulide
Oxaprozin
Phenylbutazone
Piroxicam
Pranoprofen
Rofecoxib
Salsalate
Sulindac
Tenoxicam
Tolmetin
Valdecoxib

Nucleoside analog reverse transcriptase inhibitor
Abacavir
Bictegravir/Emtricitabine/Tenofovir Alafenamide
Cobicistat/Elvitegravir/Emtricitabine/Tenofovir Alafenamide
Cobicistat/Elvitegravir/Emtricitabine/Tenofovir Disoproxil
Didanosine
Emtricitabine

Emtricitabine/Rilpivirine/ Tenofovir Alafenamide
Lamivudine
Stavudine
Telbivudine
Tenofovir Disoproxil
Zalcitabine
Zidovudine

Oligonucleotide
Defibrotide

Opiate agonist
Codeine
Heroin
Hydrocodone
Hydromorphone
Loperamide
Meperidine
Methadone
Morphine
Nalbuphine
Oxycodone
Oxymorphone
Pentazocine
Propoxyphene
Sufentanil
Tramadol

Phosphodiesterase inhibitor
Apremilast
Avanafil
Cilostazol
Inamrinone
Milrinone
Roflumilast
Sildenafil
Tadalafil
Vardenafil

Programmed death receptor-1 (PD-1) inhibitor
Nivolumab
Pembrolizumab

Prostaglandin
Alprostadil
Dinoprostone
Iloprost
Treprostinil
Unoprostone

Prostaglandin analog
Bimatoprost
Gemeprost
Latanoprost
Tafluprost
Travoprost

Proton pump inhibitor (PPI)
Dexlansoprazole
Esomeprazole
Lansoprazole
Omeprazole
Pantoprazole
Rabeprazole

Retinoid
Acitretin
Adapalene
Alitretinoin
Bexarotene
Clindamycin/Tretinoin
Isotretinoin
Tretinoin

Selective estrogen receptor modulator (SERM)
Chlorotrianisene
Clomiphene
Ospemifene
Raloxifene
Tamoxifen
Tibolone
Toremifene

Selective serotonin reuptake inhibitor (SSRI)
Citalopram
Escitalopram
Fluoxetine
Fluvoxamine
Paroxetine Hydrochloride
Paroxetine Mesylate
Sertraline

Serotonin
Buspirone
Sibutramine

serotonin receptor agonist
Almotriptan
Eletriptan
Frovatriptan
Lorcaserin
Rizatriptan
Sumatriptan
Vortioxetine
Zolmitriptan

serotonin receptor antagonist
Naratriptan
Vortioxetine

serotonin reuptake inhibitor
Duloxetine
Trazodone
Vortioxetine

serotonin type 3 receptor antagonist
Alosetron
Dolasetron
Granisetron
Netupitant & Palonosetron
Ondansetron
Palonosetron

serotonin type 4 receptor agonist
Tegaserod

serotonin-norepinephrine reuptake inhibitor
Desvenlafaxine
Levomilnacipran
Venlafaxine
Vilazodone

Statin
Atorvastatin
Fluvastatin
Lovastatin
Pitavastatin
Pravastatin
Rosuvastatin
Simvastatin

Sulfonylurea
Acetohexamide
Chlorpropamide
Gliclazide
Glimepiride
Glipizide
Glyburide
Tolazamide
Tolazoline
Tolbutamide

Topoisomerase 1 inhibitor
Irinotecan
Topotecan

Topoisomerase 2 inhibitor
Etoposide
Teniposide

Trace element
Arsenic
Selenium
Sulfites
Zinc

Tyrosine kinase inhibitor
Afatinib
Axitinib
Bosutinib
Brigatinib
Cabozantinib
Ceritinib
Crizotinib
Dasatinib
Erlotinib
Gefitinib
Imatinib
Lapatinib
Leflunomide
Lenvatinib
Nilotinib
Nintedanib
Pazopanib
Ponatinib
Regorafenib
Sorafenib
Sunitinib
Vandetanib

Vaccine
Anthrax Vaccine
BCG Vaccine
Cholera Vaccine
Diphtheria Antitoxin
Hemophilus B Vaccine
Hepatitis A Vaccine
Hepatitis B Vaccine
Human Papillomavirus (HPV) Vaccine
Human Papillomavirus Vaccine (Bivalent)
Inactivated Polio Vaccine
Influenza Vaccine
Japanese Encephalitis Vaccine
Measles, Mumps & Rubella (MMR) Virus Vaccine
Meningococcal Group B Vaccine
Meningococcal Groups C & Y & Haemophilus B Tetanus Toxoid Conjugate Vaccine
Pandemic Influenza Vaccine (H1N1)
Pneumococcal Vaccine
Sipuleucel-T
Smallpox Vaccine
Typhoid Vaccine
Varicella Vaccine
Yellow Fever Vaccine
Zoster Vaccine

Vasodilator
Ambrisentan
Amyl Nitrite
Astragalus Root
Benazepril
Bosentan
Captopril
Cilazapril
Diazoxide
Enalapril
Fosinopril
Hydralazine
Iloprost
Isosorbide Dinitrate
Isosorbide Mononitrate
Minoxidil
Nesiritide
Nitroglycerin
Nitroprusside
Prenylamine
Quinapril
Ramipril
Trandolapril

peripheral
Cilostazol
Papaverine
Pentoxifylline
Peppermint

Vitamin
Ascorbic Acid
Beta-Carotene
Cyanocobalamin
Ergocalciferol
Folic Acid
Niacin
Niacinamide
Pantothenic Acid
Phytonadione
Pyridoxine
Riboflavin
Thiamine
Vitamin A
Vitamin E

Vitamin D receptor agonist
Dihydrotachysterol
Doxercalciferol
Paricalcitol

Xanthine alkaloid
Aminophylline
Caffeine
Green Tea
Pentoxifylline

Table 1 – Reported genetic associations with cutaneous adverse drug reactions

Felix L. Chan[1], Neil H. Shear[2], Roni P. Dodiuk-Gad[2,3,4]

[1]Mississauga Academy of Medicine, Faculty of Medicine, University of Toronto, Mississauga, ON, Canada
[2]Division of Dermatology, Department of Medicine, Sunnybrook Health Sciences Centre, University of Toronto, Toronto, ON, Canada
[3]The Ruth and Bruce Rappaport Faculty of Medicine, Technion Institute of Technology, Israel
[4]Department of Dermatology, Emek Medical Centre, Israel

Allele	Reaction	Ethnic population	Sensitivity (%)	Specificity (%)	PPV	NPV	Est.	Ref.
ANTIBIOTICS / ANTI-INFLAMMATORY								
Dapsone								
HLA-B*13:01	DRESS	Chinese	85.5-90	85.7-93.1	7.8	99.8		[1–4]
HLA-B*13:01	DRESS	Thai						[4,5]
HLA-B*13:01	SJS/TEN	Thai						[4,5]
ANTIBIOTICS, SULFONAMIDES								
Sulfamethoxazole								
HLA-A*29	SJS/TEN	Caucasian/European						[6]
HLA-A*30	FDE	Turkish						[7]
HLA-A*30-B*13-C*06	FDE	Turkish						[7]
HLA-B*12	SJS/TEN	Caucasian/European						[6]
HLA-B*38	SJS/TEN	Caucasian/European						[8]
HLA-DR*07	SJS/TEN	Caucasian/European						[6]
ANTICONVULSANTS								
Carbamazepine								
HLA-A*24:02	SJS/TEN	Chinese (Han)						[9]
HLA-A*31	DRESS	Japanese						[10]
HLA-A*31	EM	Japanese						[10]
HLA-A*31	MPE	Japanese						[10]
HLA-A*31	SJS/TEN	Japanese						[10]
HLA-A*31:01	DRESS	Caucasian/European	70	96.1	0.89	99.98		[11,12]
HLA-A*31:01	DRESS	Chinese (Han)	50	95.8	0.59	99.97		[12,13]
HLA-A*31:01	DRESS	Japanese	60.7	87.5			A	[14]
HLA-A*31:01	DRESS	Korean						[15]
HLA-A*31:01	MPE	Caucasian/European						[11]
HLA-A*31:01	MPE	Chinese (Han)						[13,16]
HLA-A*31:01	SJS/TEN	Caucasian/European						[11,17]
HLA-A*31:01	SJS/TEN	Chinese (Han)						[17]
HLA-A*31:01	SJS/TEN	Japanese	60.7	87.5			A	[14,17]
HLA-A*31:01	SJS/TEN	Korean						[17]
HLA-B*15:02	MPE	Thai						[18]

Allele	Reaction	Ethnic population	Sensitivity (%)	Specificity (%)	PPV	NPV	Est.	Ref.
HLA-B*15:02	SJS/TEN	Chinese						[19]
HLA-B*15:02	SJS/TEN	Chinese (Han)	72.2-100	86.3-95.8	3.4-9	92-100		[9,12,13,17,20–28]
HLA-B*15:02	SJS/TEN	Indian						[29]
HLA-B*15:02	SJS/TEN	Korean						[22]
HLA-B*15:02	SJS/TEN	Malaysian	96	88	1.8	100	B	[17,19,22]
HLA-B*15:02	SJS/TEN	Thai	88.1-100	75-88.1	1.92	99.96		[18,22,30–32]
HLA-B*15:11	SJS/TEN	Chinese (Han)						[9,33]
HLA-B*15:11	SJS/TEN	Japanese						[33]
HLA-B*15:11	SJS/TEN	Korean						[33]
HLA-B*15:11	SJS/TEN	Thai						[33]
HLA-B*15:11	SJS/TEN	Vietnamese						[33]
HLA-B*15:21	SJS/TEN	Thai						[18]
HLA-B*51:01	DRESS	Chinese (Han)						[13]
HLA-B*51:01	MPE	Chinese (Han)						[13]
HLA-B*58:01	DRESS	Thai						[18]
HLA-B*58:01	MPE	Thai						[18]
HLA-DRB1*14:05	MPE	Chinese (Han)						[34]
Lamotrigine								
HLA-A*02:07	DRESS	Thai						[35]
HLA-A*02:07	MPE	Thai						[35]
HLA-A*02:07	SJS/TEN	Thai						[35]
HLA-A*24:02 / HLA-C*01:02	MPE	Korean						[36]
HLA-A*30:01	MPE	Chinese (Han)						[34]
HLA-A*31:01	DRESS	Korean						[37]
HLA-A*31:01	SJS/TEN	Korean						[37]
HLA-A*33:03	MPE	Thai						[35]
HLA-A*68:01	DRESS	Caucasian/European						[38]
HLA-A*68:01	SJS/TEN	Caucasian/European						[38]
HLA-B*13:02	MPE	Chinese (Han)						[34]
HLA-B*15:02	DRESS	Thai						[35]
HLA-B*15:02	MPE	Thai						[35]
HLA-B*15:02	SJS/TEN	Chinese (Han)	29.4	89.7				[21,25,39]
HLA-B*15:02	SJS/TEN	Thai						[35]
HLA-B*38	SJS/TEN	Caucasian/European						[8]
HLA-B*44:03	MPE	Thai						[35]

Allele	Reaction	Ethnic population	Sensitivity (%)	Specificity (%)	PPV	NPV	Est.	Ref.
HLA-B*58:01	DRESS	Caucasian/European						[38]
HLA-B*58:01	SJS/TEN	Caucasian/European						[38]
HLA-C*07:18	DRESS	Caucasian/European						[38]
HLA-C*07:18	SJS/TEN	Caucasian/European						[38]
HLA-DQB1*06:09	DRESS	Caucasian/European						[38]
HLA-DQB1*06:09	SJS/TEN	Caucasian/European						[38]
HLA-DRB1*13:01	DRESS	Caucasian/European						[38]
HLA-DRB1*13:01	SJS/TEN	Caucasian/European						[38]
Oxcarbazepine								
HLA-B*15:02	MPE	Chinese (Han)						[40]
HLA-B*15:02	SJS/TEN	Chinese (Han)						[16]
HLA-B*38:02	MPE	Chinese (Han)						[41]
Phenobarbital								
CYP2C19*2	DRESS	Thai						[42]
CYP2C19*2	SJS/TEN	Thai						[42]
HLA-B*51:01	SJS/TEN	Japanese						[43]
Phenytoin								
CYP2C9*3	DRESS	Chinese (Han)						[44]
CYP2C9*3	DRESS	Japanese						[44]
CYP2C9*3	DRESS	Malaysian						[44]
CYP2C9*3	SJS/TEN	Chinese (Han)						[44]
CYP2C9*3	SJS/TEN	Japanese						[44]
CYP2C9*3	SJS/TEN	Malaysian						[44]
CYP2C9*3	SJS/TEN	Thai						[45]
HLA-B*13:01	SJS/TEN	Chinese (Han)						[16]
HLA-B*15:02	SJS/TEN	Chinese (Han)	36.6	87.2				[16,21,25]
HLA-B*15:02	SJS/TEN	Malaysian						[46]
HLA-B*15:02	SJS/TEN	Thai						[30]
HLA-B*15:13	DRESS	Malaysian						[46]
HLA-B*15:13	SJS/TEN	Malaysian	53.8	90.6				[46]
HLA-B*56:02	SJS/TEN	Thai						[45]
HLA-C*08:01	SJS/TEN	Chinese (Han)						[16]
HLA-DRB1*16:02	SJS/TEN	Chinese (Han)						[16]
Zonisamide								
HLA-A*02:07	SJS/TEN	Japanese						[43]
				ANTIRETROVIRALS				
Nevirapine								
CYP2B6 T983C	SJS/TEN	African (Malawian, Ugandan)						[47]

Allele	Reaction	Ethnic population	Sensitivity (%)	Specificity (%)	PPV	NPV	Est.	Ref.
CYP2B6 T983C	SJS/TEN	African (Mozambique)						[48]
HLA-C*04	DRESS	Chinese (Han)						[49]
HLA-C*04	SJS/TEN	African (Malawian)			2.6	99.2		[50]
HLA-C*04:01 (rs5010528)	SJS/TEN	African (Sub-Saharan)			2.8	42.4		[51]
HLA-C*08	DRESS	Japanese						[52]
HLA-C*08:02 / HLA-B*14:02	DRESS	Caucasian/European (Sardinian)						[53]
HLA-DRB1*01:01	DRESS	Caucasian/European						[54]
ANTIRETROVIRALS, NUCLEOSIDE ANALOG REVERSE TRANSCRIPTASE INHIBITORS								
Abacavir								
HLA-B*57:01	HSS	African/African descent	100	99	50	100		[55,56]
HLA-B*57:01	HSS	Caucasian/European	100	96	66	100		[55–59]
HLA-B*57:01	HSS	Hispanic	26	99	96	60		[56]
CARBONIC ANHYDRASE INHIBITORS								
Acetazolamide								
HLA-B*59	SJS/TEN	Korean						[60]
Methazolamide								
HLA-B*59	SJS/TEN	Japanese						[61]
HLA-B*59:01	SJS/TEN	Chinese (Han)	87.5	63.3				[62]
HLA-B*59:01	SJS/TEN	Korean						[63]
HLA-C*01:02	SJS/TEN	Chinese (Han)						[62]
HLA-C*01:02	SJS/TEN	Korean						[63]
DISEASE-MODIFYING ANTIRHEUMATIC DRUGS (DMARDS)								
Sulfasalazine								
HLA-B*13:01	DRESS	Chinese (Han)	66.7	86.7				[64]
NON-STEROIDAL INFLAMMATORY (NSAID)								
Isoxicam, Piroxicam								
HLA-A*02	SJS/TEN	Caucasian/European						[6]
HLA-B*12	SJS/TEN	Caucasian/European						[6]
Oxicams								
HLA-B*73	SJS/TEN	Caucasian/European						[8]
XANTHINE OXIDASE INHIBITORS								
Allopurinol								
HLA-A*33:03	DRESS	Korean	88	73.7	0.8	99.96	A	[65]
HLA-A*33:03	SJS/TEN	Korean	88	73.7	0.8	99.96	A	[65]
HLA-B*58:01	DRESS	Caucasian/European						[66–68]

Allele	Reaction	Ethnic population	Sensitivity (%)	Specificity (%)	PPV	NPV	Est.	Ref.
HLA-B*58:01	DRESS	Caucasian/European (Portuguese)						[69]
HLA-B*58:01	DRESS	Chinese (Han)	84-100	82-88.9	1.6-5	100	A	[67,68,70–74]
HLA-B*58:01	DRESS	Japanese						[67,68]
HLA-B*58:01	DRESS	Korean	92-100	89.5-90.7	2.06	99.98	A	[65,67,68,75]
HLA-B*58:01	DRESS	Thai						[67,68]
HLA-B*58:01	MPE	Chinese (Han)	100	88.89			A	[67,68,71]
HLA-B*58:01	MPE	European						[67]
HLA-B*58:01	MPE	Japanese						[67]
HLA-B*58:01	MPE	Korean						[67]
HLA-B*58:01	MPE	Thai						[67]
HLA-B*58:01	SJS/TEN	Asian, East						[66]
HLA-B*58:01	SJS/TEN	Asian, South						[66]
HLA-B*58:01	SJS/TEN	Caucasian/European	50-60			95	B	[8,67,68,76, 77]
HLA-B*58:01	SJS/TEN	Caucasian/European (Portuguese)						[69]
HLA-B*58:01	SJS/TEN	Caucasian/European (Sardinian)						[78]
HLA-B*58:01	SJS/TEN	Chinese (Han)	84-100	82-88.89	1.6-5	100	A	[67,68,70–74,76,77]
HLA-B*58:01	SJS/TEN	Japanese	50-60			99	B	[67,68,76, 77,79]
HLA-B*58:01	SJS/TEN	Korean	92-100	89.5-90.7	2.06	99.98	A	[65,67,68, 75,76]
HLA-B*58:01	SJS/TEN	Thai	100	87	1.52	100		[67,68,76,80]
HLA-C*03:02	DRESS	Korean	92	87.7	1.77	99.98	A	[65]
HLA-C*03:02	SJS/TEN	Korean	92	87.7	1.77	99.98	A	[65]
rs2734583	DRESS	Thai	90.6	86.0			A	[81]
rs2734583	SJS/TEN	Thai	90.6	86.0			A	[81]
rs2734583 (*BAT1*); rs3094011 (*HCP5*); GA005234 (*MICC*)	SJS/TEN	Japanese						[82]
rs3099844	DRESS	Thai	90.6	85.0			A	[81]
rs3099844	SJS/TEN	Thai	90.6	85.0			A	[81]
rs9263726	DRESS	Thai	90.6	82.4			A	[81]
rs9263726	SJS/TEN	Thai	90.6	82.4			A	[81]
rs9263726 (*PSORS1C1*)	SJS/TEN	Japanese						[82]

A – Sensitivities, specificities, PPVs, and NPVs include or are based on data from studies which analyzed multiple cutaneous reactions (e.g. SJS/TEN, DRESS, MPE, EM, etc.) as a group. If data does not have a range, it is derived from a single study and should be considered as an estimate.

B – Sensitivities, specificities, PPVs, and NPVs include or are based on on data from studies which analyzed multiple ethnicities (e.g. Chinese (Han), Japanese, Korean, Thai, Caucasian/European, etc.) as a group. If data does not have a range, it is derived from a single study and should be considered as an estimate.
DRESS, drug reaction with eosinophilia and systemic symptoms; EM, erythema multiforme; FDE, fixed drug eruption; HSS, hypersensitivity syndrome; MPE, maculopapular exanthema; NPV, negative predictive value; PPV, positive predictive value; SJS/TEN, Stevens-Johnson syndrome/toxic epidermal necrolysis

The category DRESS includes drug-induced hypersensitivity syndrome (DIHS) and hypersensitivity syndrome (HSS), excluding abacavir HSS.

References

1. Wang H, Yan L, Zhang G, Chen X, Yang J, Li M, *et al*. Association between HLA-B*1301 and Dapsone-Induced Hypersensitivity Reactions among Leprosy Patients in China. *J. Invest. Dermatol*. 2013;**133**(11):2642–4.
2. Zhang F-R, Liu H, Irwanto A, Fu X-A, Li Y, Yu G-Q, *et al*. *HLA-B*13:01* and the Dapsone Hypersensitivity Syndrome. *N. Engl. J. Med. [Internet]* 2013;**369**(17):1620–8. Available from: http://www.nejm.org/doi/10.1056/NEJMoa1213096
3. Chen WT, Wang CW, Lu CW, Chen CB, Lee HE, Hung SI, *et al*. The Function of HLA-B*13:01 Involved in the Pathomechanism of Dapsone-Induced Severe Cutaneous Adverse Reactions. *J. Invest. Dermatol*. The Authors; 2018;
4. Tangamornsuksan W, Lohitnavy M. Association between HLA-B*1301 and dapsone-induced cutaneous adverse drug reactions a systematic review and meta-analysis. *JAMA Dermatology* 2018;**154**(4):441–6.
5. Tempark T, Satapornpong P, Rerknimitr P, Nakkam N, Saksit N, Wattanakrai P, *et al*. Dapsone-induced severe cutaneous adverse drug reactions are strongly linked with HLA-B 13:01 allele in the Thai population. *Pharmacogenet. Genomics* 2017;**27**(12):429–37.
6. Roujeau JC, Huynh TN, Bracq C EA. Genetic susceptibility to toxic epidermal necrolysis. *Arch Dermatol*. 1987;**123**(9):1171–1173.
7. Özkaya-Bayazit E, Akar U. Fixed drug eruption induced by trimethoprim-sulfamethoxazole: Evidence for a link to HLA-A30 B13 Cw6 haplotype. *J. Am. Acad. Dermatol*. 2001;**45**(5):712–7.
8. Lonjou C, Borot N, Sekula P, Ledger N, Thomas L, Halevy S, *et al*. A European study of HLA-B in Stevens-Johnson syndrome and toxic epidermal necrolysis related to five high-risk drugs. *Pharmacogenet. Genomics* 2008;**18**(2):99–107.
9. Shi YW, Min FL, Qin B, Zou X, Liu XR, Gao MM, *et al*. Association between HLA and Stevens-Johnson Syndrome Induced by Carbamazepine in Southern Han Chinese: Genetic Markers besides B*1502? *Basic Clin. Pharmacol. Toxicol*. 2012;**111**(1):58–64.
10. Niihara H, Kakamu T, Fujita Y, Kaneko S, Morita E. HLA-A31 strongly associates with carbamazepine-induced adverse drug reactions but not with carbamazepine-induced lymphocyte proliferation in a Japanese population. *J. Dermatol*. 2012;**39**(7):594–601.
11. McCormack M, Alfirevic A, Bourgeois S, Farrell JJ, Kasperaviciute D, Carrington M, *et al*. HLA-A*3101 and Carbamazepine-Induced Hypersensitivity Reactions in Europeans. *N. Engl. J. Med. [Internet]* 2011 Mar 24;**364**(12):1134–43. Available from: http://www.nejm.org/doi/abs/10.1056/NEJMoa1013297
12. Genin E, Chen D-P, Hung S-I, Sekula P, Schumacher M, Chang P-Y, *et al*. HLA-A*31:01 and different types of carbamazepine-induced severe cutaneous adverse reactions: an international study and meta-analysis. *Pharmacogenomics J. [Internet]* 2014;**14**(3):281–8. Available from: http://www.nature.com/doifinder/10.1038/tpj.2013.40
13. Hsiao YH, Hui RCY, Wu T, Chang WC, Hsih MS, Yang CH, *et al*. Genotype-phenotype association between HLA and carbamazepine-induced hypersensitivity reactions: Strength and clinical correlations. *J. Dermatol. Sci. [Internet]* Japanese Society for Investigative Dermatology; 2014;**73**(2):101–9. Available from: http://dx.doi.org/10.1016/j.jdermsci.2013.10.003
14. Ozeki T, Mushiroda T, Yowang A, Takahashi A, Kubo M, Shirakata Y, *et al*. Genome-wide association study identifies HLA-A*3101 allele as a genetic risk factor for carbamazepine-induced cutaneous adverse drug reactions in Japanese population. *Hum. Mol. Genet*. 2011;**20**(5):1034–41.
15. Kim SH, Lee KW, Song WJ, Kim SH, Jee YK, Lee SM, *et al*. Carbamazepine-induced severe cutaneous adverse reactions and HLA genotypes in Koreans. *Epilepsy Res. [Internet]* Elsevier B.V.; 2011;**97**(1–2):190–7. Available from: http://dx.doi.org/10.1016/j.eplepsyres.2011.08.010
16. Hung S, Chung W, Liu Z, Chen C, Hsih M, Hui RC, *et al*. Common risk allele in aromatic antiepileptic-drug induced Stevens – Johnson syndrome and toxic epidermal necrolysis in Han Chinese. *Pharmacogenomics* 2010;**11**(3):349–56.
17. Yip VL, Marson AG, Jorgensen AL, Pirmohamed M, Alfirevic A. HLA genotype and carbamazepine-induced cutaneous adverse drug reactions: A systematic review. *Clin. Pharmacol. Ther*. 2012;**92**(6):757–65.
18. Sukasem C, Chaichan C, Nakkrut T, Satapornpong P, Jaruthamsophon K, Jantararoungtong T, *et al*. Association between HLA-B Alleles and Carbamazepine-Induced Maculopapular Exanthema and Severe Cutaneous Reactions in Thai Patients. *J. Immunol. Res*. 2018;**2018**.
19. Then S-M, Rani ZZM, Raymond AA, Ratnaningrum S, Jamal R. Frequency of the HLA-B*1502 allele contributing to carbamazepine-induced hypersensitivity reactions in a cohort of Malaysian epilepsy patients. *Asian Pacific J. allergy Immunol*. Thailand; 2011 Sep;**29**(3):290–3.
20. Zhang Y, Wang J, Zhao L-M, Peng W, Shen G-Q, Xue L, *et al*. Strong association between HLA-B*1502 and carbamazepine-induced Stevens-Johnson syndrome and toxic epidermal necrolysis in mainland Han Chinese patients. *Eur. J. Clin. Pharmacol. [Internet]* 2011;**67**(9):885–7. Available from: http://link.springer.com/10.1007/s00228-011-1009-4
21. Cheung Y-K, Cheng S-H, Chan EJM, Lo S V., Ng MHL, Kwan P. HLA-B alleles associated with severe cutaneous reactions to antiepileptic drugs in Han Chinese. *Epilepsia [Internet]* 2013;**54**(7):1307–14. Available from: http://doi.wiley.com/10.1111/epi.12217
22. Tangamornsuksan W, Chaiyakunapruk N, Somkrua R, Lohitnavy M, Tassaneeyakul W. Relationship Between the *HLA-B*1502* Allele and Carbamazepine-Induced Stevens-Johnson Syndrome and Toxic Epidermal Necrolysis. *JAMA Dermatology [Internet]* 2013;**149**(9):1025. Available from: http://archderm.jamanetwork.com/article.aspx?doi=10.1001/jamadermatol.2013.4114
23. Chung WH, Hung SI, Hong HS, Hsih MS, Yang LC, Ho HC, *et al*. A marker for Stevens-Johnson syndrome. *Nature* England; 2004 Apr;**428**(6982):486.
24. Hung S-I, Chung W-H, Jee S-H, Chen W-C, Chang Y-T, Lee W-R, *et al*. Genetic susceptibility to carbamazepine-induced cutaneous adverse drug reactions. *Pharmacogenet. Genomics [Internet]* 2006;**16**(4):297–306. Available from: http://content.wkhealth.com/linkback/openurl?sid=WKPTLP:landingpage&an=01213011-200604000-00008
25. Man CBL, Kwan P, Baum L, Yu E, Lau KM, Cheng ASH, *et al*. Association between HLA-B*1502 allele and antiepileptic drug-induced cutaneous reactions in Han Chinese. *Epilepsia* 2007;**48**(5):1015–8.
26. Wu XT, Hu FY, An DM, Yan B, Jiang X, Kwan P, *et al*. Association between carbamazepine-induced cutaneous adverse drug reactions and the HLA-B*1502 allele among patients in central China. *Epilepsy Behav*. 2010;**19**(3):405–8.

27. Chen P, Lin J-J, Lu C-S, Ong C-T, Hsieh PF, Yang C-C, *et al*. Carbamazepine-Induced Toxic Effects and HLA-B*1502 Screening in Taiwan. *N. Engl. J. Med. [Internet]* 2011;**364**(12):1126–33. Available from: http://www.nejm.org/doi/abs/10.1056/NEJMoa1009717
28. Wang Q, Zhou JQ, Zhou LM, Chen ZY, Fang ZY, Chen S Da, *et al*. Association between HLA-B*1502 allele and carbamazepine-induced severe cutaneous adverse reactions in Han people of southern China mainland. *Seizure [Internet]* BEA Trading Ltd; 2011;**20**(6):446–8. Available from: http://dx.doi.org/10.1016/j.seizure.2011.02.003
29. Mehta T, Prajapati L, Mittal B, Joshi C, Sheth J, Patel D, *et al*. Association of HLA-BFNx01502 allele and carbamazepine-induced Stevens-Johnson syndrome among Indians. *Indian J. Dermatol. Venereol. Leprol. [Internet]* 2009;**75**(6):579. Available from: http://www.ijdvl.com/text.asp? 2009/75/6/579/57718
30. Locharernkul C, Loplumlert J, Limotai C, Korkij W, Desudchit T, Tongkobpetch S, *et al*. Carbamazepine and phenytoin induced Stevens-Johnson syndrome is associated with HLA-B*1502 allele in Thai population. *Epilepsia* 2008;**49**(12):2087–91.
31. Tassaneeyakul W, Tiamkao S, Jantararoungtong T, Chen P, Lin SY, Chen WH, *et al*. Association between HLA-B*1502 and carbamazepine-induced severe cutaneous adverse drug reactions in a Thai population. *Epilepsia* 2010;**51**(5):926–30.
32. Kulkantrakorn K, Tassaneeyakul W, Tiamkao S, Jantararoungtong T, Prabmechai N, Vannaprasaht S, *et al*. HLA-B*1502 Strongly Predicts Carbamazepine-Induced Stevens-Johnson Syndrome and Toxic Epidermal Necrolysis in Thai Patients with Neuropathic Pain. *Pain Pract*. 2012;**12**(3):202–8.
33. Wang Q, Sun S, Xie M, Zhao K, Li X, Zhao Z. Association between the HLA-B alleles and carbamazepine-induced SJS/TEN: A meta-analysis. *Epilepsy Res*. Elsevier B.V.; 2017.
34. Li LJ, Hu FY, Wu XT, An DM, Yan B, Zhou D. Predictive markers for carbamazepine and lamotrigine-induced maculopapular exanthema in Han Chinese. *Epilepsy Res. [Internet]* Elsevier B.V.; 2013;**106**(1–2):296–300. Available from: http://dx.doi.org/10.1016/j.eplepsyres.2013.05.004
35. Koomdee N, Pratoomwun J, Jantararoungtong T, Theeramoke V, Tassaneeyakul W, Klaewsongkram J, *et al*. Association of HLA-A and HLA-B alleles with lamotrigine-induced cutaneous adverse drug reactions in the Thai population. *Front. Pharmacol*. 2017;**8**(NOV):1–7.
36. Moon J, Park HK, Chu K, Sunwoo JS, Byun JI, Lim JA, *et al*. The HLA-A 2402/Cw 0102 haplotype is associated with lamotrigine-induced maculopapular eruption in the Korean population. *Epilepsia* 2015;**56**(10):e161–7.
37. Kim B-K, Jung J-W, Kim T-B, Chang Y-S, Park H-S, Moon J, *et al*. HLA-A*31:01 and lamotrigine-induced severe cutaneous adverse drug reactions in a Korean population. *Ann. Allergy. Asthma Immunol*. United States; 2017 May;**118**(5):629–30.
38. Kazeem GR, Cox C, Aponte J, Messenheimer J, Brazell C, Nelsen AC, *et al*. High-resolution HLA genotyping and severe cutaneous adverse reactions in lamotrigine-treated patients. *Pharmacogenet. Genomics* 2009;**19**(9):661–5.
39. Zeng T, Long YS, Min FL, Liao WP, Shi YW. Association of HLA-B*1502 allele with lamotrigine-induced Stevens-Johnson syndrome and toxic epidermal necrolysis in Han Chinese subjects: A meta-analysis. *Int. J. Dermatol*. 2015;**54**(4):488–93.
40. Hu FY, Wu XT, An DM, Yan B, Stefan H, Zhou D. Pilot association study of oxcarbazepine-induced mild cutaneous adverse reactions with HLA-B*1502 allele in Chinese Han population. *Seizure [Internet]* BEA Trading Ltd; 2011;**20**(2):160–2. Available from: http://dx.doi.org/10.1016/j.seizure.2010.11.014
41. Lv YD, Min FL, Liao WP, He N, Zeng T, Ma DH, *et al*. The association between oxcarbazepine-induced maculopapular eruption and HLA-B alleles in a Northern Han Chinese population. *BMC Neurol*. 2013;**13**.
42. Manuyakorn W, Siripool K, Kamchaisatian W, Pakakasama S, Visudtibhan A, Vilaiyuk S, *et al*. Phenobarbital-induced severe cutaneous adverse drug reactions are associated with CYP2C19*2 in Thai children. *Pediatr. Allergy Immunol*. 2013;**24**(3):299–303.
43. Kaniwa N, Sugiyama E, Saito Y, Kurose K, Maekawa K, Hasegawa R, *et al*. Specific HLA types are associated with antiepileptic drug-induced Stevens-Johnson syndrome and toxic epidermal necrolysis in Japanese subjects. *Pharmacogenomics* England; 2013 Nov;**14**(15):1821–31.
44. Chung W-H, Chang W-C, Lee Y-S, Wu Y-Y, Yang C-H, Ho H-C, *et al*. Genetic Variants Associated With Phenytoin-Related Severe Cutaneous Adverse Reactions. *Jama [Internet]* 2014;**312**(5):525. Available from: http://jama.jamanetwork.com/article.aspx?doi=10.1001/jama.2014.7859
45. Tassaneeyakul W, Prabmeechai N, Sukasem C, Kongpan T, Konyoung P, Chumworathayi P, *et al*. Associations between HLA class i and cytochrome P450 2C9 genetic polymorphisms and phenytoin-related severe cutaneous adverse reactions in a Thai population. *Pharmacogenet. Genomics* 2016;**26**(5):225–34.
46. Chang CC, Ng CC, Too CL, Choon SE, Lee CK, Chung WH, *et al*. Association of HLA-B 15:13 and HLA-B 15:02 with phenytoin-induced severe cutaneous adverse reactions in a Malay population. *Pharmacogenomics J*. 2017;**17**(2):170–3.
47. Carr DF, Chaponda M, Castro EMC, Jorgensen AL, Khoo S, Van Oosterhout JJ, et *al*. CYP2B6 c.983T>C polymorphism is associated with nevirapine hypersensitivity in Malawian and Ugandan HIV populations. *J. Antimicrob. Chemother.* 2014;**69**(12):3329–34.
48. Ciccacci C, Di Fusco D, Marazzi MC, Zimba I, Erba F, Novelli G, *et al*. Association between CYP2B6 polymorphisms and Nevirapine-induced SJS/TEN: A pharmacogenetics study. *Eur. J. Clin. Pharmacol*. 2013;**69**(11):1909–16.
49. Gao S, Gui X, Liang K, Liu Z, Hu J, Dong B. HLA-Dependent Hypersensitivity Reaction to Nevirapine in Chinese Han HIV-Infected Patients. *AIDS Res. Hum. Retroviruses [Internet]* 2012;**28**(6):540–3. Available from: http://online.liebertpub.com/doi/abs/10.1089/aid.2011.0107
50. Carr DF, Chaponda M, Jorgensen AL, Castro EC, Van Oosterhout JJ, Khoo SH, et *al*. Association of human leukocyte antigen alleles and nevirapine hypersensitivity in a Malawian HIV-infected population. *Clin. Infect. Dis*. 2013;**56**(9):1330–9.
51. Carr DF, Bourgeois S, Chaponda M, Takeshita LY, Morris AP, Cornejo Castro EM, et *al*. Genome-wide association study of nevirapine hypersensitivity in a sub-Saharan African HIV-infected population. *J. Antimicrob. Chemother.* 2017;**72**(4):1152–62.
52. Gatanaga H, Yazaki H, Tanuma J, Honda M, Genka I, Teruya K, *et al*. HLA-Cw8 primarily associated with hypersensitivity to nevirapine. *AIDS* England; 2007. p. 264–5.
53. Littera R, Carcassi C, Masala A, Piano P, Serra P, Ortu F, *et al*. HLA-dependent hypersensitivity to nevirapine in Sardinian HIV patients. *Aids* 2006;**20**(12):1621–6.
54. Martin AM, Nolan D, James I, Cameron P, Keller J, Moore C, *et al*. Predisposition to nevirapine hypersensitivity associated with HLA-DRB1*0101 and abrogated by low CD4 T-cell counts. *AIDS* England; 2005 Jan;**19**(1):97–9.
55. Saag M, Balu R, Phillips E, Brachman P, Martorell C, Burman W, et *al*. High Sensitivity of Human Leukocyte Antigen–B*5701 as a Marker for Immunologically Confirmed Abacavir Hypersensitivity in White and Black Patients. *Clin. Infect. Dis. [Internet]* 2008;**46**(7):1111–8. Available from: https://academic.oup.com/cid/article-lookup/doi/10.1086/529382
56. Sousa-Pinto B, Pinto-Ramos J, Correia C, Gonçalves-Costa G, Gomes L, Gil-Mata S, *et al*. Pharmacogenetics of abacavir hypersensitivity: A systematic review and meta-analysis of the association with HLA-B 57:01. *J. Allergy Clin. Immunol*. 2015;**136**(4):1092–1094e3.
57. Hetherington S, Hughes AR, Mosteller M, Shortino D, Baker KL, Spreen W, et *al*. Genetic variations in HLA-B region and hypersensitivity reactions to abacavir Tamoxifen for breast cancer among hysterectomised women For personal use . Only reproduce with permission from The Lancet Publishing Group . 2002;**359**:1121–2.
58. Mallal S, Nolan D, Witt C, Masel G, Martin AM, Moore C, *et al*. Association between presence of HLA-B*5701, HLA-DR7, and HLA-DQ3 and hypersensitivity to HIV-1 reverse-transcriptase inhibitor abacavir. *Lancet (London, England)* England; 2002 Mar;**359**(9308):727–32.

59. Mallal S, Phillips E, Carosi G, Molina J-M, Workman C, Toma iè J, *et al.* HLA-B*5701 Screening for Hypersensitivity to Abacavir. *N. Engl. J. Med.* 2009;

60. Her Y, Kil MS, Park JH, Kim CW, Kim SS. Stevens-Johnson syndrome induced by acetazolamide. *J. Dermatol. [Internet]* 2011;**38**(3):272–5. Available from: http://www.ncbi.nlm.nih.gov/pubmed/21342230

61. Shirato S, Kagaya F, Suzuki Y, Jouhou S. Stevens-Johnson syndrome induced by methazolamide treatment. *Arch. Ophthalmol.* United States; 1997 Apr;**115**(4):550–3.

62. Yang F, Xuan J, Chen J, Zhong H, Luo H, Zhou P, *et al.* HLA-B 59:01: A marker for Stevens-Johnson syndrome/toxic epidermal necrolysis caused by methazolamide in Han Chinese. *Pharmacogenomics J.* 2016;**16**(1):83–7.

63. Kim S-H, Kim M, Lee KW, Kim S-H, Kang H-R, Park H-W, *et al.* HLA-B*5901 is strongly associated with methazolamide-induced Stevens-Johnson syndrome/toxic epidermal necrolysis. *Pharmacogenomics* England; 2010 Jun;**11**(6):879–84.

64. Yang F, Gu B, Zhang L, Xuan J, Luo H, Zhou P, *et al.* HLA-B*13:01 is associated with salazosulfapyridine-induced drug rash with eosinophilia and systemic symptoms in Chinese Han population. *Pharmacogenomics* England; 2014 Aug;**15**(11):1461–9.

65. Kang HR, Jee YK, Kim YS, Lee CH, Jung JW, Kim SH, *et al.* Positive and negative associations of HLA class i alleles with allopurinol-induced SCARs in Koreans. *Pharmacogenet. Genomics* 2011;**21**(5):303–7.

66. Lee MH, Stocker SL, Anderson J, Phillips EJ, Nolan D, Williams KM, *et al.* Initiating allopurinol therapy: Do we need to know the patient's human leucocyte antigen status? *Intern. Med. J.* 2012;**42**(4):411–6.

67. Jarjour S, Barrette M, Normand V, Rouleau JL, Dubé MP, De Denus S. Genetic markers associated with cutaneous adverse drug reactions to allopurinol: A systematic review. *Pharmacogenomics* England; 2015;**16**(7):755–67.

68. Ng CY, Yeh YT, Wang CW, Hung SI, Yang CH, Chang YC, *et al.* Impact of the HLA-B'58:01 Allele and Renal Impairment on Allopurinol-Induced Cutaneous Adverse Reactions. *J. Invest. Dermatol.* The Authors; 2016;**136**(7):1373–81.

69. Gonçalo M, Coutinho I, Teixeira V, Gameiro AR, Brites MM, Nunes R, *et al.* HLA-B*58:01 is a risk factor for allopurinol-induced DRESS and Stevens-Johnson syndrome/toxic epidermal necrolysis in a Portuguese population. *Br. J. Dermatol.* 2013;**169**(3):660–5.

70. Hung S-I, Chung W-H, Liou L-B, Chu C-C, Lin M, Huang H-P, *et al.* HLA-B*5801 allele as a genetic marker for severe cutaneous adverse reactions caused by allopurinol. *Proc. Natl. Acad. Sci. [Internet]* 2005;**102**(11):4134–9. Available from: http://www.pnas.org/cgi/doi/10.1073/pnas.0409500102

71. Cao ZH, Wei ZY, Zhu QY, Zhang JY, Yang L, Qin SY, *et al.* HLA-B*58:01 allele is associated with augmented risk for both mild and severe cutaneous adverse reactions induced by allopurinol in Han Chinese. *Pharmacogenomics* 2012;**13**(10):1193–201.

72. Chiu MLS, Hu M, Ng MHL, Yeung CK, Chan JCY, Chang MM, *et al.* Association between HLA-B*58:01 allele and severe cutaneous adverse reactions with allopurinol in Han Chinese in Hong Kong. *Br. J. Dermatol.* 2012;**167**(1):44–9.

73. Cheng L, Xiong Y, Qin CZ, Zhang W, Chen XP, Li J, *et al.* HLA-B 58:01 is strongly associated with allopurinol-induced severe cutaneous adverse reactions in Han Chinese patients: A multicentre retrospective case-control clinical study. *Br. J. Dermatol.* 2015;**173**(2):555–8.

74. Ko TM, Tsai CY, Chen SY, Chen KS, Yu KH, Chu CS, *et al.* Use of HLA-B 58:01 genotyping to prevent allopurinol induced severe cutaneous adverse reactions in Taiwan: National prospective cohort study. *BMJ [Internet]* 2015;**351**:h4848. Available from: http://www.bmj.com/lookup/doi/10.1136/bmj.h4848

75. Jung JW, Song WJ, Kim YS, Joo KW, Lee KW, Kim SH, *et al.* HLA-B58 can help the clinical decision on starting allopurinol in patients with chronic renal insufficiency. *Nephrol. Dial. Transplant.* 2011;**26**(11):3567–72.

76. Somkrua R, Eickman EE, Saokaew S, Lohitnavy M, Chaiyakunapruk N. Association of HLA-B*5801 allele and allopurinol-induced stevens johnson syndrome and toxic epidermal necrolysis: A systematic review and meta-analysis. *BMC Med. Genet. [Internet]* BioMed Central Ltd; 2011;**12**(1):118. Available from: http://www.biomedcentral.com/1471-2350/12/118

77. Yu K-H, Yu C-Y, Fang Y-F. Diagnostic utility of HLA-B*5801 screening in severe allopurinol hypersensitivity syndrome: an updated systematic review and meta-analysis. *Int. J. Rheum. Dis.* England; 2017 Sep;**20**(9):1057–71.

78. Atzori L, Pinna AL, Mantovani L, Ferreli C, Pau M, Mulargia M, *et al.* Cutaneous adverse drug reactions to allopurinol: 10 year observational survey of the dermatology department - Cagliari University (Italy). *J. Eur. Acad. Dermatology Venereol.* 2012;**26**(11):1424–30.

79. Kaniwa N, Saito Y, Aihara M, Matsunaga K, Tohkin M, Kurose K, *et al.* HLA-B locus in Japanese patients with anti-epileptics and allopurinol-related Stevens-Johnson syndrome and toxic epidermal necrolysis. *Pharmacogenomics* England; 2008 Nov;**9**(11):1617–22.

80. Tassaneeyakul W, Jantararoungtong T, Chen P, Lin P-Y, Tiamkao S, Khunarkornsiri U, *et al.* Strong association between HLA-B*5801 and allopurinol-induced Stevens–Johnson syndrome and toxic epidermal necrolysis in a Thai population. *Pharmacogenet. Genomics [Internet]* 2009;**19**(9):704–9. Available from: http://content.wkhealth.com/linkback/openurl?sid=WKPTLP:landingpage&an=01213011-200909000-00006

81. Saksit N, Nakkam N, Konyoung P, Khunarkornsiri U, Tasseneeyakul W, Chumworathayi P, *et al.* Comparison between the HLA-B 58: 01 Allele and Single-Nucleotide Polymorphisms in Chromosome 6 for Prediction of Allopurinol-Induced Severe Cutaneous Adverse Reactions. *J. Immunol. Res.* 2017;**2017**.

82. Tohkin M, Kaniwa N, Saito Y, Sugiyama E, Kurose K, Nishikawa J, *et al.* A whole-genome association study of major determinants for allopurinol-related Stevens-Johnson syndrome and toxic epidermal necrolysis in Japanese patients. *Pharmacogenomics J. [Internet]* Nature Publishing Group; 2013;**13**(1):60–9. Available from: http://dx.doi.org/10.1038/tpj.2011.41

Table 2 – Recommendations from various sources regarding genetic screening to prevent cutaneous adverse drug reactions

Felix L. Chan[1], Neil H. Shear[2], Roni P. Dodiuk-Gad[2,3,4]
[1]Mississauga Academy of Medicine, Faculty of Medicine, University of Toronto, Mississauga, ON, Canada
[2]Division of Dermatology, Department of Medicine, Sunnybrook Health Sciences Centre, University of Toronto, Toronto, ON, Canada
[3]The Ruth and Bruce Rappaport Faculty of Medicine, Technion Institute of Technology, Israel
[4]Department of Dermatology, Emek Medical Centre, Israel

Allele	Source	Recommendations	Ref.
		ANTICONVULSANTS	
Carbamazepine			
HLA-A*31:01	Canadian Pharmacogenomics Network for Drug Safety (2014)	Genotype patients of all ancestries prior to prescribing carbamazepine. Use alternative medications if HLA-A*31:01-positive, accounting for cross-reactivities.	[1]
	Clinical Pharmacogenetics Implementation Consortium (2018)	Avoid use of carbamazepine in HLA-A*31:01-positive patients.	[2]
HLA-B*15:02	U.S. Food and Drug Administration (2007)	Genotype patients of Asian descent prior to prescribing carbamazepine. HLA-B*15:02-positive patients should not be treated with carbamazepine or anticonvulsants associated with SJS/TEN unless the expected benefit outweighs risks.	[3,4]
	Health Canada (2008)	Consider genotyping genetically at-risk patients.	[5]
	Hong Kong (2008)	Genotyping prior to prescribing carbamazepine was implemented as a system-wide mandatory policy in 2008. Carbamazepine is to be prescribed only for HLA-B*15:02-negative patients.	[6,7]
	UK Medicines and Healthcare Products Regulatory Agency (2008)	Genotype patients of Han Chinese, Hong Kong Chinese, or Thai ethnic origin prior to prescribing carbamazepine. HLA-B*15:02-positive patients should not be prescribed carbamazepine unless benefits clearly outweigh risks.	[8]
	Taiwan National Health Insurance (2010)	Since 2010, national health insurance covers expense of genotyping for HLA-B*15:02 in patients initiating carbamazepine.	[9]
	Singapore Health Sciences Authority (2013)	Genotyping prior to prescribing carbamazepine is considered the standard of care. Avoid use of carbamazepine in carriers of HLA-B*15:02. A 75% subsidy for genotype testing is provided for low-income patients.	[10,11]
	Clinical Pharmacogenetics Implementation Consortium (2014, 2018)	Avoid using carbamazepine in HLA-B*15:02-positive patients.	[2,12]
	Canadian Pharmacogenomics Network for Drug Safety (2014)	Genotype patients from ethnic populations where HLA-B*15:02 is prevalent (e.g. Chinese, Thai, Indian, Malay, Filipino, Indonesian) prior to prescribing carbamazepine. Use alternative medications if HLA-B*15:02 positive, accounting for cross-reactivities.	[1]
	Thailand (2014)	Since 2014, genotyping for HLA-B*15:02 covered under national universal healthcare system.	[13]
Oxcarbazepine			
HLA-B*15:02	Clinical Pharmacogenetics Implementation Consortium (2018)	Avoid use of oxcarbazepine in HLA-B*15:02-positive patients.	[2]
Phenytoin			
CYP2C9*3	Clinical Pharmacogenetics Implementation Consortium (2014)	Consider dose reduction and adjustment of maintenance doses of phenytoin according to therapeutic drug monitoring for CY2C9*2 and CYP2C9*3-positive patients.	[14]
HLA-B*15:02	Singapore Health Sciences Authority (2013)	Avoid prescribing if patient is HLA-B*15:02-positive.	[10]

Allele	Source	Recommendations	Ref.
ANTIRETROVIRALS, NUCLEOSIDE ANALOG REVERSE TRANSCRIPTASE INHIBITORS			
Abacavir			
HLA-B*57:01	U.S. Food and Drug Administration (2008)	All patients should be screened for HLA-B*57:01 prior to initiating abacavir. Avoid use of abacavir in HLA-B*57:01-positive patients.	[15]
	European Medicines Agency (2009)	Genotype patients irrespective of ethnic origin prior to initiating abacavir. Avoid use of abacavir in HLA-B*57:01-positive patients.	[16]
	Clinical Pharmacogenetics Implementation Consortium (2012)	Genotype all abacavir-naive patients before initiating abacavir. Avoid use of abacavir if patient is HLA-B*57:01-positive or has signs/symptoms of hypersensitivity.	[17]
XANTHINE OXIDASE INHIBITORS			
Allopurinol			
HLA-B*58:01	Clinical Pharmacogenetics Implementation Consortium (2012, 2016)	Avoid prescribing allopurinol to HLA-B*58:01-positive patients.	[18,19]
	2012 American College of Rheumatology Guidelines for Management of Gout (2012)	Consider genotyping subpopulations at higher risk for severe AHS (e.g. Koreans with stage 3 or worse CKD, and all Han Chinese and Thai patients) prior to prescribing allopurinol.	[20]
	Taiwan Department of Health (2012)	Genotype for HLA-B*58:01 prior to use of allopurinol.	[19]
	Singapore Health Sciences Authority (2016)	Consider genotyping patients with pre-existing risk factors for allopurinol-induced SCAR such as renal impairment.	[21]
	Hong Kong Department of Health Drug Office (2016)	Consider genotyping patients with pre-existing risk factors for allopurinol-induced SCAR such as renal impairment.	[22]

References

1. Amstutz U, Shear NH, Rieder MJ, Hwang S, Fung V, Nakamura H, et al. Recommendations for HLA-B15:02 and HLA-A31:01 genetic testing to reduce the risk of carbamazepine-induced hypersensitivity reactions. *Epilepsia* 2014;**55**(4):496–506.
2. Phillips EJ, Sukasem C, Whirl-Carrillo M, Müller DJ, Dunnenberger HM, Chantratita W, et al. Clinical Pharmacogenetics Implementation Consortium Guideline for HLA Genotype and Use of Carbamazepine and Oxcarbazepine: 2017 Update. *Clin. Pharmacol. Ther.* 2018;**103**(4):574–81.
3. U.S. FDA. Information for Healthcare Professionals: Dangerous or Even Fatal Skin Reactions – Carbamazepine (marketed as Carbatrol, Equetro, Tegretol, and generics) [Internet]. 2007. p. 1–4. Available from: https://www.fda.gov/Drugs/DrugSafety/PostmarketDrugSafetyInformationforPatientsandProviders/ucm124718.htm
4. Ferrell PBJ, McLeod HL. Carbamazepine, HLA-B*1502 and risk of Stevens-Johnson syndrome and toxic epidermal necrolysis: US FDA recommendations. *Pharmacogenomics* England; 2008 Oct;**9**(10):1543–6.
5. Health Canada. Health Canada Endorsed Important Safety Information on TEGRETOL (carbamazepine) [Internet]. *Recalls Saf. Alerts* 2008 [cited 2018 Jan 1]. Available from: http://www.healthycanadians.gc.ca/recall-alert-rappel-avis/hc-sc/2008/14522a-eng.php
6. The Chinese University of Hong Kong. Re: Genetic testing prior to prescription of carbamazepine [Internet]. 2008. Available from: www.cuhk.edu.hk/med/paf/ups/HLA-B-1502.pdf%0A
7. Chen Z, Liew D. Effects of a HLA-B * 15 : 02 screening policy on antiepileptic drug use and severe skin reactions. *Neurology* 2014;**83**:1–8.
8. UK MHRA. Carbamazepine: genetic testing recommended in some Asian populations. *Drug Saf.* Updat. 2008;**1**(9):2–4.
9. Phillips EJ, Chung W, Mockenhaupt M, Roujeau J, Mallal SA, Bs MB. NIH Public Access. *J. Allergy Clin. Immunol.* 2011;**127**:60–6.
10. Singapore HSA. HLA-B*1502 genotype testing: Towards safer use of carbamazepine [Internet]. 2016. Available from: http://www.hsa.gov.sg/content/hsa/en/Health_Products_Regulation/Safety_Information_and_Product_Recalls/Product_Safety_Alerts/2013/hla-b_1502_genotype.html
11. Sung C. Genetically-mediated Serious Skin Rash: Singapore Health Sciences Authority Experience. *Res. Dir. Genet. Stevens-Johnson Syndr. Epidermal Necrolysis [Internet]* Bethesda, MD: NIH National Human Genome Research Institute; 2015. p. 1–20. Available from: https://www.genome.gov/27560487/research-directions-in-geneticallymediated-stevensjohnson-syndrometoxic-epidermal-necrolysis/
12. Leckband SG, Kelsoe JR, Dunnenberger HM, Jr ALG, Tran E, Berger R, et al. Guideline Summary: Clinical Pharmacogenetics Implementation Consortium guidelines for HLA-B genotype and abacavir dosing. [Clinical Pharmacogenetics Implementation Consortium]. *info@guideline.gov (NGC) [Internet]* 2013;(February):1–5. Available from: http://guideline.gov/content.aspx?f=rss&id=39535
13. Chantratita W. Implementing Genomics in Clinical Practice/Healthcare: Thailand. *Res. Dir. Genet. Stevens-Johnson Syndr. Epidermal Necrolysis [Internet]* Bethesda, MD: NIH National Human Genome Research Institute; 2015. p. 1–47. Available from: https://www.genome.gov/27560487/research-directions-in-geneticallymediated-stevensjohnson-syndrometoxic-epidermal-necrolysis/
14. Caudle KE, Rettie AE, Smith LH, Mintzer S, Lee MTM, Klein TE. Clinical Pharmacogenetics Implementation Consortium (CPIC) Guidelines for CYP2C9 and HLA-B Genotype and Phenytoin Dosing. 2014;**96**(5):1–28.
15. U.S. FDA. Labels for NDA 020977 (Ziagen) [Internet]. 2018. p. 1–32. Available from: https://www.fda.gov/Drugs/ScienceResearch/ucm572698.htm
16. European Medicines Agency. EPAR summary for the public: Ziagen (Abacavir) [Internet]. 2016 [cited 2018 Jan 1]. p. 1–3. Available from: http://www.ema.europa.eu/ema/index.jsp%3Fcurl%3Dpages/medicines/human/medicines/000252/human_med_001179.jsp%26mid%3DWC0b01ac058001d124

17. Martin MA, Klein TE, Dong BJ, Pirmohamed M, Haas DW, Kroetz DL. Clinical Pharmacogenetics Implementation Consortium Guidelines for HLA-B Genotype and Abacavir Dosing. *Clin. Pharmacol. Ther.* 2012. p. 734–8.
18. Saito Y, Stamp LK, Caudle KE, Hershfield MS, McDonagh EM, Callaghan JT, et al. CPIC: Clinical Pharmacogenetics Implementation Consortium of the Pharmacogenomics Research Network. *Clin. Pharmacol. Ther.* 2016;**99**(1):36–7.
19. Hershfield MS, Callaghan JT, Tassaneeyakul W, Mushiroda T, Thorn CF, Klein TE, et al. Clinical pharmacogenetics implementation consortium guidelines for human leukocyte antigen-b genotype and allopurinol dosing. *Clin. Pharmacol. Ther.* 2013;**93**(2):153–8.
20. Khanna D, Fitzgerald JD, Khanna PP, Bae S, Singh MK, Neogi T, et al. 2012 American college of rheumatology guidelines for management of gout. part 1: Systematic nonpharmacologic and pharmacologic therapeutic approaches to hyperuricemia. *Arthritis Care Res.* 2012;**64**(10):1431–46.
21. Singapore HSA. Allopurinol-induced serious cutaneous adverse reactions and the role of genotyping [Internet]. 2016. Available from: http://www.hsa.gov.sg/content/hsa/en/Health_Products_Regulation/Safety_Information_and_Product_Recalls/Product_Safety_Alerts/2016/allopurinol-inducedseriouscutaneousadversereactionsandtheroleofg.html
22. Hong Kong Department of Health. Singapore: Allopurinol-induced serious cutaneous adverse reactions and the role of genotyping [Internet]. *Saf. Alerts Prod. Recalls* 2016 [cited 2018 Jan 1]. Available from: https://www.drugoffice.gov.hk/eps/news/showNews/newsTitle/pharmaceutical_trade/2016-09-22/en/26856.html

Concordance of Synonyms and Trade Names with Generic Drug Names

Synonym/Trade name	Generic
13-cis-retinoic acid	isotretinoin
3,4-methylenedioxymethamphetamine	MDMA
3TC	lamivudine
4-aminopyridine	dalfampridine
4-demethoxydaunorubicin	idarubicin
4-DMDR	idarubicin
5-aminosalicylic acid	mesalamine
5-ASA	mesalamine
5-aza-2'-deoxycytidine	decitabine
5-fluorouracil	fluorouracil
6-mercaptopurine	mercaptopurine
6-MP	mercaptopurine

A

Synonym/Trade name	Generic
A-Acido	tretinoin
A-Gram	amoxicillin
Abaprim	trimethoprim
Abbocillin	penicillin V
Abelcet	amphotericin B
Aberal	tretinoin
Aberela	tretinoin
Abetol	labetalol
Abilify	aripiprazole
Abilitat	aripiprazole
Abraxane	paclitaxel
Abrifam	rifampin
Abstral	fentanyl
Ac-De	dactinomycin
Acaren	vitamin A
Accolate	zafirlukast
AccuNeb	albuterol
Accupril	quinapril
Accuprin	quinapril
Accupro	quinapril
Accuretic	hydrochlorothiazide, quinapril
Accutane	isotretinoin
Acenor-M	fosinopril
Acenorm	captopril
Aceon	perindopril
Acepril	captopril
Acerbon	lisinopril
Acertil	perindopril
Acetazolam	acetazolamide
acetylsalicylic acid	aspirin
Acfol	folic acid
aciclovir	acyclovir
Acid A Vit	tretinoin
Acidulated phosphate fluoride	fluorides
Acifur	acyclovir
Acimox	amoxicillin
Aciphex	rabeprazole
Aclasta	zoledronate
Aclinda	clindamycin
Acnamino	minocycline
Acnavit	tretinoin
Acon	vitamin A
Act-3	ibuprofen
ACT	dactinomycin
Acta	tretinoin
Actacode	codeine
Actemra	tocilizumab
ActHIB	Hemophilus B vaccine
Actigall	ursodiol
Actilyse	alteplase
Actimmune	interferon gamma
actinomycin-D	dactinomycin
Actiprofen	ibuprofen
Actiq	fentanyl
Activacin	alteplase
Activase	alteplase
Actonel	risedronate
Actos	pioglitazone
Acuitel	quinapril
Acular	ketorolac
Acupril	quinapril
ACV	acyclovir
Acyclo-V	acyclovir
acycloguanosine	acyclovir
Acyvir	acyclovir
Aczone	dapsone
Adalat	nifedipine
Adalate	nifedipine
Adant	hyaluronic acid
Adapin	doxepin
Adaquin	quinine
Adasuve	loxapine
Adcetris	brentuximab vedotin
Adcirca	tadalafil
Adderall	dextroamphetamine
Addyi	flibanserin
Adempas	riociguat
Adenic	adenosine
Adeno-Jec	adenosine
Adenocard	adenosine
Adenocur	adenosine
Adenoject	adenosine
Adenoscan	adenosine
Adiblastine	doxorubicin
Adipex-P	phentermine
Adipine	nifedipine
Adlyxin	lixisenatide

Adocor	captopril
Adofen	fluoxetine
Adoxa	doxycycline
Adrecar	adenosine
Adrenaclick	epinephrine
Adrenalin	epinephrine
adrenaline	epinephrine
Adriablastine	doxorubicin
Adriacin	doxorubicin
Adriamycin	doxorubicin
Adriblatina	doxorubicin
Adsorbocarbine	pilocarpine
Adumbran	oxazepam
Adursall	ursodiol
Advantan	methylprednisolone
Advicor	lovastatin, niacin
Advil	ibuprofen
Aerolate	aminophylline
Aerovent	aldesleukin
Afaxin	vitamin A
Afinitor	everolimus
Aflodac	sulindac
Aflorix	miconazole
Afluria	influenza vaccine
Afstyla	antihemophilic factor
Aggrenox	aspirin, dipyridamole
Agilect	rasagiline
Agisolvan	acetylcysteine
Agrippal	influenza vaccine
AH3 N	hydroxyzine
Airol	tretinoin
AK-Chlor	chloramphenicol
Ak-Zol	acetazolamide
Akarpine	pilocarpine
Akatinol	memantine
Aknemin	minocycline
Aknemycin Plus	tretinoin
AKTob Ophthalmic	tobramycin
Akynzeo	netupitant & palonosetron
AL-R	chlorpheniramine
Alapril	lisinopril
Alavert	loratadine
Albenza	albendazole
Albiotic	lincomycin
Alcloxidine	chlorhexidine
Alcomicinx	gentamicin
Aldactazide	hydrochlorothiazide, spironolactone
Aldactone	spironolactone
Aldara	imiquimod
Aldoclor	methyldopa
Aldocumar	warfarin
Aldomet	methyldopa
Aldopur	spironolactone
Aldoril	hydrochlorothiazide, methyldopa
Alecensa	alectinib
Alendronic acid	alendronate
Alepsal	phenobarbital
Alercet	cetirizine
Alerid	cetirizine
Alertec	modafinil
Alesse	oral contraceptives
Aleve	naproxen
Alexan	cytarabine
Alfadil	doxazosin
Alfatil	cefaclor
Alferon N	interferon alfa
Alfotax	cefotaxime
Algocetil	sulindac
Alimta	pemetrexed
Alinia	nitazoxanide
Aliqopa	copanlisib
Alka-Seltzer	aspirin
Alkeran	melphalan
all-trans-retinoic acid	tretinoin
Allegra-D	pseudoephedrine
Allegra	fexofenadine
Allegron	nortriptyline
Aller-Chlor	chlorpheniramine
Allerdryl	diphenhydramine
Allerglobuline	immune globulin IV
Allermax	diphenhydramine
Allermin	diphenhydramine
Alli	orlistat
Allo 300	allopurinol
Allo-Puren	allopurinol
Alloprin	allopurinol
Allvoran	diclofenac
Almarytm	flecainide
Almatol	spironolactone
Almodan	amoxicillin
Almogran	almotriptan
Aloid	miconazole
Alopexy	minoxidil
Alora	estradiol
Aloxi	palonosetron
alpha tocopherol	vitamin E
Alphagan P	brimonidine
Alphapress	hydralazine
Alprim	trimethoprim
Alprox	alprazolam
Alquingel	tretinoin
Alrheumat	ketoprofen
Alrheumun	ketoprofen
Alsuma	sumatriptan
Altace	ramipril
Alten	tretinoin
Alti-Diltiazem	diltiazem
Alti-Doxepin	doxepin
Alti-Ipratropium	ipratropium
Alti-Minocycline	minocycline
Alti-MPA	medroxyprogesterone
Alti-Trazodone	trazodone
Altocor	lovastatin
Altoprev	lovastatin
Alunbrig	brigatinib
Aluvira	lopinavir
Alveolex	acetylcysteine
Amaryl	glimepiride
Ambi	hydroquinone
Ambien	zolpidem
AmBisome	amphotericin B
Amdepin	amlodipine

Ameluz	aminolevulinic acid
amethopterin	methotrexate
Ametycine	mitomycin
Amfipen	ampicillin
Amias	candesartan
Amicacina	amikacin
Amicasil	amikacin
Amikacin sulfate	amikacin
Amikal	amiloride
Amikan	amikacin
Amineurin	amitriptyline
Aminophyllin	aminophylline
Amipress	labetalol
Amisalen	procainamide
Amitiza	lubiprostone
Amjevita	adalimumab
Amlodin	amlodipine
Amlogard	amlodipine
Amlopin	amlodipine
Amlor	amlodipine
Amnesteem	isotretinoin
Amodex	amoxicillin
Amodopa	methyldopa
Amoxan	amoxapine
Amoxapine	amoxapine
Amoxil	amoxicillin
amoxycillin	amoxicillin
Amphocin	amphotericin B
Amphotec	amphotericin B
Ampicin	ampicillin
Amprace	enalapril
Ampyra	dalfampridine
Amrix	cyclobenzaprine
Amterene	triamterene
Amuno	indomethacin
Amycil	mebendazole
Anacin-3	acetaminophen
Anacin	aspirin
Anacobin	cyanocobalamin
Anafranil Retard	clomipramine
Anafranil	clomipramine
Anamantle HC	lidocaine
Anamorph	morphine
Anaprox	naproxen
Anaspaz	hyoscyamine
Anatensol	fluphenazine
Anaxanil	hydroxyzine
Anco	ibuprofen
Andro LA	testosterone
Androcur	cyproterone
Androderm	testosterone
AndroGel	testosterone
Android	methyltestosterone
Andronaq	testosterone
Androral	methyltestosterone
Andrumin	dimenhydrinate
Anectine	succinylcholine
Aneol	ketoprofen
Anergan	promethazine
Anestacon	lidocaine
Angilol	propranolol
Angiomax	bivalirudin
Angioverin	papaverine
Anitrim	co-trimoxazole
Annovera	segesterone acetate
Ansaid	flurbiprofen
Ansail	buspirone
Antabus	disulfiram
Antabuse	disulfiram
Antagonil	nicardipine
Antaxone	naltrexone
antegren	natalizumab
Anten	doxepin
Antepsin	sucralfate
Antiflog	piroxicam
Antilak	etodolac
Antilirium	physostigmine
Antipressan	atenolol
Antra	omeprazole
Antrex	leucovorin
Apacef	cefotetan
APAP	acetaminophen
Apatef	cefotetan
Apdormin	hydralazine
Apekumarol	dicumarol
Aphtiria	lindane
Apidra	insulin glulisine
APO-Alpraz	alprazolam
Apo-Amoxi	amoxicillin
Apo-Atenol	atenolol
Apo-Bisoprolol	bisoprolol
Apo-Bromocriptine	bromocriptine
Apo-Buspirone	buspirone
APO-Capto	captopril
Apo-Carbamazepine	carbamazepine
Apo-Cefaclor	cefaclor
Apo-Cephalex	cephalexin
Apo-Cimetidine	cimetidine
Apo-Clomipramine	clomipramine
Apo-Diclo	diclofenac
Apo-Doxy	doxycycline
Apo-Enalapril	enalapril
Apo-Ethambutol	ethambutol
Apo-Famotidine	famotidine
Apo-Fenofibrate	fenofibrate
Apo-Fluoxetine	fluoxetine
Apo-Fluphenazine	fluphenazine
Apo-Flurbiprofen	flurbiprofen
Apo-Fluvoxamine	fluvoxamine
Apo-Folic	folic acid
Apo-Furosemide	furosemide
Apo-Gain	minoxidil
Apo-Hydro	hydrochlorothiazide
Apo-Imipramine	imipramine
Apo-Indomethacin	indomethacin
Apo-ISDN	isosorbide dinitrate
Apo-Lorazepam	lorazepam
Apo-Lovastatin	lovastatin
Apo-Metformin	metformin
Apo-Metronidazole	metronidazole
Apo-Minocycline	minocycline
Apo-Nadolol	nadolol

Apo-Nicotinamide	niacin
Apo-Nifed	nifedipine
Apo-Nortriptyline	nortriptyline
Apo-Oxazepam	oxazepam
Apo-Pen	penicillin V
Apo-Pentoxifylline	pentoxifylline
Apo-Perphenazine	perphenazine
Apo-Piroxicam	piroxicam
Apo-Propranolol	propranolol
Apo-Ranitidine	ranitidine
Apo-Selegiline	selegiline
Apo-Sulfatrim	co-trimoxazole
APO-Sulin	sulindac
Apo-Tamox	tamoxifen
Apo-Temazepam	temazepam
Apo-Tetra	tetracycline
Apo-Trimip	trimipramine
APO-Verap	verapamil
Apocard	flecainide
Aponal	doxepin
Apranax	naproxen
Apresazide	hydralazine
Apresolin	hydralazine
Apresoline	hydralazine
Aprical	nifedipine
Aprovel	irbesartan
Apsifen	ibuprofen
Apsolol	propranolol
Aptiom	eslicarbazepine
Aptivus	tipranavir
Aquachloral	chloral hydrate
Aquamid	hyaluronic acid
Aquamycetin	chloramphenicol
Aquarius	ketoconazole
Aquasol A	vitamin A
Aquasol E	vitamin E
ara-C	cytarabine
Arabitin	cytarabine
Arace	cytarabine
Aracytine	cytarabine
Aragest 5	medroxyprogesterone
Aralen	chloroquine
Aranesp	darbepoetin alfa
Aratac	amiodarone
Arcapta Neohaler	indacaterol
Aredia	pamidronate
Arestin	minocycline
Argesic-SA	salsalate
Aricept Evess	donepezil
Aricept	donepezil
Arimidex	anastrozole
Aristada	aripiprazole
Arixtra	fondaparinux
Aromasin	exemestane
Arovit	vitamin A
Arpamyl LP	verapamil
Arsacol	ursodiol
Artal	pentoxifylline
Artamin	penicillamine
Artecoll	collagen (bovine)
Artha-G	salsalate

Arthaxan	nabumetone
Arthro-Aid	glucosamine
Arthrocine	sulindac
Arthrotec	diclofenac, misoprostol
Artifar	carisoprodol
ARTZ	hyaluronic acid
Arythmol	propafenone
Arzerra	ofatumumab
ASA	aspirin
Asacol	mesalamine
Asacolitin	mesalamine
Asclera	polidocanol
Ascriptin	aspirin
Asendis	amoxapine
Aside	etoposide
Asig	quinapril
Asmaven	albuterol
Aspergum	aspirin
Aspro	aspirin
ASS	aspirin
Assival	diazepam
AsthmaHaler	epinephrine
Astramorph	morphine
Atabrine	quinacrine
Atacand HCT	hydrochlorothiazide
Atacand	candesartan
Ataline	terbutaline
Atarax	hydroxyzine
AteHexal	atenolol
Atelvia	risedronate
Atem	aldesleukin
Atendol	atenolol
Atisuril	allopurinol, salsalate
Ativan	lorazepam
Atosil	promethazine
ATP	adenosine
ATRA	tretinoin
Atragen	tretinoin
Atrenta	artesunate
Atreol	carbamazepine
Atridox	doxycycline
Atripla	efavirenz, emtricitabine, tenofovir disoproxil
Atronase	aldesleukin
Atropine Martinet	atropine sulfate
Atropt	atropine sulfate
Atrovent	ipratropium
Atruline	sertraline
Aubagio	teriflunomide
Audazol	omeprazole
Augmentin	amoxicillin
Austedo	deutetrabenazine
Autologen	collagen (bovine)
Auvi-Q	epinephrine
Avage	tazarotene
Avalide	hydrochlorothiazide, irbesartan
Avandamet	metformin, rosiglitazone
Avandaryl	glimepiride, rosiglitazone
Avandia	rosiglitazone
Avapro	irbesartan
Avastin	bevacizumab
Avaxim	hepatitis A vaccine

Avelox	moxifloxacin
Aventyl	nortriptyline
Aviane	oral contraceptives
Avinza	morphine
Avipur	vitamin A
Avirax	acyclovir
Avita	tretinoin
Avitcid	tretinoin
Avitene	collagen (bovine)
Avitin	vitamin A
Avitoin	tretinoin
Avloclor	chloroquine
Avlosulfon	dapsone
Avodart	dutasteride
Avonex	interferon beta
Avycaz	ceftazidime & avibactam
Axerol	vitamin A
Axert	almotriptan
Axoban	ranitidine
Aygestin	progestins
Azamedac	azathioprine
Azamune	azathioprine
Azantac	ranitidine
Azasan	azathioprine
AzaSite	azithromycin
Azatrilem	azathioprine
Azenil	azithromycin
azidothymidine	zidovudine
Azilect	rasagiline
Azitrocin	azithromycin
Azitromax	azithromycin
Azol	danazol
Azopt	brinzolamide
AZT	zidovudine
Azucimet	cimetidine
Azulfidine	sulfasalazine
Azupamil	verapamil
Azupentat	pentoxifylline
Azutranquil	oxazepam
Azzalure	botulinum toxin (A & B)

B

Bacille Calmette-Guerin	BCG vaccine
Baclofen	baclofen
Baclon	baclofen
Baclosal	baclofen
Bacomine	hydrocodone
Bactelan	co-trimoxazole
Bactin	trimethoprim
Bactocill	oxacillin
Bactocin	ofloxacin
Bactoscrub	chlorhexidine
BactoShield	chlorhexidine
Bactrim	co-trimoxazole, sulfamethoxazole, trimethoprim
Baklofen	baclofen
BAL5788	ceftobiprole
Balcoran	vancomycin
Balminil	dextromethorphan, pseudoephedrine
Ban-Tuss HC	hydrocodone
Banophen	diphenhydramine
Bantenol	mebendazole
Baraclude	entecavir
Barazan	norfloxacin
Barbilixir	phenobarbital
Barbita	phenobarbital
Barbital	phenobarbital
Barclyd	clonidine
Basaglar	insulin glargine
Basoquin	amodiaquine
Batrizol	co-trimoxazole
Bavencio	avelumab
Baxan	cefadroxil
Baxdela	delafloxacin
Baxo	piroxicam
Baygam	immune globulin IV
Baymycard	nisoldipine
BB	clindamycin
Beatryl	fentanyl
Becenun	carmustine
Beconase AQ	beclomethasone
Begrivac	influenza vaccine
Behapront	phentermine
Beleodaq	belinostat
Belladenal	atropine sulfate
Bellafill	collagen (bovine)
Bellergal-S	atropine sulfate
Beloc-Zoc	metoprolol
Belsomra	suvorexant
Belviq	lorcaserin
Benadryl	diphenhydramine, pseudoephedrine
Benahist	diphenhydramine
Benaxima	cefotaxime
Benaxona	ceftriaxone
Bencid	probenecid
Benecid	probenecid
Benhex Cream	lindane
Benicar	olmesartan
Benuryl	probenecid
Benylin	dextromethorphan, diphenhydramine
Benzaclin	clindamycin
Benzamin	cyclobenzaprine
Benzylpenicillin	penicillin G
Beriglobulin	immune globulin IV
Berkatens	verapamil
Berlthyrox	levothyroxine
Berubigen	cyanocobalamin
Bespar	buspirone
Beta-Adalat	atenolol
Beta-Cardone	sotalol
Betades	sotalol
Betaferon	interferon beta
Betaloc	metoprolol
Betanis	mirabegron
Betapace	sotalol
Betasept	chlorhexidine
Betaseron	interferon beta
Betazok	metoprolol
Betolvex	cyanocobalamin
Betoptic [Ophthalmic]	betaxolol
Betoptic S	betaxolol
Betoptima	betaxolol
Bevyxxa	betrixaban

Bex	aspirin
Bexsero	meningococcal group B vaccine
BG-12	dimethyl fumarate
Bi-Profenid	ketoprofen
Biaxin HP	clarithromycin
Biaxin	clarithromycin
Bicide	lindane
Biclin	amikacin
BiCNU	carmustine
Bidocef	cefadroxil
Biklin	amikacin
Biliepar	ursodiol
Bilim	tamoxifen
Biltricide	praziquantel
Bimaran	trazodone
Binocrit	epoetin alfa
Binosto	alendronate
Binotal	ampicillin
Bio E	vitamin E
Bio-Well	lindane
Biocet	cephalexin
Biocoryl	procainamide
Biofanal	nystatin
Biosint	cefotaxime
BioThrax	anthrax vaccine
Biozolene	fluconazole
Biron	buspirone
Bismatrol	bismuth
Bismuth Iodoform Paraffin Paste (BIPP)	bismuth
Bismuth subcitrate	bismuth
Bismuth subgallate	bismuth
Bismuth sucralfate	bismuth
Bleminol	allopurinol
Blenoxane	bleomycin
bleo	bleomycin
Bleocin	bleomycin
Bleomycine	bleomycin
Bleomycinum	bleomycin
Blephamide	prednisolone
Blincyto	blinatumomab
BLM	bleomycin
Blocan	cimetidine
Bobsule	hydroxyzine
Bocouture	botulinum toxin (A & B)
Bolutol	gemfibrozil
Bondronat	ibandronate
Boniva	ibandronate
Bonnox	promethazine
Bonzol	danazol
Botox	botulinum toxin (A & B)
Braftovi	encorafenib
Brek	loperamide
Brethine	terbutaline
Brevibloc	esmolol
Brevicon	oral contraceptives
Bricanyl	terbutaline
Bridion	sugammadex
Brilinta	ticagrelor
Brisdelle	paroxetine mesylate
Bristopen	oxacillin
Britiazem	diltiazem
BritLofex	lofexidine
Briviact	brivaracetam
Brocadopa	levodopa
Bromed	bromocriptine
Bromfed	pseudoephedrine
Broncho-Spray	albuterol
Bronitin	epinephrine
Bronkaid	epinephrine
Bronkodyl	aminophylline
Brothine	terbutaline
Brovana	arformoterol
Brufen	ibuprofen
Bucaril	terbutaline
Bufigen	nalbuphine
Busetal	disulfiram
Busirone	buspirone
BuSpar	buspirone
Bustab	buspirone
Butaline	terbutaline
Butibel	atropine sulfate
Bydureon	exenatide
Byetta	exenatide
Bystolic	nebivolol
Byvalson	nebivolol, valsartan

C

Caduet	amlodipine, atorvastatin
Calamine	zinc
Calan	verapamil
Calcicard	diltiazem
calcidiol	calcifediol
Calcidrine	codeine
Calcilat	nifedipine
Calcilean	heparin
Calcimar	calcitonin
Calciparin	heparin
calcipotriene	calcipotriol
Calm-X	dimenhydrinate
Calquence	acalabrutinib
Caltine	calcitonin
Calypsol	ketamine
Cambia	diclofenac
Camochin	amodiaquine
Camoquin	amodiaquine
Camoquinal	amodiaquine
Campath	alemtuzumab
Camptosar	irinotecan
Canasa	mesalamine
Cancidas	caspofungin
Candio-Hermal	nystatin
cannabis	marihuana
Caplenal	allopurinol
Capoten	captopril
Capozide	captopril, hydrochlorothiazide
Caprelsa	vandetanib
Caprilon	tranexamic acid
Caprin	aspirin, heparin
Captolane	captopril
Captoril	captopril
Carac	fluorouracil
Carace	lisinopril

Carafate	sucralfate
Carbatrol	carbamazepine
Carbex	selegiline
carbidopa	levodopa
Carbolith	lithium
Carbometyx	cabozantinib
Carboplat	carboplatin
Carbosap	anthrax vaccine
Carbosin	carboplatin
Carcinil	leuprolide
Cardem	celiprolol
Cardene	nicardipine
Cardicor	bisoprolol
Cardigox	digoxin
Cardine	quinidine
Cardiosteril	dopamine
Cardizem	diltiazem
Cardol	sotalol
Cardoxan	doxazosin
Cardoxin	dipyridamole
Cardular	doxazosin
Cardura	doxazosin
Carisoma	carisoprodol
Carmubris	carmustine
Cartia-XT	diltiazem
Casodex	bicalutamide
Cassadan	alprazolam
Cataflam	diclofenac
Catapres	clonidine
Catapresan	clonidine
Caved-S	bismuth
Caverject	alprostadil
CDDP	cisplatin
Cebenicol	chloramphenicol
Cebutid	flurbiprofen
CEC 500	cefaclor
Ceclor	cefaclor
Cedocard	isosorbide dinitrate
Cedrox	cefadroxil
Cefabiocin	cefaclor
cefalexin	cephalexin
Cefamox	cefadroxil
Cefaxim	cefotaxime
Cefaxona	ceftriaxone
Cefaxone	ceftriaxone
Ceforal	cephalexin
Cefotan	cefotetan
Cefotax	cefotaxime
Cefspan	cefixime
Ceftazim	ceftazidime
Ceftenon	cefotetan
Ceftin	cefuroxime
Cefuril	cefuroxime
Celebrex	celecoxib
Celectol	celiprolol
Celexa	citalopram
Celipres	celiprolol
Celipro	celiprolol
CellCept	mycophenolate
Cellmusin	estramustine
Celol	celiprolol
Celsentri	maraviroc
Celupan	naltrexone
Celvapan	pandemic influenza vaccine (H1N1)
Cemidon	isoniazid
Centedrin	methylphenidate
Cepan	cefotetan
Cepazine	cefuroxime
Cephoral	cefixime
Ceporex	cephalexin
Ceporexine	cephalexin
Ceptaz	ceftazidime
Cerdelga	eliglustat
Cerepax	temazepam
Certican	everolimus
Cerubidine	daunorubicin
Cervarix	human papillomavirus vaccine (bivalent)
Cervidel	dinoprostone
Cerviprime	dinoprostone
Cerviprost	dinoprostone
Cesamet	nabilone
Cetrine	cetirizine
Cetrotide	cetrorelix
Cezin	cetirizine
Champix	varenicline
Chantix	varenicline
Chemet	succimer
Cheracol-D	dextromethorphan
Cheracol	codeine
Chibro-Atropine	atropine sulfate
Chibroxin	norfloxacin
Chibroxine	norfloxacin
Chibroxol	norfloxacin
Chinine	quinine
Chitosamine	glucosamine
Chlo-Amine	chlorpheniramine
Chlor-Pro	chlorpheniramine
Chlor-Trimeton	chlorpheniramine
Chlor-Tripolon	chlorpheniramine
Chloractil	chlorpromazine
Chloraldurat	chloral hydrate
Chlorate	chlorpheniramine
Chlorazin	chlorpromazine
Chlorhexamed	chlorhexidine
Chloroptic	chloramphenicol
chlorphenamine	chlorpheniramine
Chlorpromanyl	chlorpromazine
Chlorquin	chloroquine
Chol-Less	cholestyramine
Cholacid	ursodiol
Cholbam	cholic acid
Choledyl	aminophylline
Cholestagel	colesevelam
Cholit-Ursan	ursodiol
Cholofalk	ursodiol
Chronovera	verapamil
Cialis	tadalafil
Cibacalcine	calcitonin
Cibace	benazepril
Cibacen	benazepril
Cibacene	benazepril
Ciclosporin	cyclosporine

Cidomycin	gentamicin
Ciflox	ciprofloxacin
Cillimicina	lincomycin
Cillimycin	lincomycin
Ciloxan Ophthalmic	ciprofloxacin
Cimedine	cimetidine
Cimehexal	cimetidine
Cimogal	ciprofloxacin
Cimzia	certolizumab
Cin-Quin	quinidine
Cinqair	reslizumab
Ciplox	ciprofloxacin
Cipramil	citalopram
Cipro	ciprofloxacin
Ciprobay Uro	ciprofloxacin
Cipromycin	ciprofloxacin
Ciproxin	ciprofloxacin
Cisplatyl	cisplatin
Cisticid	praziquantel
Citanest	prilocaine
Citax	immune globulin IV
Citosulfan	busulfan
Citrec	leucovorin
citrovorum factor	leucovorin
Ciuk	cimetidine
Civeran	loratadine
Clacine	clarithromycin
Claforan	cefotaxime
Clamoxyl	amoxicillin
Claragine	aspirin
Claratyne	loratadine
Claravis	isotretinoin
Clarinex	desloratadine
Clarith	clarithromycin
Claritin-D	loratadine
Claritin	loratadine
Claritine	loratadine
Clarus	isotretinoin
Classen	mercaptopurine
Clasynar	calcitonin
Claversal	mesalamine
Cleocin-T	clindamycin
Cleocin	clindamycin
Cleridium	dipyridamole
Clexane	enoxaparin
Climara	estradiol
Clindacin	clindamycin
Clindagel	clindamycin
Clindets	clindamycin
Clinofem	medroxyprogesterone
Clinoril	sulindac
Cloben	cyclobenzaprine
Clofen	baclofen
Clofranil	clomipramine
Clonex	clonazepam
Clont	metronidazole
Clopress	clomipramine
Closerin	cycloserine
Closerina	cycloserine
Closin	promethazine
Clothia	hydrochlorothiazide

Clozaril	clozapine
club drug	MDMA
Coartem	artemether/lumefantrine
Cobex	cyanocobalamin
Cobutolin	albuterol
Codamine	hydrocodone
Codicept	codeine
Codiforton	codeine
Colazal	balsalazide
Colazide	balsalazide
ColBenemid	colchicine
Colchiquim	colchicine
Colcrys	colchicine
Cold-Eeze	zinc
Coledos	ursodiol
Colestrol	cholestyramine
Colgout	colchicine
Colo-Fresh	bismuth
Colo-Pleon	sulfasalazine
Combivent	albuterol, ipratropium
Combivir	lamivudine, zidovudine
Cometriq	cabozantinib
Compazine	prochlorperazine
Complera	emtricitabine, tenofovir disoproxil
Compoz	diphenhydramine
Comtan	entacapone
Comtess	entacapone
Comvax	Hemophilus B vaccine, hepatitis B vaccine, influenza vaccine
Concerta	methylphenidate
Concor	bisoprolol
Consolan	nabumetone
Consupren	cyclosporine
Contalgin	morphine
Contergan	thalidomide
Contigen	collagen (bovine)
Contramal	tramadol
Contrave	naltrexone
Convon	terbutaline
Copaxone	glatiramer
Copegus	ribavirin
copolymer-1	glatiramer
Coracten	nifedipine
Coradur	isosorbide dinitrate
Corax	chlordiazepoxide
Corbionax	amiodarone
Cordarex	amiodarone
Cordarone X	amiodarone
Cordarone	amiodarone
Cordes VAS	tretinoin
Cordiax	celiprolol
Cordilox	verapamil
Coreg	carvedilol
Corflene	flecainide
Corgard	nadolol
Coric	lisinopril
Coricidin D	aspirin
Corifam	rifampin
Corlanor	ivabradine
Corogal	nifedipine
Coronarine	dipyridamole

Corophyllin	aminophylline
Corotrend	nifedipine
Coroxin	dipyridamole
Corsodyl	chlorhexidine
Cortastat	dexamethasone
Cortone	cortisone
Cortosporin	neomycin
Corvert	ibutilide
Corzide	nadolol
Cosentyx	secukinumab
Cosmegen Lyovac	dactinomycin
Cosmegen	dactinomycin
Cosopt	dorzolamide
Cotellic	cobimetinib
Cotempla	methylphenidate
Cotrim	co-trimoxazole
Coumadin	warfarin
Coumadine	warfarin
Covera-HS	verapamil
Coversum	perindopril
Coversyl	perindopril
Cozaar	losartan
CPM	cyclophosphamide
Cranoc	fluvastatin
Crasnitin	asparaginase
Cresemba	isavuconazonium sulfate
Crestor	rosuvastatin
Crixivan	indinavir
Cryocriptina	bromocriptine
Cryodoxin	sulfadoxine
Cryptaz	nitazoxanide
Crystamine	cyanocobalamin
Crystapen	penicillin G
Crysti-12	cyanocobalamin
CsA	cyclosporine
CTX	cyclophosphamide
Cubicin	daptomycin
Curantyl N	dipyridamole
Curretab	progestins
Cuvitru	immune globulin sc
Cuvposa	glycopyrrolate
CyA	cyclosporine
Cyanoject	cyanocobalamin
Cyben	cyclobenzaprine
Cycloblastin	cyclophosphamide
Cyclomen	danazol
Cyclomycin	cycloserine
Cyclorine	cycloserine
Cyclostin	cyclophosphamide
Cycosin	cycloserine
Cyklokapron	tranexamic acid
Cymbalta	duloxetine
Cynomel	liothyronine
Cyomin	cyanocobalamin
Cyramza	ramucirumab
Cystrin	oxybutynin
CYT	cyclophosphamide
Cytamen	cyanocobalamin
Cytarbel	cytarabine
Cytomel	liothyronine
Cytosar-U	cytarabine

Cytosar	cytarabine
Cytospaz	hyoscyamine
Cytotec	misoprostol
Cytoxan	cyclophosphamide

D

D-Amp	ampicillin
D-Penamine	penicillamine
D-Zol	danazol
D4T	stavudine
Dacatic	dacarbazine
Dacogen	decitabine
Dagan	nicardipine
Daipres	clonidine
Daklinza	daclatasvir
Daktarin	miconazole
Dalacin C	clindamycin
Dalacin	clindamycin
Dalacine	clindamycin
Daliresp	roflumilast
Dalisol	folic acid
Danocrine	danazol
Danol	danazol
Dantamacrin	dantrolene
Dantrium	dantrolene
Dantrolen	dantrolene
Daonil	glyburide
Dapa-tabs	indapamide
Dapatum D25	fluphenazine
Dapotum D	fluphenazine
Dapson-Fatol	dapsone
Dapson	dapsone
Daraprim	pyrimethamine
Darvocet-N	acetaminophen
Darvon Compound	aspirin
Darzalex	daratumumab
daunomycin	daunorubicin
DaunoXome	daunorubicin
Davedax	reboxetine
Davesol	lindane
Davitamon E	vitamin E
Daxas	roflumilast
Daypro	oxaprozin
Daytrana	methylphenidate
Dazamide	acetazolamide
DDAVP	desmopressin
ddC	zalcitabine
De-Nol	bismuth
Deca-Durabolin	nandrolone
Decadron	dexamethasone
Decentan	perphenazine
Deconsal	pseudoephedrine
Decrelip	gemfibrozil
Dedralen	doxazosin
Defanyl	amoxapine
Defiltran	acetazolamide
Defirin	desmopressin
Defitelio	defibrotide
Deflam	oxaprozin
Dehydrobenzperidol	droperidol
Delatest	testosterone

Delatestryl	testosterone
Delice	lindane
Delstrigo	doravirine/lamiduvine/tenofovir disoproxil
Delsym	dextromethorphan
Delta-Cortef	prednisolone
Delta-Lutin	progestins
Deltasone	prednisone
Deltazen	diltiazem
Delursan	ursodiol
Demadex	torsemide
Demerol	meperidine
Demolox	amoxapine
Demulen	oral contraceptives
Denan	simvastatin
Densul	methyldopa
Dentipatch	lidocaine
Denzapine	clozapine
Depacon	valproic acid
Depade	naltrexone
Depakene	valproic acid
Depakote	valproic acid
Depen	penicillamine
Depo-Provera	medroxyprogesterone
DepoCyt	cytarabine
Deprax	trazodone
deprenyl	selegiline
Derm A	tretinoin
DermaDeep	hyaluronic acid
DermaFlex	lidocaine
Dermairol	tretinoin
DermaLive	hyaluronic acid
Dermalogen	collagen (bovine)
Dermojuventus	tretinoin
Desconex	loxapine
Descovy	emtricitabine, tenofovir alafenamide
Deseril	methysergide
Desernil	methysergide
Deserril	methysergide
Deseryl	methysergide
Desferal	deferoxamine
Desferin	deferoxamine
Desirel	trazodone
Desmospray	desmopressin
Desocol	ursodiol
Desogen	oral contraceptives
Desoxil	ursodiol
Desoxyn	methamphetamine
Destolit	ursodiol
Desyrel	trazodone
Detensol	propranolol
Deticene	dacarbazine
Detimedac	dacarbazine
Detrol	tolterodine
Detulin	vitamin E
Deurcil	ursodiol
Devrom	bismuth
Dexacine	neomycin
Dexambutol	ethambutol
Dexamphetamine	dextroamphetamine
Dexamphetamini	dextroamphetamine
Dexedrine	dextroamphetamine
Dexilant	dexlansoprazole
Dexo	ursodiol
Dexone	dexamethasone
Dextrostat	dextroamphetamine
DHC-Continus	dihydrocodeine
Di-Hydran	phenytoin
Diabeta	glyburide
Diabex	metformin
Diacomit	stiripentol
Diaformin	metformin
Dialar	diazepam
Diamox	acetazolamide
Diapax	diazepam
Diar-Aid	loperamide
Diarr-Eze	loperamide
Diarrol	triamterene
Diarstop-L	loperamide
Diastat	diazepam
Diatracin	vancomycin
Diazemuls	diazepam
Diazid	isoniazid
Dibloc	carvedilol
Diblocin	doxazosin
Dibrondrin	diphenhydramine
DIC	dacarbazine
Dichlotride	hydrochlorothiazide
Dicolmax	diclofenac
Dicumarol	dicumarol
Dicumol	dicumarol
dideoxycytidine	zalcitabine
Didronate	etidronate
Didronel	etidronate
Differin	adapalene
Diflucan	fluconazole
Diformin	metformin
Difosfen	etidronate
Digacin	digoxin
Digoxine	digoxin
Dilacor XR	diltiazem
Dilanorm	celiprolol
Dilantin	phenytoin
Dilatrate-SR	isosorbide dinitrate
Dilatrend	carvedilol
Dilaudid-HP	hydromorphone
Dilaudid	hydromorphone
Dilocaine	lidocaine
Dilrene	diltiazem
Diltahexal	diltiazem
Diltia-XT	diltiazem
Dimetabs	dimenhydrinate
dimethyl (E) butenedioate	dimethyl fumarate
Diminex	phentermine
Dimitone	carvedilol
Dimodan	disopyramide
Dinol	etidronate
Diocarpine	pilocarpine
Diochloram	chloramphenicol
Diogent	gentamicin
Dionephrine	phenylephrine
Diotame	bismuth
Diovan HCT	hydrochlorothiazide, valsartan

Diovan	valsartan
Diphenylan	phenytoin
diphenylhydantoin	phenytoin
Diphos	etidronate
Dipridacot	dipyridamole
Diprivan	propofol
Diram	spironolactone
Dirythmin SA	disopyramide
Disalgesic	salsalate
Discoid	furosemide
Disonorm	disopyramide
Disprin	aspirin
Distaclor	cefaclor
Distamine	penicillamine
Distaval	thalidomide
Distocide	praziquantel
Ditropan	oxybutynin
Diu-Melsin	hydrochlorothiazide
Diuchlor H	hydrochlorothiazide
Diuramid	acetazolamide
Diuteren	triamterene
divalproex	valproic acid
Divigel	estradiol
Dixarit	clonidine
Dizac	diazepam
DMSA	succimer
DNR	daunorubicin
Dobetin	cyanocobalamin
Doblexan	piroxicam
Dolac	ketorolac
Dolantin	meperidine
Dolce	vitamin A
Dolestan	diphenhydramine
Dolestine	meperidine
Dolophine	methadone
Dolosal	meperidine
Dom-Baclofen	baclofen
Dom-Fluoxetine	fluoxetine
Domical	amitriptyline
Doneurin	doxepin
Donnagel	atropine sulfate
Donnamar	hyoscyamine
Donnatal	atropine sulfate
Donnazyme	atropine sulfate
Dopaflex	levodopa
Dopamet	methyldopa
Dopamin AWD	dopamine
Dopamin	dopamine
Doparl	levodopa
Dopastat	dopamine
Doptelet	avatrombopag
Dormicum	midazolam
Doryx	doxycycline
Dostinex	cabergoline
Dovonex	calcipotriol
Doxil	doxorubicin
Doximed	doxycycline
Doxy-100	doxycycline
Doxycin	doxycycline
Doxytec	doxycycline
Dozic	haloperidol
DPH	phenytoin
Dramamine	dimenhydrinate
Dridase	oxybutynin
Drogenil	flutamide
Droleptan	droperidol
Droperidol	droperidol
Droxia	hydroxyurea
Droxine	levothyroxine
Dryptal	furosemide
Dryvax	smallpox vaccine
DTIC-Dome	dacarbazine
DTIC	dacarbazine
Duboisine	hyoscyamine
Ducene	diazepam
Duexis	famotidine
Dulera	formoterol
Dumirox	fluvoxamine
Dumyrox	fluvoxamine
Dunate	artesunate
Duoneb	albuterol, ipratropium
Duopa	levodopa
Dura-Vent	phenylephrine
Duracef	cefadroxil
Duraclon	clonidine
Duragesic	fentanyl
Duralith	lithium
Duralutin	progestins
Durametacin	indomethacin
Duramorph	morphine
Duraperidol	haloperidol
Duraprox	oxaprozin
Durater	famotidine
Duratest	testosterone
Duratuss	hydrocodone
Durazepam	oxazepam
Durazolam	lorazepam
Durbis	disopyramide
Duricef	cefadroxil
Durlaza	aspirin
Duzallo	allopurinol, lesinurad
Dyazide	hydrochlorothiazide, triamterene
Dyloject	diclofenac
Dymenalgit	naproxen
Dyna-Hex	chlorhexidine
Dynacil	fosinopril
Dynacin	minocycline
Dynacirc SRO	isradipine
DynaCirc	isradipine
Dynatra	dopamine
Dyrenium	triamterene
Dysman	mefenamic acid
Dyspamet	cimetidine
Dysport	botulinum toxin (A & B)
Dytac	triamterene

E

E Perle	vitamin E
E-Mycin	erythromycin
E-Pam	diazepam
E-Vitamin Succinate	vitamin E
E102	tartrazine

E	MDMA
Ebixa	memantine
Ebufac	ibuprofen
Ecalta	anidulafungin
Ecomucyl	acetylcysteine
Economycin	tetracycline
Ecotrin	aspirin
Ecridoxan	etodolac
ecstasy	MDMA
Ectaprim	co-trimoxazole
Ectasule	ephedrine
ED-SPAZ	hyoscyamine
Edenol	furosemide
Edex	alprostadil
Edisylate	prochlorperazine
Edolan	etodolac
Edronax	reboxetine
EES	erythromycin
Efedron	ephedrine
Eferox	levothyroxine
Effexor XL	venlafaxine
Effexor	venlafaxine
Effient	prasugrel
Efracea	doxycycline
Efudex	fluorouracil
Efudix	fluorouracil
Efurix	fluorouracil
Egacene Durettes	hyoscyamine
Egazil	hyoscyamine
ELA-Max	lidocaine
Elavil	amitriptyline
Eldeprine	selegiline
Eldepryl	selegiline
Elderin	etodolac
Eldopal	levodopa
Elentol	lindane
Elepsia XR	levetiracetam
Elestrin	estradiol
Elidel	pimecrolimus
Eligard	leuprolide
Eliquis	apixaban
Elisor	pravastatin
Elixophyllin	aminophylline
Ellence	epirubicin
Elobact	cefuroxime
Eloctate	antihemophilic factor
Elorgan	pentoxifylline
Eloxatin	oxaliplatin
Elspar	asparaginase
Eltor 120	pseudoephedrine
Eltroxin	levothyroxine
EMB	ethambutol
Embolin	dicumarol
Emcor	bisoprolol
Emcyt	estramustine
Emend	aprepitant
Emeset	ondansetron
Emeside	ethosuximide
Emflaza	deflazacort
EMLA	lidocaine
Emorhalt	tranexamic acid
Empirin	aspirin
Empliciti	elotuzumab
Emquin	chloroquine
Emsam	selegiline
Emselex	darifenacin
Emtriva	emtricitabine
Enablex	darifenacin
Enaladil	enalapril
Enantone	leuprolide
Enapren	enalapril
Enarmon	methyltestosterone
Enbrel	etanercept
Encore	acetylcysteine
Endeavor	zotarolimus
Endep	amitriptyline
Endobulin	immune globulin IV
Endocodone	oxycodone
Endoxan	cyclophosphamide
Endoxana	cyclophosphamide
Ener-B	cyanocobalamin
Engerix B	hepatitis B vaccine
Entex HC	hydrocodone
Entex	pseudoephedrine
Entresto	sacubitril/valsartan
Entumin	clozapine
Entumine	clozapine
Entyvio	vedolizumab
Envarsus XR	tacrolimus
Epanutin	phenytoin
Epaxal	hepatitis A vaccine
Epclusa	sofosbuvir & velpatasvir
Ephedsol	ephedrine
Ephynal	vitamin E
Epi E-Z Pen	epinephrine
Epi-Aberel	tretinoin
Epidiolex	cannabidiol
Epiduo	adapalene
Epifrin	epinephrine
Epimorph	morphine
Epipen	epinephrine
Epitol	carbamazepine
Epivir	lamivudine
EPO	epoetin alfa
Epogen	epoetin alfa
Epoxitin	epoetin alfa
Eppy	epinephrine
Eppystabil	epinephrine
Eprex	epoetin alfa
Eprolin	vitamin E
Eptadone	methadone
Epzicom	abacavir, lamivudine
Equagesic	aspirin
Equibar	methyldopa
Eramycin	erythromycin
Eraxis	anidulafungin
Erbaprelina	pyrimethamine
Erbitux	cetuximab
Ercar	carboplatin
Ercoquin	hydroxychloroquine
Erelzi	etanercept
Ergomar	ergotamine

Ergometrine	ergometrine
Ergostat	ergotamine
Erivedge	vismodegib
Ery-Ped	erythromycin
Ery-Tab	erythromycin
Eryc	erythromycin
Erypar	erythromycin
Erypo	epoetin alfa
Erythrocin	erythromycin
erythropoiesis stimulating protein	darbepoetin alfa
erythropoietin	epoetin alfa
Eryzole	erythromycin
Esbriet	pirfenidone
Esclim	estradiol
eserine	physostigmine
Esidrex	hydrochlorothiazide
Eskalith	lithium
Esmino	chlorpromazine
Esperal	disulfiram
Estazor	ursodiol
Esteprim	co-trimoxazole
Estrace	estradiol
Estraderm	estradiol
Estratest	methyltestosterone
Estring	estradiol
Estrogel	estradiol
Estrostep	oral contraceptives
Etapiam	ethambutol
Ethinyl Estradiol	segesterone acetate
Ethymal	ethosuximide
Etibi	ethambutol
Etopos	etoposide
Etosid	etoposide
Etrafon	perphenazine
Eucrisa	crisaborole
Eudigox	digoxin
Eudyna	tretinoin
Euflex	flutamide
Euflexxa	hyaluronic acid
Euglucan	glyburide
Euglucon	glyburide
Euhypnos	temazepam
Eulexin	flutamide
Eulexine	flutamide
Eupen	amoxicillin
Euphyllin	aminophylline
Evamist	estradiol
Evista	raloxifene
Evitocor	atenolol
Evomela	melphalan
Evotaz	atazanavir
Evoxac	cevimeline
Evra	oral contraceptives
Evzio	naloxone
Exacyl	tranexamic acid
Exalgo	hydromorphone
Excedrin	acetaminophen, aspirin
Exelon	rivastigmine
Exforge	amlodipine, valsartan
Exidine Scrub	chlorhexidine
Exjade	deferasirox
Exocine	ofloxacin
Exodus	nicotine
Exomuc	acetylcysteine
Extavia	interferon beta
Eylea	aflibercept
Ezetrol	ezetimibe

F

Fabior	tazarotene
Fabrol	acetylcysteine
Falciquin	artesunate
Famodil	famotidine
Famoxal	famotidine
Famvir	famciclovir
Fanapt	iloperidone
Fansidar	pyrimethamine, sulfadoxine
Fareston	toremifene
Farmablastina	doxorubicin
Farmagard	nadolol
Farxiga	dapagliflozin
Farydak	panobinostat
Faverin	fluvoxamine
Favoxil	fluvoxamine
FazaClo	clozapine
FD&C yellow No.5	tartrazine
Felden	piroxicam
Feldene	piroxicam
Femara	letrozole
Fempatch	estradiol
Fenac	diclofenac
Fentanest	fentanyl
Fentazin	perphenazine
Fenytoin	phenytoin
Feraheme	ferumoxytol
Ferndex	dextroamphetamine
Ferriprox	deferiprone
Fetzima	levomilnacipran
Fevarin	fluvoxamine
Fexmid	cyclobenzaprine
Fibrel	collagen (bovine)
Fibrocit	gemfibrozil
Fiorinal	aspirin
fisalamine	mesalamine
Fisamox	amoxicillin
Fixime	cefixime
Flagyl	metronidazole
Flanax	naproxen
Flavoquin	amodiaquine
Flecaine	flecainide
Flector Patch	diclofenac
Flexeril	cyclobenzaprine
Flexiban	cyclobenzaprine
Flexitec	cyclobenzaprine
Flexyx	flucloxacillin
Flobasin	ofloxacin
Flodine	folic acid
Flolan	epoprostenol
Flomax	tamsulosin
Flopen	flucloxacillin
Florazole	metronidazole
Florid	miconazole

Florocycline	tetracycline
Floxan	ofloxacin
Floxapen	flucloxacillin
Floxil	ofloxacin
Floxin	ofloxacin
Floxstat	ofloxacin
Fluad	influenza vaccine
Fluarix	influenza vaccine
Flucazol	fluconazole
Flucinom	flutamide
Fluclox	flucloxacillin
Fluctin	fluoxetine
Fluctine	fluoxetine
Fludac	fluoxetine
Fludara	fludarabine
Fludecate	fluphenazine
Fludex	indapamide
Fluimucil	acetylcysteine
Flukacide	praziquantel
Fluken	flutamide
Flukezol	fluconazole
Flulem	flutamide
FluMist	influenza vaccine
Fluorophosphate	fluorides
Fluoroplex	fluorouracil
Fluorouracil Injection, USP	fluorouracil
Fluoxac	fluoxetine
Fluoxeren	fluoxetine
Flurix	influenza vaccine
Flurofen	flurbiprofen
Flurozin	flurbiprofen
Fluviral	influenza vaccine
Fluxil	fluoxetine
Fluzone	fluconazole, influenza vaccine
Focalin	dexmethylphenidate
Focetria	pandemic influenza vaccine (H1N1)
folacin	folic acid
folate	folic acid
Folina	folic acid
folinic acid	leucovorin
Folinsyre	folic acid
Folitab	folic acid
Folsan	folic acid
Fontex	fluoxetine
Foradil	formoterol
Formula-Q	quinine
Forsteo	teriparatide
Fortamet	metformin
Fortaz	ceftazidime
Forteo	teriparatide
Fortesta	testosterone
Fortipine	nifedipine
Fortum	ceftazidime
Forvade	cidofovir
Fosalan	alendronate
Fosamax	alendronate
Fosinorm	fosinopril
Foxsalepsin	carbamazepine
Fozitec	fosinopril
Fragmin	dalteparin
Fragmine	dalteparin
Fraurs	ursodiol
Frenal	pimozide
Froben	flurbiprofen
Froxal	cefuroxime
Frusid	furosemide
Fugerel	flutamide
Fulcin	griseofulvin
Fulvicin	griseofulvin
Fulvina P/G	griseofulvin
Fulyzaq	crofelemer
Fumaderm	dimethyl fumarate
Funcort	miconazole
Fungarest	ketoconazole
Fungata	fluconazole
Fungilin	amphotericin B
Fungizone	amphotericin B
Fungoid Tincture	miconazole
Fungoral	ketoconazole
Furadantin	nitrofurantoin
Furadantina	nitrofurantoin
Furadoine	nitrofurantoin
Furalan	nitrofurantoin
Furan	nitrofurantoin
Furobactina	nitrofurantoin
Furorese	furosemide
Furoside	furosemide
Fusid	furosemide
Fuzeon	enfuvirtide
Fycompa	perampanel

G

G-Well	lindane
GAB	lindane
Gabbroral	paromomycin
Gabitril	tiagabine
Gablofen	baclofen
Gabrilen Retard	ketoprofen
Gabroral	paromomycin
Galafold	migalastat hydrochloride
Galecin	clindamycin
Galedol	diclofenac
Galmax	ursodiol
Galzin	zinc
Gamabenceno	lindane
Gamafine	immune globulin IV
Gamastan	immune globulin IV
Gambex	lindane
Gamene	lindane
Gamikal	amikacin
Gamimune	immune globulin IV
Gamma 16	immune globulin IV
gamma benzene hexachloride	lindane
Gammabulin	immune globulin IV
Gammagard	immune globulin IV
Gammalin	lindane
Gammar PIV	immune globulin IV
Gammer-IV	immune globulin IV
Gammonayiv	immune globulin IV
Gamunex	immune globulin IV
Ganor	famotidine
Garamycin	gentamicin

Garatec	gentamicin
Gardasil	human papillomavirus (HPV) vaccine
Gardenal	phenobarbital
Gastro	famotidine
Gastrodyn	glycopyrrolate
Gastroloc	omeprazole
Gastrosed	hyoscyamine
Gattex	teduglutide
Gazyva	obinutuzumab
GBH	lindane
Geangin	verapamil
Gelnique	oxybutynin
Gelprin	aspirin
Geluprane	acetaminophen
Gemicina	neomycin
Gemlipid	gemfibrozil
Gemzar	gemcitabine
Gen-Baclofen	baclofen
Gen-Fibro	gemfibrozil
Gen-Metformin	metformin
Gen-XENE	clorazepate
Genabid	papaverine
Genahist	diphenhydramine
Genin	quinine
Genoptic	gentamicin
Genora	oral contraceptives
Genoxal	cyclophosphamide
Genpril	ibuprofen
Gentacidin	gentamicin
Gentalline	gentamicin
Gentalol	gentamicin
Genvoya	cobicistat/elvitegravir/emtricitabine/tenofovir alafenamide
Geodon	ziprasidone
Geroxalen	methoxsalen
Gestapuran	medroxyprogesterone
Gesterol 50	progestins
Gevilon Uno	gemfibrozil
Gilenya	fingolimod
Gilex	doxepin
Gilotrif	afatinib
Glatopa	glatiramer
Gleevec	imatinib
Gliadel Wafer	carmustine
glibenclamide	glyburide
Glibenese	glipizide
Glimel	glyburide
Glioten	enalapril
Glipid	glipizide
Glivec	imatinib
Glucagon Emergency Kit	glucagon
Glucal	glyburide
Glucobay	acarbose
Glucomet	metformin
Glucophage	metformin
Glucosamine sulfate	glucosamine
Glucotrol	glipizide
Glucovance	glyburide, metformin
Gluquine	quinidine
glybenclamide	glyburide
glyceryl trinitrate	nitroglycerin
glycopyrronium bromide	glycopyrrolate
Glyde	glipizide
Glynase	glyburide
Glypressin	terlipressin
Glyxambi	empagliflozin, linagliptin
GoNitro	nitroglycerin
Goodnight	promethazine
Gopten	trandolapril
Goutnil	colchicine
Gralise	gabapentin
grass	marihuana
Green-Alpha	interferon alfa
Grifulvin V	griseofulvin
Gris-PEG	griseofulvin
Grisefuline	griseofulvin
Griseostatin	griseofulvin
Grisovin	griseofulvin
Guiatuss AC	codeine
Gynodiol	estradiol

H

Habitrol Patch	nicotine
Haemiton	clonidine
Haemopressin	terlipressin
Hairgaine	minoxidil
Halaven	eribulin
Haldol	haloperidol
Halfprin	aspirin
Haloper	haloperidol
Halotussin	codeine
Haltran	ibuprofen
Hamarin	allopurinol
Harkoseride	lacosamide
Harvoni	ledipasvir & sofosbuvir
hashish	marihuana
Havrix	hepatitis A vaccine
Heitrin	terazosin
Helidac	bismuth, tetracycline
Heliopar	chloroquine
Helminzole	mebendazole
Heloxatin	oxaliplatin
Hemangeol	propranolol
Hemi-Daonil	glyburide
Hemovas	pentoxifylline
Henexal	furosemide
Hep-Flush	heparin
Hep-Lock	heparin
Hepalean	heparin
Heparin-Leo	heparin
Heparine	heparin
Hepsera	adefovir
Herceptin	trastuzumab
Herklin	lindane
Herpefug	acyclovir
Hetlioz	tasimelteon
hexachlorocyclohexane	lindane
Hexadrol	dexamethasone
Hexicid	lindane
Hexit	lindane
Hexol	chlorhexidine
Hibiclens	chlorhexidine

Hibident	chlorhexidine
Hibidil	chlorhexidine
Hibiscrub	chlorhexidine
Hibistat	chlorhexidine
Hibitane	chlorhexidine
HibMenCY	meningococcal groups C & Y & Haemophilus B tetanus toxoid conjugate vaccine
HibTITER	Hemophilus B vaccine
Histantil	promethazine
Hitrin	terazosin
Hivid	zalcitabine
Hizentra	immune globulin sc
Holoxan	ifosfamide
Horizant	gabapentin
HPV4	human papillomavirus (HPV) vaccine
Huberplex	chlordiazepoxide
Humagel	paromomycin
Humatin	paromomycin
Humira	adalimumab
Hyalgan	hyaluronic acid
hyaluronidase	hyaluronic acid
Hybloc	labetalol
Hycamtin	topotecan
Hyco	hyoscyamine
Hycosol SI	hyoscyamine
Hycotuss	hydrocodone
Hydeltrasol	prednisolone
Hydopa	methyldopa
Hydrea	hydroxyurea
Hydrogen fluoride [HF]	fluorides
Hydromet	hydrocodone
Hydrosaluric	hydrochlorothiazide
HydroStat IR	hydromorphone
hydroxycarbamide	hydroxyurea
hydroxydaunomycin	doxorubicin
Hylaform	hyaluronic acid
Hylan G-F 20	hyaluronic acid
Hylutin	progestins
Hynorex Retard	lithium
Hyospaz	hyoscyamine
Hypolar	nifedipine
Hysingla ER	hydrocodone
Hytrin	terazosin
Hytrine	terazosin
Hytrinex	terazosin
Hyzaar	hydrochlorothiazide, losartan

I

IB-Stat	hyoscyamine
ibandronic acid	ibandronate
Ibrance	palbociclib
Idamycin	idarubicin
Idhifa	enasidenib
Idotrim	trimethoprim
Ifex	ifosfamide
IFN	interferon alfa
Ifoxan	ifosfamide
IG Gamma	immune globulin IV
IGIM	immune globulin IV
IGIV	immune globulin IV
Iktorivil	clonazepam
IL-2	aldesleukin
Ilaris	canakinumab
Ilosone	erythromycin
Ilotycin	erythromycin
Imbrilon	indomethacin
Imbruvica	ibrutinib
Imdur	isosorbide mononitrate
Imfinzi	durvalumab
Imidol	imipramine
Imigran	sumatriptan
Imipramin	imipramine
Imitrex	sumatriptan
Imlygic	talimogene laherparepvec
Imodium	loperamide
Imossel	loperamide
Imovane	eszopiclone
Imovax	influenza vaccine
Implanta	cyclosporine
Impril	imipramine
Imuprin	azathioprine
Imuran	azathioprine
Imurek	azathioprine
Imurel	azathioprine
Inapsin	droperidol
Inapsine	droperidol
Incivek	telaprevir
Incruse	umeclidinium
Inderal LA	propranolol
Inderal	propranolol
Inderide	hydrochlorothiazide
Indochron	indomethacin
Indocin	indomethacin
Indolar SR	indomethacin
indometacin	indomethacin
Indotec	indomethacin
Inegy	simvastatin
INF	interferon alfa
Infergen	interferon alfa
Inflamase	prednisolone
Inflectra	infliximab
Inflexal V	influenza vaccine
Influsome	influenza vaccine
Infumorph	morphine
Infurin	nitrofurantoin
Ingrezza	valbenazine
INH	isoniazid
Inhibitron	omeprazole
Inlyta	axitinib
Innofem	estradiol
Innohep	tinzaparin
Innopran XL	propranolol
Innovace	enalapril
Insomnal	diphenhydramine
Integrex	reboxetine
Integrilin	eptifibatide
Intelence	etravirine
Intercon	oral contraceptives
Interglobin	immune globulin IV
interleukin-2	aldesleukin
Intron A	interferon alfa
Introna	interferon alfa

Introne	interferon alfa
Intropin	dopamine
Invanz	ertapenem
Invega	paliperidone
Invirase	saquinavir
Invivac	influenza vaccine
Invokamet	canagliflozin, metformin
Invokana	canagliflozin
Ionamin	phentermine
Iopidine	apraclonidine
Ipamix	indapamide
Ipolab	labetalol
Ipral	trimethoprim
Ipratropium Steri-Neb	ipratropium
Iquix	levofloxacin
Iremofar	hydroxyzine
Irenor	reboxetine
Iressa	gefitinib
Isavuconazole	isavuconazonium sulfate
Isentress	raltegravir
Ismipur	mercaptopurine
Ismo	isosorbide mononitrate
Ismotic	isosorbide
Isobac	co-trimoxazole
Isoptin	verapamil
Isoptine	verapamil
Isopto Atropine	atropine sulfate
Isopto Eserine	physostigmine
Isopto Pilocarpine	pilocarpine
Isopto-Epinal	epinephrine
Isopto	atropine sulfate
Isordil	isosorbide dinitrate
Isorythm	disopyramide
Isotamine	isoniazid
Isotrex	isotretinoin
Isox	itraconazole
Isozid	isoniazid
Istin	amlodipine
Istodax	romidepsin
Istubol	tamoxifen
Italnik	ciprofloxacin
Itranax	itraconazole
Itrin	terazosin
IV Globulin-S	immune globulin IV
Iveegam	immune globulin IV
IVIG	immune globulin IV
Ixiaro	Japanese encepahlitis vaccine
Izba	travoprost

J

Jacutin	lindane
Jadelle	levonorgestrel
Jadenu	deferasirox
Jalyn	dutasteride, tamsulosin
Janumet	metformin, sitagliptin
Januvia	sitagliptin
Jardiance	empagliflozin
Jenamicin	gentamicin
Jetrea	ocriplasmin
Jezil	gemfibrozil
Jodatum	potassium iodide
Jodid	potassium iodide
Jublia	efinaconazole
Juluca	dolutegravir
Jumex	selegiline
Jurnista	hydromorphone
Juvederm	hyaluronic acid
Juxtapid	lomitapide

K

Kabikinase	streptokinase
Kadcyla	trastuzumab emtansine
Kadian	morphine
Kalcide	praziquantel
Kaletra	lopinavir, ritonavir
Kalium	potassium iodide
Kallmiren	buspirone
Kalma	alprazolam
Kalten	atenolol
Kaluril	amiloride
Kalydeco	ivacaftor
Kanamicina	kanamycin
Kanamycine	kanamycin
Kanamytrex	kanamycin
Kanbine	amikacin
Kanescin	kanamycin
Kannasyn	kanamycin
Kantrex	kanamycin
Kanuma	sebelipase alfa
Kaywan	phytonadione
Kcentra	prothrombin complex concentrate (human)
Keduril	ketoprofen
Kefarol	cephalexin
Keflex	cephalexin
Kefolor	cefaclor
Keftab	cephalexin
Kelac	ketorolac
Kelatin	penicillamine
Kenaprol	metoprolol
Kengreal	cangrelor
Kenzoflex	ciprofloxacin
Kepivance	palifermin
Keppra	levetiracetam
Kerlon	betaxolol
Kerlone	betaxolol
Kerydin	tavaborole
Kessar	tamoxifen
Ketalar	ketamine
Ketalin	ketamine
Ketanest	ketamine
Ketoderm	ketoconazole
Ketoisidin	ketoconazole
Ketolar	ketamine
Ketonic	ketorolac
Kevadon	thalidomide
Keytruda	pembrolizumab
Khedezla	desvenlafaxine
KI	potassium iodide
Kidrolase	asparaginase
Kie	potassium iodide
Kildane	lindane
Kineret	anakinra

Kinidin	quinidine
Kisqali	ribociclib
Klacid	clarithromycin
Klaricid	clarithromycin
Klexane	enoxaparin
Klonopin	clonazepam
Kloramfenicol	chloramphenicol
Klozapol	clozapine
Kodapan	carbamazepine
Koffex	dextromethorphan
Kolkicin	colchicine
Konakion	phytonadione
Konicine	colchicine
Korec	quinapril
Korlym	mifepristone
Kovaltry	antihemophilic factor
Kovanaze	tetracaine & oxymetazoline
KP-E	dinoprostone
Kredex	carvedilol
Krenosin	adenosine
Krenosine	adenosine
Krintafel	tafenoquine
Kripton	bromocriptine
Krystexxa	pegloticase
Kwell	lindane
Kwildane	lindane
Kybella	deoxycholic acid
Kyleena	levonorgestrel
Kyprolis	carfilzomib

L

L-asparaginase	asparaginase
L-Cysteine	acetylcysteine
L-deprenyl	selegiline
L-dopa	levodopa
L-DOPS	droxidopa
L-Gent	gentamicin
L-Polamidon	methadone
L-thyroxine sodium	levothyroxine
Labrocol	labetalol
Ladogal	danazol
Lagaquin	chloroquine
lambrolizumab	pembrolizumab
Lamictal	lamotrigine
Lamisil	terbinafine
Lamocot	diphenoxylate
Landsen	clonazepam
Lanicor	digoxin
Lanoxin	digoxin
Lantarel	methotrexate
Lantus	insulin glargine
Lapole	flurbiprofen
Laraflex	naproxen
Larapam	piroxicam
Largactil	chlorpromazine
Lariam	mefloquine
Laricam	mefloquine
Laroferon	interferon alfa
Laroxyl	amitriptyline
Lartruvo	olaratumab
Lasilix	furosemide
Lasix	furosemide
Laspar	asparaginase
Lastet	etoposide
Latisse	bimatoprost
Latuda	lurasidone
Laubeel	lorazepam
Lebic	baclofen
Lederfolin	leucovorin
Ledertrexate	methotrexate
Ledoxina	cyclophosphamide
Lenal	temazepam
Lencid	lindane
Lenoxin	digoxin
Lentizol	amitriptyline
Lentorsil	ursodiol
Lenvima	lenvatinib
Leponex	clozapine
Leptanal	fentanyl
Leptopsique	perphenazine
Lescol	fluvastatin
Letairis	ambrisentan
Leucovorin	leucovorin
Leukerin	mercaptopurine
Leukosulfan	busulfan
Leunase	asparaginase
Leuprorelin	leuprolide
Leustatin	cladribine
Levanxene	temazepam
Levaquin	levofloxacin
Levate	amitriptyline
Levbid	hyoscyamine
Levemir	insulin detemir
Levitra	vardenafil
Levlen	oral contraceptives
Levlite	oral contraceptives
Levo-T	levothyroxine
Levodopa-Woelm	levodopa
Levora	oral contraceptives
Levothyroid	levothyroxine
Levothyrox	levothyroxine
Levoxyl	levothyroxine
Levsin/SL	hyoscyamine
Levsin	hyoscyamine
Levsinex	hyoscyamine
Levulan Kerastick	aminolevulinic acid
Lexapro	escitalopram
Lexin	carbamazepine
Lexinor	norfloxacin
Lexiva	fosamprenavir
Lexpec	folic acid
Lexxel	enalapril
Lialda	mesalamine
Libritabs	chlordiazepoxide
Librium	chlordiazepoxide
Lidaprim	trimethoprim
Lidifen	ibuprofen
Lidodan	lidocaine
Lidoderm	lidocaine
Lidoject-2	lidocaine
Lifaton B_{12}	cyanocobalamin
lignocaine	lidocaine

Likudin M	griseofulvin
Limbitrol	amitriptyline, chlordiazepoxide
Lin-Amnox	amoxicillin
Lincocin	lincomycin
Lincocine	lincomycin
Linzess	linaclotide
Liocarpina	pilocarpine
Lioresal	baclofen
Lipex	simvastatin
Lipitor	atorvastatin
Liponorm	simvastatin
Lipostat	pravastatin
Liptruzet	atorvastatin, ezetimibe
Lipur	gemfibrozil
Liquemin	heparin
Liquiprin	acetaminophen
Liroken	diclofenac
Lisino	loratadine
Lismol	cholestyramine
Litalir	hydroxyurea
Litanin	ursodiol
Lithicarb	lithium
Lithizine	lithium
Lithobid	lithium
Lithonate	lithium
Lithotabs	lithium
Litocure	ursodiol
Litoff	ursodiol
Litursol	ursodiol
Livalo	pitavastatin
Lo/Ovral	oral contraceptives
Locion-V	lindane
Locol	fluvastatin
Lodales	simvastatin
Lodimol	dipyridamole
Lodine	etodolac
Loestrin	oral contraceptives
Lofene	atropine sulfate, diphenoxylate
Logastric	omeprazole
Logen	atropine sulfate, diphenoxylate
Lokelma	sodium zirconium cyclosilicate
Lomaira	phentermine
Lomanate	atropine sulfate, diphenoxylate
Lomarin	dimenhydrinate
Lomir SRO	isradipine
Lomir	isradipine
Lomotil	atropine sulfate, diphenoxylate
Lomper	mebendazole
Lonazep	clonazepam
Lonine	etodolac
Loniten	minoxidil
Lonolox	minoxidil
Lonoten	minoxidil
Lonox	diphenoxylate
Lonsurf	trifluridine & tipiracil
Lop-Dia	loperamide
Loperhoe	loperamide
Lopid	gemfibrozil
Lopirin	captopril
Lopressor	hydrochlorothiazide, metoprolol
Lopril	captopril
Lorastine	loratadine
Lorcet	acetaminophen
Lorexane	lindane
Lortab	hydrocodone
Losec	omeprazole
Lotensin HCT	benazepril, hydrochlorothiazide
Lotensin	benazepril, hydrochlorothiazide
Lotrel	amlodipine, benazepril
Lovalip	lovastatin
Lovenox	enoxaparin
Low-Quel	diphenoxylate
Loxapac	loxapine
Loxen	nicardipine
Loxitane	loxapine
Lozapin	clozapine
Lozide	indapamide
Lozol	indapamide
Lucassin	terlipressin
Lucemyra	lofexidine
Lucentis	ranibizumab
Lucrin	leuprolide
Lugol's solution	potassium iodide
Lukadin	amikacin
Lumigan	bimatoprost
Luminal	phenobarbital
Luminaletten	phenobarbital
Lunelle	medroxyprogesterone, oral contraceptives
Lunesta	eszopiclone
Lupron Depot-Ped	leuprolide
Lupron	leuprolide
Lustra	hydroquinone
Luvox	fluvoxamine
Luzu	luliconazole
Lyeton	ursodiol
Lynparza	olaparib
Lyovac	dactinomycin
Lyple	alprostadil
Lyrica	pregabalin
Lyrinel	oxybutynin
Lysalgo	mefenamic acid
Lysatec rt-PA	alteplase
Lyxumia	lixisenatide

M

M-KYA	quinine
Maalox Anti-Diarrheal	loperamide
Maalox	loperamide
MabCampath	alemtuzumab
Mablin	busulfan
MabThera	rituximab
Macladin	clarithromycin
Macrobid	nitrofurantoin
Macrodantin	nitrofurantoin
Macugen	pegaptanib
Malarivon	chloroquine
Malarone	atovaquone/proguanil
Malocide	pyrimethamine, sulfadoxine
Maloprim	dapsone
Mamofen	tamoxifen
Mapap	acetaminophen
Marax	ephedrine, hydroxyzine

Marcillin	ampicillin
Mareen	doxepin
Marevan	warfarin
marijuana	marihuana
Marinol	dronabinol
Marmine	dimenhydrinate
Marthritic	salsalate
Masmoran	hydroxyzine
Maveral	fluvoxamine
Mavik	trandolapril
Maxalt	rizatriptan
Maxcef	cefepime
Maxidone	hydrocodone
Maxiphed	pseudoephedrine
Maxipime	cefepime
Maxitrol	neomycin
Maxtrex	methotrexate
Maxzide	hydrochlorothiazide, triamterene
Mazepine	carbamazepine
Measurin	aspirin
Mebensole	mebendazole
Med-Glibe	glyburide
Medamor	amiloride
Medianox	chloral hydrate
MedihalerEpi	epinephrine
Medilium	chlordiazepoxide
Medimet	methyldopa
Medipren	ibuprofen
Medispaz	hyoscyamine
Medrol	methylprednisolone
Mefac	mefenamic acid
Mefic	mefenamic acid
Megace	progestins
Megacillin	penicillin G
Mekinist	trametinib
Mektovi	binimetinib
Meladinine	methoxsalen
Melizide	glipizide
Menabol	stanozolol
Menhibrix	meningococcal groups C & Y & Haemophilus B tetanus toxoid conjugate vaccine
Menostar	estradiol
mepacrine	quinacrine
Mephaquin	mefloquine
Mephaquine	mefloquine
Mephenon	methadone
Mephyton	phytonadione
Merabis	spironolactone
Merlit	lorazepam
Meronem	meropenem
Merrem IV	meropenem
mesalazine	mesalamine
Mesasal	mesalamine
Mestacine	minocycline
Mestatin	nystatin
Mestinon	pyridostigmine
Metadate CD	methylphenidate
Metadon	methadone
Metaglip	glipizide, metformin
Metandren	methyltestosterone
Metex	methotrexate

Metforal	metformin
Methadose	methadone
Methipox	sulfadoxine
Methoprim	trimethoprim
Methylin	methylphenidate
methylmorphine	codeine
Meticorten	prednisone
Metomin	metformin
Metrocream	metronidazole
MetroGel	metronidazole
Metrolotion	metronidazole
Metrolyl	metronidazole
Mevacor	lovastatin
Meval	diazepam
Mevinacor	lovastatin
Mevinolin	lovastatin
Miacalcic	calcitonin
Miacalcin	calcitonin
Miacin	amikacin
Miaquin	amodiaquine
Micardis	hydrochlorothiazide, telmisartan
Micotef	miconazole
Micronase	glyburide
Micronor	progestins
Microzide	hydrochlorothiazide
Midamor	amiloride
Midol 220	ibuprofen
Midoride	amiloride
Mifeprex	mifepristone
Miglucan	glyburide
Mindiab	glipizide
Mindol	mebendazole
Minidiab	glipizide
Miniprostin E(2)	dinoprostone
Minirin	desmopressin
Minitran	nitroglycerin
Minobese-Forte	phentermine
Minocin	minocycline
Minoclir 50	minocycline
Minodiab	glipizide
Minogalen	minocycline
Minomycin	minocycline
Minoximen	minoxidil
Minprog	alprostadil
Minurin	desmopressin
Miocarpine	pilocarpine
Miracol	miconazole
Mirapex	pramipexole
Mircette	oral contraceptives
Mirena	levonorgestrel
Mirvaso	brimonidine
Misulban	busulfan
mitomycin-C	mitomycin
Mitomycin	mitomycin
Mitomycine	mitomycin
Mitoxana	ifosfamide
Mitran	chlordiazepoxide
Mobic	meloxicam
Mobilin	sulindac
Modamide	amiloride
Modecate	fluphenazine

Modicon	oral contraceptives
Moditen	fluphenazine
Moduretic	amiloride, hydrochlorothiazide
Molelant	cefotaxime
Molipaxin	trazodone
molly	MDMA
Monazole-7	miconazole
Monistat	miconazole
Mono-Gesic	salsalate
Monocor	bisoprolol
Monodox	doxycycline
Monoflam	diclofenac
Monofluorophosphate [MFP]	fluorides
Monoket	isosorbide mononitrate
Mononate	artesunate
Monopril	fosinopril
Monotrim	trimethoprim
Mopral	omeprazole
Morcomine	hydrocodone
Moronal	nystatin
Morphabond	morphine
Morphine-HP	morphine
MOS	morphine
Moscontin	morphine
Motiax	famotidine
Motifene	diclofenac
Motrin	ibuprofen
Movantik	naloxegol
Movergan	selegiline
Moxacef	cefadroxil
Moxeza	moxifloxacin
Moxidectin	moxidectin
MS Contin	morphine
MS-IR	morphine
MS/S	morphine
MSIR Oral	morphine
MST Continus	morphine
MTC	mitomycin
MTX	methotrexate
Mucofillin	acetylcysteine
Mucolit	acetylcysteine
Mucolitico	acetylcysteine
Mucoloid	acetylcysteine
Mucomiste	acetylcysteine
Mucomyst-10	acetylcysteine
Mucomyst	acetylcysteine
Mucosil-10	acetylcysteine
Mulpleta	lusutrombopag
Multaq	dronedarone
Multipax	hydroxyzine
Multum	chlordiazepoxide
Murelax	oxazepam
Muse	alprostadil
Mustargen	mechlorethamine
Mustine Hydrochloride Boots	mechlorethamine
mustine	mechlorethamine
Mutamycin	mitomycin
Myambutol	ethambutol
Mycamine	micafungin
Myciguent	neomycin
Mycobax	BCG vaccine
Mycobutin	rifabutin
Mycol	metoprolol
Mycology-II	nystatin
mycophenolate mofetil, mycophenolate sodium	mycophenolate
Mycostatin	nystatin
Mydayis	dextroamphetamine
Myfortic	mycophenolate
Mylanta AR	famotidine
Myleran	busulfan
Mylocel	hydroxyurea
Mynocine	minocycline
Myobloc	botulinum toxin (A & B)
Myolax	carisoprodol
Myrbetriq	mirabegron

N

N-acetyl-glucosamine (NAG)	glucosamine
N-acetylcysteine	acetylcysteine
Nabuser	nabumetone
NAC	acetylcysteine
Nadic	nadolol
Nalcryn SP	nalbuphine
Nalorex	naltrexone
Nalpin	naloxone
Namenda	memantine
Naplin	indapamide
Naprelan	naproxen
Naprogesic	naproxen
Napron X	naproxen
Naprosyn	naproxen
Naprosyne	naproxen
Narcan	naloxone
Narcanti	naloxone
Narcotan	naloxone
Narilet	aldesleukin
Narol	buspirone
Nascobal	cyanocobalamin
Natesto	testosterone
Natrilix	indapamide
Nauseatol	dimenhydrinate
Nausicalm	dimenhydrinate
Navelbine	vinorelbine
Naxen	naproxen
Nazoltec	ketoconazole
Nebilet	nebivolol
NebuPent	pentamidine
Necon	oral contraceptives
NEE	oral contraceptives
Nelova	oral contraceptives
Nemasol	mebendazole
Nemexin	naltrexone
Neo-Synephrine	phenylephrine
Neomicina	neomycin
Neomycine Diamant	neomycin
Neopap	acetaminophen
Neoral	cyclosporine
Neosar	cyclophosphamide
Neosporin	neomycin
Neosulf	neomycin
Neotigason	acitretin
NEPA	netupitant & palonosetron

Nephronex	nitrofurantoin
Nergadan	lovastatin
Nerlynx	neratinib
Nesina	alogliptin
Neupro	rotigotine
Neurap	pimozide
Neurobloc	botulinum toxin (A & B)
Neurontin	gabapentin
Neurosine	buspirone
Nexavar	sorafenib
Nexiclon	clonidine
Nexium	esomeprazole
Nia-Bid	niacin
Niac	niacin
Niacels	niacin
Niacinamide	niacinamide
Niacor	niacin
Niaspan	niacin
Nicabate	nicotine
Nicardal	nicardipine
Nico-Vert	dimenhydrinate
Nicobid	niacin
Nicobion	niacin
Nicodel	nicardipine
Nicoderm	nicotine
Nicolan	nicotine
Nicorette Plus	nicotine
Nicorette	nicotine
Nicotibine	isoniazid
nicotinamide	niacinamide
Nicotinell-TTS	nicotine
Nicotinex	niacin
nicotinic acid	niacin
Nicotrans	nicotine
Nicotrol	nicotine
Nicovital	niacin
Nicozid	isoniazid
Nida Gel	metronidazole
Nifecor	nifedipine
Nifedipress	nifedipine
Nikofrenon	nicotine
Ninlaro	ixazomib
Niotal	zolpidem
Nirulid	amiloride
Nistaquim	nystatin
Nitro-Dur	nitroglycerin
NitroBid	nitroglycerin
Nitrocap	nitroglycerin
Nitrocine	nitroglycerin
Nitrodur	nitroglycerin
nitrogen mustard	mechlorethamine
Nitroglin	nitroglycerin
nitroglycerol	nitroglycerin
Nitrolingual	nitroglycerin
Nitromist	nitroglycerin
Nitronal	nitroglycerin
Nitrospan	nitroglycerin
Nitrostat	nitroglycerin
Nitrumon	carmustine
Nivemycin	neomycin
Nizoral	ketoconazole
Nobegyl	salsalate
Nocbin	disulfiram
Noctec	chloral hydrate
Noctiva	desmopressin
Nodine	ketorolac
Nolvadex	tamoxifen
Nor-QD	progestins
Norboral	glyburide
Norco	hydrocodone
Nordette	oral contraceptives
Norebox	reboxetine
Norethin	oral contraceptives
Norfenon	propafenone
Norgesic	aspirin
Norinyl	oral contraceptives
Noritate	metronidazole
Noritren	nortriptyline
Norlutate	progestins
Norlutin	progestins
Normison	temazepam
Normorytmin	propafenone
Normozide	labetalol
Noroxin	norfloxacin
Norpace	disopyramide
Norphyl	aminophylline
Norplant	levonorgestrel
Norpress	nortriptyline
Northera	droxidopa
Nortrilen	nortriptyline
Norvas	amlodipine
Norvasc	amlodipine
Norvir	ritonavir
Noten	atenolol
Novahistine DH	codeine
Novahistine	phenylephrine
Novamin	prochlorperazine
Novamoxin	amoxicillin
Novantrone	mitoxantrone
Novapen-VK	penicillin V
Novasen	aspirin
Novazam	diazepam
Novitropan	oxybutynin
Novo-Atenol	atenolol
Novo-AZT	zidovudine
Novo-Chlorpromazine	chlorpromazine
Novo-Cycloprine	cyclobenzaprine
Novo-Digoxin	digoxin
Novo-Dipiradol	dipyridamole
Novo-Doxepin	doxepin
Novo-Doxylin	doxycycline
Novo-Flutamide	flutamide
Novo-Furan	nitrofurantoin
Novo-Hylazin	hydralazine
Novo-Ipramide	ipratropium
Novo-Keto	ketoprofen
Novo-Lexin	cephalexin
Novo-Medrone	medroxyprogesterone
Novo-Metformin	metformin
Novo-Naprox	naproxen
Novo-Pramine	imipramine
Novo-Purol	allopurinol

Novo-Selegiline	selegiline
Novo-Semide	furosemide
Novo-Spiroton	spironolactone
Novo-Sundac	sulindac
Novo-Zolamide	acetazolamide
Novochlorhydrate	chloral hydrate
Novocimetine	cimetidine
Novoclopate	clorazepate
Novofen	tamoxifen
NovoLog	insulin aspart
Novomit	prochlorperazine
Novopen-G	penicillin G
Novopoxide	chlordiazepoxide
NovoRapid	insulin aspart
Novotriptyn	amitriptyline
Novoxapam	oxazepam
Noxafil	posaconazole
NTG	nitroglycerin
Nu-Alprax	alprazolam
Nu-Amoxi	amoxicillin
Nu-Atenol	atenolol
Nu-Baclo	baclofen
Nu-Buspirone	buspirone
Nu-Capto	captopril
Nu-Cimet	cimetidine
Nu-Clonidine	clonidine
Nu-Diclo	diclofenac
Nu-Diltiaz	diltiazem
Nu-Doxycycline	doxycycline
Nu-Famotidine	famotidine
Nu-Flurprofen	flurbiprofen
Nu-Gemfibrozil	gemfibrozil
Nu-Hydral	hydralazine
Nu-Indo	indomethacin
Nu-Loraz	lorazepam
Nu-Medopa	methyldopa
Nu-Naprox	naproxen
Nu-Nifed	nifedipine
Nu-Pirox	piroxicam
Nu-Ranit	ranitidine
Nu-Temazepam	temazepam
Nu-Verap	verapamil
Nubain SP	nalbuphine
Nubain	nalbuphine
Nucala	mepolizumab
Nucofed	codeine
Nucynta ER	tapentadol
Nucynta	tapentadol
Nulev	hyoscyamine
Nulojix	belatacept
Nuplazid	pimavanserin
Nuprin	ibuprofen
Nuvigil	armodafinil
Nyaderm	nystatin
Nystacid	nystatin
Nystan	nystatin
Nystex	nystatin
Nytol	diphenhydramine

O

Ocaliva	obeticholic acid
Octagam	immune globulin IV
Octocaine	lidocaine
Octostim	desmopressin
Ocuflox	ofloxacin
Ocumycin	gentamicin
Ocusert Pilo	pilocarpine
Odefsey	emtricitabine/rilpivirine/tenofovir alafenamide
Odomzo	sonidegib
Odrik	trandolapril
Ofev	nintedanib
Ofirmev	acetaminophen
Oflocet	ofloxacin
Oflocin	ofloxacin
Oforta	fludarabine
Oftalmotrisol-T	tobramycin
Oleomycetin	chloramphenicol
Oleptro	trazodone
Olmetec	olmesartan
Olumiant	baricitinib
Olysio	simeprevir
Omed	omeprazole
Omegaven	fish oil triglycerides
Omnicef	cefdinir
OmniHIB	Hemophilus B vaccine
OMS Oral	morphine
Onbrez Breezhaler	indacaterol
Oncaspar	pegaspargase
Onco-Carbide	hydroxyurea
Oncocarbin	carboplatin
Oncoden	ondansetron
oncovin	vincristine
Onglyza	saxagliptin
Onicit	palonosetron
Onivyde	irinotecan
Onmel	itraconazole
Onpattro	patisiran
Onzetra Xsail	sumatriptan
Opana	oxymorphone
Opdivo	nivolumab
Ophthochlor	chloramphenicol
Opistan	meperidine
Opizone	naltrexone
Opsumit	macitentan
Optenyl	papaverine
Optipres	betaxolol
Optovit-E	vitamin E
Oracea	doxycycline
Oracefal	cefadroxil
Oramorph SR	morphine
Oranor	norfloxacin
Oranyst	nystatin
Orap	pimozide
Oravig	miconazole
Orbactiv	oritavancin
Orencia	abatacept
Orientomycin	cycloserine
Orilissa	elagolix sodium
Oritaxim	cefotaxime
Orkambi	lumacaftor/ivacaftor
Ormazine	chlorpromazine
Ornade	chlorpheniramine

Ornidyl	eflornithine
Oroken	cefixime
Ortho Tri-Cyclen	oral contraceptives
Ortho-Cept	oral contraceptives
Ortho-Cyclen	oral contraceptives
Ortho-Novum	oral contraceptives
Orthovisc	hyaluronic acid
Orudis	ketoprofen
Oruvail	ketoprofen
Osiren	spironolactone
Ospen	penicillin V
Ospexin	cephalexin
Osphena	ospemifene
Osteum	etidronate
Otarex	hydroxyzine
Otezla	apremilast
Otrexup	methotrexate
Otrivine	xylometazoline
Ovcon	oral contraceptives
Ovral	oral contraceptives
Ovrette	progestins
Oxiklorin	hydroxychloroquine
Oxpam	oxazepam
Oxsoralen	methoxsalen, psoralens
Oxsoralon	methoxsalen
Oxtellar XR	oxcarbazepine
Oxyban	oxybutynin
Oxybutyn	oxybutynin
OxyContin	oxycodone
Oxydess	dextroamphetamine
OxyIR	oxycodone
Oxytrol	oxybutynin
Ozoken	omeprazole
Ozurdex	dexamethasone

P

Pacerone	amiodarone
Pacifen	baclofen
Paclimer	paclitaxel
Palaron	aminophylline
Palexia	tapentadol
Palladone	hydromorphone
Palmitate A	vitamin A
Palux	alprostadil
Pameion	papaverine
Pamelor	nortriptyline
Pamid	indapamide
Pamprin	ibuprofen
Panadol	acetaminophen
Panbesy	phentermine
Panbesyl	phentermine
Pandemrix	pandemic influenza vaccine (H1N1)
Panglobulin	immune globulin IV
Panoral	cefaclor
Panretin	alitretinoin
Pantelmin	mebendazole
Panuric	probenecid
Papaverine 60	papaverine
Papaverini	papaverine
paracetamol	acetaminophen
Paraplatin	carboplatin
Paraplatine	carboplatin
Parilac	bromocriptine
Parizac	omeprazole
Parkemed	mefenamic acid
Parlodel	bromocriptine
Parsabiv	etelcalcetide
Parvolex	acetylcysteine
Pasmex	hyoscyamine
Pasotomin	prochlorperazine
Pavabid	papaverine
Pavagen	papaverine
Pavased	papaverine
Pavatine	papaverine
Paveral	codeine
Paxene	paclitaxel
Paxil CR	paroxetine hydrochloride
Paxil	paroxetine hydrochloride
Paxistil	hydroxyzine
Paxtibi	nortriptyline
PCC	prothrombin complex concentrate (human)
PCE	erythromycin
PCV	pneumococcal vaccine
Pedi-Dri	nystatin
Pediapred	prednisolone
Pediatrix	hepatitis B vaccine
Pediazole	erythromycin
PedivaxHIB	Hemophilus B vaccine
Pegasys	PEG-interferon
PegIntron	PEG-interferon
Penbeta	penicillin V
Penbritin	ampicillin
Pendramine	penicillamine
Pennsaid	diclofenac
Penstabil	ampicillin
Pentacarinat	pentamidine
Pentaglobin	immune globulin IV
Pentam 300	pentamidine
Pentamycetin	chloramphenicol
Pentasa SR	mesalamine
Pentasa	mesalamine
Pentazine	promethazine
Pentoxi	pentoxifylline
Pentoxil	pentoxifylline
Pepcid	famotidine
Pepcidine	famotidine
Pepdul	famotidine
Pepeom Amide	niacin
Peptard	hyoscyamine
Peptaron	ursodiol
Pepto-Bismol	bismuth
Peptol	cimetidine
Peratsin	perphenazine
Percocet	acetaminophen, oxycodone
Percogesic	acetaminophen
Perforomist	formoterol
Peridex	chlorhexidine
Peridol	haloperidol
PerioChip	chlorhexidine
Periogard	chlorhexidine
Periostat	doxycycline
Perlane	hyaluronic acid

Perlutex	medroxyprogesterone
Perphenan	perphenazine
Persantin	dipyridamole
Persantine	dipyridamole
Pertussin	dextromethorphan
Petar	ketamine
pethidine	meperidine
Petidin	meperidine
Petnidan	ethosuximide
Pexal	pentoxifylline
PGE	alprostadil
Phenaemal	phenobarbital
Phenaphen	acetaminophen
Phenazine	promethazine
Phenergan	promethazine
Phenetron	chlorpheniramine
Phenhydan	phenytoin
phenobarbitone	phenobarbital
Phenoxymethylpenicillin	penicillin V
phenylethylmalonylurea	phenobarbital
Phenytek	phenytoin
phenytoin sodium	phenytoin
Pheryl-E	vitamin E
Phyllocontin	aminophylline
Phyllotemp	aminophylline
Phytomenadione	phytonadione
Picato	ingenol mebutate
Pidilat	nifedipine
Pifeltro	doravirine
Pilo Grin	pilocarpine
Pilogel	pilocarpine
Pilopine	pilocarpine
Pilopt	pilocarpine
Pimodac	pimozide
Pink Bismuth	bismuth
Pirimecidan	pyrimethamine
Pitocin	oxytocin
Placil	clomipramine
Plan B	levonorgestrel
Planphylline	aminophylline
Planum	temazepam
Plaquenil	hydroxychloroquine
Plaquinol	hydroxychloroquine
Plasmotrim	artesunate
Plasticin	cisplatin
Platiblastin	cisplatin
Platinex	cisplatin
Platinol-AQ	cisplatin
Platinol	cisplatin
Platistil	cisplatin
Plavix	clopidogrel
Plegridy	interferon beta
Pletal	cilostazol
Plurimen	selegiline
PMS-Baclofen	baclofen
PMS-Cholestyramine	cholestyramine
PMS-Isoniazid	isoniazid
PMS-Lindane	lindane
PncOMP	pneumococcal vaccine
Pneumovax II	pneumococcal vaccine
Pnu-Immune	pneumococcal vaccine
Polinal	methyldopa
Poly-Pred	neomycin
Polygam S/D	immune globulin IV
Polygris	griseofulvin
Polytrim	trimethoprim
Pomalyst	pomalidomide
Ponstan	mefenamic acid
Ponstel	mefenamic acid
Ponstyl	mefenamic acid
Portrazza	necitumumab
pot	marihuana
Potiga	ezogabine
PPV	pneumococcal vaccine
Pradaxa	dabigatran
Praluent	alirocumab
Prandin E2	dinoprostone
Pravachol	pravastatin
Pravasin	pravastatin
Pravasine	pravastatin
Pravidel	bromocriptine
Praxbind	idarucizumab
Praxiten	oxazepam
Prazite	praziquantel
Pre-Par	ritodrine
Precaptil	captopril
Precose	acarbose
Pred-G	gentamicin
Prefrin Liquifilm	phenylephrine
Prelone	prednisolone
Premphase	medroxyprogesterone
Prempro	medroxyprogesterone
Prepidil	dinoprostone
Pres	enalapril
Prescal	isradipine
Presinol	methyldopa
Presoken	diltiazem
Presolol	labetalol
Prestalia	amlodipine, perindopril
Pretz-D	ephedrine
Prevacid	lansoprazole
Prevalite	cholestyramine
Preveon	adefovir
Prevnar	pneumococcal vaccine
Prevpac	amoxicillin
Prexum	perindopril
Prezcobix	darunavir
Prezista	darunavir
Priadel	lithium
Pridemon	tranexamic acid
Prilosec	omeprazole
Primacor	milrinone
Primafen	cefotaxime
Primatene Mist	epinephrine
Primatene	epinephrine
Primiprost	dinoprostone
Primonil	imipramine
Primosept	trimethoprim
Primsol	trimethoprim
Principen	ampicillin
Princol	lincomycin
Prinil	lisinopril

Prinivil	lisinopril
Prinzide	hydrochlorothiazide, lisinopril
Pristiq	desvenlafaxine
Pro-Amox	amoxicillin
Pro-Ampi	ampicillin
Pro-Cure	finasteride
Pro-Depo	progestins
Pro-Trin	co-trimoxazole
Probalan	probenecid
Probuphine	buprenorphine
Procan SR	procainamide
Procan	procainamide
Procanbid	procainamide
Procardia	nifedipine
Procid	probenecid
Procoralan	ivabradine
Procren Depot	leuprolide
Procrin	leuprolide
Procrit	epoetin alfa
Procytox	cyclophosphamide
Prodac	nabumetone
Prodopa	methyldopa
Prodox	progestins
Profen	ibuprofen
Proflex	ibuprofen
Progestaject	progestins
Progevera	medroxyprogesterone
Prograf	tacrolimus
ProHIBIT	Hemophilus B vaccine
Prolaken	metoprolol
Proleukin	aldesleukin
Prolex-D	phenylephrine
Prolex-DH	hydrocodone
Prolia	denosumab
Prolift	reboxetine
Prolixin	fluphenazine
Promacta	eltrombopag
Prometh-50	promethazine
Promine	procainamide
Pronestyl	procainamide
Propachem	hydrocodone
Propaphenin	chlorpromazine
Propecia	finasteride
Propess	dinoprostone
Prorazin	prochlorperazine
Proscar 5	finasteride
Proscar	finasteride
prostaglandin E_1	alprostadil
Prostaphlin	oxacillin
Prostarmon	dinoprostone
Prostigmin	neostigmine
Prostin E2	dinoprostone
Prostin VR	alprostadil, dinoprostone
Prostin	dinoprostone
Prostine VR	alprostadil
Prostine	dinoprostone
Prostivas	alprostadil
Prothiazine	promethazine
Protium	pantoprazole
Protogen	dapsone
Protonix	pantoprazole
Protopam	pralidoxime
Protopic	tacrolimus
Proventil	albuterol
Provera	medroxyprogesterone, progestins
Provigil	modafinil
Prozac	fluoxetine
Prozin	chlorpromazine
Pryleugan	imipramine
Psicofar	chlordiazepoxide
Pulmicort Turbuhaler	budesonide
Punktyl	lorazepam
Puri-Nethol	mercaptopurine
Purinethol	mercaptopurine
Purinol	allopurinol
Puvasoralen	methoxsalen
Pyknolepsinum	ethosuximide
Pyoredol	phenytoin
Pyrethia	promethazine

Q

Q-Vel	quinine
Qnasl	beclomethasone
Qsymia	phentermine, topiramate
Qtern	dapagliflozin, saxagliptin
Qualaquin	quinine
Quantalan	cholestyramine
Qudexy	topiramate
Quellada	lindane
Quensyl	hydroxychloroquine
Querto	carvedilol
Questran Lite	cholestyramine
Questran	cholestyramine
Quibron	aminophylline
Quiess	hydroxyzine
Quinalan	quinidine
Quinate	quinidine
Quinazil	quinapril
Quini Durules	quinidine
Quinoctal	quinine
Quinora	quinidine
Quinsan	quinine
Quinsul	quinine
Quintasa	mesalamine
Quiphile	quinine
Quixin	levofloxacin
Qvar	beclomethasone

R

Ra-223 dichloride	radium-223 dichloride
Radicava	edaravone
Radiesse	calcium hydroxylapatite
Ralovera	medroxyprogesterone
Ralozam	alprazolam
Ramicin	rifampin
Randikan	kanamycin
Ranexa	ranolazine
Raniben	ranitidine
Raniplex	ranitidine
Ranisen	ranitidine
Ranvil	nicardipine

Rapaflo	silodosin
Rapamune	sirolimus
rapamycin	sirolimus
Rapivab	peramivir
Rasuvo	methotrexate
Rayaldee	calcifediol
Razadyne	galantamine
Reactine	cetirizine
Rebetol	ribavirin
Rebetron	interferon alfa, ribavirin
Rebif	interferon beta
Reclast	zoledronate
Recombivax HB	hepatitis B vaccine
Rectiv	nitroglycerin
Redisol	cyanocobalamin
Redusa	phentermine
Refobacin	gentamicin
Refolinin	leucovorin
Refusal	disulfiram
Regaine	minoxidil
Regitin	phentolamine
Regitine	phentolamine
Regonol	pyridostigmine
Relafen	nabumetone
Relenza	zanamivir
Relief	tretinoin
Relif	nabumetone
Relifex	nabumetone
Relpax	eletriptan
Remeron	mirtazapine
Remethan	diclofenac
Remicade	infliximab
Reminyl	galantamine
Renflexis	infliximab
Renitec	enalapril
Reniten	enalapril
Renova	tretinoin
Repatha	evolocumab
Reposans-10	chlordiazepoxide
Requip	ropinirole
Rescufolin	leucovorin
Rescuvolin	leucovorin
Resmin	diphenhydramine
Respirol	terbutaline
Respontin	ipratropium
Restasis	cyclosporine
Restoril	temazepam
Restylane Fine Lines	hyaluronic acid
retigabine	ezogabine
Retin-A Micro	tretinoin
Retinoic Acid	tretinoin
Retinova	tretinoin
Retrovir	zidovudine
Revapole	mebendazole
Revatio	sildenafil
ReVia	naltrexone
Revimine	dopamine
Reviten	triamterene
Revlimid	lenalidomide
Revolade	eltrombopag
Revonto	dantrolene
Rexulti	brexpiprazole
Reyataz	atazanavir
Rezine	hydroxyzine
rFVIIIFc	antihemophilic factor
Rheumatrex	methotrexate
Rhinocort	budesonide
Rhodacine	indomethacin
Rhodis	ketoprofen
Rhofade	oxymetazoline
Rhonal	aspirin
Rhotrimine	trimipramine
Rhovail	ketoprofen
Rhythmin	procainamide
Ride	amiloride
Ridene	nicardipine
Rifadin	rifampin
Rifaldin	rifampin
Rifamate	isoniazid
Rifamed	rifampin
rifampicin	rifampin
Rifater	isoniazid
Rilatine	methylphenidate
Rimactane	rifampin
Rimpin	rifampin
Rimycin	rifampin
Rinatec	ipratropium
Riomet	metformin
Risperdal Consta	risperidone
Risperdal	risperidone
Ritalin	methylphenidate
Ritmocamid	procainamide
Ritmolol	metoprolol
Rituxan	rituximab
Rivotril	clonazepam
RMS	morphine
Roaccutan	isotretinoin
Roaccutane	isotretinoin
Roacutan	isotretinoin
Roacuttan	isotretinoin
Robaxisal	aspirin
Robidrine	pseudoephedrine
Robimycin	erythromycin
Robinul	glycopyrrolate
Robitussin AC	codeine
Robitussin-CF	pseudoephedrine
Robitussin	dextromethorphan
Rocefin	ceftriaxone
Rocephalin	ceftriaxone
Rocephin	ceftriaxone
Roceron-A	interferon alfa
Rofact	rifampin
Roferon-A	interferon alfa
Rogaine	minoxidil
Rogal	piroxicam
Rogitene	phentolamine
Rogitine	phentolamine
Rotarix	rotavirus vaccine
RotaTeq	rotavirus vaccine
Roubac	co-trimoxazole
Rovacor	lovastatin
Rowasa	mesalamine

Roxanol	morphine
Roxicodone	oxycodone
Rozerem	ramelteon
Rtsun	artesunate
Ru-Tuss	hydrocodone
Rubesol-1000	cyanocobalamin
Rubex	doxorubicin
rubidomycin	daunorubicin
Rubifen	methylphenidate
Rubraca	rucaparib
Rubramin	cyanocobalamin
Rufen	ibuprofen
Ryanodex	dantrolene
Rybix ODT	tramadol
Rydapt	midostaurin
Rydene	nicardipine
Rynatan	phenylephrine
Rynatuss	ephedrine
Rytary	levodopa
Rythmex	propafenone
Rythmol	propafenone
Rytmonorm	propafenone
Ryzodeg	insulin aspart, insulin degludec

S

S-1	tegafur/gimeracil/oteracil
S-2	epinephrine
Sabril	vigabatrin
Sacbexyl	lindane
Saccharin	saccharin
Saflutan	tafluprost
Salagen	pilocarpine
salazopyrin	sulfasalazine
Salbulin	albuterol
salbutamol	albuterol
Salflex	salsalate
Salgesic	salsalate
salicylazosulfapyridine	sulfasalazine
Salina	salsalate
Salisulf	sulfasalazine
Salmagne	labetalol
Salofalk	mesalamine
Sandimmun	cyclosporine
Sandimmune	cyclosporine
Sandoglobulin	immune globulin IV
Sandoglobulina	immune globulin IV
Sandoglobuline	immune globulin IV
Sandostatin	octreotide
Sandostatina	octreotide
Sandostatine	octreotide
Sanoma	carisoprodol
Sansert	methysergide
Saphris	asenapine
Sarafem	fluoxetine
Sarconyl	lindane
Saridine	sulfasalazine
Saroten	amitriptyline
SAS-500	sulfasalazine
Savaysa	edoxaban
Savella	milnacipran
Savlon	chlorhexidine
Saxenda	liraglutide
Scabecid	lindane
Scabene	lindane
Scabex	lindane
Scabi	lindane
Scabisan	lindane
SCIG	immune globulin sc
Sebomin	minocycline
Sebvio	telbivudine
Sedanazin	gentamicin
Sediat	diphenhydramine
Seebri Neohaler	glycopyrrolate
Selectin	pravastatin
Selectol	celiprolol
Selektine	pravastatin
Selipran	pravastatin
Seloken-Zok	metoprolol
Selozok	metoprolol
Selzentry	maraviroc
Sendoxan	cyclophosphamide
Septra	co-trimoxazole, sulfamethoxazole, trimethoprim
Ser-Ap-Es	hydralazine
Serax	oxazepam
Serenace	haloperidol
Serepax	oxazepam
Serocryptin	bromocriptine
Seromycin	cycloserine
Seroquel	quetiapine
Seroxat	paroxetine hydrochloride
Serozide	etoposide
Sesamol	flucloxacillin
Setamine	hyoscyamine
Sevredol	morphine
Sideril	trazodone
Sigacefal	cefaclor
Sigafam	famotidine
Silenor	doxepin
Silgard	human papillomavirus (HPV) vaccine
Silicofluoride	fluorides
Simatin	ethosuximide
Simcor	niacin, simvastatin
Simovil	simvastatin
Simplene	epinephrine
Simponi	golimumab
Simulect	basiliximab
Sinaplin	ampicillin
Sinemet	levodopa
Singulair	montelukast
Sinomin	sulfamethoxazole
Sinosid	paromomycin
Sinquan	doxepin
Sintodian	droperidol
Sinutab	acetaminophen
Siran	acetylcysteine
Sirdalud	tizanidine
Sirtal	carbamazepine
Sirturo	bedaquiline
Sitavig	acyclovir
Sivastin	simvastatin
Sivextro	tedizolid
Sizopin	clozapine

Skelaxin	metaxalone
Sklice	ivermectin
Slo-Bid	aminophylline
Slo-Niacin	niacin
SMX-TMP	co-trimoxazole
SMZ-TMP	co-trimoxazole
Sno Pilo	pilocarpine
Sobelin	clindamycin
Sodium fluoride [NaF]	fluorides
Sodium monofluorophosphate	fluorides
Sodol	carisoprodol
Solage	tretinoin
Solaraze Gel	diclofenac
Solcodein	codeine
Solesorin	hydralazine
Solfoton	phenobarbital
Solgol	nadolol
Soliqua	insulin glargine, lixisenatide
Soliris	eculizumab
Solis	diazepam
Solium	chlordiazepoxide
Solodyn	minocycline
Solpurin	probenecid
Solu-Medrol	methylprednisolone
Solutrat	ursodiol
Solvex	reboxetine
Soma Compound	aspirin
Soma	carisoprodol
Somadril	carisoprodol
Somatuline Autogel	lanreotide
Somatuline Depot	lanreotide
Somatuline LA	lanreotide
Somavert	pegvisomant
Sominex 2	diphenhydramine
Somnox	chloral hydrate
Somophyllin	aminophylline
Sonata	zaleplon
Soolantra	ivermectin
Sopamycetin	chloramphenicol
Sorbitrate	isosorbide dinitrate
Soriatane	acitretin
Soridol	carisoprodol
Sorine	sotalol
Sostril	ranitidine
Sotacor	sotalol
Sotahexal	sotalol
Sotalex	sotalol
Sotilen	piroxicam
Sotret	isotretinoin
Sovaldi	sofosbuvir
Spectro Gram	chlorhexidine
Spersacarpine	pilocarpine
Spinax	baclofen
Spinraza	nusinersen
Spiriva	tiotropium
Spiroctan	spironolactone
Spirosine	cefotaxime
Splenda	sucralose
Sporacid	itraconazole
Sporal	itraconazole
Sporanox	itraconazole

Sprycel	dasatinib
SSKI	potassium iodide
Stable	hydralazine
Stalevo	entacapone, levodopa
Stamaril	yellow fever vaccine
Stambutol	ethambutol
Stangyl	trimipramine
Stannous fluoride [SF]	fluorides
Stapenor	oxacillin
Staril	fosinopril
Starlix	nateglinide
Statex	morphine
Steclin	tetracycline
SteiVAA	tretinoin
Stelara	ustekinumab
Stella	prochlorperazine
Stemetil	prochlorperazine
Stendra	avanafil
Stieva-A	tretinoin
Stilnoct	zolpidem
Stilnox	zolpidem
Stimate	desmopressin
Stiolto Respimat	olodaterol, tiotropium
Stomedine	cimetidine
Stopit	loperamide
Storzine	pilocarpine
Strattera	atomoxetine
Strensiq	asfotase alfa
Streptase	streptokinase
Streptomycin	streptomycin
Stribild	cobicistat/elvitegravir/emtricitabine/tenofovir disoproxil
Striverdi Respimat	olodaterol
Stromba	stanozolol
Stromectol	ivermectin
Strumazol	methimazole
Stubit	nicotine
Sublimaze	fentanyl
Suboxone	buprenorphine, naloxone
Subutex	buprenorphine
Sucrabest	sucralfate
Sucrets	dextromethorphan
Sudafed	pseudoephedrine
Sular	nisoldipine
Sulcrate	sucralfate
Sulene	sulindac
sulfamethoxazole-trimethoprim	co-trimoxazole
Sulfatrim	co-trimoxazole
Sulfazine	sulfasalazine
Sulfona	dapsone
Sulfur hexafluoride [SF6]	fluorides
Sulic	sulindac
Sulmidine	clonidine
Suloril	sulindac
Suloton	triamterene
Sumacef	cefadroxil
Sumavel DosePro	sumatriptan
Sumontil	trimipramine
Sumycin	tetracycline
Supartz	hyaluronic acid
Supeudol	oxycodone

Suppress	dextromethorphan
Supradol	naproxen
Supran	cefixime
Suprax	cefixime
Suprenza	phentermine
Supressin	doxazosin
Suretin	tazarotene
Surmontil	trimipramine
Sustiva	efavirenz
Sutent	sunitinib
suxamethonium	succinylcholine
Sweet'N Low	saccharin
Sylatron	PEG-interferon
Symbicort	budesonide, formoterol
Symbol	misoprostol
Symbyax	fluoxetine, olanzapine
Symjepi	epinephrine
Symproic	naldemedine
Syn-Minocycline	minocycline
Syn-Nadolol	nadolol
Synagis	palivizumab
Syndros	dronabinol
Synflex	naproxen
Synjardy	empagliflozin, metformin
Synthroid	levothyroxine
Syntocinon	oxytocin
Syraprim	trimethoprim
Syscor	nisoldipine
Sytobex	cyanocobalamin

T

T-20	enfuvirtide
T-DM1	trastuzumab emtansine
T-VEC	talimogene laherparepvec
T_3 sodium	liothyronine
T_3	liothyronine
T_4	levothyroxine
Tabalom	ibuprofen
Tabco	flecainide
Tabrin	ofloxacin
Tacex	ceftriaxone
Tachydaron	amiodarone
Tadol	tramadol
Tafil	alprazolam
Tafinlar	dabrafenib
Taflutan	tafluprost
Tagal	ceftazidime
Tagamet	cimetidine
Tagrisso	osimertinib
Taks	diclofenac
Taloken	ceftazidime
Taltz	ixekizumab
Talwin Compound	aspirin
Talwin-NX	naloxone
Tamaxin	tamoxifen
Tambocor	flecainide
Tamiflu	oseltamivir, pandemic influenza vaccine (H1N1)
Tamofen	tamoxifen
Tamoxan	tamoxifen
Tanzeum	albiglutide
Tapazole	methimazole
Tapros	leuprolide
Taravid	ofloxacin
Tarceva	erlotinib
Targiniq	naloxone, oxycodone
Targocid	teicoplanin
Targretin	bexarotene
Tarka	trandolapril, verapamil
Taro-Ampicillin Trihydrate	ampicillin
Taro-Atenol	atenolol
Tasigna	nilotinib
Taucor	lovastatin
Tavanic	levofloxacin
Tavor	lorazepam
Taxagon	trazodone
Taxol	paclitaxel
Taxotere	docetaxel
Taxus	tamoxifen
Tazicef	ceftazidime
Tazorac	tazarotene
Tecentriq	atezolizumab
Tecfidera	dimethyl fumarate
Technivie	ombitasvir/paritaprevir/ritonavir
Tecoplanin	teicoplanin
Tecprazin	praziquantel
Teczem	diltiazem, enalapril
Tedolan	etodolac
Tefamin	aminophylline
Teflaro	ceftaroline fosamil
Teflin	tetracycline
Tega-Cert	dimenhydrinate
Tega-Vert	dimenhydrinate
Tegretol XR	carbamazepine
Tegretol	carbamazepine
Teichomycin-A2	teicoplanin
Tekamlo	amlodipine
Tekturna HCT	hydrochlorothiazide
Telachlor	chlorpheniramine
Teldrin	chlorpheniramine
Teline	tetracycline
Temazepam	temazepam
Tementil	prochlorperazine
Temesta	lorazepam
Temgesic	buprenorphine
Temodar	temozolomide
Tenif	atenolol, nifedipine
Teniken	praziquantel
Tenolin	atenolol
Tenoret 50	atenolol
Tenoretic	atenolol
Tenormin	atenolol
Tenormine	atenolol
Tensin	spironolactone
Tensipine MR	nifedipine
Tensopril	lisinopril
Teralithe	lithium
Teril	carbamazepine
Terlipressin	terlipressin
Ternalax	tizanidine
Ternelin	tizanidine
Tertroxin	liothyronine
Tesavel	sitagliptin

Testandro	testosterone
Testim	testosterone
Testoderm	testosterone
Teston	methyltestosterone
Testopel	testosterone
Testotonic 'B'	methyltestosterone
Testovis	methyltestosterone
Testred	methyltestosterone
Tetradin	disulfiram
tetrahydrocannabinol	dronabinol
Tetramig	tetracycline
Teveten HCT	hydrochlorothiazide
Teveten	eprosartan
Texate	methotrexate
Teysuno	tegafur/gimeracil/oteracil
Thacapzol	methimazole
Thalomid	thalidomide
THC	dronabinol
Theo-Dur	aminophylline
theophylline ethylenediamine	aminophylline
Thevier	levothyroxine
Thiamazol	methimazole
thiamazole	methimazole
Thinex	lindane
Thioprine	azathioprine
Thorazine	chlorpromazine
Thyroid-Block	potassium iodide
Thyronine	liothyronine
Thyrozol	methimazole
tiabendazole	thiabendazole
Tiamate	diltiazem
Tiazac	diltiazem
Tibinide	isoniazid
Tibsovo	ivosidenib
TICE BCG	BCG vaccine
Tidocol	mesalamine
Tiempe	trimethoprim
Tifomycine	chloramphenicol
Tilazem	diltiazem
Tildiem	diltiazem
Timonil	carbamazepine
Titus	lorazepam
Tivicay	dolutegravir
TMP-SMX	co-trimoxazole
TMP-SMZ	co-trimoxazole
TOBI	tobramycin
Tobra	tobramycin
TobraDex	tobramycin
Tobrex	tobramycin
Tofranil	imipramine
Tolak	fluorouracil
Toloxim	mebendazole
Topadol	ketorolac
Topamax	topiramate
Topicycline	tetracycline
Toprol XL	metoprolol
Toradol	ketorolac
Torem	torsemide
Toremonil	hydroxychloroquine
Torental	pentoxifylline
Torisel	temsirolimus
Torolac	ketorolac
Torvin	ketorolac
Totacillin	ampicillin
Totapen	ampicillin
Toviaz	fesoterodine
tPA	alteplase
Tpoxx	tecovirimat
Tracleer	bosentan
Tradjenta	linagliptin
Tradol	tramadol
Tramal	tramadol
Tramed	tramadol
Tramol	tramadol
Trandate	labetalol
Transderm-Nitro	nitroglycerin
Transene	clorazepate
Transtec	buprenorphine
Tranxal	clorazepate
Tranxen	clorazepate
Tranxene	clorazepate
Tranxilen	clorazepate
Tranxilium	clorazepate
Trasamlon	tranexamic acid
Travatan Z	travoprost
Travatan	travoprost
Travel Tabs	dimenhydrinate
Trazalon	trazodone
Tremfya	guselkumab
Trendar	ibuprofen
Trental	pentoxifylline
Tresiba	insulin degludec
Trexan	naltrexone
Tri-Levlen	oral contraceptives
Tri-Norinyl	oral contraceptives
Triadapin	doxepin
Triaken	ceftriaxone
Triaminic DM	dextromethorphan
Triaminic	chlorpheniramine
Trian	triamterene
Triasox	thiabendazole
Triavil	perphenazine
Tricodein	codeine
Tricor	fenofibrate
Tridil	nitroglycerin
Tridol	tramadol
Triflucan	fluconazole
Trijodthyronin BC N	liothyronine
Trikacide	metronidazole
Trilafon	perphenazine
Trileptal	oxcarbazepine
Trilifan Retard	perphenazine
Trimopan	trimethoprim
Trimox	amoxicillin
Trimzol	co-trimoxazole
Trinalin	pseudoephedrine
Trintellix (formerly Brintellix)	vortioxetine
Triomin	perphenazine
Triostat	liothyronine
Triphasil	oral contraceptives
Triprim	trimethoprim
Triptone	dimenhydrinate

Trisoralen	psoralens
Trisulfa	co-trimoxazole
Tritace	ramipril
Triumeq	abacavir, dolutegravir, lamivudine
Trivora	oral contraceptives
Triz	cetirizine
Trizivir	abacavir, lamivudine, zidovudine
Trobalt	ezogabine
Trocal	dextromethorphan
Trokendi XR	topiramate
Tronoxal	ifosfamide
Tropax	oxybutynin
Tropium	chlordiazepoxide
Tropyn Z	atropine sulfate
Troxyca	naltrexone, oxycodone
Trulance	plecanatide
Trulicity	dulaglutide
Trumenba	meningococcal group B vaccine
Truphylline	aminophylline
Trusopt	dorzolamide
Truvada	emtricitabine, tenofovir disoproxil
Tryptanol	amitriptyline
Tryptizol	amitriptyline
TS-1	tegafur/gimeracil/oteracil
Tussar-2	codeine
Tussgen	hydrocodone
Tussi-12D	phenylephrine
Tussi-Organidin	codeine
Tussionex	hydrocodone
Tussogest	hydrocodone
Twinrix	hepatitis B vaccine
Tykerb	lapatinib
Tylenol	acetaminophen
Tylox	oxycodone
Tymlos	abaloparatide
Typherix	typhoid vaccine
Typhim Vi	typhoid vaccine
Tysabri	natalizumab
Tyzeka	telbivudine

U

UDC Hexal	ursodiol
UDC	ursodiol
UDCA	ursodiol
Udrik	trandolapril
Uducil	cytarabine
Ulcar	sucralfate
Ulcedine	cimetidine
Ulcogant	sucralfate
Ulcol	sulfasalazine
Ulcyte	sucralfate
Uloric	febuxostat
Ulsen	omeprazole
Ultra-MOP	methoxsalen
Ultracet	tramadol
Ultram	tramadol
Umbradol	salsalate
Umine	phentermine
Unasyn	ampicillin/sulbactam
Unat	torsemide
Uniflox	ciprofloxacin
Unimazole	methimazole
Unimetone	nabumetone
Uniparin	heparin
Uniretic	hydrochlorothiazide
Unithroid	levothyroxine
Unitrim	trimethoprim
Unituxin	dinutuximab
Unizuric	allopurinol
Uptravi	selexipag
Urbal	sucralfate
Urdox	ursodiol
Urem	ibuprofen
Urex	furosemide
Urief	silodosin
Urised	atropine sulfate, hyoscyamine
Uritol	furosemide
Uro-cephoral	cefixime
Urobak	sulfamethoxazole
Urocid	probenecid
Urofuran	nitrofurantoin
Uromax	oxybutynin
Uroxatral	alfuzosin
Urozide	hydrochlorothiazide
Urso 250	ursodiol
Urso Forte	ursodiol
Urso Heumann	ursodiol
Urso Vinas	ursodiol
Ursochol	ursodiol
ursodeoxycholic acid	ursodiol
Ursofal	ursodiol
Ursofalk	ursodiol
Ursoflor	ursodiol
Ursogal	ursodiol
Ursolac	ursodiol
Ursolism	ursodiol
Ursolvan	ursodiol
Urson	ursodiol
Ursoproge	ursodiol
Ursosan	ursodiol
Ursotan	ursodiol
USCA	ursodiol
Utibron Neohaler	glycopyrrolate, indacaterol
Utinor	norfloxacin
Utradol	etodolac

V

V-cillin K	penicillin V
Vacanyl	terbutaline
Vagifem	estradiol
Valadol	acetaminophen
Valcyte	valganciclovir
Valdrene	diphenhydramine
Valium	diazepam
Valni XL	nifedipine
Valodex	tamoxifen
valproate sodium	valproic acid
Valtrex	valacyclovir
Valturna	valsartan
Vamate	hydroxyzine
Vanatrip	amitriptyline
Vanceril	beclomethasone

Vancocin	vancomycin
Vancotil	loperamide
Vandazole	metronidazole
Vaniqa	eflornithine
Vanmicina	vancomycin
Vanquish	aspirin
Vaprisol	conivaptan
Vaqta	hepatitis A vaccine
Varilrix	varicella vaccine
Variquel	terlipressin
Varithena	polidocanol
Varivax	varicella vaccine
Varsan	lindane
Varubi	rolapitant
Vascal	isradipine
Vaseretic	enalapril, hydrochlorothiazide
Vasopril	fosinopril
Vasotec	enalapril
Vaxchora	cholera vaccine
Vaxigrip	influenza vaccine
Veclam	clarithromycin
Vectibix	panitumumab
Velban	vinblastine
Velbe	vinblastine
Velcade	bortezomib
Veletri	epoprostenol
Velodan	loratadine
Velsar	vinblastine
Velsay	naproxen
Veltassa	patiromer
Vemlidy	tenofovir alafenamide
Venclexta	venetoclax
Venoglobulin	immune globulin IV
Ventolin	albuterol
Ventoline	albuterol
VePesid	etoposide
Vepeside	etoposide
Veraken	verapamil
Verelan	verapamil
Vermicol	mebendazole
Vermox	mebendazole
Versed	midazolam
Vertab	dimenhydrinate
Vertigon	prochlorperazine
Verzenio	abemaciclib
Vesanoid	tretinoin
Vesicare	solifenacin
Vestra	reboxetine
Vfend	voriconazole
Viadur	leuprolide
Viaflex	heparin
Viagra	sildenafil
Viberzi	eluxadoline
Vibra-Tabs	doxycycline
Vibramycin-D	doxycycline
Vicapan N	cyanocobalamin
Vicard	terazosin
Vicks Formula 44	dextromethorphan
Vicks Vatronol	ephedrine
Vicodin	acetaminophen, hydrocodone
Vicoprofen	hydrocodone, ibuprofen

Victoza	liraglutide
Victrelis	boceprevir
Vidaza	azacitidine
Videx	didanosine
Vidopen	ampicillin
Viekira Pak	ombitasvir/paritaprevir/ritonavir
Viekira XR	dasabuvir/ombitasvir/paritaprevir/ritonavir
Viekirax	ombitasvir/paritaprevir/ritonavir
Viibryd	vilazodone
Vimizim	elosulfase alfa
Vimpat	lacosamide
Vincasar	vincristine
Viracept	nelfinavir
Viramid	ribavirin
Viramune	nevirapine
Virazid	ribavirin
Virazole	ribavirin
Viread	tenofovir disoproxil
Virilon	methyltestosterone
Virlix	cetirizine
Viromone	methyltestosterone
Vistabel	botulinum toxin (A & B)
Vistacarpin	pilocarpine
Vistaril	hydroxyzine
Vistide	cidofovir
Visudyne	verteporfin
Vita Plus E	vitamin E
Vita-E	vitamin E
Vitak	phytonadione
vitamin B_{12}	cyanocobalamin
vitamin B_3	niacin, niacinamide
vitamin B_9	folic acid
vitamin K_1	phytonadione
Vitamin K	phytonadione
Vitatropine	atropine sulfate
Vitec	vitamin E
Vitrase	hyaluronic acid
Vivaglobin	immune globulin sc
Vivatec	lisinopril
Vivelle-Dot	estradiol
Vivelle	estradiol
Vividyl	nortriptyline
Vivitrex	naltrexone
Vivitrol	naltrexone
Vivol	diazepam
Vivotif	typhoid vaccine
Vogan	vitamin A
Volibris	ambrisentan
Volmax	albuterol
Voltaren	diclofenac
Voltarene	diclofenac
Voltarol	diclofenac
Vomacur	dimenhydrinate
Vomex A	dimenhydrinate
Vomisen	dimenhydrinate
Vonum	indomethacin
Vozet	levocetirizine
VP-TEC	etoposide
Vraylar	cariprazine
Vytorin	ezetimibe, simvastatin
Vyvanse	lisdexamfetamine

W

Waran	warfarin
Warfilone	warfarin
Waytrax	ceftazidime
Wehamine	dimenhydrinate
Welchol	colesevelam
Wellbutrin	bupropion
Welldorm	chloral hydrate
Wigrettes	ergotamine
Winobanin	danazol
Winstrol	stanozolol
Wintrocin	erythromycin
Wyamicin S	erythromycin

X

X	MDMA
Xadago	safinamide
Xalatan	latanoprost
Xalkori	crizotinib
Xanax	alprazolam
Xanef	enalapril
Xarelto	rivaroxaban
Xatral	alfuzosin
Xelevia	sitagliptin
Xeljanz	tofacitinib
Xeloda	capecitabine
Xenical	orlistat
Xeomin	botulinum toxin (A & B)
Xerava	eravacycline
Xgeva	denosumab
Xifaxan	rifaximin
Xifaxanta	rifaximin
Xigduo XR	dapagliflozin, metformin
Xiidra	lifitegrast
Xofigo	radium-223 dichloride
Xolair	omalizumab
Xomolix	droperidol
Xozal	levocetirizine
Xtampza ER	oxycodone
Xtandi	enzalutamide
Xtoro	finafloxacin
Xultophy	insulin degludec, liraglutide
Xusal	levocetirizine
xylocaine	lidocaine
Xylocard	lidocaine
Xyzal	levocetirizine

Y

Yamatetan	cefotetan
Yasmin	oral contraceptives
Yaz	oral contraceptives
Yectamid	amikacin
Yentreve	duloxetine
Yervoy	ipilimumab
YF-VAX	yellow fever vaccine
Yosprala	aspirin, omeprazole
Yuma	hydroxychloroquine
Yurelax	cyclobenzaprine

Z

Zaltrap	aflibercept
Zanaflex	tizanidine
Zanosar	streptozocin
Zantab	ranitidine
Zantac-C	ranitidine
Zantac	ranitidine
Zantic	ranitidine
Zantryl	phentermine
Zapex	oxazepam
Zaponex	clozapine
Zariviz	cefotaxime
Zarondan	ethosuximide
Zarontin	ethosuximide
Zavedos	idarubicin
Zebeta	bisoprolol
Zebinix	eslicarbazepine
Zecuity	sumatriptan
Zedolac	etodolac
Zefone	ceftriaxone
Zeftera	ceftobiprole
Zejula	niraparib
Zelapar	selegiline
Zelboraf	vemurafenib
Zemdri	plazomicin
Zenapax	daclizumab
Zentropil	phenytoin
Zeos	loratadine
Zepatier	elbasvir & grazoprevir
Zerbaxa	ceftolozane & tazobactam
Zerit	stavudine
Zestoretic	hydrochlorothiazide, lisinopril
Zestril	lisinopril
Zetia	ezetimibe
Zeto	azithromycin
Ziac	bisoprolol, hydrochlorothiazide
Ziagen	abacavir
Zicam	zinc
Zimovane	eszopiclone
Zinacef	cefuroxime
Zinacet	cefuroxime
Zinat	cefuroxime
Zinbryta	daclizumab
Zinnat	cefuroxime
Zinplava	bezlotoxumab
Zioptan	tafluprost
Zipan	tramadol
Zipsor	diclofenac
Zirtin	cetirizine
Zithromax	azithromycin
Zitromax	azithromycin
ziv-aflibercept	aflibercept
Zmax	azithromycin
Zocor	simvastatin
Zocord	simvastatin
Zofran	ondansetron
Zofron	ondansetron
Zohydro ER	hydrocodone
Zoldan-A	danazol
Zole	miconazole
zoledronic acid	zoledronate

Zolinza	vorinostat
Zoloft	sertraline
ZoMaxx Drug-Eluting Coronary Stent	zotarolimus
Zometa	zoledronate
Zomig	zolmitriptan
Zonegran	zonisamide
Zontivity	vorapaxar
Zorac	tazarotene
Zorbenal-G	tetracycline
Zoref	cefuroxime
Zoroxin	norfloxacin
Zortress	everolimus
Zorvolex	diclofenac
Zostavax	zoster vaccine
Zosyn	piperacillin/tazobactam
Zovia	oral contraceptives
Zovirax	acyclovir
Zumalin	lincomycin
Zunden	piroxicam
Zuplenz	ondansetron
Zurampic	lesinurad
Zyban	bupropion
Zyclara	imiquimod
Zyclir	acyclovir
Zydelig	idelalisib
Zyderm	collagen (bovine)
Zydone	hydrocodone
Zyflo	zileuton
Zyloprim	allopurinol
Zyloric	allopurinol
Zymerol	cimetidine
Zynox	naloxone
Zyplast	collagen (bovine)
Zyprexa Relprevv	olanzapine
Zyprexa	olanzapine
Zyrtec	cetirizine
Zytiga	abiraterone
Zyvox	linezolid